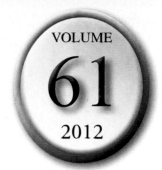

VOLUME
61
2012

INSTRUCTIONAL COURSE LECTURES

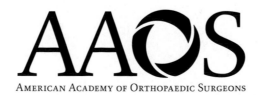

AMERICAN ACADEMY OF ORTHOPAEDIC SURGEONS

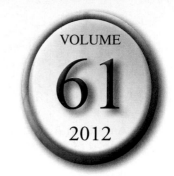

VOLUME

61
2012

INSTRUCTIONAL COURSE LECTURES

Edited by

Paul Tornetta III, MD
Professor and Vice Chairman
Director of Orthopaedic Trauma
Department of Orthopaedic Surgery
Boston University Medical Center
Boston, Massachusetts

Mark W. Pagnano, MD
Professor of Orthopedics
Department of Orthopedic Surgery
Mayo Clinic College of Medicine
Rochester, Minnesota

Published 2012 by the
American Academy
of Orthopaedic Surgeons
6300 North River Road
Rosemont, IL 60018

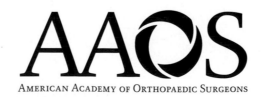

AMERICAN ACADEMY OF ORTHOPAEDIC SURGEONS

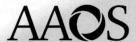

AAOS
AMERICAN ACADEMY OF ORTHOPAEDIC SURGEONS

Instructional Course Lectures Volume 61
American Academy of Orthopaedic Surgeons

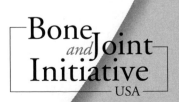

Contributors

Geoffrey D. Abrams, MD
Resident, Department of Orthopaedic Surgery, Stanford University, Stanford, California

Jeffrey S. Abrams, MD
Attending Surgeon, Department of Surgery, University Medical at Princeton, Princeton, New Jersey

Julie E. Adams, MD
Assistant Professor, Department of Orthopaedic Surgery, University of Minnesota, Minneapolis, Minnesota

Jesse Affonso, MD
Clinical Fellow, Division of Shoulder Surgery, Department of Orthopaedic Surgery, Johns Hopkins University School of Medicine, Baltimore, Maryland

Samuel G. Agnew, MD, FACS
Partner, Senior Consultant, Orthopaedic Trauma Practice Consultants, Lutz, Florida

Christopher S. Ahmad, MD
Associate Professor, Department of Orthopaedic Surgery, Columbia University Medical Center, New York, New York

Behrooz A. Akbarnia, MD
Medical Director, San Diego Center for Spinal Disorders, La Jolla, California

Paul E. Beaulé, MD, FRCSC
Associate Professor, Head of Adult Reconstruction, Division of Orthopaedic Surgery, University of Ottawa, Ottawa, Ontario, Canada

Keith R. Berend, MD
Clinical Assistant Professor, Department of Orthopaedics, The Ohio State University, New Albany, Ohio

Michael E. Berend, MD
Orthopaedic Surgeon, Center for Hip and Knee Surgery, St. Francis Medical Group, Mooresville, Indiana

Mohit Bhandari, MD, FRCSC
Chair, Division of Surgery, McMaster University, Hamilton, Ontario, Canada

Randy R. Bindra, MD, FRCS
Professor of Orthopaedic Surgery, Departments of Orthopaedic Surgery and Rehabilitation, Stritch School of Medicine, Loyola University, Chicago, Illinois

Robert H. Blotter, MD
Orthopaedic Surgery Associates of Marquette, Marquette, Michigan

Joseph A. Bosco III, MD
Vice Chair of Clinical Affairs, Department of Orthopaedics, New York University Hospital for Joint Diseases, New York, New York

Thomas D. Brown, PhD
Richard and Janice Johnston Chair of Orthopaedic Biomechanics, Departments of Orthopaedics and Rehabilitation, University of Iowa, Iowa City, Iowa

Jacob M. Buchowski, MD
Assistant Professor of Orthopaedic and Neurological Surgery, Director, Center for Spinal Tumors, Department of Orthopaedic Surgery, Washington University, St. Louis, Missouri

Stephen S. Burkhart, MD
Fellowship Director, The San Antonio Orthopaedic Group, San Antonio, Texas

David F. Dalury, MD
Chief, Adult Reconstruction Surgery, Department of Orthopedics, St. Joseph Hospital, Towson, Maryland

Craig J. Della Valle, MD
Orthopaedic Surgeon, Department of Joint Replacement, Midwest Orthopaedics at Rush, Chicago, Illinois

Patrick J. Denard, MD
Fellow, San Antonio Orthopaedic Group, San Antonio, Texas

Douglas R. Dirschl, MD
Professor and Chairman, Department of Orthopaedics, University of North Carolina, Chapel Hill, North Carolina

Adam S. Dowrick, PhD
Research Fellow, Department of Orthopaedic Surgery, The Alfred Hospital, Melbourne, Victoria, Australia

Gerard A. Engh, MD
Director, Knee Research, Anderson Orthopaedic Institute, Alexandria, Virginia

Jill A. Erickson, PA-C
Physician Assistant, Department of Orthopaedics, University of Utah, Salt Lake City, Utah

A. Reed Estes, MD
Clinical Fellow, Department of Orthopaedics, Division of Sports Medicine, Children's Hospital of Boston, Boston, Massachusetts

Wolfgang Fitz, MD
Associate Orthopaedic Surgeon, Department of Orthopaedic Surgery, Brigham and Women's Hospital, Chestnut Hill, Massachusetts

Evan L. Flatow, MD
Lasker Professor and Chairman, Department of Orthopaedic Surgery, Mt. Sinai Medical Center, New York, New York

Mark A. Frankle, MD
Chief, Shoulder and Elbow Service, Department of Upper Extremity Surgery, Florida Orthopaedic Institute, Tampa, Florida

Kevin L. Garvin, MD
Professor and Chairman, Department of Orthopaedic Surgery and Rehabilitation, University of Nebraska Medical Center, Omaha, Nebraska

Juan Garzon-Muvdi, MD
Clinical Research Fellow, Division of Shoulder Surgery, Department of Orthopaedic Surgery, The Johns Hopkins University School of Medicine, Baltimore, Maryland

Trevor Gaskill, MD
Fellow, Department of Orthopaedic Surgery, Steadman Philippon Research Institute, Vail, Colorado

William B. Geissler, MD
Professor and Chief, Division of Hand and Upper Extremity Surgery, Department of Orthopaedic Surgery, University of Mississippi Medical Center, Jackson, Mississippi

Christian Gerber, MD
Professor and Chair, Department of Orthopaedics, University of Zurich, Zurich, Switzerland

Steven D. Glassman, MD
Professor, Department of Orthopaedics, University of Louisville, Louisville, Kentucky

Kevin L. Harreld, MD
Shoulder and Elbow Fellow, Florida Orthopaedic Institute, Tampa, Florida

Curtis W. Hartman, MD
Assistant Professor, Department of Orthopaedic Surgery and Rehabilitation, University of Nebraska Medical Center, Omaha, Nebraska

Richard J. Hawkins, MD
Orthopaedic Surgeon, Steadman Hawkins Clinic of the Carolinas, Greenville Hospital System, Greenville, South Carolina

Patrick D.G. Henry, MD, FRCSC
Clinical Fellow, Division of Orthopaedics, Department of Surgery, St. Michael's Hospital, University of Toronto, Toronto, Ontario, Canada

Alan Hilibrand, MD
Professor of Orthopaedic Surgery and Neurosurgery, Director of Medical Education, Rothman Institute, Thomas Jefferson University Hospital, Philadelphia, Pennsylvania

Stephanie H. Hsu, MD
Orthopedic Surgery Fellow, Department of Orthopedic Surgery, New York Presbyterian Hospital, Columbia University, New York, New York

Wellington K. Hsu, MD
Assistant Professor, Department of Orthopaedic Surgery and Department of Neurological Surgery, Northwestern University Feinberg School of Medicine, Chicago, Illinois

Jason M. Hurst, MD
Associate, Joint Implant Surgeons, Mount Carmel Health System, New Albany, Ohio

Ramon L. Jimenez, MD
Monterey Peninsula Orthopaedic and Sports Medicine Institute, Monterey, California

Riyaz H. Jinnah, MD, FRCS
Professor, Department of Orthopaedic Surgery, Wake Forest School of Medicine, Winston-Salem, North Carolina

William A. Jiranek, MD, FACS
Chief, Adult Reconstruction Section, Department of Orthopaedics, Virginia Commonwealth University, Richmond, Virginia

Clifford B. Jones, MD, FACS
Clinical Professor, Michigan State University, College of Human Medicine, Orthopaedic Associates of Michigan, Grand Rapids, Michigan

Gregory Katz, BS
New York University Hospital for Joint Diseases, New York, New York

Young-Jo Kim, MD, PhD
Associate Professor of Orthopaedic Surgery, Department of Orthopaedic Surgery, Children's Hospital Boston, Boston, Massachusetts

Michael J. Kissenberth, MD
Orthopedic Surgeon, Steadman Hawkins Clinic of the Carolinas, Greenville Hospital System, Greenville, South Carolina

Frank M. Klenke, MD, PhD
Senior Physician, Department of Orthopedic Surgery, Inselspital, Bern University Hospital, Bern, Switzerland

Beau S. Konigsberg, MD
Assistant Professor, Department of Orthopaedic Surgery and Rehabilitation, University of Nebraska Medical Center, Omaha, Nebraska

Paul K. Kosmatka, MD
Orthopedic Trauma Surgeon, Department of Orthopedics, Essentia Health, Duluth, Minnesota

John C. Kurylo, MD
Orthopaedic Surgery Resident, Department of Orthopaedic Surgery, Boston University Medical Center, Boston, Massachusetts

William D. Lanzinger, MD
Hand Surgery Fellow, Department of Orthopaedic Surgery and Rehabilitation, Stritch School of Medicine, Loyola University, Chicago, Illinois

Christopher M. Larson, MD
Director of Arthroscopic Hip Joint Preservation, Minnesota Orthopedic Sports Medicine Institute, Twin Cities Orthopedics, Edina, Minnesota

Lawrence G. Lenke, MD
Jerome J. Gilden Endowed Professor of Orthopaedic Surgery, Professor of Neurological Surgery, Department of Orthopaedic Surgery, Washington University School of Medicine, St. Louis, Missouri

William N. Levine, MD
Vice Chairman and Professor, Department of Orthopaedic Surgery, Columbia University Medical Center, New York, New York

Valerae O. Lewis, MD
Associate Professor, Department of Orthopaedic Oncology, MD Anderson Cancer Center, Houston, Texas

Jay R. Lieberman, MD
Director, New England Musculoskeletal Institute, Professor and Chairman, Department of Orthopaedic Surgery, University of Connecticut Health Center, Farmington, Connecticut

Frank A. Liporace, MD
Director of New Jersey Medical School Orthopaedic Trauma Fellowship, Associate Professor of Orthopaedic Surgery, Division of Orthopaedic Trauma, Department of Orthopaedic Surgery, New Jersey Medical School, Newark, New Jersey

Adolph V. Lombardi Jr, MD, FACS
President of Joint Implant Surgeons, Clinical Assistant Professor, Department of Orthopaedics and Department of Biomedical Engineering, The Ohio State University, New Albany, Ohio

Jess H. Lonner, MD
Associate Professor of Orthopaedic Surgery, Rothman Institute, Thomas Jefferson University, Bryn Mawr Hospital, Bryn Mawr, Pennsylvania

Jason A. Lowe, MD
Assistant Professor, Department of Orthopaedic Surgery, University of Alabama at Birmingham, Birmingham, Alabama

William B. Macaulay, MD
Chief of Adult Reconstruction, Anne Youle Stein Professor, College of Physicians and Surgeons, Director of the Center for Hip and Knee Replacement, Department of Orthopaedics, Columbia University, New York, New York

Steven J. MacDonald, MD, FRCSC
Professor of Orthopaedic Surgery, University of Western Ontario, London, Ontario, Canada

David A. McCall, MD
Resident Physician, Stanford University Hospital and Clinics, Stanford University, Stanford, California

Edward G. McFarland, MD
Wayne H. Lewis Professor of Orthopaedic and Shoulder Surgery, Department of Orthopaedic Surgery, Johns Hopkins University School of Medicine, Baltimore, Maryland

Michael D. McKee, MD, FRCSC
Professor, Division of Orthopaedics, Department of Surgery, St. Michael's Hospital and the University of Toronto, Toronto, Ontario, Canada

Robbin C. McKee
Research Student, Division of Orthopaedics, Department of Surgery, St. Michael's Hospital and the University of Toronto, Toronto, Ontario, Canada

Toni M. McLaurin, MD
Assistant Professor, Department of Orthopaedics, New York University Hospital for Joint Diseases, New York, New York

Samir Mehta, MD
Chief, Division of Orthopaedic Trauma, Department of Orthopaedic Surgery, Hospital of the University of Pennsylvania, Philadelphia, Pennsylvania

Lyle J. Micheli, MD
Director, Division of Sports Medicine, Children's Hospital Boston, Boston, Massachusetts

Mark M. Mikhael, MD
Clinical Instructor, Orthopaedic Surgery, University of California Los Angeles Comprehensive Spine Center, Santa Monica, California

Matthew D. Milewski, MD
Sports Medicine Fellow, Department of Orthopaedics, University of Virginia, Charlottesville, Virginia

Mark D. Miller, MD
S. Ward Casscells Professor of Orthopaedic Surgery, Department of Orthopaedic Surgery, University of Virginia, Charlottesville, Virginia

Peter J. Millett, MD, MSc
Orthopaedic Surgeon, Steadman Philippon Research Institute, Vail, Colorado

Bernard F. Morrey, MD
Consultant, Department of Orthopaedic Surgery, Mayo Clinic, Rochester, Minnesota

Carol D. Morris, MD
Attending Surgeon, Orthopaedic Service, Memorial Sloan-Kettering Cancer Center, New York, New York

Brian H. Mullis, MD
Chief, Orthopaedic Trauma Service, Department of Orthopaedics, Indiana University School of Medicine, Indianapolis, Indiana

Andrew S. Neviaser, MD
Shoulder Reconstruction Fellow, Department of Orthopaedic Surgery, Mt. Sinai Medical Center, New York, New York

Gregory P. Nicholson, MD
Associate Professor, Department of Orthopaedic Surgery, Rush University Medical Center, Chicago, Illinois

William T. Obremskey, MD
Chief, Orthopedic Trauma, Department of Orthopedics, Vanderbilt University, Nashville, Tennessee

Reza Omid, MD
Fellow in Shoulder and Elbow Surgery, Shoulder and Elbow Service, Department of Orthopaedic Surgery, Washington University School of Medicine, St. Louis, Missouri

Norman Y. Otsuka, MD
Joseph E. Milgram Professor of Orthopaedic Surgery, New York University Hospital for Joint Diseases, New York University Langone Medical Center, New York, New York

Mark W. Pagnano, MD
Professor of Orthopedics, Department of
Orthopedic Surgery, Mayo Clinic College of
Medicine, Rochester, Minnesota

Michael R. Pagnotto, MD
Adult Lower Extremity Reconstruction Fellow,
Department of Orthopedic Surgery, Mayo Clinic,
Rochester, Minnesota

David M. Panicek, MD
Vice Chair for Clinical Affairs in Radiology,
Department of Radiology, Memorial Sloan-
Kettering Cancer Center, New York, New York

Billy K. Parsley, MD
Orthopaedic Surgeon, Appalachian Orthopaedic
Associates, Kingsport, Tennessee

Theodore W. Parsons III, MD, FACS
Professor and Chairman, Department of
Orthopaedic Surgery, Henry Ford Hospital,
Detroit, Michigan

Joshua C. Patt, MD, MPH
Department of Orthopaedic Surgery, Carolinas
Medical Center, Charlotte, North Carolina

Christopher E. Pelt, MD
Visiting Instructor, Department of Orthopaedics,
University of Utah, Salt Lake City, Utah

Joseph H. Perra, MD
Staff Surgeon, Twin Cities Spine Center,
Minneapolis, Minnesota

Christopher L. Peters, MD
Professor and Medical Director of Adult
Reconstruction and Hip Preservation, Department
of Orthopaedics, University of Utah, Salt Lake City,
Utah

Jason Phillips, MD
Sports Medicine Surgical Fellow, Steadman Hawkins
Clinic of the Carolinas, Greenville Hospital System,
Greenville, South Carolina

Stephan G. Pill, MD, MSPT
Sports Medicine Surgical Fellow, Steadman Hawkins
Clinic of the Carolinas, Greenville Hospital System,
Greenville, South Carolina

Michael S. Pinzur, MD
Professor of Orthopaedic Surgery, Department of
Orthopaedic Surgery, Loyola University Health
System, Maywood, Illinois

Brian L. Puskas, MD
Shoulder and Elbow Fellow, Department of
Orthopaedic Surgery, Tampa General Hospital,
Florida Orthopaedic Institute, Tampa, Florida

Kawan S. Rakhra, MD, FRCPC
Musculoskeletal Radiologist, Department of
Diagnostic Imaging, The Ottawa Hospital, Ottawa,
Ontario, Canada

Mark C. Reilly, MD
Chief, Division of Orthopaedic Trauma,
Department of Orthopaedic Surgery, New Jersey
Medical School, Newark, New Jersey

John A. Repicci, DDS, MD
Orthopedic Surgeon, Department of Joint
Reconstruction and Orthopedics, Kenmore Mercy
Hospital, Buffalo, New York

Anthony S. Rhorer, MD
Director, Orthopaedic Trauma, Sonoran
Orthopaedic Trauma Surgeons, Scottsdale
Healthcare, Scottsdale, Arizona

Peter S. Rose, MD
Consultant Surgeon, Department of Orthopedic
Surgery, Mayo Clinic, Rochester, Minnesota

Guy J. Rudin, MD
Orthopedic Surgeon, Twin Cities Orthopedics,
Minneapolis, Minnesota

Marc R. Safran, MD
Professor, Department of Orthopedic Surgery,
Stanford University, Stanford, California

Vincent James Sammarco, MD
Fellowship Director, Foot and Ankle, Cincinnati
Sports Medicine and Orthopaedic Center,
Cincinnati, Ohio

Joaquin Sanchez-Sotelo, MD, PhD
Consultant and Associate Professor, Department
of Orthopaedic Surgery, Mayo Clinic, Rochester,
Minnesota

Timothy G. Sanders, MD
Director of Education and Research, Department of Radiology, NationalRad, Weston, Florida

Frank J. Schwab, MD
Chief, Spinal Deformity Service, Department of Orthopaedic Surgery, New York University Hospital for Joint Diseases, New York, New York

Joseph H. Schwab, MD
Instructor, Department of Orthopedic Surgery, Massachusetts General Hospital, Boston, Massachusetts

Giles R. Scuderi, MD
Director, Insall Scott Kelly Institute for Orthopaedics and Sports Medicine, New York, New York

Klaus A. Siebenrock, MD
Professor of Orthopedics, Department of Orthopedic Surgery, Inselspital, Bern University Hospital, Bern, Switzerland

David J. Slutsky, MD, FRCSC
Associate Professor, David Geffen University of California Los Angeles School of Medicine, Department of Orthopedics, Harbor–University of California Los Angeles Medical Center, The Hand and Wrist Institute, Torrance, California

Jeremy S. Smith, MD
Fellow, Department of Spine Surgery, Thomas Jefferson University, Rothman Institute, Philadelphia, Pennsylvania

Frederick S. Song, MD
Attending Surgeon, Department of Surgery, University Medical Center at Princeton, Princeton, New Jersey

Hillard T. Spencer, MD
Pediatric Orthopaedic/Spine Fellow, Department of Orthopaedic Surgery, Children's Hospital Boston, Boston, Massachusetts

Paul D. Sponseller, MD
Professor, Department of Orthopaedic Surgery, Johns Hopkins Medical Institutions, Baltimore, Maryland

Scott M. Sporer, MD
Assistant Professor, Department of Orthopaedic Surgery, Rush University Medical Center, Chicago, Illinois

David Stelzeneder, MD
Research Fellow, Department of Orthopedic Surgery, Children's Hospital Boston, Boston, Massachusetts

David W. Stoller, MD
Director, National Orthopedic Imaging Associates and MRI, California Pacific Medical Center, San Francisco, California

Benjamin M. Stronach, MD
Visiting Instructor, Department of Orthopaedics, University of Utah, Salt Lake City, Utah

Daniel J. Sucato, MD
Staff Orthopaedist, Professor, Department of Orthopaedic Surgery, Texas Scottish Rite Hospital for Children, Dallas, Texas

Nirmal C. Tejwani, MD
Associate Professor, Department of Orthopaedics, New York University Hospital for Joint Diseases, New York, New York

Vernon T. Tolo, MD
Chief Emeritus, Children's Orthopaedic Center, Children's Hospital Los Angeles, Los Angeles, California

Paul Tornetta III, MD
Professor and Vice Chairman, Director of Orthopaedic Trauma, Department of Orthopaedic Surgery, Boston University Medical Center, Boston, Massachusetts

Oliver A.J. van der Meijden, MD
Research Scholar, Department of Orthopaedic Surgery, Steadman Philippon Research Institute, Vail, Colorado

Kelly G. Vince, MD, FRCSC
Consultant Orthopedic Surgeon, Northland District Health Board, Whangarei Hospital, Whangarei, Northland, New Zealand

Gilles Walch, MD
Centre Orthopaedique Santy, Hopital Prive Jean Mermoz, Lyon, France

Jeffrey C. Wang, MD
Professor of Orthopaedic and Neurosurgery, University of California Los Angeles Comprehensive Spine Center, Santa Monica, California

Christopher F. Wolf, MD
Clinical Instructor, Orthopaedic Surgery, University of California Los Angeles Comprehensive Spine Center, Santa Monica, California

Philip R. Wolinsky, MD
Chief of Orthopaedic Trauma Service, Vice Chairman, Department of Orthopaedic Surgery, University of California, Davis, Sacramento, California

Adam L. Wollowick, MD
Assistant Professor, Department of Orthopaedic Surgery, Albert Einstein College of Medicine, Bronx, New York

Dane K. Wukich, MD
Associate Professor of Orthopaedic Surgery, Chief, Division of Foot and Ankle Surgery, University of Pittsburgh Medical Center, Pittsburgh, Pennsylvania

Ken Yamaguchi, MD
Sam and Marilyn Fox Distinguished Professor of Orthopaedic Surgery, Chief, Shoulder and Elbow Service, Department of Orthopaedic Surgery, Washington University School of Medicine, St. Louis, Missouri

Brad J. Yoo, MD
Assistant Professor, Department of Orthopaedics, University of California, Davis Medical Center, Sacramento, California

Richard S. Yoon, MD
Resident, Department of Orthopaedic Surgery, New York University Hospital for Joint Diseases, New York, New York

Preface

The instructional course lectures presented each year at the American Academy of Orthopaedic Surgeons Annual Meeting have long been recognized as an excellent educational resource for orthopaedic surgeons. The faculty for these courses is dedicated to providing their fellow surgeons with current research, treatments, and techniques that will expand orthopaedic knowledge and improve care for patients with musculoskeletal disorders and injuries. *Instructional Course Lectures, Volume 61* continues in the proud educational tradition of the preceding 60 volumes, with 48 excellent chapters selected from the many outstanding courses presented at the 2011 AAOS Annual Meeting in San Diego.

I want to express my sincere appreciation to the more than 130 authors who took the time to organize, write, and illustrate their Annual Meeting presentations. The short amount of time between the past meeting and the publication of this volume is a testament to their dedication to the field of orthopaedics and their generosity in sharing their knowledge and experience. I especially would like to thank my assistant editor, Mark W. Pagnano, MD, for his help in providing peer review for the manuscripts in ICL 61.

It has been my privilege to serve as the Chairman of the 2011 AAOS Instructional Courses Committee and the editor for this publication. For their dedicated work in reviewing and selecting the lectures and symposia presented at the AAOS Annual Meeting, thanks goes to Kenneth A. Egol, MD; Mary I. O'Connor, MD; Robert A. Hart, MD; Mark W. Pagnano, MD; and Dempsey S. Springfield, MD. As in past years, Kathie Niesen, Education Manager, deserves recognition for the invaluable guidance and direction she provides to the members of Instructional Courses Committee.

Publication of *Instructional Course Lectures, Volume 61,* would not be possible without the efforts of the AAOS staff, including Marilyn L. Fox, PhD, director of the publications department; Lisa Claxton Moore, managing editor; and Kathleen A. Anderson, senior editor. Reid L. Stanton, manager of electronic media, and his staff deserve credit and thanks for organizing the DVD material, which enhances this volume.

Our hope in putting together this volume is to advance the knowledge of practicing physicians and residents to better care for our patients. This book is geared toward improving outcomes for those under our care.

I would like to dedicate ICL 61 to my mother, Phyllis, who found the best in people, had compassion for all, and whose insight, guidance, and love have always made me believe that anything is possible.

Paul Tornetta III, MD
Boston, Massachusetts

Table of Contents

Section 3: Elbow

Section 4: Adult Reconstruction: Hip

Section 5: Adult Reconstruction: Knee

Trauma

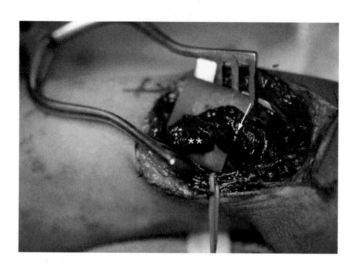

Initial Management and Classification of Pelvic Fractures

John C. Kurylo, MD

Paul Tornetta III, MD

Abstract

Pelvic fractures represent a significant transfer of kinetic energy to the body, and more than 80% of patients with unstable pelvic fractures have additional musculoskeletal injuries. A systematic approach with prompt intervention is critical in the initial management of patients with pelvic fractures. If intra-abdominal bleeding is suspected, diagnostic peritoneal lavage, focused assessment with sonography for trauma, or a CT examination is usually performed. CT angiography and interventional radiographic angiography are useful tools for determining the location of bleeding and the amount of blood loss. Patients presenting in extremis should undergo immediate pelvic stabilization and laparotomy with pelvic packing if indicated. Stable patients can undergo CT angiography. If a large pelvic hematoma or contrast blush is present, extraperitoneal packing or angiography can be performed based on the availability of the needed subspecialists. The orthopaedic surgeon provides prompt stabilization using external immobilizers, external fixation, or traction. The bladder, urethra, and nerve roots have an intimate location within the pelvis and are predisposed to injury in patients with pelvic fractures. Appropriately identifying associated abdominal, urologic, or neurologic injuries will provide important opportunities to reduce patient morbidity and improve long-term outcomes.

Instr Course Lect 2012;61:3-18.

Whether occurring in a hemodynamically stable or unstable patient, pelvic fractures are caused by a significant transfer of kinetic energy to the body. The fractured pelvis may represent the single bony injury in a patient with multiple traumatic organ injuries; however, more than 80% of patients with unstable pelvic fractures have additional musculoskeletal injuries.[1-3] Management of the trauma patient with a pelvic fracture requires a multidisciplinary approach to reduce morbidity/mortality and provide optimal timely care.[4,5]

Mortality

Even with expeditious management of pelvic fractures, the mortality rate ranges from 15% to 25% for closed fractures.[6] In an analysis of two different level 1 trauma centers, Sathy et al[7] evaluated more than 63,000 trauma patients and found a mortality rate of 8.4% to 13.6% for patients with pelvic fractures, compared with 2.4% to 4.5% for those without pelvic fractures. The odds ratio of mortality for patients with a pelvic fracture compared to those without a pelvic fracture is 2.0, similar to the odds ratio for patients who sustain an abdominal injury.

Open pelvic fractures are one of the most devastating injuries in musculoskeletal trauma. Open pelvic fractures are rare, accounting for only 2% to 4% of all pelvic fractures; however, the mortality rate for open pelvic fractures ranges from 15% to 80%.[8] An open pelvic fracture is present when there is direct communication between the fracture and the external skin, rectum, or vagina (**Figure 1**). Open pelvic fractures can range from a small puncture wound over the anterosuperior iliac

Neither Dr. Kurylo nor any immediate family member has received anything of value from or owns stock in a commercial company or institution related directly or indirectly to the subject of this chapter. Dr. Tornetta or an immediate family member has received royalties from Smith & Nephew; serves as a paid consultant to Smith & Nephew; and serves as a board member, owner, officer, or committee member of the American Orthopaedic Association.

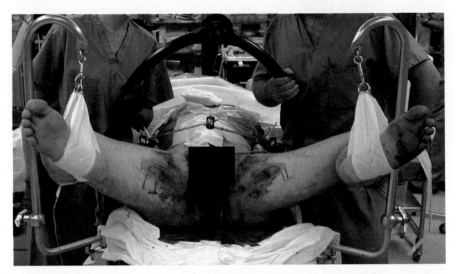

Figure 1 Photograph of a patient with an open pelvic fracture. Obvious disruption of the perineum and genital area is seen.

crest to a large pelvic disruption that injures the external perineum.[9,10] The incidence of open pelvic fractures is higher in children (12.9%) than in adults (2% to 4%). This is believed to result from the greater plasticity of the immature pelvic ring, which requires a higher applied force to cause a pediatric pelvic fracture.[11]

The age of the trauma patient plays a critical role in survival. In patients older than 60 years, Starr et al[12] reported a predicted mortality of 11%, with a sensitivity and specificity of 26% and 91%, respectively. The mortality rate is higher in patients older than 55 years compared with younger patients, 12.3% versus 2.3%, respectively; older patients are also expected to have a longer hospital stay.[6]

It is believed that the actual mortality rate associated with a pelvic fracture or trauma involving the pelvis is much higher when prehospital deaths are taken into account. In a review by Adams et al[13] of 392 "rapid fatalities" based on records from a coroner's office and medical examiner's office, it was determined that 25% of patients who died in the field from traumatic causes had a pelvic fracture, and more

than 50% of those patients had unstable pelvic fractures. It was also found that pedestrians and motorcyclists were twice as likely to sustain a pelvic fracture, and the severity of the pelvic fracture correlated with the increasing speed of the vehicle involved in the crash.[13] Based on prior published survivorship studies of pelvic fractures, pelvic injuries tend to be more severe in victims who do not survive to hospitalization. The study indicates that the current estimation of mortality after a pelvic fracture may actually be lower than reported because patients who die in the field are excluded from most analyses. For example, Eastridge et al[14] reported that 38 of 231 patients (16.5%) died on arrival or very shortly after arrival at the emergency department before receiving any medical intervention.

In patients with multiple injuries and a pelvic injury, the pelvic fracture is usually not the primary cause of death. Studies reported that the pelvic fracture was the precipitating cause of death in 13% of patients, and patients who died had an injury severity score that implicated at least one additional major visceral injury.[15,16] Sepsis, acute

respiratory distress syndrome, coagulopathy, wound infection, pneumonia, and urinary tract infection are common complications (in addition to death) seen in almost one third of patients with blunt trauma pelvic fractures.[17]

In the acute phase of care, it is crucial to identify risk factors for morbidity and mortality. Retrospective analyses of surviving patients compared with those who died have shown that blood pressure, initial trauma score on presentation, revised trauma score, and transfusion requirements correlate with survival. One of the first investigations into predictors of mortality in patients with pelvic fractures was done in 1984 by Mucha and Farnell.[18] In evaluating 34 deaths, the authors reported a 3.4% mortality in patients who presented with a systolic blood pressure higher than 90 and 42% in those presenting with a systolic blood pressure less than 90. A 2002 study reported that an initial systolic blood pressure less than 90 and a revised trauma score of less than 11 are associated with increased mortality, transfusion requirements, the use of pelvic arteriography, and later complications.[12] Shock on arrival at the emergency department predicted mortality with 27% sensitivity and 96% specificity.[12] The revised trauma score assigns a number from 0 to 4, with 0 being the worst and 4 being the best, for the patient's systolic blood pressure on arrival, Glasgow Coma Score, and respiratory rate. These numbers are then entered into an algorithm to determine the probability of survival.[19] A revised trauma score of less than 11 predicts mortality with a 58% sensitivity and 92% specificity.[10] Patients with a base deficit (a lack of bicarbonate in the blood caused by respiratory or metabolic acidosis or alkalosis) of –5 mmol/L or less are more likely to die[20] (**Table 1**).

Table 1

Factors Associated With Increased Rates of Mortality in Patients With Pelvic Fractures

Systolic blood pressure < 90 mm Hg on arrival at the emergency department
Revised trauma score < 11
Blood transfusion requirement
Base deficit ≤ –5

Table 2

Young and Burgess Pelvic Fracture Classification System

APC-I	Minor opening of symphysis and SI joint anteriorly
APC-II	Opening of anterior SI joint, intact posterior SI ligaments
APC-III	Complete disruption of SI joint
LC-I	Sacral fracture on the side of impact
LC-II	Crescent fracture on the side of impact
LC-III	Type I or II LC injury with opening rotation of contralateral hemipelvis
VS	Vertical displacement of hemipelvis with symphysis diastasis or rami fractures anterior, iliac wing, sacral fracture, or SI dislocation posterior

APC = anteroposterior compression, LC = lateral compression, VS = vertical shear, SI = sacroiliac

Classification

On arrival to the emergency department, chest and AP pelvis radiographs of the patient should be taken in accordance with Advanced Trauma Life Support guidelines to provide an immediate and valuable tool for determining the mechanism of injury and to help predict resuscitation needs.[21] Because the pelvis is a ring structure, significant disruption and displacement of one area is accompanied by the same forces in another area, resulting in both bone and ligamentous disruptions. The sacroiliac (SI) joints are the strongest joints in the body and resist both vertical and anteroposterior displacement. The pubic symphysis is the weakest link in the pelvic ring, supplying only 15% of intrinsic pelvic stability.[22] The pelvic floor muscles and ligaments also contribute to pelvic stability. Initial emergency department radiographs of the pelvis have been shown to be only 68% sensitive for identifying all fractures, although large fractures that lead to instability are almost always seen.[23] Fifty percent to 69% of patients with unstable pelvic fractures seen on the initial AP pelvic radiograph will require four or more units of blood, 36% to 55% will have an intra-abdominal injury, and 6% to 18% will have a pelvic arterial injury.[24]

Multiple pelvic fracture classification schemes are presented in the orthopaedic literature.[25,26] The Orthopaedic Trauma Association pelvic fracture classification, which is loosely based on the Young-Burgess classification system, states that a type A pelvic fracture denotes a pelvic injury with a stable posterior ring. Type B injuries have partial stability, with the fracture rotationally unstable but vertically stable. A type C injury indicates that vertical shear has occurred, resulting in rotational and vertical instability.[13] In the Young and Burgess classification system, pelvic fractures are divided into four groups: anteroposterior compression (APC), lateral compression (LC), vertical shear (VS), and combined mechanical injury.[27,28] The first two groups are further categorized according to the severity of injury based on the energy imparted to the pelvis. This part of the classification system is based on a study of 210 pelvic fractures in which the authors found that the plane of the anterior ring disruption indicated the direction of the force imparted on the pelvis (**Table 2**).

It is necessary to understand the pelvic anatomy to correctly understand the different classification systems and how that guides the subsequent management of pelvic injuries. The bony pelvic ring is composed of the sacrum posteriorly, which connects to the two hemipelves via anterior, intra-articular, and posterior SI ligaments. The sacrospinous and sacrotuberous ligaments also contribute to the stability of the posterior pelvic ring. The posterior pelvis and sacrum are the keystone elements of the pelvis because they provide structural support that dictates the stability of the entire pelvic ring (**Figure 2**). The anterior pelvic ring is held in place via the pubic symphysis, which provides 15% of the total pelvic ring stability.[29] Disruption of the bony or ligamentous structures can result in a vascular injury because of the intimate association of these structures. Specifically, the internal iliac vessels and their branches (iliolumbar, lateral sacral, superior gluteal, obturator, and inferior gluteal) are at risk for arterial and venous injury resulting in severe hemorrhage. The bladder, urethra, and vagina are directly posterior to the pubic symphysis, placing them at risk for injury when the pelvis undergoes a significant deforming force.

The Young and Burgess classification is the most useful system for correlating the injury mechanism with a fracture pattern and associated bodily injuries (**Figure 3**). APC injuries are rotational injuries that "open the book" of the pelvis through the symphysis. Although described as APC injuries, it is likely that most of these injuries are caused by aggressive external rotation of the limb, such as occurs in a motorcycle or snowmobile crash. As the energy increases, the symphysis separates (APC-I injuries), the pelvic

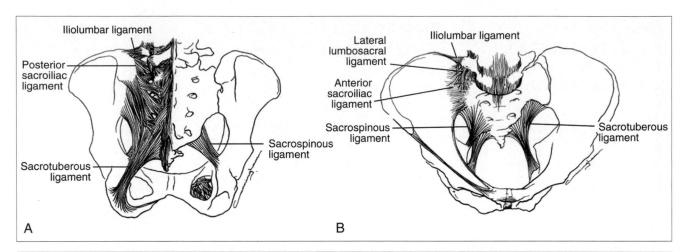

Figure 2 Illustrations of the major posterior (**A**) and anterior (**B**) stabilizing ligamentous structures of the pelvic ring. (Reproduced with permission from Hak DJ, Smith WR, Suzuki T: Management of hemorrhage in life-threatening pelvic fracture. *J Am Acad Orthop Surg* 2009;7:447-457.)

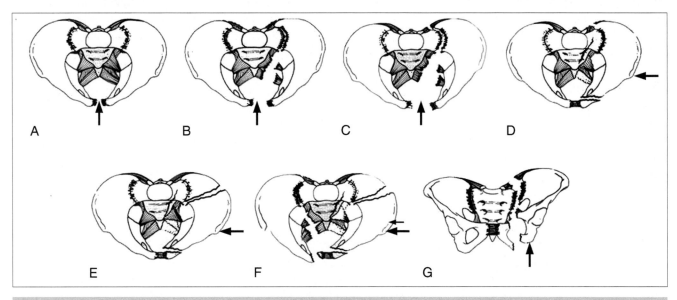

Figure 3 Illustration of the Young-Burgess classification of pelvic fractures. **A**, APC-I. **B**, APC-II. **C**, APC-III. **D**, LC-I. **E**, LC-II. **F**, LC-III. **G**, VS fracture. The arrow in each panel indicates the direction of force producing the fracture pattern. (Copyright Jesse B. Jupiter, MD, Boston, MA and Bruce D. Browner, MD, Farmington, CT.)

floor with its associated sacrospinous ligaments tears, and the SI joint opens anteriorly (APC-II injuries). If enough energy is present, then the SI joint completely ruptures, including the strong posterior SI ligaments (APC-III injuries). The difference in the APC-II and APC-III patterns is the total loss of the posterior attachment of the sacrum and ilium. This is best seen with CT. An APC-II injury demonstrates an anterior opening but with an intact posterior hinge (**Figure 4**), whereas an APC-III injury has widening of the entire SI joint (**Figure 5**). APC injuries are associated with spleen, liver, and bowel injuries. With the increasing severity of the APC injury, the risk of abdominal organ injury increases. The most important concern with APC injuries is blood loss from tearing of the pelvic floor and associated vasculature. Although the pelvic volume is mathematically increased, this volume represents only a small portion of the possible blood loss. Most of the blood loss extends proximally into the retroperitoneum and distally into the legs via the torn pelvic floor.

LC type I and II injuries are characterized by an oblique anterior ring fracture and are associated with decreasing pelvic volume, intraperitoneal or in-

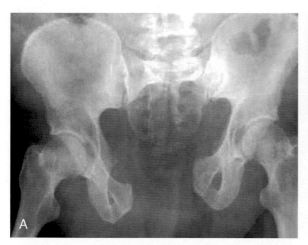
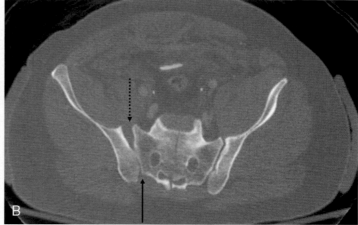

Figure 4   Radiograph (**A**) and CT scan (**B**) showing an APC-II pelvic injury. The dotted line on the CT scan shows the opening of anterior SI joint. The solid line shows the posterior SI joint acting as a hinge.

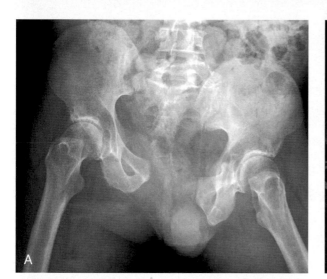
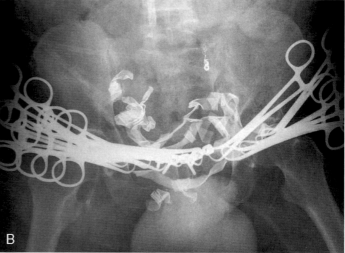

Figure 5   **A,** Preoperative AP radiograph of an APC-III pelvic injury. **B,** Postoperative radiograph after pelvic packing, open reduction and internal fixation of the pubic symphysis, and angiography.

trathoracic hemorrhage, and a high incidence of head and chest injury, which is predictable because the typical patient sustaining an LC pelvic injury is in a car struck from the side. The impact causes injury to the chest and head as the patient is accelerated against the inside of the car (**Figure 6**). In an LC-I type fracture, anterior sacral compression fractures occur on the side of impact. This fracture pattern is stable because the posterior tension bands remain intact. By increasing the LC force, the anterior sacrum acts as the pivot point, and a

crescent iliac wing fracture occurs (LC-II pattern). The LC-III fracture is often described as a rollover fracture because it occurs when an automobile rolls over, causing one hemipelvis to internally rotate and the other to externally rotate (**Figure 7**); however, these fractures occur more commonly when a pedestrian is struck by a vehicle. Because one hemipelvis externally rotates and tears the pelvic floor, these injuries are severely unstable and are more like APC injuries with associated retroperitoneal hemorrhage and vascular injury.

VS injuries, which are often associated with massive blood loss, have an initial cephalad displacement that is not seen in APC injuries (**Figure 8**). These injuries, which commonly occur after a fall from a height, may show either symphyseal separation or vertical rami fractures as the anterior injury and SI dislocation or sacral fracture as the posterior injury.

Combined mechanical injuries may incorporate two or more injury patterns. The incidence of pelvic fracture with associated brain injury is 37% to

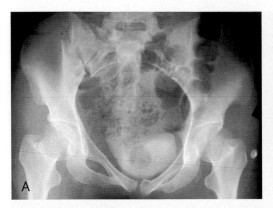
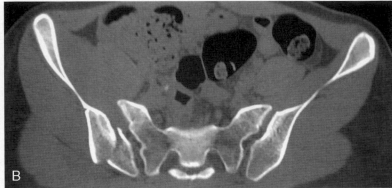

Figure 6 Radiograph (**A**) and CT scan (**B**) of a LC-II pelvic fracture pattern.

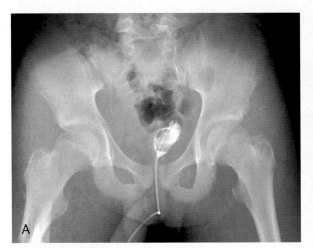
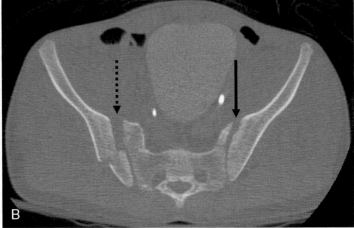

Figure 7 Radiograph (**A**) and CT scan (**B**) of the LC-III fracture pattern. Dotted line with arrow on the CT scan shows a fracture-dislocation of the right SI joint. Solid line with arrow shows anterior compression of the left anterior SI joint.

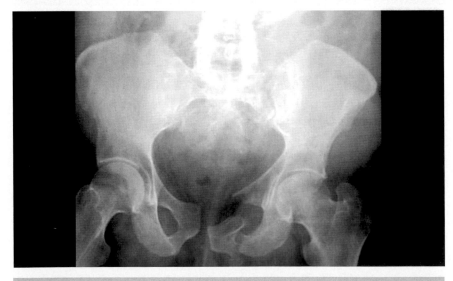

Figure 8 AP radiograph of a patient with a VS pelvic fracture with an L5 nerve root palsy.

50%; associated thoracic injury, 25% to 66%; and associated abdominal injury, 42% to 51%.[3,24,25,30,31]

Initial Management

The initial management of the trauma patient should follow Advanced Trauma Life Support guidelines. The physical examination and portable AP pelvis radiograph are often the key elements in diagnosing associated injuries and improving the patient's chance of survival. The following ABCs of trauma care should be initiated: A, airway maintenance with cervical spine control; B, breathing and ventilation; C, circulation with hemorrhage control; D, disability evaluation (neurologic status), and E, exposure and environmental control (completely undress the patient but prevent hypothermia).

The first physical examination should be performed by the most experienced treating physician in a cranial-caudal order that screens for obvious injuries, especially sources of major blood loss in the regions of the head, chest, abdomen, pelvis, and limbs. After the primary survey is completed, pelvic stability may be assessed by gently yet firmly compressing and distracting the iliac wings. This examination is typically unnecessary if a good AP radiograph is available, and it should be remembered that manipulation of an unstable pelvic ring can be harmful. If manipulated, any increased mobility is a sign of gross instability. For the more thorough secondary survey, a high level of suspicion is mandatory for pelvic soft-tissue injury because clinical findings can be inconsistent, and missed injuries are common. A study of 100 patients transferred to a tertiary trauma center in England found that 7 pelvic fractures and 3 bladder/urethral injuries were missed, 5 hips were dislocated, and 1 patient had an undiagnosed open pelvic fracture.[32] Because the intimate relationship of the pelvic soft tissues to the bony ring can result in injuries such as rectal, vaginal, urogenital, or vascular lesions, the examination should include inspection of the perianal tissues, the vaginal vault, and the digital rectum.[8] A palpable hematoma over the perineum (Destot sign), above the inguinal ligament, or on the proximal thigh indicates a possible pelvic fracture with associated bleeding. The Grey Turner sign, ecchymosis in the flank, is associated with retroperitoneal hemorrhage.[33]

Patient resuscitation begins by placing at least two large-caliber, 16-gauge, intravenous catheters in the upper extremities for administration of fluids or blood. If routine intravenous access is not possible, central venous access may be required. Immediately after intravenous access is established, before delivering fluids or blood, hematology, blood chemistry, clotting factor evaluation, typing and cross-matching, and pregnancy test and toxicology laboratory results should be obtained. Studies have shown that a state of underresuscitated shock leads to systemic inflammatory response syndrome, eventual irreversible body-wide ischemia, and multiple organ dysfunction syndrome, followed by death.[34-38] As indicators of shock, elevated lactate levels and base deficits directly correlate with mortality in patients with pelvic trauma.[20,39] Measuring the patient's temperature is also important because hypothermia can affect blood pressure and the heart rate. If a source of hemorrhage has been identified and the patient is in shock, hemostatic or damage control resuscitation is promptly administered with the transfusion of packed red blood cells, fresh frozen plasma, and platelets, ideally in a 1:1:1 (pack) ratio using type-specific products unless the patient is completely unresponsive. Using this ratio of blood products has been shown to improve survival in patients requiring massive transfusions.[34-38] In patients with a hemodynamically unstable pelvic fracture, statistically significant independent predictors of mortality are systolic blood pressure less than 90 after receiving 2 L of intravenous fluid, a high injury severity score, age older than 60 years, and transfusion requirements during hospitalization.[40]

Pelvic Bleeding

Locating the source of bleeding, whether from the pelvis itself, the vasculature, or abdominal contents, is of paramount importance. The question arises regarding which of several modalities should be used to identify the bleeding—angiography, diagnostic peritoneal lavage, CT, or ultrasound.

Velmahos et al[41] showed that angiographic embolization is safe and effective in 94% of patients; however, mortality after angiographic treatment remains high unless it is completed within 3 hours.[42] Most studies on angiography predated rapid external immobilization as it is currently performed; if angiography follows current techniques, it is likely to be more effective. Most importantly, if the patient is hemodynamically unstable, older than 55 years, and does not have a long-bone fracture, there is a 95% predictive risk of active bleeding. Of all patients who underwent an angiogram, 4% had recurrent bleeding and 5% had a complication caused by the procedure[20,42-45] (**Table 3**).

Historically, diagnostic peritoneal lavage (41% sensitivity, 99% specificity, 94% positive predicative value, and 95% negative predicative value) has been the standard in most trauma centers.[46] However, diagnostic peritoneal lavage is associated with a high number of false-positive results, nontherapeutic laparotomy, and a negative impact on outcome.[2,14,47] In the United States, it is used only for unstable patients in a setting in which ultrasound is not available or the patient cannot safely undergo CT. For the stable patient with suspected intra-abdominal injury, CT examination (95% sensitivity, 95% specificity) has largely supplanted diagnostic peritoneal lavage.[48] In Europe, ultrasonography (90% sensitivity; 95% specificity) is the screening tool of choice.[48] Patients who appear to have significant hemoperitoneum as determined by ultrasound and/or diagnostic peritoneal lavage are transferred to the operating room for abdominal exploration and pelvic fixation with treatment of associated injuries.

Table 3					
Summary of Angiogram Data					
Author	No. of Pelvic Fractures	No. of Patients Undergoing Angiography	Bleeding Site Identified	Successful Embolization	Overall Mortality in Patients Undergoing Angiography
Matalon et al[43]	324	28 (8.6%)	71%	64%	50%
Panetta et al[44]	31	31	100%	87.5%	35.5%
Allen et al[20]	675	14 (2%)	N/A	N/A	50%
Wong et al[45]	507	17 (3.5%)	N/A	100%	18%
Agolini et al[42]	806	35 (4.3%)	43%	100%	0% within 3 hours
N/A = not available					

Indicators of major hemorrhage in a patient with a pelvic fracture are a presenting hematocrit level less than 30%, heart rate greater than 130, a displaced obturator ring fracture, or a symphyseal diastasis.[49] Even with a stable pelvic fracture pattern, all patients who present with a systolic blood pressure less than 90, hematocrit level of 30% or lower, and the presence of a pelvic hematoma on CT scan will require a blood transfusion and possibly an intervention to control bleeding within the first 24 hours after admission.[50] Hemorrhage from the cancellous bone surfaces of the pelvis and the presacral venous plexus may contribute to hypotension.[51,52] In 10% to 15% of patients, the hemorrhage is arterial, and the pudendal and superior gluteal arteries are the most commonly identified source of arterial bleeding at arteriography.[22] Patients presenting in extremis with a posterior fracture along the SI joints may have a disruption of a main iliac trunk. This is a rare injury occurring in less than 1% of patients.[53,54] Patients with higher energy injuries (APC-II, APC-III, LC-III, VS, or combined mechanism) are more likely to receive a blood transfusion (44%) than other patients with other fracture types (8.5%).[55]

CT angiography and interventional radiographic angiography are useful tools in determining the location of bleeding and the amount of blood loss in a patient with a pelvic fracture. A CT angiogram provides a three-dimensional image that allows the volumes of pelvic hemorrhage to be calculated. The sensitivity of active bleeding on contrast CT showing a significant arterial bleed was 80%; specificity, 98%; positive predicative value, 80%; and negative predicative value, 98%.[56] Siegel et al[57] reported on 58 high-energy trauma patients and demonstrated that CT angiography had a 100% negative predictive value for arterial bleeding requiring therapeutic angiography. Positive findings correlated well with the anatomic location of the pelvic injury and had a 70% positive predictive value for angiographically treatable bleeding.[57] Based on the very high negative predictive values in these two independent studies, it can be confidently assumed that no active arterial hemorrhage is present if a patient does not have evidence of bleeding on a CT angiogram.

On average, patients with a pelvic fracture will have 149 mL of fracture-related hemorrhage.[58] Diligence is required in determining the amount of pelvic fracture-related hemorrhage to decide if interventional radiographic angiography is needed. Patients with a pelvic blood volume greater than 500 mL on CT scanning have almost a 5 times increased risk that arterial bleeding will be found on a formal angiogram.[58] Only one study showed an-giography to be 100% effective in reducing mortality.[42] Although the applications of angiography are limited, it is still useful in a select group of patients. In patients with uncontrolled hypotension, the bleeding source can be identified 78% of the time.[59] For patients with an identifiable vascular injury, more than 50% will have more than one bleeding site, and some bleeding sites may not be on the injured side.[60] For select patients in whom subselective pelvic embolization is unsuccessful in controlling bleeding, temporary angiographic embolization of bilateral internal iliac arteries can be performed. Velmahos et al[61] demonstrated that after performing such a procedure, clinical and radiographic bleeding was successfully controlled in 90% of patients. Posterior arterial bleeding, either internal iliac or its posterior branches, is statistically more common in patients with unstable posterior pelvic fractures. The superior gluteal artery is the most commonly injured vessel associated with posterior pelvic fractures. Anterior arterial bleeding from the pudendal or obturator arteries is more common in patients with LC injuries. The pudendal artery is the most commonly injured vessel in LC injuries.[60] Although angiography is relatively successful in treating pelvic bleeding, the time spent to perform the angiographic evaluation and treatment may compromise the overall management of the patient, specifically external stabilization of the pelvis. Thus, it has been recommended that skeletal stabilization occur before any angiographic studies and, if indicated, laparotomy be used to manage intraperitoneal blood loss before pelvic angiography.[59]

External Immobilization

The orthopaedic surgeon plays an important role in the initial management of unstable pelvic injuries by providing initial stabilization using external immobilizers, external fixation, or traction. This role is especially important in cases of abdominal bleeding, when the pelvis is stabilized before any intervention. Pelvic skeletal stability can be achieved with a sheet wrapped circumferentially around the pelvis, a pelvic binder, a C-clamp, or an external fixator. Reduction and stabilization of pelvic fractures prevents further blood loss by limiting the bleeding from the fracture fragments and reducing the pelvic volume. For every 1 cm widening of the pubic symphysis, there is a 4.6% increase in the volume of the true pelvis; and for every 1 cm displacement at the SI joint, there is a 3.1% increase in true pelvic volume.[62] In most patients, the bleeding source is the injured sacral venous plexus or bone surfaces; providing stability helps to tamponade the hemorrhage.[63-65] Although the pelvic volume is decreased, the benefit of reducing motion and allowing the low-pressure system to clot and maintain the clot is likely the most important benefit of external immobilization. In a recent comparison of three different pelvic compression devices—the Pelvic Binder (Pelvic Binder Inc, Dallas, TX), the SAM Sling (SAM Medical Products, Wilsonville, OR), and the T-POD (T-Pod, Bio-cybernetics International, La Verne, CA)—each device provided sufficient reduction in both partially stable

and unstable pelvic fractures without overreducing the pelvis.[66] When placing external immobilization on the pelvis, it is important to recognize the type of fracture pattern. Using external immobilization for unilateral LC patterns can cause further internal rotation of the hemipelvis and result in increased fracture diastases, which should be avoided. At Boston University Medical Center, pelvic skeletal stability in the trauma bay is provided with an anteriorly placed C-clamp, as described by Richard and Tornetta,[67] or using the sheeting method, as described by Routt et al.[68] A longitudinally folded bed sheet is applied circumferentially around the pelvis with a gel pad placed on each greater trochanter. The sheet is securely held in place by clamping the sheet anteriorly. The sheet should be wide but not tight over the pelvis and tight over the proximal thighs. A gel pad is also placed between the medial malleoli of the ankles, and the ankles are circumferentially wrapped with an elastic bandage. This technique provides a quick, inexpensive, and effective method of providing pelvic stability. Additionally, the sheet can be positioned so that the pelvis is still being compressed while more rigid fixation is applied using an external fixator or a C-clamp.[68]

Some form of external pelvic stabilization (a noninvasive method, an external fixator, or a C-clamp) is indicated when a fracture pattern results in increased pelvic volume (APC-II, APC-III, LC-III, or VS patterns). Of note, VS patterns may respond best to longitudinal skeletal traction, which should be applied as soon as feasible. The external immobilization will address hemodynamic instability via anterior compression of the pelvic ring. This method will provide adequate temporary anterior ring stabilization but may not fully address posterior ring displacement. A relative indica-

tion for pelvic external fixation is skeletal instability, as seen in LC-II injury patterns. In addition to providing pelvic stability and reducing pelvic volume, external immobilization will allow patient mobilization and can provide definitive treatment in certain circumstances. Contraindications for using a bony external fixator include an inability to control pelvic volume, as seen in iliac and acetabular fractures, and a treating physician who is inexperienced with the procedure. Most surgeons no longer use pin placement in the iliac crests and now favor placing pins along the pelvic brim, the so-called Hannover frame[69,70] (**Figure 9**).

The pelvic C-clamp was designed to provide direct reduction and compression of sacral fractures and SI dislocations;[71] however, it has been adapted to be placed anteriorly two finger breadths below the anterosuperior iliac spine to close the pelvic volume (**Figure 10**). The simple design can be applied in less than 10 minutes and can be placed in the emergency department, interventional radiology suite, or operating room. Importantly, because of its design, the C-clamp does not interfere with the ability to carry out subsequent laparotomy or other required abdominal procedures. Historically, the C-clamp was used acutely to rapidly stabilize the posterior pelvic ring at the SI joints in hypotensive patients. This method, however, requires fluoroscopy and can be time consuming. A recent study by Richard and Tornetta[67] showed that anterior placement of the C-clamp raised the systolic blood pressure on average 23 mm Hg in patients with a systolic blood pressure lower than 90 mm Hg. The authors also demonstrated that symphyseal separation could be reduced from a mean of 4.5 cm (range, 3 to 9 cm) to less than 2 cm in all cases, and the C-clamp could be easily draped for any angiogram or abdominal surgical procedure. In a study of 30 patients treated with the pelvic C-clamp, the initial reduction was appropriate in 66% of the patients, and the anatomy of the pelvic ring was adequately restored.[72] There were no complications directly related to the C-clamp.

Pelvic Packing

Extraperitoneal pelvic packing is a rapid method for controlling pelvic fracture-related hemorrhage that may supplant the need for emergent angiography.[1] Prior to performing pelvic packing, external immobilization of the pelvis is needed to avoid losing the final restraint to external rotation of the ring and to help control the torn pelvic floor and vasculature. To perform extraperitoneal pelvic packing, a 6- to 8-cm midline incision is made from the symphysis pubis and is extended cranially. The linea alba is incised, and the peritoneum is left intact. The pelvic hematoma has often dissected the preperitoneal and prevesical space to the presacral region. After delivering the hematoma, three surgical laparotomy sponges are placed on each side of the true pelvis below the pelvic brim to tamponade bleeding. These are pushed tightly all the way to the SI joints. The fascia and skin are then closed, and the packs are removed after 24 to 48 hours. The total time for the packing procedure should be less than 20 minutes.[73] Even with successful pelvic packing, there is a high rate of arterial injury.[1] Smith et al[73] and Tötterman et al[74] recommend that following packing, the patient with persistent hypotension should undergo pelvic angiography or surgical exploration to gain direct control of presumed arterial bleeding. Because the standard laparotomy exposure will not allow access to the true or lesser pelvis, the incision must be extended distally. When packing is performed, it may be possible to do minimal and expeditious open reduction and internal fixation of simple anterior ring injuries, such as a symphyseal separation.

Associated Pelvic Injuries

Like the delicate vasculature of the pelvis, the bladder and the urethra have an intimate location within the pelvis

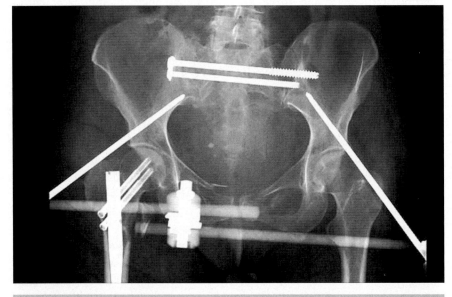

Figure 9 AP radiograph showing placement of supra-acetabular external fixator pins.

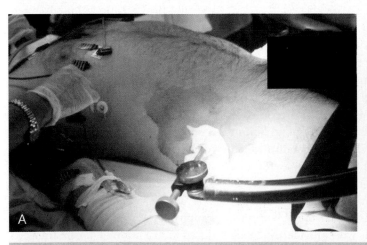
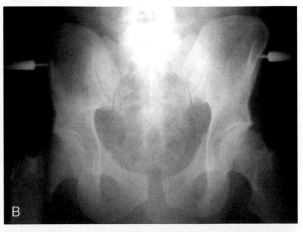

Figure 10 Photograph (**A**) and radiograph (**B**) show anterior placement of the C-clamp. The radiograph shows the large area available for the performance of abdominal surgical procedures. Direct reduction of the pelvic ring can be seen.

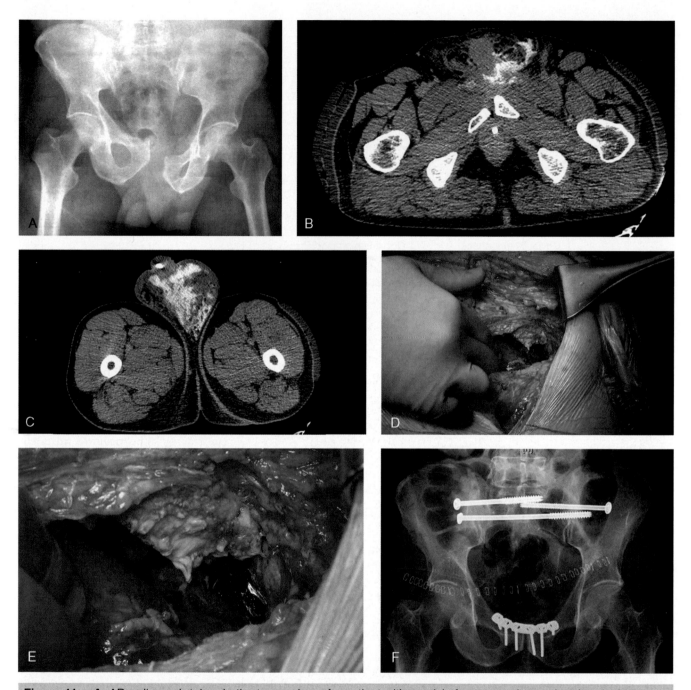

Figure 11   **A,** AP radiograph taken in the trauma bay of a patient with a pelvic fracture and associated urologic trauma. **B** and **C,** CT cystograms showing extravasation of contrast around the urethra into the scrotum. **D** and **E,** Intraoperative photographs showing a bladder rupture with an associated pelvic fracture. **F,** Postoperative radiograph showing anterior and posterior pelvic ring fixation.

that predisposes them to injury with a pelvic fracture. The incidence of urologic trauma after pelvic fracture is approximately 16%, and these injuries range from bladder contusions (manifesting as microscopic hematuria) to bladder rupture and urethral injuries.[75] Zingg et al[76] reported that 35 of 44 posterior urethral injuries occurred with an LC-type pelvic fracture pattern. Bladder rupture most commonly occurs with a full bladder at the time of injury and is typically extraperitoneal (**Figure 11**). A bladder injury with a concomitant urethral tear is possible. Dunstan and Bircher[77] reported on the urologic pitfalls in unstable pelvic fractures and made several

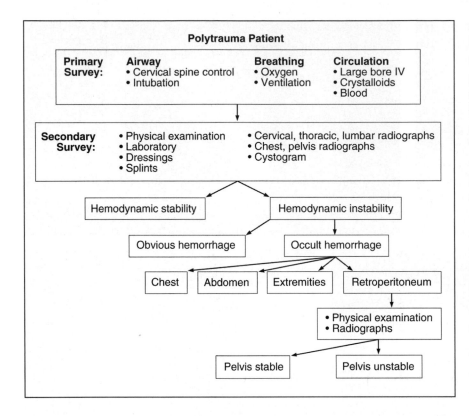

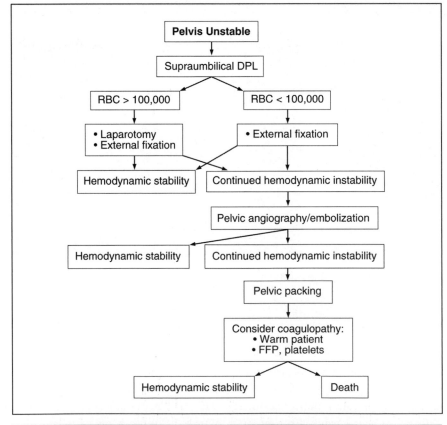

Figure 12 Algorithm for initial pelvic fracture management. RBC = red blood cells, DPL = diagnostic peritoneal lavage, FFP = fresh frozen plasma, IV = intravenous.

recommendations. (1) Genitourinary injury should be assumed in all patients with pelvic fractures until proven otherwise. (2) High-energy shearing injuries and transverse or pubic ramus fractures should increase this suspicion. (3) Retrograde combined urethrocystograms may require up to 450 mL of contrast to demonstrate a leak, and true oblique with postwashout radiographs should be obtained. (4) The ability to pass a catheter in the resuscitation room does not exclude a urethral tear. Unless the patient is in extremis, a retrograde urethrogram should be performed on all male patients with a pelvic fracture. If this important step is missed, then it should be performed later as tolerated. Pericatheter urethrograms have been recommended in this scenario but are difficult to perform and not as accurate, so it is best to perform a true urethrogram before anterior pelvic skeletal reconstruction. The suggested treatment of intraperitoneal bladder ruptures is to repair the bladder, whereas extraperitoneal ruptures require repair only if the anterior ring is surgically repaired. Typically, diversion is sufficient if the pelvis is treated nonsurgically. There is approximately a 10% infection rate with genital urinary repair and orthopaedic pelvic fixation.[76]

Nerve injury is also common in pelvic fractures, with an overall incidence of 10%; the highest rates occur with sacral fractures and posterior ring displacement. More than 50% of vertically unstable pelvic fractures have an accompanying nerve injury, which is typically a nerve root avulsion. LC fracture patterns will have impingement of the nerve roots, whereas the APC fracture pattern will have nerve root avulsions. Reilly el al[78] reviewed 83 unstable pelvic injuries and reported that 21% had a neurologic injury, of which 37% were sensory only and 63% were sensory and motor. All patients had some recovery, and only 58% had complete recovery, with the L5 nerve the least likely to resolve. Two studies examined the functional outcomes of treated unstable pelvic fractures and found that 66% of patients had returned to their original jobs, and 63% had no pain or pain only with strenuous activity.[79,80] Twenty-seven percent of the patients had lower extremity weakness, and 13% had sexual problems. These findings illustrate the importance of a thorough sensory examination from L4 to the lower sacral nerve roots, as well as an examination of the sphincter tone and perianal sensation, because early urologic consultation and cystometry studies may be indicated in the future.

A systematic approach with prompt action is essential for the initial management of a pelvic fracture. It must be determined if the patient is hemodynamically and skeletally stable. The need for additional workup for bleeding (focused assessment with sonography for trauma, diagnostic peritoneal lavage, or CT) and the presence of any associated urologic or neurologic injury also should be determined. Applying an algorithm that takes all these points into account is critical (**Figure 12**).

Summary

Hemorrhage must be stopped urgently to improve the chance of survival in a patient with an unstable pelvic fracture. This is best accomplished by a multidisciplinary team at a level I trauma center. Hemodynamic stability is initially provided via external pelvic immobilization with concurrent aggressive fluid and blood resuscitation. Associated injuries should be identified by a thorough yet expeditious head-to-toe physical examination. If abdominal bleeding is suspected, a focused assessment with sonography for trauma, CT examination, or diagnos-

tic peritoneal lavage is usually performed. Patients presenting in extremis should undergo immediate pelvic stabilization and laparotomy, with pelvic packing if indicated. Stable patients can undergo CT angiography. If a large pelvic hematoma or contrast blush is seen, extraperitoneal packing or angiography can be performed based on the availability of the needed subspecialists. The role of the orthopaedic surgeon is critical in providing pelvic stability. The importance of identifying associated abdominal, urologic, or neurologic injuries will provide important opportunities to improve patient morbidity and long-term outcomes.

References

1. Cothren CC, Osborn PM, Moore EE, Morgan SJ, Johnson JL, Smith WR: Preperitonal pelvic packing for hemodynamically unstable pelvic fractures: A paradigm shift. *J Trauma* 2007;62(4): 834-839, discussion 839-842.

2. Gustavo Parreira J, Coimbra R, Rasslan S, Oliveira A, Fregoneze M, Mercadante M: The role of associated injuries on outcome of blunt trauma patients sustaining pelvic fractures. *Injury* 2000; 31(9):677-682.

3. McMurtry R, Walton D, Dickinson D, Kellam J, Tile M: Pelvic disruption in the polytraumatized patient: A management protocol. *Clin Orthop Relat Res* 1980;151: 22-30.

4. Turen CH, Dube MA, LeCroy MC: Approach to the polytraumatized patient with musculoskeletal injuries. *J Am Acad Orthop Surg* 1999;7(3):154-165.

5. Biffl WL, Smith WR, Moore EE, et al: Evolution of a multidisciplinary clinical pathway for the management of unstable patients with pelvic fractures. *Ann Surg* 2001;233(6):843-850.

6. O'Brien DP, Luchette FA, Pereira SJ, et al: Pelvic fracture in the elderly is associated with increased mortality. *Surgery* 2002;132(4): 710-714, discussion 714-715.

7. Sathy AK, Starr AJ, Smith WR, et al: The effect of pelvic fracture on mortality after trauma: An analysis of 63,000 trauma patients. *J Bone Joint Surg Am* 2009; 91(12):2803-2810.

8. Grotz MR, Allami MK, Harwood P, Pape HC, Krettek C, Giannoudis PV: Open pelvic fractures: Epidemiology, current concepts of management and outcome. *Injury* 2005;36(1):1-13.

9. Jones AL, Powell JN, Kellam JF, McCormack RG, Dust W, Wimmer P: Open pelvic fractures: A multicenter retrospective analysis. *Orthop Clin North Am* 1997; 28(3):345-350.

10. Faringer PD, Mullins RJ, Feliciano PD, Duwelius PJ, Trunkey DD: Selective fecal diversion in complex open pelvic fractures from blunt trauma. *Arch Surg* 1994;129(9):958-963, discussion 963-964.

11. Mosheiff R, Suchar A, Porat S, Shmushkevich A, Segal D, Liebergall M: The "crushed open pelvis" in children. *Injury* 1999;30 (Suppl 2):B14-B18.

12. Starr AJ, Griffin DR, Reinert CM, et al: Pelvic ring disruptions: Prediction of associated injuries, transfusion requirement, pelvic arteriography, complications, and mortality. *J Orthop Trauma* 2002; 16(8):553-561.

13. Adams JE, Davis GG, Alexander CB, Alonso JE: Pelvic trauma in rapidly fatal motor vehicle accidents. *J Orthop Trauma* 2003; 17(6):406-410.

14. Eastridge BJ, Starr A, Minei JP, O'Keefe GE, Scalea TM: The importance of fracture pattern in guiding therapeutic decision-making in patients with hemorrhagic shock and pelvic ring dis-

ruptions. *J Trauma* 2002;53(3):446-450, discussion 450-451.

15. Baker SP, O'Neill B, Haddon W Jr, Long WB: The injury severity score: A method for describing patients with multiple injuries and evaluating emergency care. *J Trauma* 1974;14(3):187-196.

16. Rittmeister M, Lindsey RW, Kohl HW III: Pelvic fracture among polytrauma decedents: Trauma-based mortality with pelvic fracture. A case series of 74 patients. *Arch Orthop Trauma Surg* 2001;121(1-2):43-49.

17. Poole GV, Ward EF, Griswold JA, Muakkassa FF, Hsu HS: Complications of pelvic fractures from blunt trauma. *Am Surg* 1992;58(4):225-231.

18. Mucha P Jr, Farnell MB: Analysis of pelvic fracture management. *J Trauma* 1984;24(5):379-386.

19. Champion HR, Sacco WJ, Copes WS, Gann DS, Gennarelli TA, Flanagan ME: A revision of the Trauma Score. *J Trauma* 1989;29(5):623-629.

20. Allen CF, Goslar PW, Barry M, Christiansen T: Management guidelines for hypotensive pelvic fracture patients. *Am Surg* 2000;66(8):735-738.

21. *Advanced Trauma Life Support Program for Doctors,* ed 6. Chicago, IL, American College of Surgeons, 1997.

22. Durkin A, Sagi HC, Durham R, Flint L: Contemporary management of pelvic fractures. *Am J Surg* 2006;192(2):211-223.

23. Guillamondegui OD, Pryor JP, Gracias VH, Gupta R, Reilly PM, Schwab CW: Pelvic radiography in blunt trauma resuscitation: A diminishing role. *J Trauma* 2002;53(6):1043-1047.

24. Cryer HM, Miller FB, Evers BM, Rouben LR, Seligson DL: Pelvic fracture classification: Correlation with hemorrhage. *J Trauma* 1988;28(7):973-980.

25. Pennal GF, Tile M, Waddell JP, Garside H: Pelvic disruption: Assessment and classification. *Clin Orthop Relat Res* 1980;151:12-21.

26. Dalal SA, Burgess AR, Siegel JH, et al: Pelvic fracture in multiple trauma: Classification by mechanism is key to pattern of organ injury, resuscitative requirements, and outcome. *J Trauma* 1989;29(7):981-1000, discussion 1000-1002.

27. Burgess AR, Eastridge BJ, Young JW, et al: Pelvic ring disruptions: Effective classification system and treatment protocols. *J Trauma* 1990;30(7):848-856.

28. Young JW, Burgess AR, Brumback RJ, Poka A: Pelvic fractures: Value of plain radiography in early assessment and management. *Radiology* 1986;160(2):445-451.

29. Vrahas M, Hern TC, Diangelo D, Kellam J, Tile M: Ligamentous contributions to pelvic stability. *Orthopedics* 1995;18(3):271-274.

30. Evers BM, Cryer HM, Miller FB: Pelvic fracture hemorrhage: Priorities in management. *Arch Surg* 1989;124(4):422-424.

31. Rothenberger DA, Fischer RP, Strate RG, Velasco R, Perry JF Jr: The mortality associated with pelvic fractures. *Surgery* 1978;84(3):356-361.

32. Ward DA, Bircher MD: The early management of pelvic and acetabular fractures. *Injury* 1996;27(Suppl 1):S-A24-8.

33. Turner GG: Local discoloration of abdominal wall as a sign of acute pancreatitis. *Br J Surg* 1920;7:394-395.

34. Shoemaker WC, Appel PL, Kram HB: Role of oxygen debt in the development of organ failure sepsis, and death in high-risk surgical patients. *Chest* 1992;102(1):208-215.

35. Davis JW, Parks SN, Kaups KL, Gladen HE, O'Donnell-Nicol S: Admission base deficit predicts transfusion requirements and risk

of complications. *J Trauma* 1996;41(5):769-774.

36. Shoemaker WC, Appel PL, Kram HB, Waxman K, Lee TS: Prospective trial of supranormal values of survivors as therapeutic goals in high-risk surgical patients. *Chest* 1988;94(6):1176-1186.

37. Gennarelli TA, Champion HR, Sacco WJ, Copes WS, Alves WM: Mortality of patients with head injury and extracranial injury treated in trauma centers. *J Trauma* 1989;29(9):1193-1201, discussion 1201-1202.

38. Price DJ, Murray A: The influence of hypoxia and hypotension on recovery from head injury. *Injury* 1972;3(4):218-224.

39. Heetveld MJ, Harris I, Schlaphoff G, Balogh Z, D'Amours SK, Sugrue M: Hemodynamically unstable pelvic fractures: Recent care and new guidelines. *World J Surg* 2004;28(9):904-909.

40. Smith W, Williams A, Agudelo J, et al: Early predictors of mortality in hemodynamically unstable pelvis fractures. *J Orthop Trauma* 2007;21(1):31-37.

41. Velmahos GC, Toutouzas KG, Vassiliu P, et al: A prospective study on the safety and efficacy of angiographic embolization for pelvic and visceral injuries. *J Trauma* 2002;53(2):303-308, discussion 308.

42. Agolini SF, Shah K, Jaffe J, Newcomb J, Rhodes M, Reed JF III: Arterial embolization is a rapid and effective technique for controlling pelvic fracture hemorrhage. *J Trauma* 1997;43(3):395-399.

43. Matalon TS, Athanasoulis CA, Margolies MN, et al: Hemorrhage with pelvic fractures: Efficacy of transcatheter embolization. *AJR Am J Roentgenol* 1979;133(5):859-864.

44. Panetta T, Sclafani SJ, Goldstein AS, Phillips TF, Shaftan GW: Percutaneous transcatheter embo-

lization for massive bleeding from pelvic fractures. *J Trauma* 1985; 25(11):1021-1029.

45. Wong YC, Wang LJ, Ng CJ, Tseng IC, See LC: Mortality after successful transcatheter arterial embolization in patients with unstable pelvic fractures: Rate of blood transfusion as a predictive factor. *J Trauma* 2000;49(1): 71-75.

46. Natarajan B, Gupta PK, Cemaj S, Sorensen M, Hatzoudis GI, Forse RA: FAST scan: Is it worth doing in hemodynamically stable blunt trauma patients? *Surgery* 2010; 148(4):695-700, discussion 700-701.

47. Hubbard SG, Bivins BA, Sachatello CR, Griffen WO Jr: Diagnostic errors with peritoneal lavage in patients with pelvic fractures. *Arch Surg* 1979;114(7):844-846.

48. Liu M, Lee CH, P'eng FK: Prospective comparison of diagnostic peritoneal lavage, computed tomographic scanning, and ultrasonography for the diagnosis of blunt abdominal trauma. *J Trauma* 1993;35(2):267-270.

49. Blackmore CC, Cummings P, Jurkovich GJ, Linnau KF, Hoffer EK, Rivara FP: Predicting major hemorrhage in patients with pelvic fracture. *J Trauma* 2006; 61(2):346-352.

50. Bramos A, Velmahos GC, Butt UM, Fikry K, Smith RM, Chang Y: Predictors of bleeding from stable pelvic fractures. *Arch Surg* 2011;146(4):407-411.

51. Huittinen VM, Slätis P: Postmortem angiography and dissection of the hypogastric artery in pelvic fractures. *Surgery* 1973;73(3): 454-462.

52. Slätis P, Karaharju EO: External fixation of unstable pelvic fractures: Experiences in 22 patients treated with a trapezoid compression frame. *Clin Orthop Relat Res* 1980;151:73-80.

53. Kataoka Y, Maekawa K, Nishimaki H, Yamamoto S, Soma K: Iliac vein injuries in hemodynamically unstable patients with pelvic fracture caused by blunt trauma. *J Trauma* 2005;58(4):704-708, discussion 708-710.

54. Smith K, Ben-Menachem Y, Duke JH Jr, Hill GL: The superior gluteal: An artery at risk in blunt pelvic trauma. *J Trauma* 1976;16(4):273-279.

55. Magnussen RA, Tressler MA, Obremskey WT, Kregor PJ: Predicting blood loss in isolated pelvic and acetabular high-energy trauma. *J Orthop Trauma* 2007; 21(9):603-607.

56. Stephen DJ, Kreder HJ, Day AC, et al: Early detection of arterial bleeding in acute pelvic trauma. *J Trauma* 1999;47(4):638-642.

57. Siegel J, Tornetta P III, Burke P, Kaseje N, Agarwal S, Soto J, Anderson S: CT angiography for pelvic trauma predicts angiographically treatable arterial bleeding. Orthopaedic Trauma Association 23rd Annual Meeting, 2007. Polytrauma paper #14. http://www.hwbf.org/ota/am/ota07/otapa/OTA070214.htm. Accessed May 31, 2011.

58. Blackmore CC, Jurkovich GJ, Linnau KF, Cummings P, Hoffer EK, Rivara FP: Assessment of volume of hemorrhage and outcome from pelvic fracture. *Arch Surg* 2003;138(5):504-508, discussion 508-509.

59. Cook RE, Keating JF, Gillespie I: The role of angiography in the management of haemorrhage from major fractures of the pelvis. *J Bone Joint Surg Br* 2002;84(2): 178-182.

60. O'Neill PA, Riina J, Sclafani S, Tornetta P III: Angiographic findings in pelvic fractures. *Clin Orthop Relat Res* 1996;329:60-67.

61. Velmahos GC, Chahwan S, Hanks SE, et al: Angiographic embolization of bilateral internal iliac arteries to control life-threatening hemorrhage after blunt trauma to the pelvis. *Am Surg* 2000;66(9):858-862.

62. Moss MC, Bircher MD: Volume changes within the true pelvis during disruption of the pelvic ring: Where does the haemorrhage go? *Injury* 1996;27(Suppl 1): S-A21-3.

63. Krieg JC, Mohr M, Ellis TJ, Simpson TS, Madey SM, Bottlang M: Emergent stabilization of pelvic ring injuries by controlled circumferential compression: A clinical trial. *J Trauma* 2005; 59(3):659-664.

64. Stover MD, Summers HD, Ghanayem AJ, Wilber JH: Three-dimensional analysis of pelvic volume in an unstable pelvic fracture. *J Trauma* 2006;61(4): 905-908.

65. Croce MA, Magnotti LJ, Savage SA, Wood GW II, Fabian TC: Emergent pelvic fixation in patients with exsanguinating pelvic fractures. *J Am Coll Surg* 2007; 204(5):935-939, discussion 940-942.

66. Knops SP, Schep NW, Spoor CW, et al: Comparison of three different pelvic circumferential compression devices: A biomechanical cadaver study. *J Bone Joint Surg Am* 2011;93(3): 230-240.

67. Richard MJ, Tornetta P III: Emergent management of APC-2 pelvic ring injuries with an anteriorly placed C-clamp. *J Orthop Trauma* 2009;23(5):322-326.

68. Routt ML Jr, Falicov A, Woodhouse E, Schildhauer TA: Circumferential pelvic antishock sheeting: A temporary resuscitation aid. *J Orthop Trauma* 2002; 16(1):45-48.

69. Gardner MJ, Nork SE: Stabilization of unstable pelvic fractures with supraacetabular compression external fixation. *J Orthop Trauma* 2007;21(4):269-273.

70. Gardner MJ, Kendoff D, Oster-meier S, et al: Sacroiliac joint compression using an anterior pelvic compressor: A mechanical study in synthetic bone. *J Orthop Trauma* 2007;21(7):435-441.

71. Ganz R, Krushell RJ, Jakob RP, Küffer J: The antishock pelvic clamp. *Clin Orthop Relat Res* 1991;267:71-78.

72. Heini PF, Witt J, Ganz R: The pelvic C-clamp for the emergency treatment of unstable pelvic ring injuries: A report on clinical experience of 30 cases. *Injury* 1996; 27(Suppl 1):S-A38-45.

73. Smith WR, Moore EE, Osborn P, et al: Retroperitoneal packing as a resuscitation technique for hemodynamically unstable patients with pelvic fractures: Report of two representative cases and a description of technique. *J Trauma* 2005;59(6):1510-1514.

74. Tötterman A, Madsen JE, Skaga NO, Røise O: Extraperitoneal pelvic packing: A salvage procedure to control massive traumatic pelvic hemorrhage. *J Trauma* 2007;62(4):843-852.

75. Starr AJ, Malekzadeh AS: Fractures of the pelvic ring, in Bucholz RW, Heckman JD, Court-Brown C, eds: *Rockwood and Green's Fractures in Adults,* ed 6. New York, NY, Lippincott Williams & Wilkins, 2006, pp 1583–1664.

76. Zingg EJ, Casanova GA, Isler B, Sohn M: Pelvic fractures and traumatic lesions of the posterior urethra. *Eur Urol* 1990;18(1):27-32.

77. Dunstan E, Bircher M: Urological pitfalls in unstable pelvic fractures. *Injury* 2000;31(5):379-382.

78. Reilly MC, Zinar DM, Matta JM: Neurologic injuries in pelvic ring fractures. *Clin Orthop Relat Res* 1996;329:28-36.

79. Tornetta P III, Dickson K, Matta JM: Outcome of rotationally unstable pelvic ring injuries treated operatively. *Clin Orthop Relat Res* 1996;329:147-151.

80. Tornetta P III, Matta JM: Outcome of operatively treated unstable posterior pelvic ring disruptions. *Clin Orthop Relat Res* 1996; 329:186-193.

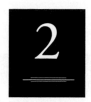

Techniques of Anterior Pelvic Fixation

Brian H. Mullis, MD

Abstract

Although definitive fixation of anterior pelvic ring injuries is usually referred to an orthopaedic trauma surgeon or a surgeon proficient in pelvic surgery, all orthopaedic surgeons should be familiar with the initial management and resuscitation of patients with high-energy pelvic ring injuries. The initial treatment may be limited to sheet or binder application in the emergency department to allow transfer of the patient to a trauma center or the application of an external fixator by an on-call surgeon, even though that surgeon may not be responsible for definitive fixation. It is important to understand the general principles and approaches used at the time of definitive surgery because decisions made by the initial treating physician may affect (or limit) the ability of the orthopaedic traumatologist to provide definitive care.

Instr Course Lect 2012;61:19-25

The primary weight-bearing forces are transmitted to the axial skeleton through the posterior pelvic ring, but the anterior ring augments the stability of the posterior ring, acting as a strut in single-leg stance and preventing external rotation caused by tension in double-leg stance. Typical indications for fixation of the anterior ring include symphyseal disruption resulting in a rotationally unstable pelvic ring (anteroposterior compression type II [APC-II] fractures; see chapter 1 for more information on pelvic fracture classification systems) or to augment the stability of the ring after fixation of the posterior ring caused by either rotationally or vertically unstable injuries. Many times, the anterior ring may appear to be stable based on static plain radiographs. Stress radiography of the anterior ring should be done following posterior ring fixation to ensure that the anterior ring is stable.

Even if the initially treating orthopaedic surgeon will not be providing definitive treatment for the pelvic ring injury, it is necessary to be familiar with the techniques for definitive fixation because decisions made emergently may affect future surgery. This chapter will present pearls and pitfalls for both emergent and definitive management of anterior pelvic ring injuries.

Emergent Management of Unstable Anterior Ring Injuries

Gross instability of the anterior ring indicates instability of the posterior ring as well. Emergent treatment should focus on resuscitation of the patient. For an unstable external rotation injury (APC-II or APC-III), a sheet or binder can be emergently applied (**Figure 1**). The lower extremities should first be internally rotated and taped together at the knees and feet to prevent further external rotation moments across the anterior ring (**Figure 2**). Cervical spine precautions should be maintained, and the patient should be log rolled to prevent further spinal injury. The sheet or binder should be placed at the level of the greater trochanters (**Figure 3**). This allows general surgeons to have access to the abdomen because many of these patients may require emergent exploratory laparotomy; it also allows access to the perineum and rectum because up to 15% of patients with pelvic ring injuries also have a urologic injury. Alternatively, a C-clamp can be applied in the emergency department, but this procedure should be performed only by a surgeon familiar with pelvic anatomy because there may be significant distortion of the pelvis after injury, and inadvertent placement of the C-clamp

Dr. Mullis or an immediate family member is a member of a speakers' bureau or has made paid presentations on behalf of Medtronic; has received research or institutional support from Amgen and Synthes; and serves as a board member, owner, officer, or committee member of the Orthopaedic Trauma Association.

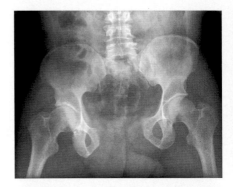

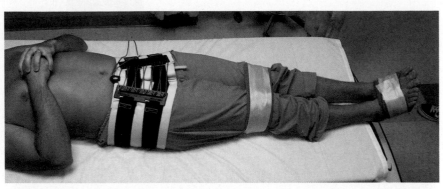

Figure 1   AP radiograph of a typical APC injury requiring application of a sheet or binder in the emergency department to help with patient resuscitation.

Figure 2   A pelvic binder is applied and centered on the greater trochanter with the feet and knees taped together in internal rotation to prevent external rotation moments across the pelvis.

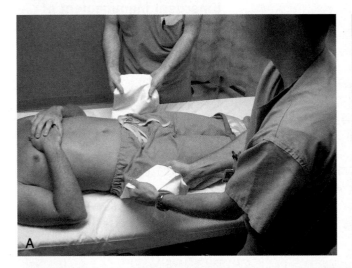

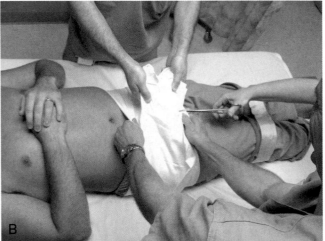

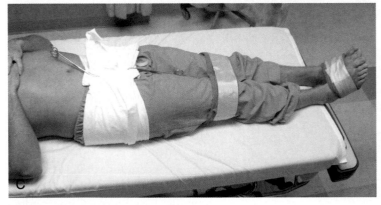

Figure 3   A sheet can be applied in the same manner as a pelvic binder. The feet and knees of the patient are taped together in internal rotation. **A,** The sheet is applied centered on the greater trochanter. **B,** The end of the sheet is grasped from the opposite side, and each assistant pulls to apply an internal rotation moment. A third assistant clamps each end of the sheet. **C,** Photograph showing appropriate placement of the sheet and internal rotation of the legs.

could result in further injury.[1] A rectal examination should be performed to rule out an open wound communicating with the pelvic fracture. If such a wound is present, an emergent diverting colostomy is needed, with washout of the rectal vault. Consultation with the urologic service is needed if a urologic injury is present. If a suprapubic catheter is to be placed, it should be tunneled to prevent contamination from an anterior approach, which will be needed for definitive fixation of the anterior ring.

External Fixation

External fixation is appropriate in the initial resuscitation and management of the patient with an unstable pelvic ring injury. It should be noted that external fixation does nothing to control the posterior ring; in fact, it can even

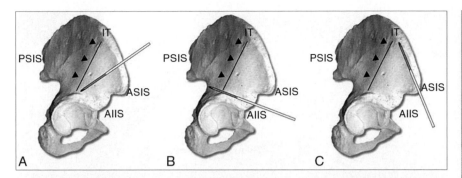

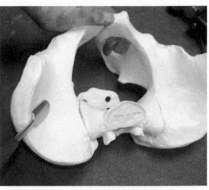

Figure 4 Illustrations showing basic pin placement options. Anterosuperior (**A**), anteroinferior (**B**), and subcristal (**C**) pin placements are shown. Anterosuperior and anteroinferior pin placements are the most commonly used. ASIS = anterosuperior iliac spine, AIIS = anteroinferior iliac spine, PSIS = posterosuperior iliac spine.

Figure 5 A periosteal elevator can be used to elevate the iliacus and help guide the anterosuperior pin placement because these are typically placed percutaneously.

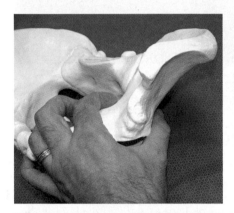

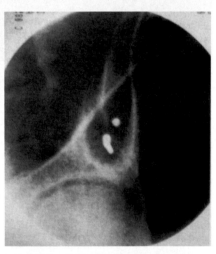

Figure 6 The corridor used for the anteroinferior external fixation pins is the sciatic buttress shown here, which is running above the acetabulum back to the posterosuperior iliac spine.

Figure 7 The obturator outlet or "teepee" view shows the radiographic corridor that corresponds to Figure 4. (Courtesy of Marvin Tile, MD, Toronto, Canada)

cause further displacement of the posterior ring.[2] This should be considered if there is a vertically unstable posterior ring injury because skeletal traction may still be needed in addition to the external fixator to prevent further migration of the pelvic ring before definitive fixation. External fixation is not as stable as internal fixation with plates and is uncomfortable for the awake and alert patient. For this reason, it usually serves as an initial resuscitation tool (or an intraoperative reduction tool) until internal fixation can be performed. In cases of gross contamination or in patients with head injuries

that require augmentation of internal fixation, the external fixator may be kept in place until the anterior ring injury is healed.

Basic pin placement options for external fixation are anterosuperior (laterally based frame), anteroinferior (anterior or Hannover frame), or subcristal (rarely used)[3] (**Figure 4**). Anterosuperior pins are easily placed without fluoroscopy because the iliac crest and anterosuperior iliac spine can be used as landmarks. Typically, the pins are placed 2 to 3 cm posterior to

the anterosuperior iliac spine. A periosteal elevator can be used to elevate the iliacus to help determine the appropriate direction for the pins (**Figure 5**). Two to three Schanz pins should be used for each side of the pelvis. Care should be taken because it is easy to penetrate the inner or outer table with the pins. The drill can be initially placed on forward to start the pin track, but then placing the drill on reverse helps the surgeon feel contact with the inner or outer table without easy penetration. The final frame should be constructed to allow access to the abdomen and the perineum.

The anteroinferior frame is more dependent on fluoroscopy for proper placement, but only one Schanz pin is needed on either side and should be placed at the level of the anteroinferior iliac spine. The corridor for pin placement is the sciatic buttress (**Figure 6**), a large area of bone located above the acetabulum running to the posterosuperior iliac spine. The obturator outlet and iliac oblique views are needed to see this corridor. The obturator outlet view "looks down the barrel" of the sciatic buttress[4] (**Figure 7**). The iliac oblique view is needed to prevent penetration of the greater sciatic notch. Final frame construction is done to allow

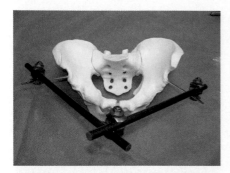

Figure 8 Photograph of a typical anteroinferior frame placed on a sawbones. Access should be available to both the abdomen and the perineum.

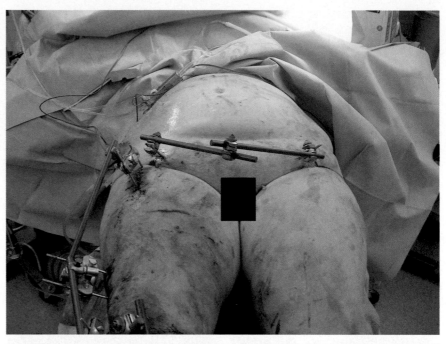

Figure 9 Photograph of a multitrauma patient with an anterior pelvic frame applied, leaving access to the abdomen and the perineum.

access to the abdomen and the perineum (**Figures 8** and **9**).

Internal Fixation

Internal fixation of the anterior ring should usually be reserved for the traumatologist or surgeon experienced in pelvic surgery. Even an apparently simple symphyseal dislocation indicates a significant posterior ring injury, which may necessitate an open or percutaneous posterior approach before a posterior ring reduction is blocked by an anterior approach and fixation. Preoperative planning is imperative. A pelvis sawbones can be placed in a clear, sterile isolation bag to help with three-dimensional spatial recognition. A Foley catheter should be placed to decompress the bladder, and the bladder should be protected at all times during surgery, usually with a malleable retractor. A standard transverse Pfannenstiel incision is used for symphyseal dislocations. For anterior ring fractures or fracture-dislocations requiring open reduction, an ilioinguinal or modified Stoppa approach is typically used. Deep dissection usually consists of splitting the rectus abdominis longitudinally, although to improve exposure, the rectus abdominis can be removed from its attachment to the pubis (many times the initial injury will have avulsed one side of the

rectus abdominis). This has the potential to further destabilize the anterior ring and should be repaired following fixation.[5] A malleable retractor is gently placed to protect the bladder, but care should be taken to avoid aggressive retraction, which can place the patient at risk for further urologic injury.

As dissection is carried around the lateral aspect of the anterior ring, the hip is flexed to take pressure off the iliopsoas and femoral vessels and nerve. Special pelvic instrumentation can be useful during this part of the dissection, especially if there is more limited visualization such as when using a modified Stoppa approach. Care should be taken as the corona mortis may be present up to 40% of the time and will be encountered at the level of the pectineal fossa[4] (**Figure 10**). There are always pubic branches in this area, but a true corona mortis indicates an aberrant takeoff of the obturator artery from the external iliac or inferior epigastric artery, which will require ligation (not by electrocautery but by vas-

cular clips or tie) because life-threatening bleeding can occur if the corona mortis is severed and retracts. In this case, emergent packing should be performed with immediate embolization of the vessel by interventional radiology if the vessel cannot be controlled by open means.

As dissection is carried past the pectineal fossa, a Hohmann retractor can be placed in the pectineal fossa to aid visualization (the hip should remain flexed). Dissection can be carried over the pectineal ridge back to the sacroiliac joint with a small malleable retractor typically placed at the sacroiliac joint to aid in visualization. Excellent visualization can be afforded even through a modified Stoppa approach.[6]

Once exposure is obtained, reduction can be performed using several techniques. Placing (or prepping in a previously placed frame) an anterior frame may be useful for significantly displaced fractures. Of note, for grossly displaced fractures, it may be necessary to reduce the posterior ring first be-

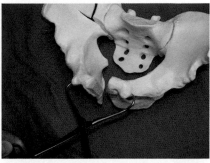

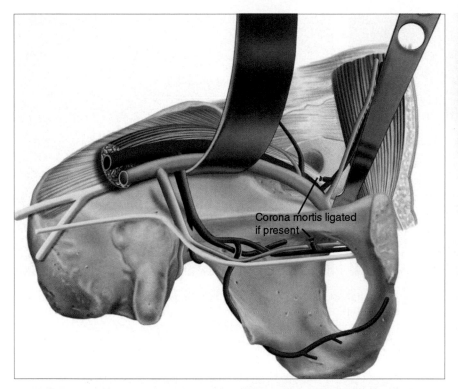

Figure 10   Illustration showing the corona mortis running over the pectineal fossa after ligation. (Reproduced with permission from Sagi H, Afsari A, Dziadosz D: The anterior intra-pelvic (modified Rives-Stoppa) approach for fixation of acetabular fractures. *J Orthop Trauma* 2010;24:263-270.)

Figure 11   Photograph of a Weber clamp with the tines placed at the pubic tubercle to obtain reduction. Alternatively, the clamp could be placed at the obturator ring, but care should be taken because this placement can pose an increased risk for neurovascular injury.

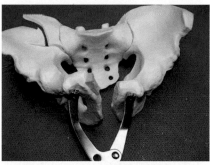

Figure 12   A Jungbluth clamp can be used to reduce the anterior ring. Note that screws have been placed laterally to allow access for medial screws through a symphyseal plate after reduction is obtained.

cause fixing the anterior ring may result in a displaced posterior pelvic injury, which has been shown to be associated with worse outcomes.[7] Once the anterior ring has been brought to a "near" reduction, a Weber clamp can be used to fine-tune the reduction until it is anatomic. The tines of the clamp are placed on the pubic tubercle (**Figure 11**) or within the obturator ring itself (care should be taken with this placement to prevent further neurovascular insult). An alternative instrument is the Jungbluth clamp, which requires further soft-tissue stripping for anterior placement and is a more aggressive reduction tool than the Weber clamp (**Figure 12**).

Once reduction is achieved, precontoured plates are available for symphyseal dislocation fixation, but standard pelvic reconstruction plates can still be used for dislocations and are

necessary for anterior ring fractures. Two-hole plates should not be used for symphyseal dislocations because they have a high failure rate and result in pelvic malunion.[8] For anterior ring fracture-dislocations, it is typically easier to first fix one of the motion segments before spanning both with a single plate (**Figure 13**).

The sharp tip of the ball-tipped pusher or Picador can be machined off so that it can be used to help buttress pelvic reconstruction plates in situ as fixation is carried around the anterior ring (**Figure 14**). Care should be taken when placing screws in this area to avoid penetrating the acetabulum. If fluoroscopy is not immediately available, a sterile esophageal stethoscope can be placed along the quadrilateral plate to listen for grinding within the joint, indicating aberrant screw placement.

Percutaneous internal fixation may be appropriate if an anatomic reduction can be achieved by closed means. Indications for percutaneous internal fixation include unstable nondisplaced or minimally displaced anterior ring fractures. Percutaneous fixation has a 15% failure rate (even when performed by experts), with elderly patients, females, and those with medial fractures at increased risk.[9] A combination of obturator outlet and iliac inlet views have been recommended, although in the experience of this chapter's author the true inlet view is sufficient and easier to obtain in com-

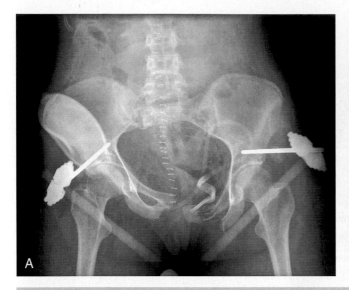

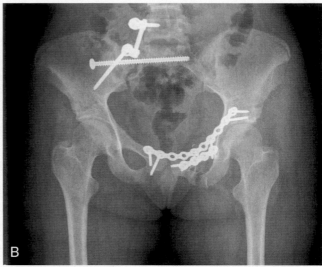

Figure 13 **A,** Radiograph of the pelvis showing the initial application of an external fixator for a fracture-dislocation of the anterior ring (with associated posterior ring involvement). **B,** Radiograph of the pelvis showing two plates that were used given the two motion segments. A short plate was first used to cross and control the fracture, and then a longer pelvic reconstruction plate was used to span both motion segments of the anterior ring after reduction was obtained.

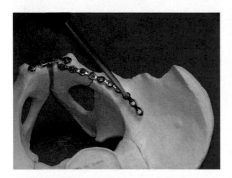

Figure 14 A Picador or ball-tipped pusher can be used to help buttress pelvic reconstruction plates in situ if the spiked tip is machined off.

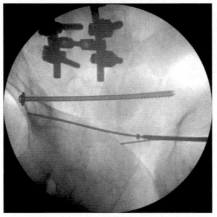

Figure 15 Obturator outlet view shows the ramus screw passes well outside the hip joint.

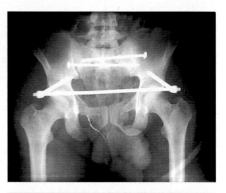

Figure 16 Radiograph showing the infix technique with pedicle screws placed down the sciatic buttress corridor and a rod tunneled subcutaneously connecting the two sides (Courtesy of Karl Shively, MD, Indiana University School of Medicine, Indianapolis, IN).

bination with the obturator outlet view. The iliac inlet or inlet view is used only to focus on the anterior ring corridor because it is normal for the screw to appear to penetrate the joint; however, the screw must not penetrate the joint on the obturator outlet view (**Figure 15**).

Another recently described percutaneous internal technique uses spine instrumentation to perform internal fixation outside the pelvis, or "infix."[10] This frame uses the same sciatic buttress corridor as the anterior external frame, with placement of pedicle

screws starting at the anteroinferior iliac spine and using iliac oblique and obturator outlet views. The pedicle screws are left several centimeters proud from the bone to allow subcutaneous passage of the bar. The bar connecting the pedicle screws runs close to the femoral artery and is tunneled subcutaneously (**Figure 16**). Removal of the implants approximately 5 months postoperatively is recommended. Complications with this technique include

heterotopic ossification and lateral femoral cutaneous nerve palsy. A high failure rate for symphyseal dislocations using this technique was recently reported (A Starr, MD, Baltimore, MD, unpublished data presented at the Pelvic Master Course, 2010). Care should be used in adopting this technique because there are only early experiences and indications are still evolving.

Summary

All orthopaedic surgeons should be able to provide emergent care to patients with pelvic ring injuries. This care may be limited to sheet or binder application, but most surgeons should be able to safely place an external fixator. There are multiple techniques for the application of external fixators. Proficiency in all the techniques is not required for an individual surgeon, but a surgeon should choose an effective technique that he or she can perform quickly and safely as part of the resuscitation efforts for a patient with a high-energy pelvic ring injury. Surgeons who have limited experience in treating pelvic injuries should usually refer definitive treatment to a traumatologist or a surgeon proficient in pelvic surgery.

References

1. Richard MJ, Tornetta P III: Emergent management of APC-2 pelvic ring injuries with an anteriorly placed C-clamp. *J Orthop Trauma* 2009;23(5):322-326.

2. Dickson KF, Matta JM: Skeletal deformity after anterior external fixation of the pelvis. *J Orthop Trauma* 2009;23(5):327-332.

3. Solomon LB, Pohl AP, Chehade MJ, Malcolm AM, Howie DW, Henneberg M: Surgical anatomy for pelvic external fixation. *Clin Anat* 2008;21(7):674-682.

4. Tile M, ed: *Fractures of the Pelvis and Acetabulum*, ed 3. Philadelphia, PA, Lippincott Williams & Wilkins, 2003.

5. Ghanayem AJ, Wilber JH, Lieberman JM, Motta AO: The effect of laparotomy and external fixator stabilization on pelvic volume in an unstable pelvic injury. *J Trauma* 1995;38(3):396-400, discussion 400-401.

6. Sagi HC, Afsari A, Dziadosz D: The anterior intra-pelvic (modified Rives-Stoppa) approach for fixation of acetabular fractures. *J Orthop Trauma* 2010;24(5): 263-270.

7. Mullis BH, Sagi HC: Minimum 1-year follow-up for patients with vertical shear sacroiliac joint dislocations treated with iliosacral screws: Does joint ankylosis or anatomic reduction contribute to functional outcome? *J Orthop Trauma* 2008;22(5):293-298.

8. Sagi HC, Papp S: Comparative radiographic and clinical outcome of two-hole and multi-hole symphyseal plating. *J Orthop Trauma* 2008;22(6):373-378.

9. Starr AJ, Nakatani T, Reinert CM, Cederberg K: Superior pubic ramus fractures fixed with percutaneous screws: What predicts fixation failure? *J Orthop Trauma* 2008;22(2):81-87.

10. Vaidya R, Tonnos F, Colen R, Sethi A: Minimally invasive treatment of unstable pelvic ring injuries with an internal anterior fixator (INFIX) and posterior iliosacral screws. COA Annual Meeting, 2009. http://www.coa-aco.org/images/stories/meetings/whistler_09/COA_11_Trauma_Lower_2.pdf. Accessed May 25, 2011.

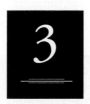

Posterior Pelvic Ring Injuries: When to Perform Open Reduction and Internal Fixation

Clifford B. Jones, MD, FACS

Abstract

Unstable posterior pelvic ring injuries are commonly treated with percutaneous iliosacral screw fixation. Despite the efficiency of the minimally invasive technique, complications and failures occur. To maximize reduction quality and fixation stability, open techniques for pelvic ring fixation exist. Timing, approaches, clamp positioning, and implant options determine the effectiveness of the open techniques.

Instr Course Lect 2012;61:27-38.

Pelvic ring injuries result from high-energy trauma. Most pelvic ring injuries are stable and are treated nonsurgically. Unstable pelvic ring injuries with posterior displacement usually require reduction and internal fixation for optimal outcomes. Percutaneous sacroiliac (SI) fixation should be performed by surgeons experienced in treating pelvic ring injuries. This type of fixation uses fluoroscopic imaging and is appropriate for fractures amenable to closed reduction. An open approach to the posterior ring is usually used to treat displaced SI joint dislocations or fracture-dislocations (crescent fractures); fractures with marked comminution of the posterior ring, which lessens stability and reduction; transfo-raminal fractures with foraminal encroachment and neural injury; and fractures requiring delayed fixation.

Anatomy

Osseous Structure

The pelvic ring consists of the sacrum attached to the paired ilium. The sacral anatomy is rhomboid shaped and articulates with the ilium as a keystone in both the axial and the coronal planes. The pelvis is rotated in the sagittal plane approximately 45° to the spine and axis of the body. The sacrum consists of four to five fused segments. Upper sacral morphology can be varied and dysmorphic, which can interfere with imaging and fixation.[1-5] The osseous elements thicken at periarticu-lar surfaces (the SI joint), perisymphyseal areas, and corridors (iliac buttress, sciatic buttress); this aids fixation.

Ligamentous Supports

Strong intraosseous SI ligaments stabilize the SI joint. To a lesser degree, the posterior and anterior SI ligaments support the joint and are a predictor of instability if avulsed posteriorly (crescent fracture or sacral avulsions) or anteriorly (**Figure 1**). The iliolumbar ligament traverses the lumbar traverse processes to the posterior iliac wing. The L5 inferior facet is intimately involved and attaches to the pelvis via the facet capsule and ligaments.

Vascular Anatomy

Blood is supplied to the pelvic ring via branches from the internal and external iliac vessels. Many vessels create the lumbosacral venous plexus and can be damaged in pelvic ring injuries. The superior gluteal artery and vein exit via the sciatic notch posteriorly and cranially. These vessels supply the gluteus medius, the gluteus minimus, and the tensor fascia lata. The superior gluteal artery is frequently damaged in displaced unstable pelvic ring injuries. The inferior gluteal artery supplies the gluteus maximus.

Dr. Jones or an immediate family member is a member of a speakers' bureau or has made paid presentations on behalf of the AONA; serves as a board member, owner, officer, or committee member of the American Academy of Orthopaedic Surgeons Coding Coverage Reimbursement Committee, the American Orthopaedic Association Own the Bone Board, the Mid-American Orthopaedic Association Bylaws Committee, the Orthopaedic Trauma Association Outcomes and Classification Committee; and is the president of the Michigan Orthopaedic Society.

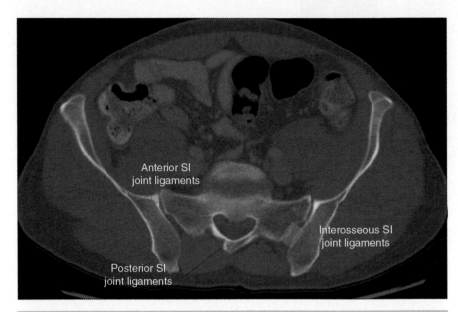

Anterior SI
joint ligaments

Interosseous SI
joint ligaments

Posterior SI
joint ligaments

Figure 1   Axial CT scan demonstrates the landmarks of the important posterior pelvic ligamentous anatomy (blue areas indicate locations of the ligaments).

Neural Anatomy

The spinal cord terminates into the filum terminale and lumbosacral nerve roots at the L1 level. The L2-L3 nerve roots join to form the lateral femoral cutaneous nerve running along the rectus muscle laterally and exiting the pelvis near the anterior superior iliac spine under the ligament. The L2-L4 nerve roots join to form the femoral nerve running along the lateral portion of the iliopsoas muscle. The L5 nerve root runs from posterior to anterior along the anterior portion of the sacral ala approximately 2 cm medial to the SI joint. Injury to the L5-S3 nerve roots, commonly termed the lumbosacral plexus, can result in varying degrees of neural damage. The sacral nerve roots exit via the sacral foramina both ventrally and dorsally. With sacral dysmorphism, small osseous tunnels place sacral nerve roots at high risk for injury during screw fixation. Subtle sacral injuries can manifest as urinary retention and saddle numbness. With displaced transforaminal sacral injuries, comminution and osseous fragments can injure the sacral nerve roots.

Pelvic Imaging

Pelvic imaging is performed with radiographs and/or CT. Traditional views include inlet (rotation, symphyseal integrity, anterior or posterior translation) and outlet (cephalad or caudal displacement and rotation) images. Outlet-obturator oblique (sciatic buttress), obturator oblique, and iliac oblique Judet images also can assist in pelvic ring assessment and fixation.[6]

Injury Patterns

The Letournel classification of acetabular fractures describes injury patterns.[7] The Tile classification system describes the rotational and axial stability of the injury (types A, B, and C).[8,9] The Young-Burgess classification describes the injury mechanism (lateral compression [LC], anteroposterior compression [APC], axial shear, combined mechanical injury) and associated injuries.[10-12] The Orthopaedic Trauma Association (OTA)/AO classification describes the injury based on displacement of the posterior arch (type A, none; type B, incomplete; and type C, complete). The Denis classification delineates the location of the sacral injury (type I, alar; type II, transforaminal; and type III, body) and associated neural injury (type I, 6%; type II, 28%; and type III, 58%).[13] The Roy-Camille classification system further delineates sacral fractures (type I, minimally displaced; type II, angulated; type III, translated; and type IV, burst/comminuted).[14] The Isler classification describes the sacral fracture in relationship to the L5 facet and the sacral facet.[15]

Surgical Indications for Posterior Ring Fixation

In general, vertically unstable fracture patterns, displacement greater than 1 cm, dislocations, complete posterior ring injuries, sacral injuries with osseous neural encroachment, and posterior injuries extending into the L5 articulation are considered unstable and require fixation with or without reduction. SI joint dislocations disrupt the SI ligaments and are associated with anterior ring fractures or symphyseal disruption (Tile type B and C injuries, Young-Burgess APC injuries, and OTA type B and C injuries). A true ligament disruption presents as a dislocation or anterior gapping with varying degrees of rotational angulation. A fracture-dislocation or a crescent fracture-dislocation results in a SI joint disruption with a displaced posterior ilium fracture (Tile type B and C injuries; Young-Burgess APC, LC, or vertical sheer patterns; and AO type 61C2 fractures). Larger crescent fracture fragments hinder or obviate potential percutaneous iliosacral screw placement. Ilium fractures (Young-Burgess LC-II or LC-III, OTA types B and C) are difficult to reduce via indirect methods and usually require open reduction and internal fixation. Sacral fractures with displacement, foraminal fracture fragments with or without neural injury, L5 facet injuries, and upper segment sacral dysmorphism usually require open reduction, possible decompression, and surgical fixation. If a patient is not surgically treated within 5 to 7 days of injury, a hematoma may form; therefore, delaying fixation usually requires open approaches to remove the organized hematoma or callus and reduce the fracture to prevent incomplete and suboptimal reduction quality.

Contraindications to an Open Approach

There are relatively few contraindications to an open surgical approach for treating pelvic ring injuries. Degloving injuries such as Morel-Lavallee lesions often require excisional débridement of the necrotic fat and contained hematoma[16] (**Figure 2**). Because the hematoma contents have been found to be colonized with bacteria,[17] operating through a degloving zone may cause further damage to the compromised skin and muscle and may increase

infection rates. Stabilizing the osseous and soft-tissue structures in a degloving injury may decrease further tissue damage and infection. For patient resuscitation, pelvic ring injuries associated with arterial injuries and hypotension are treated with angiographic occlusion of the bleeding. If the angiographically occluded vessel (for exam-

ple, the superior gluteal artery) supplies the gluteal compartment, elevating the periosteum during exposure of a posterior ilium fracture will devitalize the gluteal compartment, and it will become necrotic (**Figure 3**). Wound breakdown and infection may develop.

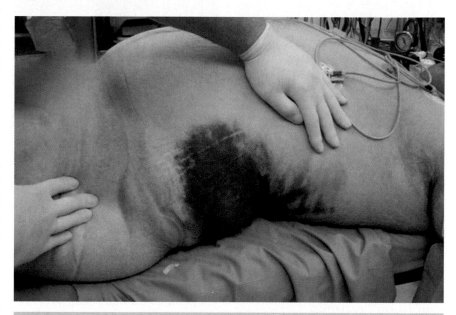

Figure 2   Clinical photograph of a patient with a Morel-Lavallee degloving lesion and unstable pelvic ring injury caused by a side-impact automobile collision.

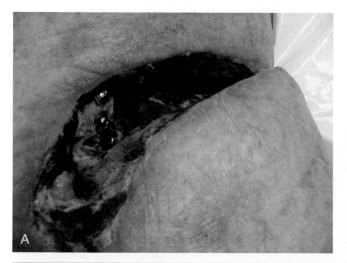 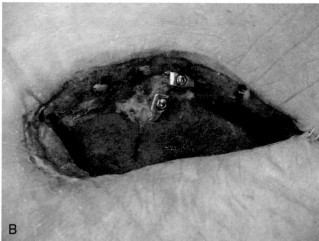

Figure 3   **A,** Clinical photograph of a posterior infected wound with necrotic gluteal muscle that occurred after a pelvic crush injury. An unstable crescent fracture-dislocation resulted and required angiographic coiling for a superior gluteal arterial injury. **B,** Clinical photograph taken 5 weeks after the patient was treated with a posterior approach, gluteal elevation, and plate application. The wound was initially closed with subcutaneous dissolvable sutures and staples.

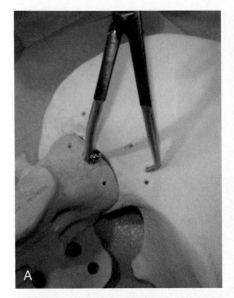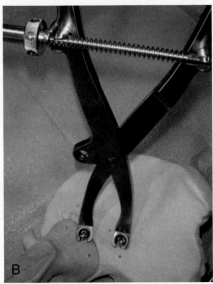

Figure 4 Photographs of a sawbones model showing anterior SI joint clamp application with screw insertion assistance (**A**) and anterior SI joint clamp application with dual screw insertion assistance and pelvic clamp application (**B**).

Approaches, Reduction Techniques, and Fixation Options

Anterior Approach to SI Joint and Ilium Fractures

The anterior approach to the SI joint or the ilium is via the lateral window of the ilioinguinal or iliac approach. The patient is positioned supine on a radiolucent table. Placing pillows below the knees allows relaxation of the iliopsoas muscle and enhances inner iliac wing exposure. Elevating the pelvis and thorax will improve exposure and allow easier insertion of percutaneous iliosacral screws. The fluoroscopic base is placed at the end of the table near the patient's feet, whereas the imaging unit will enter and exit perpendicular to the patient opposite the side of surgery. Draping should begin proximal to the iliac crest and extend to the proximal thighs. The exposure is usually performed in conjunction with other anterior ring or acetabular approaches. The incision parallels the iliac crest, preferably 2 to 3 cm caudad to the external oblique insertion. The external

oblique is then elevated sharply from the iliac crest, proximally to the internal oblique, and distally just proximal to the anterior superior iliac spine to avoid lateral femoral cutaneous nerve injury. The iliopsoas muscle is elevated bluntly from the inner iliac wing. The use of a lap sponge in conjunction with a Cobb elevator allows for efficient periosteal elevation and reduces bleeding. A blunt Hohmann retractor placed through the sciatic notch avoiding the sciatic nerve and above the sacral alar area allows excellent exposure. To avoid L5 nerve root injury, dissection is limited to approximately 2 cm medial to the sacral portion of the SI joint.

The SI joint is débrided of debris and cartilaginous fragments. Many reductions of SI dislocations are aided by anterior pelvic ring or acetabular reduction and fixation, which should be performed first. The ability to place and angle an inner pelvic clamp may be limited in morbidly obese patients or nonrelaxed anesthetized patients (not paralyzed). The clamp placement

is enhanced with unicortical drill hole or screw placement on either side of the SI joint (**Figure 4**). The hole or screw used for the clamp is placed within the midportion of the sacrum and the corresponding ilium in the anterior-posterior plane to enhance symmetric reduction and compressive forces while avoiding potential plate positioning with 90-90 fixation. Clamp reduction also can be performed by using a large pelvic reduction clamp or a forceps placed at the midportion of the sacrum (same position as previously described without the need for a drill hole or a screw) and along the outer pelvic wing (**Figure 5**). Creating a small fascial elevation and tunnel to slide the arm of the clamp assists in placement. The outer table clamp position should avoid the superior gluteal artery and entrance site for potential percutaneous SI screw placement. Placing a 5.0 mm Schanz pin into the inner table of the iliac buttress will fine-tune the hemipelvis mobilization and reduction. Appropriate SI joint reduction should be confirmed with inlet and outlet fluoroscopic images because of variations in joint anatomy and SI joint osteophytes. Once the SI joint is reduced, percutaneous SI screw placement or plate application can be performed. The plate application is performed using two 3.5-mm reconstruction plates (three- or four-hole) applied in a 90-90 position (**Figure 6**). The 90-90 position enhances the reduction stability compared with parallel plate application and optimizes the thickened bone windows of the ilium (sciatic buttress caudally and posterior ilium cranially). Screw insertion should parallel the SI joint along the sacral side to enhance screw length and avoid errant transforaminal placement.

Ilium fractures extending into the sciatic notch or the SI joint are approached via the iliac window. The re-

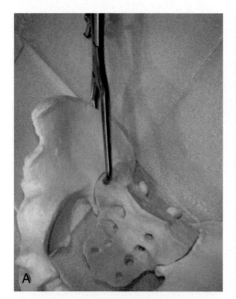

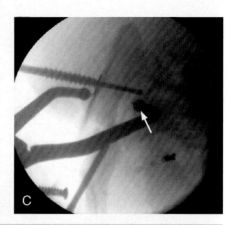

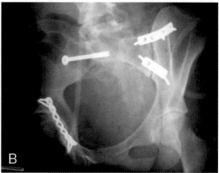

Figure 5   Anterior (**A**) and posterior (**B**) views of a King Tong (Synthes, Paoli, PA) pelvic clamp application for SI joint reduction. **C,** Intraoperative C-arm view of the pelvic clamp application and percutaneous iliosacral screw insertion. The arrow shows the point of sacral contact with the clamp.

duction maneuvers are similar to those previously described but have the advantage of direct visualization. Plate application uses osseous thickenings inferiorly with the sciatic buttress and superiorly with the iliac wing. Plates can be used at both locations but usually are inserted inferiorly, whereas intraosseous screw placement is reserved for the iliac wing portion. Drilling is done in the oscillating position to diminish violation of the cortical table and enhance intraosseous screw insertion.

Closure is performed in layers over a drain. This chapter's author prefers reattachment of the muscle to the iliac wing using five to six vertical mattress transosseous sutures (No. 2.0 Ethibond; Ethicon, Johnson and Johnson, New Brunswick, NJ). Skin is reapproximated with 3.0 nylon sutures using Allgower-Donati sutures.[18]

Posterior Approach to the Sacrum

Whenever possible, anterior pelvic ring reduction and fixation should be performed to enhance posterior ring

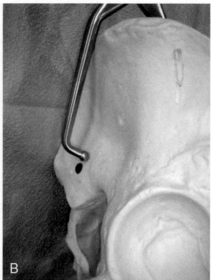

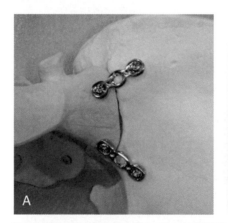

Figure 6   **A,** Sawbones model with a 90-90, 3.5-mm reconstruction plate applied across the SI joint. **B,** Obturator oblique Judet radiograph of an unstable pelvic ring injury treated with 90-90 plate fixation of an unstable left SI joint disruption.

reduction and stability. The patient is placed prone on a radiolucent table with laminectomy rolls, the arms are placed in a relaxed forward-flexed position, and protection is provided for the patient's eyes (**Figure 7**). An impervious drape is used before prepping to seal the perirectal area. Draping should extend proximally to the iliac crest and the L4 level, distally to the proximal femur, and anteriorly to the anterior half

of the femur (**Figure 8**). This preparation allows for percutaneous SI screw placement, plating, and the lumbopelvic instrumentation of all posterior pelvic ring lesions.

The posterior approaches are midline and paramedian (**Figure 9**). The midline approach is better for bilateral pelvic ring involvement, lumbopelvic fixation or extension to the spine, and sacral foraminal decompression. The

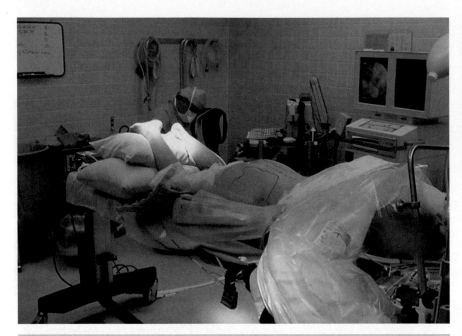

Figure 7 The patient is positioned prone on a radiolucent table with laminectomy rolls and eye protection, and the arms are placed in a relaxed forward-flexed position in preparation for the posterior pelvic approach.

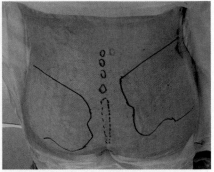

Figure 8 Draping is used to seal the perirectal area in preparation for the posterior pelvic approach. The markings on the drape are proximal to the lumbar spine, lateral to the anterior half of the pelvis, and distal to the buttocks and proximal femur.

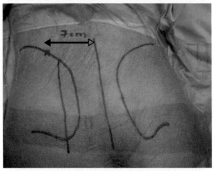

Figure 9 Markings on the drape for the posterior pelvic approach delineate the posterior pelvic anatomy in relationship to the paramedian (solid arrowhead) and midline (open arrowhead) approaches.

paramedian approach is better for unilateral pelvic ring injuries, crescent fractures, and SI joint injuries. The rule of creating full-thickness flaps extends to both approaches. The midline approach extends from the L5 level to the distal extent of the sacrum. After reaching the sacral spinous processes, the fascia is elevated laterally to the posterior SI joint ligaments. It is important to be aware of posterior cortical defects or thin sacral canal bone (as in spina bifida occulta) to avoid dural or nerve root injury. The paramedian approach begins 1 to 2 cm lateral to the posterior iliac crest. After reaching the gluteal fascia, the dissection is directed medially to the posterior ilium for SI joint or sacral fractures and medially to the gluteal attachments for crescent fractures. Proximal dissection should avoid gluteal nerve injury proximal to the iliac crest. Distal dissection should avoid injury to the superior gluteal artery and the superior gluteal nerve exiting the sciatic notch posteriorly.

The crescent fracture can be reduced with the aid of joysticks and femoral traction, but it is best reduced and compressed with a Weber tenaculum clamp placed laterally along the posterior ilium and medially on the crescent or the sacral spinous process. Compression can be achieved with a Weber tenaculum clamp placed laterally along the posterior ilium and medially on the crescent or the sacral spinous process. The reduction quality is checked with direct visualization, fluoroscopy, and direct palpation inferiorly and anteriorly. Fracture stabilization is performed with interfragmentary screws placed posterior to anterior, percutaneous SI screw placement, or posterior plating. Large crescent fracture fragments hinder or obviate SI screw placement. Laterally applied plating is performed with a one third tubular or 3.5 mm reconstruction plate with four to five holes. The plate is positioned inferiorly at the posterior inferior iliac spine. The plate is bent 90° at the posterior ilium to al-

low for a medullary screw (50 to 60 mm) within the sciatic buttress and then tensioned laterally with two to three screws (22 to 26 mm) within the plate and across the sciatic buttress. Additional intramedullary or plate fixation depends on bone quality, comminution, and additional anterior fixation. Closure is performed over a drain, in layers, and covering the plate (**Figure 10**). The skin is closed with Allgower-Donati sutures.

The SI joint disruption is débrided of chondral debris. Reduction is assisted with a 5.0-mm Schanz pin in the posterior inferior iliac spine for rotation and translation, while compression is performed with a Weber clamp laterally along the posterior ilium and the sacral spinous process. The quality of the reduction is checked with direct visualization, fluoroscopy, and direct palpation inferiorly and anteriorly. Fixation is usually accomplished with percutaneous SI screw placement.

Sacral fractures are approached via a paramedian or a midline approach. Femoral traction should be continued intraoperatively to achieve axial reduction. Transforaminal fracture debris is removed. If minor amounts of bone are removed, reduction is assisted with a 5.0-mm Schanz pin in the posterior inferior iliac spine for rotation and translation, while compression is performed with a Weber clamp laterally along the posterior ilium and the sacral spinous process. The inferior portion of the fracture line exiting at the S3-S4 level is used for the fracture read and reduction. If large amounts of bone are removed creating an unstable reduction, lumbopelvic or triangular fixation should be considered. Fracture reduction quality is confirmed with cranial sacral alar and/or L5-S1 facet reduction. Overcompression of clamp or screw fixation should be avoided.

Posterior Sacral Fixation Options

Biomechanical Analysis of Posterior Pelvic Fixation

A biomechanical study was done to determine the stiffness of several different posterior pelvic ring fixation options and combinations.[19] A single SI screw, tension band plate, or two sacral bars had the least stiffness in gapping. The group with intermediate stiffness consisted of a tension band plate in combination with a single SI screw, and one or two sacral bars in combination with a single SI screw. The stiffest fixation group was two anterior SI

plates, two SI screws, and two anterior SI plates in combination with a single SI screw. For rotation, the group with the least stiffness was a single SI screw, two SI plates, a tension band plate with or without an SI screw, and one or two sacral bars. The group with intermediate rotational stiffness consisted of one or two sacral bars in combination with an SI screw. The rotationally stiffest group consisted of two SI screws and two SI plates with an SI screw. In another biomechanical study, some of the posterior fixation options previously described increased pelvic ring stiffness during single-leg stance to levels comparable with an intact pelvic ring.[20] Internal fixation options and decisions should be based on the skill of the surgeon, fracture-injury patterns, associated injuries, and reduction quality.

Percutaneous Iliosacral Screws

Upper sacral dysmorphism decreases the size of the S1 safe zone.[1,2,21-23] Malreduction of the sacrum impedes the sacral safe zone size and stability.[24] Therefore, accurate reduction of the SI joint injury and sacral fractures is important (**Figure 11**). SI screw fixation can be performed with the patient supine or prone. The use of SI screw fixation is indicated for correcting SI joint injuries, crescent fracture-dislocations, sacral fractures, and sacral U-shaped injuries.[5,21,22,25-27] An S2 iliosacral screw individually or in addition to an S1 iliosacral screw can aid fixation options and stability.[28,29]

Sacral Bars and Transiliac Screws

Sacral bars or transiliac screws for pelvic fixation are indicated for SI joint disruptions and sacral fractures, although their use has become uncommon because of the use of percutaneous SI screws and lumbopelvic fixation. Sacral bars are inserted through the thickened portions of the

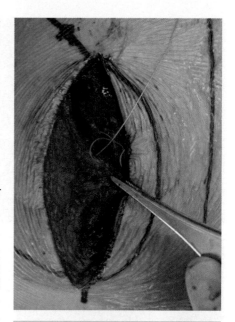

Figure 10 Photograph showing gluteal muscle-fascial closure over the posterior ilium with a posterior pelvic approach used to treat a crescent fracture-dislocation with plate application.

posterior ilium at the posterior superior iliac spine and the posterior inferior iliac spine.[30] The bar should be posterior to the sacrum and the L5 lamina to avoid neural injury.[31] The bars have threaded end caps to allow for compression and stability. Fully threaded 7.0- to 8.0-mm screws also can be used.

Transiliac and Tension Band Plate

Transiliac or tension band plating are indicated for sacral fractures. The plate can be used in combination with an SI screw to improve biomechanical stability. The plate is a 3.5- or 4.5-mm reconstruction or dynamic compression plate of 12 to 14 holes placed dorsally along the posterior ilium (**Figure 12**). If the plate is placed caudally over the posterior inferior iliac spine, a 60- to 80-mm medullary screw can be inserted in the sciatic buttress along with additional 22- to 26-mm screw fixation through the plate at either end. The plate is bent approximately 35° to 45° just lateral to either iliac crest to

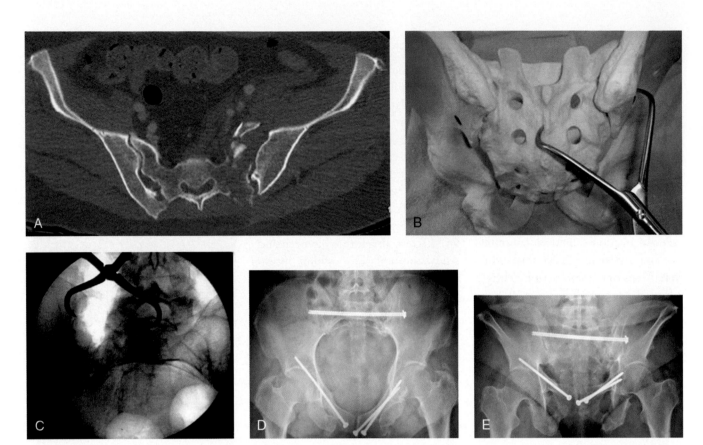

Figure 11 **A,** Axial CT scan of an unstable, irreducible, comminuted sacral alar fracture in a 64-year-old woman injured in a motor vehicle collision. Saw bones (**B**) and intraoperative fluoroscopic image (**C**) show a posterior pelvic ring Weber clamp applied from the sacral spine to the posterior aspect of the ilium. Final radiographic inlet (**D**) and outlet (**E**) images of the pelvic ring treated with anatomic open reduction, percutaneous iliosacral screw application, and bilateral retrograde percutaneous ramus screw insertion.

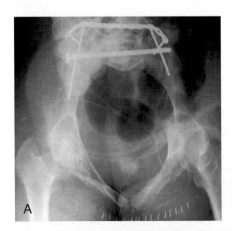
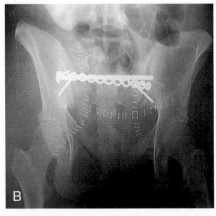

Figure 12 Inlet (**A**) and outlet (**B**) postoperative images of an unstable pelvic ring fracture treated with percutaneous iliosacral screw application and tension band plate application with a 3.5-mm 12-hole reconstruction plate.

assure proper contouring. If a ridge is removed from the posterior inferior iliac spine, the plate will be applied flush to the posterior cortex and lessen plate prominence and irritation.[32,33]

Sacral Plating

Sacral plating is indicated for vertical or horizontal sacral fractures. Plate fixation is usually performed using a midline incision. Prone positioning of the patient will sometimes help reduce the flexion deformity of the fracture. The fracture is usually impacted anteriorly. Decompression of the sacral canal reduces risks to neural structures during fracture reduction. The plate is positioned lateral to the sacral pedicles and foramina. Plate fixation is performed with 2.7- or 3.5-mm reconstruction or locked reconstruction plates with six to eight holes (**Figure 13**). Bicortical fixation is preferred cranially (24 to 30 mm) and caudally (12 to 16 mm).

Lumbopelvic and Triangular Fixation

Indications for lumbopelvic or triangular fixation include a small upper safe zone screw placement, extensive bony removal for sacral nerve root decompression, combined sacral and spinal injuries, and unstable posterior pelvic ring injuries.[6,34-39] Lumbopelvic fixation consists of L5 pedicle screw (45 to 50 mm × 5.0 to 6.0 mm) fixation connected to a sciatic buttress pedicle screw (110 to 130 mm × 7.0 to 8.0 mm) via a rod[36] (Universal Spinal System; Synthes, Paoli, PA). Triangular fixation consists of lumbopelvic fixation in addition to an iliosacral screw[6,34,38] (**Figure 14**). Midline approaches are preferred. The transforaminal or sacral canal fragments are removed. If the fracture is markedly displaced vertically or sagittally, the surgeon should be prepared to repair or cover the dural tear. Once the neural elements are decompressed, the fracture reduction is performed. The Universal Spinal System allows joystick reduction for axial length and rotation via the pedicle screw handles. Compression is facilitated with Weber clamp fixation from the ilium to the sacral spinous process. If the L5 facet is disrupted, extension of lumbar fixation to the L4 or contralateral pedicles is useful. There has been controversy concerning removal of hardware secondary to irritation and nonfused L5 to sacrum fixation. Removing some of the medial portion of the posterior inferior iliac spine allows recession of the sciatic buttress pedicle screw and potentially lessens posterior soft-tissue irritation. Ligamentous and/or facet injuries may benefit from simultaneous arthrodesis (**Figure 15**).

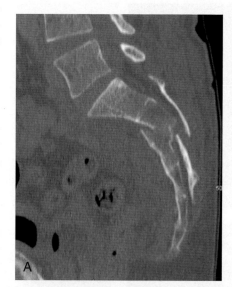
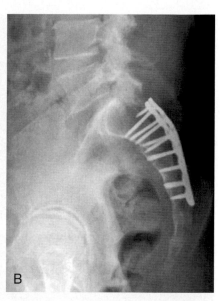

Figure 13   **A,** Lateral sacral CT image of a sacral U-shaped fracture in a 38-year-old man who fell from a height, resulting in kyphosis, translation, and cauda equina. **B,** This unstable injury with neurologic damage was treated with open decompression, reduction, and bilateral sacral alar plate fixation.

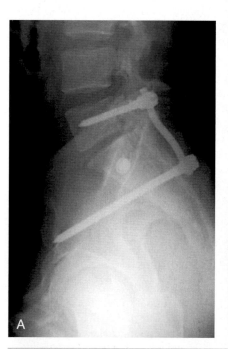
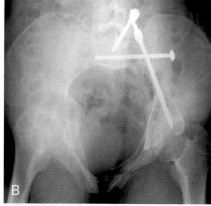
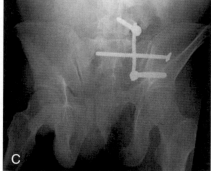

Figure 14   Radiographic inlet (**A**), outlet (**B**), and lateral (**C**) images of triangular lumbopelvic fixation.

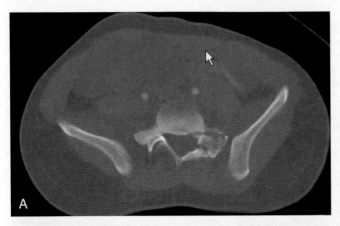

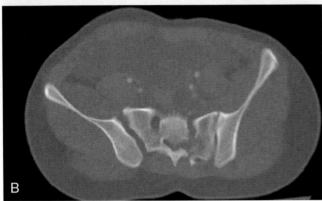

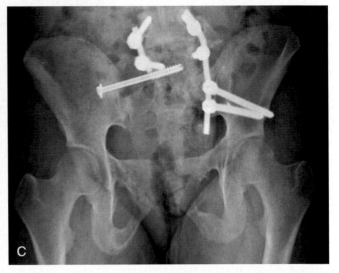

Figure 15 Injury axial CT scan of a L5-S1 facet injury (**A**) and comminuted transforaminal sacral fracture (**B**) in a 19-year-old woman involved in a motor vehicle collision. **C,** The lumbosacral plexus injury was treated with lumbopelvic fixation with extension to the L5-S1 level, arthrodesis of L5-S1, and contralateral SI joint percutaneous iliosacral screw fixation.

Discussion

Early reduction and stabilization of unstable pelvic ring injuries is encouraged.[40] Accurate reduction of fracture fragments enhances fixation safety and stability.[24] An increased risk of infection is noted with posterior pelvic fixation in combination with Morel-Lavellee degloving lesions.[33,41] Implant prominence should be avoided to diminish soft-tissue irritation and implant removal.[32,33,41] With modern fixation methods and soft-tissue handling, acceptable rates of soft-tissue complications can be expected.[42]

Summary

Although percutaneous iliosacral screw fixation is a common treatment for posterior pelvic ring injuries, complications and failures occur with this approach. Open techniques, which can maximize the quality of the reduction and the stability of the fixation, are available treatment options. The success of open techniques is affected by timing, the approach used, clamp positioning, and implant choices.

References

1. Conflitti JM, Graves ML, Chip Routt ML Jr : Radiographic quantification and analysis of dysmorphic upper sacral osseous anatomy and associated iliosacral screw insertions. *J Orthop Trauma* 2010; 24(10):630-636.

2. Farrell ED, Gardner MJ, Krieg JC, Chip Routt ML Jr: The upper sacral nerve root tunnel: An anatomic and clinical study. *J Orthop Trauma* 2009;23(5):333-339.

3. Gardner MJ, Morshed S, Nork SE, Ricci WM, Chip Routt ML Jr: Quantification of the upper and second sacral segment safe zones in normal and dysmorphic sacra. *J Orthop Trauma* 2010; 24(10):622-629.

4. Guyton GP, Mann RA, Kreiger LE, Mendel T, Kahan J: Cumulative industrial trauma as an etiology of seven common disorders in the foot and ankle: What is the evidence? *Foot Ankle Int* 2000; 21(12):1047-1056.

5. Routt ML Jr, Simonian PT, Mills WJ: Iliosacral screw fixation: Early

complications of the percutaneous technique. *J Orthop Trauma* 1997;11(8):584-589.

6. Schildhauer TA, Ledoux WR, Chapman JR, Henley MB, Tencer AF, Routt ML Jr: Triangular osteosynthesis and iliosacral screw fixation for unstable sacral fractures: A cadaveric and biomechanical evaluation under cyclic loads. *J Orthop Trauma* 2003; 17(1):22-31.

7. Letournel E: Pelvic fractures. *Injury* 1978;10(2):145-148.

8. Tile M: Pelvic fractures: Operative versus nonoperative treatment. *Orthop Clin North Am* 1980; 11(3):423-464.

9. Tile M: Acute Pelvic Fractures: I. Causation and classification. *J Am Acad Orthop Surg* 1996;4(3):143-151.

10. Burgess AR, Eastridge BJ, Young JW, et al: Pelvic ring disruptions: Effective classification system and treatment protocols. *J Trauma* 1990;30(7):848-856.

11. Dalal SA, Burgess AR, Siegel JH, et al: Pelvic fracture in multiple trauma: Classification by mechanism is key to pattern of organ injury, resuscitative requirements, and outcome. *J Trauma* 1989; 29(7):981-1000, discussion 1000-1002.

12. Young JW, Burgess AR, Brumback RJ, Poka A: Pelvic fractures: Value of plain radiography in early assessment and management. *Radiology* 1986;160(2):445-451.

13. Denis F, Davis S, Comfort T: Sacral fractures: An important problem. Retrospective analysis of 236 cases. *Clin Orthop Relat Res* 1988;227:67-81.

14. Roy-Camille R, Saillant G, Gagna G, Mazel C: Transverse fracture of the upper sacrum: Suicidal jumper's fracture. *Spine (Phila Pa 1976)* 1985;10(9):838-845.

15. Isler B: Lumbosacral lesions associated with pelvic ring injuries. *J Orthop Trauma* 1990;4(1):1-6.

16. Tseng S, Tornetta P III: Percutaneous management of Morel-Lavallee lesions. *J Bone Joint Surg Am* 2006;88(1):92-96.

17. Hak DJ, Olson SA, Matta JM: Diagnosis and management of closed internal degloving injuries associated with pelvic and acetabular fractures: The Morel-Lavallée lesion. *J Trauma* 1997; 42(6):1046-1051.

18. Sagi HC, Papp S, Dipasquale T: The effect of suture pattern and tension on cutaneous blood flow as assessed by laser Doppler flowmetry in a pig model. *J Orthop Trauma* 2008;22(3):171-175.

19. Yinger K, Scalise J, Olson SA, Bay BK, Finkemeier CG: Biomechanical comparison of posterior pelvic ring fixation. *J Orthop Trauma* 2003;17(7):481-487.

20. Comstock CP, van der Meulen MC, Goodman SB: Biomechanical comparison of posterior internal fixation techniques for unstable pelvic fractures. *J Orthop Trauma* 1996;10(8):517-522.

21. Routt ML Jr, Kregor PJ, Simonian PT, Mayo KA: Early results of percutaneous iliosacral screws placed with the patient in the supine position. *J Orthop Trauma* 1995;9(3):207-214.

22. Routt ML Jr, Simonian PT: Closed reduction and percutaneous skeletal fixation of sacral fractures. *Clin Orthop Relat Res* 1996; 329:121-128.

23. Routt ML Jr, Simonian PT, Agnew SG, Mann FA: Radiographic recognition of the sacral alar slope for optimal placement of iliosacral screws: A cadaveric and clinical study. *J Orthop Trauma* 1996; 10(3):171-177.

24. Reilly MC, Bono CM, Litkouhi B, Sirkin M, Behrens FF: The effect of sacral fracture malreduction on the safe placement of iliosacral screws. *J Orthop Trauma* 2003;17(2):88-94.

25. Barei DP, Bellabarba C, Mills WJ, Routt ML Jr: Percutaneous management of unstable pelvic ring disruptions. *Injury* 2001; 32(Suppl 1):SA33-SA44.

26. Nork SE, Jones CB, Harding SP, Mirza SK, Routt ML Jr: Percutaneous stabilization of U-shaped sacral fractures using iliosacral screws: Technique and early results. *J Orthop Trauma* 2001; 15(4):238-246.

27. Routt ML Jr, Nork SE, Mills WJ: Percutaneous fixation of pelvic ring disruptions. *Clin Orthop Relat Res* 2000;375:15-29.

28. Moed BR, Geer BL: S2 iliosacral screw fixation for disruptions of the posterior pelvic ring: A report of 49 cases. *J Orthop Trauma* 2006;20(6):378-383.

29. van Zwienen CM, van den Bosch EW, Snijders CJ, Kleinrensink GJ, van Vugt AB: Biomechanical comparison of sacroiliac screw techniques for unstable pelvic ring fractures. *J Orthop Trauma* 2004; 18(9):589-595.

30. Atlíhan D, Bozkurt M, Turanlí S, Doğan M, Tekdemir I, Elhan A: Anatomy of the posterior iliac crest as a reference to sacral bar insertion. *Clin Orthop Relat Res* 2004;418:141-145.

31. Leggon RE, Meister B, Lindsey RW: Inadvertent sacral bar transfixation of the cauda equina. *J Orthop Trauma* 2002;16(2): 127-130.

32. Krappinger D, Larndorfer R, Struve P, Rosenberger R, Arora R, Blauth M: Minimally invasive transiliac plate osteosynthesis for type C injuries of the pelvic ring: A clinical and radiological follow-up. *J Orthop Trauma* 2007;21(9): 595-602.

33. Suzuki T, Hak DJ, Ziran BH, et al: Outcome and complications of posterior transiliac plating for vertically unstable sacral fractures. *Injury* 2009;40(4):405-409.

34. Sagi HC: Technical aspects and recommended treatment algorithms in triangular osteosynthesis and spinopelvic fixation for vertical shear transforaminal sacral fractures. *J Orthop Trauma* 2009; 23(5):354-360.

35. Sagi HC, Militano U, Caron T, Lindvall E: A comprehensive analysis with minimum 1-year follow-up of vertically unstable transforaminal sacral fractures treated with triangular osteosynthesis. *J Orthop Trauma* 2009; 23(5):313-319, discussion 319-321.

36. Schildhauer TA, Bellabarba C, Nork SE, Barei DP, Routt ML Jr, Chapman JR: Decompression and lumbopelvic fixation for sacral fracture-dislocations with spinopelvic dissociation. *J Orthop Trauma* 2006;20(7):447-457.

37. Schildhauer TA, Bellabarba C, Selznick HS, McRoberts D, Vedder NB, Chapman JR: Unstable pediatric sacral fracture with bone loss caused by a high-energy gunshot injury. *J Trauma* 2007;63(4): E95-E99.

38. Schildhauer TA, Josten C, Muhr G: Triangular osteosynthesis of vertically unstable sacrum fractures: A new concept allowing early weight-bearing. *J Orthop Trauma* 1998;12(5):307-314.

39. Vaccaro AR, Kim DH, Brodke DS, et al: Diagnosis and management of thoracolumbar spine fractures. *Instr Course Lect* 2004;53: 359-373.

40. Barei DP, Shafer BL, Beingessner DM, Gardner MJ, Nork SE, Routt ML: The impact of open reduction internal fixation on acute pain management in unstable pelvic ring injuries. *J Trauma* 2010;68(4):949-953.

41. Bellabarba C, Schildhauer TA, Vaccaro AR, Chapman JR: Complications associated with surgical stabilization of high-grade sacral fracture dislocations with spinopelvic instability. *Spine (Phila Pa 1976)* 2006;31(11, Suppl):S80-S88, discussion S104.

42. Stover MD, Sims SH, Templeman DC, Merkle P, Matta JM: Is the posterior approach to pelvic ring injuries associated with a high rate of soft tissue complications? *Orthopaedic Trauma Association, Annual Meeting*. Vancouver, British Columbia; 1998. http://www.hwbf.org/ota/am/ota98/otapa/OTA98101.htm. Accessed August 25, 2011.

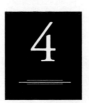

Surgical Techniques for Complex Proximal Tibial Fractures

Jason A. Lowe, MD
Nirmal Tejwani, MD
Brad J. Yoo, MD
Philip R. Wolinsky, MD

Abstract

In managing complex proximal tibia fractures, several options are available to the treating surgeon. Closed management with or without external fixation, formal open reduction and internal fixation, and intramedullary nail fixation have been described in the literature. There is a lack of consensus regarding the optimal treatment method for complex bicondylar patterns or proximal metadiaphyseal fractures with or without involvement of the articular surface. It is helpful to review the standard and alternative surgical approaches to bicondylar tibial plateau fractures and to be aware of the intramedullary nail as an alternative approach for complex proximal metadiaphyseal patterns.

Instr Course Lect 2012;61:39-51.

Traditional and Alternative Surgical Approaches to the Tibial Plateau: How to Select Them

Any surgical approach for fracture fixation should facilitate visualization of fracture fragments and allow the application of optimal fixation devices and soft-tissue repair. Treatment goals applied to tibial plateau fractures include anatomic articular surface reduction, restoration of the anatomic axis, and preservation of the menisci. The approach should not devitalize soft tissues or cause further injury to surrounding structures. An ideal surgical dissection encompasses these principles and permits early joint motion.

The midline longitudinal incision is the favored approach to the knee joint because this incision facilitates knee replacement if needed in the future. Surgical exposure for complex injuries (bicondylar fractures) requiring dual fixation needs large medial and lateral flaps that add to soft-tissue complications. Other surgical approaches allowing a more direct approach to the fracture to decrease the risk of soft-tissue injury from excessive retraction or periosteal stripping are available. When one incision does not adequately expose the fracture, it is better to use a dual incision than a single midline exposure.[1-3]

Anterolateral Approach

The anterolateral approach is used for the most commonly seen tibial plateau fractures (Schatzker types I, II, and III).[4] It is also used for the lateral part of a dual-incision approach needed for internal fixation of a bicolumnar fracture. The incision is centered on the

Dr. Lowe or an immediate family member serves as an unpaid consultant to Synthes; has received research or institutional support from Synthes; and has received nonincome support (such as equipment or services), commercially derived honoraria, or other non—research-related funding (such as paid travel) from Synthes. Dr. Tejwani or an immediate family member has received royalties from Biomet; is a member of a speakers' bureau or has made paid presentations on behalf of Zimmer and Stryker; serves as a paid consultant to Zimmer and Stryker; and serves as a board member, owner, officer, or committee member of the American Academy of Orthopaedic Surgeons. Neither Dr. Yoo nor any immediate family member has received anything of value from or owns stock in a commercial company or institution related directly or indirectly to the subject of this chapter. Dr. Wolinsky or an immediate family member serves as a paid consultant to Biomet and Zimmer; has received research or institutional support from Synthes; and serves as a board member, owner, officer, or committee member of the Orthopaedic Trauma Association and the American Academy of Orthopaedic Surgeons.

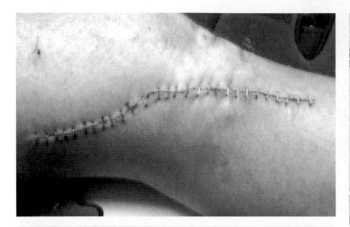

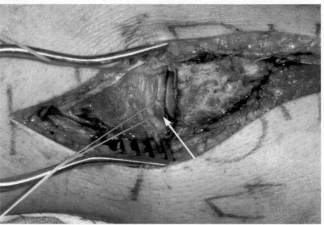

Figure 1 Clinical photograph of a patient's right knee with the lazy-S incision used for internal fixation of a lateral proximal tibial fracture.

Figure 2 Clinical photograph of a patient's right knee with retention sutures in the lateral meniscus (arrow) of a submeniscal arthrotomy.

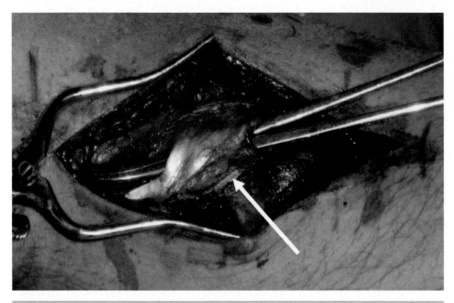

Figure 3 Clinical photograph of a patient's left knee with a medial incision (patient's head is to the left). The tendons of the pes anserinus (arrow) are seen over the clamp.

Gerdy tubercle and is shaped like a lazy S or a hockey stick. The fascia is elevated off the tibial tubercle to expose the lateral tibial plateau. The knee capsule is incised, and a submeniscal arthrotomy allows visualization of the articular surface (**Figures 1** and **2**). In addition to visualization of the articular surface, this approach allows repair of any meniscal tears.

Medial Approach

The medial approach is used for a medial tibial plateau fracture (Schatzker type IV) or as part of a dual approach to the plateau. The incision parallels the posteromedial border of the proximal part of the tibia. The pes anserinus is elevated, the fracture reduced, and fixation implants are placed beneath the pes anserinus. The pes anserinus

may either be retracted (**Figure 3**) or incised, with repair after fracture fixation. The medial meniscus cannot be elevated as is possible with the lateral meniscus; therefore, the limitation of this approach is the limited visualization of the articular surface of the medial plateau. Also, access to the posterior plateau is limited, but the medial approach can be converted to a posteromedial approach.

Anterior Approach With Tibial Tubercle Osteotomy

The advantage of the anterior approach with osteotomy of the tibial tubercle is that the tibial plateau and the intercondylar notch are completely exposed, allowing reattachment or primary suture of the cruciate ligaments.[5] This approach is rarely used, and most complex, bicondylar fractures are now treated with dual incisions.

Posteromedial Approach

Medial tibial plateau fractures extending to the posterior aspect of the tibial plateau, posterior metaphyseal fractures, or those that require a buttress on the posteromedial cortex are best fixed with use of the posteromedial approach. Fragment-specific fixation of the medial plateau is recommended over stabilization with a laterally based locking construct.[6] To obtain optimal fixation of bicondylar fractures, a dual-plating technique is recommended, with one plate fixing the medial fragment and the other fixing the lateral plateau. Medial plateau fractures may be medial or posteromedial, with each requiring a plate to be, ideally, placed at the apex of the fracture (fragment specific).

The patient can be positioned prone or supine.[7] An incision is made over the posteromedial aspect of the knee (**Figure 4**). Dissection between the medial head of the gastrocnemius muscle and the semitendinosus muscle allows exposure of the semimembranosus muscle, which is detached for better access to the posterior aspect of the tibia. Visualization of the articular surface is limited, but, if necessary, visualization can be improved with a longitudinal split in the medial collateral ligament and the capsule. Through this incision, visualization of the articular cartilage can aid in congruent joint reduction.

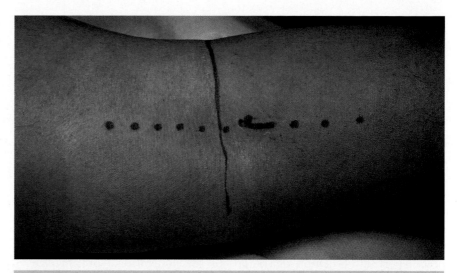

Figure 4 Clinical photograph of a patient's right knee. With the patient in the prone position, the solid line identifies the level of the knee joint, with the femur to the left. The dotted line illustrates an incision for a posteromedial incision.

Posterior Approach

An isolated posterior shear fracture, a posterior cruciate ligament avulsion fracture with a large osseous fragment, or a posterior fracture-dislocation is best exposed with a posterior approach.[8,9] A z-shaped incision across the flexor crease is used. The deep tissue planes are between the medial head of the gastrocnemius and the semimembranosus muscles or between the two heads of the gastrocnemius muscle with protection of the neurovascular structures. The medial or lateral head of the gastrocnemius muscle may be partially detached if it is necessary to improve exposure, enable fracture reduction, or insert fixation on the posterior rim.

Extended Lateral Approach With Fibular Osteotomy

The Lobenhoffer approach is used to expose fractures of the lateral tibial plateau that extend posteriorly when the head of the fibula limits the exposure.[10,11] The skin incision is made along the course of the peroneal nerve, posterior to the fibular head. After dissection, the common peroneal nerve is protected and an osteotomy of the fibula at the junction of the head and neck is performed, leaving the proximal attachments intact. This allows exposure of the tibial plateau from anterior to posterior.

Another way to approach the posterolateral plateau is without a fibular osteotomy.[10] Absence of an osteotomy makes it more difficult to visualize the tibial fracture at the level of the fibular head; however, this approach is preferred because it avoids the risk of a nonunion at the fibular osteotomy site.

Medial Tibial Plateau Reduction

A shearing force produces a coronal plane fracture comprising approximately 25% of the medial articular surface.[12] This fragment is seen on a lateral radiograph, but the full extent of articular involvement is best appreciated on sagittal CT images. Because the medial collateral ligament prevents a submeniscal arthrotomy, reduction of the medial joint line is often obtained indirectly with anatomic restoration of the medial cortex. If there is a question about the accuracy of the reduction of the articular surface of the medial plateau, a longitudinal incision is made in the medial collateral ligament, where the fracture enters the medial aspect of the joint. Anatomic reduction is confirmed by aligning the articular cartilage of each fragment while the cortex is reduced with a well-placed Weber clamp perpendicular to the fracture. This white-white read of the medial plateau articular cartilage augments the accuracy of reduction.

Medial Plateau Fixation

Surgical stabilization of isolated medial plateau fractures (Schatzker type IV) is accomplished with an undercontoured, nonlocking, flexible plate (one third T-plate or reconstruction plate) applied as a buttress. Fixation of the medial plateau in Schatzker type V and VI fractures is more controversial. Stabilization can be accomplished with locking screws placed through a laterally based implant alone or stabilized with a medial plate as part of a dual plating construct (medial and lateral plate).[13-17] Biomechanical and clinical data support both techniques. Although lateral-only locked plates reduce surgical time, reduce blood loss, and limit soft-tissue stripping, a high rate of articular subsistence (26%) has been reported.[13-17] Displacement of the medial fragment can result in knee instability, pain, and posttraumatic osteoarthritis.[12] This chapter's authors, therefore, recommend fragment-specific fixation of the posteromedial and lateral plateau through a two-incision approach for bicondylar tibial plateau fractures. Fragment-specific fixation of the medial plateau avoids inadequate purchase of the posteromedial fragment observed with lateral-only locking screws.[6,16-18] The benefit of added fracture stability is offset by greater surgical time and higher postoperative infection rates. Current reports have demonstrated postoperative infection rates of 8.4% with dual plating compared with 1.6% with lateral-only fixation.[13,14] In the absence of a prospective, randomized, controlled trial comparing these surgical approaches, the need for anatomic reduction of the joint surface and adequate stabilization of the medial plateau takes precedence.

Lateral Plateau Articular Reduction

High-energy bicondylar tibial fractures are typically associated with articular surface impaction of the lateral plateau. Successful restoration of the lateral aspect of the joint requires adequate visualization and an array of reduction techniques. A submeniscal arthrotomy and a laterally based femoral distractor improve visualization of the articular surface when needed. A single Schanz pin is placed into the femoral metaphysis, parallel to the joint line, and a second Schanz pin is placed in the tibia, distal to planned plate placement location.[19] Care must be used with placement of a lateral tibial pin so as to not injure the neurovascular structures of the anterior compartment.[20] Applying distraction opens the joint and enhances visualization of the lateral plateau. Retraction of the posterolateral or anterolateral fragments (opening the door) can allow even more visualization.

Mobile articular pieces are reduced with a dental pick or a small (0.45- to 0.62-mm) wire and are temporarily stabilized with Kirschner wires. Impacted articular fragments must be mobilized from surrounding cancellous bone before they can be reduced. A 0.25- to 0.50-inch (0.64- to 1.3-cm) osteotome or bone tamp is used to elevate 1.0 to 1.5 cm of cancellous bone with the articular segment. Once levered into position, the fragment is stabilized with Kirschner wires. With the impacted segment reduced and secured with wire fixation, bone voids can be filled with graft material and the lateral segment can be reduced (closing the door). The medial and lateral plateaus can be reduced and compressed with a periarticular reduction clamp.[19]

The contained defect of a pure depression fracture cannot be reduced without an osteotomy. If there is an incomplete fracture, the articular segment is accessed by completing the fracture and reducing the articular fragment as previously described. If there is no cortical fracture, articular reduction is done with one of two techniques. The anterior compartment is released from the metaphyseal flare for both. One technique is to use the Dynamic Hip Screw (DHS; Synthes, Paoli, PA) set and fluoroscopic visualization. The guidewire is directed from the lateral tibial metaphysis toward the impacted segment. The cortex is then opened with the cannulated 11-mm reamer from the DHS system. Bone tamps are introduced and used to tap the articular segment into place. The articular reduction is confirmed by direct visualization through the submeniscal arthrotomy. Alternatively, a lateral osteotomy is made with drill holes (2.0-mm drill-bit) in a diamond pattern, with the drill holes connected with use of a 0.25-inch (0.64-cm) osteotome. The articular segment is reduced as just described. With either technique, the articular fragments can be supported with Kirschner wires and bone graft before definitive fixation.

Lateral Plateau Fixation

Surgical stabilization of the lateral plateau must maintain reduction and rigid fixation of the articular segment to a well-aligned tibial shaft. The joint surface is stabilized with multiple parallel screws placed just beneath the subchondral bone. These rafting screws support the reduced articular surface fragments and can be the proximal screws of a 3.5-mm or a 4.5-mm, precontoured periarticular plate or with minifragment (2.4- or 2.7-mm) screws. Minifragment screws and plates are favored for articular comminution with fragments having minimal subchondral bone or when the proximal screws in the precontoured plate are not subchondral.

The articular segment is reduced to the shaft with traction (a manual or femoral distractor). First, the plate is fixed to the proximal segment with bicortical screws (locked or nonlocked) inserted parallel to the joint.[21] The plate is reduced to the tibial shaft with a bicortical screw or a so-called whirlybird push-pull type of device. It is important to ensure that this does not

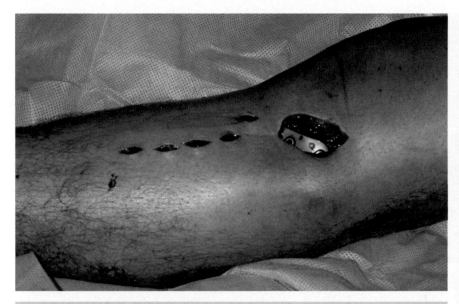

Figure 5 Clinical intraoperative photograph of a patient's left knee showing incisions for minimally invasive plate osteosynthesis.

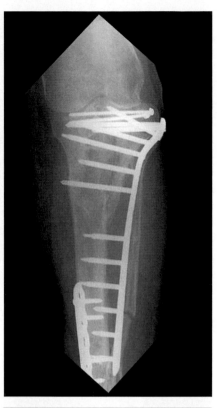

Figure 6 AP radiograph of a knee illustrating the inability of locking screws to reduce the valgus malalignment in the coronal plane. As a result, a valgus malunion, with the plate poorly apposed to the tibia, is observed.

malreduce the fracture in the coronal plane, and locking screws should not be placed in the distal segment until the alignment is correct.[22]

Minimally Invasive Plate Osteosynthesis

The proximal tibial anatomy and fracture pattern must be clearly understood if precontoured plates are used with minimally invasive techniques. The articular surface is visualized with a small arthrotomy, and percutaneous techniques are used for screw placement into the tibial shaft (**Figure 5**). Care must be taken when this technique is used for plates longer than 11 holes because the neurovascular bundles in the anterior and lateral compartments are at risk.[12,23]

Locking Screws

Locking screws increase construct rigidity, but they should be placed bicortically.[21,24] They are useful in severely osteoporotic bone, substantial metaphyseal-diaphyseal comminution, or short-segment periarticular and/or

intra-articular fractures. Malunion has been a problem, and it is necessary to pay meticulous attention to fracture reduction before placement of locking screws[25] (**Figure 6**).

Intramedullary Nailing of Proximal Tibial Fractures

The use of an intramedullary nail for fracture stabilization is appealing. The insertion point of an intramedullary nail is remote from the fracture site (minimizing vascular disruption of the fracture fragments), the implants are centrally located, and tibial diaphyseal fractures have a high rate of union and a low rate of complications. As a result, the use of intramedullary nailing for tibial fractures has expanded from midshaft diaphyseal fractures to proximal fractures.[26-32] Intramedullary nail fixation is technically more demanding for proximal tibial fractures than for diaphyseal fractures. Unlike intramedullary nailing of a diaphyseal fracture, placement of the intramedullary nail does not reduce a proximal tibial fracture, and malreductions of proximal

tibial fractures with intramedullary nail fixation are reported to be as high as 84%.[27,33-36]

The typical deformity caused by intramedullary nailing of proximal tibial fractures is valgus and apex anterior angulation with anterior translation of the proximal fragment (**Figure 7**). The valgus deformity is caused by an imbalance of muscle forces on the proximal fragment and is accentuated when the insertion point is too medial or directed laterally. The tip of the nail can abut the lateral cortex, causing the proximal fragment to rotate into a valgus position[34,35,37] (**Figure 8**). The apex anterior deformity results from a combination of the pull of the patellar tendon,[34] a distal insertion site, or a posteriorly directed nail that deflects

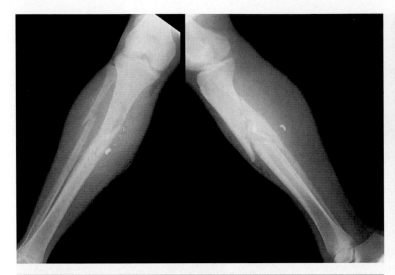

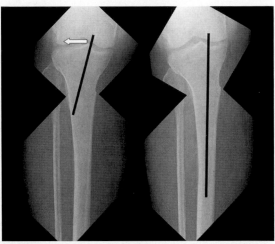

Figure 7 AP (left) and lateral (right) radiographs of an extra-articular proximal tibial fracture showing the most common deformities (valgus and procurvatum) observed in these fractures.

Figure 8 AP radiographs showing how a medial starting site produces a valgus deformity as the intramedullary device enters the tibial diaphysis.

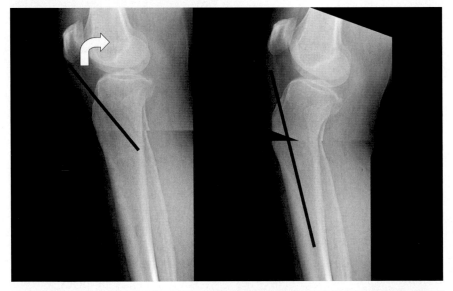

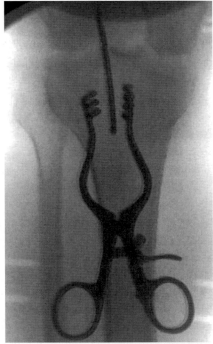

Figure 9 Lateral radiographs showing how an inferior starting site and posterior nail trajectory produce a procurvatum deformity of the proximal segment as the nail enters the diaphysis.

Figure 10 AP radiograph showing an appropriate starting site, just medial to the lateral tibial spine and in line with the mechanical axis.

off the posterior tibial cortex and rotates the proximal fragment (**Figure 9**). Nails with an accentuated distal Herzog bend may translate the proximal fragment anteriorly, described by Henley et al[38] as the wedge effect.

To prevent malalignment of proximal tibial fractures during intramedullary nailing, the starting point should

be properly placed; the fracture should be reduced before guidewire placement, reaming, and nail insertion; and the reduction should be held until all of the locking bolts have been inserted.

The Proper Starting Point
Fluoroscopic imaging is used to obtain good AP and lateral C-arm images of the knee. The starting point on the AP

radiograph is in line with the medial border of the lateral tibial spine (**Figure 10**). The insertion site on the lateral radiograph is slightly anterior to the anterior margin of the articular

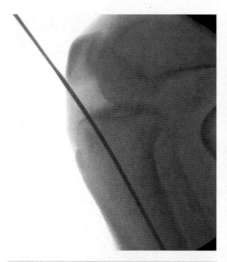

Figure 11 Lateral radiograph showing a correctly selected starting site and wire trajectory. The wire is just anterior to the articular margin and directed parallel to the anterior tibial cortex.

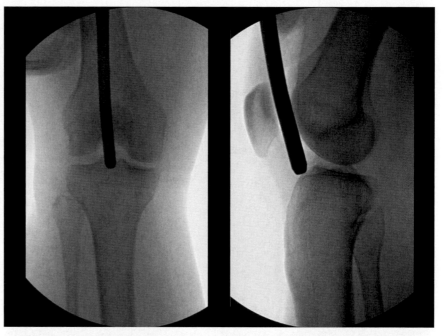

Figure 12 AP (left) and lateral (right) radiographs with a protection sleeve for a retropatellar tibial nail centered at an appropriate starting site.

surface. The guidewire and nail are inserted as parallel to the anterior cortex as possible (**Figure 11**).

Fracture Reduction Techniques

Extended Leg Position

It is critical to reduce the fracture and maintain the reduction during fracture fixation. The intraoperative position of the leg affects fracture reduction. When the knee is maximally flexed, which facilitates collinear insertion of the nail with the anterior tibial cortex, the pull of the patellar tendon increases the apex anterior deformity. When this occurs, the apex deformity can be limited by placing the instrumentation in the leg with minimal knee flexion.[39] Originally, semiextended nailing was performed through a large medial parapatellar incision; however, it can now be done with a small suprapatellar incision. The instruments and nail are passed through protective sleeves, posterior to the patella to the proximal part of the tibia[16] (**Figure 12**). Recent studies have suggested this technique can be used with-

out injury to the patella or femoral articular cartilage, the menisci, or the anterior cruciate ligament.[16,18,40] No outcomes data are available for this technique.

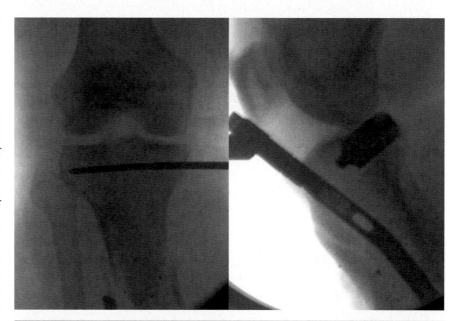

Figure 13 AP (left) and lateral (right) radiographs with a proximal Schanz pin for the AO distractor, appropriately placed parallel to the articular surface (left) and posterior to the nail path (right).

Use of a Femoral Distractor or an External Fixation Frame

A universal distractor or an external fixator can be used to obtain and maintain fracture reduction. With use

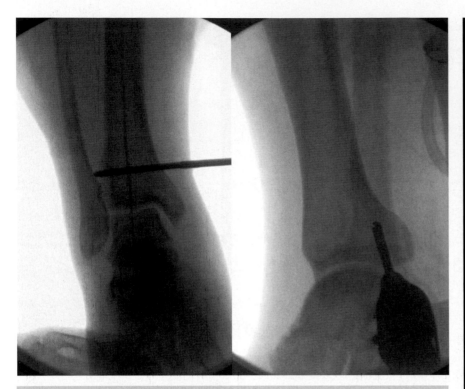

Figure 14 AP (left) and lateral (right) radiographs showing an appropriately placed distal Schanz pin inserted parallel to the ankle joint and posterior to the nail path.

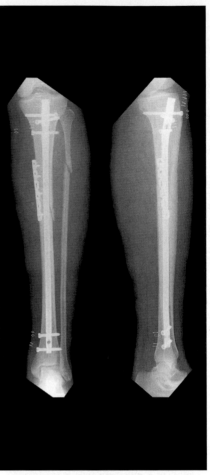

Figure 15 AP (left) and lateral (right) radiographs with a provisional locking plate on the posteromedial tibial cortex. Unicortical locking screws are used so as to not obstruct insertion of reamers or the intramedullary implant.

of fluoroscopic imaging, a proximal Schanz pin is inserted from the medial side of the proximal part of the tibia posterior to the planned intramedullary nail path (**Figure 13**), and a distal Schanz pin is placed medially in the posterior malleolus (behind the nail) or at the level of the physeal scar (**Figure 14**). The pins should be inserted parallel to the proximal and distal joint lines. Application of traction through the frame until the pins are parallel typically results in adequate reduction.[34,41]

Temporary Plate Fixation

A small plate can be used as a temporary reduction device.[29,42] The plate may be placed on the medial or lateral tibial border, but the medial border is better because the medial side of the fracture is often less comminuted. The medial incision is positioned posterior to the posterior borders of the tibia so that if the incision fails to heal, no bone will be exposed (**Figure 15**). Minimal deep dissection is needed, and the plate is placed over intact periosteum. Unicortical screws are used so the reamer and nail can pass. After insertion of the nail and all interlocking screws, the plate may be removed or the screws on the proximal side of the fracture may be taken out. The plate then acts as a buttress construct, preventing a deformity from recurring while permitting relative motion at the fracture site.

Blocking Screws

So-called blocking or Poller screws can be used during intramedullary nailing of proximal tibial fractures. They are placed preemptively in an effort to prevent a deformity or as a so-called bailout after deformity has occurred. They are used to narrow the canal, to create a path, or as an artificial cortex for the nail to pass down.[28,33,43]

Blocking screws are inserted perpendicular to the plane of the deformity, on the concave side of the deformity, within the more mobile fracture segment. For example, with a valgus deformity, the screw is placed from anterior to posterior, on the lateral side of the instrument path, and in the proximal segment (**Figure 16**). The screw functions as a so-called artificial cortex.

Blocking screws also can be used for an anterior malalignment. The blocking screw is placed slightly posterior to

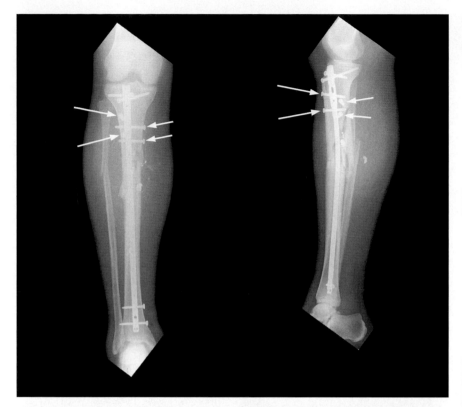

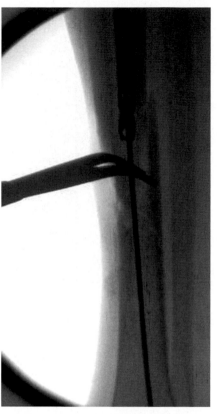

Figure 16 AP (left) and lateral (right) radiographs showing proper positioning of blocking screws to aid in fracture reduction and strengthen the implant construct. Anterior-posterior screws placed lateral to the nail (long arrows) prevent valgus deformation, and medial-lateral screws placed posterior to the nail (short arrows) prevent procurvatum.

Figure 17 Intraoperative lateral radiograph with a Weber clamp placed percutaneously to hold the reduction during nail insertion.

the midline, from medial to lateral, in the proximal fragment (**Figure 16**). As a nail is inserted, it contacts the blocking screw, extending the proximal fragment and decreasing the apex anterior deformity. The screw should not be placed in the midline because nail passage may be blocked by the screw.

Percutaneous Clamps

The orientation of a fracture line may allow percutaneous placement of a reduction clamp to obtain and maintain the reduction (**Figure 17**). The use of clamps has not been shown to increase infection rates.[44]

Implant Selection

It is important to know the implants to ensure that at least two locking screws can be placed in the proximal segment.

The distance from the end of the nail to the locking bolts determines how far proximal or distal fracture lines can extend and still be stabilized by the intramedullary nail. The number and orientation of the proximal and distal interlocking bolts vary by implant. Oblique bolts have demonstrated more stability than transverse bolts in resisting coronal plane deformity but not axial or torsional stability.[38] The combination of oblique and transverse interlocking screws increases construct stability.[45,46] Intramedullary devices with a distal Herzog bend may accentuate a sagittal plane deformity because, as the Herzog bend contacts the posterior cortex, it can create a so-called wedge effect and translate the proximal segment anteriorly[38] (**Figure 18**).

Complications and Pitfalls

Knee pain, after intramedullary nailing of the tibia, affects 60% to 70% of patients.[47-50] The anterior knee pain is exacerbated by kneeling, squatting, stair climbing, or high-performance athletic activities. Implant removal after fracture union has had inconsistent results with regard to relieving anterior knee pain. There is no difference in the prevalence of knee pain when a transpatellar or parapatellar incision is used.

The prevalence of malunion has been reported to be as high as 84%.[36] With use of the techniques described in this chapter, malunion rates have been reduced to between 8% and 23%.[28,29,31] Strict attention to surgical technique and the use of reduction aids decrease the prevalence of malreduction.

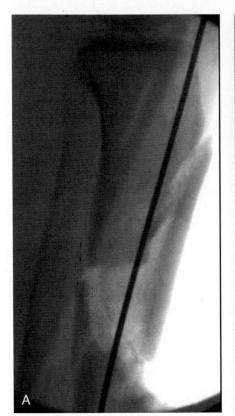
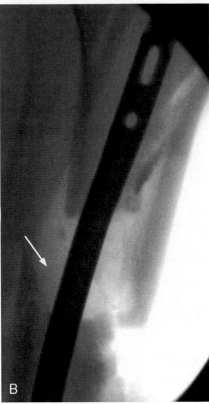

Figure 18 **A,** Lateral intraoperative radiograph with a well-positioned guide-wire (parallel to the anterior cortex) during reaming. **B,** Insertion of a nail with a low Herzog bend (arrow) showing displacement of the proximal fragment as it contacts the posterior cortex.

Infections and nonunions are most commonly associated with open and/or comminuted fractures.[29,31,36,42,51] Ultimate union rates of 91% to 100% have been reported, but the union rate following primary fixation is approximately 77%.[28,29,36,42] Lindvall et al[31] reported a 100% union rate for closed tibial fractures and a 23% rate of nonunion for open fractures stabilized with an intramedullary nail.

Patient-specific contraindications to the use of an intramedullary nail include open physes, intramedullary canals too narrow to allow insertion of a nail, preexisting canal deformities, knee contractures, and so-called blocking hardware such as an ipsilateral knee replacement or knee fusion. Fracture-specific contraindications to the use of an intramedullary nail in-

clude substantial intra-articular involvement and short extra-articular segments that preclude placement of at least two interlocking screws.[6]

Nails Compared With Plates

A literature meta-analysis found a trend toward an increased prevalence of malunion after intramedullary nailing compared with plate and screw osteosynthesis ($P = 0.06$) but a lower infection rate after intramedullary nailing ($P < 0.05$).[52] Lindvall et al[31] also demonstrated a trend toward a higher malunion rate for intramedullary nailing ($P = 0.103$), a threefold increased rate of hardware removal after plate and screw fixation, and no difference in implant failure between these two techniques. Both intramedullary nails and plates can be inserted with

use of surgical techniques that respect the local soft-tissue biology. These techniques optimize fracture-healing and contribute to a high rate of fracture union for both surgical procedures.[27,29,52,53]

Implant failure has been reported for both intramedullary nails and plates.[35,36,53] Early studies of intramedullary nails had implant failure rates as high as 25%, whereas only 2.6% of plates failed.[36,53] Many early failures of intramedullary nails involved small-diameter locking bolts.[24] More recent literature has demonstrated similar prevalences of implant failure for intramedullary nails and plates.[2,28,31,34,54,55]

Summary

Extra-articular proximal tibial fractures are technically demanding fractures to treat. Fixation with an intramedullary nail requires a firm understanding of the anatomy of the proximal part of the tibia, the fracture pattern, the deforming forces, and the implant system. The prevalence of malreduction can be reduced with use of meticulous surgical technique, a correct nail insertion site, and adjuvant reduction aids. The rates of postoperative infection and nonunion are related more to the nature of the injury (open and comminuted) than to the implant. Patients should be educated on the occurrence of postoperative functional knee pain, which seems to occur more commonly in younger, more active patients.

References

1. Barei DP, Nork SE, Mills WJ, Coles CP, Henley MB, Benirschke SK: Functional outcomes of severe bicondylar tibial plateau fractures treated with dual incisions and medial and lateral plates. *J Bone Joint Surg Am* 2006; 88(8):1713-1721.

2. Egol KA, Tejwani NC, Capla EL, Wolinsky PL, Koval KJ: Staged management of high-energy proximal tibia fractures (OTA types 41): The results of a prospective, standardized protocol. *J Orthop Trauma* 2005;19(7):448-455, discussion 456.

3. Georgiadis GM: Combined anterior and posterior approaches for complex tibial plateau fractures. *J Bone Joint Surg Br* 1994;76(2): 285-289.

4. Schatzker J, McBroom R, Bruce D: The tibial plateau fracture: The Toronto experience 1968–1975. *Clin Orthop Relat Res* 1979;138: 94-104.

5. Fernandez DL: Anterior approach to the knee with osteotomy of the tibial tubercle for bicondylar tibial fractures. *J Bone Joint Surg Am* 1988;70(2):208-219.

6. Barei DP, O'Mara TJ, Taitsman LA, Dunbar RP, Nork SE: Frequency and fracture morphology of the posteromedial fragment in bicondylar tibial plateau fracture patterns. *J Orthop Trauma* 2008; 22(3):176-182.

7. Weil YA, Gardner MJ, Boraiah S, Helfet DL, Lorich DG: Posteromedial supine approach for reduction and fixation of medial and bicondylar tibial plateau fractures. *J Orthop Trauma* 2008;22(5): 357-362.

8. Fakler JK, Ryzewicz M, Hartshorn C, Morgan SJ, Stahel PF, Smith WR: Optimizing the management of Moore type I postero-medial split fracture dislocations of the tibial head: Description of the Lobenhoffer approach. *J Orthop Trauma* 2007;21(5):330-336.

9. Galla M, Lobenhoffer P: The direct, dorsal approach to the treatment of unstable tibial posteromedial fracture-dislocations. *Unfallchirurg* 2003;106(3): 241-247.

10. Solomon LB, Stevenson AW, Baird RP, Pohl AP: Posterolateral transfibular approach to tibial plateau fractures: Technique, results, and rationale. *J Orthop Trauma* 2010;24(8):505-514.

11. Tao J, Hang DH, Wang QG, et al: The posterolateral shearing tibial plateau fracture: Treatment and results via a modified posterolateral approach. *Knee* 2008;15(6): 473-479.

12. Higgins TF, Kemper D, Klatt J: Incidence and morphology of the posteromedial fragment in bicondylar tibial plateau fractures. *J Orthop Trauma* 2009;23(1):45-51.

13. Gosling T, Schandelmaier P, Muller M, Hankemeier S, Wagner M, Krettek C: Single lateral locked screw plating of bicondylar tibial plateau fractures. *Clin Orthop Relat Res* 2005;439:207-214.

14. Gösling T, Schandelmaier P, Marti A, Hufner T, Partenheimer A, Krettek C: Less invasive stabilization of complex tibial plateau fractures: A biomechanical evaluation of a unilateral locked screw plate and double plating. *J Orthop Trauma* 2004;18(8):546-551.

15. Barei DP, Taitsman LA, Beingessner D, Dunbar RP, Nork SE: Open diaphyseal long bone fractures: A reduction method using devitalized or extruded osseous fragments. *J Orthop Trauma* 2007;21(8):574-578.

16. Eastman J, Tseng S, Lo E, Li CS, Yoo B, Lee M: Retropatellar technique for intramedullary nailing of proximal tibia fractures: A cadaveric assessment. *J Orthop Trauma* 2010;24(11):672-676.

17. Higgins TF, Klatt J, Bachus KN: Biomechanical analysis of bicondylar tibial plateau fixation: How does lateral locking plate fixation compare to dual plate fixation? *J Orthop Trauma* 2007;21(5): 301-306.

18. Eastman JG, Tseng SS, Lee MA, Yoo BJ: The retropatellar portal as an alternative site for tibial nail insertion: A cadaveric study. *J Orthop Trauma* 2010;24(11): 659-664.

19. Koval KJ, Sanders R, Borrelli J, Helfet D, DiPasquale T, Mast JW: Indirect reduction and percutaneous screw fixation of displaced tibial plateau fractures. *J Orthop Trauma* 1992;6(3):340-346.

20. Pichler W, Grechenig W, Tesch NP, Weinberg AM, Heidari N, Clement H: The risk of iatrogenic injury to the deep peroneal nerve in minimally invasive osteosynthesis of the tibia with the less invasive stabilisation system: A cadaver study. *J Bone Joint Surg Br* 2009; 91(3):385-387.

21. Dougherty PJ, Kim DG, Meisterling S, Wybo C, Yeni Y: Biomechanical comparison of bicortical versus unicortical screw placement of proximal tibia locking plates: A cadaveric model. *J Orthop Trauma* 2008;22(6):399-403.

22. Oh JK, Sahu D, Hwang JH, Cho JW, Oh CW: Technical pitfall while reducing the mismatch between LCP PLT and upper end tibia in proximal tibia fractures. *Arch Orthop Trauma Surg* 2010; 130(6):759-763.

23. Musahl V, Tarkin I, Kobbe P, Tzioupis C, Siska PA, Pape HC: New trends and techniques in open reduction and internal fixation of fractures of the tibial plateau. *J Bone Joint Surg Br* 2009; 91(4):426-433.

24. Gautier E, Sommer C: Guidelines for the clinical application of the LCP. *Injury* 2003;34(Suppl 2): B63-B76.

25. Marsh JL, Muehling V, Dirschl D, Hurwitz S, Brown TD, Nepola J: Tibial plafond fractures treated by articulated external fixation: A randomized trial of postoperative motion versus nonmotion. *J Orthop Trauma* 2006;20(8): 536-541.

26. Krettek C, Schandelmaier P, Tscherne H: Nonreamed interlocking nailing of closed tibial

fractures with severe soft tissue injury. *Clin Orthop Relat Res* 1995;315:34-47.

27. Bolhofner BR: Indirect reduction and composite fixation of extraarticular proximal tibial fractures. *Clin Orthop Relat Res* 1995;315:75-83.

28. Ricci WM, O'Boyle M, Borrelli J, Bellabarba C, Sanders R: Fractures of the proximal third of the tibial shaft treated with intramedullary nails and blocking screws. *J Orthop Trauma* 2001;15(4):264-270.

29. Nork SE, Barei DP, Schildhauer TA, et al: Intramedullary nailing of proximal quarter tibial fractures. *J Orthop Trauma* 2006;20(8):523-528.

30. Vidyadhara S, Sharath KR: Prospective study of the clinicoradiological outcome of interlocked nailing in proximal third tibial shaft fractures. *Injury* 2006;37(6):536-542.

31. Lindvall E, Sanders R, Dipasquale T, Herscovici D, Haidukewych G, Sagi C: Intramedullary nailing versus percutaneous locked plating of extra-articular proximal tibial fractures: Comparison of 56 cases. *J Orthop Trauma* 2009;23(7):485-492.

32. Nork SE, Schwartz AK, Agel J, Holt SK, Schrick JL, Winquist RA: Intramedullary nailing of distal metaphyseal tibial fractures. *J Bone Joint Surg Am* 2005;87(6):1213-1221.

33. Krettek C, Stephan C, Schandelmaier P, Richter M, Pape HC, Miclau T: The use of Poller screws as blocking screws in stabilising tibial fractures treated with small diameter intramedullary nails. *J Bone Joint Surg Br* 1999;81(6):963-968.

34. Buehler KC, Green J, Woll TS, Duwelius PJ: A technique for intramedullary nailing of proximal third tibia fractures. *J Orthop Trauma* 1997;11(3):218-223.

35. Freedman EL, Johnson EE: Radiographic analysis of tibial fracture malalignment following intramedullary nailing. *Clin Orthop Relat Res* 1995;315:25-33.

36. Lang GJ, Cohen BE, Bosse MJ, Kellam JF: Proximal third tibial shaft fractures: Should they be nailed? *Clin Orthop Relat Res* 1995;315:64-74.

37. Weninger P, Tschabitscher M, Traxler H, Pfafl V, Hertz H: Intramedullary nailing of proximal tibia fractures: An anatomical study comparing three lateral starting points for nail insertion. *Injury* 2010;41(2):220-225.

38. Henley MB, Meier M, Tencer AF: Influences of some design parameters on the biomechanics of the unreamed tibial intramedullary nail. *J Orthop Trauma* 1993;7(4):311-319.

39. Tornetta P III, Collins E: Semiextended position of intramedullary nailing of the proximal tibia. *Clin Orthop Relat Res* 1996;328:185-189.

40. Gelbke MK, Coombs D, Powell S, DiPasquale TG: Suprapatellar versus infra-patellar intramedullary nail insertion of the tibia: A cadaveric model for comparison of patellofemoral contact pressures and forces. *J Orthop Trauma* 2010;24(11):665-671.

41. Wysocki RW, Kapotas JS, Virkus WW: Intramedullary nailing of proximal and distal one-third tibial shaft fractures with intraoperative two-pin external fixation. *J Trauma* 2009;66(4):1135-1139.

42. Dunbar RP, Nork SE, Barei DP, Mills WJ: Provisional plating of type III open tibia fractures prior to intramedullary nailing. *J Orthop Trauma* 2005;19(6):412-414.

43. Shahulhameed A, Roberts CS, Ojike NI: Technique for precise placement of poller screws with intramedullary nailing of metaphyseal fractures of the femur and the tibia. *Injury* 2011;42(2):136-139.

44. Tang P, Gates C, Hawes J, Vogt M, Prayson MJ: Does open reduction increase the chance of infection during intramedullary nailing of closed tibial shaft fractures? *J Orthop Trauma* 2006;20(5):317-322.

45. Laflamme GY, Heimlich D, Stephen D, Kreder HJ, Whyne CM: Proximal tibial fracture stability with intramedullary nail fixation using oblique interlocking screws. *J Orthop Trauma* 2003;17(7):496-502.

46. Hansen M, Blum J, Mehler D, Hessmann MH, Rommens PM: Double or triple interlocking when nailing proximal tibial fractures? A biomechanical investigation. *Arch Orthop Trauma Surg* 2009;129(12):1715-1719.

47. Court-Brown CM, Gustilo T, Shaw AD: Knee pain after intramedullary tibial nailing: Its incidence, etiology, and outcome. *J Orthop Trauma* 1997;11(2):103-105.

48. Keating JF, Orfaly R, O'Brien PJ: Knee pain after tibial nailing. *J Orthop Trauma* 1997;11(1):10-13.

49. Toivanen JA, Väistö O, Kannus P, Latvala K, Honkonen SE, Järvinen MJ: Anterior knee pain after intramedullary nailing of fractures of the tibial shaft: A prospective, randomized study comparing two different nail-insertion techniques. *J Bone Joint Surg Am* 2002;84-A(4):580-585.

50. Karladani AH, Ericsson PA, Granhed H, Karlsson L, Nyberg P: Tibial intramedullary nails: Should they be removed? A retrospective study of 71 patients. *Acta Orthop* 2007;78(5):668-671.

51. Gaebler C, Berger U, Schandelmaier P, et al: Rates and odds ratios for complications in closed and open tibial fractures treated with unreamed, small diameter

tibial nails: A multicenter analysis of 467 cases. *J Orthop Trauma* 2001;15(6):415-423.

52. Bhandari M, Audige L, Ellis T, Hanson B; Evidence-Based Orthopaedic Trauma Working Group: Operative treatment of extra-articular proximal tibial fractures. *J Orthop Trauma* 2003; 17(8):591-595.

53. Cole PA, Zlowodzki M, Kregor PJ: Treatment of proximal tibia fractures using the less invasive stabilization system: Surgical experience and early clinical results in 77 fractures. *J Orthop Trauma* 2004;18(8):528-535.

54. Stannard JP, Wilson TC, Volgas DA, Alonso JE: The less invasive stabilization system in the treatment of complex fractures of the tibial plateau: Short-term results. *J Orthop Trauma* 2004;18(8): 552-558.

55. Ricci WM, Rudzki JR, Borrelli J Jr: Treatment of complex proximal tibia fractures with the less invasive skeletal stabilization system. *J Orthop Trauma* 2004; 18(8):521-527.

Staged Treatment and Associated Complications of Pilon Fractures

Frank A. Liporace, MD

Samir Mehta, MD

Anthony S. Rhorer, MD

Richard S. Yoon, MD

Mark C. Reilly, MD

Abstract

Historically, the treatment and outcomes related to pilon fractures have been variable despite anatomic reduction and fixation. Early results with treatment via early primary open reduction and internal fixation yielded mixed clinical outcomes, especially suboptimal complication rates, including infection, malunion, and nonunion. Treatment with external fixation also exhibited similar outcomes with mixed support reported in the literature. Despite continued controversy, the advent of newer implant technologies, improved surgical techniques, and management with a staged protocol have resulted in encouraging clinical outcomes with minimization of postoperative complications. Crucial decisions made during treatment can help to maximize outcomes while minimizing complication rates. Particular attention to the fracture pattern with radiographic guidance can help direct surgical decision making with appropriate care given to optimize soft-tissue status. A variety of available incisions can facilitate proper bony and articular reduction. During the late and failed stages of fracture management, additional treatment options include external ring fixation, arthrodesis, and arthroplasty. As complications arise, meticulous, prompt care can help to achieve the best possible outcomes.

Instr Course Lect 2012;61:53-70.

Named after its characteristic shape, the pilon or plafond fracture pattern is defined by intra-articular involvement of the distal tibia with metaphyseal extension.[1-3] Although pilon fractures account for only a small percentage of tibial and lower extremity injuries, more than 30% of pilon fractures are caused by high-energy injury mechanisms and are often associated with concomitant polytrauma with the presence of open wounds, degloving injuries, and severe soft-tissue trauma. These circumstances make injury management difficult.[4-9]

Historically, treatment involved early acute open reduction and internal fixation (ORIF), which led to dismal clinical outcomes and high complication rates[4,6,8,10-13] (**Table 1**). In

Dr. Liporace or an immediate family member is a member of a speakers' bureau or has made paid presentations on behalf of DePuy, Osteotech, Synthes, and Smith & Nephew; serves as a paid consultant to DePuy, Osteotech, Synthes, Smith & Nephew, and Stryker; serves as an unpaid consultant to AO North America; and has received research or institutional support from Synthes, Smith & Nephew, and Acumed. Dr. Mehta or an immediate family member is a member of a speakers' bureau or has made paid presentations on behalf of Zimmer, Smith & Nephew, and AO North America; serves as a paid consultant to Smith & Nephew and Synthes; has received research or institutional support from Amgen, Medtronic, and Smith & Nephew; and serves as a board member, owner, officer, or committee member of the Pennsylvania Orthopaedic Society. Dr. Rhorer or an immediate family member is a member of a speakers' bureau or has made paid presentations on behalf of Smith & Nephew; serves as a paid consultant to Smith & Nephew; has received research or institutional support from Smith & Nephew; and has received nonincome support (such as equipment or services), commercially derived honoraria, or other non–research-related funding (such as paid travel) from Synthes. Neither Dr. Yoon nor any immediate family member has received anything of value from or owns stock in a commercial company or institution related directly or indirectly to the subject of this chapter. Dr. Reilly or an immediate family member is a member of a speakers' bureau or has made paid presentations on behalf of Synthes, Smith & Nephew, and Stryker; and serves as a board member, owner, officer, or committee member of the AO Foundation.

Table 1

Summary Regarding Treatment and Complications for Pilon Fractures

Author (Year)	Management/Treatment	Number of Fractures	Reported Complications and Rates
Bourne et al[4] (1983)	Primary ORIF	42	Infection: 4.8% Nonunion/malunion: 33%
Teeny and Wiss[13] (1993)	Primary ORIF	60	Major complication: 50% (at least one of the following: skin slough, wound dehiscence, infection, nonunion, malunion, or implant failure)
Helfet et al[6] (1994)	Primary ORIF	34	Pin tract infection: 2.9% Deep infection: 5.9% Malunion: 8.8%
White et al[33] (2010)	Primary ORIF Within 48 hours: 98%	95	Wound dehiscence or deep infection: 6% Delayed or nonunion: 6%
Marsh et al[18] (1991)	External fixation (unilateral)	101	Reoperations: 5% Infection: 6% Loss of reduction during external fixation: 21% Malunion: 3%
Tornetta et al[19] (1993)	Limited internal fixation, hybrid external fixation	26	Superficial infection: 3.8% Deep infection: 3.8% Pin tract infection: 12% Malunion: 3.8%
Bone et al[16] (1993)	Delta-framed external fixation	20	Infection: 0% Delayed union/nonunion: 15% Malunion: 4.8%
Barbieri et al[15] (1996)	Hybrid external fixation	37	Skin slough: 2.7% Pin tract infection: 13.5% Deep infection: 8.1% Nonunion: 8.1% Loss of reduction during external fixation: 8.1%

Wyrsch et al[20] (1996)	Randomized controlled trial: primary ORIF versus external fixation (with and without limited internal fixation)	ORIF: 18
		External fixation: 20
			ORIF:
			  wound dehiscence/infection: 67%
			  amputation: 17%
			External fixation:
			  nerve injury: 5%
			  pin tract infection: 5%
			  deep infection: 5%
			  malunion: 5%

Anglen[14] (1999)	Comparative, ORIF versus hybrid external fixation (some soft-tissue optimization in both groups via temporizing external fixation)	ORIF: 19
		External fixation: 29
			ORIF:
			  amputation: 5.3%
			  skin slough: 5.3%
			  sensory deficit: 5.3%
			External fixation:
			  wire site infection: 24%
			  half-pin site infection: 10.3%
			  wound healing problems: 10.3%
			  tethered flexor tendon: 3.4%
			  nerve deficit: 3.4%
			  nonunion: 21%

Sirkin et al[67] (1999)	Staged protocol, soft-tissue optimization	Closed: 30
		Open: 19
			Closed:
			  partial-thickness skin necrosis: 17%
			  osteomyelitis: 3.4%
			Open:
			  wound dehiscence: 5.2%
			  osteomyelitis: 5.2%

Patterson and Cole[31] (1999)	Staged protocol, soft-tissue optimization	22	Infections/soft-tissue complications: 0% Malunion: 4% Nonunion: 4%
Grose et al[5] (2007)	Staged protocol, soft-tissue optimization, lateral approach study	44	Deep infection: 4.5% Wound dehiscence: 4.5% Nonunion: 9%
Boraiah et al[69] (2010)	Staged protocol, soft-tissue optimization	59 (all open)	Amputation: 1.7% Deep infection: 3% Superficial infection: 5%

ORIF = open reduction and internal fixation.

an effort to minimize soft-tissue complications, limited approaches and treatments involving external fixation resulted in minimal improvement and generated little enthusiasm.[13-21] However, with the implementation of a delayed, staged surgical treatment protocol, along with improvements in imaging, implant technology, and surgical technique, complication rates have decreased with a coinciding improvement in clinical and functional outcomes.[5,7,9,22-32] Although it has been suggested that early definitive ORIF can achieve results comparable to those of staged protocols, it should be stressed that definitive ORIF should be performed by experienced trauma surgeons and may not be appropriate in all cases.[33] Experts have indicated that a delay in definitive treatment is necessary for some patients.[33] In the late and failed stages of treatment, options become more limited as complications, including infections, malunions, and nonunions, become more prevalent and difficult to manage. At this juncture, external fixation, ankle arthrodesis, and ankle arthroplasty become more viable options.[34-46]

This chapter reviews the current state of the decision-making process, staging, and the choice of surgical options for the definitive treatment of pilon fractures and associated complications, especially in the late and failed stages of fracture management.

Imaging and Classification

Initial assessment and thorough preoperative planning begins with radiographic imaging. Analysis of the fracture pattern is performed with the three standard views of the ankle (AP, lateral, and mortise), along with centered, orthogonal views above and below the joint, which are needed because of the high rate of concomitant polytrauma in patients with pilon frac-

tures. Full-length tibia and fibula radiographs can provide information on general alignment.[2,4,9,10] In select patients, radiographs of the contralateral limb also can be helpful to provide a template for reconstruction for more complex pilon fractures and detect any preexisting anatomic or congenital variants that indicate a different "normal" baseline.

Theoretically, fracture classification systems are a tool for communication and providing information relative to treatment decisions and prognoses; however, to achieve those goals, the system must allow consistent, reliable, and reproducible classification of various fracture patterns. Rüedi and Allgöwer[12] offered the original foundation for pilon fracture classification, indicating three fracture types that increased in severity from low-energy, nondisplaced fractures of the tibia plafond to high-energy, severely comminuted and impacted articular fracture patterns. However, poor reliability and agreement have been reported.[47-49]

Based on plain radiographs alone, Martin et al[48] reported poor interobserver reliability of the Rüedi and Allgöwer classification system, with mean kappa values of 0.46 for all observers, 0.38 for more experienced observers, and 0.56 for less experienced observers. Similarly, Dirschl and Adams[47] reported a mean kappa value of 0.46, which indicated poor reliability. Removing the data from third-year residents resulted in a slight increase in the kappa value to 0.52.

Minimal improvements to classification agreement were observed with the development of the AO/Orthopaedic Trauma Association (OTA) classification system. Despite exhibiting higher reliability than the Rüedi and Allgöwer system, only moderate agreement between observers has been reported.[12,47,48,50] Regarding fracture type, group agreement, and

subgroup agreement, Swiontkowski et al[50] reported only modest values, with agreement occurring 57%, 43%, and 41% of the time, respectively. Despite the use of CT, Ramappa et al[49] reported similar reliability and agreement values for both the Rüedi and Allgöwer and AO/OTA classification systems.

Realizing the inherent difficulty in stratifying outcomes based on unreliable classification systems, DeCoster et al[51] developed a rank order method, classifying patients based on injury severity and reduction quality. The results exhibited 94% agreement in ranking the severity of the articular surface, 89% agreement in ranking the severity of the fracture pattern, 89% agreement in ranking the reduction considering only the articular surface, and 88% agreement in ranking the reduction when considering the entire fracture pattern.

Although orthopaedic surgeons might not agree on the specific classification of the pilon fracture pattern presented, there is reliably high agreement on assessing the severity of the injury and in determining the quality of a poor or good fracture reduction.

Decision Making in the Initial Period

Management in the immediate period following a pilon fracture should focus on expedited medical optimization and clearance and soft-tissue stabilization. Important considerations include the presence of an open wound and/or a vascular injury.[52,53] A history of diabetes or smoking also may be a crucial consideration in decision making and in avoiding potential wound complications.[11,33,54,55] In patients with primarily indirect ankle fractures and complicated diabetes (diabetes associated with end organ damage), Wukich et al[56] reported a 3.8 times increased risk of overall complications and a

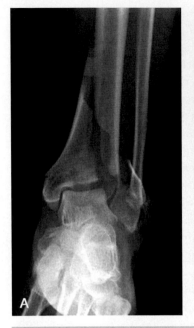
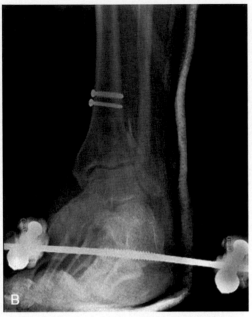

Figure 1 Preoperative (**A**) and postoperative (**B**) radiographs showing restoration of length, alignment, and rotation with ORIF to protect soft tissues, and simplify the pilon fracture for later definitive reconstruction.

5 times increased risk of revision surgery when compared with patients with ankle fractures and tightly controlled diabetes. A recent meta-analysis analyzing 6 randomized trials and 15 observational studies reported a significant decrease in total complications, wound complications, and pulmonary complications with prolonged smoking cessation.[55]

The amount of energy absorbed in the fracture is indicated by the degree of comminution, the Tscherne class of injury, and the presence of significant open wounds or a fibular fracture. The presence of a fibular fracture provides clues into the mechanism of injury and fracture pattern.[57] A fibular fracture typically is associated with higher energy injuries; however, if the injury is known to have been caused by a high-energy mechanism, the presence of the fracture contributes information on the direction of the mechanism (typically a valgus and an axial load).[57] Conversely, the absence of a fibular fracture or a tension failure of the fibula is associated with an injury pattern caused by a varus and an axial load.[57]

Following medical clearance and before definitive fixation, temporizing the extremity and restoring the mechanical axis, length, and alignment are pivotal to soft-tissue stabilization. Dunbar et al[58] described a technique that offered early, limited ORIF for AO/OTA type C fractures that typically present with a long, oblique metadiaphyseal spike. The authors presented data to suggest that early, limited restoration of length, alignment, and rotation with ORIF of the oblique fracture spike not only provides soft-tissue protection but also helps to simplify later definitive reconstruction without an increase in wound breakdown or complications (**Figure 1**).

It has been popularized that acute fibular fixation provides safe restoration of length in the initial period without an increased risk of complications.[7,53] However, preoperative planning, including determination of the "workhorse" surgical incision is of paramount importance, especially when considering additional incisions with an appropriate skin bridge.[7,33,59] Many surgeons have recommended a minimum 7-cm skin bridge to minimize soft-tissue and wound complications.[45,60,61] However, in a recent prospective study using at least two skin incisions with an average width of 5.9 cm, Howard et al[59] reported a low rate of soft-tissue complications in 42 patients with 46 pilon fractures. In essence, the "workhorse" incision is the main distal tibial incision that will allow definitive ORIF, even if smaller ancillary incisions are used.[7] However, it is important to understand that the ratio of the length of the incision to the width of the skin bridge is directly related to the soft-tissue complication rate.[7]

If the surgeon is unsure of the length of the "workhorse" incision or is not providing definitive treatment, it may be prudent to defer fibular fixation until an external fixator has been placed to restore the general mechanical axis and length and obtain a CT scan. In such instances, the application of a simple joint-spanning external fixator can achieve the initial goals and decrease the initial surgical time (**Figure 2**). This chapter's authors typically use a delta frame construct with two 5.0-mm pins in the tibial shaft placed out of the zone of injury and a 6.0-mm calcaneal transfixation pin in the posterior tuberosity of the calcaneus. Posterior splint supplementation or supplementary 4.0-mm metatarsal pins attached to the main delta frame can be used to maintain a plantigrade foot and avoid anteriorly prominent metaphyseal spikes of bone, which may cause deep soft-tissue pressure while waiting for definitive internal fixation.[7,13,15,16,18,19,61]

Knowledge gained during the past five decades makes it compelling to

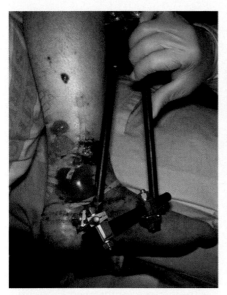

Figure 2 A spanning external fixator can help achieve the initial goals of restoring the mechanical axis and length and stabilizing the bone as the soft-tissue swelling subsides.

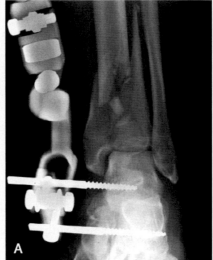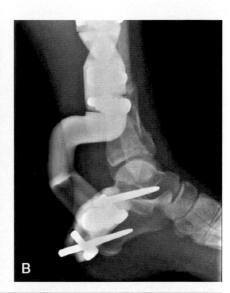

Figure 3 AP (**A**) and lateral (**B**) radiographic views of a pilon fracture after external fixation.

consider using multiple small incisions and staging definitive fixation procedures from the time of the initial external fixator application. This may require more than two total procedures based on the experience of this chapter's authors and is relative to the quality of the soft tissue. This may be the best method to decrease complications and potentially improve outcomes for patients with these injuries.

The anatomic placement of fixator pins is paramount. Proximally, pin placement should be just distal to the tibial tubercle to avoid the proximal metadiaphyseal extent of the zone of injury, which will require surgical manipulation at the time of the definitive procedure. Distally, pin placement may be transcalcaneal to construct a delta frame or medially through the talar neck and the medial calcaneus (**Figure 3**). The lateral plantar nerve, the most posterior lateral plantar nerve, and the medial calcaneal nerve should be avoided during transcalcaneal external fixator pin placement.[62] When

considering medially based external fixators, close monitoring of the status of the medial talar neck pin is needed because infection in this pin may cause contamination within close proximity to the distal tibial incisions or the ankle joint.

Decision Making for Surgical Timing

It had been suggested that definitive surgical management within 6 hours of injury can be safe. However, on re-evaluation and in the setting of high-energy injury mechanisms, ORIF undertaken in the acute period has yielded suboptimal results with high complication rates and poor clinical outcomes.[4,10-13,61] It has been shown that the risks of soft-tissue impairment caused by inflammatory processes is highest for up to 6 days after injury.[63]

Proponents of definitive external fixator constructs have cited slight improvements.[14-16,20] In a prospective, randomized study comparing external fixation to ORIF, Wyrsch et al[20] reported superior results in the cohort treated with external fixation; however, the ORIF cohort was operated on within 3 to 5 days of injury, whereas

the external fixator cohort with limited open fixation was definitively treated more than 7 days after injury.[20] The importance of soft-tissue management has been emphasized.[64,65] The Tscherne soft-tissue classification system offers graded indicators of severe soft-tissue damage ranging from minimal superficial abrasions and degloving injuries to deep muscular and subcutaneous fat contusions, vascular injury, and compartment syndrome.[64] Despite determining two safe surgical windows—an early period within 6 hours after injury and a late period between 6 and 12 days after injury—surgery during this high risk period still exhibited consistently high complication rates and subpar clinical results.[13,20,64-66]

Staged management protocols have yielded improved results, with lower complication rates and improved clinical outcomes.[5,7,30,67] Sirkin et al,[7] using a staged protocol that consisted of acute external fixation and delayed definitive reconstruction, placed particular focus on soft-tissue optimization. The authors waited from 7 to 14 days for edema to subside, as indicated by subsidence with the presence of skin wrinkling.[7] Applying this staged protocol on the management of 56 pilon fractures, the authors reported two deep infections and the healing of all surgical wounds, which represented complication rates significantly lower than those of previous reports.[7,13,20]

The presence of blisters, which occur at a relatively high rate in pilon fractures, offer clues to the timing of definitive management.[20,68] In patients with blood-filled blisters, which indicate a complete separation of the dermis from the epidermis, Giordano and Koval[68] recommended waiting for full reepithelialization before surgical intervention. Resolution of edema is often indicated by the absence of shiny skin, with normal skin creases or wrinkles predominately exposed. Staging treatment and waiting for soft-tissue optimization has achieved favorable results in a more recent study that evaluated ORIF in open 59 pilon fractures.[69] Boraiah et al[69] reported excellent clinical outcomes at a minimum 2-year follow-up with 88% union and 9% delayed union, with only three deep infections, two superficial infections, and one amputation after a failed free-flap transfer.

Despite the success of the staged protocol, some surgeons remain proponents for early ORIF. White et al[33] performed ORIF within 48 hours in 95 patients with tibial pilon fractures and reported good clinical outcomes at 1-year follow-up. The authors reported an overall 19% complication rate in open and closed type C fractures and excluded fractures with "local soft-tissue factors" that were not specifically defined. In closed fractures, the complication rate was only 2.7%. Of note, the authors stress that the procedure must be done in "the right setting" and that all the resources must be available. They advise that early ORIF should not be done if resources are not available or if the patients present late or beyond an early treatment window. The authors suggest that medical judgment is needed.[33] It is important to note that the study included only patients who were deemed appropriate for the procedure; no guidance was provided on the criteria used to select suitable patients.

When planning for definitive fixation, CT is an invaluable tool. To best define the articular fragments and the definitive surgical approaches that may be required, this chapter's authors recommend that a CT scan should be obtained after external fixation is used to restore the length and mechanical axis of the extremity. Acquiring appropriate length with temporizing external fixation will disimpact the talus from the distal tibia and allow for better visualization of the articular injury.

Information on the specific areas of articular involvement, comminution, and impaction not seen on plain radiographs can be seen on CT scans[32] (**Figure 4,** A and B). Tornetta and Gorup[32] studied the impact of CT on the management of pilon fractures and reported that information from CT changed management decisions in 64% of the patients. The operating surgeons reported that information derived from the CTs bettered their understanding of the fracture pattern in 82% of patients and shortened the surgical time in 77% of patients.[32] Analysis of the surrounding soft tissues via soft-tissue windows on the CT scans also can provide valuable information, such as potentially entrapped tendinous or neurovascular structures (**Figure 4,** C and D).

Decision Making for Definitive Management

Over the past 40 to 50 years, the original principles set forth by Rüedi and Allgöwer[12] concerning pilon fracture management and reconstruction have not drastically changed.[70] The treatment algorithm, which emphasizes restoration of length with fibular reconstruction, reconstruction of the metaphyseal shell and articular joint, bone grafting, and a medial buttress to stabilize the metaphysis to the diaphysis reconstruction, still applies. Some advances in surgical approach options and implant technology have helped surgeons achieve those goals.[5,22,24,26-29,58,71]

Standard Approach

The standard approach to the tibial plafond is described as a two-incision technique—an anteromedial incision for the tibia and a posterolateral incision for the fibula.[12,70,72] However, depending on preoperative planning with CT identification of the major fracture fragments and lines and remembering to use an adequate skin bridge, additional surgical approaches can be used to maximize exposure and address specific articular issues.[7,27-29,32,59]

Anterior Approaches

Anterior approaches to the tibial plafond are based on the principle of reconstruction from posterior to anterior after "opening the book."[71-73] Use of the posterolateral (Volkmann) fragment as the "constant fragment" often relies on the assumption that the fibula was anatomically and stably reduced in terms of alignment, length, and rotation.[2,73] Each anterior approach (anteromedial, anterolateral, and direct anterior) has unique advantages and disadvantages.

With any of the anterior approaches, an external fixator or femoral distractor can be helpful to aid in evaluating and reducing articular fragments (**Figure 5**). It should be remembered that relative to the midsagittal plane of the tibia, the position of the transcalcaneal pin in a delta frame can

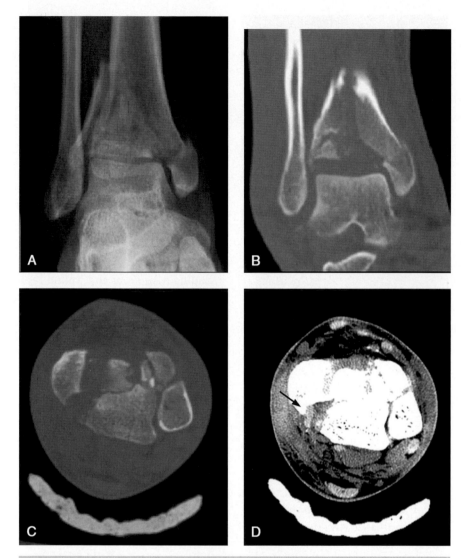

Figure 4 Surgical planning can be enhanced as degrees of comminution, impaction, or displacement not seen on a plain radiograph (**A**) can be seen on a CT scan (**B**). Bone windows (**C**) may be enhanced with soft-tissue windows (**D**), which may reveal entrapped tendinous or neurovascular structures such as the posterior tibialis tendon and flexor digitorum longus tendon (arrow).

cause a dorsiflexion moment of the foot with significant attempted distraction. This can inhibit direct visualization of the joint when there is significant anterior or central comminution. When the femoral distractor is applied with a pin in the talar neck and a pin in the tibia, a plantar flexion moment will yield excellent visualization of the joint; however, after the articular surface is stabilized, excessive distraction must be removed to allow appropriate reduction of the metadiaphyseal component that may have been deformed in the sagittal plane with the distractor. When applying the distractor, care must be taken to have the talar neck pin parallel to the superior dome of the talus to avoid "dialing-in" a coronal plane deformity.

Anteromedial Approach
The classic anteromedial approach described by Tile is typically used for AO/OTA type 43B and C fractures.[6,61,70,72,73] Starting approxi-mately 5 cm proximal to the tibiotalar joint line and just lateral to the tibial crest, the anteromedial incision can extend distally to form around the medial malleolus or continue distally with the tibialis anterior tendon toward the talonavicular joint.[2,73,74] Care must be taken to avoid violating the tibialis anterior tendon sheath because, unlike the tendon itself, it will readily accept grafts (especially in the case of wound dehiscence).[75] Preservation of the periosteum in an already vascularly tenuous area is a high priority. Although this incision offers good access for medial and anterior hardware application, it does not allow ready access to the anterolateral (Tillaux-Chaput) fragment[71,73] (**Figure 6**).

Anterolateral Approach
The Böhler anterolateral approach to the tibial plafond allows direct access to the Tillaux-Chaput fragment left by the anteromedial approach.[22,27] Depending on concomitant foot and ankle injuries, the approach can be extended to provide direct visualization of the anterior talar dome and talar neck and lateral talonavicular, subtalar, and calcaneocuboid joints.[27] The incision is in line with the fourth metatarsal when the foot is in neutral dorsiflexion, and it starts 5 cm proximal to the tibiotalar joint.[27] Identifying and protecting the superficial peroneal nerve branches are imperative.[27] The origin of the extensor digitorum brevis is divided, reflecting it distally. The dorsalis pedis and the deep peroneal nerve are reflected medially, and the capsule is incised to provide access to the ankle joint. Herscovici et al[27] described this incision, noting that, if needed, the incision could be extended in both the proximal and distal directions with maintenance of straightforward closure and without an increase in wound complications. Although some surgeons have criticized the

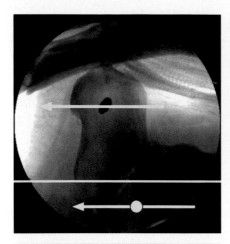

Figure 5 With an anterior approach, a femoral distractor or an external fixator can assist in achieving length and visualization. However, important consideration must be paid to the potential plantar flexion moments (right arrow) or dorsiflexion moments (left arrow) when manipulating along the midsagittal axis (central line).

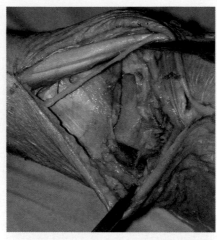

Figure 6 The anteromedial incision offers access for medial and anterior hardware application, but does not allow ready access to the anterolateral (Tillaux-Chaput) fragment.

approach because of a lack of access to posterior fracture elements, Mehta et al[30] described successful total articular reconstruction with a bony distractor, headlamp, and intraoperative imaging via the anterolateral and a second more medially based incision. Grose et al,[5] using an alternative extensile approach from the lateral plafond and crossing medially to reach the anterior, reported good results and low complication rates, especially regarding deep infection (4.5%) and wound dehiscence (4.5%).

Direct Anterior Approach

The direct anterior approach can provide access to both the anteromedial and anterolateral fragments of a pilon fracture with a straightforward linear incision centered over the tibiotalar joint. The approach is centered between the malleoli, with protection of the superficial peroneal nerve. The incision is developed between the extensor digitorum longus (EDL) and extensor hallucis longus (EHL), with

protection of the deep neurovascular bundle using medial retraction. Traditionally used for ankle arthrodesis, the direct anterior approach can be used to treat pilon fractures and, if necessary, for future fusion (**Figure 7**). In a recent retrospective review of 49 pilon fractures, McCann et al[76] reported low complication rates with minimal soft-tissue disturbance with the direct anterior approach.

Posterior Approaches

Posterior approaches to the pilon are used in select situations when the goals cannot be accomplished using the anterior approaches. Of note, direct articular reduction is not possible and relies on cortical reduction and fluoroscopic assistance.[29,65,77] Benefits of the posterolateral incision are its use in rebuilding the constant fragment, especially if it has significant impaction and/or rotation[2,29,73] (**Figure 8**). Rebuilding the constant fragment also can convert a C-type fracture to a B-type fracture. The surgeon can use an anterior approach to rebuild the plafond from posterior to anterior.[58] Attention must be given to correcting

the sagittal plane deformity of articular fragments because direct joint visualization is not possible with the posterior approach; the surgeon must rely on fluoroscopic and direct cortical readings.

Posterolateral Approach

The posterolateral approach, which exploits the interval between the lateral and the posterior compartment musculature, was believed to offer a lower complication rate;[2,29,73] however, Bhattacharyya et al[77] noted a high complication rate with this approach, including nonunions and wound healing problems leading to fusions and suboptimal clinical outcomes. Of note, the authors attempted complete fixation tibial pilon fractures through the one surgical approach.[77] When required, the posterolateral tibia can be addressed between the peroneus longus and the flexor hallucis longus, while the fibula can be addressed posteriorly by going anterior to the peroneus brevis.

Posteromedial Approach

The posteromedial approach is helpful when treating tendon or neurovascular bundle entrapment.[28] The incision is made at the midpoint between the medial malleolus and the posteromedial aspect of the Achilles tendon. Identification of the tendinous and neurovascular structures is paramount to allow safe development of intervals based on the fracture pattern. Using both a posteromedial and a posterolateral approach on the same patient should be done with caution because of the relative proximity of the approaches and the need for extensive deep surgical dissection. Typically, most of the posterior aspect of the distal tibia can be addressed through either approach; the area requiring more direct manipulation should be chosen. In select situations when a small window is required

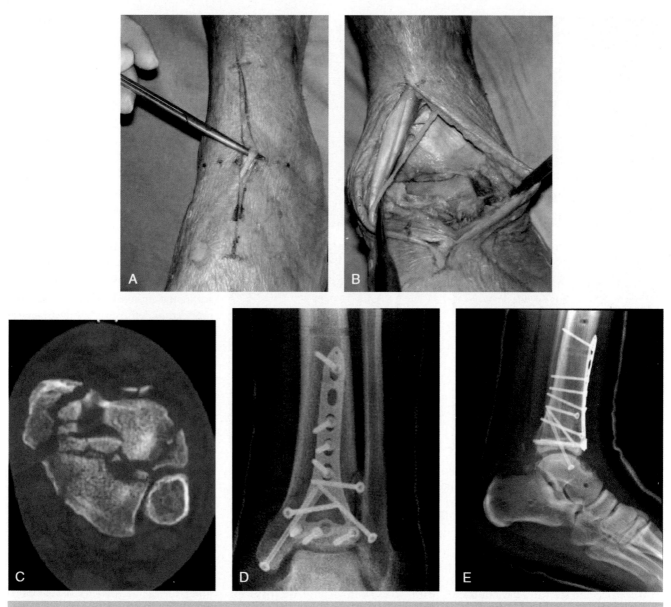

Figure 7   The direct anterior approach can be used to treat pilon fractures. **A,** An incision should be made at the center of the mortise, providing access to the anteromedial and anterolateral aspects of the joint. The branches of the superficial peroneal nerve should be avoided, and the extensor retinaculum should be incised. **B,** Intervals include the EHL/tibialis anterior, EHL/EDL, and the EDL/peroneus tertius. Note that proximal to the tibiotalar joint, the neurovascular bundle lies between EHL/tibialis anterior but distal to the tibiotalar joint. The bundle lies between the EHL and the EDL. The anterior ankle capsule and the intra-articular fat is excised to expose the joint. **C,** At times, the fracture pattern and location can dictate the use of a direct anterior approach. AP (**D**) and lateral (**E**) radiographs of definitive ORIF via a direct anterior approach. Using the direct anterior approach can help facilitate future ankle fusion if needed.

for the placement of a reduction aid, the use of both approaches can be considered.

Discussion

The multitude of surgical approaches and advancements in small fragment, mini-fragment, and bioabsorbable fix-ation have provided improvements in specifically treating articular fragments in previously unreconstructable fractures.[22-25,28,29,53,78] Locking-plate constructs may obviate the need for bone grafting in select patients and provide added stability in patients with comminuted fractures or osteoporo-sis.[2] Such fixed-angle constructs can help decrease the number of plates required based on the fracture pattern and comminution while providing adequate stability to allow for protracted healing.

Future implant modifications may further improve the clinical results.

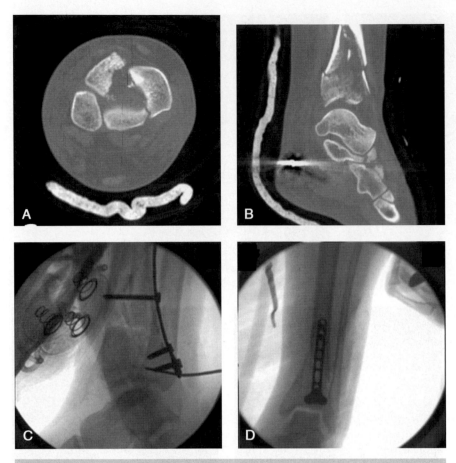

Figure 8 **A** and **B,** The posterolateral incision allows for reconstruction of the constant fragment, especially if it has significant impaction and/or rotation. Derotation (**C**) and rebuilding (**D**) of the constant fragment with limited fixation can act as a bridge to staged anterior ORIF.

The role of intramedullary nailing (IMN) for pilon fractures has not been extensively studied. In a study of the results of IMN for distal tibial fractures, Vallier et al[79] found complication and union rates comparable to plating. When considering limited ORIF with IMN for fixation of fractures of the plafond, careful study of the CT scan and understanding the fracture is imperative. Stable articular reduction and independent screw fixation are required, while leaving access for appropriate placement of an IMN. This technique is recommended only for simple articular fractures without impaction when performed by an experienced surgeon. The metaphyseal defects should be addressed primarily with bone graft to limit the risks for nonunion.[40,80] However, in select patients with "unreconstructable" pilon fractures, severe soft-tissue injuries, or significant comorbidities precluding safe direct fixation, external ring fixation can be considered.

External Ring Fixation

The application of external ring fixation for pilon fractures requires careful patient selection, extensive knowledge of fixation constructs, familiarity with the ring fixation system being used, comprehensive knowledge of the cross-sectional anatomy, and diligent postoperative maintenance.[41] External ring fixation can serve as a limb-salvage technique in scenarios where extensive internal fixation is not an option and thus should be used judiciously.[34,81]

External ring fixation for pilon fractures is indicated if the patient is not amenable to standard stable internal fixation or in the setting of combined limited ORIF.[46,81,82] Ring fixation is best suited to patients with severe soft-tissue injuries who are not candidates for plastic reconstructive surgery, such as free vascularized muscle transfers or rotational flaps. Ring fixation is also an excellent modality for late reconstruction and salvage of pilon fractures with segmental bone loss, infection, and preexisting deformity.[83] Advantages of ring fixation in pilon fracture management include earlier weight bearing, the ability to make postoperative frame adjustments, better soft-tissue management, and no complications relating to retained hardware.[84]

Many parts and components must be assembled to build a stable construct. Pilon fracture frames will typically consist of two rings. The proximal ring should always be placed above the zone of injury, which can be in the proximal third of the tibia. This ring can be stabilized to bone with bicortical half pins or fine wires. The entire inner surface of the ring should be at least 3 cm from any skin or soft tissue to allow adequate expansion after swelling. Half-pin and thin wire placement techniques are of utmost importance. Improperly placed pins and wires will result in loosening, soft-tissue infection, and potentially even osteomyelitis. A small stab incision large enough to allow placement of the drill tip, followed by careful drilling of both cortices of bone is imperative. Bone should not be drilled so aggressively as to allow smoke or burnt bone. Irrigation and cleaning of the drill flutes should be done frequently to prevent necrosis of the bone around the edge of the hole. Once the proximal ring has been fastened to the half pins, the distal ring may be applied around the fracture. The metaphyseal bone is often not amenable to half-pin fixation secondary to comminution and bone destruction. The distal segments therefore are held by thin wires at an optimal 60° angle from one another. If internal fixation of the joint is not used, the articular surface can be reduced and stabilized with olive wires. The olive wires are tensioned from one side and create a vector of force that compresses the bone fragments together (**Figure 9**). Similarly, olive wires and smooth wires can be used to suspend the metaphyseal bone and the joint surface under the diaphysis in the correct anatomic and mechanical axis.

Regardless of the decision to fix the joint either with minimal internal fixation or with wires alone, it is always necessary to perform an open reduction of the joint with the goal of anatomic reduction. In cases where there is severe comminution of the joint and metaphysis and fixation with thin wires is tenuous, the application of a foot plate can be helpful. The foot plate is connected to the distal ring, and the hind foot and forefoot are connected to the foot plate using thin wires and olive wires. The foot should be held in a plantar-flexed position, especially during application of the forefoot wires.

Many ring fixation systems offer 0.5 rings and 0.625 rings that can be used to afford access to soft tissue and allow movement of the ankle joint. For example, a 0.625 ring can be placed with the open portion over the dorsum of the foot, thus allowing the patient to dorsiflex the ankle without impinging on the ring. Similarly, a ring opening can be oriented to allow access to a suture line, a traumatic wound, or a muscle flap.

Delicate, meticulous management

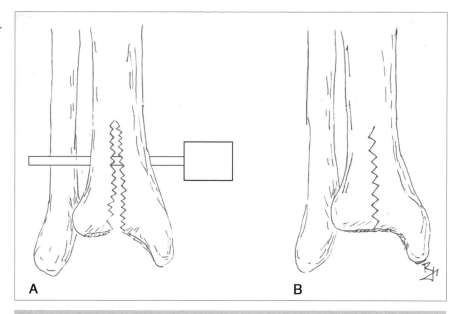

Figure 9   **A,** Olive wires can be tensioned from one side using a tensioner (shown as box) to create a vector to assist in bone compression. **B,** The bone after compression.

in the postoperative period following ring fixation is crucial to a successful outcome. Compressive dressings are applied, and the patient is kept on bed rest for 48 hours, with strict elevation of the extremity. Intravenous antibiotics should continue for 24 hours postoperatively, and appropriate thromboembolic prophylaxis should be used. On postoperative day 2, pin care should begin. Daily showering of the external fixator with soap and water followed by scrubbing the pin sites with povidone iodine or chlorhexidine is safe and effective. Hydrogen peroxide is not recommended for pin care. Weight bearing in the frame should take place only after there is radiographic evidence of union of the articular fracture, which can occur as early as 8 weeks. Close follow-up in the first 6 to 12 weeks is necessary to prevent pin tract infections and noncompliance with frame maintenance.

Initially, radiographs should be made every 2 to 4 weeks to ensure that there is no loss of reduction or migration of wires through comminuted

bone. To prevent loss of a pin or a wire, pin tract infections should be treated with oral antibiotics, with coverage for staphylococcus, and monitored closely. In infections that are recalcitrant to oral antibiotics, pins and wires should be removed to prevent the development of osteomyelitis. If a frame is needed for more than 3 months, at least one pin or wire should be removed during the course of treatment. Despite the scarcity of data, with meticulous care and proper management, external ring fixation can provide a viable treatment option in the setting of salvage, a pilon fracture with severe soft-tissue injury, or in the late or failed stages of definitive fracture management.

Decision Making for Managing Complications

There are many potential complications resulting from the surgical treatment of tibial pilon fractures.[45,85] Early complications of the definitive management of pilon fractures include surgical wound dehiscence, postoperative infection, malreduction, and loss of fixation.[45] Late complications include chronic infection, nonunion, malunion, and posttraumatic arthritis.[45] Infection is potentially the most devastating complication.[86]

In the early postoperative period, the most common wound complication is superficial surgical wound necrosis without dehiscence.[45,87] This condition can be treated with standard local wound care and soft-tissue rest with temporary splint or cast immobilization. If associated with wound erythema, there may be a role for systemic oral antibiotics. Wound culture of the partial thickness skin slough is not generally indicated and will likely result in only normal skin flora being isolated. Close observation of the wound is required to expeditiously identify a deep wound infection.[86]

If a surgical wound dehiscence is identified, the patient should be treated with urgent surgical débridement.[86] The tenuous soft-tissue envelope surrounding the distal tibia often makes reclosure of the surgical wound unlikely. The wound should be cleansed, deep cultures taken, and the stability of the fracture implants assessed. Although grossly loose and incompetent implants should be removed, bone stability is critical to controlling the integrity of the soft tissues, and competent hardware should be retained. There may be a role for negative-pressure wound management if the surgical wound cannot be fully approximated.[45]

Deep wound infection also requires surgical treatment, frequently with serial irrigation and débridement procedures performed every 48 to 72 hours until no further purulence is identified and no devitalized or necrotic tissue is present.[45,87] Negative-pressure wound management or local antibiotic therapy with impregnated polymethyl methacrylate beads is used in combination with systemic antibiotic therapy based on the findings from the wound cultures. Typically, systemic antibiotics are given for 6 weeks, followed by serial erythrocyte sedimentation rate and C-reactive protein analyses to guide the appropriate duration of the therapy. Definitive soft-tissue management with rotational or free-tissue transfer may be needed; a surgeon familiar with such procedures should be consulted early in the treatment process to appropriately coordinate the reconstruction.[88]

Late or chronic infections after pilon fracture surgery are generally associated with osteomyelitis and contaminated surgical implants.[45] The implants usually cannot be retained if successful sterilization of the bone is to be achieved. All devitalized and necrotic bone should be removed. Cortical saucerization with a high-speed burr should be performed, and a thorough bony débridement may require reaming of the intramedullary canal. Large bony defects may be filled with an antibiotic-impregnated cement spacer.[45,87] In rare instances of gross osseous instability, hardware may be exchanged or retained; removal of the hardware with spanning external fixation also can be considered until the infection has subsided and definitive internal fixation can be reapplied.

Malunions or nonunions after pilon fracture surgery may pose complex reconstructive problems.[86,89] The deformity must be characterized and understood. Is the deformity extra-articular or intra-articular? What is the sagittal and coronal alignment? Is there a rotational malalignment? What is the relationship of the tibial articular surface to that of the distal fibula? What is the degree of axial shortening? It is also important to evaluate the soft-tissue status around the distal tibia, and it is critical to assess the viability (salvageability) of the joint. Often, the articular surface of the pilon fracture has united, and the nonunion or malunion is largely extra-articular. If the articular surface is reasonably well aligned, an extra-articular correction of the deformity or nonunion may be performed. The choice of correcting such a deformity in a single stage or by gradual correction will be determined by the integrity of the soft tissues and their tolerance to surgical intervention. The selection of nail fixation, plate fixation, or external fixation should be made with consideration of the distance of the deformity from the articular surface, the viability of the bone at the nonunion/malunion site, the patency of the medullary canal, and the effect on the bone of prior implants and surgeries. Resultant bone defects after the correction of the deformity may require treatment with morcellized or structural bone grafts. Large complex deformities, particularly in compromised soft tissues, may be best treated with gradual correction and distraction osteogenesis.

The treatment of intra-articular malunion or nonunion requires a careful assessment of the viability of the ankle joint. Well-positioned radiographs and CT are used to assess the congruence of the joint surfaces and the degree of union between fracture fragments. MRI may be used to assess the degree of articular damage and chondral injury but is less useful when there is retained hardware from a prior fracture or nonunion surgery. Staging arthroscopy may be used to evaluate the chondral surface in circumstances where other diagnostic imaging studies have failed to provide sufficient information for surgical planning and decision making. Joint mobility and the degree of soft-tissue contracture around the ankle must be carefully assessed. Correction of bony deformity without soft-tissue balancing is likely to lead to a poor outcome. Achilles tendon lengthening and the release of joint contractures may be done either as part of the surgical approach or as a separate part of the procedure. In difficult situations, bony union may have to be achieved first and a secondary subsequent soft-tissue surgery performed later; however, the treatment of both components simultaneously is generally preferred.[45,90]

In general, the treatment of intra-articular nonunion or malunions after pilon fracture is generally reserved for partial articular fractures[76] (**Figure 10**). The correction of a complete articular nonunion, while possible, is generally exceedingly difficult because the vascularity of each articular fragment must be maintained during the osteotomy, realignment, and fixation. Partial articular nonunions or malunions require osteotomy and mobilization of the displaced articular fragment and reduction of the articular surface (**Figure 11, **A*). There may be resultant gaps in the articular reconstruction, but the goal is to provide a congruent joint surface with as minimal a residual irregularity as possible (**Figure 11, **B* and *C*). Stable interfragmentary compressive fixation is required and is often supplemented by buttress plate fixation (**Figure 12**). Intercalary allograft or tricortical autograft may be necessary if stable

fixation cannot be achieved by compression alone.

The most common long-term complication after a tibial pilon fracture is posttraumatic arthritis.[45,85] Radiographic findings of posttraumatic arthritis may not always correlate with the patient's symptoms or reported disability. The initial management of the

symptomatic patient should include nonsteroidal anti-inflammatory drugs, shoe wear modification, or activity modification. A heel lift may provide some initial relief to the patient with limited dorsiflexion caused by anterior tibiotalar osteophyte formation. A rocker-bottom sole or an Arizona brace may provide symptomatic relief

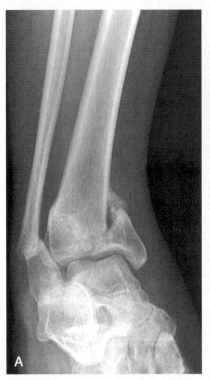
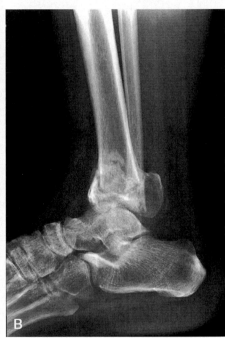

Figure 10   AP (**A**) and lateral (**B**) radiographs of a pilon fracture malunion 7 months after the initial injury.

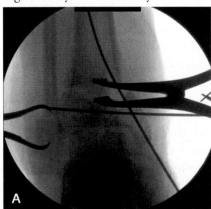
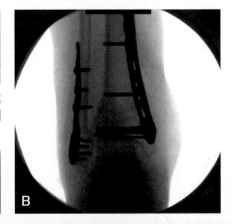
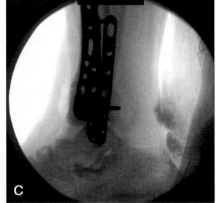

Figure 11   **A,** Intraoperative fluoroscopic view of the restoration of alignment and the articular joint surface. AP (**B**) and lateral (**C**) intraoperative views of definitive ORIF.

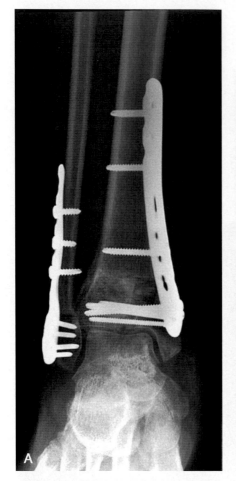

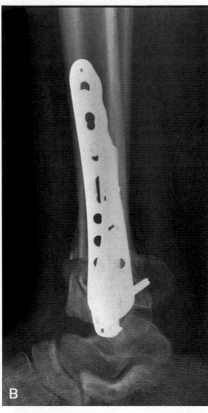

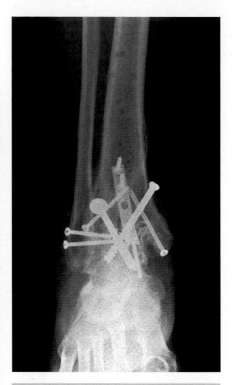

Figure 12 AP (**A**) and lateral (**B**) radiographs of a pilon fracture at 3-month follow-up with corrected and articular alignment.

Figure 13 AP radiograph following ankle arthrodesis for posttraumatic arthritis 2 years after definitive ORIF for a pilon fracture.

for the relatively stiff, painful ankle. Intra-articular steroid injections may provide temporary symptomatic relief but are typically used sparingly. Arthroscopy generally plays a role only in the patient with symptomatic impingement; the resection of anterior osteophytes may temporarily relieve symptoms and improve ambulation.[45] The long-term results are uncertain. Although distraction arthroplasty with or without fascial interposition has been advocated, there are no large series reporting long-term relief of symptoms with this technique.[45]

The most reliable treatment of end-stage posttraumatic ankle arthritis is arthrodesis[35,36,38,39,91] (**Figure 13**). This is generally performed as an open

procedure because of the presence of previously placed fracture hardware. Retained implants are generally removed, erosions or subchondral cysts are grafted, and the deformity is corrected to establish proper position for foot placement. Generally, the recommended position for arthrodesis is with a plantigrade foot, slight hindfoot valgus, external rotation equivalent to the patient's contralateral limb, and a translation of the talus posteriorly under the plafond to improve gait mechanics. Motion in the subtalar joint and midtarsal joints should be preserved if possible, and a careful assessment of arthritic changes, particularly in the subtalar joint, should be performed. Selective injection of the sub-

talar joint as a diagnostic procedure may help the surgeon determine whether radiographic changes in the subtalar joint are sufficiently symptomatic to warrant treatment at the time of ankle arthrodesis. In posttraumatic situations, the surgical approach and the technique for arthrodesis is generally determined on the basis of prior incisions, the compromise of soft-tissue flaps, the location of previously placed implants, and any residual deformity.[39] The presence of infection and osteonecrotic bone may necessitate a staged procedure with removal of the implants, débridement, and placement of an antibiotic spacer followed by second-stage definitive arthrodesis.[35] Arthrodesis in the presence of significant deformity may require acute shortening to avoid soft-tissue coverage. Subsequent limb lengthening may be performed if the resultant limb-length inequality is unacceptable to the patient. Alternatively, gradual deformity correction may be combined with the arthrodesis and limb lengthening with of the use of multiplanar external fixation and distraction osteogenesis.[92,93]

Short- and intermediate-term outcomes are generally good after arthrodesis, with patients reporting a significant reduction in pain and improvement in gait; however, the development of symptomatic degenerative arthritis in the subtalar, transverse tarsal, and midtarsal joints may be reported with long-term follow-up.[36,39] Patients almost universally report functional limitations secondary to pain.[35,36,39,91]

Ankle arthroplasty is another option for the treatment of symptomatic posttraumatic ankle arthritis.[37,43,44] It is generally reserved for patients with minimal deformity, a healthy soft-tissue envelope, and no history of prior infection.[94] Vascularized bone, a healed fracture, and minimal residual implant defects are considered prerequisites for this procedure.[94] Many surgeons recommend a staged treatment protocol for these injuries, with initial removal of the hardware, a biopsy to rule out infection, and an assessment of bone viability followed by a second-stage definitive arthroplasty. The results of total ankle arthroplasty for posttraumatic arthritis are generally inferior to those of arthrodesis.[44] In most studies, an increased incidence of major complications is generally reported after arthroplasty, and satisfaction is equivalent to that after arthrodesis.[43] The major reoperation rate for complications after the procedures is substantially higher after arthroplasty, although the need for subtalar arthrodesis has been reported to be lower.[44] At the present time, most authors generally do not recommend total ankle arthroplasty over arthrodesis for posttraumatic ankle arthritis after a

pilon fracture. It is hoped that continued improvements in implant design and longevity will lead to improved outcomes and expanded indications for the procedure.

Ankle arthrodesis remains the mainstay of treatment of the failed pilon fracture. Osteotomy and joint salvage of the nonunited or malunited fracture is an uncommon situation and is generally reserved for partial articular injuries or those in which the articular surface has united in a reasonable position. The role of arthroplasty is uncertain and remains investigational, with longer term follow-up required to arrive at a definitive, efficacious conclusion.

Summary

Even though staged protocols and advancements in technique and technology have evolved, the original principles regarding pilon fracture management remain unchanged. Restoration of length with fibular fixation, reconstruction of the articular surface, bone grafting, and buttressing of the metadiaphyseal reconstruction remain the foundation of optimal management. Treatment modifications include a better understanding of the importance of soft-tissue management, with particular focus on soft-tissue edema and blister resolution. Strategic preoperative planning with the use of CT and selection of appropriately bridged surgical incisions may facilitate an easier perioperative period and desired postoperative outcome. To stage the subsequent incision, the surgeon who provides definitive treatment should initiate the first "workhorse" incision. Knowing the pros and cons of each surgical approach will improve the chances of achieving the desired clinical results. Future protocol changes, implant technologies, and the role of IMN in the management of pilon fractures may be the subjects of

further research, but the principles of pilon restoration will most likely remain the same. External ring fixators are complicated but are viable options for treating unsalvageable, severely injured pilon fractures and are a useful tool for fracture management in the late and failed stages of treatment. Treating complications requires careful attention to wound management to avoid infection, malunion, and nonunion. If complications arise, arthrodesis remains the mainstay of management. The efficacy of ankle arthroplasty awaits improved clinical and longer term survival data.

References

1. Michelson J, Moskovitz P, Labropoulos P: The nomenclature for intra-articular vertical impact fractures of the tibial plafond: Pilon versus pylon. *Foot Ankle Int* 2004; 25(3):149-150.

2. Browner BD, Jupiter J, Levine A, Trafton P, Krettek C: *Skeletal Trauma: Basic Science, Management, and Reconstruction.* Philadelphia, PA, Elsevier, 2009, vol 2.

3. Destot E: *Traumataismes du pied et rayons x malleoles, astragale, calcaneum, avant-pied.* Paris, France, Masson, 1911.

4. Bourne RB, Rorabeck CH, Macnab J: Intra-articular fractures of the distal tibia: The pilon fracture. *J Trauma* 1983;23(7): 591-596.

5. Grose A, Gardner MJ, Hettrich C, et al: Open reduction and internal fixation of tibial pilon fractures using a lateral approach. *J Orthop Trauma* 2007;21(8): 530-537.

6. Helfet DL, Koval K, Pappas J, Sanders RW, DiPasquale T: Intraarticular "pilon" fracture of the tibia. *Clin Orthop Relat Res* 1994; 298:221-228.

7. Sirkin M, Sanders R, DiPasquale T, Herscovici D Jr: A staged pro-

tocol for soft tissue management in the treatment of complex pilon fractures. *J Orthop Trauma* 2004; 18(8 Suppl):S32-S38.

8. Babis GC, Vayanos ED, Papaioannou N, Pantazopoulos T: Results of surgical treatment of tibial plafond fractures. *Clin Orthop Relat Res* 1997;341:99-105.

9. Egol KA, Wolinsky P, Koval KJ: Open reduction and internal fixation of tibial pilon fractures. *Foot Ankle Clin* 2000;5(4):873-885.

10. Bourne RB: Pylon fractures of the distal tibia. *Clin Orthop Relat Res* 1989;240:42-46.

11. Ovadia DN, Beals RK: Fractures of the tibial plafond. *J Bone Joint Surg Am* 1986;68(4):543-551.

12. Rüedi TP, Allgöwer M: The operative treatment of intra-articular fractures of the lower end of the tibia. *Clin Orthop Relat Res* 1979; 138:105-110.

13. Teeny SM, Wiss DA: Open reduction and internal fixation of tibial plafond fractures: Variables contributing to poor results and complications. *Clin Orthop Relat Res* 1993;292:108-117.

14. Anglen JO: Early outcome of hybrid external fixation for fracture of the distal tibia. *J Orthop Trauma* 1999;13(2):92-97.

15. Barbieri R, Schenk R, Koval K, Aurori K, Aurori B: Hybrid external fixation in the treatment of tibial plafond fractures. *Clin Orthop Relat Res* 1996;332:16-22.

16. Bone L, Stegemann P, McNamara K, Seibel R: External fixation of severely comminuted and open tibial pilon fractures. *Clin Orthop Relat Res* 1993;292:101-107.

17. Marsh JL, Bonar S, Nepola JV, Decoster TA, Hurwitz SR: Use of an articulated external fixator for fractures of the tibial plafond. *J Bone Joint Surg Am* 1995; 77(10):1498-1509.

18. Marsh JL, Nepola JV, Wuest TK, Osteen D, Cox K, Oppen-

heim W: Unilateral external fixation until healing with the dynamic axial fixator for severe open tibial fractures. *J Orthop Trauma* 1991;5(3):341-348.

19. Tornetta P III, Weiner L, Bergman M, et al: Pilon fractures: Treatment with combined internal and external fixation. *J Orthop Trauma* 1993;7(6):489-496.

20. Wyrsch B, McFerran MA, McAndrew M, et al: Operative treatment of fractures of the tibial plafond: A randomized, prospective study. *J Bone Joint Surg Am* 1996; 78(11):1646-1657.

21. Dickson KF, Montgomery S, Field J: High energy plafond fractures treated by a spanning external fixator initially and followed by a second stage open reduction internal fixation of the articular surface: Preliminary report. *Injury* 2001;32(Suppl 4):SD92-SD98.

22. Assal M, Ray A, Stern R: The extensile approach for the operative treatment of high-energy pilon fractures: Surgical technique and soft-tissue healing. *J Orthop Trauma* 2007;21(3):198-206.

23. Blauth M, Bastian L, Krettek C, Knop C, Evans S: Surgical options for the treatment of severe tibial pilon fractures: A study of three techniques. *J Orthop Trauma* 2001;15(3):153-160.

24. Borens O, Kloen P, Richmond J, Roederer G, Levine DS, Helfet DL: Minimally invasive treatment of pilon fractures with a low profile plate: Preliminary results in 17 cases. *Arch Orthop Trauma Surg* 2009;129(5):649-659.

25. Borrelli J Jr, Prickett W, Song E, Becker D, Ricci W: Extraosseous blood supply of the tibia and the effects of different plating techniques: A human cadaveric study. *J Orthop Trauma* 2002;16(10): 691-695.

26. Chen L, O'Shea K, Early JS: The use of medial and lateral surgical approaches for the treatment of

tibial plafond fractures. *J Orthop Trauma* 2007;21(3):207-211.

27. Herscovici D Jr, Sanders RW, Infante A, DiPasquale T: Bohler incision: An extensile anterolateral approach to the foot and ankle. *J Orthop Trauma* 2000;14(6): 429-432.

28. Kao KF, Huang PJ, Chen YW, Cheng YM, Lin SY, Ko SH: Postero-medio-anterior approach of the ankle for the pilon fracture. *Injury* 2000;31(2):71-74.

29. Konrath GA, Hopkins G II: Posterolateral approach for tibial pilon fractures: A report of two cases. *J Orthop Trauma* 1999; 13(8):586-589.

30. Mehta S, Gardner MJ, Barei DP, Benirschke SK, Nork SE: Reduction strategies through the anterolateral exposure for fixation of type B and C pilon fractures. *J Orthop Trauma* 2011;25(2): 116-122.

31. Patterson MJ, Cole JD: Two-staged delayed open reduction and internal fixation of severe pilon fractures. *J Orthop Trauma* 1999; 13(2):85-91.

32. Tornetta P III, Gorup J: Axial computed tomography of pilon fractures. *Clin Orthop Relat Res* 1996;323:273-276.

33. White TO, Guy P, Cooke CJ, et al: The results of early primary open reduction and internal fixation for treatment of OTA 43.C-type tibial pilon fractures: A cohort study. *J Orthop Trauma* 2010;24(12):757-763.

34. Bozkurt M, Ocguder DA, Ugurlu M, Kalkan T: Tibial pilon fracture repair using Ilizarov external fixation, capsuloligamentotaxis, and early rehabilitation of the ankle. *J Foot Ankle Surg* 2008;47(4): 302-306.

35. Cierny G III, Cook WG, Mader JT: Ankle arthrodesis in the presence of ongoing sepsis: Indications, methods, and results. *Orthop Clin North Am* 1989;20(4): 709-721.

36. Coester LM, Saltzman CL, Leupold J, Pontarelli W: Long-term results following ankle arthrodesis for post-traumatic arthritis. *J Bone Joint Surg Am* 2001;83-A(2):219-228.

37. Knecht SI, Estin M, Callaghan JJ, et al: The Agility total ankle arthroplasty: Seven to sixteen-year follow-up. *J Bone Joint Surg Am* 2004;86-A(6):1161-1171.

38. Morgan SJ, Thordarson DB, Shepherd LE: Salvage of tibial pilon fractures using fusion of the ankle with a 90 degrees cannulated blade-plate: A preliminary report. *Foot Ankle Int* 1999;20(6):375-378.

39. Morrey BF, Wiedeman GP Jr: Complications and long-term results of ankle arthrodeses following trauma. *J Bone Joint Surg Am* 1980;62(5):777-784.

40. Niikura T, Miwa M, Sakai Y, et al: Ankle arthrodesis using antegrade intramedullary nail for salvage of nonreconstructable tibial pilon fractures. *Orthopedics* 2009;32(8):611.

41. Ristiniemi J: External fixation of tibial pilon fractures and fracture healing. *Acta Orthop Suppl* 2007;78(326):3, 5-34.

42. Rosen H: The treatment of nonunions and pseudarthroses of the humeral shaft. *Orthop Clin North Am* 1990;21(4):725-742.

43. Saltzman CL, Mann RA, Ahrens JE, et al: Prospective controlled trial of STAR total ankle replacement versus ankle fusion: Initial results. *Foot Ankle Int* 2009;30(7):579-596.

44. SooHoo NF, Zingmond DS, Ko CY: Comparison of reoperation rates following ankle arthrodesis and total ankle arthroplasty. *J Bone Joint Surg Am* 2007;89(10):2143-2149.

45. Thordarson DB: Complications after treatment of tibial pilon fractures: Prevention and management strategies. *J Am Acad Orthop Surg* 2000;8(4):253-265.

46. Vidyadhara S, Rao SK: Ilizarov treatment of complex tibial pilon fractures. *Int Orthop* 2006;30(2):113-117.

47. Dirschl DR, Adams GL: A critical assessment of factors influencing reliability in the classification of fractures, using fractures of the tibial plafond as a model. *J Orthop Trauma* 1997;11(7):471-476.

48. Martin JS, Marsh JL, Bonar SK, DeCoster TA, Found EM, Brandser EA: Assessment of the AO/ASIF fracture classification for the distal tibia. *J Orthop Trauma* 1997;11(7):477-483.

49. Ramappa M, Bajwa A, Singh A, Mackenney P, Hui A, Port A: Interobserver and intraobserver variations in tibial pilon fracture classification systems. *Foot (Edinb)* 2010;20(2-3):61-63.

50. Swiontkowski MF, Sands AK, Agel J, Diab M, Schwappach JR, Kreder HJ: Interobserver variation in the AO/OTA fracture classification system for pilon fractures: Is there a problem? *J Orthop Trauma* 1997;11(7):467-470.

51. DeCoster TA, Willis MC, Marsh JL, et al: Rank order analysis of tibial plafond fractures: Does injury or reduction predict outcome? *Foot Ankle Int* 1999;20(1):44-49.

52. Gustilo RB, Anderson JT: Prevention of infection in the treatment of one thousand and twenty-five open fractures of long bones: Retrospective and prospective analyses. *J Bone Joint Surg Am* 1976;58(4):453-458.

53. Sirkin M, Sanders R: The treatment of pilon fractures. *Orthop Clin North Am* 2001;32(1):91-102.

54. Mehta SK, Breitbart EA, Berberian WS, Liporace FA, Lin SS: Bone and wound healing in the diabetic patient. *Foot Ankle Clin* 2010;15(3):411-437.

55. Mills E, Eyawo O, Lockhart I, Kelly S, Wu P, Ebbert JO: Smoking cessation reduces postoperative complications: A systematic review and meta-analysis. *Am J Med* 2011;124(2):144-154, e8.

56. Wukich DK, Joseph A, Ryan M, Ramirez C, Irrgang JJ: Outcomes of ankle fractures in patients with uncomplicated versus complicated diabetes. *Foot Ankle Int* 2011;32(2):120-130.

57. Barei DP, Nork SE, Bellabarba C, Sangeorzan BJ: Is the absence of an ipsilateral fibular fracture predictive of increased radiographic tibial pilon fracture severity? *J Orthop Trauma* 2006;20(1):6-10.

58. Dunbar RP, Barei DP, Kubiak EN, Nork SE, Henley MB: Early limited internal fixation of diaphyseal extensions in select pilon fractures: Upgrading AO/OTA type C fractures to AO/OTA type B. *J Orthop Trauma* 2008;22(6):426-429.

59. Howard JL, Agel J, Barei DP, Benirschke SK, Nork SE: A prospective study evaluating incision placement and wound healing for tibial plafond fractures. *J Orthop Trauma* 2008;22(5):299-305, discussion 305-306.

60. Bonar SK, Marsh JL: Tibial plafond fractures: Changing principles of treatment. *J Am Acad Orthop Surg* 1994;2(6):297-305.

61. Mast JW, Spiegel PG, Pappas JN: Fractures of the tibial pilon. *Clin Orthop Relat Res* 1988;230:68-82.

62. Casey D, McConnell T, Parekh S, Tornetta P III: Percutaneous pin placement in the medial calcaneus: Is anywhere safe? *J Orthop Trauma* 2002;16(1):26-29.

63. Wagner HE, Jakob RP: Plate osteosynthesis in bicondylar fractures of the tibial head. *Unfallchirurg* 1986;89(7):304-311.

64. Tscherne H, Gotzen L, eds: *Fractures with Soft Tissue Injuries*. Berlin, Germany, Springer-Verlag, 1984.

65. Tscherne H, Schatzker J, eds: *Major Fractures of the Pilon, the Talus,*

and the Calcaneus. Heidelberg, Germany, Springer-Verlag, 1993.

66. McFerran MA, Smith SW, Boulas HJ, Schwartz HS: Complications encountered in the treatment of pilon fractures. *J Orthop Trauma* 1992;6(2):195-200.

67. Sirkin M, Sanders R, DiPasquale T, Herscovici D Jr: A staged protocol for soft tissue management in the treatment of complex pilon fractures. *J Orthop Trauma* 1999; 13(2):78-84.

68. Giordano CP, Koval KJ: Treatment of fracture blisters: A prospective study of 53 cases. *J Orthop Trauma* 1995;9(2):171-176.

69. Boraiah S, Kemp TJ, Erwteman A, Lucas PA, Asprinio DE: Outcome following open reduction and internal fixation of open pilon fractures. *J Bone Joint Surg Am* 2010;92(2):346-352.

70. Rüedi T, Matter P, Allgöwer M: Intra-articular fractures of the distal tibial end. *Helv Chir Acta* 1968;35(5):556-582.

71. Müller FJ, Nerlich M: Tibial pilon fractures. *Acta Chir Orthop Traumatol Cech* 2010;77(4): 266-276.

72. Tscherne H, Schatzker J, eds: *Manual of Internal Fixation Techniques Recommended by the AO Group.* New York, NY, Springer Verlag, 1979.

73. Schatzker J, Tile M: *The Rationale of Operative Fracture Care,* ed 3. Berlin, Germany, Springer-Verlag, 2005.

74. Borrelli J Jr, Catalano L: Open reduction and internal fixation of pilon fractures. *J Orthop Trauma* 1999;13(8):573-582.

75. Gould JS: Reconstruction of soft tissue injuries of the foot and ankle with microsurgical techniques. *Orthopedics* 1987;10(1):151-157.

76. McCann PA, Jackson M, Mitchell ST, Atkins RM: Complications of definitive open reduction and internal fixation of pilon fractures of the distal tibia. *Int Orthop* 2011;35(3):413-418.

77. Bhattacharyya T, Crichlow R, Gobezie R, Kim E, Vrahas MS: Complications associated with the posterolateral approach for pilon fractures. *J Orthop Trauma* 2006; 20(2):104-107.

78. Hazarika S, Chakravarthy J, Cooper J: Minimally invasive locking plate osteosynthesis for fractures of the distal tibia: Results in 20 patients. *Injury* 2006;37(9): 877-887.

79. Vallier HA, Le TT, Bedi A: Radiographic and clinical comparisons of distal tibia shaft fractures (4 to 11 cm proximal to the plafond): Plating versus intramedullary nailing. *J Orthop Trauma* 2008;22(5):307-311.

80. Gagneux E, Gerard F, Garbuio P, Vichard P: Treatment of complex fractures of the ankle and their sequellae using trans-plantar intramedullary nailing. *Acta Orthop Belg* 1997;63(4):294-304.

81. Pugh KJ, Wolinsky PR, McAndrew MP, Johnson KD: Tibial pilon fractures: A comparison of treatment methods. *J Trauma* 1999;47(5):937-941.

82. Leung F, Kwok HY, Pun TS, Chow SP: Limited open reduction and Ilizarov external fixation in the treatment of distal tibial fractures. *Injury* 2004;35(3):278-283.

83. McDonald MG, Burgess RC, Bolano LE, Nicholls PJ: Ilizarov treatment of pilon fractures. *Clin Orthop Relat Res* 1996;325: 232-238.

84. Zarek S, Othman M, Macias J: The Ilizarov method in the treatment of pilon fractures. *Ortop Traumatol Rehabil* 2002;4(4): 427-433.

85. Resch H, Benedetto KP, Pechlaner S: Development of post-traumatic arthrosis following pilon tibial fractures. *Unfallchirurg* 1986;89(1):8-15.

86. Mader JT, Shirtliff M, Calhoun JH: Staging and staging application in osteomyelitis. *Clin Infect Dis* 1997;25(6):1303-1309.

87. Pollak AN, McCarthy ML, Bess RS, Agel J, Swiontkowski MF: Outcomes after treatment of high-energy tibial plafond fractures. *J Bone Joint Surg Am* 2003; 85-A(10):1893-1900.

88. Zalavras CG, Patzakis MJ, Thordarson DB, Shah S, Sherman R, Holtom P: Infected fractures of the distal tibial metaphysis and plafond: Achievement of limb salvage with free muscle flaps, bone grafting, and ankle fusion. *Clin Orthop Relat Res* 2004;427: 57-62.

89. Feldman DS, Shin SS, Madan S, Koval KJ: Correction of tibial malunion and nonunion with six-axis analysis deformity correction using the Taylor Spatial Frame. *J Orthop Trauma* 2003; 17(8):549-554.

90. Trumble TE, Benirschke SK, Vedder NB: Use of radial forearm flaps to treat complications of closed pilon fractures. *J Orthop Trauma* 1992;6(3):358-365.

91. Moore TJ, Prince R, Pochatko D, Smith JW, Fleming S: Retrograde intramedullary nailing for ankle arthrodesis. *Foot Ankle Int* 1995; 16(7):433-436.

92. Paley D, Chaudray M, Pirone AM, Lentz P, Kautz D: Treatment of malunions and mal-nonunions of the femur and tibia by detailed preoperative planning and the Ilizarov techniques. *Orthop Clin North Am* 1990;21(4):667-691.

93. Tetsworth KD, Paley D: Accuracy of correction of complex lower-extremity deformities by the Ilizarov method. *Clin Orthop Relat Res* 1994;301:102-110.

94. Clare MP, Sanders RW: Preoperative considerations in ankle replacement surgery. *Foot Ankle Clin* 2002;7(4):709-720.

Scaphoid Fractures: What's Hot, What's Not

William B. Geissler, MD
Julie E. Adams, MD
Randy R. Bindra, MD, FRCS
William D. Lanzinger, MD
David J. Slutsky, MD, FRCSC

Abstract

The scaphoid is the most commonly fractured carpal bone of the wrist. It is an unusual carpal bone in that it bridges both the proximal and the distal rows; this subjects it to continuous shearing and bending forces. Approximately 80% of the scaphoid is covered by cartilage, which limits its ligamentous attachment and vascular supply.

Most scaphoid fractures occur at the waist. Acute stable fractures or incomplete fractures of the scaphoid may be treated nonsurgically; a high rate of union can be expected. However, there is considerable debate about the type of immobilization needed. Although closed treatment of stable wrist fractures of the scaphoid achieve a high rate of healing, prolonged cast immobilization may lead to complications, including muscle atrophy, possible joint contracture, and disuse osteopenia. Because of this, internal fixation of minimally displaced fractures of the scaphoid has recently become popular.

There is consensus in the literature that nonunion of the scaphoid and proximal pole fractures should be treated surgically. In the past several decades, percutaneous arthroscopic techniques of scaphoid stabilization, which minimize surgical morbidity, have become popular. There also has been a significant improvement in the management of difficult scaphoid nonunions, with or without deformity. Improved techniques include open and dorsal approaches and vascularized bone grafting of resistant scaphoid nonunions.

Declining in popularity is the prolonged immobilization of unstable fractures when surgical stabilization may have been a better treatment option.

Instr Course Lect 2012;61:71-84.

The scaphoid is the most commonly fractured carpal bone, accounting for between 60% and 70% of all carpal fractures. Approximately 80% of the surface of the scaphoid is covered by cartilage, which limits its ligamentous attachment and vascular supply. Most scaphoid fractures occur at the waist. Acute stable fractures or incomplete fractures of the scaphoid may be treated nonsurgically, resulting in a high rate of fracture union. Although closed treatment of stable fractures of the scaphoid is associated with a high rate of healing, this method requires prolonged cast immobilization, which may lead to muscle atrophy, possible joint contracture, disuse osteopenia, and potential financial hardship. Because of this, internal fixation of minimally displaced fractures of the scaphoid has become popular. There is a consensus that scaphoid nonunions

Dr. Geissler or an immediate family member has received royalties from Acumed, Arthrex, Medartis, and Springer; is a member of a speakers' bureau or has made paid presentations on behalf of Acumed, Arthrex, Medartis, and Ascension; serves as a paid consultant to or is an employee of Acumed and Ascension; and owns stock or stock options in Tornier. Dr. Adams or an immediate family member has received royalties from DePuy and serves as a paid consultant to or is an employee of Arthrex, DePuy, and Wright Medical Technology. Dr. Bindra or an immediate family member serves as a board member, owner, officer, or committee member of the American Association for Hand Surgery and the American Society for Surgery of the Hand; has received royalties from Tornier; is a member of a speakers' bureau or has made paid presentations on behalf of Auxilium and Integra NeuroSciences; and serves as a paid consultant to or is an employee of Acumed and Integra LifeSciences. Dr. Slutsky or an immediate family member serves as a board member, owner, officer, or committee member of the American Society for Surgery of the Hand and owns stock or stock options in South Bay Hand Surgery. Neither Dr. Lanzinger nor any immediate family member has received anything of value from or owns stock in a commercial company or institution related directly or indirectly to the subject of this chapter.

and fractures of the proximal pole of the scaphoid should be treated surgically. What is hot in the management of scaphoid fractures is the development of percutaneous arthroscopic techniques of scaphoid stabilization that minimize surgical morbidity. In addition, what is hot in scaphoid fracture treatment is a significant improvement in the treatment of difficult scaphoid nonunions with the use of vascularized bone grafts. What is not hot in scaphoid fracture treatment is prolonged immobilization for unstable fractures when surgical stabilization may have been the best option. This chapter will describe percutaneous and arthroscopic reduction, mini dorsal and open volar approaches to the scaphoid, and vascularized bone grafting for resistant scaphoid fracture nonunions.

Prevalence, Anatomy, and Classification of Scaphoid Fractures

Prevalence

The scaphoid is the most commonly fractured carpal bone and accounts for 60% to 70% of all carpal fractures. Most scaphoid fractures are relatively low-energy injuries and usually occur in young men.

Anatomy

The scaphoid bone is the only carpal bone that bridges both the proximal and distal rows, thereby being subjected to continuous shearing and bending forces. Approximately 80% of the surface of the scaphoid is covered by cartilage, which limits ligamentous attachments and its vascular supply. Gelberman and Menon[1] studied the blood supply of the carpus in 15 fresh cadaver specimens using injection techniques. They found the primary blood supply to the scaphoid was from the radial artery. Seventy percent to 80% of interosseous vascularity in

the entire proximal pole is from branches of the radial artery entering along the dorsal ridge of the scaphoid along the scaphoid waist. Because of the dependence of the scaphoid on a single dominant artery, the proximal pole is uniquely susceptible to osteonecrosis after injury.

Most scaphoid fractures occur at the waist and result from wrist hyperextension to greater than 95°. Placing the wrist in extreme dorsiflexion and ulnar deviation causes fractures to the scaphoid waist as the scaphoid impinges on the dorsal rim of the radius.[2] Fractures of the proximal pole of the scaphoid result from dorsal subluxation during forced hyperextension.[2] Heinzelmann et al,[2] using microcomputed tomography (micro CT), found that the scaphoid bone is most dense at the proximal pole where the trabecular bone is thickest and more tightly packed. The trabeculae are thinnest and more sparsely distributed at the scaphoid waist; this is where most fractures occur.

Classification

Scaphoid fractures have been classified by many methods, including stability, location of the fracture site, and fracture plane. Russe[3] classified fractures of the scaphoid as horizontal oblique, transverse, and vertically oblique. He noted that oblique fractures were unstable and were difficult to control with cast immobilization. Herbert and Fisher[4] classified scaphoid fractures according to their stability. Type A fractures were considered stable and included incomplete fractures or fractures of the scaphoid tubercle. Type B fractures were unstable acute fractures, with type B1 being a distal oblique fracture; type B2, a complete fracture at the waist; type B3, a proximal pole fracture; and type B4, a transscaphoid perilunate fracture-dislocation. Type C fractures resulted in delayed union,

and type D fractures represented established nonunions, including type D1 fibrous union and type D2 pseudarthrosis. They noted that all other fractures except type A were potentially unstable.

Cooney et al[5] further defined unstable fracture patterns. These include fractures displaced more than 1 mm, a lateral intrascaphoid angle greater than 35°, bone loss or comminution, a perilunate fracture-dislocation, dorsal intercalated segmental instability alignment, and proximal pole fractures.

Geissler and Slade[6] published a radiographic classification of scaphoid nonunions (**Table 1**).

Management of Acute Scaphoid Fractures

Distal Pole Fractures

Distal pole fractures of the scaphoid are generally treated nonsurgically. The distal pole of the scaphoid is well vascularized, and distal pole fractures of the scaphoid have a high union rate after 6 to 8 weeks of immobilization in a short arm cast. Distal pole fractures generally fall into two groups: group I, avulsion fractures from the radial palmar lip of the scaphoid tuberosity; and group II, impaction fractures of the radial half of the distal scaphoid articular surface. If displaced, these impacted fractures may need to be surgically stabilized.

Proximal Pole Fractures

Both displaced and nondisplaced fractures of the proximal pole are considered unstable and cannot be reliably treated nonsurgically because of the small fracture fragment size and tenuous blood supply. Because of the intra-articular location, synovial fluid can block fracture healing, and the proximal location of the fracture leads to large lever-arm stress across the fracture site. Rettig and Raskin[7] reported a 100% healing rate of 17 proximal pole

Table 1

Radiographic Classification System of Geissler and Slade[6] for Scaphoid Nonunion

Classification	Description
Class I	Scaphoid fractures with a 4- to 12-week delayed presentation for treatment
Class II	Fibrous union: minimal fracture line at nonunion interface; no cyst or sclerosis
Class III	Minimal sclerosis: ≤ 1 mm of bone resorption at nonunion interface
Class IV	Cystic formation and sclerosis: bone resorption of > 1 mm but < 5 mm at nonunion interface; cyst; no deformity visible on lateral radiograph
Class V	Deformity and/or pseudarthrosis: ≥ 5 mm of bone resorption at nonunion interface; cyst; fragment motion; deformity visible on lateral radiograph
Class VI	Wrist arthrosis: scaphoid nonunion with radiocarpal and/or midcarpal arthrosis
Special circumstances	Proximal pole nonunion: The proximal pole of the scaphoid has a tenuous blood supply and a mechanical disadvantage, which places it at greater risk of delayed or failed union. Because of these difficulties, this injury requires aggressive treatment to ensure successful healing.
	Osteonecrosis: Scaphoid nonunion with osteonecrosis is suggested by MRI, demonstrating a decrease or absence of vascularity of one or both poles. Bone biopsy can confirm necrosis. Intraoperative inspection of the scaphoid for punctate bleeding is considered definitive.
	Ligament injury: Ligament injury is suggested by static and dynamic imaging of the carpal bones. Arthroscopy is the most sensitive tool for detecting carpal ligament injury.

Table 2

Algorithm for Management of Acute Scaphoid Fractures

Acute Scaphoid Fracture Type	Treatment
Stable fractures, nondisplaced	
Tubercle fracture	Short arm cast for 6 to 8 weeks
Distal third fracture and/or incomplete fracture	Short arm cast for 6 to 8 weeks
Waist fracture	Long arm thumb spica cast for 6 weeks, short arm cast for 6 weeks or until CT confirms healing; especially for pediatric patients, sedentary or low-demand patients, or patients with a preference for nonsurgical treatment
	Percutaneous or open internal fixation; especially for active and young patients performing manual labor, athletes, patients with high-demand occupations, or patients with a preference for early range of motion
Proximal pole fracture, nondisplaced	Percutaneous or open internal fixation
Unstable fractures	
Displacement > 1 mm	Dorsal percutaneous or open screw fixation
Lateral intrascaphoid angle > 35°	Dorsal percutaneous or open screw fixation
Bone loss or comminution	Dorsal percutaneous or open screw fixation
Perilunate fracture-dislocation	Dorsal intercalated segmental instability alignment

fractures treated acutely with screw fixation through a dorsal approach.

Waist Fractures

Acute stable fractures or incomplete fractures of the scaphoid waist may be treated nonsurgically with a high rate of union (**Table 2**). There is no agreement in the literature regarding the position of mobilization or the type of cast because truly stable fractures of the scaphoid may be treated by a variety of methods (thumb spica cast, wrist extension cast, wrist neutral cast, and ulnar deviation cast) with nearly equivalent results. Historic literature suggests that the union rate after cast treatment approaches 85% to 95%; however, studies with radiographs made 6 to 12 months after injury or CT evaluation show lower rates of union. At a follow-up period of 1 year from injury, Terkelsen and Jepsen[8] reported 10 nonunions in 92 scaphoid waist fractures that were treated with removable splints or long arm casts.

Delaying treatment reduces the likelihood of union of stable scaphoid waist fractures. In a series of 285 scaphoid fractures, Langhoff and

Table 3

Algorithm for Management of Scaphoid Fracture Nonunion

Type of Fracture	Treatment
Delayed union	Percutaneous or open rigid fixation with a headless compression screw
Established nonunion	Open repair and bone grafting
Fibrous nonunion, waist	Dorsal for proximal pole fracture, volar for waist fracture
Sclerotic nonunion, waist	Dorsal for proximal pole fracture, volar for waist fracture
Humpback nonunion, waist	Volar approach and corticocancellous wedge graft
Proximal pole nonunion, nonischemic	Dorsal approach; percutaneous or open bone grafting and fixation with headless screw; lock midcarpal joint with mini-screw or sandwich proximal fragment between lunate and scaphoid waist with headless screw
Vascular nonunion, waist or proximal pole	Vascularized bone graft: dorsal or palmar approach

Andersen[9] reported that, if fractures were treated more than 4 weeks after injury, there was a substantially increased risk of delayed union or nonunion. Up to 25% of scaphoid fractures are not visible on initial radiographs. Because a failure to treat a stable scaphoid fracture for 4 weeks increases the nonunion rate, all clinically suspected scaphoid fractures should be treated as fractures, with the limb immobilized in a short arm cast, until the cause of symptoms is clarified. Follow-up radiographs with the cast removed are obtained 10 to 14 days after the initial cast has been applied. MRI is the most reliable modality for the diagnosis of acute and occult fractures and is able to identify a scaphoid fracture within 24 hours of injury.[2]

Although closed treatment of stable waist fractures of the scaphoid has a high rate of fracture union, prolonged cast immobilization may lead to muscle atrophy, joint contracture, disuse osteopenia, and potential financial hardship. Closed treatment of scaphoid waist fractures may require cast immobilization for 3 to 6 months. The economic cost of surgical versus nonsurgical treatment of stable scaphoid waist fractures has been well studied in the literature. Arora et al[10] compared two groups of patients with stable scaphoid fractures. One group was treated with plaster immobilization, and the other was treated with internal screw fixation. Internal screw fixation of nondisplaced scaphoid fractures was associated with a shorter time to osseous union, and patients returned to work an average of 7 weeks earlier than those treated with cast immobilization. In this study, the cost of surgical management was lower.

Davis et al[11] conducted a cost analysis to compare open reduction with cast immobilization for the treatment of acute nondisplaced midwaist scaphoid fractures. A mathematical model was developed to calculate the outcomes and the cost of open reduction compared with cast immobilization with estimated Medicare reimbursement rates and the cost of lost productivity estimated by average wages obtained from the US Bureau of Labor Statistics. They found that open reduction with internal fixation offered greater quality-adjusted life-years than casting. Open reduction and internal fixation was less costly than casting ($7,940 versus $13,851 per patient, respectively) because of the longer period of lost productivity with casting.

There is strong consensus in the literature that nonunion of the scaphoid should be treated surgically (**Table 3**). Management of scaphoid nonunion depends on the scaphoid alignment, bone loss, presence of a humpback deformity, carpal collapse, and osteonecrosis. Nonunion of the scaphoid leads to a predictable humpback deformity with flexion of the distal pole.

Fractures of the scaphoid continue to be a challenging injury for surgeons to treat. What is hot in the management of scaphoid fractures over the past two decades is the development of percutaneous and arthroscopic techniques of scaphoid stabilization that minimize surgical morbidity. However, potential complications exist. This chapter will describe techniques to lower the complication rate. What is hot in scaphoid treatment is the substantial improvement in the treatment of difficult scaphoid nonunions, with or without deformity. This includes open and dorsal approaches to the scaphoid and vascularized bone grafting of resistant scaphoid nonunions. What is not hot in scaphoid management is prolonged immobilization for unstable fractures when surgical stabilization may have been the best option and complications from an arthroscopic or open procedure that potentially could have been avoided. This discussion aims to help the surgeon define the indications for surgical management in a patient with a fracture of the scaphoid, and, when surgical fixation is indicated, to define whether an arthroscopic or an open technique is the best option.

Volar Percutaneous Technique

Haddad and Goddard[12] popularized the volar percutaneous technique. The patient is positioned supine with the thumb suspended in a Chinese finger trap. Placing the thumb under suspension allows ulnar deviation of the wrist, which improves surgical access to the distal pole of the scaphoid. Under fluoroscopic guidance, a longitudinal 0.5-cm–long skin incision is made over the distal radial aspect of the scaphoid, and a percutaneous guidewire is inserted into the scaphotrapezial joint and advanced proximally and dorsally across the fracture site. The position of the guidewire is easily checked by rotating the forearm under fluoroscopy. This technique provides an almost 360° view of the position of the guidewire within the scaphoid. The length of the guidewire within the scaphoid is determined by placing a second guidewire next to the initial one and measuring the difference between the two. A drill is then inserted through the soft-tissue protector, the scaphoid is reamed, and a headless cannulated screw is inserted.

This technique is straightforward and requires minimal specialized equipment. The disadvantage is that the screw may be placed slightly oblique to a fracture line in the midwaist portion of the scaphoid.

Dorsal Percutaneous Approach

Slade et al[13] popularized the dorsal percutaneous approach. The wrist is flexed and pronated under fluoroscopy until the proximal and distal poles of the scaphoid are aligned to form a perfect cylinder. Continuous fluoroscopy is recommended as the wrist is flexed and pronated to obtain a true ring sign as the proximal and distal poles are aligned. Under fluoroscopy, a 14-gauge needle is placed percutaneously in the center of the ring sign and parallel to the fluoroscopic beam. A guidewire is inserted through the 14-gauge needle and driven across the central axis of the scaphoid until it comes in contact with the distal cortex of the scaphoid. It is important not to extend the wrist because this may bend the guidewire. A second guidewire is then placed parallel to the first so that it touches the proximal pole of the scaphoid, and the difference in length of the two guidewires is measured to determine the length of the screw. The authors recommended the use of a screw 4 mm shorter than what is measured to allow compression at the fracture site.[13] The goal is to place a screw the length of the scaphoid to compress the fracture and resist lever-arm bending forces.

The primary guidewire is then advanced volarly until it is flush with the proximal pole of the scaphoid dorsally and the wrist is extended. The radiocarpal and midcarpal spaces are evaluated arthroscopically for any associated soft-tissue injuries. The arthroscope is placed in the midcarpal space to evaluate the fracture reduction and may be adjusted. The wrist is then flexed, and the guidewire is advanced dorsally, exiting the skin. A portion of the guidewire is to be left outside the volar and dorsal aspects of the wrist in case of wire breakage. Blunt dissection is continued around the guidewire dorsally to minimize the risk of soft-tissue injury to the extensor tendon as the scaphoid is reamed and the screw is inserted.

The advantage of the dorsal approach is that the screw can be inserted down the central axis of the scaphoid. The disadvantage of the dorsal approach is that, as the wrist is hyperflexed, the unstable scaphoid fracture may displace to create a humpback deformity.

Arthroscopic Reduction (The Geissler Technique)

The Geissler technique can be used for acute scaphoid fractures and selected scaphoid nonunions.[14] The hand is initially suspended in a traction tower (Acumed, Hillsboro, OR) at 30° of wrist flexion. The arthroscope is initially placed in the 3-4 portal (between the extensor pollicis longus [EPL] and the extensor digitorum tendons) to evaluate any associated soft-tissue injuries. The arthroscope is then transferred into the 6-R portal (**Figure 1**). A 14-gauge needle is inserted through the 3-4 portal, and the scapholunate interosseous ligament is palpated at its junction with the proximal pole of the scaphoid (**Figure 2**). The junction of the scapholunate interosseous ligament with the proximal pole of the scaphoid along its middle third is the ideal starting point, and the needle is inserted there. The traction tower is flexed at its base, and the starting point of the needle is evaluated under fluoroscopy. The needle is simply aimed toward the thumb under fluoroscopy, and a guidewire is advanced through the needle and down the central axis of the scaphoid to abut the distal pole (**Figure 3**). The position of the guidewire is evaluated under fluoroscopic guidance by rotating the forearm in the traction tower (**Figure 4**). A second guidewire is placed against the proximal pole of the scaphoid to determine the length of the screw. A screw that is at least 4 mm shorter than the length measured is used.

The reduction of the scaphoid is evaluated with the arthroscope in the midcarpal portals. The traction tower may be flexed, extended, and deviated either radially or ulnarly to further reduce the fracture. After the fracture is reduced, the guidewire is aimed proximally into the proximal pole of the scaphoid and out the dorsum of the

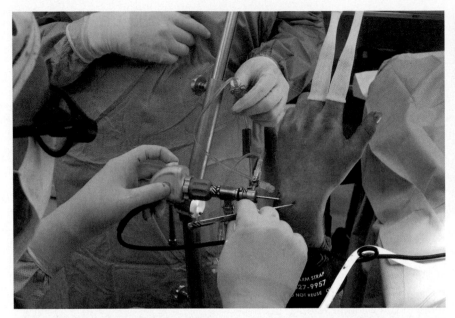

Figure 1 The hand is suspended in 10 lb of traction in a traction tower, with the wrist in approximately 30° of flexion. The arthroscope is placed in the 6-R portal, and a probe is inserted into the 3-4 portal to palpate the scapholunate interosseous ligament at its junction with the proximal pole of the scaphoid.

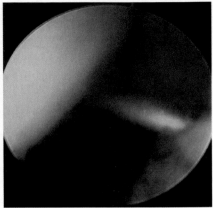

Figure 2 Arthroscopic view of a 14-gauge needle inserted through the 3-4 portal as it impales the proximal pole of the scaphoid. In this manner, the exact starting point of the guidewire and initial screw placement can be directly visualized arthroscopically.

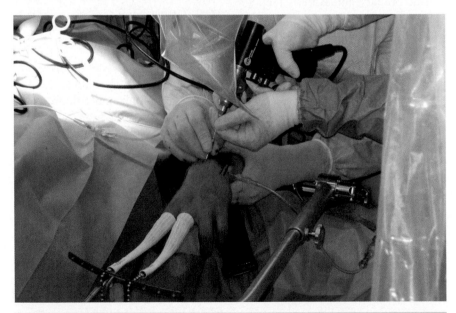

Figure 3 The wrist arthroscopy traction tower is flexed down, the needle is aimed toward the thumb, and the guidewire is placed.

wrist. The scaphoid is then reamed, and a headless cannulated screw is placed (**Figures 5** and **6**). It is important to arthroscopically evaluate the radiocarpal space after screw insertion to ensure that the screw is inserted completely within the scaphoid and is not protruding proximally, which would injure the articular cartilage of the distal portion of the radius.

The advantage of this technique is that it allows direct visualization and reduction of the scaphoid fracture, the precise insertion point for the guidewire is identified, and the wrist is not hyperflexed, which could displace the fracture. Associated soft-tissue injuries that may occur with a fracture of the scaphoid may be detected and can be managed at the same time.

Arthroscopic Management of Selected Scaphoid Nonunions

Slade et al[13] described their use of Slade's dorsal percutaneous fixation technique in 15 patients with stable fibrous nonunions of the scaphoid. All patients underwent percutaneous dorsal fixation with a headless cannulated screw and no accessory bone grafting. All fractures healed in an average of 3 months. Twelve of 15 patients had excellent results according to the modified Mayo wrist scale. Dorsal percutaneous fixation without bone grafting was recommended for patients with a stable fibrous nonunion and no signs of a humpback deformity. This technique may be used in scaphoid nonunion types I to III, as proposed by the authors.

For patients who have a cystic scaphoid nonunion without a humpback deformity (type IV), percutaneous cancellous bone grafting or injection of demineralized bone matrix may be used. With the Geissler technique, a guidewire is inserted down the central axis of the scaphoid, and the scaphoid is reamed through a soft-tissue protector. A bone biopsy needle filled with demineralized bone matrix putty is placed over the guidewire and inserted through the reamed scaphoid directly into the nonunion site. The demineralized bone matrix is then injected through the bone biopsy needle directly into the central hole of the scaphoid at the nonunion site. Following injection of the demineralized bone matrix, the guidewire is advanced back through the bone biopsy needle, from volar to dorsal, and out the dorsum of the wrist. A headless cannulated screw is then inserted over the guidewire across the fracture site, and the radiocarpal and midcarpal spaces are reevaluated arthroscopically.

Geissler and Slade[6] reported on the use of the Geissler technique in 15 patients with cystic scaphoid nonunions without humpback deformity; fracture union was obtained in 14 of the patients.

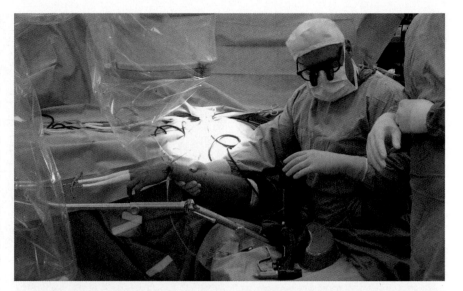

Figure 4   The position of the guidewire is then checked under fluoroscopic guidance in the posteroanterior, oblique, and lateral planes to ensure that it has been placed within the central axis of the scaphoid.

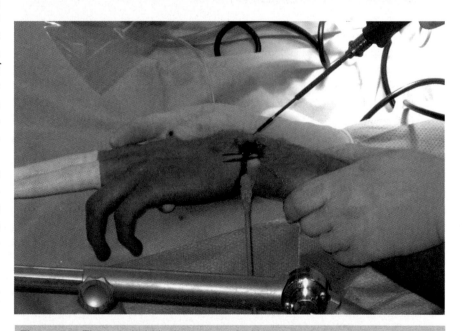

Figure 5   The scaphoid is then reamed with a cannulated reamer, and a headless cannulated screw is placed over the guidewire.

 Video 6.1: Arthroscopically Assisted Fixation and Percutaneous Grafting of Scaphoid Nonunions. William B. Geissler, MD (6 min)

Mini-Open Technique

The mini-open dorsal technique is a modification of the dorsal percutaneous technique that was popularized by Slade et al[15] The entry point for the guidewire is identified by an open incision, making this a simpler technique.

Indications and Contraindications
The dorsal mini-open technique can be used for the fixation of acute nondisplaced scaphoid waist fractures and proximal pole fractures. Augmented with bone grafting, the technique can be used for the treatment of delayed union and scaphoid nonunion without

collapse. In displaced fractures, the percutaneous technique can be used only if the scaphoid can be reduced by percutaneous manipulation with Kirschner wires. Fractures of the distal third of the scaphoid should be fixed from the volar approach to ensure more screw purchase in the smaller fragment.

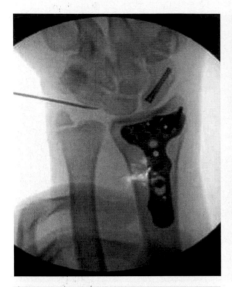

Figure 6 Intraoperative fluoroscopy is used to confirm placement of the screw in the central axis of the scaphoid.

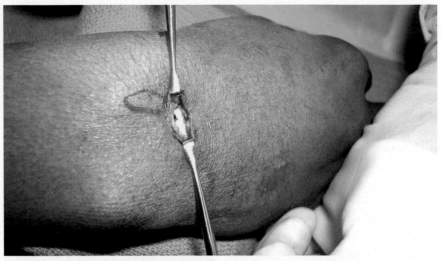

Figure 7 A 1-cm long, longitudinal incision is made on the ulnar aspect of the Lister tubercle. The EPL is retracted radially, and the extensor digitorum communis tendon is retracted ulnarly, thus exposing the dorsal capsule. This incision corresponds to the 3-4 portal on arthroscopy.

Surgical Technique

The following landmarks are identified by palpation and are marked on the skin: scaphoid tuberosity on the palmar aspect, tip of the radial styloid on the radial aspect, and the Lister tubercle on the dorsum of the radius. These three landmarks help to identify the spatial orientation of the scaphoid on the surface and facilitate guidewire placement. A longitudinal skin incision, approximately 1 cm in length, is placed over the radiocarpal joint radial to the Lister tubercle and extending along the radial border of the third metacarpal (**Figure 7**). The incision corresponds to the 3-4 wrist arthroscopy portal. The EPL tendon is identified and released for a distance of 2 cm to allow retraction of the EPL radially. The fascia over the extensor digitorum communis tendon in the fourth compartment is incised longitudinally. By placing retractors between the EPL tendon radially and the extensor digitorum communis tendons ulnarly, the underlying radiocarpal joint capsule is exposed at the level of the scapholunate articulation.

A limited longitudinal capsulotomy is performed along the long axis of the incision, taking care to avoid plunging the scalpel blade into the scapholunate interosseous ligament. The articular surface of the scaphoid is immediately visible, and it is possible to identify the dorsal portion of the scapholunate interosseous ligament and its insertion on the scaphoid pole. The wrist is flexed over a bolster of three rolled towels. The starting point for a central guidewire is located 3 mm radial to the insertion of the proximal membranous portion of the scapholunate ligament origin. A soft-tissue protector or a 14-gauge intravenous cannula is placed at this point and directed to a point 5 mm distal to the scaphoid tuberosity. The appropriate guidewire is inserted through the cannula until it tents the skin on the palm at the intended exit point. The direction of the guidewire may be checked fluoroscopically on a lateral radiograph with the wrist pronated to 45°. A small stab incision may be necessary to facilitate the exiting of the wire on the palmar surface (**Figure 8**). A second guidewire is inserted

4 mm from the first, and the more central of the two wires is selected, with the second wire used to prevent fracture displacement during drilling and screw insertion.

The wires are then withdrawn through the palmar wound until they lie flush within the articular surface of the scaphoid. The wrist is extended for imaging (**Figure 9**). The more optimal wire is selected for drilling the screw track. The selected guidewire is drilled back into the scaphoid in a retrograde direction under fluoroscopic control until it lies within the scaphoid at the scaphotrapezial joint. The length of the guidewire within the scaphoid is measured. A screw that is 4 mm shorter than this measurement is selected.

The wire is driven back in an antegrade direction to exit at the palm to have access to both ends of the wire in case of breakage. A cannulated drill is inserted over the guidewire, and the screw track is prepared by hand or by power drilling. The selected cannulated screw is then manually inserted over the wire until the screw lies 2 mm beneath the articular surface.

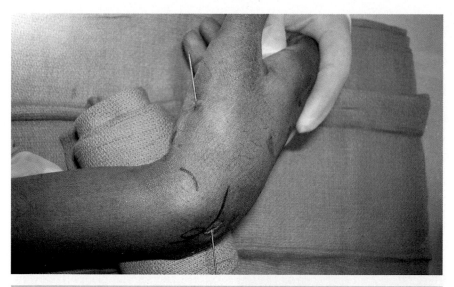

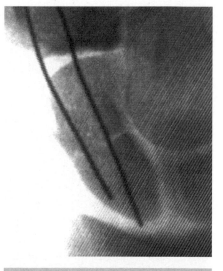

Figure 8 A Kirschner wire is drilled through the central axis of the scaphoid while flexing the wrist. A second guidewire will then be inserted 4 mm from and parallel to this position.

Figure 9 Positioning of the wires is verified with the use of a portable image intensifier or mini C-arm in both PA lateral views. The more optimal wire is selected for drilling the screw track.

The capsulotomy is left open, and the skin edges are approximated. The wrist is immobilized in a short arm plaster splint, and frequent digital range-of-motion exercises are initiated. The patient is fitted with a removable wrist splint and given instructions for a home exercise program of wrist and hand mobilization to be performed several times a day, with the wrist out of the splint, starting 2 weeks postoperatively (**Figure 10**).

Open Treatment of Scaphoid Fractures and Nonunions

Open techniques for fixation of scaphoid fractures are indicated for acute displaced scaphoid fractures that cannot be reduced by closed means, comminuted acute fractures, and many but not all scaphoid nonunions.[6]

Surgical Approaches

The volar approach is typically used for distal third or midwaist fractures or nonunions of the scaphoid. This approach is particularly useful to correct a humpback deformity of the scaph-

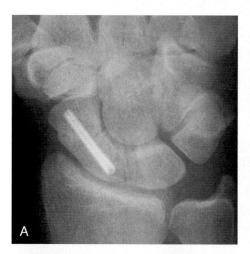

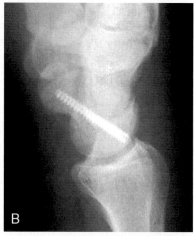

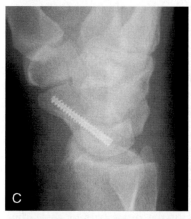

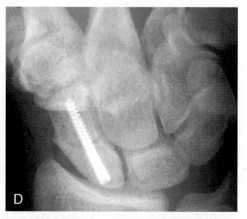

Figure 10 A through **D,** Postoperative scaphoid series of radiographs demonstrate central screw placement within the scaphoid with the mini-open technique.

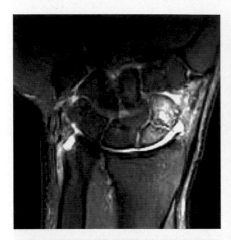

Figure 11 MRI scan of the wrist of a 20-year-old man with rheumatoid arthritis who presented with a 9-month history of wrist pain following a fall on the wrist. Scaphoid waist nonunion with cystic resorption is shown.

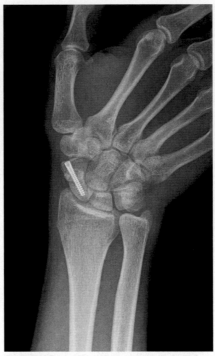

Figure 12 Radiograph of the wrist of the patient in Figure 11 after open reduction and internal fixation with iliac crest bone graft and the placement of a compression screw.

oid. The important dorsal blood supply is left undisturbed, and a good view of the volar surface of the scaphoid is facilitated. Care is taken to preserve and repair the volar carpal ligaments to avoid instability. The use of a structural corticocancellous bone graft can restore carpal height and correct a humpback deformity.

A longitudinal incision is made over the flexor carpi radialis tendon. Distally, the incision is curved obliquely toward the scaphoid tubercle. The flexor carpi radialis tendon is retracted ulnarly, and the dissection proceeds through the floor of the flexor carpi radialis tendon sheath ulnar to the radial artery. The capsule is opened between the long radiolunate ligament and the radioscaphocapitate ligament. The fracture site is exposed for reduction or curetting and/or bone grafting as needed. Structural bone graft may be placed for correction of a humpback deformity, or a vascularized bone graft may be used. It is sometimes helpful to insert 0.045- or 0.054-inch (1.1 or 1.4 mm) Kirschner wires into the proximal and distal fragments to use as

joysticks for manipulating the fragments. The radial surface of the capitate is used as a template for reduction and, by moving the Kirschner wires divergently, the nonunion site can be exposed for curettage and preparation of the nonunion site for bone grafting.

Several nonvascular bone grafting techniques are noted, as follows. The Matti-Russe bone graft technique involves the creation of cavities in the proximal and the distal fragments to accept placement of a strip of corticocancellous bone, which is then wedged into place. This provides intrinsic stability, which may be sufficient alone or may be augmented with Kirschner wires. This technique is not appropriate in the presence of osteonecrosis of the proximal pole or a humpback deformity.[16] Reported union rates have ranged from 54% to 92%. The technique described by Fernandez involves

the use of a wedge-shaped corticocancellous graft, usually from the iliac crest, to restore alignment in a humpback deformity.[5] Fixation is applied to secure the graft and nonunion site. Union rates have been reported to be greater than 94%.[5]

The screw can easily be placed from distal to proximal. To improve the starting point, the proximal volar portion of the trapezium may be removed, thus allowing the surgeon to place the guide pin and screw in a more centralized starting point. A guide pin is directed in a 45° plane to the forearm in both the coronal and sagittal planes. Following completion of scaphoid bone grafting and fixation, final radiographic images are assessed, and the capsule is repaired (**Figures 11** and **12**).

A dorsal approach is most useful for proximal pole fractures and preserves the volar carpal ligaments. In addition, exposure of the scapholunate ligament is facilitated to address any injury there. There are concerns about disruption of the blood supply to the scaphoid, particularly in the setting of nonunions. The incision may be longitudinal or transverse and is centered over the Lister tubercle. The surgical approach is as described previously in the mini-open technique.

Pedicled Vascularized Bone Grafts for Scaphoid Nonunions

The emergence of vascularized bone grafts has changed the treatment of scaphoid nonunions. Their use can lead to a faster rate of union, and they improve the viability of the proximal pole. They can also provide an alternative to a salvage procedure with previously failed conventional bone grafting. A variety of grafts with a vascular pedicle from the dorsal and volar aspects of the distal part of the radius have been described, as well as a graft from the thumb metacarpal with a vascular pedicle (**Figures 13** through **15**).

Indications

Some general indications for the use of vascularized bone grafts are osteonecrosis of the proximal pole, symptomatic proximal pole nonunion, displaced proximal pole fractures, and failed traditional bone grafting. Some authors, however, use this type of graft for any scaphoid nonunion.

Absolute Contraindications

The following are contraindications to the use of vascular pedicle flaps based on the radius and thumb metacarpal: (1) radiocarpal and midcarpal arthritis caused by a scaphoid nonunion advanced collapse wrist, and stage II/III (radiocarpal/midcarpal arthritis) and (2) damage to the radial artery, first dorsal metacarpal artery, or dorsal carpal arch.

Relative contraindications to the procedure include previous surgery on or injury to the dorsal aspect of the wrist or distal part of the radius, which might impair the blood supply to the dorsal capsule. Caution is needed when treating patients who are smokers.

Vascularized Bone Grafts with 1,2 Intercompartmental Supraretinacular Artery

In 1991, Zaidemberg et al[17] described a bone graft source from the dorsoradial aspect of the radius with a vascular pedicle based on an ascending irrigating branch of the radial artery. The authors reported a 100% union rate in 11 patients who had a scaphoid nonunion treated with this graft, at an average time to union of 6.2 weeks. The blood supply to the dorsal aspect of the carpus has been extensively described by Sheetz et al.[18] They described several pedicles from which potential vascularized bone grafts may be harvested from the dorsum of the distal aspect of the radius. The most common of these pedicles is the 1,2 intercompartmental

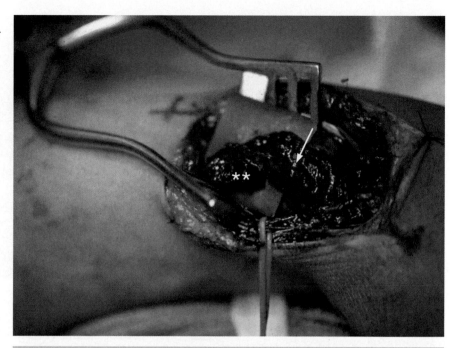

Figure 13 Vascularized bone graft (asterisks) with vascular pedicle (arrow) on the 1,2 intercompartmental supraretinacular artery. (Courtesy of David Slutsky, MD, Torrance, CA.)

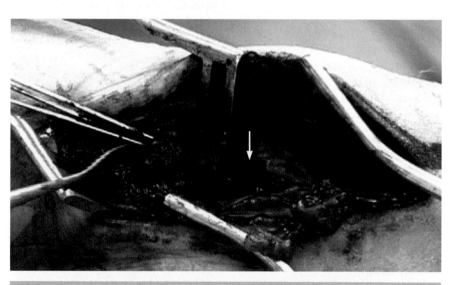

Figure 14 Volar aspect of the right wrist, showing distraction of the scaphoid nonunion site (arrow) with preplaced Kirschner wires in the distal pole (upper left). (Courtesy of David Slutsky, MD, Torrance, CA.)

supraretinacular artery, which is the term now used for the ascending irrigating branch of the radial artery.

Anatomy

The 1,2 intercompartmental supraretinacular artery branches from the radial artery at an average of 1.9 mm proximal to the radial styloid (range, –6.3 to 3.2 mm). The internal diameter of the vessel averages 0.30 mm (range, 0.14 to 0.58 mm). The pedicle length averages 22.5 mm (range, 15 to 31 mm). The graft is located approximately

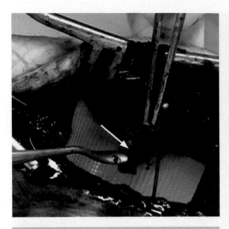

Figure 15   Volar vascularized bone graft (arrow) is elevated on the volar carpal artery pedicle held with the forceps. (Courtesy of David Slutsky, MD, Torrance, CA.)

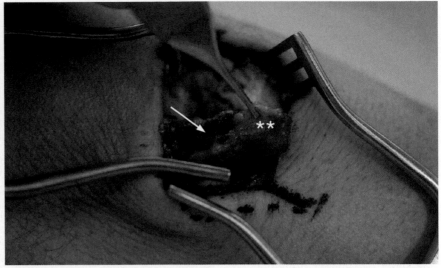

Figure 16   Dorsal view of a left wrist showing a vascularized bone graft (asterisks) pedicled on a strip of dorsal capsule (arrow). (Courtesy of David Slutsky, MD, Torrance, CA.)

10 mm (range, 8 to 18 mm) proximal to the articular surface, where it incorporates the largest number of perforator vessels.

Advantages and Disadvantages

This graft can be used as an onlay graft to act as a vascular pedicle or a structural strut graft to maintain the scaphoid length. It has a constant artery with a long pedicle. Because it is rotated 180°, the pedicle is vulnerable to kinking. Dissection of the pedicle can be tedious, and impingement and thrombosis of the pedicle over the radial styloid can occur when attempting to pass the graft volarly. It is prudent to perform a limited radial styloidectomy to decrease tension on the pedicle and facilitate volar passage.

Volar Carpal Artery Vascularized Bone Graft

Anatomy

This vascularized bone graft was initially described by Kuhlmann et al[19] and was recently popularized by Mathoulin et al.[20] The vascularized bone graft is harvested from the volar ulnar metaphysis of the distal part of the radius. It is nourished by the volar

carpal artery, which has a diameter of 0.5 to 1.0 mm. This artery originates from the radial artery at the level of the radial styloid and traverses the palmar aspect of the distal part of the radius along the distal edge of the pronator quadratus muscle. It forms a T-shaped anastomosis with the anterior interosseous artery. The average vascular pedicle length is 3 cm (range, 2 to 4.6 cm).

Advantages and Disadvantages

This vascularized bone graft has a long pedicle that is consistently present, and harvesting the volar carpal artery does not interfere with the dorsal blood supply. It is ideal for scaphoid nonunions with a humpback deformity because the volar approach provides good access to the nonunion site for débridement and simplifies the insertion of a volar wedge-shaped graft to restore scaphoid height. It is a small graft, however, and is technically difficult to raise. It cannot be used for nonunions of the distal third of the scaphoid. Because it is immediately adjacent to the radiocarpal joint, there

is a risk of fracture into the radiocarpal joint or the sigmoid notch.

Capsular-Based Vascularized Bone Graft

Anatomy

This vascularized bone graft, which was originally described by Sotereanos et al,[21] is an axial pattern flap based on the fourth extracompartment artery of the dorsal carpal arch, which extends between the anterior or posterior interosseous artery proximally and the dorsal carpal arch or fifth extracompartment artery distally. The average pedicle diameter is 0.4 mm. The pedicle length ranges between 1 and 2 cm and easily reaches the proximal third of the scaphoid (**Figures 16** through **18**).

Advantages and Disadvantages

The vascularized bone graft is based on a constant artery, and the flap is easy to dissect. The graft needs to rotate only 10° to 30° on the pedicle to reach the scaphoid, which lowers the risk of arterial kinking. A disadvantage is that it has a relatively short pedicle; hence the graft is useful only for proximal third nonunions. It can be used as an onlay

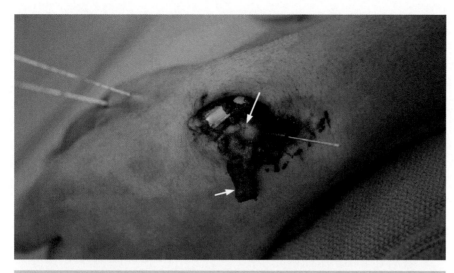

Figure 17 Intraoperative photograph illustrating the proximity of the capsular graft (vascularized bone graft [short arrow]) to the nonunion site while a headless compression screw is inserted into the proximal pole to stabilize the nonunion site (long arrow). (Courtesy of David Slutsky, MD, Torrance, CA.)

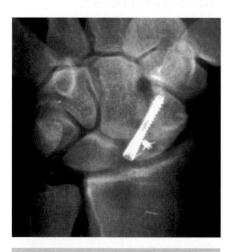

Figure 18 AP radiograph showing the relative ulnar position of the headless screw and the bone anchor that is used to prevent graft extrusion. (Courtesy of David Slutsky, MD, Torrance, CA.)

graft only, and there is the risk of a radiocarpal articular fracture.

 Video 6.2: Capsular-Based Vascularized Distal Radius Graft for Scaphoid Nonunions. David J. Slutsky, MD (5 min)

Vascularized Thumb Metacarpal Graft

Anatomy

This vascularized bone graft, as described by Bertelli et al,[22] is based on the radial branch of the first dorsal metacarpal artery. The average vessel diameter is 1 mm. The pedicle arises from the radial artery 5 to 10 mm proximal to the trapeziometacarpal joint and continues along the radial third of the dorsal side of the thumb metacarpal. The vascularized bone graft is harvested from the metacarpal head, resulting in a pedicle length of approximately 50 mm.

Advantages and Disadvantages

The pedicle can be quite long and is based on a constant artery. It can be used as an onlay or a structural graft. The pedicle is rotated 180°, which can lead to kinking. It leaves a large donor-site defect, which can lead to fracture, and it is technically difficult.

Summary

Fractures of the scaphoid are common injuries. There are several treatment options available, including percutane-

ous, arthroscopic, and open volar and dorsal approaches. There are advantages and disadvantages associated with each technique, and the surgeon should select what is most comfortable based on his or her experience. In addition, for resistant scaphoid nonunions, there are multiple vascularized bone grafting techniques to obtain union in these difficult fractures.

References

1. Gelberman RH, Menon J: The vascularity of the scaphoid bone. *J Hand Surg Am* 1980;5(5): 508-513.

2. Heinzelmann AD, Archer G, Bindra RR: Anthropometry of the human scaphoid. *J Hand Surg Am* 2007;32(7):1005-1008.

3. Russe O: Fracture of the carpal navicular: Diagnosis, nonoperative treatment, and operative treatment. *J Bone Joint Surg Am* 1960;42-A:759-768.

4. Herbert TJ, Fisher WE: Management of the fractured scaphoid using a new bone screw. *J Bone Joint Surg Br* 1984;66(1): 114-123.

5. Cooney WP, Dobyns JH, Linscheid RL: Fractures of the scaphoid: A rational approach to management. *Clin Orthop Relat Res* 1980;149:90-97.

6. Geissler WB, Slade JF: Fractures of the carpal bones, in Wolfe SW, Hotchkiss RN, Peterson WC, Kozin SH, eds: *Green's Operative Hand Surgery*, ed 6. Philadelphia, PA, Elsevier, 2010, vol 1, pp 639-707.

7. Rettig ME, Raskin KB: Retrograde compression screw fixation of acute proximal pole scaphoid fractures. *J Hand Surg Am* 1999; 24(6):1206-1210.

8. Terkelsen CJ, Jepsen JM: Treatment of scaphoid fractures with a removable cast. *Acta Orthop Scand* 1988;59(4):452-453.

9. Langhoff O, Andersen JL: Consequences of late immobilization of scaphoid fractures. *J Hand Surg Br* 1988;13(1):77-79.

10. Arora R, Gschwentner M, Krappinger D, Lutz M, Blauth M, Gabl M: Fixation of nondisplaced scaphoid fractures: Making treatment cost effective. Prospective controlled trial. *Arch Orthop Trauma Surg* 2007; 127(1):39-46.

11. Davis EN, Chung KC, Kotsis SV, Lau FH, Vijan S: A cost/utility analysis of open reduction and internal fixation versus cast immobilization for acute nondisplaced mid-waist scaphoid fractures. *Plast Reconstr Surg* 2006;117(4):1223-1238.

12. Haddad FS, Goddard NJ: Acute percutaneous scaphoid fixation: A pilot study. *J Bone Joint Surg Br* 1998;80(1):95-99.

13. Slade JF III, Geissler WB, Gutow AP, Merrell GA: Percutaneous internal fixation of selected scaphoid nonunions with an arthroscopically assisted dorsal approach. *J Bone Joint Surg Am* 2003;85-A(Suppl 4):20-32.

14. Geissler WB, Hammit MD: Arthroscopic aided fixation of scaphoid fractures. *Hand Clin* 2001; 17(4):575-588, viii.

15. Slade JF III, Grauer JN, Mahoney JD: Arthroscopic reduction and percutaneous fixation of scaphoid fractures with a novel dorsal technique. *Orthop Clin North Am* 2001;32(2):247-261.

16. Green DP: The effect of avascular necrosis on Russe bone grafting for scaphoid nonunion. *J Hand Surg Am* 1985;10(5):597-605.

17. Zaidemberg C, Siebert JW, Angrigiani C: A new vascularized bone graft for scaphoid nonunion. *J Hand Surg Am* 1991;16(3): 474-478.

18. Sheetz KK, Bishop AT, Berger RA: The arterial blood supply of the distal radius and ulna and its potential use in vascularized pedicled bone grafts. *J Hand Surg Am* 1995;20(6):902-914.

19. Kuhlmann JN, Mimoun M, Boabighi A, Baux S: Vascularized bone graft pedicled on the volar carpal artery for non-union of the scaphoid. *J Hand Surg Br* 1987; 12(2):203-210.

20. Mathoulin C, Haerle M, Vandeputte G: Vascularized bone graft in carpal bone reconstruction. *Ann Chir Plast Esthet* 2005; 50(1):43-48.

21. Sotereanos DG, Darlis NA, Dailiana ZH, Sarris IK, Malizos KN: A capsular-based vascularized distal radius graft for proximal pole scaphoid pseudarthrosis. *J Hand Surg Am* 2006;31(4):580-587.

22. Bertelli JA, Tacca CP, Rost JR: Thumb metacarpal vascularized bone graft in long-standing scaphoid nonunion: A useful graft via dorsal or palmar approach. A cohort study of 24 patients. *J Hand Surg Am* 2004;29(6): 1089-1097.

Video References

6.1: Geissler WB: Video. *Arthroscopically Assisted Fixation and Percutaneous Grafting of Scaphoid Nonunions.* Jackson, MS, 2011.

6.2: Slutsky DJ: Video. *Capsular-Based Vascularized Distal Radius Graft for Scaphoid Nonunion.* Torrance, CA, 2011.

Shoulder

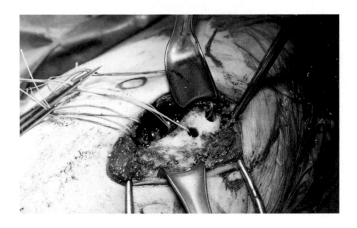

Surgical Anatomy of the Shoulder

Peter J. Millett, MD, MSc
Olivier A.J. van der Meijden, MD
Trevor Gaskill, MD

Abstract

The glenohumeral articulation is a versatile joint that requires a complex integration of bony ligamentous, musculotendinous, and neurovascular structures for proper function. Injuries resulting from dysfunction are common and potentially debilitating. Many of these injuries can be managed nonsurgically; however, if surgical treatment is indicated, a thorough knowledge of the anatomy of the shoulder girdle is critical. It is important for the surgeon to be aware of commonly used arthroscopic and surgical approaches to the glenohumeral joint along with anatomic structures at risk with each surgical approach and methods of avoiding injury.

Instr Course Lect 2012;61:87-95.

Surgical Anatomy

Bony Structures

The shoulder complex comprises several bony structures that play an important role in normal shoulder function. The clavicle is the only bony attachment that connects the glenohumeral joint to the axial skeleton. Its articulation with the sternum and acromial process allows the clavicle to function as a strut, suspending the glenohumeral joint from the axial skeleton. The broad, flat acromion is the most lateral part of the scapula and articulates with the clavicle through the diarthrodial acromioclavicular joint and also serves as an attachment site for several muscles and ligaments.

The coracoid process is an excellent landmark for many shoulder procedures. It lies medial and anterior to the glenohumeral joint and is the attachment site for the conjoined tendon of the coracobrachialis muscle and short head of the biceps muscles. The coracoacromial ligament connects the coracoid and anterolateral acromion, thereby forming the coracoacromial arch. The proximal humerus consists of the head, the surgical and anatomic neck, and the greater (lateral) and lesser (anteromedial) tuberosities. The tuberosities form attachment sites for the rotator cuff muscles, and the bicipital groove lies between them.

The glenohumeral articulation is a ball-and-socket joint formed by the shallow glenoid and the large humeral head. This lack of bony containment is unique to the glenohumeral joint and provides a wide range of motion; however, it also makes the joint prone to instability. The surrounding ligaments and muscles substantially contribute to glenohumeral stability.

Soft-Tissue Structures

The labrum surrounds the glenoid and functions to deepen the glenohumeral socket and provides an attachment site for the glenohumeral ligaments. The superior glenohumeral ligament originates at the superior glenoid tubercle and blends with the anterior rotator cuff musculature and coracohumeral ligament to form the bicep pulley near the bicipital groove. The middle glenohumeral ligament runs from the anterior labrum to the lesser tuberosity, and the inferior glenohumeral ligament connects the inferior glenoid to

Dr. Millett or an immediate family member has received royalties from Arthrex; serves as a paid consultant to Arthrex and Arthrocare; owns stock or stock options in Game Ready and VuMedi; and has received research or institutional support from Arthrex, Arthrocare, OrthoRehab, Ossur Americas, Siemens Medical Solutions USA, and Smith & Nephew. Dr. van der Meijden or an immediate family member has received nonincome support (such as equipment or services), commercially derived honoraria, or other non-research–related funding (such as paid travel) from Arthrex. Neither Dr. Gaskill nor any immediate family member has received anything of value from or owns stock in a commercial company or institution related directly or indirectly to the subject of this chapter.

the inferior humerus. Each glenohumeral ligament is believed to contribute to glenohumeral stability in various positions of glenohumeral motion.

Shoulder Musculature

Glenohumeral motion and stability are directly linked to the surrounding musculature. The deltoid consists of anterior, lateral, and posterior components separated by fibrous raphes. Its proximal attachment is to the lateral third of the clavicle anteriorly, the lateral acromion, and the scapular spine posteriorly. The deltoid muscle is innervated by branches of the axillary nerve and inserts at the deltoid tuberosity of the lateral humerus. Its primary function is abduction, flexion, and extension of the shoulder.

The coracobrachialis muscle and pectoralis major muscle lie medial to the deltoid. The two heads of the pectoralis major originate from the clavicle and sternum and insert lateral to the bicipital groove of the humerus. The pectoralis major is innervated by the medial and lateral pectoral nerves and functions primarily as a humeral adductor. The coracobrachialis and the short head of the biceps lie deep to the pectoralis major and deltoid. They originate from the coracoid process and are innervated by the musculocutaneous nerve. The coracobrachialis and the short head of the biceps serve as an important landmark for shoulder surgery because the brachial plexus and vascular structures lie just medial and deep to them.

The rotator cuff musculature exists deep to the deltoid muscle and surrounds the glenohumeral joint. It is composed of four muscles that play an important role in glenohumeral motion and dynamic shoulder stability. The subscapularis originates from the undersurface of the scapula and inserts at the lesser tuberosity. It is innervated by the upper and lower subscapular nerves and functions to internally rotate the humerus. In collaboration with the infraspinatus, the subscapularis inferiorly depresses the humerus, thereby preventing acromial impingement when the deltoid is activated. The infraspinatus and teres minor originate from the posterior scapula and insert at the greater tuberosity. They primarily function by providing an external rotation moment at different degrees of glenohumeral abduction and are innervated by the suprascapular and axillary nerve, respectively. The supraspinatus is also innervated by the suprascapular nerve and inserts at the greater humeral tuberosity. It is responsible for initiating glenohumeral abduction, which allows the deltoid to function more efficiently.

Neural Structures

The axillary nerve innervates the deltoid and teres minor muscles. It originates from the posterior cord of the brachial plexus and runs along the anterior aspect of the subscapularis muscle before passing under the inferior border of the subscapularis medial to the coracoid process. The axillary nerve forms two major branches as it passes under the inferior glenohumeral capsule and exits through the quadrangular space. One branch innervates the teres minor and posterior deltoid, and the other branch winds around the proximal humerus to innervate the lateral and anterior deltoid. In this lateral position, the average distance from the acromion to the axillary nerve is approximately 5 to 7 cm.[1-3]

The musculocutaneous nerve originates from the lateral cord of the brachial plexus and enters the muscle belly of the coracobrachialis an average of 4 to 8 cm distal to the tip of the coracoid process. From this location the nerve exits the coracobrachialis and traverses the interval between the biceps and brachialis muscles. Although the musculocutaneous nerve is not frequently encountered during surgical approaches to the glenohumeral joint, it can be injured by indiscriminant retraction of the conjoined tendon.

The suprascapular nerve originates from the upper trunk of the brachial plexus and passes beneath the trapezius muscle before it passes through the suprascapular notch along the superior edge of the scapula. It is likely most vulnerable to injury along the superior margin of the glenoid before entering the infraspinatus fossa.

Vascular Structures

The blood supply of the shoulder girdle is derived primarily from branches of the subclavian and axillary arteries. The suprascapular artery accompanies the suprascapular nerve and vein over the superior edge of the scapula. In contrast to the suprascapular nerve, the suprascapular artery passes over the transverse scapular ligament and must be protected during suprascapular nerve release. The thoracoacromial branch of the axillary artery follows the course of the coracoacromial ligament and can be injured near this location. If injury occurs, the artery usually can be easily cauterized arthroscopically. The anterior and posterior circumflex humeral arteries encircle the humerus deep to the deltoid. The posterior circumflex artery accompanies the axillary nerve and posterior circumflex vein, whereas the anterior circumflex artery arises deep to the coracobrachialis and runs along the inferior border of the subscapularis. This vessel is frequently encountered with a deltopectoral approach and is ligated before subscapularis mobilization.[4-6]

Surgical Anatomic Layers

Cooper et al[7] described the anatomy of the shoulder as consisting of four layers. Layer 1 consists of the deltoid and pectoralis major muscle bellies. Layer 2 is formed by the clavipectoral fascia, the conjoined tendon, and the coracoacromial ligament anteriorly and is posteriorly continuous with the clavipectoral fascia, with the posterior scapular fascia overlying the infraspinatus and the teres minor muscles. The third layer is composed of the deep layer of the subdeltoid bursa and underlying rotator cuff. Layer 4 is formed by the capsule of the glenohumeral joint.

Open Surgical Approaches to the Shoulder Joint

Deltopectoral Approach
Indications
The indications for a deltopectoral approach to the shoulder joint have decreased considerably over the past two decades because of the evolution of advanced arthroscopic techniques; however, this extensile approach continues to serve as a workhorse approach because it allows access to many areas of the shoulder. Currently, the deltopectoral approach is primarily used for reduction and internal fixation of proximal humerus fractures, to treat bony glenoid injuries, and in shoulder arthroplasty procedures. It can also be used to perform an inferior capsular shift, or in Bankart repair, bicep tenodesis, or rotator cuff repair if the procedure cannot be accomplished arthroscopically.

Technique
The deltopectoral approach is classically performed with the patient in the modified beach chair position. Standard procedures are used to prepare the patient, and the involved extremity is prepped free. A skin incision is made beginning just inferior to the clavicle and passes along the lateral border of the coracoid process. The incision is extended distally along the deltopectoral interval approximately 10 to 12 cm. The subcutaneous tissue is di-

vided, and the cephalic vein should be identified.

The cephalic vein marks the internervous plane between the deltoid and pectoralis major muscles, which are innervated by the axillary and pectoral nerves, respectively.[8] The cephalic vein should be carefully mobilized and may be retracted either medially or laterally. More branches requiring ligation are encountered if the cephalic vein is mobilized from the deltoid and retracted medially; however, the vein is likely easier to protect in this location. The pectoralis major is retracted medially, and the deltoid is retracted laterally to expose the clavipectoral fascia investing the strap muscles and subscapularis. After developing the subdeltoid and subpectoral spaces, a self-retaining retractor can be placed.

The clavipectoral fascia is incised from the inferior margin of the coracoacromial ligament inferiorly along the lateral border of the conjoined tendons of the coracoid process. A subcoracoid plane is then developed bluntly to identify the axillary nerve medially as it passes inferior to the subscapularis muscle. Care should be taken while retracting the conjoined tendon to prevent neurapraxia of the musculocutaneous nerve that enters the coracobrachialis muscle 5 to 8 cm distal to the coracoid process.

The arm is externally rotated, thereby tensioning the subscapularis muscle and increasing the distance between its lesser tuberosity attachment and the axillary nerve along its inferomedial border. The inferior margin of the subscapularis is marked by a triad of small vessels that must be ligated before reflecting the subscapularis insertion. The rotator interval can be incised along the inferior border of the supraspinatus tendon to provide access to the glenohumeral joint. The lesser tuberosity is identified, and the sub-

scapularis insertion is removed sharply, leaving a 1-cm stump for reattachment, or, alternatively, the lesser tuberosity may be removed with a small fleck of bone. Removal of the bone provides bone-to-bone healing that can be radiographically monitored. Regardless of the technique, it is usually possible to separate the capsule from the overlying subscapularis tendon if desired. A capsulotomy is then preformed, and access to the anterior glenohumeral joint is established (**Figure 1**).

Structures at Risk
Several neurovascular structures may be at risk with a deltopectoral approach. The cephalic vein lies within the deltopectoral interval and is an excellent landmark for its identification. It can be mobilized either medially or laterally as the interval is opened. Lateral retraction is often easier to accomplish because fewer tributaries requiring ligation are encountered entering the pectoralis compared with the deltoid. However, the vessel is more frequently injured intraoperatively with lateral mobilization because of the placement of the deltoid retractor. Although efforts are made to preserve this vessel if possible, it can be ligated if it is injured.

The musculocutaneous and axillary nerves are also occasionally injured during the deltopectoral approach. The musculocutaneous nerve is infrequently directly encountered during the surgical approach as it enters the coracobrachialis 5 to 8 cm distal to the coracoid and medial to the typical surgical exposure. Nevertheless, a traction injury can occur with exuberant traction of the conjoined tendon. Adequate subcoracoid mobilization and moderated retraction are usually successful in preventing a traction neurapraxia. The axillary nerve is also at risk during this approach. It should

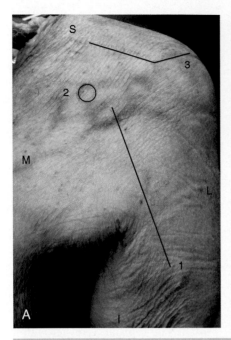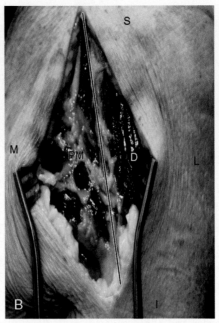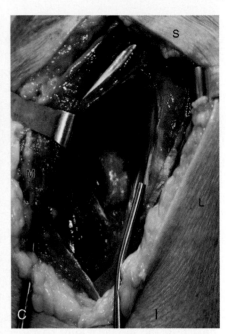

Figure 1 The deltopectoral approach to the shoulder joint demonstrated on a left cadaver shoulder. M = medial, L = lateral, S = superior, I = inferior. **A,** Markings show the skin incision (1), the coracoid process (2), and the anterior and lateral rim of the acromion (3). **B,** Markings show the pectoralis major (PM) muscle medially and the deltoid (D) muscle laterally. **C,** After performing a capsulotomy, the anterior glenohumeral joint is exposed by retracting the joint capsule and the surrounding musculature.

always be identified inferior and medial to the coracoid process after the clavipectoral fascia is incised. It can typically be palpated running inferior to the subscapularis in this location. Injury can also occur along the inferior glenoid. Several cadaver studies have reported that the nerve is within 10 to 15 mm of the inferior glenoid and can be within 2 to 3 mm of the inferior capsular pouch. Care should be taken in performing an inferior capsular release for shoulder arthroplasty or when taking tucks of capsular tissue during a capsular shift procedure. Damage to this nerve can cause dramatic functional limitations if the deltoid is completely denervated.[4-6]

Lateral Deltoid-Splitting Approach

Indications

The lateral deltoid-splitting approach provides exposure of the lateral aspect of the humeral head and rotator cuff. It is not a traditional extensile approach because of the proximity to the axillary nerve inferiorly. The lateral deltoid-splitting approach is primarily limited to rotator cuff repair and surgical fixation of greater tuberosity fractures or simple, two-part proximal humerus fractures. More recently, it is occasionally used for reverse shoulder arthroplasty if the superior rotator cuff is absent.

Technique

The patient is typically placed in the modified beach chair position and the involved extremity is prepped free. A 5-cm skin incision is made from the anterolateral tip of the acromion and extended inferiorly along the lateral aspect of the deltoid. Subcutaneous tissue is divided, and the deltoid is identified. The deltoid is split in line with its fibers from the acromion distally but should not be extended more than 5 cm from the acromion to avoid injury to the axillary nerve. The deltoid

may be split between any of its fibers, but the raphe dividing the anterior and the lateral deltoid provides a relatively avascular plane to expose underlying structures. Retraction of the deltoid musculature reveals the subdeltoid portion of the subacromial bursa. Removal of this bursa provides access to the underlying rotator cuff musculature, greater tuberosity, and subacromial space (**Figure 2**).

Structures at Risk

The primary structure at risk during the lateral deltoid-splitting approach is the lateral continuation of the axillary nerve along the inferior margin of the incision. On average, this portion of the axillary nerve is located 5 to 7 cm distal to the lateral border of the acromion deep to the deltoid muscle. If the deltoid split is not extended more than 5 cm distal to the acromion, injury to the axillary nerve is unlikely. Injury to the nerve in this location can poten-

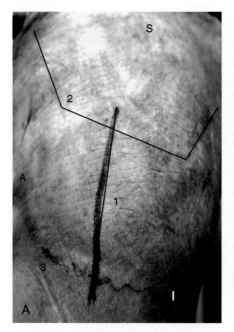
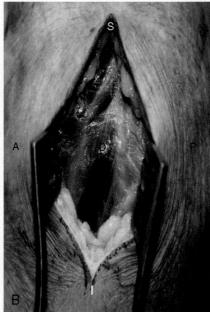
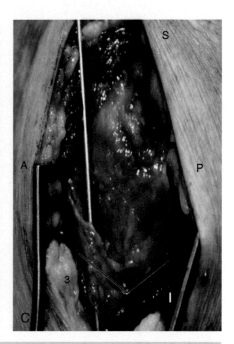

Figure 2 Lateral deltoid-splitting approach demonstrated on a left cadaver shoulder. A = anterior, P = posterior, S = superior, I = inferior. **A,** Markings show the skin incision (1), the lateral aspect of the acromion (2), and the suspected site of axillary nerve (3). **B,** Markings show the deltoid muscle (D) after the skin is incised and the subcutaneous tissue is divided. **C,** Markings show the suspected site of the axillary nerve (3) after splitting and retracting the deltoid muscle.

tially cause denervation of the lateral or anterior deltoid and numbness along the lateral deltoid.[4-6]

Posterior Glenohumeral Approach

Indications

The indications for a posterior approach to the glenohumeral joint have decreased as advanced arthroscopic techniques have emerged. This approach is still frequently used to treat recurrent posterior shoulder dislocations, either by performing a posteroinferior capsular shift or with bony reconstruction of the posterior glenoid deficiency. In certain circumstances, the posterior approach may also be used to perform a glenoid osteotomy or for internal fixation of scapular or glenoid fractures.

Technique

A posterior approach to the glenohumeral joint may be performed with the patient in the modified beach chair or

the lateral decubitus positions. The involved extremity is prepped and draped free. A linear incision is made approximately 2 cm medial to the posterolateral border of the acromion. The incision is begun just inferior to the spine of the scapula and extended distally approximately 7 to 8 cm. The subcutaneous tissues are divided, thereby exposing the posterior deltoid and underlying musculature.

The arm is abducted and externally rotated slightly to relax the posterior deltoid. This technique allows the deltoid to be retracted laterally to expose the underlying teres minor and major musculature medially and the long head of the triceps more laterally. An internervous plane exists between the infraspinatus (suprascapular nerve) and teres minor (axillary nerve) muscles. This interval is developed by retracting the infraspinatus superiorly and the teres minor inferiorly to expose the posterior glenohumeral joint capsule. The capsule is tagged and in-

cised and provides access to the posterior glenoid and humerus (**Figure 3**).

Structures at Risk

Two structures are primarily at risk using the posterior approach to the glenohumeral joint. The axillary nerve emerges from the quadrilateral space between the teres major and minor muscles as it proceeds along the lateral aspect of the humerus deep to the deltoid. If dissection is inadvertently carried through the teres minor and teres major interval, injury to the axillary nerve or the posterior circumflex humeral artery may occur. It is important to precisely identify the appropriate surgical interval between the infraspinatus and teres minor to avoid iatrogenic injury to these structures. Less commonly, the suprascapular nerve can be injured beneath the infraspinatus medial to the glenoid. Although the suprascapular nerve can be injured if dissection proceeds too medially, it is primarily injured by exuberant retrac-

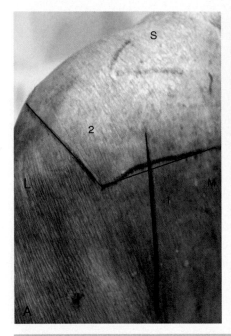 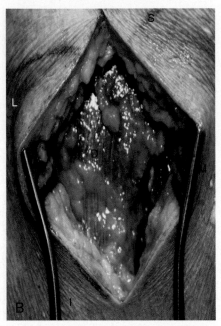 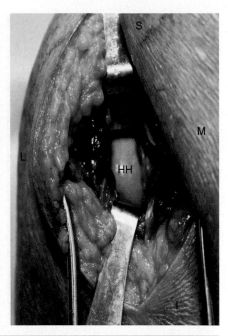

Figure 3 Posterior approach to the glenohumeral joint demonstrated on a left cadaver shoulder. M = medial, L = lateral, S = superior, I = inferior. **A,** Markings show the skin incision (1) and the lateral aspect of the acromion (2). **B,** Markings show the deltoid muscle (D) after the skin is incised and the subcutaneous tissue is divided. **C,** Markings show the posterior aspect of the humeral head (HH) after incision of the posterior joint capsule.

tion of the muscle. Careful mobilization and retraction of the infraspinatus and teres minor will minimize the risk of traction injury to the nerve.[4-6]

Arthroscopic Treatment Considerations
Relevant Anatomy
Arthroscopic shoulder surgery has dramatically improved the diagnosis and treatment of shoulder injuries. Anatomically, the shallow ball-and-socket joint and sizable capsule make the joint ideal for arthroscopic treatment; however, the thick muscular layers and the presence of neurovascular structures require accurate portal placement.

A thorough knowledge of the anatomy of the surrounding neurovascular structures is important to the shoulder arthroscopist. Anteriorly, the neurovascular structures at risk for injury with aberrant portal placement include the axillary and musculocutaneous nerves, the cephalic vein, and the

thoracoacromial artery. The axillary and musculocutaneous nerves both lie medial and distal to the coracoid process. If portals are placed superior or lateral to the coracoid, the axillary and musculocutaneous nerves are unlikely to be injured. Lateral portal placement, however, risks injury to the cephalic vein running within the deltopectoral interval. If the anterior portal is placed within the rotator interval, risk to the cephalic vein is minimal. Branches of the thoracoacromial artery also may be injured with superiorly placed portals used to enter the subacromial space near the coracoacromial ligament. If these branches are inadvertently damaged, they are usually easily coagulated arthroscopically.

Posterior portal placement also puts several neurovascular structures at risk. The axillary nerve exits the axillary pouch through the quadrangular space and courses around the proximal humerus deep to the deltoid at 6 to 7 cm (on average) distal to the acromion.

Only very inferior posterior portal placement should put the nerve at risk in this location. The suprascapular nerve innervates the supraspinatus and infraspinatus muscles. It runs through the suprascapular notch medial to the coracoclavicular ligaments, enters the supraspinatus fossa deep to its muscle belly, wraps lateral to the scapular spine, and terminates within the infraspinatus fossa. The suprascapular nerve may be at risk with posterior portal placement situated several centimeters medial to its ideal location.

Standard Portal Placement
Indications
As advanced arthroscopic techniques emerge and instrumentation improves, more procedures that have traditionally been performed open can be accomplished arthroscopically. Current indications for arthroscopic treatment include rotator cuff tears, long head of the biceps and superior labral injuries, labral detachment, and arthrofibrosis

of the shoulder. More recent arthroscopic applications include suprascapular nerve decompression and transcapular axillary nerve and brachial plexus exploration.

Basic Technique

A basic understanding of the principles of arthroscopic portal placement is important to facilitate safe portal placement. Anatomic landmarks should be used to estimate the appropriate portal location. Because the anatomy of each patient will differ slightly, an 18-gauge spinal needle should be used to confirm (before making the skin incision) that the location of the portal is appropriate to treat the suspected glenohumeral injury. Next, a No. 11 blade scalpel is used to make a 5- to 6-mm incision just through the skin and subcutaneous tissue. Because arthroscopic portals are placed blindly, a blunt trocar should always used. This method provides an added measure of security when placing portals in close proximity to neurovascular structures.

Although outside-in portal placement techniques are most commonly used, familiarity with inside-out techniques may occasionally be useful. After an initial arthroscopic portal is established, a switching stick or other device can be advanced from the interior to the exterior of the joint to localize other arthroscopic portals. This technique is most frequently used to establish anterior portals after a standard posterior portal is established. The disadvantage to this technique is that secondary portal placement is constrained by the placement of the initial portal. Therefore, there is less freedom for portal placement compared with outside-in techniques. When placing portals in sensitive areas close to neurovascular structures, a Seldinger-type technique can be used. A guidewire or switching stick is placed, and cannulated dilators are sequentially passed before placing the working portal cannula.

Specific Portal Techniques

Knowledge of bony landmarks of the shoulder will aid the surgeon in portal placement (**Figure 4**).

Anterior and Posterior Portals

In a manner similar to that used in other shoulder procedures, the patient is placed in the modified beach chair position. Standard methods are used to prepare the patient, and the extremity is draped free. The posterior and anterior portals are commonly used in shoulder surgery and are interchangeable as viewing and working portals. The posterior portal is typically established first for visualization of the glenohumeral joint. This portal is traditionally placed 2 cm inferior to and 1 cm lateral to the posteroinferior border of the acromion; however, portal placement will vary based on the expected intra-articular pathology. Using the coracoid as a guide, the arthroscopic trocar is introduced into the glenohumeral joint. The posterocentral portal differs slightly in that it is placed in line with the glenoid, allowing easier passage of the arthroscope anteriorly if necessary. Although the trocar may pass between the infraspinatus and teres minor, it more frequently travels through the substance of the infraspinatus muscle.[9]

The anterior portal is typically placed half the distance between the coracoid process and anterolateral acromion, although its placement should again be modified based on intra-articular pathology. Typically, a spinal needle is used to localize the portal within the rotator interval before cannula insertion. Although most glenohumeral joint pathology can be treated through these portals (**Figure 5**), several others are frequently used for more specialized tasks.

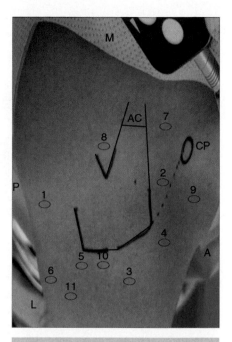

Figure 4 Superior view of a left shoulder with bony landmarks and possible portal placements marked. M = medial, L= lateral, A = anterior, P = posterior, CP = coracoid process, AC = acromioclavicular joint, 1 = standard posterior portal, 2 = standard anterior portal, 3 = standard lateral portal, 4 = anterolateral portal, 5 = posterolateral portal, 6 = posteroinferolateral portal, 7 = subclavian portal, 8 = Neviaser portal, 9 = anteroinferior portal, 10 = portal of Wilmington, 11 = trans-rotator cuff portal.

Lateral Portals

Anterolateral and posterolateral portals are frequently used to provide access to the subacromial space to perform an arthroscopic rotator cuff repair, subacromial decompression, acromioplasty, or suprascapular nerve decompression. These portals are typically located approximately 2 cm distal to the lateral border of the acromion and 1 cm from the respective anterior or posterior corners of the acromion. No structures are jeopardized by these portals if they are not placed extremely distally, where damage can occur to the axillary nerve.

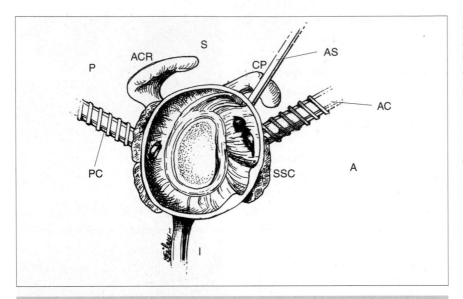

Figure 5 Illustration showing anterior and posterior intra-articular portal placement viewed laterally. The anterior portal is placed in the rotator interval between the supraspinatus and subscapularis muscle. A = anterior, P = posterior, S = superior, I = inferior, AC = anterior canula, PC = posterior canula, AS = arthroscope, ACR = acromion, CP = coracoid process, SSC = subscapularis muscle. (Reproduced from Millet PJ, Clavert P, Hatch GR III, Warner JJ: Recurrent posterior shoulder instability. *J Am Acad Orthop Surg* 2006;14(8): 464-476.)

Posteroinferolateral Portal

A posteroinferolateral portal can be placed approximately 5 to 6 cm distal to and in line with the posterolateral corner of the acromion and provides improved access to the inferior glenohumeral pouch. From this portal, inferior humeral osteophytes can be removed and inferior glenoid anchors can be placed to complete an inferior capsular shift. It can also be used to perform a transcapular axillary nerve decompression for quadrilateral space syndrome. The posteroinferior lateral portal is in close proximity to the axillary nerve as it passes through the axillary space. The axillary nerve travels anteromedially to posterolaterally as it passes beneath the glenohumeral capsule. To prevent iatrogenic injury to the axillary nerve, the portal should enter the glenohumeral joint just anterior to the posterior band of the glenohumeral ligament at the junction of its medial and middle thirds.

Subclavian Portal

The subclavian portal was created to facilitate rotator cuff repairs by allowing more direct access to rotator cuff tissues for passage of penetrating instruments. It is located 1 to 2 cm medial to the acromioclavicular joint (just medial to the coracoid process) and directly under the clavicle. The trocar is then advanced anterior and inferior to the acromioclavicular joint before entering the subacromial bursa. From this portal, rotator cuff penetrating devices can be used to pass stitches through the rotator cuff after anchors have been placed in the humeral head. Medial or inferior placement may endanger the subclavian vascular structures or the brachial plexus.

Neviaser Portal

The Neviaser portal is also known as the supraclavicular fossa portal. Its was initially described as an inflow portal, but it is also useful for arthroscopic re-

pair of superior labrum anterior and posterior lesions.[10] It is created in the soft spot defined by the clavicle anteriorly, the acromion laterally, and the scapular spine posteriorly. The portal is typically created using an outside-in technique, passing the arthroscopic trocar slightly laterally and posteriorly. Although this is a relatively safe position for portal placement, it is typically a mean distance of 24 mm from the suprascapular artery and 26 mm from the suprascapular nerve. Passing the arthroscopic trocar slightly laterally will help avoid injury to these structures because they lie more medially than the portal incision.

Anteroinferior Portal

The anteroinferior or 5-o'clock portal was developed to improve arthroscopic access for Bankart repairs. This portal provides perpendicular access to the anteroinferior glenoid for inferior anchor placement and inferior capsular shift procedures. The 5-o'clock portal was initially described using an inside-out technique with a switching stick from the standard posterior viewing portal. This results in portal placement that exits the skin in an anteroinferior position near neurovascular structures. Cadaver studies have shown the axillary artery is in closest proximity to the 5-o'clock portal and can be within 13 mm of the portal. The axillary nerve and cephalic vein are also at risk at approximately 15 and 17 mm from the trocar.[9] Some physicians recommend establishing this portal using an outside-in technique that allows a more lateral and less inferior starting point, which may provide a larger margin of safety while facilitating anteroinferior glenohumeral joint access.[11]

Port of Wilmington and Trans-Rotator Cuff Portals

A skin incision for the port of Wilmington portal is established 1 cm anterior and 1 cm lateral to the posterolateral corner of the acromion. An arthroscopic trocar is then advanced in a direction that allows approximately a 45° angle of approach to the posterosuperior glenoid and traverses the rotator cuff. A similar trans-rotator cuff portal was described by O'Brien et al.[12] Typically, this portal is made approximately 2 cm lateral and 1 cm posterior to the posterolateral acromion. This portal also passes through the rotator cuff to the posterosuperior aspect of the labrum. These portals can facilitate anchor placement and suture management of superior labrum anterior and posterior lesion repairs with a large posterior component. These approaches pose little risk to neurovascular structures, but the portals uniformly violate the supraspinatus or infraspinatus tendon—although the clinical significance is unknown.

Summary

The glenohumeral articulation is a versatile and complex joint. Bony, ligamentous, musculotendinous, and neurovascular structures each play a key role in joint function. In patients treated with arthroscopic shoulder procedures, a thorough knowledge of the surgical anatomy and approaches to the glenohumeral joint are mandatory to optimize joint function.

References

1. Bailie DS, Moseley B, Lowe WR: Surgical anatomy of the posterior shoulder: Effects of arm position and anterior-inferior capsular shift. *J Shoulder Elbow Surg* 1999; 8(4):307-313.

2. Burkhead WZ, Scheinberg RR, Box G: Surgical anatomy of the axillary nerve. *J Shoulder Elbow Surg* 1992;1:31-36.

3. Uz A, Apaydin N, Bozkurt M, Elhan A: The anatomic branch pattern of the axillary nerve. *J Shoulder Elbow Surg* 2007;16(2): 240-244.

4. Craig EV: Surgical exposures of the shoulder and elbow, in McCollister Evarts C, ed: *Surgery of the Musculoskeletal System*, ed 2. New York, NY, Churchill Livingstone, 1990, vol 2, pp 1356-1375.

5. Becker DA, Cofield RH: Anatomy and surgical approaches to the shoulder, in Morrey BF, ed: *Reconstructive Surgery of the Joints*, ed 2. New York, NY, Churchill Livingstone, 1996, vol 2, pp 705-727.

6. Campbell WC: Surgical approach to the shoulder, in Crenshaw AH, ed: *Campbell's Operative Orthopaedics,* ed 7. St. Louis, MO, CV Mosby, 1987, pp 88-98.

7. Cooper DE, O'Brien SJ, Warren RF: Supporting layers of the glenohumeral joint: An anatomic study. *Clin Orthop Relat Res* 1993; 289:144-155.

8. Zlotolow DA, Catalano LW III, Barron OA, Glickel SZ: Surgical exposures of the humerus. *J Am Acad Orthop Surg* 2006;14(13): 754-765.

9. Meyer M, Graveleau N, Hardy P, Landreau P: Anatomic risks of shoulder arthroscopy portals: Anatomic cadaveric study of 12 portals. *Arthroscopy* 2007;23(5): 529-536.

10. Neviaser TJ: Arthroscopy of the shoulder. *Orthop Clin North Am* 1987;18(3):361-372.

11. Lo IK, Lind CC, Burkhart SS: Glenohumeral arthroscopy portals established using an outside-in technique: Neurovascular anatomy at risk. *Arthroscopy* 2004; 20(6):596-602.

12. O'Brien SJ, Allen AA, Coleman SH, Drakos MC: The trans-rotator cuff approach to SLAP lesions: technical aspects for repair and a clinical follow-up of 31 patients at a minimum of 2 years. *Arthroscopy* 2002;18(4):372-377.

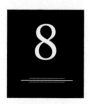

Decision Making in Massive Rotator Cuff Tears

Stephan G. Pill, MD, MSPT
Jason Phillips, MD
Michael J. Kissenberth, MD
Richard J. Hawkins, MD

Abstract

Although many definitions have been used to define massive rotator cuff tears, a tear is generally considered massive if it is greater than 5 cm in diameter. Most massive rotator cuff tears are chronic, and patients commonly present with an insidious onset of gradually worsening pain and weakness in the involved shoulder. In rare situations, patients without preexisting rotator cuff disease may experience an acute injury and present with a massive rotator cuff tear. A thorough history and physical examination is important to establish the diagnosis and determine the most appropriate treatment. Because most massive rotator cuff tears are chronic in nature, the quality of the underlying rotator cuff tissue is often poor, making repair difficult. Other treatment options include physical therapy, biceps tenotomy or tenodesis, suprascapular nerve release, rotator cuff repair with tissue augmentation, tendon transfer, and reconstruction with hemiarthroplasty or reverse shoulder arthroplasty. Integrating findings from the history, physical examination, and diagnostic imaging is the basis of clinical decision making.

Instr Course Lect 2012;61:97-111.

Many definitions have been used to describe the size of rotator cuff tears. Massive tears are typically considered 5 cm or greater in the largest dimension.[1] Some physicians consider the area when defining tear size by combining the anteroposterior and mediolateral dimensions of the tear.[2] At least two tendons are typically involved in massive tears, which may disrupt the balanced force couples required for proper shoulder function. Most massive tears occur within the posterosuperior rotator cuff, involving the supraspinatus and infraspinatus tendons. Anterosuperior tears, which also involve the subscapularis, are less common.

Massive rotator cuff tears can be challenging to manage. Patients may present with varying degrees of pain, weakness, and physical impairment. A detailed history and physical examination is paramount to establishing the correct diagnosis, formulating appropriate treatment options, and counseling patients on appropriate expectations. Imaging may help confirm the diagnosis, stage the process, identify concomitant disease, and help in management planning, which may include surgical intervention. Massive rotator cuff tears, if repaired, are associated with a high retear rate, and obtaining a tension-free repair at the time of surgery can be technically demanding, if not impossible. Other reasons for failure include poor tissue quality, tendon hypovascularity, scarring of the retracted tendons, and, importantly, fatty infiltration and atrophy of the muscles. The orthopaedic surgeon should be aware of all these factors when evaluating patients with massive rotator cuff tears.

Patient History

Patients with massive rotator cuff tears typically present with pain. The pain is

None of the following authors or any immediate family member has received anything of value from or owns stock in a commercial company or institution related directly or indirectly to the subject of this chapter: Dr. Pill, Dr. Phillips, and Dr. Kissenberth. Dr. Hawkins or an immediate family member has received royalties from DePuy and Össur; has received research or institutional support from Arthrocare, DJ Orthopaedics, Breg, Smith & Nephew, Medica, and OrthoRehab; and serves as a board member, owner, officer, or committee member of the Orthopaedic Learning Center and the Orthopaedic Research Foundation of the Carolinas.

often related to activity and worse at night. Weakness and poor function are other common symptoms. Obtaining information on the onset and progression of symptoms over time is critical in differentiating acute traumatic, chronic atraumatic, and acute-on-chronic rotator cuff tears. For example, a patient with a previously well-functioning shoulder who sustains a fall may have an acute traumatic tear. In the absence of an already degenerative rotator cuff, such a tear is rare. In general, patients with acute traumatic tears are younger than patients with chronic atraumatic tears. With an acute tear, the retracted tendon edge is less likely to be scarred, the quality of the tendon is often good, and the muscle is free from atrophy and fatty infiltration, in contrast with chronic tears. These factors may enable a robust, tension-free repair, and patients may benefit from early surgical treatment before the development of tendon, muscle, and possibly glenohumeral degeneration. However, because there is a 28% incidence of full-thickness rotator cuff tears in asymptomatic patients older than 60 years, older adults who present with a rotator cuff tear after an acute injury cannot be assumed to have normal underlying rotator cuff tissue.[3]

In contrast, a patient with worsening pain and weakness may have a chronic atraumatic or acute-on-chronic tear. Patients with an acute-on-chronic tear may present with worsening pain and decompensation of shoulder function that occurs at intervals following an acute injury. Patients with chronic atraumatic tears often present with more subtle pain and weakness that have gradually worsened over time. These patients are usually older and less active. The tendons in acute-on-chronic and chronic atraumatic tears tend to have poor tissue quality.

A thorough patient history is important to rule out other causes of shoulder pain. The history should include questions relating to the cervical spine, such as those regarding the presence of neck pain and radiculopathy. Complete past medical and social histories should be obtained to determine the patient's overall health status and activity level. Low-demand patients and those with multiple comorbidities may not be acceptable candidates for surgical treatment. Alternatively, older patients who are healthy enough for surgical treatment may achieve a more predictable functional outcome and have a better-tolerated postoperative recovery with reverse shoulder arthroplasty rather than with rotator cuff repair.[4] The patient should be preoperatively counseled about realistic expectations if a surgical repair is planned. Patients must be willing to comply with the prolonged postoperative immobilization period. Patients also should be informed about the significant risks of failure to heal and retearing the tendons.

Physical Examination

A thorough physical examination for a patient with a massive rotator cuff tear begins with an inspection of the shoulders. Patients with suspected massive rotator cuff tears should be appropriately draped to allow visualization of both shoulders. Disposable, sleeveless halter-top garments can be helpful for examining female patients. The contours of both shoulders should be compared. The involved shoulder may appear swollen from the escape of synovial fluid into the subdeltoid space. There may be atrophy in the supraspinatus or infraspinatus fossae, especially in chronic tears. Infraspinatus fossa atrophy is a hallmark of large, long-standing rotator cuff tears. Atrophy of the supraspinatus can be more difficult to evaluate because of the overlying

trapezius muscle. Patients with acute traumatic tears typically have preserved muscle bulk. A prominent humeral head may occur in patients with anterosuperior escape. A Popeye deformity, which frequently occurs in patients with a ruptured long head of the biceps tendon, may be evident.

Next, range of motion can be assessed. Passive motion is often preserved in patients with a massive rotator cuff tear, although minimal stiffness at the end ranges of motion may be present. More pronounced stiffness in massive tears is rare, suggesting frozen shoulder or, more likely, glenohumeral arthritis. Cuff tear arthropathy may develop in patients with long-standing massive rotator cuff tears. Although plain radiographs will help diagnose cuff tear arthropathy, deep bone-on-bone crepitus may be appreciated when assessing range of motion in these patients. The crepitus is exaggerated when evaluating resisted elevation. Often, active range of motion is deficient because of weakness and/or pain; however, it is not uncommon for a patient with a large or massive rotator cuff tear to have normal active range of motion.

If shoulder elevation is painful, a diagnostic injection can be useful. A subacromial injection of lidocaine may eliminate pain and allow a better assessment of rotator cuff strength. The postinjection evaluation is helpful in establishing the diagnosis and planning the next step in managing the disorder. Some patients will regain full, active range of motion after the pain is eliminated, whereas other patients may have continued weakness. This weakness may be profound if the tear extends inferior to the humeral equator, thus interrupting the coronal force couple between the deltoid and the rotator cuff. The term pseudoparalysis has been used to describe the phenomenon of not being able to elevate the arm because of a massive rotator cuff tear. Because of anterosuperior humeral head escape, a patient with pseudoparalysis will be unable to achieve any active elevation (< 30°) when asked to raise his or her arm. Pseudoparalysis is one of the hallmark signs of a large or massive rotator cuff tear, in which the patient has almost no active elevation but full passive elevation.

For patients who do not have pseudoparalysis, the Jobe empty can test can be used to isolate the supraspinatus from the deltoid (**Figure 1**). It is done with the shoulder internally rotated and elevated 90° in the scapular plane. Both shoulders can be tested simultaneously to compare strength. Weakness with an isometric break test is consistent with a supraspinatus tear. Because pain can confuse the interpretation of weakness, a lidocaine injection may be useful in painful shoulders.

Patients with rotator cuff tears often present with external rotation weakness, and a positive external rotation lag sign (ERLS) is an indication of massive rotator cuff tears (**Figure 2**). Patients with an ERLS cannot maintain external rotation of the shoulder when positioned by the examiner. An ERLS with the arm at the side has been shown to be sensitive and specific for infraspinatus fatty degeneration.[5] Hertel et al[6] found that as the size of a posterosuperior rotator cuff tear increases, so does the amount of external lag. The teres minor is another important contributor to external rotation and may hypertrophy after infraspinatus injury.[5] Walch et al[5] found a positive hornblower sign to be 100% sensitive and 93% specific for diagnosing irreparable degeneration of the teres minor on a CT scan. A patient with a positive hornblower sign has an ERLS in 90° of abduction (**Figure 2,** *D* through *F*). Similarly, Otis et al[7] used an in vitro shoulder model to demon-

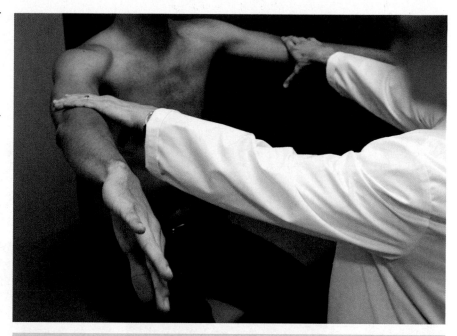

Figure 1 The Jobe empty can test is done with the shoulder internally rotated and elevated 90° in the scapular plane. Both shoulders can be tested simultaneously to better compare strength. Weakness with an isometric break test is consistent with a supraspinatus tear.

strate that the infraspinatus undergoes a decrease in its rotational moment arm in abduction; however, the teres minor maintained its moment arm with increasing abduction angles, making it a more effective external rotator in this position.

The subscapularis can be evaluated with a lift-off test, belly-press test, or bear-hug test. Patients with large tears of the subscapularis may also have increased passive external rotation of the shoulder. In 1991, Gerber and Krushell[8] described the lift-off test whereby the patient places the dorsum of his or her hand on the lower back and is asked to raise the hand off the back (**Figure 3**). The ability to actively lift the dorsum of the hand off the back constitutes a normal lift-off test, whereas the inability to lift the hand suggests subscapularis dysfunction. Patients with subscapularis dysfunction may "cheat" and lift the hand away from the back by extending the elbow with the use of the triceps instead of

the subscapularis; the examiner should not misinterpret this ability to lift the hand and conclude that the patient has a normal subscapularis. Hertel et al[6] described a modification of the lift-off test, called the internal rotation lag sign, in which the examiner passively positions the patient's hand in a lifted-off position and then releases it. The test is considered positive if the patient cannot maintain the lifted-off position. This test was found to be more sensitive than the lift-off test. Because many patients with shoulder pain or stiffness have difficulty positioning the arm behind the back, they cannot be tested with the lift-off test. To evaluate patients with pain or limited range of motion, Gerber et al[9] described the belly-press test, which evaluates the subscapularis by having the patient exert pressure with the palm of the hand on the abdomen while the shoulder is maximally internally rotated (**Figure 4**). If the elbow remains in front of the trunk and the wrist does not flex

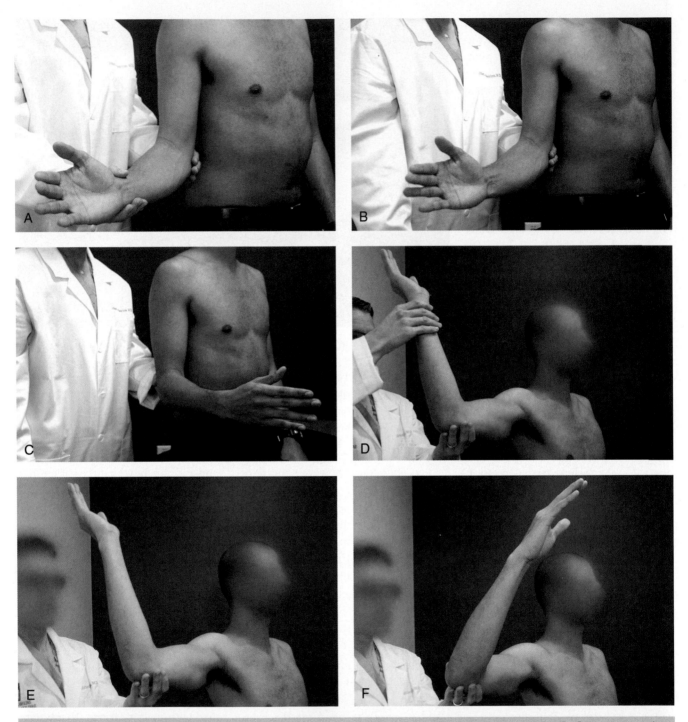

Figure 2 **A,** To test for the ERLS, the shoulder is positioned in external rotation by the examiner. **B,** Once the arm is released, a patient with an intact posterosuperior cuff can maintain the shoulder in the externally rotated position. **C,** In a patient with a large posterosuperior rotator cuff tear, the ERLS will be positive, with the arm falling into internal rotation. An ERLS with the arm at the side has been shown to be sensitive and specific for infraspinatus fatty degeneration. **D,** The ERLS can also be tested with the arm in 90° of abduction, which preferentially challenges the teres minor. **E,** A patient with an intact teres minor can maintain the position. **F,** If the arm falls into internal rotation, the patient may have a torn teres minor.

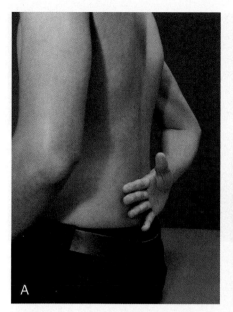
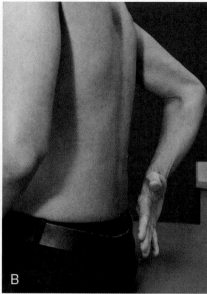
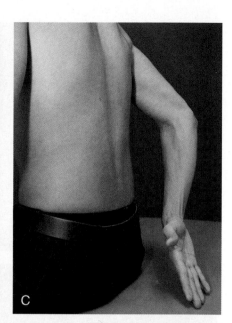

Figure 3 **A,** In the lift-off test, the patient places the dorsum of his or her hand over the lumbar spine. **B,** The patient is asked to raise the hand off his or her back. The ability to actively lift the dorsum of the hand off the back constitutes a normal lift-off test. The inability to lift the hand suggests subscapularis dysfunction. **C,** Patients with subscapularis dysfunction may "cheat" and lift the hand away from the back by extending the elbow, therefore using the triceps instead of the subscapularis.

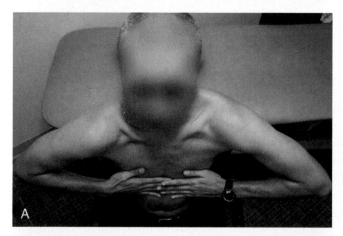
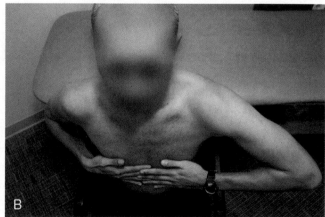
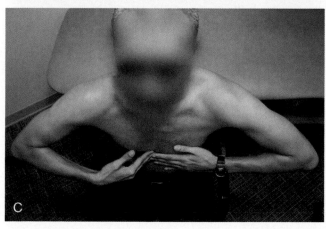

Figure 4 **A,** In the belly-press test, the patient places both hands just inferior to the xiphoid process and maximally internally rotates the shoulders while keeping the wrists straight. The patient is asked to exert pressure on the abdomen. If the elbow remains in front of the trunk and the wrist does not flex, the subscapularis tendon is considered functional and the test is normal. The test is considered positive if the patient cannot maintain maximum internal rotation, and the patient exerts pressure on the abdomen by extending the shoulder (**B**) or by flexing the wrist (**C**).

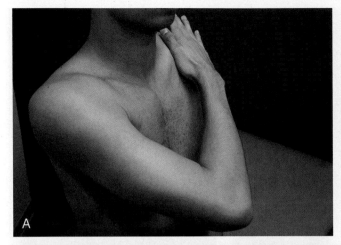

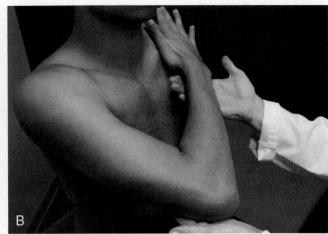

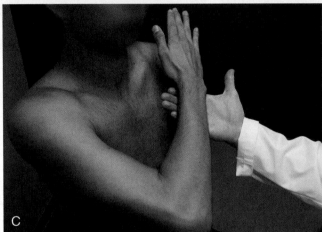

Figure 5 **A,** In a bear-hug test in 45° elevation, the patient places his or her palm on the contralateral shoulder with the fingers extended, the elbow anterior to the body, and the injured shoulder in 45° of elevation. **B,** The examiner tries to lift the patient's hand off the shoulder by applying an external rotation force perpendicular to the forearm. **C,** If the patient cannot maintain the hand on the shoulder or exhibits weakness compared with the contralateral shoulder, the patient may have a tear involving the upper portion of the subscapularis.

while pressure is exerted, the subscapularis tendon is considered functional and the test is normal. The test is considered positive if the patient cannot maintain maximum internal rotation and the patient exerts pressure on the abdomen by extending the shoulder or by flexing the wrist. More recently, Barth et al[10] described the bear-hug test in which the patient places the palm of the involved extremity on the contralateral shoulder with the fingers extended and the elbow anterior to the body (**Figure 5**). While the patient attempts to hold that position, the examiner tries to lift the patient's hand off the shoulder by applying an external rotation force perpendicular to the forearm. The test is considered positive if the patient is unable to hold the hand on the shoulder or has greater

than 20% weakness compared with the contralateral side. The authors found the bear-hug and belly-press tests to be more sensitive than the lift-off test in diagnosing subscapularis tears at the time of arthroscopy. Recent electromyographic studies showed that the bear-hug test (done with a shoulder elevation of 45°) and the belly-press test challenge the upper portion of the subscapularis, whereas the bear-hug test done in 90° of shoulder elevation and the lift-off test activate the lower aspect of the subscapularis.[11,12]

Palpation is an important component of the physical examination. Patients with chronic massive rotator cuff tears are particularly at risk for tearing in the long head of the biceps tendon. The examiner should determine if the long head of the biceps tendon is still

intact and should palpate to determine if groove tenderness is present. A positive Speed test, which consists of pain in the biceps area with resisted elevations with an extended elbow, supports the finding of biceps pathology. A patient with a chief report of pain and preserved motion may benefit from biceps tenotomy or tenodesis even if rotator cuff repair is not possible.[13] Repairing a massive rotator cuff tear in a patient with well-preserved motion and other causes of pain such as biceps tendinopathy may lead to unsatisfactory results if shoulder motion is lost. Palpation of the shoulder may also reveal tenderness at the acromioclavicular joint. Cross-body adduction is also useful for detecting acromioclavicular pathology. Patients with these findings may benefit from a distal clavicle exci-

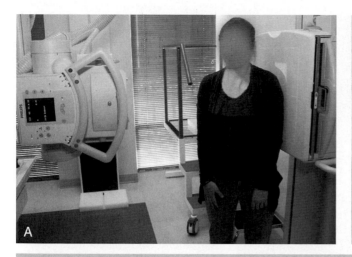
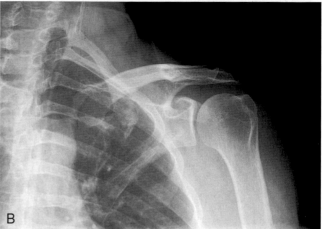

Figure 6 **A,** Photograph of patient positioning to obtain a true AP radiograph of the glenohumeral joint, which is taken at a right angle to the scapula, with the x-ray beam tilted approximately 35° to 45° toward the midline. **B,** With this view, the glenohumeral joint space and position of the humeral head in the coronal plane (acromiohumeral interval distance) can be determined.

sion at the time of surgery, especially if an acromioclavicular joint injection helps relieve pain. Codman[14] suggested that a massive rotator cuff tear may be palpated as a sulcus at the greater tuberosity. Wolf and Agrawal[15] later referred to the transdeltoid palpation of a rotator cuff tear as the rent test and found it to be 95.7% sensitive and 96.8% specific for detecting full-thickness rotator cuff tears in 109 patients undergoing shoulder arthroscopy.

Other causes for shoulder pain should be considered. The cervical spine should be evaluated because spondylosis and radiculopathy can cause pain and weakness in the shoulder. A neurologic assessment should be done to evaluate for Parsonage-Turner syndrome, brachial plexopathy, or suprascapular neuropathy. These entities can cause weakness and atrophy, which can mimic a rotator cuff tear. A diagnostic shoulder injection can be useful when it is difficult to determine the contribution of spine and shoulder pathology to the overall clinical picture.

Radiographic Evaluation

Radiographic evaluation of all patients with a suspected rotator cuff tear should include a true AP radiograph of the glenohumeral joint and axillary and supraspinatus outlet views. It is important to understand the difference between obtaining a true AP radiograph of the glenohumeral joint rather than an AP radiograph of the shoulder, which is taken in the plane of the thorax. Many AP radiographs are not true AP views and result in overlap of the humeral head on the glenoid and an oblique view of the glenoid. In contrast, a true AP radiograph of the glenohumeral joint is taken at a right angle to the scapula, with the x-ray beam tilted approximately 35° to 45° toward the midline (**Figure 6**). With this view, the glenohumeral joint space and position of the humeral head in the coronal plane are determined. The axillary radiograph is obtained with the x-ray beam directed into the patient's axilla with the arm abducted (**Figure 7**). The optimal amount of abduction is 90°; however, this amount of abduction may not be possible because of pain or stiffness. An adequate axillary radiograph is captured with as little as 40° of abduction. The supraspinatus outlet view is taken in the plane of the scapula from posterior to

anterior with a 10° caudal tilt, which provides visualization of the subacromial space (**Figure 8**).

Good-quality plain radiographs can provide much information. The presence or absence of glenohumeral arthritis is an important factor in formulating a treatment plan for patients with massive rotator cuff tears because treatment algorithms are related to the amount of degenerative changes present on both the AP and axillary radiographs. Plain films also show the position of the humeral head relative to the acromion, termed the acromiohumeral interval distance, which can be measured on true AP radiographs. Saupe et al[16] compared the acromiohumeral distance measured on plain radiographs with MRI scans. The authors showed that 90% of patients with an acromiohumeral distance less than 7 mm on true AP and supraspinatus outlet views had full-thickness tears of the supraspinatus, and 71% had atrophy of the supraspinatus. Other clues on plain radiographs that suggest a chronic process include sclerosis and cystic changes on the undersurface of the acromion; acetabularization of the anterior acromion; and hypertrophy,

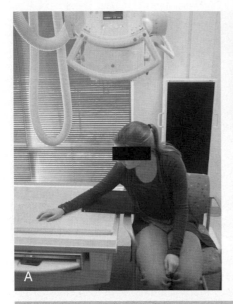

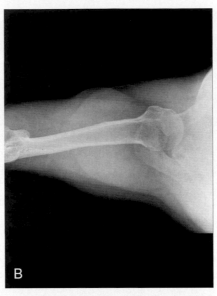

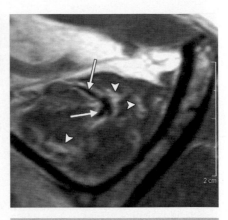

Figure 9 This sagittal MRI scan shows that the supraspinatus has Goutallier stage 2 fatty infiltration (arrows). There is still more muscle than fat (arrowheads) within the bulk of the muscle.

Figure 7 A, The axillary radiograph is performed with the x-ray beam directed into the patient's axilla with the arm abducted. B, Axillary radiograph.

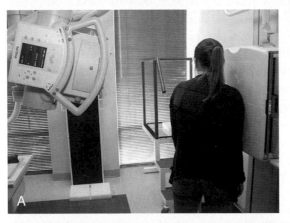

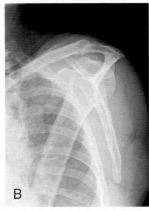

Figure 8 A, Photograph showing patient positioning for the supraspinatus outlet radiographic view, which is taken in the plane of the scapula from posterior to anterior with a 10° caudal tilt. B, This view provides visualization of the subacromial space.

sclerosis, or cystic changes in the greater tuberosity.

MRI provides vital information on rotator cuff tears such as the size of the tear on coronal and sagittal views, staging of fatty infiltration, and grading of muscle atrophy. Goutallier initially used CT images to develop his widely used staging system for quantifying the degree of fatty infiltration of the cuff muscles[17] (Figure 9). The Goutallier system is now standardized for staging fatty infiltration on sagittal MRI scans

in which the coracoid process, scapular spine, and scapular body are joined to form a Y.[18] Stage 0 represents normal muscle; stage 1 represents small streaks of fat within an otherwise normal muscle; stage 2 has more fatty infiltration, but there is still more muscle than fat; stage 3 has equal amounts of fat and muscle; and stage 4 has more fat than muscle. Studies have shown that stages 0 and 1 are found within normal, nonpathologic tissue, whereas stages 2 through 4 signify pathologic

changes within the muscle. MRI also allows grading of muscle atrophy on the same sagittal image that is used to stage fatty infiltration. Muscles are graded as having no, mild, moderate, or severe atrophy based on a line connecting the tip of the coracoid process to the scapular spine for the supraspinatus, and a line running from the tip of the inferior border of the scapular body to the midportion of the scapular spine for the infraspinatus (Figure 10). The distinction must be made between mild and moderate atrophy, with a muscle being classified as having moderate atrophy if it falls below these lines.[19] The so-called tangent sign occurs when the supraspinatus muscle belly does not cross a tangent line connecting the superior border of the scapular spine and the superior margin of the coracoid process and represents the presence of moderate to severe atrophy of the supraspinatus[20] (Figure 11).

Staging fatty infiltration and grading muscle atrophy are helpful in determining appropriate treatment of massive rotator cuff tears. The failure rates for repairing rotator cuff tears with stage 0 to 1 fatty infiltration and no to mild atrophy are 29% and 22%, respectively, whereas the failure rates in patients with stages 2 to 4 fatty infiltration and moderate to severe atrophy are 70% and 67%, respectively.[21] This represents a 2.4-fold and threefold increase in failure rates between these groups. Several other studies have shown that the retear rate is much higher for patients with advanced fatty infiltration and muscles with moderate to severe atrophy.[17,22] It is unlikely that a cuff repair is a viable option for patients with advanced degenerative changes within the muscle.

It is important to specifically evaluate the status of the teres minor on the MRI scan. Patients with stage 3 or 4 fatty infiltration of the teres minor have been shown to have worse outcomes when treated with reverse total shoulder arthroplasty compared with those who have stage 0 to 2 fatty infiltration.[23] Patients with stage 3 or 4 fatty infiltration of the teres minor showed an average loss of 7° of external rotation postoperatively compared with their preoperative range of motion, versus a net gain of 9° of external rotation in the subgroup of patients with fatty infiltration of stage 2 or less.[23] Similarly, patients with a normal or hypertrophic teres minor who were treated with an isolated biceps tenotomy or tenodesis for a massive, irreparable rotator cuff tear had statistically significant improvements in their Constant scores and active external rotation compared with patients who had an atrophied teres minor.[24]

MRI also provides information on the dimensions of the rotator cuff tear. The extent of medial retraction of the rotator cuff can be quantified on the coronal MRI scan, allowing the medial to lateral distance between the tendon edge and greater tuberosity (tear diameter) to be measured. It is important to include the most lateral extent of the rotator cuff footprint on the greater tu-

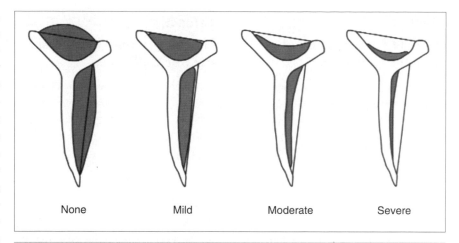

None Mild Moderate Severe

Figure 10 Illustrations showing measurements of muscle atrophy. Muscles are graded as having no, mild, moderate, or severe atrophy based on a line connecting the tip of the coracoid process to the scapular spine for the supraspinatus and a line running from the tip of the inferior border of the scapular body to the midportion of the scapular spine for the infraspinatus. (Reproduced with permission from Warner JP, Higgins L, Parsons IM, Dowdy P: Diagnosis and treatment of anterosuperior rotator cuff tears. *J Shoulder Elbow Surg* 2001;10:37-46.)

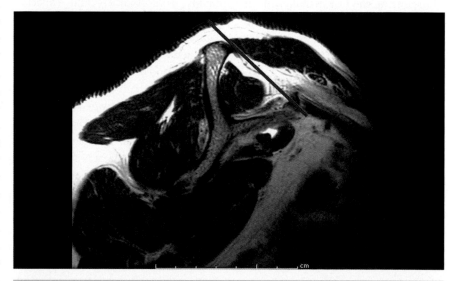

Figure 11 MRI showing moderate atrophy of the supraspinatus. The muscle belly does not cross a tangent line connecting the superior border of the scapular spine and the superior margin of the coracoid process (the tangent sign).

berosity when measuring retraction on coronal MRI scans, ensuring accurate assessment of medial retraction. Sagittal MRI scans allow measurement of the anterior-posterior extent of the tear (tear width) and also can be used to identify the number of tendons involved.

Classification

Many systems have been developed to classify rotator cuff tears, but no system is universally accepted. Rotator cuff tears can be classified based on size, the number of tendons involved, and the shape of the tear pattern. Cofield originally classified tears based on

Table 1

Cofield Classification of Rotator Cuff Tears

Small	< 1 cm
Medium	1-3 cm
Large	3-5 cm
Massive	> 5 cm

Table 2

Hamada-Fukuda Radiographic Classification of Massive Rotator Cuff Tears

Grade 1	Acromiohumeral distance > 6 mm
Grade 2	Acromiohumeral distance < 6 mm
Grade 3	Grade 2 + acetabularization of acromion
Grade 4	Grade 3 + evidence of glenohumeral arthritis
Grade 5	Grade 4 + humeral head collapse

the medial to lateral diameter of the tear and categorized tears greater than 5 cm as massive[1] (**Table 1**). Zumstein et al[25] classified rotator cuff tears as massive if they involved more than one tendon. Although there is no consensus on which classification system is best, this chapter's authors tend to classify tears based on size as determined by measuring the tear diameter on the coronal MRI scan. Most studies classify tears based on tear diameter; retear rates after rotator cuff repair appear to be proportional to tear size.[26-28] The insertional anatomy of the rotator cuff was originally described by Dugas et al;[29] however, a recent study showed the supraspinatus footprint in the Japanese population to be smaller than previously believed.[30] Therefore, because there may be variability in the size of the rotator cuff footprint between populations, quantifying the number of tendons involved in a tear based on the width of the tear alone may be an oversimplification.

The Hamada-Fukuda classification system appears to be the most widely used and accepted system for classifying massive rotator cuff tears and the subsequent development of glenohumeral arthritis[31] (**Table 2**). This staging system evaluates the natural progression of untreated massive rotator cuff tears, with the key distinction being made between stage 3 and 4 tears, with stage 4 marked by the presence of glenohumeral arthritis.

Treatment

The treatment of massive rotator cuff tears depends on many factors, including tear chronicity, fatty infiltration, muscle atrophy, the presence or absence of glenohumeral arthritis, and whether the long head of the biceps tendon is contributing to pain. The surgeon must also consider patient-related factors such as age, physical demands, comorbidities, and expectations. The patient must be willing to comply with the postoperative treatment plan, which may include a prolonged period of immobilization in the case of rotator cuff repair. This chapter's authors are unaware of any randomized controlled trials that compare the surgical options for patients with massive rotator cuff tears. However, the following scenarios present some general guidelines for managing a patient with a massive rotator cuff tear.

Nonsurgical Course

If the patient has pain-free, functional range of motion, a course of physical therapy focusing on strengthening the remaining rotator cuff may be appropriate. Frequently, a patient's range of motion is limited by pain rather than dysfunction of the rotator cuff. A subacromial injection and a detailed physical examination before and after the injection may help identify the true cause of shoulder dysfunction. In addition to having diagnostic benefits, injections can be therapeutic because they can markedly reduce pain, allow-

ing the patient to participate in a conservative physical therapy program. If a course of nonsurgical treatment is prescribed, rehabilitation should focus on strengthening both the remaining functional rotator cuff muscles and the deltoid. A recent study showed that specific retraining of the anterior deltoid resulted in significant improvements in the Constant score and forward flexion.[32] Nonsurgical treatment may be best for low-demand patients and those with significant comorbidities that preclude surgical intervention.

Biceps Tenotomy or Tenodesis

Patients with massive rotator cuff tears may report pain, loss of motion, or both. This distinction is critical to determine the most appropriate treatment. If the patient has good shoulder motion, minimal glenohumeral arthritis, and the chief symptom is pain, rotator cuff débridement and especially a biceps tenotomy can be very effective. Occasionally, a gentle smoothing of an acromial spur may be necessary, but the coracoacromial arch should be preserved in massive rotator cuff tears.

Anatomically, the long head of the biceps tendon is covered by a layer of synovial tissue that extends into the intertubercular groove of the humerus, containing both sensory and sympathetic elements within its substance, with the highest degree of innervation occurring at the tendon origin.[33,34] Thus, the biceps tendon is a primary pain generator within the shoulder. Studies have shown that performing an isolated biceps tenotomy or tenodesis in massive irreparable rotator cuff tears results in a high degree of patient satisfaction.[24,35] Most patients in these studies had good preoperative motion and no arthritis, with pain as the chief symptom. The average preoperative forward flexion was 132°, and 90% of the patients were classified as Hamada-Fukuda grade 1 or 2. Patients showed significant gains in active forward flexion and relief of pain, which resulted in an average 20-point improvement using the Constant and Murley scoring system. In a study by Walch et al,[35] the average acromiohumeral distance decreased by 1.3 mm, and there was a 30% increase in the presence of glenohumeral arthritis at an average follow-up of 57 months. In a study by Boileau et al,[24] the average acromiohumeral distance decreased by 1.1 mm, and glenohumeral arthritis developed in only one patient at an average follow-up of 35 months. Patients with teres minor atrophy had statistically significant worse functional outcomes compared with patients with a healthy teres minor. The mean Constant scores of patients with an atrophied teres minor were 10 points lower, and these patients had 22° less external rotation compared with the group with an intact teres minor. These studies provide evidence that there is a role for an isolated biceps procedure in an appropriately selected group of patients, specifically, those with a massive irreparable rotator cuff tear, minimal glenohumeral arthritis, a chief report of pain, and good shoulder range of motion. Patients should be warned that biceps tenotomy does not preclude the possibility of the development of cuff tear arthropathy. Instead, the goals of the procedure are pain relief and improved ability to perform daily tasks.

In terms of selecting biceps tenotomy versus tenodesis, a recent study found no long-term differences in elbow flexion or forearm supination strength in a group of 67 patients.[36] This chapter's authors advise patients that a tenodesis is predominantly a cosmetic procedure to prevent deformity. A recent systematic review comparing tenotomy and tenodesis found similar results, with more deformity in patients treated with tenotomy and an increased risk of postoperative bicipital pain in patients treated with tenodesis.[37] This chapter's authors prefer a tenotomy for most patients with massive tears.

Rotator Cuff Repair

When determining which patients should be treated with a rotator cuff repair, many factors should be considered. Patients should have a thorough understanding of the expected postoperative rehabilitation course and must be counseled on the possibility that the rotator cuff may not heal. Fatty infiltration and muscle atrophy are poor prognostic signs of rotator cuff healing after repair. Age is also a factor in rotator cuff healing, with patients older than 65 years having significantly lower healing rates.[38,39] Galatz et al[26] reported that 17 of 18 patients who underwent arthroscopic repair of the rotator cuff had documented evidence of failure postoperatively. Despite this high failure rate, at 1-year follow-up, patients had improvements in pain and range of motion. However, results deteriorate with time. Although an attempted repair may fail, patients can anticipate an initial improvement in pain and range of motion, but it appears unlikely that such improvements will be long lasting.

Many studies show no advantage for double-row repairs over single-row repairs; however, a recently published systematic review showed that double-row repairs had improved healing compared with single-row or transosseous repairs in tears greater than 1 cm in diameter.[28] In tears greater than 5 cm, the retear rate for double-row techniques was 41% versus 69% using single-row or transosseous repair methods.

Repair of a massive rotator cuff tear may be considered if there was an acute inciting event that led to a rapid onset of pain and shoulder dysfunction in a previously normal functioning shoulder. MRI should not show advanced muscle atrophy or fatty infiltration. The patient should understand the strict compliance needed to complete the postoperative rehabilitation protocol and should be counseled regarding the possibility that the repair could fail.

Repair With Augmentation

Various scaffolds have been proposed to augment massive rotator cuff tear repairs. The augmentation materials are intended to act as a scaffold for the ingrowth of new tissue. Many biologic tissues have been introduced, but dermis-based patches appear to show the most promising results.[40] The biomaterials are not intended to span a defect, which remains an off-label use. Without long-term, randomized controlled trials, it remains unclear if tissue augmentation improves outcome.

Suprascapular Nerve Release

Recently, there has been growing interest in the role of suprascapular nerve pathology in massive rotator cuff tears. In massive rotator cuff tears, medial retraction of the tendons may cause traction of the nerve because of the tethering that occurs at both the suprascapular and spinoglenoid notches. Albritton et al[41] showed that with as little as 2 to 3 cm of medial retraction of the supraspinatus, tension developed in the suprascapular nerve and its motor branch to the supraspinatus. Studies of massive rotator cuff tears have shown that suprascapular nerve pathology may be present and possibly reversible with rotator cuff repair.[42,43] Currently, there are few studies to support suprascapular nerve release in massive rotator cuff tears; however, preliminary results provide some early evidence that suprascapular nerve injury may be part of the overall pathologic process seen with massive rotator cuff tears.

Tendon Transfers

Younger patients with an irreparable rotator cuff tear, minimal glenohumeral arthritis, and a chief report of weakness or pain may be candidates for a tendon transfer. The most commonly used tendons for transfer are the latissimus dorsi and teres major for posterosuperior tears and the pectoralis major tendon for subscapularis tears. At an average follow-up of 53 months, Gerber et al[44] reported increased active range of motion and Constant scores from 55% to 73% in 67 patients treated with a latissimus dorsi transfer. However, worse results were found when the patients had preoperative subscapularis dysfunction. Elhassan et al[45] reported on 11 patients treated with transfer of the sternal head of the pectoralis major tendon for a massive anterosuperior rotator cuff tear. At mean follow-up of 57 months, the authors found 7 of 11 patients had decreased pain, and the Constant score increased from 28.7 preoperatively to 52.3 postoperatively. Tendon transfers remain an especially viable option for active laborers with profound weakness, especially weakness in external rotation. The patient must accept a prolonged recovery period and an extensive postoperative regimen of physical therapy.

Arthroplasty

Patients who present with a massive irreparable rotator cuff tear, multiple failed rotator cuff repairs, symptomatic rotator cuff arthropathy (RCA), and a pseudoparalytic shoulder may be candidates for arthroplasty if nonsurgical treatments have failed. Both hemiarthroplasty and reverse shoulder arthroplasty have been used to treat RCA. The results of hemiarthroplasty for RCA have been mixed, as progressive wear of the glenoid and acromion and the development of anterosuperior escape often occurs. Cuff tear hemiarthroplasty implants have increased lateral coverage to prevent painful articulation of the greater tuberosity with the undersurface of the acromion. Williams and Rockwood[46] reported 86% satisfactory results in 21 patients treated with hemiarthroplasty for RCA at a mean follow-up of 4 years. In contrast, Sanchez-Sotelo et al[47] reported that 9 of 33 patients treated with hemiarthroplasty for a massive rotator cuff tear had moderate pain at a mean follow-up of 5 years, and anterosuperior instability developed in 7 patients. Although controversial, hemiarthroplasty may have a role in RCA in younger patients after failed arthroscopic treatment, those who cannot accept the long-term complications of reverse shoulder arthroplasty, and patients with preserved overhead motion.

Because reverse shoulder arthroplasty also replaces the degenerated glenoid surface and corrects anterosuperior escape, it has the potential to provide more reliable pain relief and function. By medializing the center of rotation and tensioning the deltoid, it has the advantage over hemiarthroplasty of improving active range of motion. Although short-term results are promising, implant survivorship remains a concern, especially in young and active patients. Complication rates tend to increase dramatically in the revision setting. Guery et al[48] reported an improvement in the Constant score from 23 to 66 and an increase in active elevation from 73° to 138° at 2-year follow-up in 77 patients treated with reverse shoulder arthroplasty for RCA. However, the implant survival rate deteriorated from 91% at 5 years to 30% at 8 years. Patients with dysfunction of the teres minor had poorer outcomes with reverse shoulder arthroplasty.[23,48] In this instance, both a latissimus dorsi and teres major transfer may improve external rotation in these patients. Boileau et al[49] reported a 28° gain in active external rotation and an improved Subjective Shoulder Score from 34% to 72% in patients who received a latissimus dorsi and teres major transfer at the time of reverse shoulder arthroplasty. Mulieri et al[4] recently reported on 69 patients who were treated with reverse shoulder arthroplasty for irreparable rotator cuff tears without RCA. The authors reported a substantial reduction in pain, significant improvement in active range of motion (including increased forward flexion from 53° to 134° and increased external rotation from 27° to 51°), and survivorship of 90.7% at 52 months. These findings suggest reverse shoulder arthroplasty may be a viable salvage option for patients with persistent pain and poor function after the failure of conservative treatment.

Summary

A detailed history and physical examination often provides sufficient information to establish the diagnosis of a massive rotator cuff tear. Imaging can be obtained to confirm the diagnosis, identify associated pathology, and plan for surgical intervention. Radiographic evaluation may reveal degenerative joint disease or superior migration of the humeral head. MRI is useful in determining rotator cuff size and health of the muscle. Less active patients with irreparable rotator cuff tears, pain, and good overhead motion may be treated successfully with physical therapy or subacromial débridement; biceps tenotomy is often the best option in those with massive tears. Active patients and those with weakness often require rotator cuff reconstruction. However, poor tissue quality and scarring can be a challenge in surgical treatment. Static superior migration of the humeral head, grade 3 or 4 fatty infiltration of the rotator cuff musculature, and pseudoparalysis are poor prognostic factors for a successful repair. Patients of an appropriate age with these findings often require reverse shoulder arthroplasty to regain shoulder function. Tendon transfers may be helpful at the time of reverse shoulder arthroplasty to improve rotation. Younger patients with irreparable rotator cuff tears with chief reports of weakness without pain may benefit from isolated tendon transfers.

References

1. Cofield RH, Parvizi J, Hoffmeyer PJ, Lanzer WL, Ilstrup DM, Rowland CM: Surgical repair of chronic rotator cuff tears: A prospective long-term study. *J Bone Joint Surg Am* 2001;83-A(1): 71-77.

2. Tauro JC: Stiffness and rotator cuff tears: Incidence, arthroscopic findings, and treatment results. *Arthroscopy* 2006;22(6):581-586.

3. Sher JS, Uribe JW, Posada A, Murphy BJ, Zlatkin MB: Abnormal findings on magnetic resonance images of asymptomatic shoulders. *J Bone Joint Surg Am* 1995;77(1):10-15.

4. Mulieri P, Dunning P, Klein S, Pupello D, Frankle M: Reverse shoulder arthroplasty for the treatment of irreparable rotator cuff tear without glenohumeral arthritis. *J Bone Joint Surg Am* 2010; 92(15):2544-2556.

5. Walch G, Boulahia A, Calderone S, Robinson AH: The 'dropping' and 'hornblower's' signs in evaluation of rotator-cuff tears. *J Bone Joint Surg Br* 1998;80(4): 624-628.

6. Hertel R, Ballmer FT, Lombert SM, Gerber C: Lag signs in the diagnosis of rotator cuff rupture. *J Shoulder Elbow Surg* 1996;5(4): 307-313.

7. Otis JC, Jiang CC, Wickiewicz TL, Peterson MG, Warren RF, Santner TJ: Changes in the moment arms of the rotator cuff and deltoid muscles with abduction and rotation. *J Bone Joint Surg Am* 1994;76(5):667-676.

8. Gerber C, Krushell RJ: Isolated rupture of the tendon of the subscapularis muscle: Clinical features in 16 cases. *J Bone Joint Surg Br* 1991;73(3):389-394.

9. Gerber C, Hersche O, Farron A: Isolated rupture of the subscapularis tendon. *J Bone Joint Surg Am* 1996;78(7):1015-1023.

10. Barth JR, Burkhart SS, De Beer JF: The bear-hug test: A new and sensitive test for diagnosing a subscapularis tear. *Arthroscopy* 2006; 22(10):1076-1084.

11. Chao S, Thomas S, Yucha D, Kelly JD IV , Driban J, Swanik K: An electromyographic assessment of the "bear hug": An examination for the evaluation of the subscapularis muscle. *Arthroscopy* 2008; 24(11):1265-1270.

12. Tokish JM, Decker MJ, Ellis HB, Torry MR, Hawkins RJ: The belly-press test for the physical examination of the subscapularis muscle: Electromyographic validation and comparison to the lift-off test. *J Shoulder Elbow Surg* 2003; 12(5):427-430.

13. Szabó I, Boileau P, Walch G: The proximal biceps as a pain generator and results of tenotomy. *Sports Med Arthrosc* 2008;16(3): 180-186.

14. Codman EA: Rupture of the supraspinatus tendon: 1911. *Clin Orthop Relat Res* 1990;254:3-26.

15. Wolf EM, Agrawal V: Transdeltoid palpation (the rent test) in the diagnosis of rotator cuff tears. *J Shoulder Elbow Surg* 2001;10(5): 470-473.

16. Saupe N, Pfirrmann CW, Schmid MR, Jost B, Werner CM, Zanetti M: Association between rotator cuff abnormalities and reduced acromiohumeral distance. *AJR Am J Roentgenol* 2006;187(2): 376-382.

17. Goutallier D, Postel JM, Bernageau J, Lavau L, Voisin MC: Fatty muscle degeneration in cuff ruptures: Pre- and postoperative evaluation by CT scan. *Clin Orthop Relat Res* 1994;304:78-83.

18. Fuchs B, Weishaupt D, Zanetti M, Hodler J, Gerber C: Fatty degeneration of the muscles of the rotator cuff: Assessment by computed tomography versus magnetic resonance imaging. *J Shoulder Elbow Surg* 1999;8(6): 599-605.

19. Warner JJ, Higgins L, Parsons IM IV, Dowdy P: Diagnosis and treatment of anterosuperior rotator cuff tears. *J Shoulder Elbow Surg* 2001;10(1):37-46.

20. Zanetti M, Gerber C, Hodler J: Quantitative assessment of the muscles of the rotator cuff with magnetic resonance imaging. *Invest Radiol* 1998;33(3):163-170.

21. Gladstone JN, Bishop JY, Lo IK, Flatow EL: Fatty infiltration and atrophy of the rotator cuff do not improve after rotator cuff repair and correlate with poor functional outcome. *Am J Sports Med* 2007; 35(5):719-728.

22. Gerber C, Fuchs B, Hodler J: The results of repair of massive tears of the rotator cuff. *J Bone Joint Surg Am* 2000;82(4):505-515.

23. Simovitch RW, Helmy N, Zumstein MA, Gerber C: Impact of fatty infiltration of the teres minor

muscle on the outcome of reverse total shoulder arthroplasty. *J Bone Joint Surg Am* 2007;89(5): 934-939.

24. Boileau P, Baqué F, Valerio L, Ahrens P, Chuinard C, Trojani C: Isolated arthroscopic biceps tenotomy or tenodesis improves symptoms in patients with massive irreparable rotator cuff tears. *J Bone Joint Surg Am* 2007;89(4): 747-757.

25. Zumstein MA, Jost B, Hempel J, Hodler J, Gerber C: The clinical and structural long-term results of open repair of massive tears of the rotator cuff. *J Bone Joint Surg Am* 2008;90(11):2423-2431.

26. Galatz LM, Ball CM, Teefey SA, Middleton WD, Yamaguchi K: The outcome and repair integrity of completely arthroscopically repaired large and massive rotator cuff tears. *J Bone Joint Surg Am* 2004;86-A(2):219-224.

27. Sugaya H, Maeda K, Matsuki K, Moriishi J: Repair integrity and functional outcome after arthroscopic double-row rotator cuff repair: A prospective outcome study. *J Bone Joint Surg Am* 2007; 89(5):953-960.

28. Duquin TR, Buyea C, Bisson LJ: Which method of rotator cuff repair leads to the highest rate of structural healing? A systematic review. *Am J Sports Med* 2010; 38(4):835-841.

29. Dugas JR, Campbell DA, Warren RF, Robie BH, Millett PJ: Anatomy and dimensions of rotator cuff insertions. *J Shoulder Elbow Surg* 2002;11(5):498-503.

30. Mochizuki T, Sugaya H, Uomizu M, et al: Humeral insertion of the supraspinatus and infraspinatus: New anatomical findings regarding the footprint of the rotator cuff. *J Bone Joint Surg Am* 2008; 90(5):962-969.

31. Hamada K, Fukuda H, Mikasa M, Kobayashi Y: Roentgenographic findings in massive rotator

cuff tears: A long-term observation. *Clin Orthop Relat Res* 1990; 254:92-96.

32. Levy O, Mullett H, Roberts S, Copeland S: The role of anterior deltoid reeducation in patients with massive irreparable degenerative rotator cuff tears. *J Shoulder Elbow Surg* 2008;17(6):863-870.

33. Alpantaki K, McLaughlin D, Karagogeos D, Hadjipavlou A, Kontakis G: Sympathetic and sensory neural elements in the tendon of the long head of the biceps. *J Bone Joint Surg Am* 2005;87(7):1580-1583.

34. Cooper DE, Arnoczky SP, O'Brien SJ, Warren RF, DiCarlo E, Allen AA: Anatomy, histology, and vascularity of the glenoid labrum: An anatomical study. *J Bone Joint Surg Am* 1992;74(1): 46-52.

35. Walch G, Edwards TB, Boulahia A, Nové-Josserand L, Neyton L, Szabo I: Arthroscopic tenotomy of the long head of the biceps in the treatment of rotator cuff tears: Clinical and radiographic results of 307 cases. *J Shoulder Elbow Surg* 2005;14(3):238-246.

36. Shank JR, Singleton SB, Braun S, Kissenberth MJ, Ramappa A, Ellis H, et al: A comparison of forearm supination and elbow flexion strength in patients with long head of the biceps tenotomy or tenodesis. *Arthroscopy* 2011;27(1): 9-16.

37. Hsu AR, Ghodadra NS, Provencher CM, Lewis PB, Bach BR: Biceps tenotomy versus tenodesis: A review of clinical outcomes and biomechanical results. *J Shoulder Elbow Surg* 2011;20(2): 326-332.

38. Tashjian RZ, Hollins AM, Kim HM, et al: Factors affecting healing rates after arthroscopic double-row rotator cuff repair. *Am J Sports Med* 2010;38(12):2435-2442.

39. Boileau P, Brassart N, Watkinson DJ, Carles M, Hatzidakis AM, Krishnan SG: Arthroscopic repair of full-thickness tears of the supraspinatus: Does the tendon really heal? *J Bone Joint Surg Am* 2005;87(6):1229-1240.

40. Bond JL, Dopirak RM, Higgins J, Burns J, Snyder SJ: Arthroscopic replacement of massive, irreparable rotator cuff tears using a GraftJacket allograft: Technique and preliminary results. *Arthroscopy* 2008;24(4):403-409, e1.

41. Albritton MJ, Graham RD, Richards RS II, Basamania CJ: An anatomic study of the effects on the suprascapular nerve due to retraction of the supraspinatus muscle after a rotator cuff tear. *J Shoulder Elbow Surg* 2003;12(5): 497-500.

42. Mallon WJ, Wilson RJ, Basamania CJ: The association of suprascapular neuropathy with massive rotator cuff tears: A preliminary report. *J Shoulder Elbow Surg* 2006;15(4):395-398.

43. Costouros JG, Porramatikul M, Lie DT, Warner JJ: Reversal of suprascapular neuropathy following arthroscopic repair of massive supraspinatus and infraspinatus rotator cuff tears. *Arthroscopy* 2007;23(11):1152-1161.

44. Gerber C, Maquieira G, Espinosa N: Latissimus dorsi transfer for the treatment of irreparable rotator cuff tears. *J Bone Joint Surg Am* 2006;88(1):113-120.

45. Elhassan B, Ozbaydar M, Massimini D, Diller D, Higgins L, Warner JJ: Transfer of pectoralis major for the treatment of irreparable tears of subscapularis: Does it work? *J Bone Joint Surg Br* 2008;90(8):1059-1065.

46. Williams GR Jr, Rockwood CA Jr: Hemiarthroplasty in rotator cuff-deficient shoulders. *J Shoulder Elbow Surg* 1996;5(5): 362-367.

47. Sanchez-Sotelo J, Cofield RH, Rowland CM: Shoulder hemiarthroplasty for glenohumeral arthritis associated with severe rotator cuff deficiency. *J Bone Joint Surg Am* 2001;83(12):1814-1822.

48. Guery J, Favard L, Sirveaux F, Oudet D, Mole D, Walch G: Reverse total shoulder arthroplasty: Survivorship analysis of eighty replacements followed for five to ten years. *J Bone Joint Surg Am* 2006;88(8):1742-1747.

49. Boileau P, Chuinard C, Roussanne Y, Neyton L, Trojani C: Modified latissimus dorsi and teres major transfer through a single delto-pectoral approach for external rotation deficit of the shoulder: As an isolated procedure or with a reverse arthroplasty. *J Shoulder Elbow Surg* 2007;16(6): 671-682.

The Role of the Biceps Tendon in Massive Rotator Cuff Tears

Stephan G. Pill, MD, MSPT
Gilles Walch, MD
Richard J. Hawkins, MD
Michael J. Kissenberth, MD

Abstract

Tendinopathy of the long head of the biceps (LHB) tendon commonly occurs in patients with rotator cuff tears, and the inflammation of one head tends to lead to inflammation of the other. Many theories have been proposed regarding the function of the LHB tendon; however, its exact purpose is poorly understood. It has been described as an important stabilizer of the glenohumeral joint, a depressor of the humeral head, and as a vestigial structure. The LHB tendon can be a significant source of pain in patients with rotator cuff tears. The appropriate treatment depends on the patient's age, comorbidities, activity level, extent of disability, the presence of rotator cuff arthropathy, and the quality of the rotator cuff tissue. Conservative treatment is usually attempted first, with modalities such as nonsteroidal anti-inflammatory drugs, corticosteroid injections, physical therapy, and activity modification. If symptoms persist, biceps tenotomy or tenodesis may be combined with rotator cuff repair, depending on the quality of the rotator cuff tissue, the severity of rotator cuff arthropathy, and the willingness of the patient to comply with postoperative immobilization and rehabilitation. Even when rotator cuff repair is not possible, isolated tenotomy or tenodesis of the LHB tendon can provide substantial pain relief.

Instr Course Lect 2012;61:113-120.

Massive rotator cuff tears are often associated with lesions of the long head of the biceps (LHB) tendon, which can cause significant shoulder pain and dysfunction. Neviaser et al[1] found that the more severe the rotator cuff disease, the more severe the biceps tendinopathy. The pathology of the biceps can vary from delamination and tendinitis to subluxation, dislocation, and entrapment in the glenohumeral joint. Spontaneous rupture of the LHB tendon may occur in patients with massive rotator cuff tears and may provide pain relief after the acute symptoms subside. This chapter discusses the anatomy, diagnosis, and treatment of biceps pathology as it pertains to patients with massive rotator cuff tears.

Anatomy

Proximally, the LHB tendon attaches to the superior labrum and the supraglenoid tubercle of the glenoid. It traverses the glenohumeral joint adjacent to the rotator interval. The tendon remains extrasynovial because its sheath is an extension of the synovium of the glenohumeral joint, and it can become inflamed in conjunction with inflammatory processes that affect the rotator cuff tendons.

The coracohumeral ligament and superior glenohumeral ligament encircle the LHB tendon as it enters the bicipital groove, which is located be-

Dr. Walch or an immediate family member has received royalties from Tornier. Dr. Hawkins or an immediate family member has received royalties from DePuy and Ossur; has received research or institutional support from Arthrocare, DJ Orthopaedics, Breg, Smith & Nephew, Medica, and OrthoRehab; and serves as a board member, owner, officer, or committee member of the Orthopaedic Learning Center and the Orthopaedic Research Foundation of the Carolinas. Neither of the following authors nor any immediate family member has received anything of value from or owns stock in a commercial company or institution related directly or indirectly to the subject of this chapter: Dr. Pill and Dr. Kissenberth.

tween the greater and lesser tuberosities of the proximal humerus. Extensions of the subscapularis and supraspinatus tendons help to form a roof to the biceps sheath and provide stability for the LHB tendon to remain within the groove. All four structures (coracohumeral ligament, superior glenohumeral ligament, supraspinatus tendon, and subscapularis tendon) form a tendoligamentous sling at the proximal end of the bicipital groove, which prevents displacement of the LHB tendon. The bicipital groove is shaped like an hourglass (narrowest at the midportion). Distally in the groove, the falciform ligament, which is a fibrous extension of the sternocostal head of the pectoralis major muscle, envelops the LHB tendon.

The LHB tendon is covered by the pectoralis major muscle distal to the tuberosities and then merges with the short head of the biceps at the level of the deltoid tuberosity. Together, the short head and LHB tendons insert onto the radial tuberosity and into the fascia of the medial forearm via the bicipital aponeurosis. Recent studies have suggested that the distal biceps tendon rotates in the coronal plane, so that the slip from the LHB tendon inserts farther from the central axis of the forearm, making it a more powerful supinator of the forearm than the short head.[2] In contrast, the slip from the short head attaches distally on the radial tuberosity, making it a more powerful flexor of the elbow.[2]

Alpantaki et al[3] reported on a neuronal network of unmyelinated and thinly myelinated nerve fibers along the course of the LHB tendon, with a predominance of fibers near the tendon's origin. The blood supply to the LHB tendon comes from branches of the anterior circumflex humeral artery and labral branches from the suprascapular artery. Abrassart et al[4] recently described a relatively avascular zone in the region of the superior glenoid.

The LHB tendon can be injured at the superior labrum, within the glenohumeral joint, or within the bicipital groove. The tendon may also subluxate or dislocate out of the groove, especially when a tear of the supraspinatus or the subscapularis is present. Walch et al[5] reported a 16% incidence of subluxation or dislocation of the LHB tendon in patients with rotator cuff tears treated over a 7-year period. The biceps may also subluxate with a more subtle injury. The term hidden lesion has been used to describe a rotator interval lesion located just below an intact ligamentous pulley of the superior glenohumeral and coracohumeral ligaments, which can result in biceps subluxation.[6]

Biomechanics

The function of the LHB tendon remains uncertain. It has been described as a humeral head depressor, a shoulder stabilizer, and a vestigial structure.[7-12] Electromyographic studies have shown little activity of the LHB tendon with isolated shoulder motion, suggesting that if it contributes to shoulder stability, it must do so only when associated with elbow or forearm motion.[12] Patients with rotator cuff disease with spontaneous rupture of the LHB tendon can have dramatic pain relief and no loss of function, suggesting that the LHB tendon has little functional role in this patient population.

Clinical Presentation

A patient history and clinical examination can often identify pathology of the LHB tendon and concomitant rotator cuff disease. It is important to determine if the chief complaint is pain or weakness because this often influences surgical decision making. The presence of comorbidities, the activity level of the patient, and the extent of disability are also helpful in directing treatment.

Patients frequently report pain in the anterior shoulder that may radiate down the anterior arm. The pain is often related to activity and exacerbated by overuse. Patients may report night pain and pain with overhead activities. LHB tendon subluxation can occur with partial- or full-thickness tears of the subscapularis, which may cause painful mechanical symptoms with shoulder range of motion. These symptoms are nonspecific and present in patients with other shoulder pathologies such as impingement.

On physical examination, range of motion and rotator cuff strength are evaluated. In patients with massive rotator cuff tears, it is crucial to differentiate between pseudoparalysis and painful loss of elevation. The definition of pseudoparalysis is often debated. Some physicians consider loss of forward elevation beyond 90° or an inability to maintain the arm just above shoulder height to represent pseudoparalysis. This chapter's authors prefer to reserve the term pseudoparalysis to describe the condition of a patient who demonstrates an ineffective shrug with attempted elevation of the arm. The humeral head may subluxate anterosuperiorly between the acromion and the coracoid (**Figure 1**). A subacromial injection of lidocaine can help differentiate between true pseudoparalysis and painful loss of elevation by assessing whether active range of motion improves after pain reduction.

Biceps tendinopathy can be difficult to diagnose because of the presence of concomitant shoulder pathology. Gross deformity of the biceps muscle, known as the Popeye sign, is indicative of LHB tendon rupture (**Figure 2**). Tenderness with palpation of the bicipital groove is common, especially when combined with passive

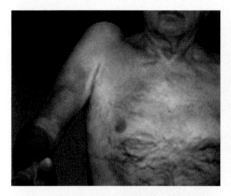

Figure 1 Clinical photograph of a patient with pseudoparalysis of the arm. An ineffective shrug results when the patient is asked to raise the arm overhead. The humeral head is escaping in an anterosuperior direction.

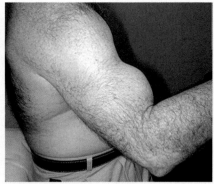

Figure 2 Photograph of a patient with Popeye deformity seen in rupture of the LHB tendon. The bulk of the biceps muscle falls distally, and the proximal arm is left with a flattened appearance.

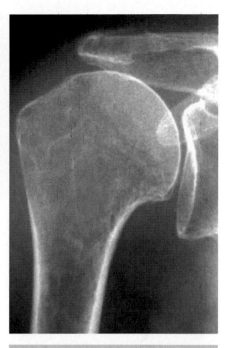

Figure 3 Glenohumeral AP radiograph shows proximal migration of the humeral head, consistent with a massive rotator cuff tear. There is a decreased acromiohumeral interval and a breech in the Moloney line.

external rotation of the shoulder. The Speed test may be positive; however, no specific test or combination of tests has a reliable positive predictive value in identifying LHB tendinitis and associated pathology. Acromioclavicular arthrosis, superior labrum anterior and posterior lesions, and rotator cuff disease also can cause positive test results. Diagnostic injections may be useful in differentiating intra-articular biceps pathology from injury within the bicipital groove. A subacromial injection may alleviate symptoms of intra-articular biceps pathology in a patient with a rotator cuff tear. In contrast, LHB tendon pathology within the groove may require an injection directed over the groove.

Radiographic examination should include a true AP radiograph of the glenohumeral joint, an axillary view, and an outlet view. These views are helpful in ruling out associated abnormalities, such as a decreased acromiohumeral interval seen in advanced rotator cuff tear arthropathy (**Figure 3**). The biceps tendon and rotator cuff can be further evaluated with MRI or ultrasonography to help determine the best surgical option and assist with preoperative patient counseling

(**Figure 4**). The functional outcome of biceps tenotomy or tenodesis is better if the infraspinatus or teres minor can provide active external rotation.[13-15]

Treatment

Many factors influence the initial treatment options for patients with massive rotator cuff tears and LHB tendinopathy, including the patient's age, activity level, medical comorbidities, and extent of disability; the presence of rotator cuff arthropathy; and the quality of the rotator cuff tissue. An initial trial of nonsurgical treatment is typically attempted and includes nonsteroidal anti-inflammatory drugs, activity modification, and physical therapy. If these treatments are unsuccessful, corticosteroid injections may be helpful. In patients with massive rotator cuff tears, a subacromial injection may alleviate symptoms from injury to the intra-articular portion of the biceps tendon. If the patient has marked tenderness in the bicipital groove without impingement signs, an injection into the soft tissues surrounding the groove may be more therapeutic. Reexamining the patient shortly after the injection can help in establishing the diagnosis.

Although nonsurgical treatment may reduce symptoms, it does not prevent progression of arthropathy if a full-thickness rotator cuff tear is present. Narrowing of the acromiohumeral interval develops within 5 years in approximately 75% of patients with full-thickness rotator cuff tears who are treated nonsurgically.[16-18] Hamada et al[19] reported that 5 of 7 patients with full-thickness rotator cuff tears treated nonsurgically progressed at least one radiographic stage of glenohumeral arthritis after a minimum of 8 years. Patients should be counseled on these risks as part of the informed consent to treatment.

Determining the most appropriate surgical treatment can be challenging. Treatment options consist of biceps tenotomy or tenodesis with or without rotator cuff repair, as well as reverse shoulder arthroplasty. The retear rate after a large or massive rotator cuff re-

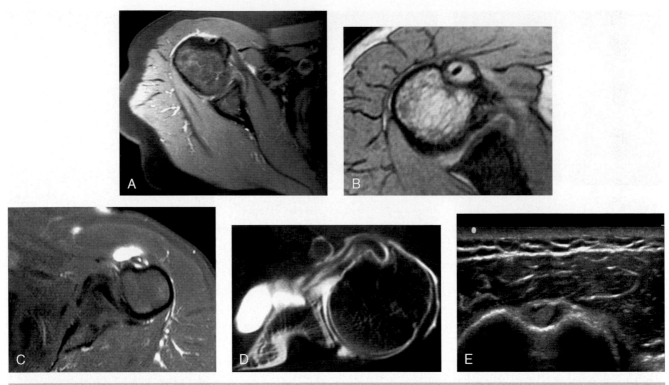

Figure 4   Axial MRI scan showing a normal (**A**) and abnormal (**B**) LHB tendon within the bicipital groove. **C,** Axial MRI scan shows intratendinous high signal consistent with tearing of the LHB within the bicipital groove. **D,** Axial MRI scan shows subluxation of the LHB out of the bicipital groove in a patient with a partial subscapularis tear. **E,** Ultrasound image shows a normal biceps tendon within the bicipital groove.

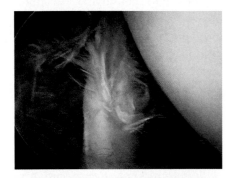

Figure 5   Intraoperative photograph of a frayed biceps tendon near its insertion on the superior labrum.

pair is considerably higher, ranging from 36% to 70%.[20,21] Determining whether a massive rotator cuff tear is worth repairing can be difficult and is often based on a combination of clinical, radiographic, and intraoperative criteria.[21,22] Fatty infiltration of the rotator cuff (Goutallier grades 3 and 4) and static proximal humeral migration are markers of poor reparability.[23,24] Attempting to repair these rotator cuff tears may result in postoperative loss of active elevation and an unsatisfied patient.[21] Even if the rotator cuff is reparable, the patient must be willing to undergo postoperative immobilization and rehabilitation after the repair.

The chief complaint is an important factor in determining the most appropriate surgical option in patients presenting with massive rotator cuff tears and LHB tendinopathy. If the patient is most affected by pain, a limited arthroscopic débridement, tuberoplasty, and biceps tenotomy or tenodesis may provide significant relief.[15,25] These patients often demonstrate nearly full active preoperative range of motion. The tendon of the LHB is often inflamed, hypertrophied, and/or erythematous at the time of surgery (**Figure 5**). The LHB tendon may develop tears, especially if it becomes unstable in the bicipital groove, and both tenotomy and tenodesis can be effective in these situations.

Arthroscopic acromioplasty has been found to be a less reliable treatment in patients with massive tears.[26-29] A subacromial injection before surgery may be prognostically helpful. Zvijac et al[29] showed that the promising early results of arthroscopic acromioplasty deteriorated with longer follow-up times. There is also a risk that an acromioplasty will destabilize the shoulder by removing the fulcrum for elevation, converting a painful functional shoulder into a painful nonfunctional shoulder with loss of active elevation. During arthroscopic débridement and biceps tenotomy, the coracoacromial ligament should be preserved and the acromion gently smoothed when a massive rotator cuff tear is present. More aggressive subacromial decompression and acromioplasty may lead to iatrogenic anterosuperior escape of the humeral head.[30,31] Some authors have reported better results with débriding and contouring the humerus (for example, tuberoplasty) rather than the acromion to preserve the integrity of the coracoacromial arch.[25,32]

If the patient's chief complaint is weakness, the biceps tendon becomes less involved in the treatment plan, and options include arthroscopic partial rotator cuff repair, repair with tissue augmentation, or tendon transfers. If the patient has an external rotation lag and hornblower sign preoperatively, tendon transfers may be required to improve external rotation.[33] If pseudoparalysis, static anterior or proximal migration of the humeral head, or advanced rotator cuff arthropathy are present, a reverse shoulder arthroplasty with biceps tenotomy or tenodesis may be the most reliable treatment to improve function and relieve pain.[34]

Tenotomy Versus Tenodesis

The outcomes of biceps tenotomy and tenodesis have been compared, and both procedures can successfully treat symptoms. Advocates of tenotomy emphasize the simplicity of the technique and the similar functional outcomes of patients.[35] Resolution of symptoms with no loss of function following spontaneous rupture of the LHB tendon in patients with rotator cuff disease further supports tenotomy. However, some authors caution against the routine practice of tenotomy because of the risk of Popeye deformity, pain in the bicipital groove if the tendon does not retract beyond the groove, and potential muscle cramping with repetitive elbow flexion or forearm supination.[13,28,36-38] These au-

thors suggest that younger patients, patients with slender arms, body builders, and those who perform repetitive supination activities may not tolerate biceps tenotomy.

Walch et al[15] reported the results of arthroscopic LHB tenotomy in 307 patients with irreparable massive rotator cuff disease and a minimum follow-up of 2 years. Patients were included in the study if they had an irreparable rotator cuff tear, which was defined as an acromiohumeral interval of less than 6 mm, grade 3 or worse fatty infiltration, or were older and unwilling to participate in the rehabilitation required after an open rotator cuff repair. The average patient age was 64 years at the time of surgery. At an average follow-up of 5 years (range, 2 to 14 years), 86.5% of the patients were either satisfied or very satisfied with the procedure. Only nine patients (3%) required another surgery (six were treated with reverse shoulder arthroplasty and three had rotator cuff repairs). The patients reported dramatic pain relief, no loss of active elevation or strength, and an improved ability to perform activities of daily living. No muscle cramping with resisted elbow flexion or forearm supination were reported, although no objective strength testing was performed. Poor results were associated with preoperative stiffness, preoperative loss of active elevation, degenerative changes in the glenohumeral joint, and fatty infiltration of the rotator cuff.

Despite encouraging clinical results, the progressive radiographic changes of rotator cuff arthropathy were unaltered when biceps tenotomy was done without rotator cuff tear repair. The acromiohumeral interval decreased from 6.6 mm to 5.3 mm ($P < 0.0001$), and 25% of the patients progressed one or two stages based on the Hamada-Fukuda classification of rotator cuff arthropathy. Rupture or

fatty infiltration of the infraspinatus was associated with decreased acromiohumeral distance (10 mm if there was no fatty infiltration versus 3.5 mm with severe fatty infiltration; $P < 0.0001$). The teres minor played a significant role in preserving the acromiohumeral distance when the infraspinatus was absent or had grade 3 or 4 fatty infiltration (1 mm with teres minor absence versus 3.7 mm with teres minor hypertrophy). The development of rotator cuff tear arthropathy was directly correlated with the patient age, the size of the rotator cuff tear, and the presence of fatty infiltration in the subscapularis.

Gill et al[39] reported a significant reduction in pain and improvement in function in 30 patients treated with biceps tenotomy, 12 of whom had a preoperative diagnosis of rotator cuff tear. In their study, 90% of the patients returned to sports participation, 97% returned to work (at 2 weeks postoperatively), and 97% did not require any pain medication by the first postoperative follow-up appointment. In contrast, Kelly et al[36] reported that 38% of the patients had fatigue discomfort in the biceps with resisted elbow flexion activities after biceps tenotomy.

In contrast, tenodesis allows for preservation of the length-tension relationship of the biceps, which may prevent postoperative muscle atrophy and fatigue cramping. Tenodesis also helps to maintain the normal contour of the biceps muscle, but the procedure can add complexity and time to the surgery. Postoperative care may be more involved following tenodesis. Also, the tenodesis screw may serve as a stress riser in the proximal humerus and can lead to fracture.[40] Tenodesis can be performed proximally with the tendon maintained within the bicipital groove, or distally, with the tendon removed from the groove. Advocates of distal fixation report that removing the

LHB tendon from the bicipital groove and excising the proximal portion of the tendon limits the potential for postoperative pain secondary to residual tenosynovitis within the biceps sheath.[41] Both open and arthroscopic tenodesis techniques have been described.[37,42]

Published studies have included comparisons of the outcomes of tenotomy and tenodesis. Boileau et al[13] reported on the outcomes of 68 patients (72 shoulders) with irreparable massive rotator cuff tears who were treated with either an isolated arthroscopic biceps tenotomy or tenodesis. The average patient age was 68 years (range, 52 to 85 years) at the time of surgery. At an average follow-up of 35 months, 78% of the patients were satisfied or very satisfied with the outcome. The average final Constant score was 66.5 points, which was 20 points higher than average preoperative scores. Similar to the results of the study by Walch et al,[15] pain reduction resulted in improved postoperative range of motion and activity level. There was no difference in the average Constant score between the tenotomy group and the tenodesis group; however, a higher prevalence of muscle belly discomfort (21% versus 9%) and Popeye deformity (62% versus 3%) was found in the tenotomy group compared with the tenodesis group. In contrast, Osbahr et al[14] reported no significant differences regarding anterior shoulder pain, muscle spasm in the biceps, and cosmetic deformities between tenotomy and tenodesis in 160 patients.

In reviewing the literature on tenotomy and tenodesis from 1966 to 2010, Hsu et al[43] found eight eligible articles involving 416 patients treated with tenotomy and 117 patients treated with tenodesis. The patients treated with tenotomy had a higher incidence of cosmetic deformity and lower load-to-

failure of the tendon. However, because of the large variability in results and the methodology of the published studies, no consensus was possible regarding tenotomy versus tenodesis for the treatment of LHB tendon lesions. Based on their findings, the authors recommended tenotomy for older patients with sedentary lifestyles, obese arms, those not concerned about cosmesis, and those not pursuing workers' compensation claims. They recommended tenodesis for patients younger than 40 years with high levels of activity, those with nonobese arms, those with concerns for cosmesis, and patients involved in workers' compensation cases. Of note, 89% of all the patients included in the studies also had rotator cuff tears.

It is debatable if patients have more weakness after tenotomy than after tenodesis. Spontaneous proximal biceps rupture is associated with a 20% loss of forearm supination strength and 8% to 20% loss of elbow flexion strength,[38] suggesting that biceps tenotomy may lead to unacceptable strength deficits in some patients. However, at a minimum follow-up of 6 months, Shank et al[35] found no statistically significant difference in isokinetic forearm supination or elbow flexion strength in 17 patients treated with tenotomy compared with 19 patients treated with tenodesis. In contrast, in a study by Wittstein et al[44] comparing 19 tenotomy patients with 16 tenodesis patients, the authors reported that the tenotomy group had decreased supination peak torque compared with the nonsurgical side and with the tenodesis group. In addition, four patients in the tenotomy group had a Popeye deformity and two patients had painful cramping. There were no significant differences in peak flexion torque or endurance testing between the groups.

Summary

The function of the LHB tendon remains poorly understood. It often acts as a pain generator in patients with massive rotator cuff tears, and its sacrifice can bring significant pain relief without a compromise in shoulder function. If rotator cuff repair is not possible and/or desirable, biceps tenotomy or tenodesis can provide favorable clinical results by reducing pain and improving functional range of motion if pain was limiting motion. Unfortunately, treatment of the biceps tendon does not inhibit the natural progressive radiographic changes of rotator cuff arthropathy that may occur with long-standing rotator cuff tears. Improved external rotation and a better functional result can be expected after biceps tenotomy or tenodesis if some of the posterior rotator cuff, particularly the teres minor, remains healthy. Many surgeons reserve the use of tenotomy for older patients and those with obese arms and perform tenodesis for younger patients, body builders, those unwilling to accept cosmetic deformity, and laborers who perform work requiring repetitive supination motions.

References

1. Neviaser TJ, Neviaser RJ, Neviaser JS, Neviaser JS: The four-in-one arthroplasty for the painful arc syndrome. *Clin Orthop Relat Res* 1982;163:107-112.

2. Eames MH, Bain GI, Fogg QA, van Riet RP: Distal biceps tendon anatomy: A cadaveric study. *J Bone Joint Surg Am* 2007;89(5): 1044-1049.

3. Alpantaki K, McLaughlin D, Karagogeos D, Hadjipavlou A, Kontakis G: Sympathetic and sensory neural elements in the tendon of the long head of the biceps. *J Bone Joint Surg Am* 2005;87(7):1580-1583.

4. Abrassart S, Stern R, Hoffmeyer P: Arterial supply of the glenoid:

An anatomic study. *J Shoulder Elbow Surg* 2006;15(2):232-238.

5. Walch G, Nové-Josserand L, Boileau P, Levigne C: Subluxations and dislocations of the tendon of the long head of the biceps. *J Shoulder Elbow Surg* 1998;7(2): 100-108.

6. Walch G, Nove-Josserand L, Levigne C, Renaud E: Tears of the supraspinatus tendon associated with "hidden" lesions of the rotator interval. *J Shoulder Elbow Surg* 1994;3(6):353-360.

7. Warner JJ, McMahon PJ: The role of the long head of the biceps brachii in superior stability of the glenohumeral joint. *J Bone Joint Surg Am* 1995;77(3):366-372.

8. Itoi E, Kuechle DK, Newman SR, Morrey BF, An KN: Stabilising function of the biceps in stable and unstable shoulders. *J Bone Joint Surg Br* 1993;75(4): 546-550.

9. McGough RL, Debski RE, Taskiran E, Fu FH, Woo SL: Mechanical properties of the long head of the biceps tendon. *Knee Surg Sports Traumatol Arthrosc* 1996; 3(4):226-229.

10. Sakurai G, Ozaki J, Tomita Y, Nishimoto K, Tamai S: Electromyographic analysis of shoulder joint function of the biceps brachii muscle during isometric contraction. *Clin Orthop Relat Res* 1998;354:123-131.

11. Yamaguchi K, Riew KD, Galatz LM, Syme JA, Neviaser RJ: Biceps activity during shoulder motion: An electromyographic analysis. *Clin Orthop Relat Res* 1997;336: 122-129.

12. Levy AS, Kelly BT, Lintner SA, Osbahr DC, Speer KP: Function of the long head of the biceps at the shoulder: Electromyographic analysis. *J Shoulder Elbow Surg* 2001;10(3):250-255.

13. Boileau P, Baqué F, Valerio L, Ahrens P, Chuinard C, Trojani C: Isolated arthroscopic biceps tenotomy or tenodesis improves symptoms in patients with massive irreparable rotator cuff tears. *J Bone Joint Surg Am* 2007;89(4): 747-757.

14. Osbahr DC, Diamond AB, Speer KP: The cosmetic appearance of the biceps muscle after long-head tenotomy versus tenodesis. *Arthroscopy* 2002;18(5):483-487.

15. Walch G, Edwards TB, Boulahia A, Nové-Josserand L, Neyton L, Szabo I: Arthroscopic tenotomy of the long head of the biceps in the treatment of rotator cuff tears: Clinical and radiographic results of 307 cases. *J Shoulder Elbow Surg* 2005;14(3):238-246.

16. Itoi E, Tabata S: Conservative treatment of rotator cuff tears. *Clin Orthop Relat Res* 1992;275: 165-173.

17. Hawkins RH, Dunlop R: Nonoperative treatment of rotator cuff tears. *Clin Orthop Relat Res* 1995; 321:178-188.

18. Bokor DJ, Hawkins RJ, Huckell GH, Angelo RL, Schickendantz MS: Results of nonoperative management of full-thickness tears of the rotator cuff. *Clin Orthop Relat Res* 1993;294:103-110.

19. Hamada K, Fukuda H, Mikasa M, Kobayashi Y: Roentgenographic findings in massive rotator cuff tears: A long-term observation. *Clin Orthop Relat Res* 1990; 254:92-96.

20. Gazielly DF, Gleyze P, Montagnon C: Functional and anatomical results after rotator cuff repair. *Clin Orthop Relat Res* 1994;304: 43-53.

21. Gerber C, Fuchs B, Hodler J: The results of repair of massive tears of the rotator cuff. *J Bone Joint Surg Am* 2000;82(4):505-515.

22. Gartsman GM, Khan M, Hammerman SM: Arthroscopic repair of full-thickness tears of the rotator cuff. *J Bone Joint Surg Am* 1998;80(6):832-840.

23. Goutallier D, Postel JM, Bernageau J, Lavau L, Voisin MC: Fatty muscle degeneration in cuff ruptures: Pre- and postoperative evaluation by CT scan. *Clin Orthop Relat Res* 1994;304:78-83.

24. Nové-Josserand L, Lévigne C, Noël E, Walch G: The acromiohumeral interval: A study of the factors influencing its height. *Rev Chir Orthop Reparatrice Appar Mot* 1996;82(5):379-385.

25. Fenlin JM Jr, Chase JM, Rushton SA, Frieman BG: Tuberoplasty: Creation of an acromiohumeral articulation: A treatment option for massive, irreparable rotator cuff tears. *J Shoulder Elbow Surg* 2002;11(2):136-142.

26. Ellman H, Kay SP, Wirth M: Arthroscopic treatment of full-thickness rotator cuff tears: 2- to 7-year follow-up study. *Arthroscopy* 1993;9(2):195-200.

27. Gartsman GM: Massive, irreparable tears of the rotator cuff: Results of operative debridement and subacromial decompression. *J Bone Joint Surg Am* 1997;79(5): 715-721.

28. Rockwood CA Jr, Williams GR Jr, Burkhead WZ Jr: Débridement of degenerative, irreparable lesions of the rotator cuff. *J Bone Joint Surg Am* 1995;77(6): 857-866.

29. Zvijac JE, Levy HJ, Lemak LJ: Arthroscopic subacromial decompression in the treatment of full thickness rotator cuff tears: A 3- to 6-year follow-up. *Arthroscopy* 1994;10(5):518-523.

30. Gartsman GM, Blair ME Jr, Noble PC, Bennett JB, Tullos HS: Arthroscopic subacromial decompression: An anatomical study. *Am J Sports Med* 1988;16(1):48-50.

31. Gartsman GM: Arthroscopic acromioplasty for lesions of the rotator cuff. *J Bone Joint Surg Am* 1990;72(2):169-180.

32. Scheibel M, Lichtenberg S, Habermeyer P: Reversed arthroscopic

subacromial decompression for massive rotator cuff tears. *J Shoulder Elbow Surg* 2004;13(3): 272-278.

33. Boileau P, Chuinard C, Roussanne Y, Neyton L, Trojani C: Modified latissimus dorsi and teres major transfer through a single delto-pectoral approach for external rotation deficit of the shoulder: As an isolated procedure or with a reverse arthroplasty. *J Shoulder Elbow Surg* 2007;16(6): 671-682.

34. Mulieri P, Dunning P, Klein S, Pupello D, Frankle M: Reverse shoulder arthroplasty for the treatment of irreparable rotator cuff tear without glenohumeral arthritis. *J Bone Joint Surg Am* 2010; 92(15):2544-2556.

35. Shank JR, Singleton SB, Braun S, et al: A comparison of forearm supination and elbow flexion strength in patients with long head of the biceps tenotomy or tenodesis. *Arthroscopy* 2011;27(1): 9-16.

36. Kelly AM, Drakos MC, Fealy S, Taylor SA, O'Brien SJ: Arthroscopic release of the long head of the biceps tendon: Functional outcome and clinical results. *Am J Sports Med* 2005;33(2):208-213.

37. Mazzocca AD, Rios CG, Romeo AA, Arciero RA: Subpectoral biceps tenodesis with interference screw fixation. *Arthroscopy* 2005; 21(7):896.

38. Mariani EM, Cofield RH, Askew LJ, Li GP, Chao EY: Rupture of the tendon of the long head of the biceps brachii: Surgical versus nonsurgical treatment. *Clin Orthop Relat Res* 1988;228:233-239.

39. Gill TJ, McIrvin E, Mair SD, Hawkins RJ: Results of biceps tenotomy for treatment of pathology of the long head of the biceps brachii. *J Shoulder Elbow Surg* 2001;10(3):247-249.

40. Reiff SN, Nho SJ, Romeo AA: Proximal humerus fracture after keyhole biceps tenodesis. *Am J Orthop (Belle Mead NJ)* 2010; 39(7):E61-E63.

41. Mazzocca AD, Bicos J, Santangelo S, Romeo AA, Arciero RA: The biomechanical evaluation of four fixation techniques for proximal biceps tenodesis. *Arthroscopy* 2005;21(11):1296-1306.

42. Boileau P, Krishnan SG, Coste JS, Walch G: Arthroscopic biceps tenodesis: A new technique using bioabsorbable interference screw fixation. *Arthroscopy* 2002;18(9): 1002-1012.

43. Hsu AR, Ghodadra NS, Provencher CM, Lewis PB, Bach BR: Biceps tenotomy versus tenodesis: A review of clinical outcomes and biomechanical results. *J Shoulder Elbow Surg* 2011;20(2): 326-332.

44. Wittstein JR, Queen R, Abbey A, Toth A, Moorman CT III: Isokinetic strength, endurance, and subjective outcomes after biceps tenotomy versus tenodesis: A postoperative study. *Am J Sports Med* 2011;39(4):857-865.

10

Arthroscopic Repair Techniques for Massive Rotator Cuff Tears

Jeffrey S. Abrams, MD
Frederick S. Song, MD

Abstract

Patients with massive rotator cuff tears present with pain, weakness, and loss of function. Candidates for arthroscopic repair include symptomatic, young, active patients; those with an acute tear or tears with early changes of atrophy; and patients willing to comply with recovery and rehabilitation processes after surgery. As massive rotator cuff tears extend, the glenohumeral articulation is destabilized, allowing superior migration. Repair of the force couples and reinforcement of the anterosuperior rotator cuff cable can restore functional elevation via the deltoid. Muscle changes, including rotator cuff atrophy and fatty infiltration, will affect shoulder strength and function. As chronic changes become more extensive (such as the absence of the acromiohumeral interval and degenerative joint changes), other repair options may be more durable. Other arthroscopic options, including partial rotator cuff closure, graft to augment the repair, and use of the long head of the biceps tendon, have been helpful in pain relief and functional gains.

Instr Course Lect 2012;61:121-130.

The frequency of rotator cuff tears in the general population increases with age. Studies have shown a 13% to 28% rate of partial- and full-thickness tears in the fifth and sixth decades of life, increasing up to 51% in patients older than 70 years.[1,2] The literature reports the occurrence of massive tears ranging from 10% to 40% of all tears.[3,4] Several definitions have been used in the literature to describe massive rotator cuff tears. The DeOrio and Cofield[5] system is widely used, with tears classified based on length in the greatest diameter (sagittal or coronal) of the tear. Tears are categorized as small (≤ 1 cm), medium (1 to 3 cm), large (3 to 5 cm), and massive (> 5 cm). Gerber et al[6] simplified the definition of a massive tear, classifying any tear involving two tendons or more as a massive tear. For the purpose of this chapter, massive rotator cuff tears are defined as tears involving two or more tendons or a multiple tendon tear retracted to the glenoid rim[7] (**Figure 1**).

As the tear margins extend in massive rotator cuff tears, it becomes more challenging for the surgeon to close the defect. Tendon fibrosis and retraction, along with rotator cuff denervation, atrophy, fatty infiltration, and tuberosity osteopenia reduce the likelihood of a successful repair. Large rotator cuff defects can lead to superior subluxation of the humeral head, which drastically changes the mechanics of the rotator cuff and disables the rotator cuff muscles above the center of rotation.[7] Articulation of the superior portion of the humeral head with the undersurface of the acromion decreases the reparability of the rotator cuff tear, although other arthroscopic procedures may improve symptoms.

Treatment Options

Patients with painful massive rotator cuff tears have surgical options ranging

Dr. Abrams or an immediate family member has received royalties from CONMED Linvatec and Arthrocare; is a member of a speakers' bureau or has made paid presentations on behalf of Mitek; serves as a paid consultant to CONMED Linvatec, Arthrocare, and Wright Medical Technology; owns stock or stock options in Arthrocare, Cayenne Medical, Core Essence Medical, KFx Medical, and Ingen Medical; and serves as a board member, owner, officer, or committee member of the Orthopaedic Learning Center Board of Directors, the Arthroscopy Association of North America Continuing Education Committee, and the American Shoulder and Elbow Surgeons. Neither Dr. Song nor any immediate family member has received anything of value from or owns stock in a commercial company or institution related directly or indirectly to the subject of this chapter.

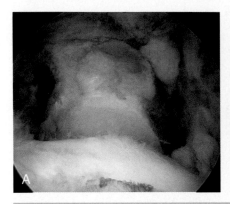
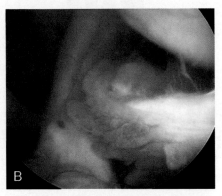

Figure 1 Arthroscopic images of a massive rotator cuff tear that includes three or more tendons (**A**) and a multitendon tear retracted back to the glenoid rim (**B**).

from arthroscopy to shoulder arthroplasty. As the acromiohumeral interval decreases to the point of articulation, and rotator cuff tear arthropathy as described by Neer et al[8] develops, reverse shoulder arthroplasty becomes the mainstay of treatment. Select patients with anterior and superior migration have shown improvement following subscapularis repair combined with supraspinatus repair. Successful repair of the disrupted force couples found in massive rotator cuff tears is often necessary to stabilize the humeral head and maintain the acromiohumeral interval.

Regardless of the surgical option, the treatment of massive rotator cuff tears remains challenging. Arthroscopic treatment allows articular joint evaluation; reduces pain and morbidity; preserves the deltoid; avoids interruption of the acromial arch; and reduces the risks of complications, including infection.[9-12] Arthroscopic techniques also provide the surgeon with better visualization and characterization of the tear, allowing for releases along the articular and bursal margins. Many studies have reported a high success rate of healing with arthroscopic rotator cuff repair of single-tendon tears.[13,14] Unfortunately, arthroscopic treatment of large and massive rotator cuff tears have not fared as well.[13-18]

Galatz et al[18] reported 17 of 18 failures of rotator cuff healing (94%) after arthroscopic repair of larger rotator cuff tears. The successful repair rates have improved as newer techniques to mobilize and fix tendons have been reported. Although the initial goal when approaching a massive rotator cuff tear is to primarily close the defect, other options are available that can lead to patient satisfaction, including biceps tenotomy, modified subacromial decompression, distal clavicle excision, partial repairs, and tissue grafting. Despite recurrent defects in one third of patients, acceptable rates of satisfaction regarding pain relief and gains in active range of motion have made arthroscopy a viable option.

Indications

It is accepted that not all massive rotator cuff tears can or should be repaired. The indications for arthroscopic repair include shoulder pain, weakness, and loss of function in a patient in whom conservative treatment has failed. The patient's ability to comply with the postoperative rehabilitation program, including sling immobilization, largely influences patient selection. Inability to comply with immobilization or to participate in a physiotherapy program is a contraindication to arthroscopic repair. Another contraindication is de-

generative arthritic changes in the glenohumeral joint. Some surgeons have included age of the patient, chronicity of the tear, advanced fatty infiltration of the rotator cuff musculature, and reduction of the acromiohumeral distance as contraindications to arthroscopic treatment. Although these factors influence rotator cuff healing, they do not necessarily define the level of patient satisfaction with the surgery. Many studies report good patient satisfaction after surgery, even when diagnostic studies show failure of rotator cuff healing.[13,14,18] It is important to counsel patients with massive rotator cuff tears regarding the likelihood of repair healing and provide information about alternative treatments that may improve function and decrease pain.

Acute and traumatic massive rotator cuff tears are often more suited for repair than chronic degenerative tears. Acute massive tears or avulsions will usually have good reducibility and elasticity with acceptable tissue quality for a primary repair. It should be recognized that these tears are different from chronic and degenerative massive rotator cuff tears, even if the tear dimensions are the same. Patients who experience a traumatic event resulting in an abrupt change in shoulder function (such as an acute tear or an acute extension of a prior chronic tear) are candidates for arthroscopic repair.

Patient Selection

History

Massive rotator cuff tears can present in several ways. The chronic degenerative tear that becomes symptomatic over time is quite different from the acute, traumatic massive tear that occurs with a dislocation. In patients with severe weakness and dysfunction, it is important to rule out other etiologies, such as a neurologic pathology. The duration of symptoms, previous treatments, and patient expectations

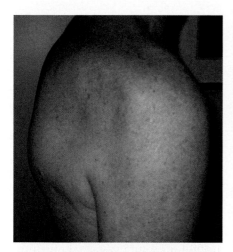

Figure 2 Clinical photograph of a patient with atrophy of the supraspinatus and infraspinatus muscles.

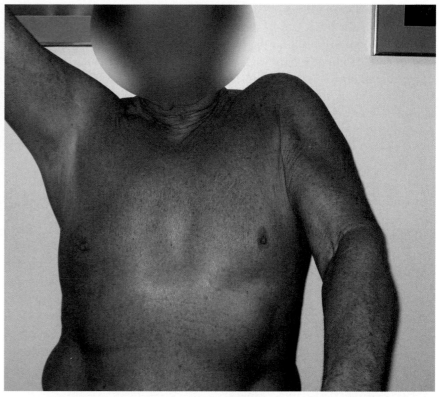

Figure 3 Clinical photograph of a patient with pseudoparalysis of the left arm exhibiting the shrug sign.

should be discussed in detail. A thorough medical history is important to identify any comorbidities, such as tobacco use, connective tissue disorders, diabetes mellitus, vascular pathology, or the use of certain medications (for example, oral steroids or immuno-modulation agents) that could affect outcomes. It is important to match patient and surgeon expectations.

Physical Examination

The physical examination begins with an inspection of the scapula of both shoulders, which should be exposed for a more thorough examination of the affected shoulder and comparisons with the contralateral shoulder. Muscular atrophy may be seen early, late, or not at all with massive tears (**Figure 2**). Infraspinatus atrophy is easier to detect based on its more superficial location compared with the supraspinatus, which lies deep to the trapezius muscle. Advanced atrophy is often irreversible and may be prognostic with regard to strength gains after surgery.

Both active and passive range of motion should be evaluated. Patients with massive rotator cuff tears often present with pseudoparalysis and weakness in rotation. Pseudoparalysis is the inability to actively elevate the extended arm above the shoulder level. Limited active forward elevation with nearly full passive motion suggests a massive rotator cuff tear (**Figure 3**). The pseudoparalysis may be acute or chronic and will indicate the degree of weakness or loss of stability of the glenohumeral joint. Maximal passive motion should be encouraged before proceeding with any surgical intervention to maximize functional outcome. Physical examination signs such as the positive belly press test, the lift-off test, or the bear-hug sign indicate subscapularis involvement. A positive hornblower sign or an external rotation deficit would suggest posterior cuff extension of the tear. During the physical examination, it is important to evaluate for other etiologies of pain, such as subacromial impingement, acromioclavicular joint arthrosis, and biceps tendon pathology, because such disorders should be addressed during surgery.

A full neurologic examination is imperative to identify any other etiologies for the patient's symptoms. Cervical pathology can often coexist with shoulder disorders and should be explored. Suprascapular nerve dysfunction can mimic physical examination findings of a massive rotator cuff tear and should be tested if the physical examination findings and imaging studies are not corroborative.

Imaging Studies

The initial diagnostic workup includes radiographs of the shoulder, including an AP view in external rotation, a transscapular outlet view, and an axillary view. Preservation of the glenohumeral joint, the acromiohumeral interval, and the anatomy of adjacent structures, including the acromion and acromioclavicular joint, can be determined. Superior migration of the humeral head, resulting in narrowing of the acromiohumeral interval to less than 5 mm in an upright radiograph, is suggestive of a chronic massive rotator cuff tear[19,20] (**Figure 4**).

Additional studies to evaluate the soft tissue are also needed, including MRI, contrast CT, or ultrasound. Ultrasound has the added benefit of be-

ing a dynamic imaging study, although it is operator dependent. These studies can help evaluate tear retraction as well as atrophy and fatty infiltration of the rotator cuff musculature. The presence of muscle atrophy and extensive fatty infiltration have been correlated to poor healing after repair[6,16,21,22] (**Figure 5**). An MRI can also identify other pathology, including cartilage defects and biceps and labral pathologies.

Techniques

The surgical treatment of a patient with a massive rotator cuff tear begins with a gentle shoulder examination under anesthesia. These patients often do not have full shoulder motion, and a gentle manipulation can help break up adhesions before the arthroscope is inserted. Patients can be placed in the lateral decubitus or beach chair position. Both positions allow conversion to an open repair if necessary. It is important to access both the anterior and the posterior aspects of the shoulder if open repair is performed.

Standard arthroscopic portals are implemented. The posterior viewing portal is placed 2 cm inferior to the

posterolateral corner of the acromion, the anterior portal is placed just inferior to the acromioclavicular joint, and the lateral portal is placed 3 cm off the lateral edge of the acromion. Several additional portals and/or percutaneous stab incisions are usually necessary for anchor placement and to aid in suture passage and management. An accessory anterior portal just lateral to the coracoid process is used for subscapularis repairs and lesser tuberosity anchor placement. The Neviaser portal is helpful for suture passage through the rotator cuff tear and for suprascapular nerve release, if indicated.

Diagnostic arthroscopy is initially performed with the arthroscope in the posterior portal. The articular surfaces are visualized, and a systematic review of the intra-articular portion of the shoulder is performed. An anterior portal is created inferior to the acromioclavicular joint. The full extent of the rotator cuff insertion can be evaluated with the arthroscope in the posterior portal followed by the anterior portal. Rotating the humeral head aids in visualizing the cuff attachment. A capsulotomy can be

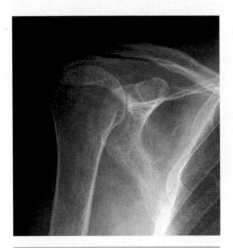

Figure 4 Radiograph in an upright patient showing fixed superior migration of the humerus.

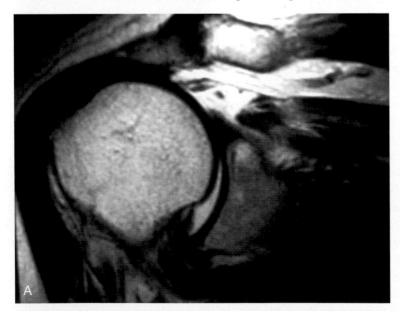
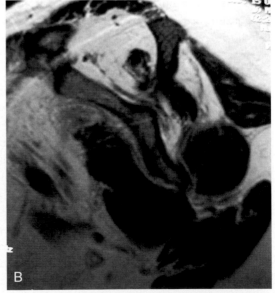

Figure 5 MRI scans of a massive rotator cuff tear. **A,** Coronal view of the retracted tear and muscle changes. **B,** Sagittal view of the scapula showing fatty changes in the supraspinatus and the infraspinatus muscles.

performed to further aid with visualization and tendon mobility.

After any ancillary procedures are completed intra-articularly, the arthroscope is placed in the subacromial space. This is initially performed through the posterior portal followed by the lateral and anterior portals to fully visualize the rotator cuff and the extent of the tear. A bursectomy may be needed for complete visualization of the tear. Caution is necessary when performing a bursectomy in a shoulder with a chronic massive rotator cuff tear to make sure viable rotator cuff tissue is not inadvertently removed with the bursa. Any adhesions, including those in the subdeltoid region, should be released for optimal visualization.

Specific Tear Patterns and Surgical Releases

Rotator cuff tears often begin in areas that attempt to restrain anterosuperior translation. Evolutionary changes occur in the superior border of the subscapularis and the leading edge of the supraspinatus, sometimes referred to as the cuff cable. With additional trauma or repetitive traction, tears can extend posteriorly and medially. Chronicity may alter the appearance of these tears, caused by interval healing to adjacent tissues. Proper reconstruction and repair requires recognition of the tear pattern and an attempt to make the repair with the least amount of tension.

Tears can be categorized as crescent shaped, L-shaped, reverse L-shaped, or large U-shaped. Surgeons should recognize the direction of the muscle fibers and perform appropriate releases to redirect the rotator cuff tendons to the proper positions on the greater tuberosity. Nonanatomic repairs, resulting in a "dog ear" deformity, may fail to heal after the return of muscular contraction during the recovery process.

Articular releases are recommended for retracted tears in patients with con-

tractures that restrict full passive range of motion. After placing the scope in the posterior articular viewing portal, the releases begin along the rotator interval. This interval exists between the anterior border of the supraspinatus and the superior border of the subscapularis. Medially retracted subscapularis tears avulse a thick band of tissue along the superior border of the tendon that comprises the biceps pulley and leading edge of the supraspinatus. This connective tissue consists of the coracohumeral ligament, medial pulley, and superior glenohumeral ligament. It is often better to preserve this strong connection and retract it laterally while opening the interval medially toward the coracoid. Articular and bursal releases of the coracohumeral ligament may avoid the need for disconnecting the subscapularis from the supraspinatus.

The scope is then placed in the anterior portal, and the tear extensions are visualized inferiorly and posteriorly. Gentle débridement can help determine the extent of tendon disruption from the tuberosities. A shaver or cutting instrument is placed in the posterior portal, and the capsule is released along the articular side of the infraspinatus and the teres minor. This release can extend into the inferior pouch if restricted, passive range of motion or chronic superior migration is suspected.

The arthroscope is then placed in the subacromial space. The initial débridement is started using the lateral portal. The débridement is directed to the anterolateral edge of the acromion, working laterally and posteriorly. The soft tissues are preserved and released from the adjacent acromion and deltoid. The intervals are opened anteriorly, laterally, and posteriorly. The scope is then placed in the lateral portal. Using the posterior portal, additional releases are performed adjacent

to the spine of the scapula. An atraumatic grasping instrument or traction sutures are placed, the tear is mobilized to define the tear pattern, and the steps of repairing to the tuberosities are planned.

Surgical Strategies

Good candidates for arthroscopic rotator cuff repair are determined based on the history, physical examination, and imaging studies. Arthroscopic evaluation and treatment goals include a complete closure of the defect. With releases as previously described, complete closure can be achieved at the time of surgery in most patients.

From an articular view via the posterior portal, the subscapularis should be mobilized via capsular releases of the middle glenohumeral ligament, with bursal release and decompression from the subcoracoid space. Decompression of the distal lateral margin of the coracoid can be achieved through an anterior portal while viewing through the "interval window" that was created. Tissue between the subscapularis and the coracoid should be removed, and the superior border of the muscle should move freely below the arch. A smooth freer or elevator can be used beneath the coracoid to release adhesions.

A series of suture anchors can be placed along the lesser tuberosity, allowing footprint coverage. If the biceps tendon is damaged, unstable, or obscuring the view, a stitch can be placed in the tendon and released from the superior labrum. Transtendon sutures are placed through the subscapularis tendon, using suture hooks and piercing grasping instruments. The superior border of the tendon is repaired with multiple sutures placed as mattress and simple sutures (**Figure 6**).

The arthroscope is replaced in the posterior portal of the subacromial space. A modified subacromial decom-

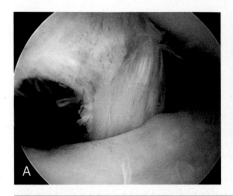
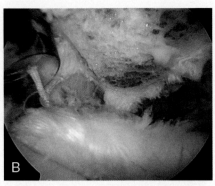

Figure 6 Arthroscopic views of a subscapularis repair. **A,** A window is created in the rotator interval of a retracted tear. **B,** Mattress suture repair and coracoid decompression is shown.

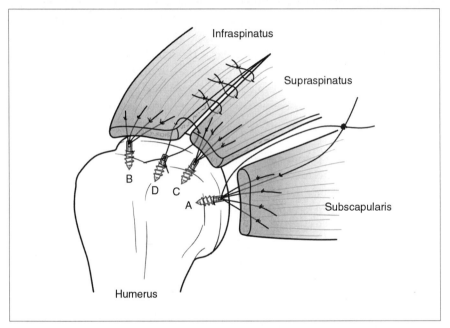

Figure 7 Illustration showing the fixation of a massive rotator cuff tear with anchors placed in the greater and lesser tuberosities. Two or three sutures per anchor (twice the number of strands as it passes through the eyelet) are placed along the tear margin. The order of anchor placement is A, B, C, and D. The subscapularis fixation through anchor A is a combination of mattress and simple sutures. The posterosuperior extension of the tear is reduced medially with mattress sutures.

convergent sutures are placed medially to reduce the L-shaped and reverse L-shaped medial extensions. Sutures adjacent to the glenoid can be tied to reduce the size of the defect. Lateral margin sutures may be left untied to allow tuberosity preparation and anchor placement. A series of anchors are placed in the greater tuberosity and are directed at repair of the supraspinatus and infraspinatus tendons (**Figure 7**). These anchors should be nonmetallic and contain two or three sutures per anchor. Follow-up imaging studies are clearer with fewer artifacts when nonmetallic anchors are used. Polyetheretherketone-absorbable, biocomposite materials are common choices for anchors. The anchors may be placed medially along the articular margin or in the middle of the tuberosity if tension is not problematic.

Suture passage is performed as mattress sutures, simple sutures, or a combination of these sutures. In tears with good elasticity, mattress sutures allow for further footprint coverage and compression with additional lateral knotless anchors. Although double-row constructs have improved tendon stability, this is not always possible with massive, retracted rotator cuff tears. Lateral-row reinforcement should be considered when possible along points of stress (the anterior margin of the supraspinatus; **Figure 8**). Additional stability of this portion of the rotator cuff will protect crescent areas of the cuff.

Patients with severe tendon retraction may develop weakness caused by suprascapular nerve angulation at the notch or the scapular spine. Tendon tear reduction along the posterior interval will often reduce this tension, improving innervation to the infraspinatus. Patients with a short supraspinatus tendon caused by tissue loss may benefit from suprascapular nerve decompression to avoid postreduction

pression can help mobilize and visualize the tear. The goal of this decompression is to create space between the tendon and the arch while preserving the coracoacromial ligament attachments. Downward-directed osteophytes are removed from the anterior edge of the acromion. The soft tissue is elevated but not removed from the anterior edge to maintain the attachment. Osteophytes below the acromioclavicular joint should be removed. The remaining distal clavicle excision can be delayed to the end of the surgery to minimize fluid extravasation.

The rotator cuff tendon margins are grasped and mobilized to identify tear patterns and allow reduction. Margin traction. With the scope in the lateral or posterior portal, the transverse ligament is released from the medial edge of the coracoid process.

 Video 10.1: Arthroscopic Repair of Massive Rotator Cuff Tears. Jeffrey S. Abrams, MD (7 min)

Arthroscopic Options for the Irreparable Massive Rotator Cuff Tear

Closure of the defect is the goal of any arthroscopic rotator cuff repair. Unfortunately, the rotator cuff tear margin cannot always be reduced and repaired in a tension-free manner, and closure of the entire defect is not possible. At this point, the surgeon has a few treatment options. A partial repair of the rotator cuff or graft augmentation can be implemented. In addition, the biceps tendon can be incorporated in either of these techniques to augment the repair.

A partial repair can help restore the transverse force couples in an irreparable, massive rotator cuff tear. In a massive U-shaped tear, side-to-side margin convergence sutures are first placed to close the medial aspect of the tear. At this point, standard suture anchors can be used to repair the anterior and posterior edges of the remaining tear if the superior rotator cuff cannot be completely closed. This type of repair can rebalance the force couples and compress the humeral head during shoulder motion, even if the superior rotator cuff has not been repaired (**Figure 9**). This construct can provide a stable fulcrum for the deltoid to act on while elevating the arm.

Burkhart et al[23] reported on 14 patients after partial rotator cuff repair. They found a significant improvement in active elevation, strength, and func-

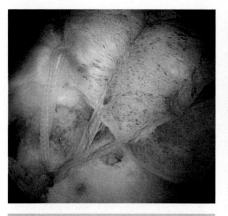

Figure 8 Arthroscopic view of a double-row reinforced repair covering the greater tuberosity of a multi-tendon tear.

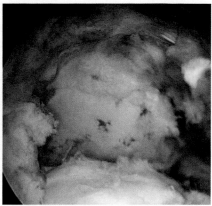

Figure 9 Arthroscopic view showing partial closure of a severely retracted rotator cuff tear with a residual supraspinatus defect.

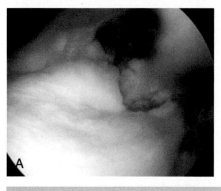 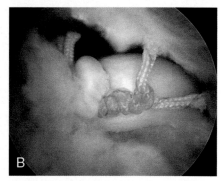

Figure 10 Augmentation of a partially closed repair of a massive rotator cuff tear with GraftJacket allograft (**A**) and using the long head of the biceps tendon (**B**).

tional outcomes after an average of 20.8 months. The results of a more recent study by Duralde and Bair[24] also demonstrated improvements with partial rotator cuff repair, with 67% excellent or good results and 33% rated as fair or poor. Although studies have shown encouraging results with partial rotator cuff repair, long-term results are lacking, and the duration of benefits is unclear.

Tissue grafts are another option for irreparable tears; varying degrees of success have been reported in the literature.[25,26] The ideal graft characteristics include strength, flexibility, and bone attachment and healing qualities similar to native tendon. Reparative

qualities are also needed so the graft can act as a scaffold for tissue ingrowth to reinforce the repair. New grafts are being introduced, but positive results have been seen with allograft tissue derived from human dermis (**Figure 10,** *A*). The biologic graft tissue creates an environment to augment the host healing response, acting as an extracellular matrix for host fibroblast infiltration. The GraftJacket (Wright Medical, Arlington, TN) is an example of prepared human dermis that has been used successfully.[27,28] Other xenografts and synthetic scaffolds have been used with varying degrees of success. Current labeling of the Food and Drug Administration permits use for tissue augmentation but not tissue substitution.

Biceps tendon augmentation is another technique that can help bridge the gap for massive rotator cuff tears that cannot be fully reduced to the footprint (**Figure 10**, *B*). The tenotomized biceps tendon can be incorporated into the posterolateral margin of the repair to further augment the repair. Cho et al[29] reviewed 37 patients who were treated with biceps tendon augmentation for massive rotator cuff tears and compared them to a randomly selected control group. The authors found that the augmentation group had fewer structural failures, equivalent clinical outcomes, and significant improvement in muscle strength. The released biceps tendon can be first attached to the posterior edge of the tear using a variety of suture passing devices, followed by reinsertion to the tuberosity footprint with a standard suture-anchor technique. Alternatively, suture limbs from the anchors could be placed through both the biceps tendon and the rotator cuff tear to reduce them both back to the footprint and hold them together. The medial sutures are passed through the rotator cuff tendon, whereas the lateral sutures can be passed through the biceps tendon. The use of biceps tendon augmentation in massive rotator cuff repairs has the added benefit of providing tenodesis for the biceps tendon as well as contributing to the repair.

Postoperative Management

Immediately following surgery, the patient's arm is placed in a padded sling with an abduction pillow. The addition of the abduction pillow reduces stress on the repair and maintains the shoulder in reduced internal rotation. This may reduce the risk of stiffness and improve the hypovascular environment for the supraspinatus.[30,31] A form of cryotherapy is typically used postoperatively for pain and edema control. The sling typically remains in place for 6 weeks depending on the integrity of the repair. During this initial period in the sling, the patient will begin active and passive range-of-motion exercises for the elbow, wrist, and hand, as well as shoulder pendulum exercises. After massive rotator cuff repairs, passive shoulder flexion is typically delayed for the first 5 weeks postoperatively to protect the repair. After 5 to 6 weeks, passive range-of-motion exercises are started in the supine position with transition to the upright position as tolerated. Internal rotation is delayed until 8 weeks after surgery because it has been demonstrated that this produces increased tension in the supraspinatus tendon.[32] Active motion commences at 10 weeks when the sling is discontinued, whereas strengthening is delayed until 12 to 16 weeks after surgery. Protective movements are emphasized, and activities and strength training are gradually increased. Return to recreational sports is often delayed for 6 months or more.

If stiffness develops, imaging should be used to evaluate the integrity of the repair. If the tendon repair is intact, a capsular release should be considered. Release of adhesions is often delayed until 9 months to optimize healing. If a repair deficiency is recognized with further imaging, additional surgical treatment based on the patient's functional status and symptoms can be considered.

Summary

A massive rotator cuff tear can occur in patients at different stages in life. Young, active individuals with an acute injury are ideally treated with an arthroscopic repair. Tendon retraction, muscle changes, and superior joint instability will develop with greater degrees of chronicity. During the early and midterm stages, the muscular effect can be salvaged if rotator cuff reconstruction can be achieved. Recognizing tear patterns and performing articular and bursal releases allows tendon repair in a high percentage of selected patients. Patients may achieve improved function and satisfaction with their surgical results with partial repairs or partial tendon healing of a persistent defect.

Several intraoperative options are available if the defect cannot be closed. A suture anchor repair of the margins of the repair may be sufficient to create a stable fulcrum for the deltoid to function. Using the biceps tendon to cross the defect and further reinforce the anterior and posterior margins of the tear is also an option. Allograft tissue may be used to assist in the reattachment of the rotator cuff to the tuberosities. Postoperative recovery after these procedures is slow, and patients should be prepared for a rehabilitation program that exceeds 6 months. Patients who choose to minimize postoperative restrictions may elect treatment with tenotomy and débridement. Those with glenohumeral arthritis or rotator cuff tear arthropathy would be better treated with arthroplasty. The arthroscopic approach to treating this difficult cohort of patients has been shown to reduce pain, increase active motion, and preserve the subacromial arch and function of the deltoid.

References

1. Sher JS, Uribe JW, Posada A, Murphy BJ, Zlatkin MB: Abnormal findings on magnetic resonance images of asymptomatic shoulders. *J Bone Joint Surg Am* 1995;77(1):10-15.

2. Tempelhof S, Rupp S, Seil R: Age-related prevalence of rotator cuff tears in asymptomatic shoulders. *J Shoulder Elbow Surg* 1999; 8(4):296-299.

3. Ellman H, Kay SP, Wirth M: Arthroscopic treatment of full-thickness rotator cuff tears: 2- to 7-year follow-up study. *Arthroscopy* 1993;9(2):195-200.

4. Ellman H, Hanker G, Bayer M: Repair of the rotator cuff: End-result study of factors influencing reconstruction. *J Bone Joint Surg Am* 1986;68(8):1136-1144.

5. DeOrio JK, Cofield RH: Results of a second attempt at surgical repair of a failed initial rotator-cuff repair. *J Bone Joint Surg Am* 1984;66(4):563-567.

6. Gerber C, Fuchs B, Hodler J: The results of repair of massive tears of the rotator cuff. *J Bone Joint Surg Am* 2000;82(4):505-515.

7. Abrams JS: Arthroscopic approach to massive rotator cuff tears. *Instr Course Lect* 2006;55:59-66.

8. Neer CS II, Craig EV, Fukuda H: Cuff-tear arthropathy. *J Bone Joint Surg Am* 1983;65(9):1232-1244.

9. Gartsman GM, Khan M, Hammerman SM: Arthroscopic repair of full-thickness tears of the rotator cuff. *J Bone Joint Surg Am* 1998;80(6):832-840.

10. Murray TF Jr, Lajtai G, Mileski RM, Snyder SJ: Arthroscopic repair of medium to large full-thickness rotator cuff tears: Outcome at 2- to 6-year follow-up. *J Shoulder Elbow Surg* 2002;11(1):19-24.

11. Wilson F, Hinov V, Adams G: Arthroscopic repair of full-thickness tears of the rotator cuff: 2- to 14-year follow-up. *Arthroscopy* 2002;18(2):136-144.

12. Burkhart SS, Danaceau SM, Pearce CE Jr: Arthroscopic rotator cuff repair: Analysis of results by tear size and by repair technique—margin convergence versus direct tendon-to-bone repair. *Arthroscopy* 2001;17(9):905-912.

13. Bishop J, Klepps S, Lo IK, Bird J, Gladstone JN, Flatow EL: Cuff integrity after arthroscopic versus open rotator cuff repair: A prospective study. *J Shoulder Elbow Surg* 2006;15(3):290-299.

14. Boileau P, Brassart N, Watkinson DJ, Carles M, Hatzidakis AM, Krishnan SG: Arthroscopic repair of full-thickness tears of the supraspinatus: Does the tendon really heal? *J Bone Joint Surg Am* 2005;87(6):1229-1240.

15. Burkhart SS, Barth JR, Richards DP, Zlatkin MB, Larsen M: Arthroscopic repair of massive rotator cuff tears with stage 3 and 4 fatty degeneration. *Arthroscopy* 2007;23(4):347-354.

16. Gladstone JN, Bishop JY, Lo IK, Flatow EL: Fatty infiltration and atrophy of the rotator cuff do not improve after rotator cuff repair and correlate with poor functional outcome. *Am J Sports Med* 2007;35(5):719-728.

17. Rockwood CA Jr, Williams GR Jr, Burkhead WZ Jr: Débridement of degenerative, irreparable lesions of the rotator cuff. *J Bone Joint Surg Am* 1995;77(6):857-866.

18. Galatz LM, Ball CM, Teefey SA, Middleton WD, Yamaguchi K: The outcome and repair integrity of completely arthroscopically repaired large and massive rotator cuff tears. *J Bone Joint Surg Am* 2004;86-A(2):219-224.

19. Weiner DS, Macnab I: Superior migration of the humeral head: A radiological aid in the diagnosis of tears of the rotator cuff. *J Bone Joint Surg Br* 1970;52(3):524-527.

20. Zingg PO, Jost B, Sukthankar A, Buhler M, Pfirrmann CW, Gerber C: Clinical and structural outcomes of nonoperative management of massive rotator cuff tears. *J Bone Joint Surg Am* 2007;89(9):1928-1934.

21. Goutallier D, Postel JM, Bernageau J, Lavau L, Voisin MC: Fatty muscle degeneration in cuff ruptures: Pre- and postoperative evaluation by CT scan. *Clin Orthop Relat Res* 1994;304:78-83.

22. Gerber C, Schneeberger AG, Hoppeler H, Meyer DC: Correlation of atrophy and fatty infiltration on strength and integrity of rotator cuff repairs: A study in thirteen patients. *J Shoulder Elbow Surg* 2007;16(6):691-696.

23. Burkhart SS, Nottage WM, Ogilvie-Harris DJ, Kohn HS, Pachelli A: Partial repair of irreparable rotator cuff tears. *Arthroscopy* 1994;10(4):363-370.

24. Duralde XA, Bair B: Massive rotator cuff tears: The result of partial rotator cuff repair. *J Shoulder Elbow Surg* 2005;14(2):121-127.

25. Derwin KA, Baker AR, Spragg RK, Leigh DR, Iannotti JP: Commercial extracellular matrix scaffolds for rotator cuff tendon repair: Biomechanical, biochemical, and cellular properties. *J Bone Joint Surg Am* 2006;88(12):2665-2672.

26. Valentin JE, Badylak JS, McCabe GP, Badylak SF: Extracellular matrix bioscaffolds for orthopaedic applications: A comparative histologic study. *J Bone Joint Surg Am* 2006;88(12):2673-2686.

27. Snyder SJ, Bond JL: Technique for arthroscopic replacement of severely damaged rotator cuff using "GraftJacket" allograft. *Oper Tech Sports Med* 2007;15(2):86-94.

28. Burkhead WZ, Schiffern SC, Krishnan SG: Use of GraftJacket as an augmentation for massive rotator cuff tears. *Semin Arthrop* 2007;18:11-18.

29. Cho NS, Yi JW, Rhee YG: Arthroscopic biceps augmentation for avoiding undue tension in repair of massive rotator cuff tears. *Arthroscopy* 2009;25(2):183-191.

30. Hatakeyama Y, Itoi E, Pradhan RL, Urayama M, Sato K: Effect of arm elevation and rotation on the strain in the repaired rotator cuff

tendon: A cadaveric study. *Am J Sports Med* 2001;29(6):788-794.

31. Rathbun JB, Macnab I: The microvascular pattern of the rotator cuff. *J Bone Joint Surg Br* 1970; 52(3):540-553.

32. McCann PD, Wootten ME, Kadaba MP, Bigliani LU: A kinematic and electromyographic study of shoulder rehabilitation exercises. *Clin Orthop Relat Res* 1993;288(288):179-188.

Video Reference

10.1: Abrams JS: Video. *Arthroscopic Repair of Massive Rotator Cuff Tears.* Princeton, NJ, 2011.

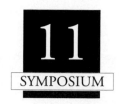

11
SYMPOSIUM

How to Minimize Complications in Shoulder Instability and Rotator Cuff Surgery

Andrew S. Neviaser, MD
Evan L. Flatow, MD
Reza Omid, MD
Ken Yamaguchi, MD
William N. Levine, MD

Abstract

Arthroscopic instability and rotator cuff repair techniques have rapidly evolved over the past decade with expanding indications; however, there has been a corresponding increase in complications. Careful attention to detail and patient selection will result in satisfactory outcomes for most patients.

Instr Course Lect 2012;61:131-141.

Surgical treatment of the unstable shoulder and rotator cuff tears has seen dramatic changes in the past decade and continues to evolve with an improved understanding of the anatomy and rapid technologic advances. Despite these improvements, the surgical treatment of shoulder instability and especially rotator cuff repairs has a high failure rate. This chapter outlines pearls and pitfalls in the surgical management of these disorders, with a specific goal of minimizing surgical complications.

Shoulder Instability

The debate surrounding the management of shoulder instability is among the oldest in medicine. In the fifth century B.C., Hippocrates wrote a prescient description of shoulder dislocations and argued that treatment (burning with a hot iron) should be directed at the inferior aspect of the shoulder rather than the superior or anterior aspects, which were the popular treatment methods at the time.[1] Modern orthopaedic surgeons have seen a shift from nonanatomic procedures complicated by stiffness (such as the Putti-Platt and the Magnuson-Stack procedures) to anatomic reconstructions with recurrence as the most common complication. Open Bankart repair, the putative gold standard for treating anterior instability, provides reliably excellent results,[2] but early attempts at arthroscopic repair were plagued by high failure rates. Advances in arthroscopic technology and an improved understanding of the pathology of instability have reduced recurrence rates after arthroscopic stabilization to rates comparable with those achieved with open repairs.[16,17] Arthroscopic soft-tissue repairs are now the most popular type of stabilization procedure. However, a subset of patients, including young patients and those with significant bone loss or hyperlaxity, remain at high risk for recurrence.[3-5] Optimal treatment should be specifically tailored to the unique character of a patient's instability, which is defined by the patient's symptoms, pathology, activity level, and desired goals of treatment. Complications arise from a failure to recognize

Dr. Flatow or an immediate family member has received royalties from Innomed and Zimmer; is a member of a speakers' bureau or has made paid presentations on behalf of Zimmer; serves as an unpaid consultant to Zimmer; has received research or institutional support from Wyeth; and serves as a board member, owner, officer, or committee member of the American Shoulder and Elbow Surgeons and the Arthroscopy Association of North America. Dr. Levine or an immediate family member serves as a board member, owner, officer, or committee member of the American Orthopaedic Association. None of the following authors or any immediate family member has received anything of value from or owns stock in a commercial company or institution related directly or indirectly to the subject of this chapter: Dr. Neviaser, Dr. Omid, and Dr. Yamaguchi.

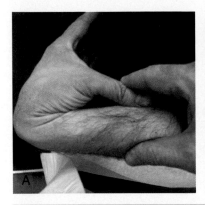
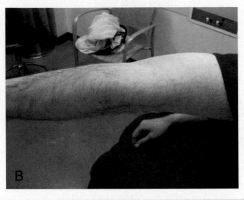
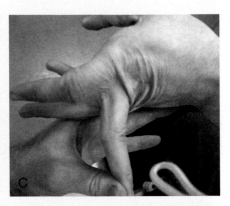

Figure 1 Preoperative assessment of the degree of laxity, such as the ability to touch the thumb to the forearm (**A**), hyperextension of the elbow (**B**), and metacarpophalangeal hyperextension (**C**) should be used to determine the amount of capsular plication included in arthroscopic shoulder stabilization surgery. Patients should be immobilized for 6 weeks after surgery. (Courtesy of Mt. Sinai Shoulder Service, New York, NY.)

contributing pathology, technical failures at the time of surgery, or inappropriate postoperative rehabilitation.

Patient Evaluation

Rather than being a dichotomous problem of traumatic unidirectional instability with a Bankart lesion or atraumatic multidirectional bilateral instability, shoulder instability encompasses a spectrum of pathologies between these two extremes. The initial patient evaluation should attempt to determine the severity of the patient's shoulder instability on the instability spectrum. The patient history should include age at onset, manner of onset (traumatic, repetitive microtraumatic, or insidious/atraumatic), magnitude (dislocation or subluxation), direction (anterior, inferior, posterior, bidirectional, or multidirectional), and the number of recurrences. Progressively less traumatic dislocation episodes can be a clue to attritional bone loss or increased joint laxity. Equally important is an understanding of the patient's activity level and expectations from treatment. Sports participation, including positions played and the level of play, should be reviewed. In a throwing athlete who requires supraphysiologic motion, interventions should be more

limited and motion maximally preserved despite the potential for recurrence. An older or more sedentary patient may benefit most from a robust repair despite the possible loss of terminal range motion. A family history of dislocations, bilateral symptoms, or ligament disorders in other joints (such as recurrent ankle sprains) may be clues to an intrinsic collagen variant and generalized laxity. Identification of voluntary dislocators can be difficult. The patient who can demonstrate his or her instability because of its severity (usually by placing the arm in an at-risk position) must be distinguished from the patient who can dislocate the shoulder for secondary gain (typically by asymmetric muscle contraction). The latter patient is not a suitable candidate for surgery, whereas the former patient should be considered for surgical treatment.

The physical examination should try to confirm the direction(s) of instability reported in the history and provide a sense of its severity. Failure to identify the direction of instability is a common cause of surgical failure and the need for revision. The anterior apprehension and relocation tests can identify anterior instability. Apprehension in the midrange of motion may

reflect the presence of significant bone loss. Posterior apprehension, or the so-called jerk test, can be used to identify posterior instability, which is important to consider if symptoms arise with the arm in forward flexion and adduction (common in some sports such as the offensive lineman position in American football). Global hyperlaxity will directly affect the surgical technique and postoperative rehabilitation and is critical to identify preoperatively. The literature provides various criteria to define hyperlaxity. Balg and Boileau[6] used external rotation in adduction beyond 85° to define anterior hyperlaxity and a positive Gagey hyperabduction test to define laxity in the inferior glenohumeral ligament. The combination of second metacarpophalangeal joint, elbow, or knee hyperextension, as well as the ability to touch the thumb to the forearm, is another standard testing maneuver (**Figure 1**). A sulcus sign that does not diminish with external rotation can indicate an inferior component in the patient's instability and global capsular laxity.

Rotator cuff strength testing is critical in patients older than 40 years with a first-time dislocation because rates of associated tears are high.[7] A

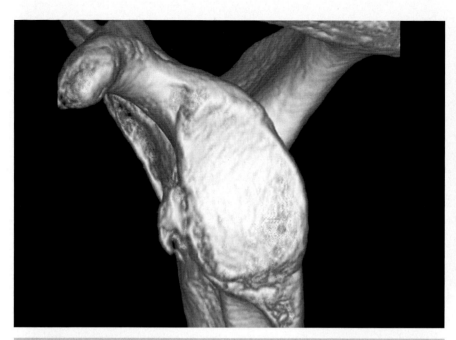

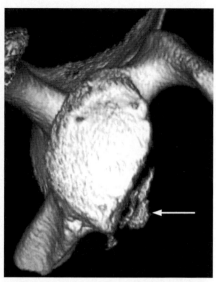

Figure 2   The inverted pear glenoid evaluation of glenoid bone loss is evaluated on a three-dimensional CT scan. (Courtesy of the Columbia University Center for Shoulder, Elbow and Sports Medicine, New York, NY.)

Figure 3   Sagittal three-dimensional CT reconstruction of the shoulder of a 25-year-old right-hand-dominant man who was previously treated with an arthroscopic stabilization procedure for a 270° labral tear. The patient had a recurrent traumatic dislocation. Note the acute anteroinferior glenoid comminuted fracture (arrow) along the suture anchor track line from the index procedure. (Courtesy of Columbia University Center for Shoulder, Elbow and Sports Medicine, New York, NY.)

complete neurologic examination will identify an uncommon neurologic injury after dislocation and should be completed for every patient.

A comprehensive history and physical examination establishes the degree and direction of instability, the tissue quality of the shoulder stabilizers, and an understanding of the patient's goals of treatment. These are crucial elements in determining the method of treatment and tailoring it to the specific patient.

Imaging

Standard radiographs are routinely obtained, including Grashey (true AP or AP in the scapular plane), axillary, and scapular Y views. Significant bone loss can typically be identified from this series, but quantification requires more advanced imaging. Loss of the antero-inferior cortical margin of the glenoid seen on a Grashey or axillary view can be a subtle indication of bone loss. MRI or magnetic resonance arthrography provides valuable information

about soft-tissue lesions as well as bone loss and should be routinely obtained. The presence of a humeral avulsion of the glenohumeral ligament lesion, a superior labrum anterior to posterior tear, or a rotator cuff tear is important to recognize preoperatively because these lesions will likely affect the prognosis and potentially the choice of surgery. An adequate assessment of bone loss can be made from MRI scans, although CT scans are more popular for this purpose.

Several studies have identified both glenoid and humeral bone loss as risk factors for failure of arthroscopic repairs.[8] The exact amount of bone loss that requires a bony reconstruction procedure remains undefined. Biomechanical studies have suggested that 20% loss of the glenoid face (around 6 mm of bone) produces significant instability.[9,10] Clinically, the presence of an inverted pear shape to the glenoid has been associated with the failure of arthroscopic stabilizations[11] (**Figure 2**). When significant bone loss is

suspected, many surgeons obtain a CT scan with three-dimensional reconstructions and humeral subtraction to best quantify the deficiency[12] (**Figure 3**). There are several methods of quantifying glenoid bone loss. The inferior two thirds portion of the glenoid is circular in shape. Bone deficiency can be determined by drawing a best-fit circle over this portion of the glenoid on the most lateral cut of a reformatted sagittal CT image. The missing bone is quantified by determining the surface area loss in the anteroinferior part of the circle.[8] Gerber and Nyffeler[13] reported that if the superior to inferior length of the glenoid deficiency was greater than the radius of the inferior glenoid, the resistance to dislocation was less than 70% that of an intact shoulder. Quantifying the size of a Hill-Sachs lesion is more difficult than measuring glenoid bone deficiency. The role of a Hill-Sachs lesion in recurrent instability is also less well defined. Hill-Sachs lesions are found in more than 75% of patients with anterior instability, and most of these lesions can be safely ignored. Burkhart et al[11] identified the engaging Hill-Sachs lesion as a potential reason for the failure of arthroscopic repairs. To engage the glenoid, the humeral lesion must be parallel to the anterior rim with the arm in a position of 90° of abduction and external rotation. It has been suggested that humeral-sided lesions evident on an external rotation AP radiographic view tend to be located more superiorly and may be more significant in the development of recurrent instability.[6] Biomechanical studies have shown that simulated Hill-Sachs lesions measuring 62.5% of the radius of the humeral head significantly decrease the distance to dislocation in external rotation and abduction. Lesions measuring 87.5% of the radius of the humeral head decrease stability in a neutral, externally rotated position.[14] Any reduction in the glenoid surface area will make engagement of the humeral-sided lesion more likely, and bone loss on either side should not be viewed in isolation.

Treatment Choices

The optimal choice of treatment for the unstable shoulder is based on the nature of the patient's pathology and his or her treatment goals. True subluxation episodes are often amenable to nonsurgical measures. After a period of rest, physical therapy is begun and should focus on improving proprioception and strengthening the dynamic stabilizers. Throwing athletes with microinstability and pain should have a rehabilitation regimen that particularly emphasizes posterior capsular stretching, scapular stabilization, and rotator cuff strengthening.

Treatment of a primary anterior shoulder dislocation remains a matter of controversy. As stated by Hovelius et al,[15] the prognosis for a nonsurgically treated primary anterior shoulder dislocation is "neither very good nor very bad." In the largest natural history study to date, 61 of 227 patients (27%) followed for 25 years eventually required surgery for persistent instability. Forty-four percent of patients younger than 22 years at the time of primary dislocation required surgical stabilization. Several smaller studies have documented recurrent instability in 92% to 95% of younger, high-demand patients after a traumatic anterior dislocation.[16,17] Comparisons of surgical and nonsurgical treatments have shown fewer recurrences in surgically treated patients.[16] Patients who present after the initial dislocation must be counseled about these risks. Considering the patient's goals for treatment is critical for management. In-season athletes who do not want to be sidelined and understand the risk of recurrence can be managed with motion-restricting bracing, can continue to play, and should be reassessed for further treatment at the end of the season.[18] Older, more sedentary patients can be given a trial of nonsurgical management with reasonable activity restrictions. Patients who wish to return to optimal function and high-risk activities are reasonable candidates for surgery.

In the absence of significant bone loss, most patients can be reliably treated with an arthroscopic soft-tissue procedure. The early arthroscopic treatment of instability resulted in high rates of failure, in part because procedures were focused solely on reattaching the avulsed labrum to its anatomic location. It is now well recognized that detachment of the anteroinferior labrum alone is insufficient to create clinically significant instability.[19] Even in the presence of a Bankart lesion, the inferior glenohumeral ligament is subjected to midsubstance strain and undergoes significant plastic deformation.[20] The pathologic process leading to shoulder instability includes repeated deformation and elongation of the inferior glenohumeral ligament and joint capsule, which must be reversed by any attempted stabilization. Inherent in successful open procedures, such as Rowe's Bankart repair and Neer's capsular shift, are reduction of the capsular volume and retensioning of the inferior glenohumeral ligament. Successful arthroscopic stabilization must address capsular laxity through capsular mobilization and imbrication. The amount of imbrication is based on the preoperative evaluation of shoulder laxity (which should be repeated under anesthesia). Failure to adequately mobilize the labrum prohibits the required inferior to superior shifting of the capsule and is a frequent cause of recurrence. This is of particular importance when addressing an anterior labrum periosteal sleeve avulsion lesion (**Figure 4**). Mobilization is adequate when the deep surface of the subscapularis muscle is identified and the labrum "floats" adjacent to the anterior face of the glenoid without external traction. A minimum of three anchors should be placed on the anteroinferior glenoid face (3 o'clock to the 6 o'clock positions in a right shoulder). If the patient has a prominent sulcus sign, a posterior plication suture can be placed at the 7:30 position to provide a posterior shift of the capsule (**Figure 5**). At the completion of the procedure, viewing from an anterosuperior portal should show the head to be centered on the glenoid, and any drive-through sign should be eliminated.

In patients who exhibit greater than 20% glenoid bone loss, a Latarjet procedure should be considered. The Latarjet procedure resists anterior dislocation by three proposed mechanisms: restoration of the glenoid anterior to posterior diameter, tensioning of the anterior capsule through repair to the stump of the coracoacromial ligament, and the sling effect of the conjoined tendon as the arm is abducted, resisting anterior translation of the humeral head. The last mechanism is likely the most critical component. Long-term studies report very low rates of recurrence, high rates of patient satisfaction, and an 83% return to preoperative level of sports participation after the Latarjet procedure.[21] Loss of external rotation, a reported complication of this procedure, can be avoided by using a subscapularis split rather than a complete or partial tenotomy. Rates of arthritis after Latarjet procedures are similar to those seen after nonsurgical treatment of instability, but graft placement is critical to avoid this complication. Placing the coracoid flush with the glenoid face most closely reproduces the mean contact pressure of native joints. No amount of lateral overhang should be tolerated because this is associated with rapid joint degeneration. Placing the coracoid in a slightly medial position relative to the face (1 to 2 mm) is acceptable.

In patients with glenoid bone loss equal to 40% of the glenoid surface or more, a Latarjet procedure will not restore sufficient bone stock. In these rare cases, cortical iliac crest grafts can be used with satisfactory results. Early reports of glenoid reconstruction with distal tibia allografts for severe bone loss are promising.[22] The cartilage on the lateral aspect of the distal tibia plafond matches the radius of curvature of the glenoid, making this a desirable choice for allograft reconstruction. No long-term results have been reported.

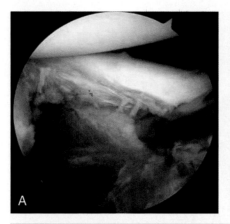
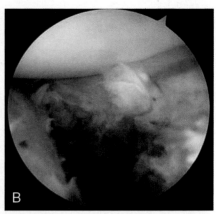

Figure 4 Adequate mobilization of the labrum is critical to relieving tension when it is reduced to the glenoid face and to adequate shifting of the capsule. **A,** The deep surface of the subscapularis should be seen arthroscopically. **B,** The labrum should "float" anterior to the glenoid face when it is adequately freed. (Courtesy of Mt. Sinai Shoulder Service, New York, NY.)

With adequate reconstitution of glenoid bone, Hill-Sachs lesions rarely require treatment. When necessary, treatment options for a large defect include bony, soft-tissue, and arthroplastic reconstructions. Miniaci[23] reported on allograft reconstruction of Hill-Sachs defects in 18 patients in whom prior anterior stabilizations had failed. The author reported no recurrence at latest follow-up, but 2 of the 18 patients had partial graft collapse. Other described techniques for large defects include filling the defect with a partial arthroplasty and remplissage or inserting the infraspinatus and posterior capsule into the defect. Small series have reported favorable results with both techniques, but further study is needed to define indications and potential complications.[24,25]

Rehabilitation

Regardless of the procedure chosen, patient-specific rehabilitation is critical to success. Stiffness following arthroscopic soft-tissue stabilization procedures occurs less frequently than after open procedures, and an initial period of immobilization is typically well tolerated. A patient should be examined at 2-week intervals following

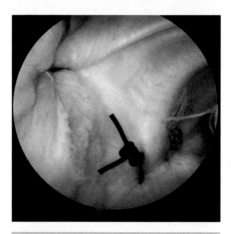

Figure 5 Arthroscopic view of a posterior tuck, which can be added via a posteroinferior suture for patients with an inferior component to their instability or hyperlaxity. (Courtesy of Mt. Sinai Shoulder Service, New York, NY.)

surgery for the first 6 weeks, and therapy should be initiated based on his or her response to the immobilization. As the initial pain from surgery subsides, patients who do not begin to regain motion should be started on a passive therapy program as early as 4 weeks after surgery. Patients who demonstrate significant laxity preoperatively, and those whose motion improves despite full-time use of a sling, can delay initi-

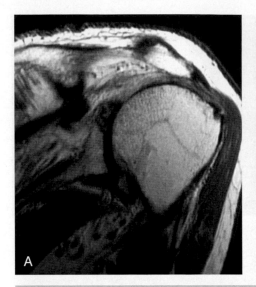

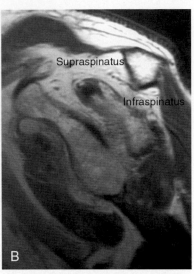

Figure 6 **A,** T1-weighted coronal MRI scan of the shoulder of a 73-year-old, right-hand-dominant man with a 5-year history of progressively worsening shoulder pain and weakness. The MRI scan shows severe atrophy and retraction of the supraspinatus with complete proximal humeral migration. **B,** T1-weighted sagittal MRI scan of the same patient showing Goutallier stage 4 atrophy of the supraspinatus and infraspinatus. (Courtesy of Columbia University Center for Shoulder, Elbow and Sports Medicine, New York, NY.)

ating therapy for 6 weeks. After this time, passive and active-assisted motion exercises are started. Strengthening and proprioceptive training begin after 3 months.

Rotator Cuff

Rotator cuff disease ranks among the most prevalent of musculoskeletal disorders, with as many as 17 million individuals in the United States at risk for disability.[26,27] Therefore, it seems intuitive that factors affecting the outcome of rotator cuff surgery are important to all orthopaedic surgeons. Complications of rotator cuff surgery include persistent pain after a repair, postoperative stiffness, deltoid compromise, and infection. The most common complication is persistent pain, which may be caused by several factors, including failure of the repair to heal or unrecognized pathology at the time of surgery. Studies suggest that healing of a rotator cuff repair may lead to better clinical outcomes;

however, no study to date has been able to conclusively prove this hypothesis.[28-31] Harryman et al[30] was the first to demonstrate the lack of healing after a rotator cuff repair with the use of ultrasound. The American Academy of Orthopaedic Surgeons recently assembled an evidence-based Clinical Practice Guideline workgroup to identify the most important questions involved in treating the rotator cuff and the best evidence available to assist orthopaedic surgeons in determining the best standard of care.[32] Unfortunately, the absence of high-quality evidence was the most important finding of this guideline process.

Although not specifically studied, many orthopaedic surgeons have noted that almost all repair failures involve a lack of healing, and few healed rotator cuff repairs remain painful. The issue is complex because a persistent or unhealed rotator cuff tear does not preclude good clinical results, although it can lead to poor

outcomes.[33-35] Many studies have highlighted the fact that patients do well without healing of the repair.[33,34] Galatz et al[33] showed that 94% of their patients had a retear; however, 72% of those patients had American Shoulder and Elbow Surgeons scores greater than 90. Jost et al[34] reported that patients with a known rerupture after rotator cuff repair still had significant improvement at long-term follow-up compared with the preoperative state. Because of such results, the necessity of repairing rotator cuff tears has been questioned. Several studies have reported that healed rotator cuff repairs result in better strength and possibly a more predictable outcome.[28-31] These findings may be most important in patients younger than 60 years. Rotator cuff disease progression has been shown to be influenced by patient age.[27] Yamaguchi et al[36] demonstrated that the presence of rotator cuff disease is highly correlated with age. Among the patients who presented with pain, the average age was 48.7 years for those with no tear, 58.7 years for those with a unilateral tear, and 67.8 years for those with a bilateral tear. There was a 50% likelihood of a bilateral tear after the age of 66 years.[36] Kartus et al[37] showed progression of partial tears to full-thickness tears in 35% of patients treated with débridement alone. A repaired rotator cuff can theoretically halt the progression of the natural history of the disease, which includes enlarging tear size, retraction, muscle atrophy, fatty infiltration, and the potential for rotator cuff arthropathy.[36]

Fatty infiltration and atrophy of the rotator cuff muscles have been described as important factors in determining the reparability of rotator cuff tears (**Figure 6**). Fatty infiltration increases with the size of tear, the location of the tear (involvement of the anterior cable), and the time elapsed after a tear has occurred.[38,39] Both clinical and experimental evidence suggests that fatty infiltration may be limited by tendon repair but not reversed.[40-42] More importantly, increased infiltration preoperatively predicts poorer postoperative results and increased retear rates.[43] Consequently, repairing tears before fatty infiltration and atrophy will likely improve overall clinical results. The ultimate goal of rotator cuff surgery remains healing of the repair.

Multiple factors are probably important in maximizing the healing potential of surgically repaired rotator cuffs. Although surgical technique is probably the focus of most surgeons, many other factors, which may be more important, deserve consideration. Such factors include biologic issues such as the age of the patient, size of the tear, chronicity of the tear, general health of the patient, and genetic factors.[44-46] Environmental factors such as work activity, rehabilitation protocol, the use of nonsteroidal anti-inflammatory drugs, and smoking are likely to be important factors.[47-49] Based on natural history information, biologic factors may be the most important in dictating the healing potential of a repair. In particular, the patient's age may be the single most important factor. Younger patients (age 55 to 60 years) may have reasonable capacity to heal, whereas a low rate of healing should be expected for physiologically older patients.[29,31,50-54] The three general categories of factors that help predict the healing potential of a rotator cuff tear are surgical technique, biology, and environmental issues. From a practical standpoint, surgeons can control all three issues, including biology. The control of biology results from careful patient selection. Once a decision has been made for surgical intervention, the surgeon can control

only for technique and environmental issues.

Multiple biomechanical studies have proven that double-row fixation has greater (1) pullout strength, (2) resistance to rotational stress, and (3) surface area for healing.[55-58] Many studies have suggested improved clinical healing with double-row fixation; however, these studies did not control for patient age or size of the tears and lacked statistical power.[75,76] In the literature, only three level I studies have been published, and none have been able to demonstrate a significant difference in the clinical outcome between single- and double-row repairs.[59-61] There are also some questions on whether these studies had sufficient power. The issue regarding whether the repair construct makes a difference in healing is still unknown; however, best evidence has not demonstrated the superiority of double-row fixation.

Given the uncertainty about the benefits of surgical technique, it may be best to consider the attributes of double-row repair within the context of biologic constraints. The best mechanical constructs (double-row constructs), conservative rehabilitation, and control of environmental factors may be more important in the younger patient with smaller tears; in this situation, the biology is optimal, and the limiting factor to healing may be the type of surgical repair or rehabilitation. These factors are less important in the older patient with a large or massive tear because the best repair and rehabilitation may still lead to a failure in healing. For this reason, early surgery should be considered in patients younger than 60 years with small- to medium-sized tears as well as acute tears (< 3 months duration).

Treatment options for failed rotator cuff repair include revision rotator cuff repair, débridement with biceps tenot-

omy, musculotendinous unit transfers, and arthroplasty. Several studies have shown that satisfactory results can be obtained with revision rotator cuff repair, but the results are inferior in comparison to primary repairs.[52,62-66] Keener et al[52] determined that healing rates can be comparable to primary repairs, but the results were again affected by age and the number of torn tendons. Clinical results were not affected by healing, and good results were possible despite the lack of cuff repair healing.

Débridement and biceps tenotomy are more popular in Europe, and some studies have reported good results by simply treating the biceps tendon. Walch et al[67] reviewed 307 cases of irreparable rotator cuff tears treated with arthroscopic biceps tenotomy. The mean Constant scores improved from 48.4 points preoperatively to 67.6 points postoperatively ($P < 0.0001$), and 87% of patients were satisfied or very satisfied with the result. Boileau et al[68] reported on 62 patients with irreparable rotator cuff tears treated with arthroscopic biceps tenotomy or tenodesis. The mean Constant scores improved from 46.3 points preoperatively to 66.5 points postoperatively ($P < 0.0001$), and 78% of patients were satisfied with the result. It must be highlighted, however, that these studies were done in the primary setting, and extrapolation of these results to the revision situation may not show similar findings.

Using tendon transfers for irreparable rotator cuff tears can provide good pain relief but usually leads to less predictable functional results. Several studies reporting on the use of latissimus dorsi transfers for irreparable posterosuperior rotator cuff tears show satisfactory pain relief; however, results are dependent on the integrity of the subscapularis and preoperative shoulder range of motion and strength.[69,70]

Warner and Parsons[71] suggested that salvage reconstruction of failed prior rotator cuff repairs yields more limited gains in patient satisfaction and function than primary latissimus dorsi transfer.

Arthroplasty for patients with rotator cuff disease has also been described. Historically, total shoulder arthroplasty has provided less than ideal results because of glenoid loosening complications. Hemiarthroplasty was the treatment of choice when arthroplasty was required in a shoulder with a deficient rotator cuff, but results were less predictable. Reasonable results could be obtained in terms of pain relief and function but depended on the preoperative status of the patient. Sanchez-Sotelo et al[72] reported on a group of patients who were treated with hemiarthroplasty for a rotator cuff-deficient arthritic shoulder. Marked pain relief was obtained in 67% of patients with slight but significant improvements in range of motion (active elevation improved from 72° preoperatively to 91° postoperatively [$P = 0.008$]). However, 27% of patients had moderate pain at rest or pain with activity. Goldberg et al[73] showed that good results could be obtained in patients with arthritic rotator cuff-deficient shoulders with hemiarthroplasty if the preoperative forward elevation was 90° or greater.

In 2004, the Food and Drug Administration approved the use of the reverse total shoulder prosthesis in the United States, and since then it has become the gold standard for the treatment of arthritic shoulders without a functional rotator cuff. Mulieri et al[74] described reverse total shoulder arthroplasty for patients with irreparable rotator cuff tears without glenohumeral arthritis. In 72 shoulders managed with a reverse shoulder arthroplasty, the American Shoulder and Elbow Surgeons scores improved from 33.3 preoperatively to 75.4 postoperatively ($P < 0.0001$); simple shoulder test scores improved from 1.6 to 6.5 ($P < 0.0001$); visual analog scores for pain improved from 6.3 to 1.9 ($P < 0.0001$); and average forward flexion improved from 53° to 134° ($P < 0.0001$). Interestingly, there was no difference between patients in the groups who did not have a previous repair versus the revision group. In the absence of multiple surgical failures or significant arthritis, an attempted revision repair was warranted.

The decision to proceed with early surgical treatment of rotator cuff tears depends on the tear size and acuity, patient age, and the presence of chronic changes to the rotator cuff and glenohumeral joint. Early repair should be undertaken for younger patients with tears at significant risk for developing chronic changes such as fatty infiltration, tear extension, humeral head migration, and arthritic changes. In surgically treated patients, reparability or healing may be maximized by appropriate early intervention, maximizing the strength of the repair with a double-row construct, cessation of smoking, the administration of nonsteroidal anti-inflammatory drugs, and conservative rehabilitation.

Summary

Successful treatment of shoulder instability and rotator cuff tears requires a comprehensive evaluation and interventions that are specifically tailored to address the individual patient's pathology and treatment goals. The results of arthroscopic stabilization have improved, and most patients who require surgery can be treated arthroscopically. Patients with significant bone loss can be reliably treated with the Latarjet procedure. Arthroscopic management of rotator cuff tears has not changed the biologic, environmental, and rehabilitation issues that continue to be critical to the ultimate outcome of these procedures. Early surgical intervention for rotator cuff tears in patients younger than 60 years is warranted to avoid the future development of an irreparable rotator cuff tear.

References

1. Rockwood CA, Matsen FA, eds: *The Shoulder*, ed 2. Philadelphia, PA, Saunders, 1998.

2. Rowe CR, Patel D, Southmayd WW: The Bankart procedure: A long-term end-result study. *J Bone Joint Surg Am* 1978;60(1):1-16.

3. Boileau P, Villalba M, Héry JY, Balg F, Ahrens P, Neyton L: Risk factors for recurrence of shoulder instability after arthroscopic Bankart repair. *J Bone Joint Surg Am* 2006;88(8):1755-1763.

4. Voos JE, Livermore RW, Feeley BT, et al; HSS Sports Medicine Service: Prospective evaluation of arthroscopic bankart repairs for anterior instability. *Am J Sports Med* 2010;38(2):302-307.

5. Porcellini G, Campi F, Pegreffi F, Castagna A, Paladini P: Predisposing factors for recurrent shoulder dislocation after arthroscopic treatment. *J Bone Joint Surg Am* 2009;91(11):2537-2542.

6. Balg F, Boileau P: The instability severity index score: A simple preoperative score to select patients for arthroscopic or open shoulder stabilisation. *J Bone Joint Surg Br* 2007;89(11):1470-1477.

7. Neviaser RJ, Neviaser TJ, Neviaser JS: Concurrent rupture of the rotator cuff and anterior dislocation of the shoulder in the older patient. *J Bone Joint Surg Am* 1988;70(9):1308-1311.

8. Piasecki DP, Verma NN, Romeo AA, Levine WN, Bach BR Jr, Provencher MT: Glenoid bone deficiency in recurrent anterior shoulder instability: Diagnosis and management. *J Am Acad Orthop Surg* 2009;17(8):482-493.

9. Itoi E, Lee SB, Berglund LJ, Berge LL, An KN: The effect of a glenoid defect on anteroinferior stability of the shoulder after Bankart repair: A cadaveric study. *J Bone Joint Surg Am* 2000;82(1):35-46.

10. Yamamoto N, Itoi E, Abe H, et al: Effect of an anterior glenoid defect on anterior shoulder stability: A cadaveric study. *Am J Sports Med* 2009;37(5):949-954.

11. Burkhart SS, Debeer JF, Tehrany AM, Parten PM: Quantifying glenoid bone loss arthroscopically in shoulder instability. *Arthroscopy* 2002;18(5):488-491.

12. Provencher MT, Arciero RA, Burkhart SS, Levine WN, Ritting AW, Romeo AA: Key factors in primary and revision surgery for shoulder instability. *Instr Course Lect* 2010;59:227-244.

13. Gerber C, Nyffeler RW: Classification of glenohumeral joint instability. *Clin Orthop Relat Res* 2002;400:65-76.

14. Kaar SG, Fening SD, Jones MH, Colbrunn RW, Miniaci A: Effect of humeral head defect size on glenohumeral stability: A cadaveric study of simulated Hill-Sachs defects. *Am J Sports Med* 2010; 38(3):594-599.

15. Hovelius L, Olofsson A, Sandström B, et al: Nonoperative treatment of primary anterior shoulder dislocation in patients forty years of age and younger: A prospective twenty-five-year follow-up. *J Bone Joint Surg Am* 2008;90(5): 945-952.

16. Kirkley A, Werstine R, Ratjek A, Griffin S: Prospective randomized clinical trial comparing the effectiveness of immediate arthroscopic stabilization versus immobilization and rehabilitation in first traumatic anterior dislocations of the shoulder: Long-term evaluation. *Arthroscopy* 2005;21(1): 55-63.

17. Larrain MV, Botto GJ, Montenegro HJ, Mauas DM: Arthroscopic repair of acute traumatic anterior shoulder dislocation in young athletes. *Arthroscopy* 2001;17(4): 373-377.

18. Buss DD, Lynch GP, Meyer CP, Huber SM, Freehill MQ: Nonoperative management for in-season athletes with anterior shoulder instability. *Am J Sports Med* 2004; 32(6):1430-1433.

19. Speer KP, Deng X, Borrero S, Torzilli PA, Altchek DA, Warren RF: Biomechanical evaluation of a simulated Bankart lesion. *J Bone Joint Surg Am* 1994;76(12):1819-1826.

20. Pollock RG, Wang VM, Bucchieri JS, et al: Effects of repetitive subfailure strains on the mechanical behavior of the inferior glenohumeral ligament. *J Shoulder Elbow Surg* 2000;9(5):427-435.

21. Young AA, Maia R, Berhouet J, Walch G: Open Latarjet procedure for management of bone loss in anterior instability of the glenohumeral joint. *J Shoulder Elbow Surg* 2011;20(2, Suppl):S61-S69.

22. Provencher MT, Ghodadra N, LeClere L, Solomon DJ, Romeo AA: Anatomic osteochondral glenoid reconstruction for recurrent glenohumeral instability with glenoid deficiency using a distal tibia allograft. *Arthroscopy* 2009;25(4): 446-452.

23. Miniaci A: Management of anterior glenohumeral instability associated with large Hill Sachs Defects. *Tech Shoulder Elbow Surg* 2004;5:170-175.

24. Moros C, Ahmad CS: Partial humeral head resurfacing and Latarjet coracoid transfer for treatment of recurrent anterior glenohumeral instability. *Orthopedics* 2009;32(8).

25. Purchase RJ, Wolf EM, Hobgood ER, Pollock ME, Smalley CC: Hill-Sachs "remplissage": An arthroscopic solution for the engaging Hill-Sachs lesion. *Arthroscopy* 2008;24(6):723-726.

26. Milgrom C, Schaffler M, Gilbert S, van Holsbeeck M: Rotator-cuff changes in asymptomatic adults: The effect of age, hand dominance and gender. *J Bone Joint Surg Br* 1995;77(2):296-298.

27. Sher JS, Uribe JW, Posada A, Murphy BJ, Zlatkin MB: Abnormal findings on magnetic resonance images of asymptomatic shoulders. *J Bone Joint Surg Am* 1995;77(1):10-15.

28. Bishop J, Klepps S, Lo IK, Bird J, Gladstone JN, Flatow EL: Cuff integrity after arthroscopic versus open rotator cuff repair: A prospective study. *J Shoulder Elbow Surg* 2006;15(3):290-299.

29. Boileau P, Brassart N, Watkinson DJ, Carles M, Hatzidakis AM, Krishnan SG: Arthroscopic repair of full-thickness tears of the supraspinatus: Does the tendon really heal? *J Bone Joint Surg Am* 2005;87(6):1229-1240.

30. Harryman DT II, Mack LA, Wang KY, Jackins SE, Richardson ML, Matsen FA III: Repairs of the rotator cuff: Correlation of functional results with integrity of the cuff. *J Bone Joint Surg Am* 1991; 73(7):982-989.

31. Nho SJ, Adler RS, Tomlinson DP, et al: Arthroscopic rotator cuff repair: Prospective evaluation with sequential ultrasonography. *Am J Sports Med* 2009;37(10):1938-1945.

32. American Academy of Orthopaedic Surgeons: *Clinical Practice Guideline on Optimizing the Management of Rotator Cuff Problems.* Rosemont, IL, American Academy of Orthopaedic Surgeons, December 2010. http://www.aaos.org/research/guidelines/RCP_guideline.pdf. Accessed April 3, 2011.

33. Galatz LM, Ball CM, Teefey SA, Middleton WD, Yamaguchi K: The outcome and repair integrity of completely arthroscopically repaired large and massive rotator

cuff tears. *J Bone Joint Surg Am* 2004;86-A(2):219-224.

34. Jost B, Pfirrmann CW, Gerber C, Switzerland Z: Clinical outcome after structural failure of rotator cuff repairs. *J Bone Joint Surg Am* 2000;82(3):304-314.

35. Jost B, Zumstein M, Pfirrmann CW, Gerber C: Long-term outcome after structural failure of rotator cuff repairs. *J Bone Joint Surg Am* 2006;88(3):472-479.

36. Yamaguchi K, Ditsios K, Middleton WD, Hildebolt CF, Galatz LM, Teefey SA: The demographic and morphological features of rotator cuff disease: A comparison of asymptomatic and symptomatic shoulders. *J Bone Joint Surg Am* 2006;88(8):1699-1704.

37. Kartus J, Kartus C, Rostgård-Christensen L, Sernert N, Read J, Perko M: Long-term clinical and ultrasound evaluation after arthroscopic acromioplasty in patients with partial rotator cuff tears. *Arthroscopy* 2006;22(1): 44-49.

38. Kim HM, Dahiya N, Teefey SA, et al: Location and initiation of degenerative rotator cuff tears: An analysis of three hundred and sixty shoulders. *J Bone Joint Surg Am* 2010;92(5):1088-1096.

39. Kim HM, Dahiya N, Teefey SA, Keener JD, Galatz LM, Yamaguchi K: Relationship of tear size and location to fatty degeneration of the rotator cuff. *J Bone Joint Surg Am* 2010;92(4):829-839.

40. Gerber C, Meyer DC, Schneeberger AG, Hoppeler H, von Rechenberg B: Effect of tendon release and delayed repair on the structure of the muscles of the rotator cuff: An experimental study in sheep. *J Bone Joint Surg Am* 2004;86-A(9):1973-1982.

41. Gladstone JN, Bishop JY, Lo IK, Flatow EL: Fatty infiltration and atrophy of the rotator cuff do not improve after rotator cuff repair and correlate with poor functional

outcome. *Am J Sports Med* 2007; 35(5):719-728.

42. Goutallier D, Postel JM, Gleyze P, Leguilloux P, Van Driessche S: Influence of cuff muscle fatty degeneration on anatomic and functional outcomes after simple suture of full-thickness tears. *J Shoulder Elbow Surg* 2003;12(6): 550-554.

43. Goutallier D, Postel JM, Bernageau J, Lavau L, Voisin MC: Fatty muscle degeneration in cuff ruptures: Pre- and postoperative evaluation by CT scan. *Clin Orthop Relat Res* 1994;304:78-83.

44. Gwilym SE, Watkins B, Cooper CD, et al: Genetic influences in the progression of tears of the rotator cuff. *J Bone Joint Surg Br* 2009;91(7):915-917.

45. Harvie P, Ostlere SJ, Teh J, et al: Genetic influences in the etiology of tears of the rotator cuff: Sibling risk of a full-thickness tear. *J Bone Joint Surg Br* 2004;86(5): 696-700.

46. Tashjian RZ, Farnham JM, Albright FS, Teerlink CC, Cannon-Albright LA: Evidence for an inherited predisposition contributing to the risk for rotator cuff disease. *J Bone Joint Surg Am* 2009;91(5):1136-1142.

47. Baumgarten KM, Gerlach D, Galatz LM, et al: Cigarette smoking increases the risk for rotator cuff tears. *Clin Orthop Relat Res* 2010;468(6):1534-1541.

48. Cohen DB, Kawamura S, Ehteshami JR, Rodeo SA: Indomethacin and celecoxib impair rotator cuff tendon-to-bone healing. *Am J Sports Med* 2006;34(3): 362-369.

49. Galatz LM, Silva MJ, Rothermich SY, Zaegel MA, Havlioglu N, Thomopoulos S: Nicotine delays tendon-to-bone healing in a rat shoulder model. *J Bone Joint Surg Am* 2006;88(9):2027-2034.

50. Charousset C, Bellaïche L, Kalra K, Petrover D: Arthroscopic repair

of full-thickness rotator cuff tears: Is there tendon healing in patients aged 65 years or older? *Arthroscopy* 2010;26(3):302-309.

51. Kamath G, Galatz LM, Keener JD, Teefey S, Middleton W, Yamaguchi K: Tendon integrity and functional outcome after arthroscopic repair of high-grade partial-thickness supraspinatus tears. *J Bone Joint Surg Am* 2009; 91(5):1055-1062.

52. Keener JD, Wei AS, Kim HM, et al: Revision arthroscopic rotator cuff repair: Repair integrity and clinical outcome. *J Bone Joint Surg Am* 2010;92(3):590-598.

53. Papadopoulos P, Karataglis D, Boutsiadis A, Fotiadou A, Christoforidis J, Christodoulou A: Functional outcome and structural integrity following mini-open repair of large and massive rotator cuff tears: A 3-5 year follow-up study. *J Shoulder Elbow Surg* 2011;20(1):131-137.

54. Tashjian RZ, Hollins AM, Kim HM, et al: Factors affecting healing rates after arthroscopic double-row rotator cuff repair. *Am J Sports Med* 2010;38(12):2435-2442.

55. Kim DH, Elattrache NS, Tibone JE, et al: Biomechanical comparison of a single-row versus double-row suture anchor technique for rotator cuff repair. *Am J Sports Med* 2006;34(3):407-414.

56. Park MC, Idjadi JA, Elattrache NS, Tibone JE, McGarry MH, Lee TQ: The effect of dynamic external rotation comparing 2 footprint-restoring rotator cuff repair techniques. *Am J Sports Med* 2008;36(5):893-900.

57. Smith CD, Alexander S, Hill AM, et al: A biomechanical comparison of single and double-row fixation in arthroscopic rotator cuff repair. *J Bone Joint Surg Am* 2006; 88(11):2425-2431.

58. Ahmad CS, Kleweno C, Jacir AM, et al: Biomechanical performance

of rotator cuff repairs with humeral rotation: A new rotator cuff repair failure model. *Am J Sports Med* 2008;36(5):888-892.

59. Burks RT, Crim J, Brown N, Fink B, Greis PE: A prospective randomized clinical trial comparing arthroscopic single- and double-row rotator cuff repair: Magnetic resonance imaging and early clinical evaluation. *Am J Sports Med* 2009;37(4):674-682.

60. Franceschi F, Ruzzini L, Longo UG, et al: Equivalent clinical results of arthroscopic single-row and double-row suture anchor repair for rotator cuff tears: A randomized controlled trial. *Am J Sports Med* 2007;35(8):1254-1260.

61. Grasso A, Milano G, Salvatore M, Falcone G, Deriu L, Fabbriciani C: Single-row versus double-row arthroscopic rotator cuff repair: A prospective randomized clinical study. *Arthroscopy* 2009;25(1):4-12.

62. Bigliani LU, Cordasco FA, McIlveen SJ, Musso ES: Operative treatment of failed repairs of the rotator cuff. *J Bone Joint Surg Am* 1992;74(10):1505-1515.

63. DeOrio JK, Cofield RH: Results of a second attempt at surgical repair of a failed initial rotator-cuff repair. *J Bone Joint Surg Am* 1984;66(4):563-567.

64. Djurasovic M, Marra G, Arroyo JS, Pollock RG, Flatow EL, Bigliani LU: Revision rotator cuff repair: Factors influencing results. *J Bone Joint Surg Am* 2001;83-A(12):1849-1855.

65. Lo IK, Burkhart SS: Arthroscopic revision of failed rotator cuff repairs: Technique and results. *Arthroscopy* 2004;20(3):250-267.

66. Neviaser RJ, Neviaser TJ: Reoperation for failed rotator cuff repair: Analysis of 50 cases. *J Shoulder Elbow Surg* 1992;1(6):283-286.

67. Walch G, Edwards TB, Boulahia A, Nové-Josserand L, Neyton L, Szabo I: Arthroscopic tenotomy of the long head of the biceps in the treatment of rotator cuff tears: Clinical and radiographic results of 307 cases. *J Shoulder Elbow Surg* 2005;14(3):238-246.

68. Boileau P, Baqué F, Valerio L, Ahrens P, Chuinard C, Trojani C: Isolated arthroscopic biceps tenotomy or tenodesis improves symptoms in patients with massive irreparable rotator cuff tears. *J Bone Joint Surg Am* 2007;89(4):747-757.

69. Gerber C, Maquieira G, Espinosa N: Latissimus dorsi transfer for the treatment of irreparable rotator cuff tears. *J Bone Joint Surg Am* 2006;88(1):113-120.

70. Iannotti JP, Hennigan S, Herzog R, et al: Latissimus dorsi tendon transfer for irreparable posterosuperior rotator cuff tears: Factors affecting outcome. *J Bone Joint Surg Am* 2006;88(2):342-348.

71. Warner JJ, Parsons IM IV: Latissimus dorsi tendon transfer: A comparative analysis of primary and salvage reconstruction of massive, irreparable rotator cuff tears. *J Shoulder Elbow Surg* 2001;10(6):514-521.

72. Sanchez-Sotelo J, Cofield RH, Rowland CM: Shoulder hemiarthroplasty for glenohumeral arthritis associated with severe rotator cuff deficiency. *J Bone Joint Surg Am* 2001;83-A(12):1814-1822.

73. Goldberg SS, Bell JE, Kim HJ, Bak SF, Levine WN, Bigliani LU: Hemiarthroplasty for the rotator cuff-deficient shoulder. *J Bone Joint Surg Am* 2008;90(3):554-559.

74. Mulieri P, Dunning P, Klein S, Pupello D, Frankle M: Reverse shoulder arthroplasty for the treatment of irreparable rotator cuff tear without glenohumeral arthritis. *J Bone Joint Surg Am* 2010;92(15):2544-2556.

75. Frank JB, ElAttrache NS, Dines JS, Blackburn A, Crues J, Tibone JE: Repair site integrity after arthroscopic transosseous-equivalent suture-bridge rotator cuff repair. *Am J Sports Med* 2008;36(8):1496-1503.

76. Toussaint B, Schnaser E, Bosley J, Lefebvre Y, Gobezie R: Early structural and functional outcomes for arthroscopic double-row transosseous-equivalent rotator cuff repair. *Am J Sports Med* 2011;39(6):1217-1225.

Massive Rotator Cuff Tears Without Arthropathy: When to Consider Reverse Shoulder Arthroplasty

Kevin L. Harreld, MD

Brian L. Puskas, MD

Mark A. Frankle, MD

Abstract

Massive rotator cuff tears often present a challenge for the treating orthopaedic surgeon. A multitude of surgical approaches have been described to manage this condition, ranging from biceps tenotomy to complex muscle transfers to reverse shoulder arthroplasty. Among these procedures, reverse shoulder arthroplasty is increasingly advocated to relieve pain and restore function; however, the exact role of this arthroplasty procedure continues to be defined, particularly in patients without any evidence of associated glenohumeral arthritis. In this patient population, the reverse shoulder prosthesis is used primarily to address the instability associated with massive rotator cuff tears, as opposed to the more common application of arthroplasty to manage cartilage disease.

Currently accepted indications for reverse shoulder arthroplasty include patients with pseudoparalysis and irreparable rotator cuff tears, with or without anterosuperior escape. Surgeons must be aware of conditions that may clinically mimic pseudoparalysis caused by a rotator cuff tear, such as axillary nerve injury, deltoid dehiscence, or cervical radiculopathy. These conditions produce deltoid insufficiency and are unlikely to benefit from a reverse shoulder arthroplasty. Caution is also warranted when considering this procedure in patients with massive rotator cuff tears in whom active forward elevation greater than 90° is preserved. These patients may achieve little benefit in range of motion and pain relief with a reverse shoulder arthroplasty.

Instr Course Lect 2012;61:143-156.

Dr. Frankle or an immediate family member has received royalties from DJ Orthopaedics; is a member of a speakers' bureau or has made paid presentations on behalf of DJ Orthopaedics; serves as a paid consultant to DJ Orthopaedics; serves as an unpaid consultant to DePuy; has received research or institutional support from DJ Orthopaedics, EBI, Eli Lilly, and Encore Medical; and has received nonincome support (such as equipment or services), commercially derived honoraria, or other non–research-related funding (such as paid travel) from DJ Orthopaedics, EBI, Eli Lilly, and Encore Medical. Neither of the following authors nor any immediate family member has received anything of value from or owns stock in a commercial company or institution related directly or indirectly to the subject of this chapter: Dr. Harreld and Dr. Puskas.

Patients with large, retracted rotator cuff tears present a surgical challenge to relieve pain and restore shoulder function. However, the term massive rotator cuff tear has been only recently adopted. The first studies to use this description, published in the late 1970s and early 1980s, focused on techniques and outcomes associated with freeze-dried rotator cuff allografts or muscle transfers.[1,2] Since then, massive rotator cuff tears have been increasingly recognized and are now a topic of particular emphasis in clinical and biomechanical research. A PubMed search yields almost 350 articles on this topic, with nearly 200 studies published within the past 5 years. Despite this increased focus, an optimal treatment has yet to be established. Current studies outline a variety of techniques to address such tears, including débridement with acromioplasty,[3,4] biceps tenotomy,[5] tenotomy with tuberoplasty,[6] partial repair,[7,8] complete arthroscopic repair,[9,10] mini-open repair,[11,12] tissue augmentation,[13,14] tendon transfer,[15,16] deltoid flap,[17,18] hemiarthroplasty,[19,20] and reverse shoulder arthroplasty.[21,22] The definition of a massive rotator cuff tear has been

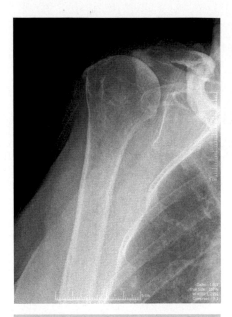

Figure 1 AP radiograph of the right shoulder showing superior migration of the humeral head, which is indicative of a massive rotator cuff tear.

inconsistent. Commonly accepted definitions include a tear size greater than 5 cm, a complete tear of at least two tendons, or both.[3,23-26] However, the more important distinction, rather than tear size or the number of tendons involved, is the healing potential of the tendon and the ability to technically achieve a satisfactory repair. A massive rotator cuff tear is not necessarily an irreparable tear.[27] Determining healing potential is critical to selecting the appropriate surgical strategy because a subset of rotator cuff tears remains irreparable.[28] Many acute tears may be quite large and may involve two or more tendons, but they may still be mobile and repairable. Conversely, smaller tears may prove to be irreparable and may represent a separate clinical entity.

Reverse shoulder arthroplasty is a well-established and reliable treatment for patients with rotator cuff tear arthropathy.[29-31] However, in the absence of cartilage disease, arthroplasty may be a less obvious decision for both the patient and the surgeon. This chapter will outline the history, indications, outcomes, and pitfalls associated with using reverse shoulder arthroplasty to manage irreparable tears without arthritis.

To understand the appropriate application of reverse shoulder arthroplasty in this patient population, the pathology and glenohumeral instability that occurs in the rotator cuff deficient shoulder must be appreciated.

Pathomechanics and Rationale of Reverse Shoulder Arthroplasty

The rotator cuff musculature acts as a dynamic stabilizer to the glenohumeral joint, centering the humeral head on the glenoid.[32-34] An intact rotator cuff creates "concavity compression," a mechanism that imparts stability to this otherwise unconstrained joint and establishes a stable fulcrum against which the deltoid can rotate the humeral head and elevate the arm.[35-37] This concept is supported by electromyographic evidence that rotator cuff contraction precedes the larger force-generating contraction of the deltoid during active arm elevation.[38] A stable fulcrum requires intact coronal and transverse muscular force couples. The subscapularis and the infraspinatus-teres muscle complex provide the transverse plane force couple, and the inferior portion of the rotator cuff on the humeral head provides the coronal plane force couple.[3,7] Minimal glenohumeral translations occur in the normal shoulder throughout arm elevation and abduction.[39-41]

In a shoulder with a rotator cuff tear, the deltoid muscle increases force generation to compensate for the loss of the abduction torque provided by the rotator cuff muscles.[42-44] The increase in deltoid force that occurs with an isolated supraspinatus tear is relatively small and compensated by cocontraction of the large adductors (latissimus dorsi and pectoralis major muscles) and remaining rotator cuff muscles. Consequently, glenohumeral stability is generally preserved.[42,45] However, as the rotator cuff tear extends posteriorly, the normal force couples are disrupted and concavity compression is lost.[45] Increasingly large deltoid abduction forces are generated, and the stabilizing effect of the remaining rotator cuff musculature is lost. Cocontraction of the adductors is no longer sufficient to counter the deltoid force. The joint reaction force vector migrates outside the glenoid rim, and instability results.[42,43,45] As a consequence of the loss of a stable fulcrum, the deltoid force no longer rotates the humeral head on the glenoid but pulls it in a superior direction[3,45,46] (**Figure 1**). This superior translation of the humeral head has previously been confirmed in several studies investigating the biomechanical effects of rotator cuff deficiency.[46-51]

Restoration of appropriate force couples may be achieved with a partial or a complete tendon repair, resulting in reestablishment of a stable fulcrum for elevation.[12,14,52-54] However, many large tears are associated with high rates of recurrent tendon defects on follow-up examinations.[11,55-57] There is evidence of an association between recurrent repair defects and postoperative strength deficits and outcome scores.[55,57-59] When appropriate force couples cannot be adequately reestablished, a stable fulcrum for humeral head rotation is not achieved. Abnormal superior translations of the humeral head persist, leading to shoulder pseudoparalysis and eventual anterosuperior escape of the humeral head. In this setting, a reverse prosthetic articulation blocks superior translation of the humerus, allows the deltoid tension to be restored, and provides stability to the glenohumeral joint. The superior pull of the deltoid is converted into a rotational moment, and elevation of the arm is restored.[30,60-62]

Video 12.1: Reverse Shoulder Arthroplasty for Massive Cuff Tears Without Arthritis. Mark A. Frankle, MD; Randall Otto, MD; Khurram Pervaiz, MD; Christopher Griffing (11 min)

History of Reverse Shoulder Arthroplasty

Early reverse shoulder arthroplasty was designed to improve clinical outcomes for patients with rotator cuff deficiency and associated glenohumeral arthritis.[63-68] Previous attempts to manage this patient population with highly constrained so-called fixed fulcrum anatomic-type designs were unsatisfactory because of the high complication rate, and these devices were eventually abandoned.[69-72] Conversely, early reverse shoulder arthroplasty series reported complication rates from 16% to 31%.[64,68] However, when reporting on failures of shoulder arthroplasty in the 1970s, authors now routinely group the higher complication rates of highly constrained anatomic devices with the lower complication rates observed with early reverse designs. Failure in both of these devices is consistently attributed to a center of rotation that is lateral to the face of the glenoid.[62,73-77]

Boileau et al[62] cited the results of two early studies on reverse devices with a lateral center of rotation in developing their argument for a medial center of rotation at the level of the glenoid face, stating that these early devices failed because of "excessive torque and shear forces at the glenoid component-bone interface." However, a careful review of these studies reveals

that such a conclusion is questionable. In the first study, there were five device failures (defined as the removal of the prosthesis) in 31 patients (16%). Three of these resulted from dislocation, one from a "wrenched shoulder," and one from persistent pain. At a mean 3.5-year follow-up, there were no reported baseplate failures.[64] Subsequently, Broström et al[78] reported on their 5-year experience in patients with rheumatoid arthritis. In this study, the authors noted increased loosening of the glenoid component, which was attributed to the constraint inherent in the device. Improved pain relief and ability to perform activities of daily living were noted in all 17 shoulders. Describing torque at the baseplate-bone interface as a uniformly causative factor in implant failure must be regarded cautiously. Alternative contributing factors may include the type of disease that is present, the degree of constraint, the adequacy of glenoid fixation, and the notable lack of bone ingrowth potential in early devices.

Modern studies of devices with a lateral center of rotation reflect a continued improvement in design with fewer reported baseplate-related complications than those seen in the early studies. In one recent study, there were 4 reported baseplate failures in 69 shoulders at a mean 52-month follow-up.[79] However, all failures occurred in an early baseplate design in which 3.5-mm nonlocking screws were used, and no failures were reported for the current locking-screw design. In a further, focused study of 96 shoulders in which a baseplate design with locking screw technology was used, no glenoid fixation failures were reported at a minimum follow-up period of 2 years.[61] In another study of patients with acquired glenoid bone defects, there was no evidence of baseplate loosening in 143 shoulders, despite the presence of abnormal gle-

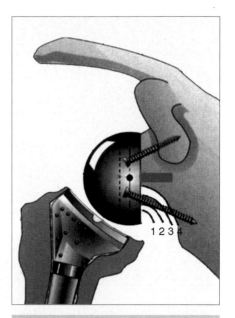

Figure 2 Classification of scapular notching as described by Sirveaux et al.[81] The defect of the bone in the inferior part of the glenoid component is classified according to the size of the defect as seen on the radiograph. A defect is classified as grade 1 when it is confined to the pillar, grade 2 when it is in contact with the lower screw, grade 3 when it is over the lower screw, and grade 4 when it extends under the baseplate. (Adapted with permission from Sirveaux F, Favard L, Oudet D, Huquet D, Walch G, Molé D: Grammont inverted total shoulder arthroplasty in the treatment of glenohumeral osteoarthritis with massive rupture of the cuff: Results of a multicentre study of 80 shoulders. *J Bone Joint Surg Br* 2004;86: 388-395.)

noids in 56 patients.[80] In contrast, current devices with a medial center of rotation have reported complication rates as high as 60%, with scapular notching (such as a defect of the inferior neck of the scapula, presumably occurring from contact with the humeral socket) frequently reported[81,82] (**Figure 2**). Both implant designs relieve pain and improve active forward elevation, and designs with both a medial and lateral center of rotation

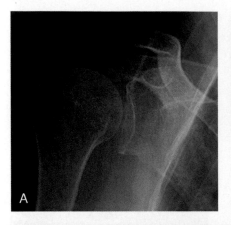
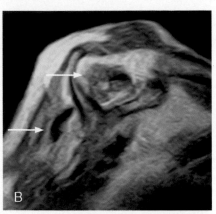
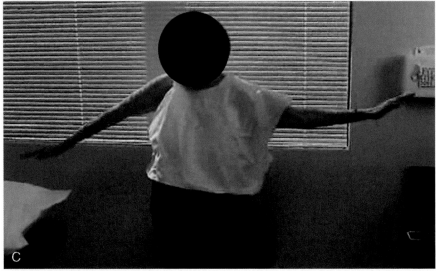

Figure 3 Scenario 1. **A,** Preoperative AP radiograph of the right shoulder demostrates no evidence of escape of the humeral head. **B,** MRI scan shows severe artophy of the supraspinatus and infraspinatus muscles (arrows). **C,** The patient has pseudoparalysis of the right shoulder on clinical examination.

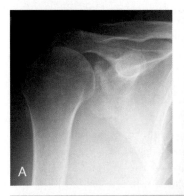
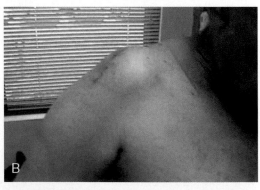

Figure 4 Scenario 2. **A,** Preoperative AP radiograph of the right shoulder shows no evidence of escape of the humeral head. **B,** Examination reveals clinically apparent anterosuperior escape of the humeral head. The prominence of the humeral head is apparent when the patient attempts to abduct the shoulder.

are widely used in the treatment of rotator-cuff deficient conditions.

Indications and Contraindications

The decision to perform a reverse shoulder arthroplasty in patients with massive rotator cuff tears without evidence of glenohumeral arthritis must be individualized. Eligible candidates for reverse shoulder arthroplasty should demonstrate forward pseudoparalysis, with active forward elevation of less than 90°, and should have weakness of the rotator cuff musculature on physical examination.[22] Often, these patients will have full, passive shoulder motion; however, some patients may exhibit stiffness on physical examination of the shoulder. This is often the result of soft-tissue contractures or scarring from previous surgery rather than glenohumeral arthritis.

The following three clinical scenarios in which application of a reverse shoulder arthroplasty would be beneficial illustrate the appropriate indications for this device.

Scenario 1

An elderly patient with comorbidities (for example, smoking or diabetes) predictive of poor healing of the rotator cuff[83-86] presents after an acute-on-chronic rotator cuff tear. The patient has pseudoparalysis (forward elevation of < 90°) and pain, and, although there is no anterosuperior escape of the humeral head, MRI reveals rotator cuff atrophy[87-90] (**Figure 3**). In this scenario, a reverse shoulder arthroplasty offers the potential for reliable return of function and relief of pain with a decreased risk of reoperation compared with attempted rotator cuff repair.

Scenario 2

A patient has a massive rotator cuff tear with pseudoparalysis, pain, and clinically (but not radiographically) evident anterosuperior escape of the humeral head (dynamic instability) (**Figure 4**).

Scenario 3

A patient has a massive rotator cuff tear with pseudoparalysis, pain, and obvious (both clinically and radiographically evident) anterosuperior escape of the humeral head[28,91-93] (**Figure 5**).

The approach of this chapter's authors to treating the patient with a massive rotator cuff tear without arthritis is summarized in the algorithm in **Figure 6**. Reverse shoulder arthroplasty is contraindicated in patients with a massive rotator cuff tear and a nonfunctional deltoid muscle. Deltoid dysfunction may be caused by cervical radiculopathy, injury from previous open rotator cuff surgery, or axillary nerve injury.

Outcomes

Early reports of reverse shoulder arthroplasty are favorable but generally include only patients with rotator cuff deficiency and associated arthrosis of the glenohumeral joint.[29-31,73,81,94-97] Although some subsequent studies stratify the study population by etiology, none of these initial reports describe outcomes based on the presence or absence of concomitant glenohumeral arthritis.[61,82,98] Werner et al[82] reported that the reoperation rate was lower and the final Constant score[99] was higher in patients who were initially treated with a primary reverse shoulder arthroplasty than in patients who were treated with a reverse shoulder arthroplasty after a prior failed rotator cuff repair or failed arthroplasty. Cuff et al[61] reported similar findings, with improved outcomes in primary use of reverse shoulder arthroplasty compared with use in revision settings. Although both of these studies suggest

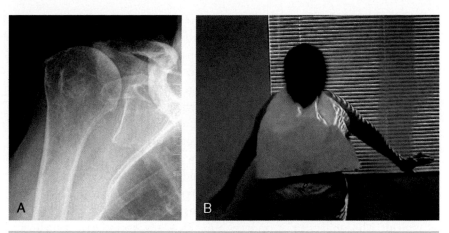

Figure 5   Scenario 3. Frank instability and escape of the humeral head in the right shoulder is apparent both radiographically (**A**) and clinically (**B**).

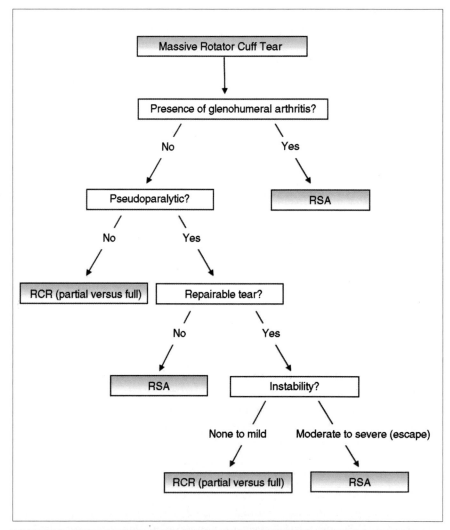

Figure 6   Algorithm for approach to a patient with a massive rotator cuff tear. RCR = rotator cuff repair, RSA = reverse shoulder arthroplasty.

a more favorable outcome after reverse shoulder arthroplasty for those patients without prior surgery for a rotator cuff tear, neither study described the degree of associated glenohumeral arthritis in these patients.

Wall et al[100] reported the outcomes after reverse shoulder arthroplasty in a subgroup of 34 shoulders with massive rotator cuff tears and no associated arthritis. There was no difference in outcomes between this group and a group of patients who underwent a primary reverse shoulder arthroplasty for the treatment of rotator cuff tear arthropathy. All patients undergoing a primary surgical procedure had a better result than those with previous failed rotator cuff surgery or failed arthroplasty.

More recently, Boileau et al[22] reported their experience with 46 shoulders in 44 patients who underwent reverse shoulder arthroplasty after failed surgical management of a rotator cuff tear. All patients had undergone only one prior surgical procedure, either attempted repair or palliative treatment (biceps tenotomy or acromioplasty). Sixty-one percent of the shoulders had radiographic evidence of glenohumeral arthritis. There was no difference in final pain scores, Constant scores, or range of motion between those with and without arthritis and no difference in the amount of improvement between the two groups. Comparing patients with a preoperative active forward elevation of less than 90° or more than 90°, there was a significant difference in the amount of improvement achieved in Constant scores and forward elevation. The group with preserved forward elevation of more than 90° preoperatively experienced a decrease in mean forward elevation from 146° to 122° after implantation of the reverse shoulder arthroplasty. They also experienced a smaller improvement in Constant scores and were generally more dissat-

isfied with their results (27%) compared with the group that had shoulder pseudoparalysis (7%).

In another report, the outcomes after reverse shoulder arthroplasty for management of an irreparable rotator cuff tear were studied in 60 shoulders (58 patients) in which there was no evidence of osteoarthritis.[79] The authors found an improvement in the total American Shoulder and Elbow Surgeons score, from 33.3 preoperatively to 75.4 postoperatively, which was similar to previously reported results in a patient population with rotator cuff deficiency and osteoarthritis.[30,101] These authors noted significant improvements in the Simple Shoulder Test score, the visual analog scores for pain and function, and the Short Form-36 physical component.[102,103] Range of motion in forward elevation improved from 53° to 134°, and external rotation improved from 27° to 51°. No significant differences were found between those patients with prior failed rotator cuff surgery and those undergoing a primary procedure. In this study population, only four patients had preserved preoperative forward flexion of more than 90°. Range of motion improved in three of these four patients. The other patient experienced a decrease in forward elevation from 95° to 90°. All four patients described their satisfaction as good or excellent. However, three complications occurred in two patients within this specific subset: baseplate failure and hematoma in one patient and postoperative dislocation in another.[79]

These studies demonstrate that, following reverse shoulder arthroplasty, equivalent improvement and final outcome may be obtained in patients with rotator cuff tears with or without associated glenohumeral osteoarthritis. Patients undergoing a primary shoulder intervention with a reverse implant tend to experience better outcomes

than those with failed prior surgery. However, the results after reverse shoulder arthroplasty in patients with preserved forward elevation of more than 90° preoperatively are not as good as those in patients with preoperative pseudoparalysis. Patients who have more preoperative forward elevation may be at an increased risk of having perioperative complications or diminished functional improvement compared with patients who have shoulder pseudoparalysis. Consequently, they may also be at risk of having lower satisfaction scores following treatment with a reverse shoulder arthroplasty.

Complications

There is some heterogeneity in studies reporting complications after reverse shoulder arthroplasty. However, a review of published series reveals sufficient commonalities to allow meaningful conclusions. The most common complication in many reports has been scapular notching.[31,81,82,104-107] However, in devices with a glenosphere with a lateral center of rotation, a much lower prevalence of scapular notching has been reported.[29,61,108] Biomechanical data also suggest that scapular notching is probably increased in devices with a medial center of rotation.[109,110] Some studies have found postoperative dislocation to be the most frequent complication.[61,82,100] Although not reported in all series, an increased infection rate, up to 16% (3 of 19 patients) in the study by Boileau et al,[31] has been reported in revision surgery.[98,100] Previous surgery is a risk factor for increased complications, reoperations, and lower implant survival rates.[82,98,100]

Postoperative fracture of the acromion is another common complication, but it is less well understood.[29,30,82] Frequently, it occurs within the acromion proper but it may occur at the base of the acromion,

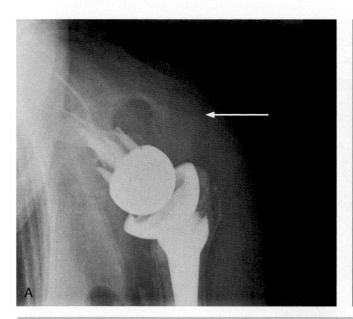
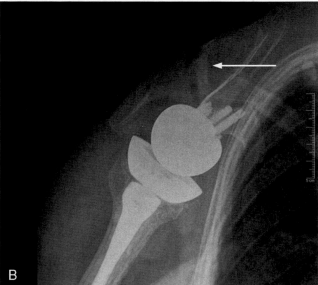

Figure 7   Acromial fracture following reverse shoulder arthroplasty. **A,** Radiograph showing a fracture (arrow) of the acromion at the location of the mesoacromion. **B,** Radiograph showing a fracture (arrow) at the base of the acromion along the scapular spine.

where it is more accurately described as a fracture of the scapular spine (**Figure** 7). A common presentation of acromial fracture is pain after a fall, a sporting activity, or a vigorous therapy session. However, a traumatic event is not necessary for fracture. A fatigue-type insufficiency fracture from over-tensioning the deltoid is one possible explanation for such fractures.[62] However, the results from one recent study could not demonstrate a correlation between the degree of humeral lengthening and postoperative acromial fracture.[111] Current studies demonstrate that, although these patients may improve from their preoperative status, ultimate functional outcome is diminished.[112,113] Preoperative acromial fracture or os acromiale does not adversely affect outcome.[113]

In a mixed group of patients with and without arthritis, Boileau et al[22] reported an 8.7% complication rate, including one glenosphere dissociation, one axillary granuloma, one postoperative periprosthetic fracture, and one instance of aseptic humeral loos-ening. There were no postoperative dislocations. Mulieri et al[79] reported a 20% complication rate in patients without associated arthritis. However, four baseplate failures were believed to be design related, and, after baseplate design modification, no further failures were reported. Excluding the baseplate failures, the complication rate was 13%. Complications included three acromial fractures, one periprosthetic humeral fracture, one dislocation, one broken screw, one hematoma, and one deep infection. The complication rates in the patient population without arthritis do not appear to be significantly different from the previously reported complication rates after reverse shoulder arthroplasty in patients with osteoarthritis.

Potential Pitfalls

Reverse shoulder arthroplasty is a reliable and successful method of treating patients with rotator cuff deficiency, particularly those with shoulder pseudoparalysis. However, pseudoparalysis presents in a varied fashion, with sud-den or progressive weakness, with or without associated pain, and with a variable history of an antecedent traumatic event. A high index of suspicion must be maintained for other conditions that may present with a pseudoparalytic shoulder. Cervical radiculopathies and deltoid dehiscence or detachment are two conditions that may mimic pseudoparalysis caused by rotator cuff deficiency, but these conditions are unlikely to be managed successfully with a reverse shoulder arthroplasty.

A thorough physical and neurologic examination of the extremity and cervical spine can differentiate a massive rotator cuff tear from cervical radiculopathy. Patients with radiculopathy usually have pain in a dermatomal distribution into the hand. Referred trapezial and periscapular pain often accompany the radicular component. Conversely, pain from a rotator cuff tear typically does not radiate distal to the elbow. Reproduction of painful symptoms with flexion and extension of the spine or with performance of the

Spurling maneuver is indicative of cervical spine pathology.

The deltoid and rotator cuff muscles are innervated predominantly from the C5 and C6 nerve roots. Typically, cervical disk herniations be-

tween C4 and C5 impinge on the C5 nerve root and may cause pain and numbness down the side of the neck, over the top of the shoulder, to the lateral aspect of the deltoid muscle. This may be associated with varying degrees of muscle weakness of the deltoid or rotator cuff muscles. A massive rotator cuff tear frequently involves the infraspinatus and teres minor muscles, resulting in more weakness in external rotation with the arm at the side or at 90° of abduction compared with the weakness seen in patients with a C5 root impingement. In an isolated C6 radiculopathy caused by a cervical disk herniation between C5 and C6, a patient may have weakness of the deltoid muscle without clinically apparent involvement of the rotator cuff muscles. Pain radiating down the lateral side of the arm and the forearm to the tip of the thumb and index finger is common. Biceps weakness in elbow flexion and supination, weakness in wrist extension, and a diminished brachioradialis reflex are signs of a cervical radiculopathy. Advanced cases of C5 or C6 nerve root compression can cause deltoid atrophy and disproportionate weakness of the trapezius. **Figures 8** and **9** demonstrate the clinical case of a

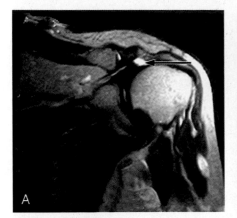 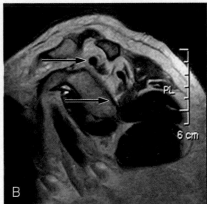
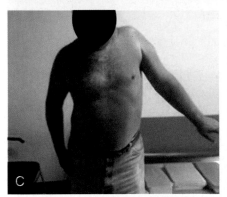 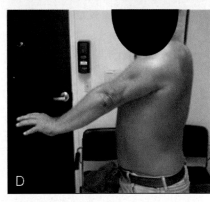
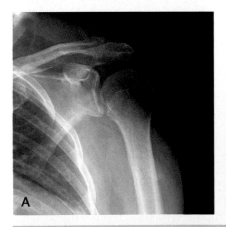 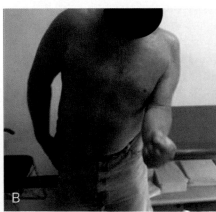

Figure 8 **A,** T2-weighted MRI scan of the left shoulder shows a large, full-thickness rotator cuff tear (arrow). **B,** MRI scan shows severe atrophy (arrows) of the supraspinatus, the infraspinatus, and the teres minor. **C** and **D,** Clinical examination suggests shoulder pseudoparalysis caused by a massive rotator cuff tear.

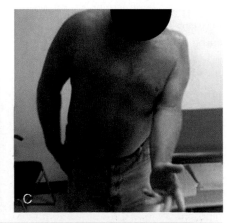

Figure 9 **A,** AP radiograph of the left shoulder shows no evidence of static superior migration of the humeral head. Further physical examination reveals a profound weakness in biceps flexion (**B**) and an inability to supinate the forearm (**C**). The patient was subsequently found to have a C6 radiculopathy and evidence of deltoid denervation. A reverse shoulder arthroplasty would be expected to provide no functional improvement in such a patient.

patient referred for evaluation for a reverse shoulder arthroplasty in whom electromyographic analysis confirmed C6 radiculopathy.

In the normal shoulder, the deltoid is responsible for more than 50% of the force necessary to elevate the arm in the plane of the scapula.[114] Consequently, deltoid dysfunction may mimic shoulder pseudoparalysis caused by rotator cuff deficiency. As this muscle is primarily responsible for powering forward elevation and abduction in the shoulder that has undergone reverse shoulder arthroplasty, it is critical to recognize a nonfunctional deltoid preoperatively. Deltoid dehiscence, proximal detachment, or axillary nerve injury can all result from prior surgery and should be considered in patients with pseudoparalysis who have a history of prior rotator cuff repair, particularly those with a prior open repair.[115-118] Whatley et al[114] described successful treatment of preoperative deltoid dysfunction in two of three patients with a deltoidplasty coupled with a reverse shoulder arthroplasty and a Nice-L'Episcopo latissimus-teres major muscle transfer.

Successful application of the reverse shoulder arthroplasty is predicated on eliminating pathologic superior translation of the humeral head and restoring a stable fulcrum for the deltoid. The preoperative ability of a patient to elevate the arm forward beyond 90° suggests the presence of intact force couples and the existence of a stable fulcrum. Special care should be taken in considering reverse shoulder arthroplasty for these patients, particularly in the absence of glenohumeral arthritis. Performing a reverse shoulder arthroplasty in this setting is associated with increased rates of patient dissatisfaction and increased risk of complications.[22,79] Diagnostic injections of local anesthetic into the glenohumeral joint in the preoperative evaluation or other procedures such as partial rotator cuff repair or biceps tenotomy should be considered rather than a reverse shoulder arthroplasty.

Summary

Reverse shoulder arthroplasty can be reliably applied to patients who are experiencing shoulder instability and pseudoparalysis from a massive rotator cuff tear. In appropriately selected patients, comparable functional improvement, pain relief, and patient satisfaction (in patients without evidence of glenohumeral arthritis as compared with those with more advanced arthropathy) can be expected. Surgeons should maintain a high index of suspicion for conditions that may mimic pseudoparalysis that is caused by a massive rotator cuff tear but that are in fact representative of underlying deltoid muscle deficiency. Particular care should be taken when considering reverse shoulder arthroplasty for treatment of a nonarthritic shoulder with a massive rotator cuff tear if the patient has preserved forward elevation of more than 90°.

References

1. Neviaser JS, Neviaser RJ, Neviaser TJ: The repair of chronic massive ruptures of the rotator cuff of the shoulder by use of a freeze-dried rotator cuff. *J Bone Joint Surg Am* 1978;60(5):681-684.

2. Cofield RH: Subscapular muscle transposition for repair of chronic rotator cuff tears. *Surg Gynecol Obstet* 1982;154(5):667-672.

3. Burkhart SS: Arthroscopic treatment of massive rotator cuff tears: Clinical results and biomechanical rationale. *Clin Orthop Relat Res* 1991;267:45-56.

4. Gartsman GM: Massive, irreparable tears of the rotator cuff: Results of operative debridement and subacromial decompression. *J Bone Joint Surg Am* 1997;79(5):715-721.

5. Walch G, Edwards TB, Boulahia A, Nové-Josserand L, Neyton L, Szabo I: Arthroscopic tenotomy of the long head of the biceps in the treatment of rotator cuff tears: Clinical and radiographic results of 307 cases. *J Shoulder Elbow Surg* 2005;14(3):238-246.

6. Verhelst L, Vandekerckhove PJ, Sergeant G, Liekens K, Van Hoonacker P, Berghs B: Reversed arthroscopic subacromial decompression for symptomatic irreparable rotator cuff tears: Mid-term follow-up results in 34 shoulders. *J Shoulder Elbow Surg* 2010;19(4):601-608.

7. Burkhart SS: Partial repair of massive rotator cuff tears: The evolution of a concept. *Orthop Clin North Am* 1997;28(1):125-132.

8. Duralde XA, Bair B: Massive rotator cuff tears: The result of partial rotator cuff repair. *J Shoulder Elbow Surg* 2005;14(2):121-127.

9. Burkhart SS, Barth JR, Richards DP, Zlatkin MB, Larsen M: Arthroscopic repair of massive rotator cuff tears with stage 3 and 4 fatty degeneration. *Arthroscopy* 2007;23(4):347-354.

10. Lafosse L, Brozska R, Toussaint B, Gobezie R: The outcome and structural integrity of arthroscopic rotator cuff repair with use of the double-row suture anchor technique. *J Bone Joint Surg Am* 2007;89(7):1533-1541.

11. Hanusch BC, Goodchild L, Finn P, Rangan A: Large and massive tears of the rotator cuff: Functional outcome and integrity of the repair after a mini-open procedure. *J Bone Joint Surg Br* 2009;91(2):201-205.

12. Papadopoulos P, Karataglis D, Boutsiadis A, Fotiadou A, Christoforidis J, Christodoulou A: Functional outcome and structural integrity following mini-open repair of large and massive

rotator cuff tears: A 3-5 year follow-up study. *J Shoulder Elbow Surg* 2011;20(1):131-137.

13. Nada AN, Debnath UK, Robinson DA, Jordan C: Treatment of massive rotator-cuff tears with a polyester ligament (Dacron) augmentation: Clinical outcome. *J Bone Joint Surg Br* 2010;92(10): 1397-1402.

14. Wong I, Burns J, Snyder S: Arthroscopic GraftJacket repair of rotator cuff tears. *J Shoulder Elbow Surg* 2010;19(2, Suppl):104-109.

15. Moursy M, Forstner R, Koller H, Resch H, Tauber M: Latissimus dorsi tendon transfer for irreparable rotator cuff tears: A modified technique to improve tendon transfer integrity. *J Bone Joint Surg Am* 2009;91(8):1924-1931.

16. Weening AA, Willems WJ: Latissimus dorsi transfer for treatment of irreparable rotator cuff tears. *Int Orthop* 2010;34(8):1239-1244.

17. Glanzmann MC, Goldhahn J, Flury M, Schwyzer HK, Simmen BR: Deltoid flap reconstruction for massive rotator cuff tears: Mid- and long-term functional and structural results. *J Shoulder Elbow Surg* 2010;19(3):439-445.

18. Lu XW, Verborgt O, Gazielly DF: Long-term outcomes after deltoid muscular flap transfer for irreparable rotator cuff tears. *J Shoulder Elbow Surg* 2008;17(5):732-737.

19. Goldberg SS, Bell JE, Kim HJ, Bak SF, Levine WN, Bigliani LU: Hemiarthroplasty for the rotator cuff-deficient shoulder. *J Bone Joint Surg Am* 2008;90(3): 554-559.

20. Sarris IK, Papadimitriou NG, Sotereanos DG: Bipolar hemiarthroplasty for chronic rotator cuff tear arthropathy. *J Arthroplasty* 2003;18(2):169-173.

21. Holcomb JO, Hebert DJ, Mighell MA, et al: Reverse shoulder arthroplasty in patients with rheu-matoid arthritis. *J Shoulder Elbow Surg* 2010;19(7):1076-1084.

22. Boileau P, Gonzalez JF, Chuinard C, Bicknell R, Walch G: Reverse total shoulder arthroplasty after failed rotator cuff surgery. *J Shoulder Elbow Surg* 2009;18(4): 600-606.

23. DeOrio JK, Cofield RH: Results of a second attempt at surgical repair of a failed initial rotator-cuff repair. *J Bone Joint Surg Am* 1984;66(4):563-567.

24. Warner JP, Krushell RJ, Masquelet A, Gerber C: Anatomy and relationships of the suprascapular nerve: Anatomical constraints to mobilization of the supraspinatus and infraspinatus muscles in the management of massive rotator-cuff tears. *J Bone Joint Surg Am* 1992;74(1):36-45.

25. Zumstein MA, Jost B, Hempel J, Hodler J, Gerber C: The clinical and structural long-term results of open repair of massive tears of the rotator cuff. *J Bone Joint Surg Am* 2008;90(11):2423-2431.

26. Rockwood CA Jr, Williams GR Jr, Burkhead WZ Jr: Débridement of degenerative, irreparable lesions of the rotator cuff. *J Bone Joint Surg Am* 1995; 77(6):857-866.

27. Bedi A, Dines J, Warren RF, Dines DM: Massive tears of the rotator cuff. *J Bone Joint Surg Am* 2010;92(9):1894-1908.

28. Davidson J, Burkhart SS: The geometric classification of rotator cuff tears: A system linking tear pattern to treatment and prognosis. *Arthroscopy* 2010;26(3): 417-424.

29. Levy JC, Virani N, Pupello D, Frankle M: Use of the reverse shoulder prosthesis for the treatment of failed hemiarthroplasty in patients with glenohumeral arthritis and rotator cuff deficiency. *J Bone Joint Surg Br* 2007;89(2): 189-195.

30. Frankle M, Siegal S, Pupello D, Saleem A, Mighell M, Vasey M: The Reverse Shoulder Prosthesis for glenohumeral arthritis associated with severe rotator cuff deficiency: A minimum two-year follow-up study of sixty patients. *J Bone Joint Surg Am* 2005;87(8): 1697-1705.

31. Boileau P, Watkinson D, Hatzidakis AM, Hovorka I: Neer Award 2005: The Grammont reverse shoulder prosthesis. Results in cuff tear arthritis, fracture sequelae, and revision arthroplasty. *J Shoulder Elbow Surg* 2006;15(5): 527-540.

32. von Eisenhart-Rothe RM, Jäger A, Englmeier KH, Vogl TJ, Graichen H: Relevance of arm position and muscle activity on three-dimensional glenohumeral translation in patients with traumatic and atraumatic shoulder instability. *Am J Sports Med* 2002;30(4): 514-522.

33. Karduna AR, Williams GR, Williams JL, Iannotti JP: Kinematics of the glenohumeral joint: Influences of muscle forces, ligamentous constraints, and articular geometry. *J Orthop Res* 1996; 14(6):986-993.

34. Ackland DC, Pandy MG: Lines of action and stabilizing potential of the shoulder musculature. *J Anat* 2009;215(2):184-197.

35. Lippitt S, Matsen F: Mechanisms of glenohumeral joint stability. *Clin Orthop Relat Res* 1993;291: 20-28.

36. Matsen FA III, Harryman DT II, Sidles JA: Mechanics of glenohumeral instability. *Clin Sports Med* 1991;10(4):783-788.

37. Saha AK: Dynamic stability of the glenohumeral joint. *Acta Orthop Scand* 1971;42(6):491-505.

38. David G, Magarey ME, Jones MA, Dvir Z, Türker KS, Sharpe M: EMG and strength correlates of selected shoulder muscles during rotations of the

glenohumeral joint. *Clin Biomech (Bristol, Avon)* 2000;15(2): 95-102.

39. Graichen H, Stammberger T, Bonel H, Karl-Hans Englmeier, Reiser M, Eckstein F: Glenohumeral translation during active and passive elevation of the shoulder: A 3D open-MRI study. *JBiomech* 2000;33(5):609-613.

40. Poppen NK, Walker PS: Normal and abnormal motion of the shoulder. *J Bone Joint Surg Am* 1976;58(2):195-201.

41. Howell SM, Galinat BJ, Renzi AJ, Marone PJ: Normal and abnormal mechanics of the glenohumeral joint in the horizontal plane. *J Bone Joint Surg Am* 1988;70(2): 227-232.

42. Steenbrink F, de Groot JH, Veeger HE, van der Helm FC, Rozing PM: Glenohumeral stability in simulated rotator cuff tears. *J Biomech* 2009;42(11):1740-1745.

43. Apreleva M, Parsons IM IV, Warner JJ, Fu FH, Woo SL: Experimental investigation of reaction forces at the glenohumeral joint during active abduction. *J Shoulder Elbow Surg* 2000;9(5): 409-417.

44. McCully SP, Suprak DN, Kosek P, Karduna AR: Suprascapular nerve block results in a compensatory increase in deltoid muscle activity. *J Biomech* 2007;40(8): 1839-1846.

45. Parsons IM, Apreleva M, Fu FH, Woo SL: The effect of rotator cuff tears on reaction forces at the glenohumeral joint. *J Orthop Res* 2002;20(3):439-446.

46. Burkhart SS: Fluoroscopic comparison of kinematic patterns in massive rotator cuff tears: A suspension bridge model. *Clin Orthop Relat Res* 1992;284:144-152.

47. Paletta GA Jr, Warner JJ, Warren RF, Deutsch A, Altchek DW: Shoulder kinematics with two-plane x-ray evaluation in patients

with anterior instability or rotator cuff tearing. *J Shoulder Elbow Surg* 1997;6(6):516-527.

48. Sharkey NA, Marder RA: The rotator cuff opposes superior translation of the humeral head. *Am J Sports Med* 1995;23(3): 270-275.

49. Thompson WO, Debski RE, Boardman ND III, et al: A biomechanical analysis of rotator cuff deficiency in a cadaveric model. *Am J Sports Med* 1996;24(3): 286-292.

50. Hurschler C, Wülker N, Mendila M: The effect of negative intraarticular pressure and rotator cuff force on glenohumeral translation during simulated active elevation. *Clin Biomech (Bristol, Avon)* 2000;15(5):306-314.

51. Su WR, Budoff JE, Luo ZP: The effect of anterosuperior rotator cuff tears on glenohumeral translation. *Arthroscopy* 2009;25(3): 282-289.

52. Burkhart SS, Danaceau SM, Pearce CE Jr: Arthroscopic rotator cuff repair: Analysis of results by tear size and by repair technique-margin convergence versus direct tendon-to-bone repair. *Arthroscopy* 2001;17(9):905-912.

53. Burkhart SS: Arthroscopic treatment of massive rotator cuff tears. *Clin Orthop Relat Res* 2001;390: 107-118.

54. Jones CK, Savoie FH III: Arthroscopic repair of large and massive rotator cuff tears. *Arthroscopy* 2003;19(6):564-571.

55. Verma NN, Dunn W, Adler RS, et al: All-arthroscopic versus mini-open rotator cuff repair: A retrospective review with minimum 2-year follow-up. *Arthroscopy* 2006;22(6):587-594.

56. Galatz LM, Ball CM, Teefey SA, Middleton WD, Yamaguchi K: The outcome and repair integrity of completely arthroscopically repaired large and massive rotator

cuff tears. *J Bone Joint Surg Am* 2004;86-A(2):219-224.

57. Liu SH, Baker CL: Arthroscopically assisted rotator cuff repair: Correlation of functional results with integrity of the cuff. *Arthroscopy* 1994;10(1):54-60.

58. Jost B, Pfirrmann CW, Gerber C, Switzerland Z: Clinical outcome after structural failure of rotator cuff repairs. *J Bone Joint Surg Am* 2000;82(3):304-314.

59. Keener JD, Wei AS, Kim HM, et al: Revision arthroscopic rotator cuff repair: Repair integrity and clinical outcome. *J Bone Joint Surg Am* 2010;92(3):590-598.

60. Grammont PM, Baulot E: Delta shoulder prosthesis for rotator cuff rupture. *Orthopedics* 1993;16(1): 65-68.

61. Cuff D, Pupello D, Virani N, Levy J, Frankle M: Reverse shoulder arthroplasty for the treatment of rotator cuff deficiency. *J Bone Joint Surg Am* 2008;90(6):1244-1251.

62. Boileau P, Watkinson DJ, Hatzidakis AM, Balg F: Grammont reverse prosthesis: Design, rationale, and biomechanics. *J Shoulder Elbow Surg* 2005;14(1, Suppl S):147S-161S.

63. Kolbel R, Rohlmann A, Bergmann G: Biomechanical considerations in the design of a semi-constrained total shoulder replacement, in Bayley I, Kessel L, eds: *Shoulder Surgery.* New York, NY, Springer, 1982, pp 144-152.

64. Bayley I, Kessel L: The Kessel total shoulder replacement, in Bayley I, Kessel L, eds: *Shoulder Surgery.* New York, NY, Springer, 1982, pp 160-164.

65. Fenlin JM Jr: Total glenohumeral joint replacement. *Orthop Clin North Am* 1975;6(2):565-583.

66. Neer CS II: Replacement arthroplasty for glenohumeral osteoarthritis. *J Bone Joint Surg Am* 1974; 56(1):1-13.

67. Neer CS II: Glenohumeral arthroplasty, in Neer CS II, ed: *Shoulder Reconstruction*. Philadelphia, PA, WB Saunders, 1990, pp 148-150.

68. Beddow F, Elloy M: Clinical experience with the Liverpool shoulder replacement, in Bayley I, Kessel L, eds: *Shoulder Surgery*. New York, NY, Springer, 1982, p 164.

69. Coughlin MJ, Morris JM, West WF: The semiconstrained total shoulder arthroplasty. *J Bone Joint Surg Am* 1979;61(4): 574-581.

70. Laurence M: Replacement arthroplasty of the rotator cuff deficient shoulder. *J Bone Joint Surg Br* 1991;73(6):916-919.

71. Lettin AW, Copeland SA, Scales JT: The Stanmore total shoulder replacement. *J Bone Joint Surg Br* 1982;64(1):47-51.

72. Post M, Jablon M: Constrained total shoulder arthroplasty: Long-term follow-up observations. *Clin Orthop Relat Res* 1983;173:109-116.

73. Boulahia A, Edwards TB, Walch G, Baratta RV: Early results of a reverse design prosthesis in the treatment of arthritis of the shoulder in elderly patients with a large rotator cuff tear. *Orthopedics* 2002;25(2):129-133.

74. Gerber C, Pennington SD, Nyffeler RW: Reverse total shoulder arthroplasty. *J Am Acad Orthop Surg* 2009;17(5):284-295.

75. Safran O, Seebauer L, Iannotti JP: Cuff deficiency arthropathy: Unconstrained and constrained shoulder arthroplasty, in Iannotti JP, Williams GR, eds: *Disorders of the Shoulder*. Philadelphia, PA, Lippincott Williams & Wilkins, 2007, vol 2, p 731.

76. Wirth MA, Rockwood CA Jr: Complications of total shoulder-replacement arthroplasty. *J Bone Joint Surg Am* 1996;78(4): 603-616.

77. Nam D, Kepler CK, Nho SJ, Craig EV, Warren RF, Wright TM: Observations on retrieved humeral polyethylene components from reverse total shoulder arthroplasty. *J Shoulder Elbow Surg* 2010;19(7): 1003-1012.

78. Broström LA, Wallensten R, Olsson E, Anderson D: The Kessel prosthesis in total shoulder arthroplasty: A five-year experience. *Clin Orthop Relat Res* 1992;277: 155-160.

79. Mulieri P, Dunning P, Klein S, Pupello D, Frankle M: Reverse shoulder arthroplasty for the treatment of irreparable rotator cuff tear without glenohumeral arthritis. *J Bone Joint Surg Am* 2010; 92(15):2544-2556.

80. Klein SM, Dunning P, Mulieri P, Pupello D, Downes K, Frankle MA: Effects of acquired glenoid bone defects on surgical technique and clinical outcomes in reverse shoulder arthroplasty. *J Bone Joint Surg Am* 2010;92(5): 1144-1154.

81. Sirveaux F, Favard L, Oudet D, Huquet D, Walch G, Molé D: Grammont inverted total shoulder arthroplasty in the treatment of glenohumeral osteoarthritis with massive rupture of the cuff: Results of a multicentre study of 80 shoulders. *J Bone Joint Surg Br* 2004;86(3):388-395.

82. Werner CM, Steinmann PA, Gilbart M, Gerber C: Treatment of painful pseudoparesis due to irreparable rotator cuff dysfunction with the Delta III reverse-ball-and-socket total shoulder prosthesis. *J Bone Joint Surg Am* 2005; 87(7):1476-1486.

83. Baumgarten KM, Gerlach D, Galatz LM, et al: Cigarette smoking increases the risk for rotator cuff tears. *Clin Orthop Relat Res* 2010;468(6):1534-1541.

84. Boileau P, Brassart N, Watkinson DJ, Carles M, Hatzidakis AM, Krishnan SG: Arthro-scopic repair of full-thickness tears of the supraspinatus: Does the tendon really heal? *J Bone Joint Surg Am* 2005;87(6):1229-1240.

85. Mallon WJ, Misamore G, Snead DS, Denton P: The impact of preoperative smoking habits on the results of rotator cuff repair. *J Shoulder Elbow Surg* 2004;13(2): 129-132.

86. Tashjian RZ, Hollins AM, Kim HM, et al: Factors affecting healing rates after arthroscopic double-row rotator cuff repair. *Am J Sports Med* 2010;38(12): 2435-2442.

87. Gladstone JN, Bishop JY, Lo IK, Flatow EL: Fatty infiltration and atrophy of the rotator cuff do not improve after rotator cuff repair and correlate with poor functional outcome. *Am J Sports Med* 2007; 35(5):719-728.

88. Goutallier D, Postel JM, Gleyze P, Leguilloux P, Van Driessche S: Influence of cuff muscle fatty degeneration on anatomic and functional outcomes after simple suture of full-thickness tears. *J Shoulder Elbow Surg* 2003;12(6):550-554.

89. Shen PH, Lien SB, Shen HC, Lee CH, Wu SS, Lin LC: Long-term functional outcomes after repair of rotator cuff tears correlated with atrophy of the supraspinatus muscles on magnetic resonance images. *J Shoulder Elbow Surg* 2008;17(1, Suppl):1S-7S.

90. Yoo JC, Ahn JH, Yang JH, Koh KH, Choi SH, Yoon YC: Correlation of arthroscopic repairability of large to massive rotator cuff tears with preoperative magnetic resonance imaging scans. *Arthroscopy* 2009;25(6):573-582.

91. Ellman H, Hanker G, Bayer M: Repair of the rotator cuff: End-result study of factors influencing reconstruction. *J Bone Joint Surg Am* 1986;68(8):1136-1144.

92. Gerber C, Fuchs B, Hodler J: The results of repair of massive tears of

the rotator cuff. *J Bone Joint Surg Am* 2000;82(4):505-515.

93. Rokito AS, Cuomo F, Gallagher MA, Zuckerman JD: Long-term functional outcome of repair of large and massive chronic tears of the rotator cuff. *J Bone Joint Surg Am* 1999;81(7):991-997.

94. Rittmeister M, Kerschbaumer F: Grammont reverse total shoulder arthroplasty in patients with rheumatoid arthritis and nonreconstructible rotator cuff lesions. *J Shoulder Elbow Surg* 2001;10(1): 17-22.

95. Favard L, Lautmann S, Sirveaux F, Oudet D, Kerjean Y, Huquet D: Hemiarthroplasty versus reverse shoulder arthroplasty in the treatment of osteoarthritis with massive rotator cuff tear. *Shoulder Prosthesis* 2000; 2000:261-268.

96. Sirveaux F, Favard L, Oudet D, Huguet D, Lautman S: Grammont inverted total shoulder arthroplasty in the treatment of glenohumeral osteoarthritis with massive and non repairable cuff rupture, in Walch G, Boileau P, Molé D, eds: *2000 Prosthèses d'épaule recul de 2 à 10 ans.* Paris, France, Sauramps Médical, 2001, pp 247-252.

97. Valenti PH, Boutens D, Nerot C: Delta III reversed prosthesis for osteoarthritis with massive rotator cuff tear: Long term results (> 5 years), in Walch G, Boileau P, Molé D, eds: *2000 Prosthèses d'épaule recul de 2 à 10 ans.* Paris, France, Sauramps Médical, 2001, pp 253-259.

98. Guery J, Favard L, Sirveaux F, Oudet D, Mole D, Walch G: Reverse total shoulder arthroplasty: Survivorship analysis of eighty replacements followed for five to ten years. *J Bone Joint Surg Am* 2006;88(8):1742-1747.

99. Constant CR, Murley AH: A clinical method of functional assessment of the shoulder. *Clin Orthop Relat Res* 1987;214:160-164.

100. Wall B, Nové-Josserand L, O'Connor DP, Edwards TB, Walch G: Reverse total shoulder arthroplasty: A review of results according to etiology. *J Bone Joint Surg Am* 2007;89(7):1476-1485.

101. Richards RR, An K-N, Bigliani LU, et al: A standardized method for the assessment of shoulder function. *J Shoulder Elbow Surg* 1994;3:347-352.

102. Lippitt SB, Harryman DT II, Matsen FA III: A practical tool for evaluating function: The simple shoulder test, in Matsen FA III, Fu FH, Hawkins RJ, eds: *The Shoulder: A Balance of Mobility and Stability.* Rosemont, IL, American Academy of Orthopaedic Surgeons, 1993, pp 501-518.

103. Roach KE, Budiman-Mak E, Songsiridej N, Lertratanakul Y: Development of a shoulder pain and disability index. *Arthritis Care Res* 1991;4(4):143-149.

104. Grassi FA, Murena L, Valli F, Alberio R: Six-year experience with the Delta III reverse shoulder prosthesis. *J Orthop Surg (Hong Kong)* 2009;17(2):151-156.

105. John M, Pap G, Angst F, et al: Short-term results after reversed shoulder arthroplasty (Delta III) in patients with rheumatoid arthritis and irreparable rotator cuff tear. *Int Orthop* 2010;34(1): 71-77.

106. Farshad M, Gerber C: Reverse total shoulder arthroplasty: From the most to the least common complication. *Int Orthop* 2010; 34(8):1075-1082.

107. Vanhove B, Beugnies A: Grammont's reverse shoulder prosthesis for rotator cuff arthropathy: A retrospective study of 32 cases. *Acta Orthop Belg* 2004;70(3): 219-225.

108. Kalouche I, Sevivas N, Wahegaonker A, Sauzieres P, Katz D, Valenti P: Reverse shoulder arthroplasty: Does reduced medialisation improve radiological and clinical results? *Acta Orthop Belg* 2009;75(2):158-166.

109. Gutiérrez S, Levy JC, Frankle MA, et al: Evaluation of abduction range of motion and avoidance of inferior scapular impingement in a reverse shoulder model. *J Shoulder Elbow Surg* 2008;17(4):608-615.

110. Nyffeler RW, Werner CM, Gerber C: Biomechanical relevance of glenoid component positioning in the reverse Delta III total shoulder prosthesis. *J Shoulder Elbow Surg* 2005;14(5):524-528.

111. Lädermann A, Williams MD, Melis B, Hoffmeyer P, Walch G: Objective evaluation of lengthening in reverse shoulder arthroplasty. *J Shoulder Elbow Surg* 2009;18(4):588-595.

112. Hattrup SJ: The influence of postoperative acromial and scapular spine fractures on the results of reverse shoulder arthroplasty. *Orthopedics* 2010;33(5):302.

113. Walch G, Mottier F, Wall B, Boileau P, Molé D, Favard L: Acromial insufficiency in reverse shoulder arthroplasties. *J Shoulder Elbow Surg* 2009;18(3):495-502.

114. Whatley AN, Fowler RL, Warner JJ, Higgins LD: Postoperative rupture of the anterolateral deltoid muscle following reverse total shoulder arthroplasty in patients who have undergone open rotator cuff repair. *J Shoulder Elbow Surg* 2011;20(1):114-122.

115. Bigliani LU, Cordasco FA, McIlveen SJ, Musso ES: Operative treatment of failed repairs of the rotator cuff. *J Bone Joint Surg Am* 1992;74(10):1505-1515.

116. Gumina S, Di Giorgio G, Perugia D, Postacchini F: Deltoid detachment consequent to open surgical repair of massive rotator cuff tears. *Int Orthop* 2008;32(1): 81-84.

117. Blazar PE, Williams GR, Iannotti JP: Spontaneous detachment of the deltoid muscle origin. *J Shoulder Elbow Surg* 1998;7(4): 389-392.

118. Morisawa K, Yamashita K, Asami A, Nishikawa H, Watanabe H: Spontaneous rupture of the deltoid muscle associated with massive tearing of the rotator cuff. *J Shoulder Elbow Surg* 1997;6(6): 556-558.

Video Reference

12.1: Frankle M, Otto R, Pervaiz K, Griffin C: Video. *Reverse Shoulder Arthroplasty for Massive Cuff Tears Without Arthritis.* Temple Terrace, FL, 2011.

Complications of the Reverse Prosthesis: Prevention and Treatment

Jesse Affonso, MD
Gregory P. Nicholson, MD
Mark A. Frankle, MD
Gilles Walch, MD
Christian Gerber, MD
Juan Garzon-Muvdi, MD
Edward G. McFarland, MD

Abstract

Reverse total shoulder arthroplasty was developed in the late 1980s for elderly patients with rotator cuff arthropathy. Several biomechanical advantages of the reverse shoulder arthroplasty result in improved deltoid function, which improves shoulder motion and function compared to other types of shoulder arthroplasty. The main indication for the reverse prosthesis is painful rotator cuff tear arthropathy. The indications for reverse shoulder arthroplasty have continued to expand since it was first performed in the United States in 2004. Although the results of reverse total shoulder arthroplasty have been generally favorable, the complication rate is higher than that of conventional total shoulder arthroplasty. Complications include those common to other shoulder procedures (infection, instability, and nerve injury) and those unique to reverse total shoulder arthroplasty (scapular notching, glenoid baseplate failure, component disassociation, and scapular stress fractures). It is helpful for orthopaedic surgeons to understand ways to avoid these complications and methods with which to treat them.

Instr Course Lect 2012;61:157-168.

In reverse total shoulder arthroplasty, first described by Grammont et al[1] in 1987, a convex articular surface is attached to the glenoid, and a concave articular surface is fixed to the proximal part of the humerus. This prosthesis was originally designed for elderly patients with rotator cuff tear arthropathy who had not been successfully treated with nonsurgical modalities. Theoretic advantages of the Grammont reverse total shoulder arthroplasty over conventional total shoulder arthroplasty for patients with a deficient rotator cuff include (1) the large glenosphere offers a greater range of

Dr. Nicholson or an immediate family member has received royalties from Innomed and Zimmer; serves as a paid consultant to Zimmer; has stock or stock options in Zimmer; and has received research support from EBI, Tornier, and Zimmer. Dr. Frankle or an immediate family member has received royalties from DJ Orthopaedics; is a member of a speakers' bureau or has made paid presentations on behalf of DJ Orthopaedics; serves as a paid consultant to DJ Orthopaedics; serves as an unpaid consultant to DePuy; has received research support from DJ Orthopaedics, EBI, Eli Lilly, and Encore Medical; and has received nonincome support (such as equipment or services), commercially derived honoraria, or other non-research–related funding (such as paid travel) from DJ Orthopaedics, EBI, Eli Lilly, and Encore Medical. Dr. Walch or an immediate family has received royalties from Tornier. Dr. Gerber or an immediate family has received royalties from Zimmer; serves as a paid consultant to Storz; has received research support from Medacta; and serves as a board member, owner, officer, or committee member of the Swiss Society of Orthopaedics and Traumatology. Dr. McFarland or an immediate family member serves as a paid consultant to DePuy Mitek and Stryker; has received research support from DJ Orthopaedics; and has received nonincome support (such as equipment or services), commercially derived honoraria, or other non-research–related funding (such as paid travel) from DJ Orthopaedics. Neither of the following authors nor any immediate family member has received anything of value from or owns stock in a commercial company or institution related directly or indirectly to the subject of this chapter: Dr. Affonso and Dr. Garzon-Muvdi.

motion than previous reverse designs; (2) the small lateral offset reduces the torque at the point of glenoid fixation; (3) medializing the center of rotation recruits more deltoid fibers for forward elevation and abduction; and (4) distalizing the humerus increases the tension on the deltoid.[1,2] These biomechanical advantages were postulated to result in an improved mechanical advantage of the deltoid, allowing it to compensate for the rotator cuff deficiency.

Indications for reverse total shoulder arthroplasty have continued to evolve since Grammont's initial work.[2-18] Current indications for this procedure include cuff tear arthropathy, rotator cuff deficient shoulders with pseudoparalysis, reconstruction after tumor resection, revision of a failed hemiarthroplasty or internal fixation with a subsequent rotator cuff deficient shoulder, and an acute three- or four-part proximal humerus fracture.[1,6,7,11,15,18] Successful implanta-

tion of a reverse total shoulder arthroplasty is contingent on a functional deltoid muscle and adequate glenoid and proximal humerus bone quality. Contraindications include patients with axillary nerve palsy, active infection, neuropathic shoulder joints, and large glenoid bone defects that are not treatable with bone grafting.

The indications for a reverse total shoulder arthroplasty differ from those for conventional total shoulder arthroplasty. Conventional anatomic total shoulder arthroplasty is minimally constrained and most often involves a stemmed humeral component with a cemented polyethylene glenoid. The primary indication for conventional total shoulder arthroplasty is an osteoarthritic glenohumeral joint that is painful and has been refractory to nonsurgical treatment. Unlike reverse total shoulder arthroplasty, conventional total shoulder arthroplasty requires an intact rotator cuff. Other indications for total shoulder arthroplasty include

inflammatory arthritis, osteonecrosis of the humeral head with subsequent glenohumeral arthritis, and posttraumatic glenohumeral arthritis. Contraindications to conventional total shoulder arthroplasty include active infection, paralysis, poor glenoid bone stock, and the lack of a rotator cuff.

Reverse total shoulder arthroplasty has been performed for nearly 25 years in Europe with promising results, but these devices were not approved by the Food and Drug Administration for use in the United States until 2004. Numerous outcome studies of reverse total shoulder arthroplasty have reported encouraging results in patients for whom there was no clearly successful procedure previously.[3-5,8,10,13,14,16,17] However, the ability to help these patients has come at the cost of a relatively high complication rate (up to 68%).[2,4,6-8,13,14,18-20] Complications include those common to other shoulder procedures (infection, instability, and nerve injury) and those unique to

Table 1
Summary of Studies on Reverse Shoulder Arthroplasty

Study (Year)	No. of Patients	Mean Patient Age (years)	Length of Follow-up (months)	Diagnosis
Valenti et al[19] (2001)	39	70	84	RCT arthropathy, failed HA or TA
Rittmeister and Kerschbaumer[13] (2001)	7 (8 shoulders)	60	54.3	Rheumatoid arthritis
Jacobs et al[20] (2001)	14	72	26	RCT arthropathy, failed HA or TA, rheumatoid arthritis
Boulahia et al[4] (2002)	16	77	35	RCT or posttraumatic arthropathy
De Wilde et al[6] (2003)	13	49	36	Tumor
Sirveaux et al[14] (2004)	80	73	44.5	RCT arthropathy
Werner et al[18] (2005)	58	68	38	RCT arthropathy, failed HA or TA
Boileau et al[2] (2005)	45	N/A	40	RCT arthropathy, fracture, failed HA or TA
Frankle et al[8] (2005)	60	71	33	RCT arthropathy, rheumatoid arthritis, posttraumatic arthropathy
De Wilde et al[7] (2005)	4	42	38	Tumor

RCT = rotator cuff tear, HA = hemiarthroplasty, TA = total arthroplasty, N/A = not available, GL = glenoid loosening, HL = humeral loosening
[a]American Shoulder and Elbow Surgeons score

reverse total shoulder arthroplasty (scapular notching, baseplate failure, component disassociation, and scapular stress fractures).

This chapter will review the most common complications associated with reverse shoulder arthroplasty and will provide information on avoiding and treating those complications.

Scapular Notching

Notching of the bone of the inferior and posterior scapular neck has been reported in 50% to 96% of reverse total shoulder arthroplasties[1,14,21-23] (**Figure 1**) (**Table 1**).[2,4,6-8,13,14,18-20] Although notching is not completely understood, it appears to result from mechanical impingement between the superomedial aspect of the humeral polyethylene insert and the inferior (and possibly the posterior) scapular neck. The Nerot system is the most commonly used scapular notching classification system and is based on radiographic evidence of the severity

and depth of the notching[19] (**Figure 2**). Scapular notching typically occurs within the first year after implantation of the prosthesis, sometimes appearing as early as a few months after implantation. It has not been established if notching progresses to an end point without further progression after a fixed amount of time. One study indicated that there is no progression of notching over time. Werner et al[18] reported that although notching occurred as early as a few months after implantation, the notching seemed to stabilize and did not progress in a high percentage (79%) of patients. Early studies reported scapular notching as a radiographic finding with no known clinical impact,[13,18-20] but one study suggested that higher grades of notching correlate with poorer functional outcomes.[14] Sirveaux et al[14] found a negative effect of scapular notching on clinical outcomes, with grade 3 and 4 notches associated with a lower Constant score.[24]

Known factors related to notching that can be controlled by the surgeon include sphere position in relationship to the superior-inferior dimensions of the glenoid, inferior tilt of the glenoid component, and the choice of implant

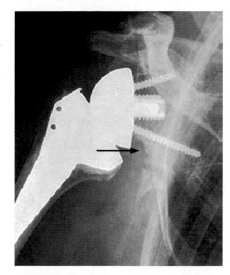

Figure 1   AP radiograph shows a high-grade notch at the inferior glenoid (arrow).

Table 1
Summary of Studies on Reverse Shoulder Arthroplasty (continued)

No. of Primary/ Revision Indications	Average Preoperative/ Postoperative Constant Score (points)	Complications	No. of Failures or Revisions
36 (92%)/3 (8%)	21/63	GL (4, 10%); infection (2, 5%)	3 (8%)
7 (100%)/0	17/63	GL (3, 38%); infection (1, 13%); acromial fracture (3, 38%)	1 (13%)
9 (64%)/5 (36%)	17.9/56.7	N/A	N/A
16 (100%)/0	22/59	GL (1, 6%); dislocation (1, 6%); phlebitis (1, 6%); hematoma (1, 6%)	2 (13%)
13 (100%)/0	39/72.5	Dislocation (4, 31%); infection (2, 15%)	1 (8%)
80 (100%)/0	22.6/65.5	GL (7, 9%); HL (1, 1%); infection (1, 1%);	3 (4%)
17 (29%)/41 (71%)	29/64	GL (3, 5%); HL (1, 2%); dislocation (5, 9%); infection (6, 10%); hematoma (12, 21%); fracture (4, 7%); nerve lesion (1, 2%); inlay dislocation (1, 2%)	6 (10%)
26 (58%)/19 (42%)	17/59[a]	HL (5, 11%); dislocation (3, 7%); infection (2, 4%); periprosthetic fracture (1, 2%); glenoid fracture (1, 2%)	10 (22%)
60 (100%)/0	34.3/68.2	GL (6, 10%); dislocation (1, 2%); infection (3, 5%); scapular fracture (1, 2%); acromial fracture (3, 5%)	7 (12%)
4 (100%)/0	(N/A)/84.5	None	0

RCT = rotator cuff tear, HA = hemiarthroplasty, TA = total arthroplasty, N/A = not available, GL = glenoid loosening, HL = humeral loosening
[a]American Shoulder and Elbow Surgeons score

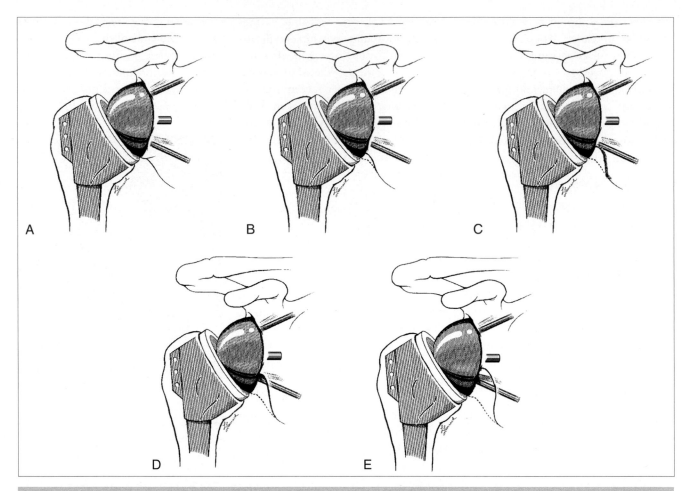

Figure 2   Illustration of the Nerot radiographic classification system for scapular notching. **A,** grade 0 (no notch). **B,** Grade 1 (small notch). **C,** Grade 2 (notch with condensation). **D,** Grade 3 (evolutive notch). **E,** Grade 4 (glenoid loosening). (Reproduced with permission from McFarland EG, Sanguanjit P, Tasaki A, Keyurapan E, Fishman EK, Fayad LM: The reverse shoulder prosthesis: A review of imaging features and complications. *Skeletal Radiol* 2006;35(7):488-496.)

design. Nyffeler et al[25] biomechanically showed that placing the glenosphere more inferiorly on the glenoid results in less mechanical impingement of the humeral component on the inferior scapular neck (and thus less notching) and increased the arc of motion of the shoulder (**Figure 3**). Inferior tilt of the glenoid component also has been shown to decrease the likelihood of scapular notching (**Figure 4**) in biomechanical and clinical studies.[14,18,21,25-28] In a clinical and radiographic evaluation of 326 consecutive reverse total shoulder arthroplasties, Lévigne et al[21] reported that the frequency of notching decreased with an increasing inferior

degree of tilt of the baseplate and sphere on the glenoid. For patients with an inferiorly inclined glenoid secondary to inferior glenoid bone loss associated with osteoarthritis, Lévigne et al[21] recommended that the baseplate be placed flush against the glenoid rim, and the glenoid should be reamed uniformly, which can help keep the baseplate inferiorly tilted. In patients with superior glenoid bone loss and a superiorly inclined glenoid, the authors recommended reaming the inferior glenoid to restore an inferior inclination to the baseplate.[21]

Design choices may have some impact on the frequency and the severity

of scapular notching. The original reverse shoulder prosthesis was designed to medialize the center of rotation as a means of decreasing shear forces between the baseplate and the underlying bone.[1,2] One design change that may affect the amount of notching is the lateralization of the center of rotation of the components.[26,27,29] Gutiérrez et al[29] studied the effect of lateralizing the center of rotation from 0 to 10 mm and found that the impingement-free range of motion in abduction was increased by approximately 32°. Frankle et al[8] used a prosthesis with a lateralized center of rotation in a cohort of 96 shoulders and found no evidence of scapular notching at a minimum 2-year follow-up.

Another suggested design change to decrease scapular notching is decreasing the neck-shaft angle of the humeral implant.[29] Many commercially available prostheses have a neck-shaft angle of approximately 155°. In a biomechanical study, Gutiérrez et al[29] found that as the humeral neck-shaft angle increased from 130° to 170°, the likelihood of inferior impingement also increased. Nicholson and Murthi[30] studied 144 patients with a reverse prosthesis with a head-neck angle of 150° created with a metallic neck-shaft angle of 143° and a polyethylene angle of 7°. The authors reported an incidence of scapular notching of only 8% at 8-month follow-up. Although notching may be more common with some designs than others, this chapter's authors are not aware of any prospective randomized trials showing the superiority of one type of prosthesis over another in relationship to notching. Newer designs may show less initial notching, but long-term follow-up is lacking for many of these prostheses.[8,30]

Despite the choice of implant, the surgeon can influence the degree of notching by placing the baseplate and the sphere more inferiorly on the glenoid along with some inferior inclination of the baseplate in relationship to the glenoid. It has not yet been determined by clinical studies if surgical technique or implant design is the most important factor in preventing scapular notching.

Instability

Instability is one of the more common complications of reverse total shoulder arthroplasty (**Table 1**) with an

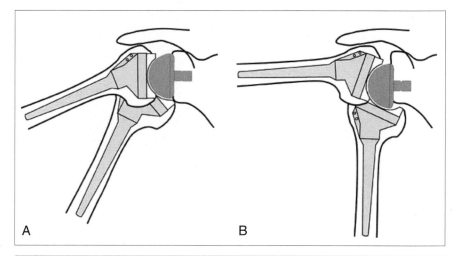

Figure 3   Placement of the glenosphere in a more inferior position on the native glenoid results in a greater arc of motion until impingement. Too much inferior placement may not allow firm fixation of the superior screw in the baseplate, which could lead to early loosening. **A,** With the glenosphere centered on the glenoid, adduction is limited by direct contact of the polyethylene cup on the inferior glenoid rim. **B,** With positioning of the glenosphere more distally, there is substantial improvement in adduction and abduction. (Reproduced with permission from Nyffeler RW, Werner CML, Gerber C: Biomechanical relevance of glenoid component positioning in the reverse Delta III total shoulder prosthesis. *J Shoulder Elbow Surg* 2005;14(5):524-528.)

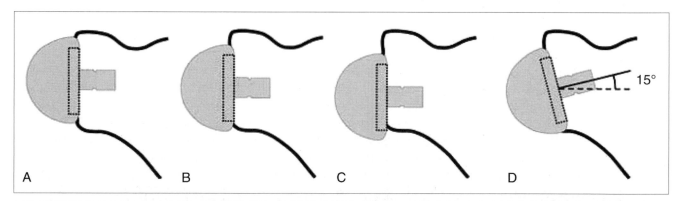

Figure 4   Various options exist for placing the glenosphere on the glenoid. **A,** Neutral, centered positioning of the glenosphere. **B,** Flush positioning of the glenosphere with the inferior rim. **C,** Extending the glenosphere beyond the inferior glenoid rim. **D,** Tilting the glenosphere downward and flush with scapular neck, which is the preferred placement for a glenosphere. (Reproduced with permission from Nyffeler RW, Werner CML, Gerber C. Biomechanical relevance of glenoid component positioning in the reverse Delta III total shoulder prosthesis. *J Shoulder Elbow Surg* 2005;14(5): 524-528.)

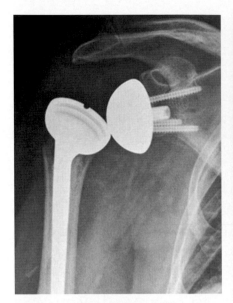

Figure 5 AP radiograph showing a dislocated reverse shoulder prosthesis.

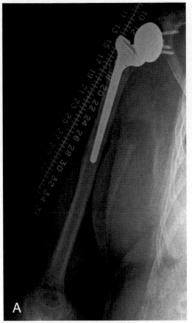
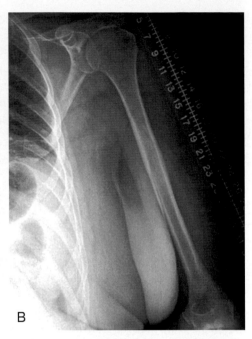

Figure 6 **A** and **B,** Radiographs of bilateral humeri with markers to assess humeral length are essential for preoperative planning in patients with extensive bone loss.

incidence in one series as high as 30%[13,14,18,31] (**Figure 5**). The major risk factor for instability of a reverse prosthesis is its use in patients undergoing revision surgery, especially when revising a failed shoulder arthroplasty to a reverse prosthesis.[32] The factors believed to be related to instability of a reverse prosthesis can be divided into three categories: patient selection factors (such as prior shoulder surgery, poor deltoid function, and compliance issues), surgical factors (such as the surgical approach, the tensioning of the implants, and subscapularis reattachment), and design factors (such as a medial or a lateral center of rotation, the depth of the polyethylene insert, the sphere diameter, and the sphere offset or asymmetry).

Patient factors can be important in the development of postoperative instability after a reverse total shoulder arthroplasty. The deltoid muscle should be functioning to achieve a stable reverse prosthesis, especially if there is a deficient soft-tissue envelope resulting from rotator cuff tears.[32] Patients with prior surgery are at a higher risk for instability than patients who have not had previous surgery.[32] The patient also should be capable of avoiding falls and following postoperative instructions. After surgery, some patients continue to position the arm behind the body in external rotation, a position that increases the risk for instability; patients at risk for falling should be treated with reverse shoulder arthroplasty only after a full discussion of the risks of fracture or instability secondary to falling.

Surgical factors that can decrease the incidence of dislocation after reverse shoulder arthroplasty include the surgical approach, correcting humeral length discrepancies, and reattaching the subscapularis tendon when it is present. The superior approach for reverse total shoulder arthroplasty has been advocated by some surgeons who have shown that instability is less frequent with this approach than with a standard deltopectoral approach.[33-35] Although the superior approach appears to confer additional stability, it is not extensile and may not allow the wider exposure of the glenoid or the proximal humerus often necessary in revision shoulder arthroplasty.

The length of the humerus at the location where the reverse prosthesis is inserted is an important factor that can affect implant instability. Nove-Josserand et al[35] have shown that in some patients humeral bone loss can be misjudged, and the humeral components can be inserted too low, especially when the humeral component has been revised. In patients with proximal humeral bone loss (such as revision cases or fracture sequelae), full-length radiographs of both humeri should be obtained to ensure proper component length[35] (**Figure 6**).

Another surgical consideration is retention of the soft-tissue envelope of the rotator cuff (when possible). Edwards et al[36] studied two cohorts of patients with reverse total shoulder arthroplasty and found that the dislocation rates for the groups with and without reattachment of the subscapularis tendon were 0% and 9.2%, respectively. Similarly, retention of the posterior rotator cuff helps the shoulder function in external rotation but likely also contributes to stability by providing some compressive force to the components.

Implant design features may also influence the incidence of shoulder instability.[1,2,26,27,29] The traditional Delta prosthesis (DePuy, Warsaw, IN) medializes the center of rotation, which may produce less shear on the glenoid baseplate but also may decrease the joint compression force. Designs that lateralize the center of rotation of the construct are purported to increase the compressive force of the deltoid on the proximal humerus, thereby increasing stability.[1,2,26,27,29]

As is the case with femoral head size in total hip arthroplasty, it has been suggested that a larger sphere size in the reverse prosthesis may decrease the ability of the shoulder to dislocate.[2,37] One biomechanical study has evaluated this issue. Gutiérrez et al,[38] using a custom testing device in the laboratory, found that the most important factors in preventing instability were the compressive force of the humerus into the sphere followed by the depth of the polyethylene insert. Based on their experimental model, the authors reported that the variable of sphere size was less important than the two other variables. However, they found that, of three sphere sizes (32, 36, and 40 mm), only the 32-mm sphere required less force to produce component instability. Whether these findings can be extrapolated to the clinical situation has not been studied, but the report by Gutiérrez et al[38] underscores the importance of evaluating the function of the nerves (specifically, the axillary nerve and brachial plexus) and muscles (specifically, the rotator cuff and del-

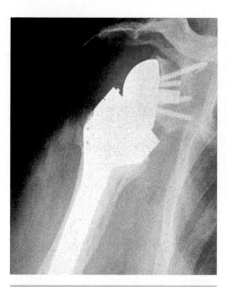

Figure 7   In patients with instability secondary to problems with humeral tensioning, metal metaphyseal extenders can be used to further increase tension on the deltoid.

toid muscles) to rule out any neurologic or muscular reason for instability in a patient with an unstable reverse shoulder prosthesis. To determine if the muscle is still functioning, electromyography or nerve conduction velocity studies may be necessary for some patients with deltoid atrophy. Radiographs should be obtained to rule out other structural reasons for the instability, such as a proximal humeral fracture, baseplate fixation failure, or component malpositioning.

After completing the evaluation of a patient with an unstable reverse shoulder prosthesis, the surgeon may attempt a closed reduction under anesthesia, which is best performed with fluoroscopic guidance. Usually, a distraction force is needed to bring the humeral component down to the level of the sphere, and the surgeon should push directly on the proximal humerus to engage the head with the sphere. The patient's arm should be positioned through a range of motion to determine which position(s) of the arm produces instability and which do not. The extremity can then be braced in a

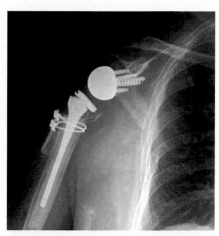

Figure 8   In revision situations with extensive proximal humeral bone loss, proximal humeral allograft can be used to restore length and tension in the deltoid muscle. (Reproduced with permission from Chacon A, Virani N, Shannon R, Levy JC, Pupello D, Frankle M: Revision arthroplasty with use of a reverse shoulder prosthesis-allograft composite. *J Bone Joint Surg Am* 2009;91(1):119-127.)

stable position for 6 weeks or more.

If instability persists despite closed reduction and immobilization, attention should be directed to correcting any soft-tissue or bony abnormalities contributing to the instability. Measuring radiographs of both extremities with a superimposed ruler or metal marker can facilitate the measurement of humeral-length discrepancy (**Figure 6**) and allows the surgeon to determine if revision surgery is needed to treat mild (< 2 cm) or larger (> 2 cm) deficits. Smaller length discrepancies may be treated by revising only the glenoid sphere to a larger sphere, with or without increasing the length of the humeral component with polyethylene or metaphyseal metal extenders before and after placing longer metaphyseal implants (**Figure 7**). In patients with large length discrepancies, it may be necessary to revise the humeral component with or without humeral allograft (**Figure 8**). In any patient with

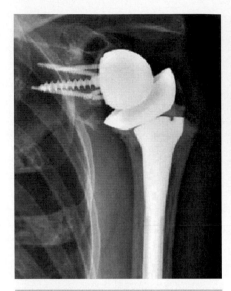

Figure 9 AP radiograph shows a broken compression screw even though serial radiographs showed no change in the position of the baseplate over time.

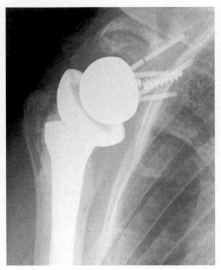

Figure 10 Radiograph shows complete failure of the baseplate with broken screws.

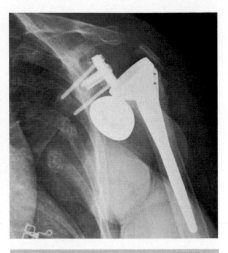

Figure 11 Radiograph shows disassociation of the glenoid sphere from the baseplate, which resulted in a painful, nonfunctioning shoulder.

instability, the soft-tissue envelope should be reconstructed as much as possible; however, in most patients, the surrounding soft tissue is scarred and immobile, and the soft-tissue envelope may not provide reliable stability to the construct.

Another option for increasing the stability of the construct is to use deeper or more constraining polyethylene components on the humeral side. Although this option is available in many current reverse prosthetic systems, there is a paucity of data concerning the effectiveness of these implants in providing shoulder stability for patients who have experienced instability. In one biomechanical study, Gutiérrez et al[38] showed that the force required to dislocate a reverse prosthesis increases as the depth of the humeral socket increases. The concerns with using deeper polyethylene inserts for reverse total shoulder procedures focus around impingement, which can result in instability, polyethylene wear, and pain.

Glenoid Baseplate Failure and Component Disassociation

Baseplate failure can take several forms, including screw fracture (**Figure 9**), screw fracture with baseplate failure (**Figure 10**), and disassociation of the baseplate and the glenoid sphere (**Figure 11**). Some of these complications are peculiar to particular reverse total shoulder implant systems, but it is not yet known if recent reverse total shoulder component design changes will eliminate some of these complications.

Gross failure of the baseplate is defined as loosening of the baseplate so that it becomes detached from the glenoid. The most common causes of baseplate detachment are poor initial fixation of the baseplate, loosening of the screws secondary to osteolysis, and infection. The relationship of the location of the center of rotation and glenoid component tilt may be a contributing factor,[26] but there are few data to support the use of one type of reverse total shoulder system over another.

Screw failure has been reported with and without loosening of the baseplate.[39] In a study of screw failures with a baseplate that could be stabilized with compression or interlocking screw fixation, Holcomb et al[39] reported that the most important factor for screw failure was not the type of screw used but the inclination and location of the baseplate on the glenoid. The authors recommended an inferior tilt of approximately 15° to provide maximum compressive force across the baseplate-glenoid interface when compared with neutral and superior tilt. However, interlocking screws may provide a more rigid construct and increase the overall stability of the implant.

Disassociation of the sphere from the baseplate has been reported for almost every type of reverse total shoulder system on the market.[3,8,17,40] One study found that the sphere appeared to be incompletely seated on the baseplate in up to 3.2% of cases.[40] Causes of incomplete seating of the sphere may include soft-tissue interposed between the sphere and the baseplate, incomplete removal of a peripheral rim of bone on the glenoid, or incorrect placement of a central screw in the sphere before impacting the sphere into position. It is important that all blood and fluids be removed from the Morse taper of the implants to allow proper surface contact of the Morse taper surfaces.

The treatment of baseplate failure depends on the cause. In many instances, the glenoid bone is too deficient to maintain another baseplate. In such cases, if future reconstruction to a reverse prosthesis of the shoulder is not possible, bone grafting the glenoid and converting the humeral side to a hemiarthroplasty is recommended. Bone grafting of the glenoid is not necessary in every case of deficient glenoid bone because a future reconstruction with a reverse prosthesis may be unlikely. If the baseplate shows screw failure alone with no other signs of movement of the baseplate, consideration should be given to early removal of the implant because a loose implant and broken screws will continue to wear away the glenoid bone.[39]

When the baseplate has failed but there is adequate bone for reconstructing the glenoid, the critical issue is to position the new implant so that it has solid fixation. In some traditional reverse prosthesis systems with a central baseplate peg, this solid fixation can be accomplished by bone grafting any glenoid bone defects and then implanting a baseplate with a longer central peg. In systems that have baseplates with central screws, the new baseplate should be placed where the screws have good purchase in bone. In some instances, doing so can be challenging if the broken screws cannot be removed (**Figure 12**). In such cases, bone grafting with blocks of bone or morcellized bone graft may be necessary and should be available at the time of surgery.

Disassociation of the sphere from the baseplate can be a devastating complication for patients. Some patients elect to live with the deformity and

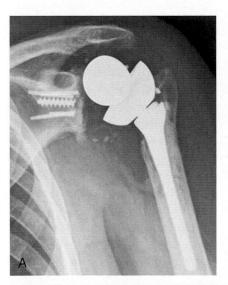
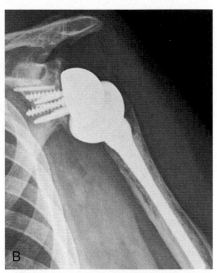

Figure 12   **A,** Radiograph of an implant with failure of all the screws. At the time of revision surgery, the screws were solidly fixed and could not be removed without extensive damage to the glenoid. **B,** The old screws were left in place, and the baseplate was repositioned so that the new screws could obtain good fixation in bone.

loss of function, but in most instances, revision of the sphere to the baseplate can be achieved with relative ease. Care must be taken to ensure the sphere can be impacted on the baseplate and no bone or soft-tissue interposition exists.

Infection

The causes of infection associated with a reverse prosthesis are multifactorial, with published rates ranging from 0% to 15.3% (mean, 5.1%).[2-18,41] The risk of infection after primary reverse shoulder arthroplasty in patients with and without previous surgery are 7% and 2%, respectively.[42]

Factors that may contribute to this relatively high rate of infection include unsuspected previous surgery-related infection, hematoma formation, and dead space. Patients who present with a painful shoulder arthroplasty are particularly at risk for an underlying infection, and it is especially important to determine preoperatively if the patient has an infection. The infection workup should include serial conventional radiographs, blood studies (such

as erythrocyte sedimentation rate and C-reactive protein level), an aspiration with cultures observed for 10 days, and, in some cases, nuclear medicine studies with tagged white blood cells.[9]

Another possible cause of infection in a reverse prosthesis is that the removal of scar tissue and malunited bone often results in a large dead space, which includes the subacromial, the joint, and the subdeltoid spaces. This dead space allows for hematoma formation, which is susceptible to bacterial colonization. Hematoma formation has been shown to be a risk factor for deep infection after conventional total shoulder arthroplasty and has been suggested to be a risk factor for reverse total shoulder arthroplasty.[9] Werner et al[18] reported postoperative hematomas in 12 of 58 patients (20.6%) undergoing primary reverse total shoulder arthroplasty. Five of the patients were treated with aspiration, and seven had an open revision procedure secondary to other concomitant complications. Although the authors concluded that aspiration and débridement should be considered for patients with hematomas, there were no infections in their patients treated without surgery.

The treatment of a deep infection involving a reverse total shoulder prosthesis has not been adequately studied, but the guidelines are similar to those for infected arthroplasties of the knee or hip. The approach to the patient and infection depends on many factors, particularly the time from implantation to the time of surgery, the virulence of the organism cultured, and the immunologic status of the patient. In the acute (< 2 weeks postoperatively) or the subacute period (2 to 6 weeks after the surgery), irrigation and débridement with polyethylene exchange and subsequent intravenous antibiotics can be attempted. If an infection presents later than 6 weeks after surgery, a two-stage reimplantation is preferred by most authors.[9,12,42,43] However, Beekman et al[43] suggested that a one-stage revision procedure can be effective for treating an infected reverse shoulder prosthesis. All infected cement and hardware should be removed at the time of surgery to successfully eradicate the infection. If a two-stage approach is used, an antibiotic spacer or antibiotic-impregnated beads should be left in the glenoid fossa to maintain space for the later reconstruction. Antibiotic therapy appropriate for the cultured organisms should be used, although the required duration of intravenous and oral therapy is controversial.[9,12]

When reimplanting a reverse prosthesis after previous implant removal, preoperative planning is necessary to determine if bone grafting of the glenoid or the humerus will be necessary. The use of antibiotic cement for securing the humeral component at the time of revision surgery is an option but not a requirement in such cases. If there is a possibility that a long revision humeral stem will be implanted, then fluoroscopy may be helpful to verify that the stem is positioned correctly in the canal and not exiting through a perforation of the humeral cortex. If there is concern that the involved extremity may be too short, then measurements of the bilateral humeri should be made with a ruler on preoperative radiographs. Intraoperatively, various humeral metaphyseal metallic and polyethylene inserts of different lengths should be available to add length as needed to properly tension the implants.

Summary

The most common complications after reverse shoulder arthroplasty are scapular notching, instability, baseplate failures, and infection. Some of these complications are avoidable using more modern implant designs, and some may be obviated by proper preoperative planning and surgical technique. The treatment of complications requires a thorough evaluation of the causes of the complication and the ability to address these variables at the time of surgery.

References

1. Grammont P, Trouilloud P, Laffay JP, Deries X: Etude et réalisation d'une nouvelle prothèse d'épaule. *Rhumatologie* 1987; 39(10):407-418.

2. Boileau P, Watkinson DJ, Hatzidakis AM, Balg F: Grammont reverse prosthesis: Design, rationale, and biomechanics. *J Shoulder Elbow Surg* 2005;14(1, Suppl S):147S-161S.

3. Boileau P, Watkinson D, Hatzidakis AM, Hovorka I: Neer Award 2005: The Grammont reverse shoulder prosthesis. Results in cuff tear arthritis, fracture sequelae, and revision arthroplasty. *J Shoulder Elbow Surg* 2006;15(5): 527-540.

4. Boulahia A, Edwards TB, Walch G, Baratta RV: Early results of a reverse design prosthesis in the treatment of arthritis of the shoulder in elderly patients with a large rotator cuff tear. *Orthopedics* 2002;25(2):129-133.

5. Cuff D, Pupello D, Virani N, Levy J, Frankle M: Reverse shoulder arthroplasty for the treatment of rotator cuff deficiency. *J Bone Joint Surg Am* 2008;90(6):1244-1251.

6. De Wilde L, Sys G, Julien Y, Van Ovost E, Poffyn B, Trouilloud P: The reversed Delta shoulder prosthesis in reconstruction of the proximal humerus after tumour resection. *Acta Orthop Belg* 2003; 69(6):495-500.

7. De Wilde LF, Plasschaert FS, Audenaert EA, Verdonk RC: Functional recovery after a reverse prosthesis for reconstruction of the proximal humerus in tumor surgery. *Clin Orthop Relat Res* 2005;430:156-162.

8. Frankle M, Siegal S, Pupello D, Saleem A, Mighell M, Vasey M: The reverse shoulder prosthesis for glenohumeral arthritis associated with severe rotator cuff deficiency: A minimum two-year follow-up study of sixty patients. *J Bone Joint Surg Am* 2005;87(8):1697-1705.

9. Gerber C, Pennington SD, Nyffeler RW: Reverse total shoulder arthroplasty. *J Am Acad Orthop Surg* 2009;17(5):284-295.

10. Guery J, Favard L, Sirveaux F, Oudet D, Mole D, Walch G: Reverse total shoulder arthroplasty: Survivorship analysis of eighty replacements followed for five to ten years. *J Bone Joint Surg Am* 2006;88(8):1742-1747.

11. Levy J, Frankle M, Mighell M, Pupello D: The use of the reverse shoulder prosthesis for the treatment of failed hemiarthroplasty for proximal humeral fracture. *J Bone Joint Surg Am* 2007;89(2): 292-300.

12. Matsen FA III, Boileau P, Walch G, Gerber C, Bicknell RT: The reverse total shoulder arthroplasty. *J Bone Joint Surg Am* 2007;89(3):660-667.

13. Rittmeister M, Kerschbaumer F: Grammont reverse total shoulder arthroplasty in patients with rheumatoid arthritis and nonreconstructible rotator cuff lesions. *J Shoulder Elbow Surg* 2001;10(1):17-22.

14. Sirveaux F, Favard L, Oudet D, Huquet D, Walch G, Molé D: Grammont inverted total shoulder arthroplasty in the treatment of glenohumeral osteoarthritis with massive rupture of the cuff: Results of a multicentre study of 80 shoulders. *J Bone Joint Surg Br* 2004;86(3):388-395.

15. Van Seymortier P, Stoffelen D, Fortems Y, Reynders P: The reverse shoulder prosthesis (Delta III) in acute shoulder fractures: Technical considerations with respect to stability. *Acta Orthop Belg* 2006;72(4):474-477.

16. Vanhove B, Beugnies A: Grammont's reverse shoulder prosthesis for rotator cuff arthropathy: A retrospective study of 32 cases. *Acta Orthop Belg* 2004;70(3):219-225.

17. Wall B, Nové-Josserand L, O'Connor DP, Edwards TB, Walch G: Reverse total shoulder arthroplasty: A review of results according to etiology. *J Bone Joint Surg Am* 2007;89(7):1476-1485.

18. Werner CM, Steinmann PA, Gilbart M, Gerber C: Treatment of painful pseudoparesis due to irreparable rotator cuff dysfunction with the Delta III reverse-ball-and-socket total shoulder prosthesis. *J Bone Joint Surg Am* 2005;87(7):1476-1486.

19. Valenti PH, Boutens D, Nerot C: Delta 3 reversed prosthesis for osteoarthritis with massive rotator cuff tear: Long-term results (> 5 years), in Walch G, Boileau P, Mole D, eds: *Shoulder Prosthesis: Two to Ten Year Follow-up*. Montpellier, France, Sauramps Medical, 2001, pp 253-259.

20. Jacobs R, Debeer P, De Smet L: Treatment of rotator cuff arthropathy with a reversed Delta shoulder prosthesis. *Acta Orthop Belg* 2001;67(4):344-347.

21. Lévigne C, Boileau P, Favard L, et al: Scapular notching in reverse shoulder arthroplasty. *J Shoulder Elbow Surg* 2008;17(6):925-935.

22. McFarland EG, Sanguanjit P, Tasaki A, Keyurapan E, Fishman EK, Fayad LM: The reverse shoulder prosthesis: A review of imaging features and complications. *Skeletal Radiol* 2006;35(7):488-496.

23. Wierks C, Skolasky RL, Ji JH, McFarland EG: Reverse total shoulder replacement: Intraoperative and early postoperative complications. *Clin Orthop Relat Res* 2009;467(1):225-234.

24. Constant CR, Murley AH: A clinical method of functional assessment of the shoulder. *Clin Orthop Relat Res* 1987;214:160-164.

25. Nyffeler RW, Werner CM, Gerber C: Biomechanical relevance of glenoid component positioning in the reverse Delta III total shoulder prosthesis. *J Shoulder Elbow Surg* 2005;14(5):524-528.

26. Gutiérrez S, Greiwe RM, Frankle MA, Siegal S, Lee WE III: Biomechanical comparison of component position and hardware failure in the reverse shoulder prosthesis. *J Shoulder Elbow Surg* 2007;16(3, Suppl):S9-S12.

27. Gutiérrez S, Levy JC, Frankle MA, et al: Evaluation of abduction range of motion and avoidance of inferior scapular impingement in a reverse shoulder model. *J Shoulder Elbow Surg* 2008;17(4):608-615.

28. Simovitch RW, Zumstein MA, Lohri E, Helmy N, Gerber C: Predictors of scapular notching in patients managed with the Delta III reverse total shoulder replacement. *J Bone Joint Surg Am* 2007;89(3):588-600.

29. Gutiérrez S, Comiskey CA IV, Luo ZP, Pupello DR, Frankle MA: Range of impingement-free abduction and adduction deficit after reverse shoulder arthroplasty: Hierarchy of surgical and implant-design-related factors. *J Bone Joint Surg Am* 2008;90(12):2606-2615.

30. Nicholson GP, Murthi AM: Trabecular metal reverse shoulder arthroplasty and the lack of scapular notching. *Clin Orthop Relat Res* 2011, in press.

31. De Wilde LF, Van Ovost E, Uyttendaele D, Verdonk R: Results of an inverted shoulder prosthesis after resection for tumor of the proximal humerus. *Rev Chir Orthop Reparatrice Appar Mot* 2002;88(4):373-378.

32. Wall B, Walch G, Jouve F, Mottier F: The reverse shoulder prosthesis for revision of failed total shoulder arthroplasty, in Walch G, Boileau P, Mole D, Favard L, Levigne C, Sirveaux F, eds: *Reverse Shoulder Arthroplasty: Clinical Results, Complications, Revision*. Montpellier, France, Sauramps Medical, 2006, pp 231-242.

33. Burkhead WZ: Why I like the superior approach, in Walch G, Boileau P, Mole D, Favard L, Levigne C, Sirveaux F, eds: *Reverse Shoulder Arthroplasty: Clinical Results, Complications, Revision*. Montpellier, France, Sauramps Medical, 2006, p 199.

34. Krishnan SG: The deltopectoral approach for primary reverse prostheses: Why I don't like it, in Walch G, Boileau P, Mole D, Favard L, Levigne C, Sirveaux F, eds: *Reverse Shoulder Arthroplasty: Clinical Results, Complications, Revision*. Montpellier, France, Sauramps Medical, 2006, p 207.

35. Nove-Josserand L, Walch G, Wall B: Instability of the reverse pros-

thesis, in Walch G, Boileau P, Mole D, Favard L, Levigne C, Sirveaux F, eds: *Reverse Shoulder Arthroplasty: Clinical Results, Complications, Revision.* Montpellier, France, Sauramps Medical, 2006, pp 247-260.

36. Edwards TB, Williams MD, Labriola JE, Elkousy HA, Gartsman GM, O'Connor DP: Subscapularis insufficiency and the risk of shoulder dislocation after reverse shoulder arthroplasty. *J Shoulder Elbow Surg* 2009;18(6):892-896.

37. Boileau P, Watkinson DJ, Hatzidakis AM, Balg F: Reverse prosthesis design, rationale and biomechanics, in Walch G, Boileau P, Mole D, Favard L, Levigne C, Sirveaux F, eds: *Reverse Shoulder Arthroplasty: Clinical Results, Complications, Revision.* Montpelier, France, Sauramps Medical, 2006, pp 22-55.

38. Gutiérrez S, Keller TS, Levy JC, Lee WE III , Luo ZP: Hierarchy of stability factors in reverse shoulder arthroplasty. *Clin Orthop Relat Res* 2008;466(3):670-676.

39. Holcomb JO, Cuff D, Petersen SA, Pupello DR, Frankle MA: Revision reverse shoulder arthroplasty for glenoid baseplate failure after primary reverse shoulder arthroplasty. *J Shoulder Elbow Surg* 2009;18(5):717-723.

40. Middernacht B, De Wilde L, Molé D, Favard L, Debeer P: Glenosphere disengagement: A potentially serious default in reverse shoulder surgery. *Clin Orthop Relat Res* 2008;466(4):892-898.

41. Cheung EV, Sperling JW, Cofield RH: Infection associated with hematoma formation after shoulder arthroplasty. *Clin Orthop Relat Res* 2008;466(6):1363-1367.

42. Jacquot N, Chuinard C, Boileau P: Results of deep infection after a reverse shoulder arthroplasty, in Walch G, Boileau P, Mole D, Favard L, Levigne C, Sirveaux F, eds: *Reverse Shoulder Arthroplasty: Clinical Results, Complications, Revision.* Montpelier, France, Sauramps Medical, 2006, pp 303-313.

43. Beekman PD, Katusic D, Berghs BM, Karelse A, De Wilde L: One-stage revision for patients with a chronically infected reverse total shoulder replacement. *J Bone Joint Surg Br* 2010;92(6):817-822.

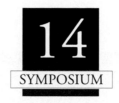

14

SYMPOSIUM

How to Minimize Complications in Acromioclavicular Joint and Clavicle Surgery

Stephanie H. Hsu, MD
Christopher S. Ahmad, MD
Patrick D.G. Henry, MD, FRCSC
Michael D. McKee, MD, FRCSC
William N. Levine, MD

Abstract

Up to 50% of all athletic shoulder injuries are acromioclavicular joint separations. The ideal treatment for type III injuries remains controversial. Current reconstruction techniques include anatomic coracoclavicular reconstructions and newly developed arthroscopic techniques. Clavicle fractures have traditionally been treated nonsurgically based largely on early reports of surgical complications, but there has been a dramatic surge in the surgical treatment of clavicle fractures over the past 5 years because of recent reports of poorer outcomes with nonsurgical management.

Instr Course Lect 2012;61:169-183.

Acromioclavicular (AC) joint separations comprise up to 50% of all athletic shoulder injuries.[1] Ideal management for type III injuries remains controversial. Although surgical techniques have evolved since the classic Weaver-Dunn coracoacromial liga-

ment transfer, complications are possible. Current techniques include anatomic coracoclavicular reconstructions and newly developed arthroscopic techniques. Clavicle fractures had traditionally been treated nonsurgically based largely on early reports of com-

plications from Neer[2] and Rowe;[3] however, surgical treatment has increased dramatically over the past 5 years because of recent reports of poorer outcomes with nonsurgical management. This chapter will focus on the indications and contraindications of surgical treatment of AC joint and clavicle injuries along with pearls and pitfalls to avoid complications.

Acromioclavicular Joint Injuries

Diagnostic Imaging

Imaging of AC joint injuries includes a true AP, a scapular outlet, and an axillary lateral view of the shoulder. An axillary view is essential to identify a type IV AC separation with posterior clavicular displacement. Appropriate radiographs such as a true AP or a serendipity view should be taken if a distal clavicle fracture, medial physeal injury in a young patient, or sternoclavicular injury is suspected. Comparison views can provide useful information concerning the coracoclavicular (CC) distance. The average distance between the coracoid process and the clavicle is

Dr. Ahmad or an immediate family member serves as a paid consultant to Acumed and Arthrex; has received research or institutional support from Stryker; and has received nonincome support (such as equipment or services), commercially derived honoraria, or other non-research–related funding (such as paid travel) from Zimmer. Dr. McKee or an immediate family member has received royalties from Stryker; is a member of a speakers' bureau or has made paid presentations on behalf of Synthes and Zimmer; serves as a paid consultant to Synthes and Zimmer; has received research or institutional support from Wright Medical Technology and Zimmer; and serves as a board member, owner, officer, or committee member of American Shoulder and Elbow Surgeons, the Orthopaedic Trauma Association, and the Canadian Orthopaedic Association. Dr. Levine or an immediate family serves as a board member, owner, officer, or committee member of the American Orthopaedic Association. Neither of the following authors nor any immediate family member has received anything of value from or owns stock in a commercial company or institution related directly or indirectly to the subject of this chapter: Dr. Hsu and Dr. Henry.

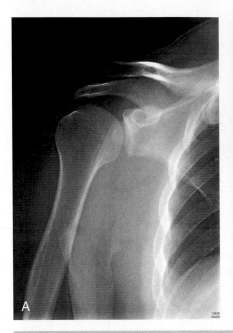

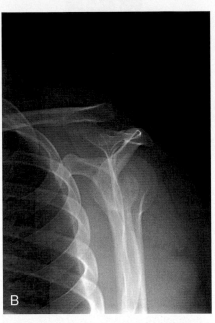

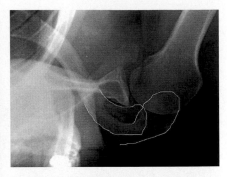

Figure 2 Axillary radiograph of a type IV AC injury. (Courtesy of Columbia University Center for Shoulder, Elbow and Sports Medicine, New York, NY.)

Figure 1 AP (**A**) and axillary (**B**) radiographs of a type III AC injury. (Courtesy of Columbia University Center for Shoulder, Elbow and Sports Medicine, New York, NY.)

1.1 to 1.3 cm.[4] If an AC dislocation is present with a normal CC distance, a coracoid process fracture should be suspected.

Classification

The Rockwood modification of the original classification systems of Tossy et al[5] and Allman[6] is most commonly used to categorize AC joint injuries into six types.[7] A type I injury is a strain of the AC ligaments with no significant instability, visible deformity, or radiographic abnormality. A type II injury involves disruption of the AC ligaments, but the CC ligaments are still intact. Radiographic changes show a widened AC joint, slight vertical displacement, and an increase in CC interspace distance. In a type III injury, both the AC and CC ligaments are torn, resulting in horizontal and vertical distal clavicle instability. Specifically, the AC joint separation is reducible with a gentle upward force on the ipsilateral elbow. Radiographs will show the AC joint dislocation (**Fig-**

ure 1). In a type IV injury, the AC and CC ligaments are torn, and the scapula is displaced inferiorly and anteriorly, resulting in the distal clavicle displacing posteriorly through or into the trapezius muscle. On examination, the anterior acromion may be prominent, and the AC joint is typically irreducible. In addition to the increased CC interspace and AC dislocation on an AP view, an axillary radiograph is important to identify the posterior displacement of the distal clavicle (**Figure 2**). In a type V injury, the deltotrapezia fascia is more extensively detached from the clavicle, and all stabilizing ligaments are disrupted. Non-weighted films show a large amount of vertical displacement (a 100% to 300% increase of CC interspace), and the joint is often irreducible. The distal clavicle may lie subcutaneously. In both type IV and V injuries, soft-tissue interposition of the deltotrapezia fascia prevents AC joint reduction. A type VI injury is a rare, high-energy injury

characterized by the distal clavicle in a subacromial or subcoracoid position. Type VI injuries may occur when the arm is hyperabducted and externally rotated at the time of injury. These injuries are often associated with clavicle and rib fractures or pneumothorax.

Associated intra-articular glenohumeral joint injuries have been reported with type III to V injuries to the AC joint. In 2009, Tischer et al[8] found an 18% rate of associated injuries in 77 patients (average age, 35 years) during diagnostic glenohumeral arthroscopy before AC reconstruction. Fourteen percent of the injuries were superior labrum anterior and posterior lesions, with few rotator cuff pathologies.

Treatment

Nonsurgical treatment is usually recommended for type I and II AC joint injuries, whereas early surgical stabilization is advocated for acute type IV to VI injuries. The treatment of type III injuries remains controversial. Several reviews and controlled trials have failed to demonstrate improved clinical outcomes with surgical reconstruction when compared with nonsurgical management.[9-14] Surgical complications and longer recovery periods and

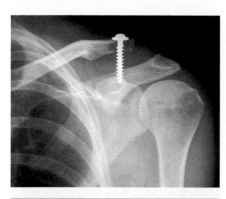

Figure 3 AP radiograph of the shoulder of a 40-year-old, right-hand-dominant man taken 6 weeks after modified Bosworth screw fixation for an AC type V separation. Complete fixation failure is shown. (Courtesy of Columbia University Center for Shoulder, Elbow and Sports Medicine, New York, NY.)

time to return to work or sports participation are also cited as reasons for selecting nonsurgical treatment.

Nonsurgical Management

Type I and II AC joint injuries do not typically require surgery and are treated with a short period of immobilization, as dictated by pain. Early range of motion is encouraged.[15] Because chronic painful symptoms may develop in up to 27% of grade I and II injuries, patients may later require surgical intervention.[16,17]

Ideal treatment of grade III injuries remains controversial. Based on the literature, nonsurgical treatment is not recommended for some patients, including young patients involved in heavy labor or high-demand overhead sports or those with AC displacement greater than 2 cm.[16-20] Studies have also demonstrated variable results with concerns for long-term sequelae in higher demand patients in whom pain, instability, deformity, mechanical symptoms, arthrosis, or scapular dyskinesis may develop.

Conversely, the belief that surgical treatment is necessary for high-demand patients has been challenged with studies showing good outcomes and the ability to recover adequate strength and endurance with nonsurgical treatment.[21-23] However, if instability and pain persist, a high-demand patient may elect surgical reconstruction. This chapter's authors prefer an initial trial of nonsurgical management with supervised physical therapy for a period of 6 to 12 weeks before surgical treatment of most type III injuries.

Surgical Management
Complications of Common Surgical Procedures

Primary fixation has consisted of Kirschner wires, plates, or screws, but concern for catastrophic pin migration to surrounding neurovascular structures and other hardware complications have minimized the use of these types of fixation.[24,25] Screws are susceptible to breaking and loosening and surrounding osteolysis or fractures (**Figure 3**). Clavicular hook-plates provide initial stability with reported good short-term results, but are also fraught with hardware complications including infection, dislocation, loosening, osteolysis, and fracture; in some instances, hardware removal is required.[26-28]

Weaver and Dunn[29] originally described the excision of the distal clavicle with coracoacromial ligament transfer. Although this was a popular surgical technique, recent studies report failure rates with loss of reduction in up to 24% of patients.[29-31] This failure rate may be attributable to the fact that the coracoacromial ligament strength is only 10% to 25% the strength of a native intact CC ligament complex, and there is a differing force vector.[32-34]

The Weaver-Dunn technique has been modified or augmented with suture anchors,[35] clavicular hook plates,[28,36] cortical buttons,[37] and other supplementary constructs. Screw fixation, synthetic ligament, suture or alternative material have also been used to reduce the AC joint.[19,38-40] Technical complications, aseptic loosening, distal clavicle osteolysis, infection, and erosion of cerclage materials through the coracoid or clavicle have been described.[27,41-43] Infection rates from 0% to 9% have been reported.

Good results have been reported for arthroscopic techniques for coracoacromial ligament transfer for acute or chronic AC dislocations.[44-46] Although arthroscopic techniques have achieved encouraging results, they are technically difficult and should be approached with caution to avoid complications such as incorrect assessment of anatomy, misplaced grafts, or poor fixation because of lack of visualization.

DeBeradino et al[46] described an arthroscopic technique using a subcoracoid button attached with nonabsorbable sutures to a clavicular washer and augmented with a soft-tissue graft; all 10 patients returned to full activity without loss of reduction. Initial enthusiasm for new techniques must be balanced with the need for long-term follow-up to detect complications not common to other techniques. For example, recent cases referred to the Columbia University Center for Shoulder, Elbow, and Sport Medicine have included button pull-through of the clavicle in first-generation TightRope (Arthrex, Naples, FL) and second-generation GraftRope (Arthrex) devices and coracoid fractures (**Figures 4** through **6**). Eccentric placement of the coracoid tunnel can increase the chances of complications related to coracoid fractures and must be avoided. If appropriate visualization is not obtained by the surgeon, conversion to an open procedure is recommended.

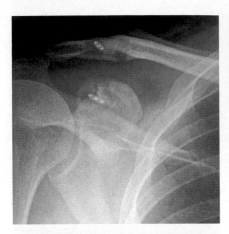

Figure 4 AP radiograph showing failure of a TightRope device with coracoid fracture and pull-through of the superior button into the clavicle. (Courtesy of Columbia University Center for Shoulder, Elbow and Sports Medicine, New York, NY.)

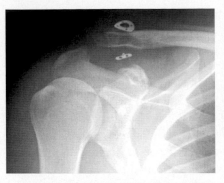

Figure 5 AP radiograph showing failure of a GraftRope device with pull-through of the inferior button through the coracoid. (Courtesy of Columbia University Center for Shoulder, Elbow and Sports Medicine, New York, NY.)

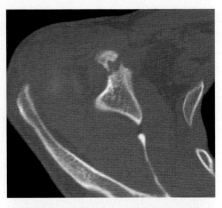

Figure 6 Axial CT scan of a coracoid fracture following arthroscopic AC joint reconstruction. (Courtesy of Columbia University Center for Shoulder, Elbow and Sports Medicine, New York, NY.)

Anatomic CC Reconstruction

Anatomic CC ligament reconstruction has been shown to have superior anatomic and biomechanical features.[18,47,48] Both single-and double-tunnel techniques have been described. Biomechanically, the use of doubled semitendinosus graft placed into a coracoid bone tunnel and secured with interference screws into two anatomically placed clavicular drill holes replicates the native anatomy and provides a superiorly stable construct.[49] The clavicular tunnels are typically 1.0 mm larger than the graft diameter. This chapter's authors prefer to use an open anatomic CC ligament complex reconstruction with semitendinosus allograft.

Distal Clavicle Excision

Recently, anatomic reconstruction of the CC ligaments has been combined with reconstruction of the AC joint capsule.[50-52] Debate continues over whether distal clavicle resection reduces overall joint stability when combined with a CC ligament complex reconstruction. Several studies suggest that retention of the distal clavicle al-

lows the AC joint and capsule to remain intact and retain stability.[53] In contrast, excision of approximately 10 mm of the distal clavicle maintains AC joint capsular attachments and should not compromise stability. In patients with preexisting AC arthrosis or chronic conditions, a distal clavicle resection may assist in reduction. The superior and posterior AC ligaments provide stability in the horizontal plane and prevent excessive posterior translation of the clavicle.[18,50,54] Careful preservation or repair should be performed to minimize the resulting instability and persistent pain caused by excessive distal clavicle resection or incompetence of the superior and posterior AC ligaments. If an excessive amount of distal clavicle has been excised and instability is present, meticulous reattachment and imbrication of the deltotrapezia fascial flaps using nonabsorbable sutures can help maintain stability.

Surgical Pearls
Clavicle Preparation

Anatomic insertions of the conoid and trapezoid ligaments are localized visually, and guide pins are placed at 30° to 45° angles to reproduce the angles of

the native ligaments. The anatomic insertion of the conoid ligament averages 46 mm medial to the AC joint on the posterior aspect of the clavicle, whereas the trapezoid averages 26 mm medial to the AC joint and more central.[18,55-57] Care is taken to remove scar tissue that may prevent full reduction between the coracoid and clavicle and at the AC joint. Failure to carefully resect this tissue may lead to an incomplete AC joint reduction and an unsatisfactory outcome.

A semitendinosus allograft, which is sized on the back table and averages from 4 to 5 mm, is typically used. A cannulated 6-mm reamer (usually 1 mm greater than the graft size to accommodate the graft and an interference screw) is drilled to create holes at 45 mm from the distal clavicle in the posterior half for the conoid tunnel and at 30 mm from the distal clavicle centrally to replicate the trapezoid insertion. Adequate distance between tunnels, usually 15 mm, aids in preventing clavicle fracture between tunnels, although fracture through tunnels has been reported[58,59] (**Figure 7**). Care should be taken to avoid penetrating the posterior or anterior cortex of the clavicle because this can cause cortical blowout. This is accomplished by careful guidewire placement in anticipation of the reamer diameter. If cortical blowout occurs, a new drill hole can be created by accepting less than anatomic placement and the possibility of clavicle fracture. Another option is conversion to a single-tunnel reconstruction technique.

Coracoid Fixation

If coracoid fixation is chosen, a full assessment of the coracoid anatomy is essential. Palpation of the medial and lateral edges with direct visualization ensures proper anchor placement or guide pin placement and drilling to prevent coracoid wall blowout, too large a tunnel, or propagation. As previously discussed, eccentric placement of a coracoid tunnel (if this technique is chosen) must be avoided to prevent coracoid fracture and loss of fixation and reduction. In general, most surgeons (including this chapter's authors) avoid drilling a tunnel in the coracoid because of the risk of fracture and instead loop the graft around the base of the coracoid.

Clavicle Fixation

The AC joint is reduced with an assistant applying upward pressure to the elbow and downward pressure on the distal clavicle. Anatomic reduction can be confirmed fluoroscopically to prevent inadequate or excessive reduction. Slight overreduction is supported because of eventual tendon graft creep. The graft is then passed though the drill holes and the conoid side is secured initially with a 5.5 × 8 mm polyetheretherketone (PEEK) tenodesis screw (Arthrex). An additional augmentation suture is passed though the cannulation of the screw. The tendon graft is cyclically tensioned, and a second 5.5 × 8 mm PEEK tenodesis screw is placed in the trapezoid tunnel to affix the graft. The nonabsorbable aug-

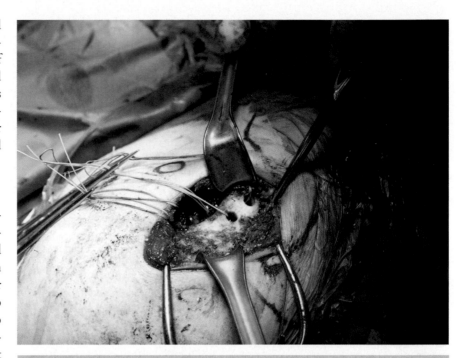

Figure 7   Intraoperative photograph of anatomic CC reconstruction with two clavicular tunnels drilled. The conoid is 45 mm from the AC joint, and the trapezoid tunnel is 30 mm from the AC joint. Note the appropriate distance between the tunnels to minimize risk of intraoperative clavicular fracture. (Courtesy of Columbia University Center for Shoulder, Elbow and Sports Medicine, New York, NY.)

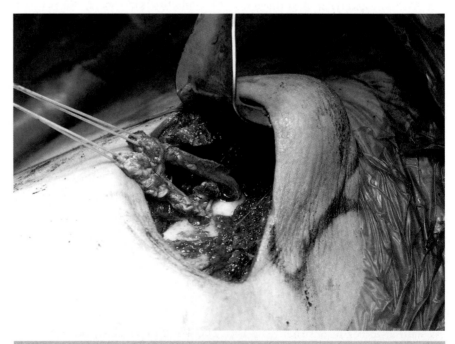

Figure 8   Intraoperative photograph of the shoulder shown in figure 7 shows reduction of the AC joint with graft in the two tunnels secured with interference screws. (Courtesy of Columbia University Center for Shoulder, Elbow and Sports Medicine, New York, NY.)

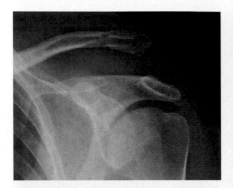

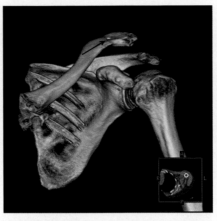

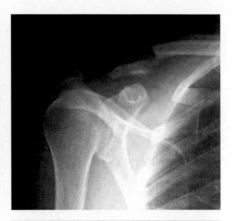

Figure 9 AP radiograph of the shoulder of a 62-year-old, right-hand-dominant man taken 8 weeks after single-tunnel allograft and Mersilene tape augmentation reconstruction for a painful, chronic type III AC joint injury. Complete failure of the reconstruction is seen. (Courtesy of Columbia University Center for Shoulder, Elbow and Sports Medicine, New York, NY.)

Figure 10 Three-dimensional CT reconstruction of the shoulder in figure 9 shows that the clavicular bone tunnel and coracoid are intact. Reconstruction failure occurred from abrasion of the allograft and Mersilene tape, which ruptured along the anterior clavicle. (Courtesy of Columbia University Center for Shoulder, Elbow and Sports Medicine, New York, NY.)

Figure 11 Postoperative AP radiograph of the shoulder of a 48-year-old, right-hand-dominant man 2.5 months after an anatomic CC reconstruction with allograft and a two-tunnel clavicular technique shows a displaced fracture through the medial conoid tunnel. Nonsurgical treatment was instituted, and healing was uneventful. (Courtesy of Columbia University Center for Shoulder, Elbow and Sports Medicine, New York, NY.)

ment sutures passed through the two tenodesis screws are then tied together to provide nonbiologic fixation of the reduction (**Figure 8**). The remaining limbs of the graft are brought across the AC joint and secured to the acromion with suture anchors or bone tunnels to provide additional AC joint stability.

Avoiding Technical Complications
Surgical Complications
Complications such as clavicle fractures or wall blowout from a drilled bone tunnel may occur intraoperatively.[58] Complications following surgical treatment may be more severe, including neurovascular damage, infection, fixation failure, fracture, the need for revision or hardware removal, and persistent pain or instability.

Single-Tunnel Complications
As with all other reconstructive techniques for AC joint injuries, single-tunnel complications include loss of fixation. A unique potential complication of this technique is that the graft

and/or augmentation devices can effectively be guillotined by wear across the anterior clavicle. A 55-year-old, right-hand dominant man was treated with a single-tunnel reconstruction for a chronic, symptomatic type III AC separation. Complete failure of the graft occurred at 8 weeks postoperatively because of rupture of the allograft and the Mersilene tape used for augmentation (WN Levine, MD, unpublished material, 2010) (**Figures 9 and 10**).

Care should be taken when performing a single-tunnel technique to ensure that there are no rough or sharp edges on the anterior clavicle at the site where the graft and/or augmentation device cross it; if necessary, a rasp should be used to smooth this area.

Double-Tunnel Complications
Clavicular fracture is the major concern with the double-tunnel technique. Two 6- to 7-mm tunnels in the clavicle create potential stress risers in

the bone. A 48-year-old, right-hand dominant man was treated with an anatomic CC reconstruction with allograft using a two-tunnel clavicular technique. A fall 2.5 months after surgery resulted in a fracture through the medial conoid tunnel (**Figure 11**). The patient was treated nonsurgically and went on to uneventful healing (WN Levine, MD, unpublished material, 2009). Despite the concerns about clavicular fracture occurring from drilling two tunnels, the reported incidence is rare, and proper attention to the technical details of the two-tunnel technique discussed in this chapter should eliminate intraoperative clavicular fracture. The two-tunnel technique is also appropriate for smaller patients; however, smaller tunnels may be needed.

Postoperative Loss of Reduction
Postoperative loss of reduction remains a concern. It is reported that up to

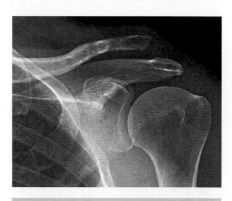

Figure 12 AP radiograph of the shoulder of a 60-year-old, left-hand-dominant woman who presented 2 years postoperatively following an anatomic CC reconstruction (double-tunnel allograft technique with interference screws). The patient had no trauma, and the graft simply stretched over time. The patient was not symptomatic and elected no further surgery. (Courtesy of Columbia University Center for Shoulder, Elbow and Sports Medicine, New York, NY.)

24% of patients have some loss of reduction after a Weaver-Dunn procedure,[29-31] whereas CC reconstructions or CC stabilizations with ligaments or implants have had greater success in maintaining AC joint reduction.[18,19,35,38,40] Despite the biomechanical advantages of the anatomic reconstructions, failures occur with loss of reduction and no bony failures (coracoid or clavicular) (**Figure 12**). If a failure occurs, it is imperative to rule out bone fractures. A three-dimensional CT reconstruction is recommended to most accurately evaluate the coracoid and clavicle for bony failure. Although long-term studies are not yet available, surgeons generally believe that anatomic CC reconstruction leads to a more reliable, predictable, and stable reconstruction.

Rehabilitation

Postoperatively, a Lerman (DonJoy Orthopaedics, Vista, CA) or Gunslinger brace (AliMed, Dedham, MA) is worn for 6 weeks to provide support beneath the elbow and relieve stress from the AC joint during healing. A progressive rehabilitation program is then started to regain range of motion and strength. This chapter's authors have not found glenohumeral stiffness to be a problem. At 8 weeks, active upright range of motion begins and scapular stabilization is emphasized. At 12 weeks, strengthening is started, and daily activities should be resumed. At 6 months, contact sports are allowed if the patient has progressed well.

Clavicle Fractures

In the 1960s, studies reported a nonunion rate of less than 1% in clavicle fractures treated nonsurgically, with a 3% to 5% nonunion rate for surgically treated fractures.[2,3] Subsequently, much of the interest in clavicle surgery was directed at treating the rare complications of nonsurgical management rather than with the surgical treatment of acute fractures. Over the past 5 years, however, the incidence of surgery for acute clavicle fractures has dramatically increased. This surge in the election of surgical treatment has been encouraged by studies reporting poorer outcomes with nonsurgical management than had been previously suspected.[60,61] In a level I study comparing treatment options for widely displaced midshaft clavicle fractures (100% displacement on AP and 45°-cephalic tilt views), patients with surgically treated fractures had a significantly lower complication rate (17%) than those who received nonsurgical treatment (43%).[62] Although the lower complication rate is an improvement, it is still a relatively high complication rate. Another study reported complication rates of up to 23% in surgically treated middle third clavicle fractures.[63] An understanding of these complications and their causes will allow surgeons to use management strategies to avoid or minimize such morbidity.

Avoiding Complications

Appropriate patient selection and choosing when to perform surgery are important. Böstman et al[63] identified fracture comminution and patient intoxication on admission as being the two most predictive factors of a complication occurring following clavicle fixation surgery. The authors stated that "the slightest suspicion of patient noncompliance must be regarded as a contraindication to surgery unless absolute conditions exist."[63] Comminution, which has the propensity to proceed to nonunion in the nonsurgically managed patient, has since been shown to be a relative indication for surgical management. Other relative indications for surgical fixation include displacement greater than 2 cm, shortening greater than 2 cm, open fractures, soft-tissue compromise, clinical deformities and/or scapular malposition, and the presence of certain associated injuries (vascular, neurologic, and ipsilateral upper extremity fractures).[64]

Infection

Infection is the most obvious complication that occurs at much higher frequency with surgical treatment versus nonsurgical management. Although the incidence of deep infection is relatively low (1.4% to 7.8%), the consequences are serious, requiring repeat surgeries, hardware removal, and a higher rate of nonunion[62,63] (**Figure 13**). The use of standard sterile technique and appropriate preoperative antibiotics can decrease the risk of infection. The chapter's authors have reduced the rate of superficial suture abscesses by using a two-layer closure with a deep layer of absorbable sutures on the myofascial layer and 3-0 nylon mattress sutures (rather than subcuta-

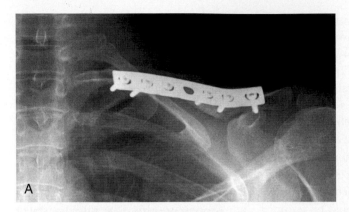
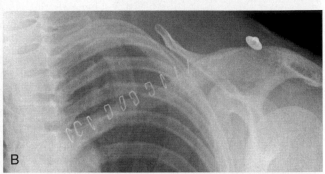

Figure 13 **A,** Radiograph of the shoulder of a patient with a draining sinus over a previously repaired clavicle fracture. **B,** Radiograph after plate removal and irrigation and débridement. The infection was eradicated. (Courtesy of Michael McKee, MD, Toronto, Ontario, Canada).

neous absorbable sutures and skin staples) on the skin.

Numbness

The most common complication of the surgical treatment of midshaft clavicle fractures is postoperative numbness of the chest wall, which can occur in up to 29% of patients.[65,66] Although many patients do not notice this numbness unless it is specifically examined, dysesthesia of the superior chest can be more distressing to female patients and may be aggravated by clothing such as bra straps. A higher percentage of patients treated nonsurgically ultimately report shoulder strap discomfort, which is related to irritation from the higher percentage of malunions and nonunions in this group of patients.[62,65,67]

Numbness is attributed to transection or traction of branches of the supraclavicular nerve. Just posterior to the sternocleidomastoid, this nerve branches into an intermediate and lateral branch, which in turn each give off two or three smaller branches that pierce the platysma and cross the lateral two thirds of the clavicle at a right angle.[68] With careful dissection, these nerves can be preserved, although it may be more difficult to achieve reduction and fixation. A 2010 study re-

ported that the incidence of postoperative numbness was reduced by using a vertical skin incision, rather than the more traditional horizontal incision along the long axis of the clavicle; scar length and satisfaction were equivalent.[66]

This chapter's authors recommend careful dissection in the subcutaneous tissue and preservation of the branches of the supraclavicular nerves; however, the final reduction or fixation should not be compromised. In many instances, preserving these nerves results in significant stretching, which can often cause symptoms similar to those encountered by transecting or applying traction to the nerves. These symptoms usually resolve with time, but patients should be advised concerning this potential complication.

Prominent Hardware and Irritation

Because the clavicle is essentially a subcutaneous bone, hardware irritation remains a problem. Hardware-related irritation is reported by more than 50% of patients.[69] In a study by Shen et al,[65] 70% of patients ultimately had plate removal. The issue of patient concern over prominent hardware has sensory, cosmetic, and psychologic elements, making it difficult to ascertain

a patient's motives for requesting hardware removal. In a randomized study involving 62 midshaft clavicle fractures plated in the superior clavicular position, 5 patients had hardware irritation leading to plate removal.[62] Anteroinferior plate position has resulted in better outcomes, with none of the 26 patients in the study by Chen et al[70] reporting symptomatic hardware irritation. Newer, precontoured, low-profile plating systems have decreased the incidence of hardware irritation problems, with irritation usually fading with time.[71]

Refracture After Plate Removal

Hardware irritation often leads to plate removal, which in turn predisposes the patient to the risk (reported rate, 0% to 8%) of refracture.[63,72] In a 1992 study of 122 surgically treated clavicle fractures, Poigenfürst et al[72] reported 4 refractures after plate removal. The authors ascribed the refractures to technical errors and recommended maintaining hardware for at least 6 months before removal and not forcibly removing interfragmentary screws. In a study of nonsurgically treated clavicle fractures, Robinson et al[61] reported that most fractures that were unhealed at 12 weeks went on to healing by 24 weeks. To allow time for re-

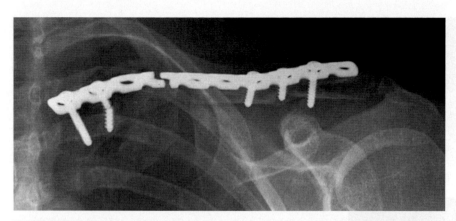

Figure 14 AP radiograph of hardware failure following inadequate fixation with a 3.5-mm reconstruction plate. (Courtesy of Michael McKee, MD, Toronto, Ontario, Canada.)

modeling, this chapter's authors recommend maintaining hardware for a minimum period of 1 year (and preferably 2 years) before removal. This protocol has achieved a refracture rate of less than 1%.

Hardware Failure

Kirschner wires in isolation should not be used to fix clavicle fractures because of their inability to resist the forces across the clavicle and the propensity for migration into dangerous locations such as the aorta.[73] Plates must have adequate strength to withstand the significant forces borne by the clavicle (**Figure 14**). One-third tubular plates have been shown to be too weak and highly susceptible to plate breakage when used in the clavicle.[63] However, a recent retrospective review of 111 patients treated with one-third tubular plates reported no episodes of breakage in a physically smaller population.[74] At this time, one-third tubular plates are considered inadequate for use in clavicle fractures. A biomechanical study by Iannotti et al[75] comparing superiorly placed 3.5-mm reconstruction plates, 3.5-mm limited contact dynamic compression plates, and 2.7-mm dynamic compression plates showed that 3.5-mm limited contact

dynamic compression plates have the greatest resistance to torsional and axial loads. Newer precontoured clavicle plates are now widely used; early clinical and laboratory testing has shown good bony conformity and low rates of implant failure.[62,71,76]

Plate position is another variable to consider, with both superior placement and anterior/inferior placement being commonly advocated positions.[77,78] Iannotti et al[75] showed that superior plating with reconstruction plates had greater biomechanical stability than anterior plating. Although this was also demonstrated in another recent study,[79] biomechanical stability has not yet been proven to provide a clinical advantage in terms of preventing hardware failure. The same study also showed improved bending failure stiffness with locking plates over superior dynamic compression plates;[79] however, another study reported that locking plates are likely unnecessary in a younger patient population.[80]

A clinical study with 40 patients showed equivalent outcomes using locking versus nonlocking reconstruction plates on midshaft clavicle fractures, with radiographic evidence of screw loosening in 3 patients in the nonlocking group and equivalent Dis-

abilities of the Arm, Shoulder and Hand scores.[80] A similar Taiwanese study with patients older than 60 years reported that the patients in the group with locking plates had significantly better results with fewer complications and faster return to work and exercise.[81]

Intramedullary fixation is a less popular but viable alternative technique to plating. Superior plating has been shown to prevent hardware loosening more effectively than intramedullary fixation in both biomechanical and clinical studies;[82-84] however, such findings are inconsistent with other studies showing minimal to no episodes of hardware complications with intramedullary fixation.[85,86] A prospective study by Lee et al[87] showed essentially no difference in the outcomes for Knowles pinning compared with plating, thus leading the authors to recommend Knowles pins over plating. Complications unique to pin fixation include skin irritation and erosion at the insertion site and telescoping of bone fragments leading to shortening when used to treat comminuted fractures.[88] Currently, most surgeons believe that intramedullary fixation provides less rigidity and has a higher incidence of hardware loosening and migration than plating. Its use in the treatment of comminuted fractures is discouraged, and special care should be taken in avoiding hardware prominence at the insertion site.[88]

If plate fixation is chosen, ideally six cortices on each side of the fracture should be engaged by screws regardless of the plate type or position.[88,89] This chapter's authors use precontoured, low-profile plates in the superior position with interfragmentary screws when the fracture pattern allows but acknowledge the advantages and good results found with anteroinferior plate positioning and have used this technique with good success.

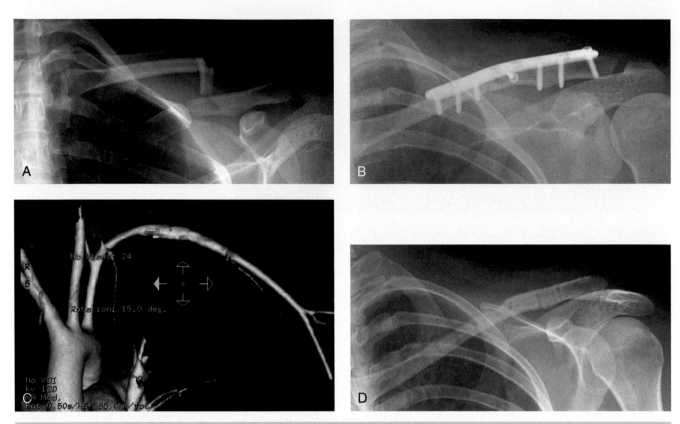

Figure 15 **A,** Radiograph of a midshaft clavicle fracture with significant comminution and displacement. **B,** Radiograph showing fracture fixation with an anatomic plate and an interfragmentary lag screw. **C,** Angiogram shows a small aneurysm in the subclavian artery; the patient presented 12 months after fracture fixation with shoulder discomfort and swelling. **D,** Radiograph of the clavicle after the patient consulted with a vascular surgeon, and the hardware was removed. Symptoms subsequently resolved. (Courtesy of Michael McKee, MD, Toronto, Ontario, Canada.)

Neurovascular Injury

Although the superficial position of the clavicle allows relative ease of access, the proximity of major vessels and nerves to the inferior border of the clavicle renders them vulnerable to insult during surgical fixation (**Figure 15**). The subclavian vein and artery are the most susceptible to injury. Complications with these vessels, including thrombosis, pseudoaneurysm, and thoracic outlet syndrome, have been reported with both nonsurgical and surgical treatment.[67,90-92] A common concern during surgery is drill or screw penetration of the artery or vein, the latter of which is located 7.5 mm beneath the clavicle.[93] One strategy to avoid penetration is the use of drill stops. With a medial clavicular thickness of 15 mm, using a drill stop of 18 mm will protect against accidental "plunging" during the drilling process.[93] A detailed analysis of safe screw trajectories in clavicle fixation used cross-sectional MRI to map spatial relationships between the clavicle and the subclavian neurovascular bundle.[94] This study demonstrated that medially the bundle is directly posterior to the clavicle, making superior-to-inferior screws safer. In the midclavicle, the bundle becomes inferior to the clavicle, making anteroposterior screws safer, and in the lateral clavicle the bundle is a safe distance inferior to the clavicle and is in little danger of iatrogenic injury.

Nonunion

Several studies have demonstrated a significantly higher nonunion rate in displaced midshaft clavicle fractures treated nonsurgically compared with surgical fixation.[62,95] For displaced fractures, a meta-analysis by Zlowodzki et al[95] showed a nonunion rate of 15.1% in the nonsurgical group and 2.2% in the group treated with plating. A randomized controlled study showed a nonunion rate of 3% with superior plating and 15% with nonsurgical treatment.[62] Nonunion in the surgically treated clavicle can be associated with infection and/or hardware failure. Accurate fracture reduction, interfragmentary compression, and solid fixation with good screw purchase are important principles to prevent nonunion. Patient factors also play a large role in the prognosis.[63] Bone grafting or bone supplements are generally not required to treat patients with acute fractures but can be helpful in treating revisions or established nonunions.

Malunion

Radiographic malunion is standard after the closed treatment of displaced clavicle fractures. However, symptomatic malunion is not as common, occurring in 15% to 20% of patients in most series.[60,62] The rate of symptomatic malunion increases as the degree of displacement increases (especially displacement greater than 2 cm). Neurologic (such as brachial plexus irritation or compression), orthopaedic (such as weakness and easy fatigability), or functional cosmetic (such as difficulty with backpacks, straps, or clothing) symptoms may occur. Electing surgical treatment for an acute fracture to prevent malunion is based on the degree of displacement and the age and activity level of the patient. Symptomatic malunion is rare in well-reduced, appropriately fixed, surgically treated clavicle fractures, with no episodes occurring in a recent study of 67 patients treated with superior plating using precontoured plates.[62] When malunion occurs, it involves some degree of implant failure, hypertrophic bone formation, or failure to achieve appropriate reduction. Clavicle fractures should be reduced with respect to length and angular displacement as well as rotatory displacement, which is a more difficult deformity to identify. Failure to properly treat a rotatory deformity can result in shoulder dyskinesia, postural complaints, and discomfort.[96,97]

In reducing the clavicle fracture, it is helpful to remember that the typical deforming forces on the medial fragment (sternocleidomastoid muscle) cause an extension-type rotation, whereas the pectoralis major muscle causes the lateral fragment to flex and rotate forward. Restoring the native anatomy during reduction is the highest priority to avoid postoperative postural or dyskinetic problems in the shoulder.

Summary

The management of AC joint injuries and clavicle fractures has evolved dramatically over the past decade. Increased awareness of the complex AC joint anatomy has led to more anatomic and biomechanically stable surgical techniques. Although complications can still occur, attention to detail and meticulous surgical technique is improving patient outcomes.

It is becoming increasingly well documented that surgical treatment improves outcomes and reduces the incidence of complications in patients with displaced and comminuted clavicle fractures. However, surgery is not a perfect solution and has inherent risks, including the usual complications intrinsic to any surgical procedure. Knowledge from current studies can aid the surgeon in educating the patient so that informed treatment decisions can be made that minimize potential complications and maximize outcomes.

References

1. Kaplan LD, Flanigan DC, Norwig J, Jost P, Bradley J: Prevalence and variance of shoulder injuries in elite collegiate football players. *Am J Sports Med* 2005;33(8): 1142-1146.

2. Neer CS II: Nonunion of the clavicle. *J Am Med Assoc* 1960; 172:1006-1011.

3. Rowe CR: An atlas of anatomy and treatment of midclavicular fractures. *Clin Orthop Relat Res* 1968;58:29-42.

4. Bearden JM, Hughston JC, Whatley GS: Acromioclavicular dislocation: Method of treatment. *J Sports Med* 1973;1(4):5-17.

5. Tossy JD, Mead NC, Sigmond HM: Acromioclavicular separations: Useful and practical classification for treatment. *Clin Orthop Relat Res* 1963;28:111-119.

6. Allman FL Jr: Fractures and ligamentous injuries of the clavicle and its articulation. *J Bone Joint Surg Am* 1967;49(4):774-784.

7. Williams GR, Nguyen VD, Rockwood CA: Classification and radiographic analysis of acromioclavicular dislocations. *Appl Radiol* 1989;18:29-34.

8. Tischer T, Salzmann GM, El-Azab H, Vogt S, Imhoff AB: Incidence of associated injuries with acute acromioclavicular joint dislocations types III through V. *Am J Sports Med* 2009;37(1):136-139.

9. Phillips AM, Smart C, Groom AF: Acromioclavicular dislocation: Conservative or surgical therapy. *Clin Orthop Relat Res* 1998;353: 10-17.

10. Spencer EE Jr: Treatment of grade III acromioclavicular joint injuries: A systematic review. *Clin Orthop Relat Res* 2007;455:38-44.

11. Ceccarelli E, Bondì R, Alviti F, Garofalo R, Miulli F, Padua R: Treatment of acute grade III acromioclavicular dislocation: A lack of evidence. *J Orthop Traumatol* 2008;9(2):105-108.

12. Tamaoki MJ, Belloti JC, Lenza M, Matsumoto MH, Gomes Dos Santos JB, Faloppa F: Surgical versus conservative interventions for treating acromioclavicular dislocation of the shoulder in adults. *Cochrane Database Syst Rev* 2010; 8(8):CD007429.

13. Larsen E, Bjerg-Nielsen A, Christensen P: Conservative or surgical treatment of acromioclavicular dislocation: A prospective, controlled, randomized study. *J Bone Joint Surg Am* 1986;68(4): 552-555.

14. Bannister GC, Wallace WA, Stableforth PG, Hutson MA: The management of acute acromiocla-

vicular dislocation: A randomised prospective controlled trial. *J Bone Joint Surg Br* 1989;71(5): 848-850.

15. Cote MP, Wojcik KE, Gomlinski G, Mazzocca AD: Rehabilitation of acromioclavicular joint separations: Operative and nonoperative considerations. *Clin Sports Med* 2010;29(2):213-228, vii.

16. Bergfeld JA, Andrish JT, Clancy WG: Evaluation of the acromioclavicular joint following first- and second-degree sprains. *Am J Sports Med* 1978;6(4):153-159.

17. Mouhsine E, Garofalo R, Crevoisier X, Farron A: Grade I and II acromioclavicular dislocations: Results of conservative treatment. *J Shoulder Elbow Surg* 2003;12(6): 599-602.

18. Carofino BC, Mazzocca AD: The anatomic coracoclavicular ligament reconstruction: Surgical technique and indications. *J Shoulder Elbow Surg* 2010; 19(2, Suppl):37-46.

19. Wei HF, Chen YF, Zeng BF, et al: Triple endobuttton technique for the treatment of acute complete acromioclavicular joint dislocations: Preliminary results. *Int Orthop* 2011;35(4):555-559.

20. Mazzocca AD, Arciero RA, Bicos J: Evaluation and treatment of acromioclavicular joint injuries. *Am J Sports Med* 2007;35(2): 316-329.

21. Glick JM, Milburn LJ, Haggerty JF, Nishimoto D: Dislocated acromioclavicular joint: Follow-up study of 35 unreduced acromioclavicular dislocations. *Am J Sports Med* 1977;5(6):264-270.

22. McFarland EG, Blivin SJ, Doehring CB, Curl LA, Silberstein C: Treatment of grade III acromioclavicular separations in professional throwing athletes: Results of a survey. *Am J Orthop (Belle Mead NJ)* 1997;26(11):771-774.

23. Wojtys EM, Nelson G: Conservative treatment of grade III acro-

mioclavicular dislocations. *Clin Orthop Relat Res* 1991;268: 112-119.

24. Sethi GK, Scott SM: Subclavian artery laceration due to migration of a Hagie pin. *Surgery* 1976; 80(5):644-646.

25. Norrell H Jr, Llewellyn RC: Migration of a threaded Steinmann pin from an acromioclavicular joint into the spinal canal: A case report. *J Bone Joint Surg Am* 1965;47:1024-1026.

26. Salem KH, Schmelz A: Treatment of Tossy III acromioclavicular joint injuries using hook plates and ligament suture. *J Orthop Trauma* 2009;23(8):565-569.

27. Chiang CL, Yang SW, Tsai MY, Kuen-Huang Chen C: Acromion osteolysis and fracture after hook plate fixation for acromioclavicular joint dislocation: A case report. *J Shoulder Elbow Surg* 2010;19(4): e13-e15.

28. Liu HH, Chou YJ, Chen CH, Chia WT, Wong CY: Surgical treatment of acute acromioclavicular joint injuries using a modified Weaver-Dunn procedure and clavicular hook plate. *Orthopedics* 2010;33(8).

29. Weaver JK, Dunn HK: Treatment of acromioclavicular injuries, especially complete acromioclavicular separation. *J Bone Joint Surg Am* 1972;54(6):1187-1194.

30. Tienen TG, Oyen JF, Eggen PJ: A modified technique of reconstruction for complete acromioclavicular dislocation: A prospective study. *Am J Sports Med* 2003; 31(5):655-659.

31. Weinstein DM, McCann PD, McIlveen SJ, Flatow EL, Bigliani LU: Surgical treatment of complete acromioclavicular dislocations. *Am J Sports Med* 1995; 23(3):324-331.

32. Harris RI, Wallace AL, Harper GD, Goldberg JA, Sonnabend DH, Walsh WR: Structural properties of the intact and the recon-

structed coracoclavicular ligament complex. *Am J Sports Med* 2000; 28(1):103-108.

33. Lee SJ, Nicholas SJ, Akizuki KH, McHugh MP, Kremenic IJ, Ben-Avi S: Reconstruction of the coracoclavicular ligaments with tendon grafts: A comparative biomechanical study. *Am J Sports Med* 2003;31(5):648-655.

34. Motamedi AR, Blevins FT, Willis MC, McNally TP, Shahinpoor M: Biomechanics of the coracoclavicular ligament complex and augmentations used in its repair and reconstruction. *Am J Sports Med* 2000;28(3):380-384.

35. Shin SJ, Yun YH, Yoo JD: Coracoclavicular ligament reconstruction for acromioclavicular dislocation using 2 suture anchors and coracoacromial ligament transfer. *Am J Sports Med* 2009;37(2): 346-351.

36. Boström Windhamre HA, von Heideken JP, Une-Larsson VE, Ekelund AL: Surgical treatment of chronic acromioclavicular dislocations: a comparative study of Weaver-Dunn augmented with PDS-braid or hook plate. *J Shoulder Elbow Surg* 2010;19(7):1040-1048.

37. Boileau P, Old J, Gastaud O, Brassart N, Roussanne Y: All-arthroscopic Weaver-Dunn-Chuinard procedure with double-button fixation for chronic acromioclavicular joint dislocation. *Arthroscopy* 2010;26(2): 149-160.

38. Lädermann A, Grosclaude M, Lübbeke A, et al: Acromioclavicular and coracoclavicular cerclage reconstruction for acute acromioclavicular joint dislocations. *J Shoulder Elbow Surg* 2011;20(3): 401-408.

39. Petersen W, Wellmann M, Rosslenbroich S, Zantop T: Minimally invasive acromioclavicular joint reconstruction (MINAR). *Oper Orthop Traumatol* 2010; 22(1):52-61.

40. Salzmann GM, Walz L, Buchmann S, Glabgly P, Venjakob A, Imhoff AB: Arthroscopically assisted 2-bundle anatomical reduction of acute acromioclavicular joint separations. *Am J Sports Med* 2010;38(6):1179-1187.

41. Fraschini G, Ciampi P, Scotti C, Ballis R, Peretti GM: Surgical treatment of chronic acromioclavicular dislocation: Comparison between two surgical procedures for anatomic reconstruction. *Injury* 2010;41(11):1103-1106.

42. Mares O, Luneau S, Staquet V, Beltrand E, Bousquet PJ, Maynou C: Acute grade III and IV acromioclavicular dislocations: Outcomes and pitfalls of reconstruction procedures using a synthetic ligament. *Orthop Traumatol Surg Res* 2010;96(7):721-726.

43. Stewart AM, Ahmad CS: Failure of acromioclavicular reconstruction using Gore-Tex graft due to aseptic foreign-body reaction and clavicle osteolysis: A case report. *J Shoulder Elbow Surg* 2004;13(5):558-561.

44. Lafosse L, Baier GP, Leuzinger J: Arthroscopic treatment of acute and chronic acromioclavicular joint dislocation. *Arthroscopy* 2005;21(8):1017.

45. Wolf EM, Pennington WT: Arthroscopic reconstruction for acromioclavicular joint dislocation. *Arthroscopy* 2001;17(5):558-563.

46. DeBerardino TM, Pensak MJ, Ferreira J, Mazzocca AD: Arthroscopic stabilization of acromioclavicular joint dislocation using the AC GraftRope system. *J Shoulder Elbow Surg* 2010;19(2, Suppl):47-52.

47. Jones HP, Lemos MJ, Schepsis AA: Salvage of failed acromioclavicular joint reconstruction using autogenous semitendinosus tendon from the knee: Surgical technique and case report. *Am J Sports Med* 2001;29(2):234-237.

48. Rios CG, Mazzocca AD: Acromioclavicular joint problems in athletes and new methods of management. *Clin Sports Med* 2008;27(4):763-788.

49. Mazzocca AD, Santangelo SA, Johnson ST, Rios CG, Dumonski ML, Arciero RA: A biomechanical evaluation of an anatomical coracoclavicular ligament reconstruction. *Am J Sports Med* 2006;34(2):236-246.

50. Klimkiewicz JJ, Williams GR, Sher JS, Karduna A, Des Jardins J, Iannotti JP: The acromioclavicular capsule as a restraint to posterior translation of the clavicle: A biomechanical analysis. *J Shoulder Elbow Surg* 1999;8(2):119-124.

51. Freedman JA, Adamson GJ, Bui C, Lee TQ: Biomechanical evaluation of the acromioclavicular capsular ligaments and reconstruction with an intramedullary free tissue graft. *Am J Sports Med* 2010;38(5):958-964.

52. Gonzalez-Lomas G, Javidan P, Lin T, Adamson GJ, Limpisvasti O, Lee TQ: Intramedullary acromioclavicular ligament reconstruction strengthens isolated coracoclavicular ligament reconstruction in acromioclavicular dislocations. *Am J Sports Med* 2010;38(10):2113-2122.

53. Flatow EL, Duralde XA, Nicholson GP, Pollock RG, Bigliani LU: Arthroscopic resection of the distal clavicle with a superior approach. *J Shoulder Elbow Surg* 1995;4(1 Pt 1):41-50.

54. Salter EG Jr, Nasca RJ, Shelley BS: Anatomical observations on the acromioclavicular joint and supporting ligaments. *Am J Sports Med* 1987;15(3):199-206.

55. Boehm TD, Kirschner S, Fischer A, Gohlke F: The relation of the coracoclavicular ligament insertion to the acromioclavicular joint: A cadaver study of relevance to lateral clavicle resection. *Acta Orthop Scand* 2003;74(6):718-721.

56. Renfree KJ, Riley MK, Wheeler D, Hentz JG, Wright TW: Ligamentous anatomy of the distal clavicle. *J Shoulder Elbow Surg* 2003;12(4):355-359.

57. Harris RI, Vu DH, Sonnabend DH, Goldberg JA, Walsh WR: Anatomic variance of the coracoclavicular ligaments. *J Shoulder Elbow Surg* 2001;10(6):585-588.

58. Turman KA, Miller CD, Miller MD: Clavicular fractures following coracoclavicular ligament reconstruction with tendon graft: A report of three cases. *J Bone Joint Surg Am* 2010;92(6):1526-1532.

59. Costic RS, Labriola JE, Rodosky MW, Debski RE: Biomechanical rationale for development of anatomical reconstructions of coracoclavicular ligaments after complete acromioclavicular joint dislocations. *Am J Sports Med* 2004;32(8):1929-1936.

60. Hill JM, McGuire MH, Crosby LA: Closed treatment of displaced middle-third fractures of the clavicle gives poor results. *J Bone Joint Surg Br* 1997;79(4):537-539.

61. Robinson CM, Court-Brown CM, McQueen MM, Wakefield AE: Estimating the risk of nonunion following nonoperative treatment of a clavicular fracture. *J Bone Joint Surg Am* 2004;86-A(7):1359-1365.

62. Canadian Orthopaedic Trauma Society: Nonoperative treatment compared with plate fixation of displaced midshaft clavicular fractures: A multicenter, randomized clinical trial. *J Bone Joint Surg Am* 2007;89(1):1-10.

63. Böstman O, Manninen M, Pihlajamäki H: Complications of plate fixation in fresh displaced midclavicular fractures. *J Trauma* 1997;43(5):778-783.

64. McKee MD: Clavicle fractures, in Bucholz RW, Heckman JD, Court-Brown CM, Tornetta P, eds: *Rockwood and Green's Fractures in Adults*, ed 7. Philadelphia,

PA, Lippincott Williams & Wilkins, 2010.

65. Shen WJ, Liu TJ, Shen YS: Plate fixation of fresh displaced mid-shaft clavicle fractures. *Injury* 1999;30(7):497-500.

66. Wang K, Dowrick A, Choi J, Rahim R, Edwards E: Post-operative numbness and patient satisfaction following plate fixation of clavicular fractures. *Injury* 2010;41(7): 939-942.

67. Shackford SR, Connolly JF: Taming of the screw: A case report and literature review of limb-threatening complications after plate osteosynthesis of a clavicular nonunion. *J Trauma* 2003;55(5): 840-843, discussion 843.

68. Havet E, Duparc F, Tobenas-Dujardin AC, Muller JM, Fréger P: Morphometric study of the shoulder and subclavicular innervation by the intermediate and lateral branches of supraclavicular nerves. *Surg Radiol Anat* 2007; 29(8):605-610.

69. Ali Khan MA, Lucas HK: Plating of fractures of the middle third of the clavicle. *Injury* 1978;9(4): 263-267.

70. Chen CE, Juhn RJ, Ko JY: Anterior-inferior plating of middle-third fractures of the clavicle. *Arch Orthop Trauma Surg* 2010;130(4):507-511.

71. Vanbeek C, Boselli KJ, Cadet ER, Ahmad CS, Levine WN: Precontoured plating of clavicle fractures: Decreased hardware-related complications? *Clin Orthop Relat Res* 2011;Mar 17. Epub.

72. Poigenfürst J, Rappold G, Fischer W: Plating of fresh clavicular fractures: Results of 122 operations. *Injury* 1992;23(4):237-241.

73. Leppilahti J, Jalovaara P: Migration of Kirschner wires following fixation of the clavicle: A report of 2 cases. *Acta Orthop Scand* 1999; 70(5):517-519.

74. Chen CH, Chen JC, Wang C, Tien YC, Chang JK, Hung SH: Semitubular plates for acutely displaced midclavicular fractures: A retrospective study of 111 patients followed for 2.5 to 6 years. *J Orthop Trauma* 2008;22(7): 463-466.

75. Iannotti MR, Crosby LA, Stafford P, Grayson G, Goulet R: Effects of plate location and selection on the stability of midshaft clavicle osteotomies: A biomechanical study. *J Shoulder Elbow Surg* 2002;11(5):457-462.

76. Huang JI, Toogood P, Chen MR, Wilber JH, Cooperman DR: Clavicular anatomy and the applicability of precontoured plates. *J Bone Joint Surg Am* 2007; 89(10):2260-2265.

77. Collinge C, Devinney S, Herscovici D, DiPasquale T, Sanders R: Anterior-inferior plate fixation of middle-third fractures and nonunions of the clavicle. *J Orthop Trauma* 2006;20(10):680-686.

78. Zenni EJ Jr, Krieg JK, Rosen MJ: Open reduction and internal fixation of clavicular fractures. *J Bone Joint Surg Am* 1981;63(1): 147-151.

79. Robertson C, Celestre P, Mahar A, Schwartz A: Reconstruction plates for stabilization of midshaft clavicle fractures: Differences between nonlocked and locked plates in two different positions. *J Shoulder Elbow Surg* 2009;18(2): 204-209.

80. Cho CH, Song KS, Min BW, Bae KC, Lee KJ: Operative treatment of clavicle midshaft fractures: Comparison between reconstruction plate and reconstruction locking compression plate. *Clin Orthop Surg* 2010;2(3):154-159.

81. Pai HT, Lee YS, Cheng CY: Surgical treatment of midclavicular fractures in the elderly: A comparison of locking and nonlocking plates. *Orthopedics* 2009;32(4):ii.

82. Golish SR, Oliviero JA, Francke EI, Miller MD: A biomechanical study of plate versus intramedullary devices for midshaft clavicle fixation. *J Orthop Surg Res* 2008; 3:28.

83. Mueller M, Rangger C, Striepens N, Burger C: Minimally invasive intramedullary nailing of midshaft clavicular fractures using titanium elastic nails. *J Trauma* 2008; 64(6):1528-1534.

84. Strauss EJ, Egol KA, France MA, Koval KJ, Zuckerman JD: Complications of intramedullary Hagie pin fixation for acute midshaft clavicle fractures. *J Shoulder Elbow Surg* 2007;16(3):280-284.

85. Chuang TY, Ho WP, Hsieh PH, Lee PC, Chen CH, Chen YJ: Closed reduction and internal fixation for acute midshaft clavicular fractures using cannulated screws. *J Trauma* 2006;60(6): 1315-1320, discussion 1320-1321.

86. Liu HH, Chang CH, Chia WT, Chen CH, Tarng YW, Wong CY: Comparison of plates versus intramedullary nails for fixation of displaced midshaft clavicular fractures. *J Trauma* 2010;69(6): E82-E87.

87. Lee YS, Huang HL, Lo TY, Hsieh YF, Huang CR: Surgical treatment of midclavicular fractures: A prospective comparison of Knowles pinning and plate fixation. *Int Orthop* 2008;32(4): 541-545.

88. Smekal V, Oberladstaetter J, Struve P, Krappinger D: Shaft fractures of the clavicle: Current concepts. *Arch Orthop Trauma Surg* 2009;129(6):807-815.

89. Jeray KJ: Acute midshaft clavicular fracture. *J Am Acad Orthop Surg* 2007;15(4):239-248.

90. Casselman F, Vanslembroek K, Verougstraete L: An unusual cause of thoracic outlet syndrome. *J Trauma* 1997;43(1):142-143.

91. Claes T, Debeer P, Bellemans J, Claes T: Deep venous thrombosis of the axillary and subclavian vein after osteosynthesis of a midshaft clavicular fracture: A case report. *Am J Sports Med* 2010;38(6):1255-1258.

92. Koss SD, Goitz HT, Redler MR, Whitehill R: Nonunion of a midshaft clavicle fracture associated with subclavian vein compression: A case report. *Orthop Rev* 1989;18(4):431-434.

93. Galley IJ, Watts AC, Bain GI: The anatomic relationship of the axillary artery and vein to the clavicle: A cadaveric study. *J Shoulder Elbow Surg* 2009;18(5):e21-e25.

94. Qin D, Zhang Q, Zhang YZ, Pan JS, Chen W: Safe drilling angles and depths for plate-screw fixation of the clavicle: Avoidance of inadvertent iatrogenic subclavian neurovascular bundle injury. *J Trauma* 2010;69(1):162-168.

95. Zlowodzki M, Zelle BA, Cole PA, Jeray K, McKee MD; Evidence-Based Orthopaedic Trauma Working Group: Treatment of acute midshaft clavicle fractures: Systematic review of 2144 fractures. *J Orthop Trauma* 2005;19(7):504-507.

96. McKee MD, Pedersen EM, Jones C, et al: Deficits following nonoperative treatment of displaced midshaft clavicular fractures. *J Bone Joint Surg Am* 2006;88(1):35-40.

97. McKee MD, Wild LM, Schemitsch EH: Midshaft malunions of the clavicle. *J Bone Joint Surg Am* 2003;85-A(5):790-797.

MRI and Arthroscopy Correlations of the Shoulder: A Case-Based Approach

Stephen S. Burkhart, MD

Timothy G. Sanders, MD

Patrick J. Denard, MD

Billy K. Parsley, MD

Abstract

Over the past three decades, shoulder arthroscopy and MRI have seen significant advancements. Initially, distinguishing between normal and pathologic anatomy was one of the greatest challenges. Radiologists and arthroscopic shoulder surgeons have provided feedback to each other based on their experiences with selected shared patients, thereby accelerating the understanding of the arthroscopic and MRI appearance of both normal and pathologic anatomy. This process has led to the current refined understanding of both the basics and subtleties of MRI and arthroscopy correlations in the shoulder. Using a case-based approach provides examples of the correlation between MRI and arthroscopic findings in selected shoulder conditions.

Instr Course Lect 2012;61:185-200.

When shoulder arthroscopy was in its infancy in the early 1980s, one of the greatest challenges was to arthroscopically differentiate between normal shoulder anatomy and pathoanatomy. Previous surgical approaches to the shoulder had been outside-in approaches that disrupted anatomic structures at each point in the exposure. In contrast, the arthroscopic approach was an inside-out approach that for the first time allowed the surgeon to see the interior of the joint without iatrogenic disruption.

As a means to help distinguish between normal anatomy and pathoanatomy, Snyder began the Shoulder Arthroscopy Study Group in the mid-1980s. Members exchanged interesting videos of arthroscopic shoulder procedures and shared ideas about normal and abnormal shoulder anatomy as well as opinions on the proper treatment for these patients. During that same period, Esch pursued similar goals with the San Diego Shoulder Course, which provided the first venue in which surgeons could learn about and share ideas about shoulder arthroscopy.

The quality of MRI of the shoulder improved significantly in the 1980s; however, before the advent of shoulder arthroscopy, the radiologist (like the surgeon using open procedures) was unable to visually confirm his or her impressions without surgical disruption of the shoulder anatomy. The advent of shoulder arthroscopy allowed radiologists and arthroscopic shoulder surgeons to provide feedback to each other based on their experiences with shared patients, thereby accelerating the understanding of the arthroscopic and MRI appearance of both normal and pathologic anatomy. This process has led to a refined understanding of both the basics and subtleties of MRI and arthroscopy correlations in the shoulder. This chapter will present examples that correlate MRI and arthroscopic findings in selected shoulder conditions.

Dr. Burkhart or an immediate family member has received royalties from Arthrex; serves as a paid consultant to Arthrex; has received research or institutional support from Arthrex; and serves as a board member, owner, officer, or committee member of the International Society of Arthroscopy, Knee Surgery, and Orthopaedic Sports Medicine and the Arthroscopy Association of North America. None of the following authors or any immediate family member has received anything of value from or owns stock in a commercial company or institution related directly or indirectly to the subject of this chapter: Dr. Sanders, Dr. Denard, and Dr. Parsley.

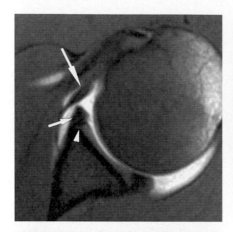

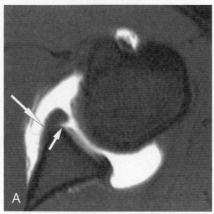

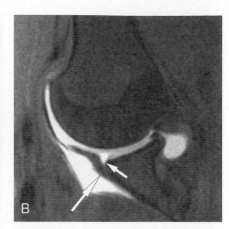

Figure 1 The normal anteroinferior labrum (short arrow) is triangular in appearance and demonstrates low signal intensity on MRI. Intermediate signal intensity hyaline cartilage (arrowhead) often partially undermines the labrum and should not be misinterpreted as a labral tear. The middle glenohumeral ligament (long arrow) is seen as a bandlike structure sitting deep to the subscapularis tendon and superficial to the anterior labrum.

Figure 2 In a Bankart or a Perthes lesion, a tear occurs in the anteroinferior labrum, while the medial scapular periosteum remains intact. The MRI appearance of a Perthes lesion is shown on standard axial (**A**) and abduction external rotation (**B**) views. Contrast (short arrows) extends partially beneath the anteroinferior labrum, whereas the medial scapular periosteum (long arrows) remains intact.

Bankart Lesions

Case Description

A 19-year-old man was tackled during a football game, resulting in injury to his dominant shoulder. The patient reported pain and instability. The physical examination provided the significant finding of a positive apprehension test in abduction and external rotation.

MRI Features

The glenoid labrum is composed of fibrocartilage and will appear dark on all MRI sequences. The anteroinferior labrum is best evaluated in the axial plane and is typically triangular in appearance. The articular cartilage of the glenoid is composed of hyaline cartilage, which has intermediate signal intensity. The area of intermediate signal intensity of the hyaline cartilage is often seen partially undermining the dark fibrocartilage. The area of cartilage undermining will have a smooth,

tapering appearance and should not be misinterpreted as a labral tear or detachment[1] (**Figure 1**).

The MRI appearance of a soft-tissue Bankart lesion will vary depending on the extent of the abnormality. Separation of the labrum from the glenoid will appear as a collection of irregular fluid or contrast extending deep to the labrum. The labrum may be displaced and is often amorphous in appearance, losing its normal triangular appearance. In a Perthes lesion, the medial scapular periosteum remains intact and the labrum will be held in near-anatomic position[2] (**Figure 2**). Medialization of a chronic labral tear, the so-called anterior labral periosteal sleeve avulsion (ALPSA) lesion, will show a medially displaced labrum that is scarred to the anterior aspect of the glenoid[3] (**Figure 3**).

Normal anatomic variants must be distinguished from a pathologic anterior labrum. The sublabral foramen is a normal anatomic variant seen as a focal detachment of the labrum in the anterosuperior quadrant and should not be misinterpreted as a labral tear. The sublabral foramen is best seen on axial im-

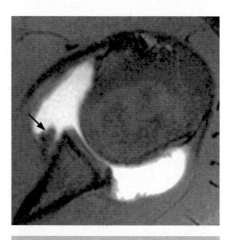

Figure 3 In an ALPSA lesion, the torn anteroinferior labrum heals medially to the glenoid neck. Axial MRI scan showing the medialized anteroinferior labrum (arrow).

ages as fluid extending completely between the labrum and the glenoid[4] (**Figure 4**). The Buford complex is composed of a thick, cordlike middle glenohumeral ligament (MGHL) combined with an absent or diminutive anterosuperior labrum. The thickened ligament should not be misinterpreted as a detached labral fragment. On axial images, the MGHL can be traced along it normal course on mul-

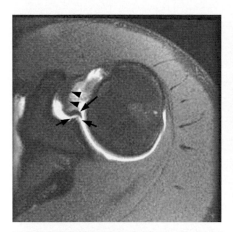

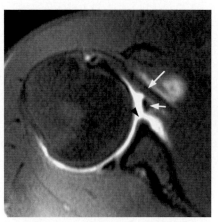

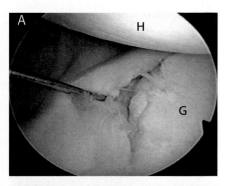

Figure 4   The sublabral foramen is a normal anatomic variant in the anterosuperior quadrant and should not be misinterpreted as a labral tear. Axial MRI scan shows the sublabral foramen (short arrows) and focal detachment of the labrum (long arrow) in the anterosuperior quadrant. The superior glenohumeral ligament (arrowheads) is also noted.

Figure 5   The Buford complex is a normal variant consisting of an absent anterosuperior labrum combined with a thick cordlike MGHL. Axial MRI scan shows the absent anterosuperior labrum (arrowhead) and cordlike MGHL (short arrow). The overlying subscapularis tendon is also noted (long arrow).

Figure 6   Arthroscopic view of a Perthes lesion from an anterosuperolateral viewing portal in a right shoulder. G = glenoid, H = humeral head.

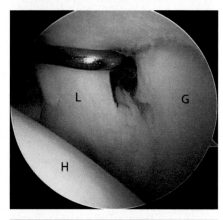

Figure 8   Arthroscopic view of the sublabral foramen through a posterior viewing portal in a left shoulder. G = glenoid, H = humeral head, L = labrum.

tiple sequential axial images[5] (**Figure 5**).

Arthroscopic Features

Arthroscopically, a typical, acute, soft-tissue Bankart lesion (Perthes lesion) will demonstrate a separation of the inferior glenohumeral ligament from the bony glenoid (**Figure 6**). The separation may extend proximally to include the middle and superior glenohumeral ligaments and the superior labrum, and it may also extend posteriorly to include the posterior labrum. In some instances, there are combined anterior, superior, and posterior labral lesions (triple labral lesions).[6]

In some patients with chronic recurrent instability, medialized healing of the Bankart (ALPSA) lesion to the anterior glenoid neck is achieved (**Figure 7**). In repairing ALPSA lesions, an elevator must be used to completely free the capsulolabral tissue from the glenoid neck so that it can "float up" to the level of the glenoid rim where it can be repaired.

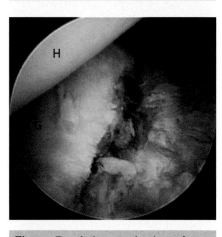

Figure 7   Arthroscopic view of a medially displaced ALPSA lesion in a left shoulder as viewed from an anterosuperolateral portal. H = humeral head, G = glenoid.

It is important not to confuse a Bankart lesion with a sublabral foramen (**Figure 8**) or a Buford complex[7] (**Figure 9**). The sublabral foramen is located superior to the midglenoid notch and is a normal variant that should not be repaired to the glenoid. The Buford complex is composed of a cordlike MGHL that attaches superiorly to the superior labrum at a point

just anterior to the biceps root in association with an absence of the anterior labrum above the midglenoid notch. The Buford complex is also a normal variant and should not be repaired to the glenoid rim.

Partial-Thickness Interstitial Tear of the Supraspinatus

Case Description

A 47-year-old man reports 6 months of lateral shoulder pain with insidious onset. The physical examination shows normal active range of motion. There is slight weakness with resisted external rotation. Hawkins and Neer signs for impingement are positive.

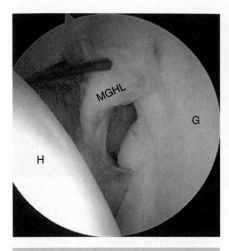

Figure 9 Arthroscopic appearance of the Buford complex from a posterior viewing portal in a left shoulder. G = glenoid, H = humeral head, MGHL = middle glenohumeral ligament.

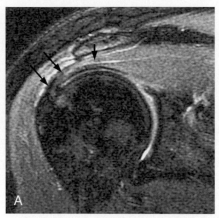

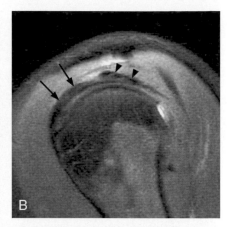

Figure 10 Normal supraspinatus tendon. Coronal (**A**) and sagittal (**B**) T2-weighted images through the glenohumeral joint demonstrate a normal low signal intensity supraspinatus tendon (long arrows). The tendon inserts onto the footprint of the greater tuberosity. The distal musculotendinous junction (short arrow) is seen on the coronal image at approximately the 12 o'clock position on the humeral head. On the sagittal image, the arrowheads indicate the infraspinatus tendon.

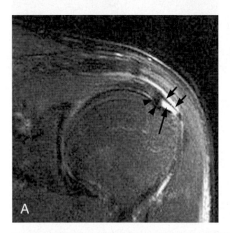

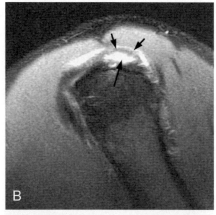

Figure 11 Coronal (**A**) and sagittal (**B**) T2-weighted images of the supraspinatus tendon demonstrate an area of fluid collection (long arrows) within the substance of the tendon, indicating a partial-thickness interstitial tear. Both the bursal (short arrows) and articular sides (arrowheads on the coronal image) of the tendon remain intact, making this tear problematic to identify at the time of arthroscopy.

MRI Features

The normal supraspinatus tendon is best seen on coronal and sagittal MRI scans and demonstrates low signal intensity on all pulse sequences. The distal musculotendinous junction is typically located at approximately the 12 o'clock position on the humeral head and distal to this level. The tendon demonstrates low signal intensity over the entire distance to its level of attachment on the footprint of the greater tuberosity (**Figure 10**).

Bright T2-weighted signal (fluid) within the expected location of the tendon is diagnostic of a tear. A partial-thickness interstitial tear is typically demonstrated on MRI as a linear fluid collection within the substance of the tendon. An interstitial tear often parallels the long axis of the tendon, and intact fibers will be noted along both the bursal and articular sides of the tear.[8] On T2-weighted sagittal images, the tear often appears as a globular area of bright T2-weighted signal within the substance of the tendon and corresponds nicely with the bubble sign seen during arthroscopy (**Figure 11**). With MRI, it is sometimes difficult to distinguish a true partial-thickness interstitial tear from a partial-thickness articular tear.[8,9]

Arthroscopic Features

The arthroscopic diagnosis of bursal-sided and articular-sided partial-thickness rotator cuff tears is straightforward; however, the diagnosis of partial-thickness interstitial cuff tears is always problematic. Arriving at this diagnosis requires both a high-quality MRI scan and arthroscopic findings that confirm an interstitial tear. The first finding that should alert the surgeon to this diagnosis is a preoperative MRI scan showing an interstitial tear.

Arthroscopically, a standard visual inspection of the intra-articular and subacromial spaces will reveal a normal-appearing rotator cuff. Two arthroscopic signs are very helpful in arriving at a diagnosis: the sliding layers and the bubble signs.[10,11] To elicit the sliding layers sign, the surgeon should first obtain an impression of the location of the interstitial tear by closely evaluating the MRI scan. A probe is then used to arthroscopically palpate that portion of the cuff (**Figure 12**). In patients with significant intrasubstance tearing, the two laminae of the rotator cuff are typically unstable and can be felt to be sliding over one another as the probe produces a combined shearing and compressive force.

Once the area of rotator cuff pathology has been localized by using MRI and the sliding layers sign, the surgeon can attempt to elicit the bubble sign. An 18-gauge spinal needle is used to penetrate the superficial lamina of the intrasubstance tear (**Figure 13, A**). The surgeon then attempts to inject sterile saline through the needle. In patients with an intact rotator cuff, significant resistance to the injection will be noted, and no saline can be injected. In patients with significant intrasubstance tearing, the saline will flow freely until the contained defect is filled, and a localized dome-shaped bubble of the superficial lamina will appear as saline is injected between the

two laminae of the rotator cuff (**Figure 13, B**). The bubble sign confirms the location and the unstable nature of the two laminae. The superficial lamina is then débrided, converting the interstitial tear to a bursal surface tear, and a suture anchor repair to the bone bed is performed (**Figure 13, C**).

Adhesive Capsulitis

Case Description
A 47-year-old woman with diabetes reports the insidious onset of restricted shoulder motion of 6-months duration. Pain is described as constant. Examination shows both active and passive restriction of shoulder range of motion.

MRI Features
On MRI scans, the normal glenohumeral joint capsule appears as a thin, band-like, linear structure measuring less than 4 mm in thickness (**Figure 14, A**). The rotator interval is a triangular-shaped space located between the anterior edge of the supraspinatus tendon and the superior leading edge of the subscapularis tendon. The coracohumeral ligament and superior glenohumeral ligament combine to form the roof of the rotator interval, which contains the intra-articular portion of the long head of

the biceps tendon and fibroadipose tissue.

Adhesive capsulitis is characterized by a synovial proliferative process that results in an increase in synovial cells, blood vessels, fibroblasts, and myoblasts within the capsule and in the region of the rotator interval. Synovial proliferation is responsible for the MRI findings of adhesive capsulitis, including thickening of the capsule (> 4 mm) in the region of the axillary pouch with pericapsular edema/enhancement; replacement of the normal fat signal within the rotator interval with inflammatory tissue and thickening of the coracohumeral ligament; a paucity of glenohumeral joint

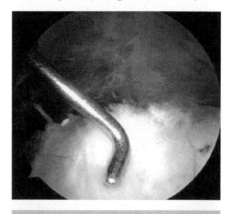

Figure 12 Arthroscopic view from the posterior subacromial portal of a left shoulder shows "sliding" of the layers of the interstitial rotator cuff tear under a hooked probe.

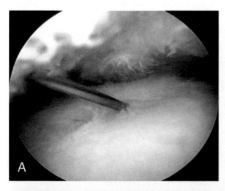
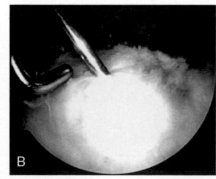
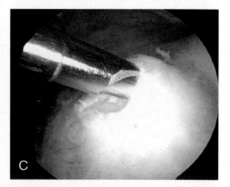

Figure 13 The bubble sign seen arthroscopically from a posterior subacromial viewing portal in a left shoulder. **A,** An 18-gauge spinal needle is inserted into the suspected defect. **B,** Saline is injected and flows into the contained rotator cuff defect, which expands and forms a bubble. **C,** Débridement with a shaver uncovers a localized area of degeneration.

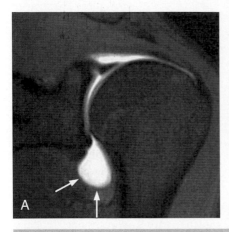
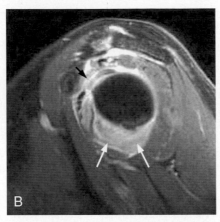
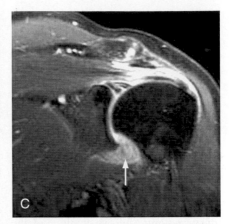

Figure 14 T1-weighted MRI scans with fat saturation following the administration of intravenous gadolinium are used to compare a normal glenohumeral joint capsule with a capsule with adhesive capsulitis. **A,** Coronal view of a normal glenohumeral joint capsule. There is a thin band-like capsule (arrows) in the region of the axillary pouch, which measures less than 4 mm in thickness. **B,** Sagittal view of a capsule with adhesive capsulitis shows marked thickening and enhancement of the capsule in the region of the axillary pouch (long arrows). There is also increased soft tissue and enhancement (short arrow) replacing the normal fat signal within the rotator interval. **C,** Coronal view shows thickening of the axillary pouch (arrow).

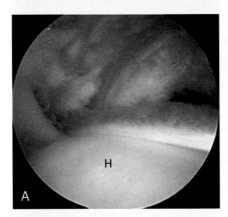
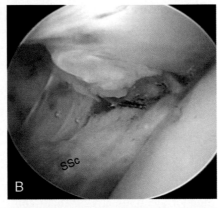

Figure 15 Arthroscopic appearance of adhesive capsulitis in a right shoulder viewed from a posterior portal. **A,** Inflamed biceps tendon with inflamed synovium. H = humeral head. **B,** The rotator interval is thickened with loss of the normal subscapularis sulcus. SSc = subscapularis.

effusion; and fluid within the bicipital tendon sheath. Although these findings can be seen on conventional MRI scans, they are usually best appreciated following the administration of intravenous gadolinium because most areas of abnormality will be enhanced[12,13] (**Figure 14,** *B* and *C*).

Arthroscopic Features

In a patient with adhesive capsulitis, examination under anesthesia will reveal passive restriction of motion that is roughly equivalent to the active loss

of motion that was apparent in the awake patient. Insertion of the arthroscope may be difficult because of the tight intra-articular space, and manual distraction of the joint by an assistant may be helpful.

On entering the joint, the surgeon will generally see an intensely red synovium resulting from the inflammatory capsulitis (**Figure 15,** *A*). Anteriorly, there is a loss of the normal redundancy of the rotator interval where it meets the top of the subscapularis ten-

don and forms a small sulcus in the normal shoulder. The subscapularis sulcus is absent in a shoulder with adhesive capsulitis (**Figure 15,** *B*).

Instead of manipulation under anesthesia, this chapter's authors prefer a sequential arthroscopic capsular release beginning with the rotator interval, then the posterior capsule, followed by the axillary capsule, and then the anterior capsule (**Figure 16**). Although the subacromial space is typically normal in adhesive capsulitis, subacromial bursoscopy and bursectomy are performed to rule out associated rotator cuff tears. It is important to recognize that postoperative stiffness (for example, after rotator cuff repair) frequently is associated with subacromial and subcoracoid adhesions, whereas these adhesions are not usually seen in adhesive capsulitis.

Osseous Bankart and Hill-Sachs Lesions

Case Description

An 18-year-old man has shoulder pain and recurrent subluxations following an anterior dislocation of his dominant shoulder. Examination shows a positive apprehension sign with the arm in abduction and external rotation.

MRI Features

An osseous Bankart lesion is shown on MRI scans as an area of disruption of the cortex along the anteroinferior margin of the glenoid. Because the cortex and the labrum both appear as low signal intensity structures on MRI, a small osseous Bankart lesion may be difficult to differentiate from a soft-tissue Bankart lesion. Larger lesions, however, are easily identified as a large displaced osseous fragment with irregularity, and the cortex of the glenoid is disrupted. All three imaging planes are useful in determining the size and extent of the osseous Bankart component[14] (**Figure 17**).

CT can be very helpful in surgical planning by defining the extent of osseous deficiency along the anteroinferior glenoid margin (**Figure 18, *A* and *B***). Sagittal CT best shows the extent of bone loss and the so-called inverted pear appearance that indicates greater than 25% loss of the inferior glenoid diameter.[15] Three-dimensional CT reconstructions have a high accuracy for predicting bone loss greater than 25%[16] (**Figure 18, *C***).

Arthroscopic Features

Although preoperative three-dimensional CT scans correctly identify significant bone loss in 92% of patients with shoulder instability, the most accurate assessment of bone loss is accomplished by arthroscopic measurement with a calibrated probe[16,17] (**Figure 19**). Because an inverted pear glenoid has greater than 25% loss of the inferior glenoid diameter, the bone deficiency requires glenoid bone grafting.[18] This chapter's authors prefer coracoid bone grafting using the modified Latarjet procedure.[19] To assess significant humeral bone loss, dynamic arthroscopy is used while viewing the glenohumeral joint through an antero-superolateral portal to detect an engaging Hill-Sachs lesion (a Hill-Sachs lesion that engages the anteroinferior glenoid rim with the shoulder in a position of abduction and external rotation) (**Figure 20**). In treating large, engaging Hill-Sachs lesions, which usually occur in association with inverted pear glenoid lesions, the Latarjet coracoid bone graft to the glenoid will prevent engagement of the Hill-Sachs lesion. This is accomplished by extending the glenoid articular arc to such a large extent that the humerus

will not externally rotate far enough to allow Hill-Sachs engagement (**Figure 21**). For a shallow Hill-Sachs lesion (< 4 mm) that is not associated with an inverted pear glenoid, this chapter's authors typically perform an arthroscopic remplissage in which the infraspinatus tendon is inset into the Hill-Sachs defect, thereby making the Hill-Sachs defect an extra-articular defect that cannot engage[20] (**Figure 22**).

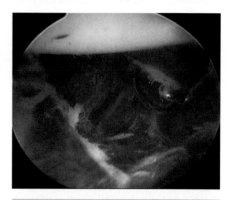

Figure 16 Arthroscopic appearance following capsular release and manipulation for adhesive capsulitis in a left shoulder viewed from an anterosuperolateral portal. The anteroinferior capsule has been divided a few millimeters from the labrum. The muscle is visualized deep to the surgically separated capsule.

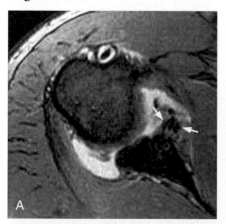
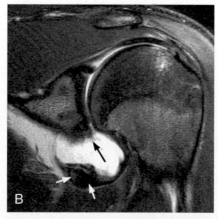
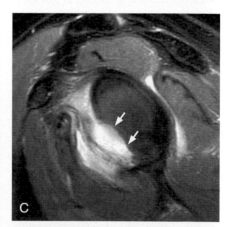

Figure 17 Axial (**A**) and coronal (**B**) T2-weighted MRI scans show a displaced osseous Bankart lesion (short arrows). On the coronal image, the cortex of the inferior glenoid rim is irregular (long arrow), indicating cortical disruption. **C,** Sagittal view demonstrates the inverted pear appearance (arrows) of the inferior glenoid rim, indicating greater than 25% loss of the inferior glenoid diameter.

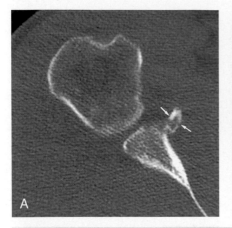
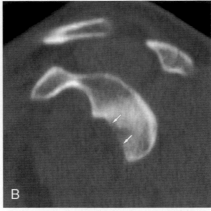
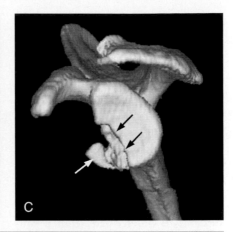

Figure 18 The appearance of an osseous Bankart lesion on CT. **A,** Axial view shows a displaced comminuted fracture (arrows) of the anterior inferior glenoid rim. Sagittal (**B**) and three-dimensional reconstruction (**C**) show the bony deficit and inverted pear appearance (short arrows) of the anterior inferior glenoid. The displaced osseous fragment (white arrow) is easily seen on the three-dimensional image.

Tear of the Upper Subscapularis and Medial Subluxation of the Long Head of the Biceps

Case Description

A 64-year-old man fell at ground level. While attempting to grab a railing to break the fall, he sustained a forced external rotation injury with his arm at his side. On examination, the bear-hug and belly-press tests were positive.

MRI Features

The intra-articular portion of the long head of the biceps tendon is normally positioned within the rotator interval and is held in place by the bicipital sling. It then exits the joint, entering the fibro-osseous tunnel of the bicipital groove at the level of the superior leading edge of the subscapularis tendon (**Figure 23,** *A*). The intra-articular portion of the long head of the biceps tendon is usually best evaluated on sagittal MRI scans, whereas the extra-articular portion of the tendon is best evaluated in the axial plane (**Figure 23,** *B*).

An interstitial or partial-thickness tear of the superior leading edge of the subscapularis tendon combined with a tear of the bicipital sling can be associated with a medial subluxation of the

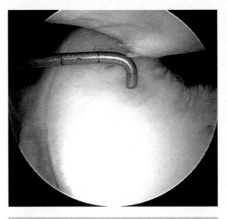

Figure 19 Arthroscopic view of a left shoulder through an anterosuperolateral portal shows the inverted pear appearance of the glenoid. The inferior aspect of the glenoid appears narrower than the superior aspect of the glenoid, and it narrows to an apex.

long head of the biceps tendon into the substance of the subscapularis tendon, the so-called hidden lesion. This lesion can be easily overlooked on both MRI scans and at the time of shoulder arthroscopy. The lesion is best seen on axial T2-weighted images with recognition of medial subluxation of the long head of the biceps tendon into the substance of the subscapularis tendon (**Figure 24**). Abnormal signal is often noted within the superior fibers

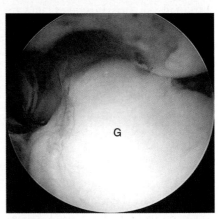

Figure 20 Arthroscopic view through an anterosuperolateral portal of a left shoulder shows an engaging Hill-Sachs lesion. The lesion is oriented parallel to the anterior rim of the glenoid (G).

of the subscapularis tendon, and the biceps tendon may also demonstrate abnormal thickening and increased T2-weighted signal intensity.[21,22]

Arthroscopic Features

Tears of the upper subscapularis can be difficult to see because they are not retracted and because the nonretracted tendon will lie against its bone bed and obscure the bare footprint on the upper part of the lesser tuberosity. This chapter's authors perform all shoulder arthroscopies with the patient in the

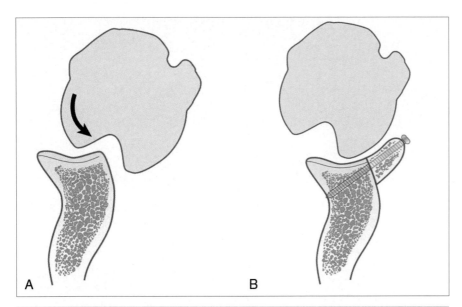

Figure 21   Schematic drawing illustrating the modified Latarjet procedure to prevent the engagement of an engaging Hill-Sachs lesion. **A,** Engaging Hill-Sachs lesion. **B,** Engagement is prevented by lengthening the glenoid articular arc.

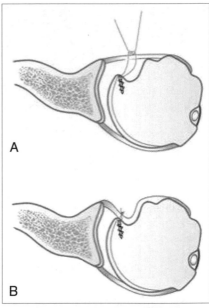

Figure 22   Schematic drawing illustrating the use of a remplissage technique to prevent the engagement of an engaging Hill-Sachs lesion in the absence of a significant glenoid defect. **A,** Engaging Hill-Sachs lesion. **B,** The remplissage technique insets the infraspinatus into the Hill-Sachs lesion, thereby making the Hill-Sachs defect an extra-articular defect that cannot engage.

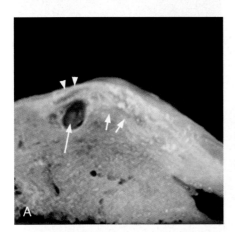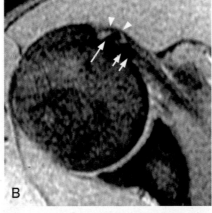

Figure 23   Cadaver section through the bicipital grove (**A**) and axial T2-weighted MRI view (**B**) show the normal position of the long head biceps tendon within the bicipital groove. The fibro-osseous tunnel of the bicipital groove (long arrow) contains the long head of the biceps tendon. The deep fibers of the subscapularis tendon insert onto the lesser tuberosity (short arrows), while the superficial fibers of the subscapularis tendon (arrowheads) form the roof of the bicipital groove inserting onto the greater tuberosity.

lateral decubitus position and have found that a manual maneuver called the posterior lever push is extremely helpful in visualizing these tears[23] (**Figure 25**). A 70°-arthroscope is also helpful to give an "aerial view" of the upper subscapularis and its footprint.

The best view is obtained with a 70°-arthroscope through a posterior viewing portal while applying a posterior force (posterior lever push) to the proximal humerus (**Figure 25, C**). Slight internal rotation of the shoulder can also help to show the bare foot-

print where the upper subscapularis had been attached. When the upper subscapularis is torn in association with a tear of the medial sling of the biceps, the biceps tendon will be subluxated or dislocated posterior to the plane of the subscapularis (**Figure 26**). If the medial sling, which is composed of the superior glenohumeral ligament and the medial head of the coracohumeral ligament, avulses along with the upper subscapularis, it forms a distinctive anatomic structure referred to as the comma sign[24] (**Figure 27**). The comma sign is useful in defining the superolateral border of the subscapularis tendon. In repairing the upper subscapularis, this chapter's authors prefer a suture anchor repair along with biceps tenodesis.[23,25] If a

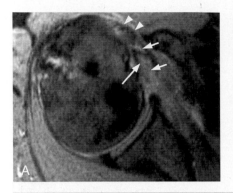 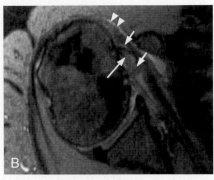 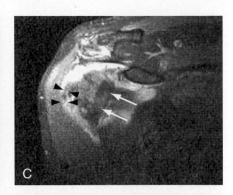

Figure 24 **A** and **B,** Sequential axial T2-weighted MRI scans through the upper subscapularis tendon demonstrate an interstitial tear of the upper subscapularis tendon (short arrows). The long head of the biceps tendon (long arrows) is thickened and edematous, indicating tendinosis with medial subluxation into the substance of the subscapularis tendon. The superficial fibers of the subscapularis tendon (arrowheads) remain intact. **C,** Coronal MRI scan shows medial subluxation of the long head of the biceps tendon (arrows). The bicipital groove (arrowheads) is the normal expected location of the long head of the biceps tendon.

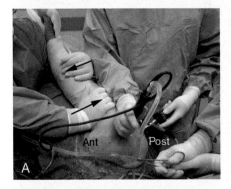 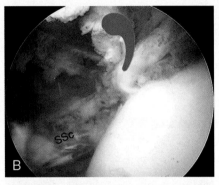 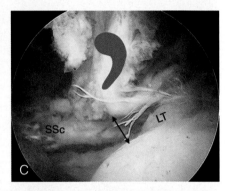

Figure 25 **A,** In the posterior lever push maneuver, an assistant simultaneously pushes the proximal humerus posteriorly and pushes the distal humerus anteriorly. Ant = anterior, Post = posterior. **B,** Standard arthroscopic view in a right shoulder from a posterior viewing portal with a 70° arthroscope before a posterior lever push maneuver. The upper tendon of the subscapularis is tightly draped across the lesser tuberosity, and the footprint is not visible. **C,** The same shoulder with a posterior lever push maneuver applied. The maneuver dramatically increases exposure of the subscapularis footprint. In **B** and **C,** note the blue comma sign. SSc = subscapularis, LT = lesser tuberosity.

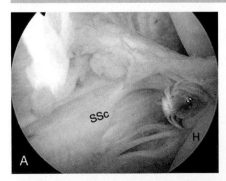 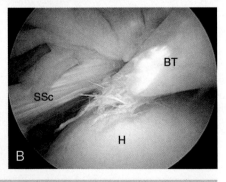

biceps tenodesis is not performed, it will resubluxate and cause failure of the subscapularis repair.

Acute Chondrolysis of the Glenohumeral Joint

Case Description

A 23-year-old man had been treated with an arthroscopic Bankart repair 1 year earlier. At 4 months postoperatively, the patient began reporting progressively worsening shoulder pain. The physical examination reveals painful global loss of motion.

Figure 26 **A,** Arthroscopic appearance of an upper subscapularis tendon in a right shoulder from a posterior viewing portal. A partial tear of the upper subscapularis is seen with the arm in 30° internal rotation. The torn fibers expose the underlying footprint of the subscapularis insertion. The medial biceps sling remains intact. **B,** Aerial view with a 70° arthroscope in a different shoulder demonstrates a degenerative and medially subluxated biceps tendon. SSc = subscapularis tendon, BT = biceps tendon, H = humeral head.

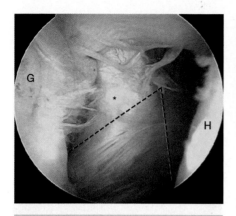

Figure 27 Arthroscopic view of a retracted subscapularis tear in a right shoulder seen through a posterior viewing portal. The comma tissue (*) marks the leading edge of the subscapularis tendon (dashed line). G = glenoid, H = humerus.

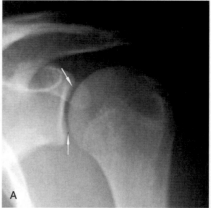 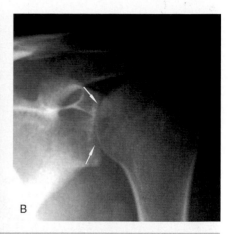

Figure 28 Radiographic features of acute chondrolysis of the glenohumeral joint. **A,** Preoperative AP radiograph showing normal glenohumeral joint space (arrows). **B,** Postoperative AP radiograph 4 months following surgery shows extensive joint-space narrowing (arrows) and minimal changes of subchondral sclerosis.

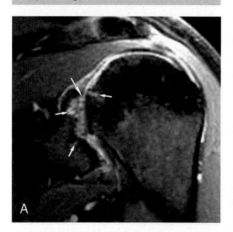 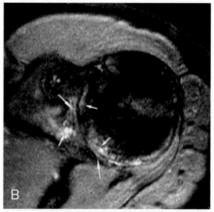 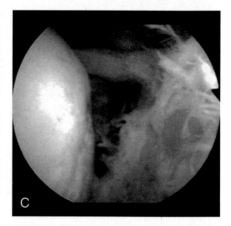

Figure 29 Coronal (**A**) and axial (**B**) T2-weighted MRI scans demonstrate marked loss of articular cartilage (long arrows) of the glenoid rim and humeral head resulting in marked joint-space narrowing in a shoulder with acute chondrolysis of the glenohumeral joint. There are minimal changes of edema and early subchondral cystic changes (short arrows) on both sides of the joint. **C,** Arthroscopic appearance of chondrolysis of the glenohumeral joint in a left shoulder seen from a posterior viewing portal. There is widespread cartilage loss with significant synovitis.

MRI Features

Acute chondrolysis of the glenohumeral joint is a disorder with rapid onset of diffuse chondrocyte cell death; it is often reported in young patients who have been recently treated with shoulder arthroscopy. The patient typically describes an insidious onset of painful, decreased shoulder range of motion that develops during the first year following reconstructive shoulder surgery. Radiographs show diffuse loss of joint space with minimal subchondral sclerosis

(**Figure 28**). MRI shows diffuse chondral loss of both the glenoid and the humeral head articular surfaces, minimal subchondral marrow signal changes, and a paucity of joint effusion[26] (**Figure 29,** *A* and *B*).

Arthroscopic Features

The causes of acute postoperative chondrolysis are probably multifactorial.[27,28] This is a devastating condition, particularly when it occurs in active teenagers or young adults.

Widespread full-thickness articular cartilage loss on both the humeral head and the glenoid are seen arthroscopically. Frequently, there is intense inflammatory synovitis with a strikingly erythematous synovium (**Figure 29,** *C*). In such instances, this chapter's authors generally recommend arthroscopic biologic resurfacing with an acellular human dermal allograft (such as Graftjacket, Wright Medical Technology, Arlington, TN; or ArthroFlex, Arthrex, Naples, FL). This treat-

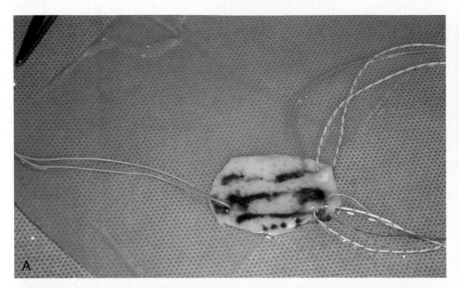

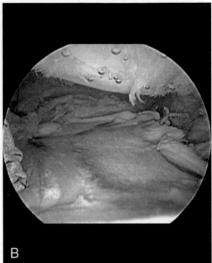

Figure 30 **A,** Extra-articular appearance of an acellular human dermal graft used for arthroscopic biologic resurfacing. **B,** Intra-articular appearance of the secured graft in a left shoulder viewed from an anterosuperolateral portal.

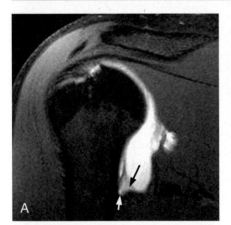

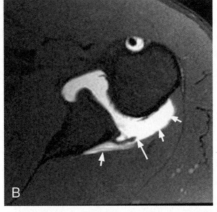

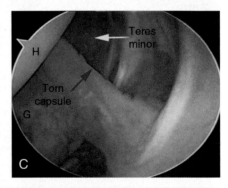

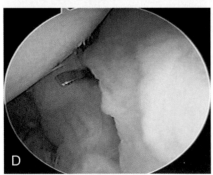

Figure 31 Coronal (**A**) and axial (**B**) T1-weighted MRI scans with fat saturation taken following injection of intra-articular gadolinium show a complete disruption (long arrows) of the posterior bundle of the inferior glenohumeral ligament in a shoulder with a reverse humeral avulsion of the glenohumeral ligament (RHAGL) lesion. Contrast (short arrows) spills through the defect and is noted to be extracapsular, indicating a disruption of the posterior capsule. **C,** Arthroscopic appearance of a RHAGL lesion in a right shoulder viewed from an anterosuperolateral portal. Capsular tearing is noted, and the teres minor, which is not normally seen, is visualized posteriorly. G = glenoid, H = humeral head. **D,** A grasper is introduced posteriorly to assess reparability.

ment achieves significant pain relief in approximately 50% of patients (SS Burkhart, MD, et al, unpublished data) (**Figure 30**). However, the duration of the pain relief is unknown. In the 50% of patients in whom pain relief is not achieved with biologic resurfacing, shoulder reconstruction is challenging because of the young age of the patients and the limited surgical options of massive osteochondral allograft transplantation or arthroplasty.

Reverse Humeral Avulsion of the Glenohumeral Ligament Lesion

A traumatic posterior shoulder subluxation occurred in a 21-year-old college football player during a game. He re-

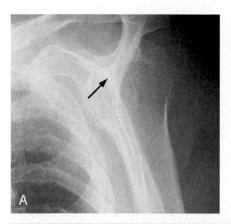
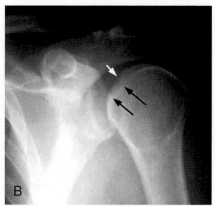
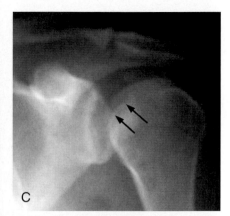

Figure 32 Plain radiographic appearance of a locked posterior shoulder dislocation. **A,** Scapular Y view shows a subtle posterior subluxation of the humeral head. The head is center posterior to the Y-shaped confluence (arrow) of the body of the scapula, the coracoid process, and the acromion process. Internal (**B**) and external (**C**) rotation views show a linear area of sclerosis (long arrows) paralleling the medial cortex of the humeral head (the so-called trough sign), indicating a reverse Hill-Sachs lesion and a previous posterior subluxation event. Subtle cortical irregularity (short arrow on the internal rotation view) seen along the medial aspect of the humeral head is also supportive evidence of a reverse Hill-Sachs lesion.

ports an inability to perform a bench press. Examination is notable for apprehension in shoulder flexion and internal rotation.

MRI Features

The inferior glenohumeral ligament is composed of an anterior bundle, the axillary pouch portion of the ligament, and the posterior bundle and plays a major role in the stability of the glenohumeral joint. The inferior glenohumeral ligament arises along the inferior margin of the glenoid rim and inserts in a cuff-like fashion on the medial aspect of the humeral neck. It is best visualized on MRI scans in the coronal and axial imaging planes; intra-articular gadolinium improves visualization of the ligament.[29]

A reverse humeral avulsion of the glenohumeral ligament (RHAGL) lesion is seen on MRI as a complete avulsion or disruption of the posterior bundle at the level of the posterior attachment to the humeral neck. When using intra-articular gadolinium, the contrast can be seen extending through the posterior capsular defect[30] (**Figure 31,** *A* and *B*).

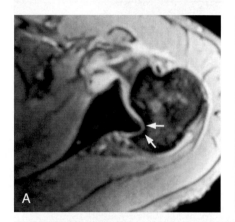
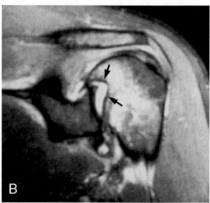

Figure 33 Axial (**A**) and coronal (**B**) T2-weighted MRI scans obtained 3 weeks following the shoulder injury in the patient in Figure 32 show a large reverse Hill-Sachs lesion (arrows) and a locked posterior dislocation of the humeral head. These findings explain the radiographic finding of the "trough" sign and the cortical irregularity of the humeral head as described in Figure 32.

Arthroscopy Features

In all patients with suspected shoulder instability, an intra-articular inspection of the joint through an anterosuperior viewing portal should be part of the arthroscopic diagnostic examination. This portal affords the best view of the glenolabral attachments and also provides the best visualization of the capsular attachments onto the humerus. Through this viewing portal, the RHAGL lesion will appear as a capsular rent, with the teres minor and the infraspinatus muscles visible through the rent (**Figure 31,** *C*). A grasper introduced through a posterior working portal can be used to reduce the RHAGL lesion and assess its reparability (**Figure 31,** *D*).

Locked Posterior Shoulder Dislocation

Case Description

A 37-year-old man fell from a junior dirt bike 3 weeks earlier onto an outstretched arm. He reports that he "felt

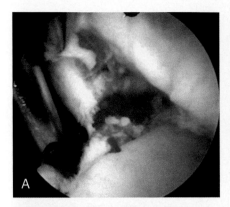

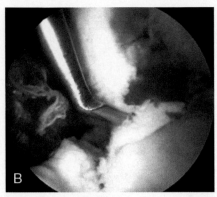

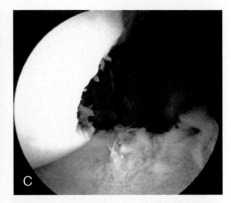

Figure 34 Locked posterior left shoulder dislocation viewed from an anterosuperolateral portal. **A,** The humeral head is dislocated posteriorly, and a reverse Hill-Sachs lesion engages the glenoid. **B,** An elevator is introduced through a posterior portal, and a shoe-horn technique is used to reduce the dislocation. **C,** Appearance after reduction.

something slip" at the time of injury. The patient went to the emergency department at the time of injury and was evaluated with radiographs, including internal and external rotation AP radiographs and a scapular Y view of the shoulder. The radiographs were interpreted as normal, and the patient was told that he had a shoulder strain and advised to "work out the stiffness."

MRI Features

Radiographic findings that suggest a locked posterior dislocation of the humeral head include fixed internal rotation of the humeral head on AP views; the presence of the trough sign, which represents the reverse osseous Hill-Sachs lesion; widening of the glenohumeral joint; and posterior positioning of the humeral head as seen on transscapular Y or axillary views[31,32] (**Figure 32**). MRI will show a wedge-shape defect along the anterior aspect of the humeral head, which indicates an impaction type injury (reverse Hill-Sachs lesion). The humeral head will demonstrate posterior subluxation, and a posterior labral tear will often be present (**Figure 33**).

Arthroscopic Features

If arthroscopy is attempted with a locked posterior dislocation, the surgeon should recognize that the hu-

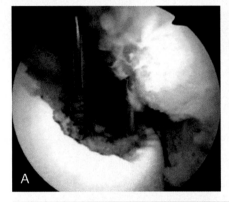

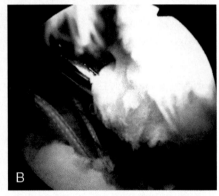

Figure 35 Arthroscopic inset of the MGHL for a reverse Hill-Sachs lesion in a left shoulder viewed from a posterior portal. **A,** An anchor is introduced from an anterior portal and placed in the reverse Hill-Sachs defect. **B,** Sutures are passed through the MGHL and then tied; this technique effectively fills the reverse Hill-Sachs defect.

meral head is displaced posteromedially and will block the establishment of a standard posterior portal. However, an anterosuperior portal just off the anterolateral edge of the acromion with a 45° posterolateral trajectory can easily be established for intra-articular viewing (**Figure 34,** *A*). Then, under direct visualization, a posterosuperior portal can be established to insert an arthroscopic elevator to assist in levering the humeral head back onto the glenoid face (**Figure 34,** *B* and *C*). After a standard arthroscopic posterior Bankart repair, the surgeon can address the reverse Hill-Sachs lesion by transferring the MGHL into the bone defect. If the

MGHL tissue is insufficient, the surgeon should consider an arthroscopic adaptation of the McLaughlin procedure, in which the upper subscapularis tendon is arthroscopically transferred into the reverse Hill-Sachs defect[33] (**Figure 35**). Either of these soft-tissue transfers (MGHL or subscapularis tendon) will prevent engagement of the bone defect onto the posterior glenoid rim by filling the defect and converting it from an intra-articular structure to an extra-articular structure.

Summary

Arthroscopic visualization of the shoulder has dramatically refined the diagnostic capabilities of MRI and vice versa. A point has been reached at which these two technologies used in concert can achieve a level of accuracy in diagnosing shoulder pathology that is unsurpassed by other means. To offer the best treatment for patients with shoulder lesions, the surgeon should be familiar with arthroscopic anatomy and pathoanatomy and its MRI correlates.

References

1. Loredo R, Longo C, Salonen D, et al: Glenoid labrum: MR imaging with histologic correlation. *Radiology* 1995;196(1):33-41.

2. Wischer TK, Bredella MA, Genant HK, Stoller DW, Bost FW, Tirman PF: Perthes lesion (a variant of the Bankart lesion): MR imaging and MR arthrographic findings with surgical correlation. *AJR Am J Roentgenol* 2002;178(1): 233-237.

3. Neviaser TJ: The anterior labro-ligamentous periosteal sleeve avulsion lesion: A cause of anterior instability of the shoulder. *Arthroscopy* 1993;9(1):17-21.

4. Palmer WE, Brown JH, Rosenthal DI: Labral-ligamentous complex of the shoulder: Evaluation with MR arthrography. *Radiology* 1994; 190(3):645-651.

5. Tirman PF, Feller JF, Palmer WE, Carroll KW, Steinbach LS, Cox I: The Buford complex: A variation of normal shoulder anatomy. MR arthrographic imaging features. *AJR Am J Roentgenol* 1996;166(4): 869-873.

6. Lo IK, Burkhart SS: Triple labral lesions: Pathology and surgical repair technique. Report of seven cases. *Arthroscopy* 2005;21(2): 186-193.

7. Williams MM, Snyder SJ, Buford D Jr: The Buford complex: The "cord-like" middle glenohumeral ligament and absent anterosupe-

rior labrum complex. A normal anatomic capsulolabral variant. *Arthroscopy* 1994;10(3):241-247.

8. Walz DM, Miller TT, Chen S, Hofman J: MR imaging of delamination tears of the rotator cuff tendons. *Skeletal Radiol* 2007; 36(5):411-416.

9. Waibl B, Buess E: Partial-thickness articular surface supraspinatus tears: A new transtendon suture technique. *Arthroscopy* 2005;21(3):376-381.

10. Burkhart SS, Lo IK, Brady PC: *Burkhart's View of the Shoulder: A Cowboy's Guide to Advanced Shoulder Arthroscopy*. Philadelphia, PA, Lippincott Williams & Wilkins, 2006.

11. Lo IK, Gonzalez DM, Burkhart SS: The bubble sign: An arthroscopic indicator of an intratendinous rotator cuff tear. *Arthroscopy* 2002;18(9):1029-1033.

12. Jung JY, Jee WH, Chun HJ, Kim YS, Chung YG, Kim JM: Adhesive capsulitis of the shoulder: Evaluation with MR arthrography. *Eur Radiol* 2006;16(4):791-796.

13. Kim KC, Rhee KJ, Shin HD: Adhesive capsulitis of the shoulder: Dimensions of the rotator interval measured with magnetic resonance arthrography. *J Shoulder Elbow Surg* 2009;18(3):437-442.

14. Beltran J, Rosenberg ZS, Chandnani VP, Cuomo F, Beltran S, Rokito A: Glenohumeral instability: Evaluation with MR arthrography. *Radiographics* 1997;17(3): 657-673.

15. Lo IK, Parten PM, Burkhart SS: The inverted pear glenoid: An indicator of significant glenoid bone loss. *Arthroscopy* 2004;20(2): 169-174.

16. Chuang TY, Adams CR, Burkhart SS: Use of preoperative three-dimensional computed tomography to quantify glenoid bone loss in shoulder instability. *Arthroscopy* 2008;24(4):376-382.

17. Burkhart SS, Debeer JF, Tehrany AM, Parten PM: Quantifying glenoid bone loss arthroscopically in shoulder instability. *Arthroscopy* 2002;18(5):488-491.

18. Burkhart SS, De Beer JF: Traumatic glenohumeral bone defects and their relationship to failure of arthroscopic Bankart repairs: Significance of the inverted-pear glenoid and the humeral engaging Hill-Sachs lesion. *Arthroscopy* 2000;16(7):677-694.

19. Burkhart SS, De Beer JF, Barth JR, Cresswell T, Roberts C, Richards DP: Results of modified Latarjet reconstruction in patients with anteroinferior instability and significant bone loss. *Arthroscopy* 2007;23(10):1033-1041.

20. Koo SS, Burkhart SS, Ochoa E: Arthroscopic double-pulley remplissage technique for engaging Hill-Sachs lesions in anterior shoulder instability repairs. *Arthroscopy* 2009;25(11):1343-1348.

21. Gleason PD, Beall DP, Sanders TG, et al: The transverse humeral ligament: A separate anatomical structure or a continuation of the osseous attachment of the rotator cuff? *Am J Sports Med* 2006;34(1): 72-77.

22. Morag Y, Jacobson JA, Shields G, et al: MR arthrography of rotator interval, long head of the biceps brachii, and biceps pulley of the shoulder. *Radiology* 2005;235(1): 21-30.

23. Burkhart SS, Brady PC: Arthroscopic subscapularis repair: Surgical tips and pearls A to Z. *Arthroscopy* 2006;22(9):1014-1027.

24. Lo IK, Burkhart SS: The comma sign: An arthroscopic guide to the torn subscapularis tendon. *Arthroscopy* 2003;19(3):334-337.

25. Lo IK, Burkhart SS: Arthroscopic biceps tenodesis using a bioabsorbable interference screw. *Arthroscopy* 2004;20(1):85-95.

26. Sanders TG, Zlatkin MB, Paruchuri NB, Higgins RW: Chondrolysis of the glenohumeral joint after arthroscopy: Findings on radiography and low-field-strength MRI. *AJR Am J Roentgenol* 2007;188(4):1094-1098.

27. Solomon DJ, Navaie M, Stedje-Larsen ET, Smith JC, Provencher MT: Glenohumeral chondrolysis after arthroscopy: A systematic review of potential contributors and causal pathways. *Arthroscopy* 2009;25(11):1329-1342.

28. Bailie DS, Ellenbecker TS: Severe chondrolysis after shoulder arthroscopy: A case series. *J Shoulder Elbow Surg* 2009;18(5):742-747.

29. Tirman PF, Steinbach LS, Feller JF, Stauffer AE: Humeral avulsion of the anterior shoulder stabilizing structures after anterior shoulder dislocation: Demonstration by MRI and MR arthrography. *Skeletal Radiol* 1996;25(8):743-748.

30. Bui-Mansfield LT, Taylor DC, Uhorchak JM, Tenuta JJ: Humeral avulsions of the glenohumeral ligament: Imaging features and a review of the literature. *AJR Am J Roentgenol* 2002;179(3):649-655.

31. Sanders TG, Jersey SL: Conventional radiography of the shoulder. *Semin Roentgenol* 2005;40(3):207-222.

32. Saupe N, White LM, Bleakney R, et al: Acute traumatic posterior shoulder dislocation: MR findings. *Radiology* 2008;248(1):185-193.

33. Krackhardt T, Schewe B, Albrecht D, Weise K: Arthroscopic fixation of the subscapularis tendon in the reverse Hill-Sachs lesion for traumatic unidirectional posterior dislocation of the shoulder. *Arthroscopy* 2006;22(2):227, e1-e227.

Elbow

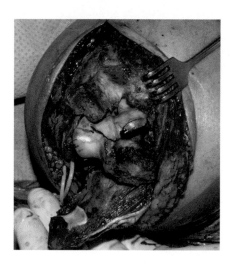

Distal Humeral Fractures: Role of Internal Fixation and Elbow Arthroplasty

Joaquin Sanchez-Sotelo, MD, PhD

Abstract

Fractures of the distal humerus can be challenging to treat. Advances in imaging, internal fixation, and arthroplasty have resulted in improved management of these injuries. Preoperative CT with three-dimensional reconstruction allows a better understanding of fracture patterns and helps the surgeon to select the best treatment options. Parallel plating techniques often provide stable internal fixation constructs, even in fractures with severe comminution. Precontoured periarticular plates facilitate internal fixation. More attention is now paid to recognizing and managing bone loss through metaphyseal shortening and/or bone grafting. Elbow arthroplasty appears to provide good early outcomes for elderly patients with severe elbow injury. Distal humeral hemiarthroplasty can be considered for elbow fractures with severe damage to the articular surface if the patient is too young and active to comply with the restrictions recommended after total elbow arthroplasty. Advances are still needed to reduce the overall complication rates associated with the treatment of distal humeral fractures.

Instr Course Lect 2012;61:203-213.

The management of distal humeral fractures has evolved over the past few years. Worldwide application of the AO principles of plate and screw fixation during the late 1980s and early 1990s remained the only breakthrough for quite some time.[1] Recent major advancements in the management of these injuries include the widespread availability of CT with three-dimensional reconstruction, recognition of the more complex articular shear fractures, understanding the benefits of the parallel-plate technique, the improved availability of precontoured periarticular plates, and the selective use of total elbow arthroplasty.[2-4] Opportunity for improvement remains, as reflected by the interest in distal humeral hemiarthroplasty for the treatment of these injuries, the controversy regarding the ideal management of the ulnar nerve during surgery, and questions on how to best manage structural bone loss. Insufficient internal fixation with Kirschner wires continues to be performed by some surgeons and can greatly compromise patient outcomes.

Evaluation

The general principles of evaluation for musculoskeletal injuries apply to distal humeral fractures, including the assessment of the soft tissues (especially in open fractures), the neurovascular status of the upper extremity, the identification of associated injuries, and adequate imaging studies. It is important to understand whether there was preexisting elbow pathology, such as inflammatory arthritis, and the anticipated physical demands on the elbow, especially when arthroplasty is considered.

AP and lateral radiographs of the elbow may be difficult to interpret because of fracture displacement and comminution (**Figure 1**). Radiographs made with the patient under traction are useful but often are not made until the patient is under anesthesia and ready for surgery. Three-dimensional reconstructions rendered from a CT scan are extremely useful in understanding the fracture pattern and planning treatment. At the Mayo Clinic, this imaging study is routinely done

Dr. Sanchez-Sotelo or an immediate family member has received royalties from Stryker and has received research or institutional support from Stryker, DePuy, and Zimmer.

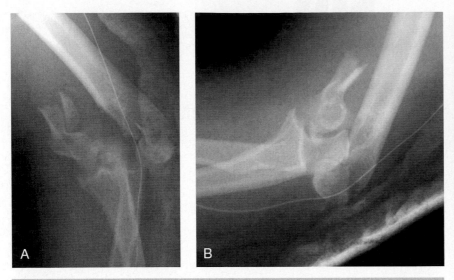

Figure 1   The precise fracture pattern on AP (**A**) and lateral (**B**) radiographs may be difficult to interpret because of fragment overlapping and displacement.

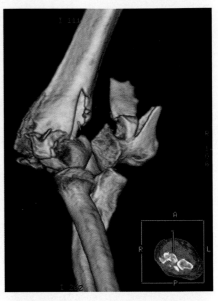

Figure 2   CT scans with three-dimensional reconstruction are helpful in decision making and surgical planning.

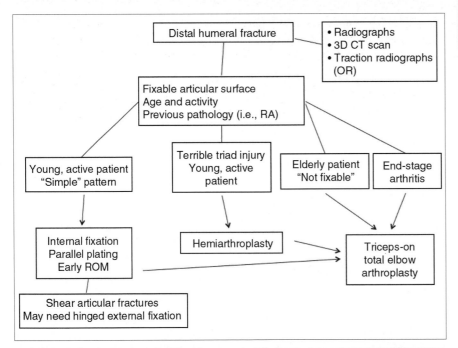

Figure 3   Treatment options for patients with distal humeral fractures. OR = operating room, 3D CT = three-dimensional CT, RA = rheumatoid arthritis, ROM = range of motion.

unless total elbow arthroplasty has already been selected for treatment (**Figure 2**).

Treatment selection should be individualized for each particular fracture and patient, but a few general guidelines may be useful (**Figure 3** and **Table 1**). Internal fixation is the treatment of choice whenever possible; the feasibility of internal fixation varies, depending on the type of fracture, the bone quality, the surgical technique, and the surgeon's experience. Elbow arthroplasty is considered very selectively for older patients with end-stage elbow arthritis before the fracture or

when the severity of destruction of the articular cartilage surface makes reliable internal fixation impossible. There is a small group of patients with severe fractures at an age when arthroplasty would have an unacceptable failure rate; hemiarthroplasty may be considered in those circumstances.[5] Internal fixation or hemiarthroplasty failures may be revised to a total elbow arthroplasty if needed. Shear fractures of the articular surface may require additional neutralization with a temporary external fixator.

Internal Fixation
Approach
Adequate surgical exposure is critical for anatomic reduction of the articular surface as well as successful internal fixation. The best exposure for most distal humeral fractures is through an olecranon osteotomy. This chapter's author favors a chevron-shaped olecranon osteotomy aimed at the bare area of the articular surface of the proximal part of the ulna (**Figure 4**). The osteot-

Table 1

Advantages and Disadvantages of Internal Fixation, Total Elbow Arthroplasty, and Distal Humeral Hemiarthroplasty for Distal Humeral Fractures

Advantages	Disadvantages
Internal fixation	
Durable	Risk of nonunion
No restrictions	Risk of posttraumatic degenerative joint disease
No prosthesis-related complications	Risk of stiffness
	Requires intensive physical therapy
Total elbow arthroplasty	
Bone union not needed	Mechanical failure
Quick return to activities of daily living	Restrictions
Easier recovery	
Avoids nonunion and degenerative joint disease	
Hemiarthroplasty	
Avoids polyethylene	Still requires internal fixation of columns
Convertible to total elbow arthroplasty	Unpredictable motion
	Unpredictable pain relief

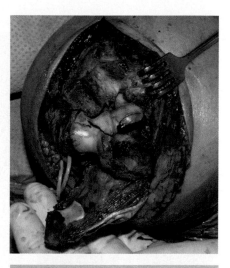

Figure 4 Olecranon osteotomy provides adequate exposure for internal fixation of distal humeral fractures.

omy is initiated with a saw and completed with an osteotome to create some irregularity at the osteotomy site, limit bone loss, and avoid inadvertent articular cartilage damage.

The olecranon osteotomy is typically secured with plate fixation or tension-band wiring with or without an intramedullary screw. Plate fixation is currently favored by most surgeons because it provides secure fixation and allows early elbow motion without the risk of osteotomy displacement and nonunion. However, when the soft tissues around the elbow are compromised, the risk of plate exposure, if wound breakdown were to happen, should be balanced against the benefits of plate fixation. Intramedullary olecranon nails have recently become commercially available and may provide the best option for osteotomy fixation; however, limited published outcome information is available.[6]

Simple fractures may occasionally be managed by exposing the distal aspect of

the humerus on both sides of the triceps; this approach is favored whenever possible. Alternatively, the extensor mechanism may be detached from its osseous attachments with use of the Bryan-Morrey[7] or triceps-reflecting anconeus pedicle[8] approaches. These approaches are especially attractive when the decision to proceed with internal fixation or arthroplasty needs to be made intraoperatively, but exposure is more limited, and the failure of triceps healing may lead to weakness in elbow extension.

Controversy remains regarding the ideal management of the ulnar nerve at the time of fixation.[9,10] This chapter's author favors subcutaneous transposition to prevent contact of the nerve with the medial plate and protect the nerve during the procedure. However, some recent studies have suggested a lower rate of postoperative neuropathy when the ulnar nerve is left in its anatomic position at the end of the procedure.[9]

Internal Fixation Technique

The preferred technique of this chapter's author for internal fixation of distal humeral fractures is the so-called parallel-plate internal fixation technique.[3] The classic AO technique recommended fixation of the articular fragments with one or two screws placed in the coronal plane followed by orthogonal plate fixation. The drawbacks of this fixation technique include limited anchorage of the plates on the distal fragments and limited compression at the supracondylar humeral level.

Biomechanical studies have shown the superiority of the parallel-plate technique, especially when bone contact is compromised[11] (**Figure 5**). After preliminary reduction of the fracture fragments with Kirschner wires, parallel plates are placed on the medial and lateral columns of the humerus, fixed distally with four to six long screws, and fixed proximally to the diaphysis after the application of supracondylar compression with clamps. The long distal screws interlock in a fixed-angle structure. Precontoured periarticular plates facilitate this technique, but the same principles may be

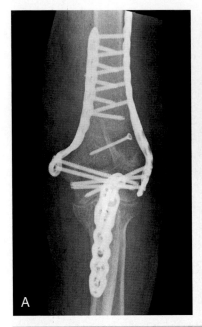
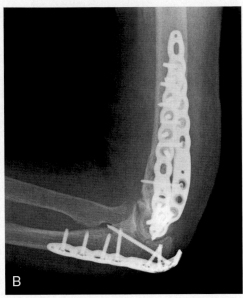

Figure 5 AP (**A**) and lateral (**B**) radiographs show the parallel plating technique for a distal humeral fracture and plate fixation of the olecranon osteotomy.

achieved with standard plates contoured intraoperatively. Locking plates may offer increased stability, but their use is limited because locked screws need a fixed trajectory in the bone, which is difficult to accomplish within the complex geometry of the distal end of the humerus.

Although orthogonal plating may offer adequate stability in simpler fractures, more complex fractures require parallel plating. Most orthopaedic surgeons do not treat a large number of distal humeral fractures each year, which makes it advisable to master one rather than two techniques.

Management of Bone Loss

Some degree of bone loss is present in many distal humeral fractures secondary to comminution. Open fractures may require removal of additional bone for adequate débridement. Depending on the severity and the location of bone loss, selective humeral shortening or bone grafting may be required.

Metaphyseal Shortening

Bone loss at the supracondylar humeral level may be addressed successfully with a moderate amount of bone shortening.[12] Humeral shortening of up to 2 cm has minimal impact on elbow biomechanics,[13] and union is more likely with bone contact in compression. The distal end of the diaphysis is contoured to match the fractured end of the articular segment. Rotational and varus-valgus malalignment of the articular segment is at risk with this technique and should be checked carefully. With shortening, the distal humeral fossae are lost, limiting elbow flexion and extension. Anterior translation of the articular segment re-creates anterior space for the coronoid and radial head in flexion. The olecranon fossa is then re-created, removing bone from the diaphysis posteriorly.

Bone Grafting

Comminution of the central aspect of the distal humeral articular surface may require bone grafting. Excessive

mediolateral compression during plate fixation leads to excessive joint-space narrowing, incongruence, stiffness, and arthritis. Fortunately, the articular cartilage of the central aspect of the trochlea is not critical, as long as the capitellum and medial trochlear cartilage are preserved. The central aspect of the trochlea may be reconstructed with a structural bone inset so that it does not reach the joint surface but restores the width of the distal end of the humerus (**Figure 6**).

Structural Bone Grafting

When the severity of columnar bone loss cannot be addressed with shortening, structural bone grafting may be required. This situation is more common in the management of distal humeral nonunion. This chapter's author favors iliac crest bone autograft, but if there is a loss of a major portion of the articular segments as well, a partial osteoarticular distal humeral allograft has occasionally been used.

Postoperative Management

Ideally, internal fixation should be stable enough to allow early unprotected rehabilitation of elbow motion. Continuous passive motion is instituted immediately if the condition of the soft tissues allows.[14] Alternatively, active-assisted elbow range-of-motion exercises may be used. Some patients have a propensity for stiffness, and static progressive splinting may be necessary for this subgroup of patients. Currently, heterotopic bone prophylaxis is not used routinely.

Outcomes

The published reports on the outcome of internal fixation for distal humeral fractures are difficult to interpret because the severity of the injuries cannot be compared, and there may be variations in the accuracy of elbow motion measurements.[15-20] Improvements in

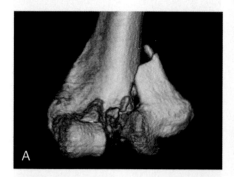
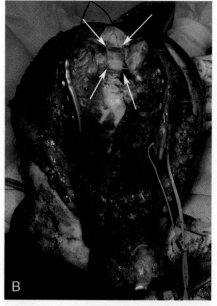
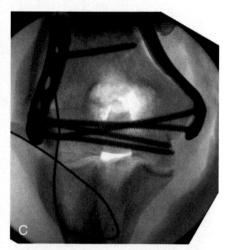

Figure 6   An elbow with comminution of the central aspect of the distal humeral articular surface. **A,** Failure to recognize central comminution as shown on this three-dimensional CT reconstruction view may lead to excessive mediolateral compression of the distal end of the humerus. **B,** Intraoperative photograph showing placement of a structural bone graft (arrows) in the area of comminution. **C,** Intraoperative fluoroscopy image showing bone graft.

fixation techniques have resulted in a decreased rate of implant failure and fracture nonunion, but elbow motion is not reliably restored in every patient. Common complications include infection, nonunion, stiffness with or without heterotopic ossification, the need for removal of the implants used for fixation of the olecranon osteotomy, and posttraumatic osteoarthritis or osteonecrosis requiring later interposition arthroplasty or elbow replacement.

The outcome of fixation with the use of a parallel-plate technique was first reported for a group of 34 elbows with severe distal humeral fractures.[3] Forty-five percent of the fractures were open, and most were classified as AO type C3. At the time of the most recent follow-up, 83% of the patients reported no or mild pain, the average elbow motion was 26° of extension to 124° of flexion, and fracture union was achieved in all but one patient who required bone grafting. Complications included deep infection in one elbow,

heterotopic ossification in five elbows, and osteonecrosis in one elbow. Later studies have confirmed the high union rate achieved with similar fixation constructs.[21,22] Higher nonunion rates have been documented with orthogonal plating compared with parallel plating.[22]

Total Elbow Arthroplasty

Rationale, Indications, and Contraindications

Joint arthroplasty is a well-accepted treatment option for fractures in other locations, such as the femoral neck or the proximal part of the humerus. The good outcomes of some elbow implants for patients with rheumatoid arthritis prompted the use of elbow replacement for distal humeral fractures.[4] Elbow arthroplasty is indicated only in a select group of elderly patients who present with either preexisting symptomatic pathology or low comminuted fractures with substantial osteopenia and severe damage to the articular surface.[23] It is contraindi-

cated in fractures amenable to stable internal fixation, open fractures, and patients with anticipated high physical demands.

This chapter's author prefers to surgically approach the joint on both sides of the triceps, remove the fractured fragments, and use a linked implant. The procedure offers several advantages: the extensor mechanism is undisturbed; no postoperative protection is required; functional elbow motion is easier to achieve; and pain and limited motion secondary to nonunion, malunion, or posttraumatic osteoarthritis are avoided. The main disadvantages are the risk of other implant-related complications and the need to limit upper-extremity use to minimize polyethylene wear and other causes of mechanical failure.

Surgical Technique

The joint is approached on both sides of the triceps muscle after ulnar nerve identification and usually transposition. Subperiosteal resection of the

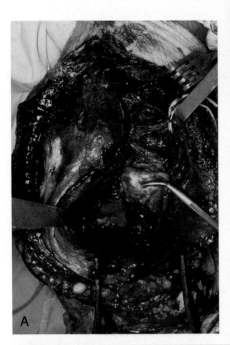

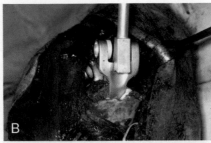

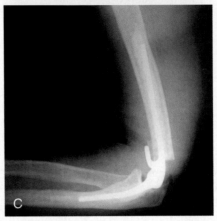

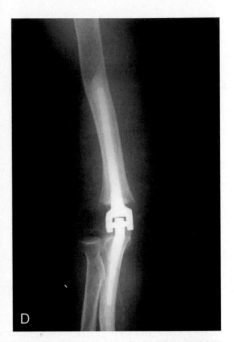

Figure 7   A total elbow arthroplasty may be the optimal treatment in some elderly patients. **A,** The fractured fragments are resected by working on either side of the triceps muscle. **B,** Canal instrumentation and implant insertion are possible through this working space without violating the extensor mechanism. Postoperative lateral (**C**) and AP (**D**) radiographs after arthroplasty.

fractured articular fragments provides a working space for broaching and implantation. Bone graft from the resected fragments is placed behind the humeral flange. Antibiotic-loaded polymethyl methacrylate is used routinely for implant fixation. The interconnecting pin can be inserted after fully seating the components. The common origins of the flexor-pronator and extensor-supinator muscles are then sutured to the triceps to seal the joint (**Figure 7**).

Postoperative Management
Postoperatively, the elbow is immobilized with an anterior splint in full extension, and the arm is elevated for 24 to 48 hours. Active range-of-motion exercises are then initiated. Most patients can be discharged from the hospital in 2 to 5 days and recover functional painless elbow motion in 2 to 3 months. Patients are placed on

weight restrictions indefinitely; they are restricted from lifting with the affected side more than 5 to 10 lb (2 to 5 kg) as a single event or more than 1 or 2 lb (0.5 to 1 kg) repetitively.

Outcomes
Cobb and Morrey[4] first reported on a series of 21 distal humeral fractures in elderly patients treated with a semiconstrained total elbow replacement. Mean range of motion was from 25° to 130°, and overall results were graded as excellent in 15 elbows and good in 5 elbows. Similar results have been reported from other centers[24-26] (**Table 2**). The Mayo Clinic experience was updated to include 43 patients followed for an average of 7 years.[21] Mean range of motion was from 24° to 132°, and the mean Mayo elbow performance score was high (93 points), but five patients required revision surgery. Interestingly, resection of the hu-

meral condyles as performed routinely in this surgical technique does not appear to adversely affect function. McKee et al[27] compared 16 elbow replacements with preservation and 16 with resection of the condyles and found no differences in motion or strength.

Two separate studies compared internal fixation and arthroplasty. Frankle et al[28] compared 24 fractures in women older than 65 years who were treated with either internal fixation or elbow replacement. Arthroplasty provided better motion and overall results. McKee et al[29] described a prospective randomized study of patients older than 65 years, with 20 elbows assigned to treatment with internal fixation and 20 assigned to arthroplasty. There were five intraoperative conversions from internal fixation to arthroplasty. Elbow arthroplasty was associated with a sub-

Table 2
Results of Total Elbow Arthroplasty for Selected Patients With Distal Humeral Fractures

Study (Year)	Number of Elbows	Mean Age (Years)	Mean Duration of Follow-up	Range of Motion	Mayo Elbow Performance Score	Complications and Reoperations
Cobb and Morrey[4] (1997)	21	72	3.3 years	25°-130°	Excellent for 15 elbows, and good for 5	Ulnar component fracture: 1
Ray et al[26] (2000)	7	82	3 years	20°-103°	Excellent for 5 elbows, and good for 2	Superficial infection: 1
Gambirasio et al[24] (2001)	10	84	17.8 months	23.5°-125°	94 (80-100)[a]	No complications
Garcia et al[25] (2002)	16	73	3 years	24°-125°	93 (80-100)[a]	No complications
Frankle et al[28] (2003)	12	72	3.75 years	15°-120°	Excellent for 11 elbows, and good for 1	Disengagement: 1; superficial infection: 2
Kamineni and Morrey[23] (2004)	43	67	7 years	24°-132°	93[a]	Revision: 5
McKee et al[29] (2009)	25	77	2 years	26°-133°	86[a]	Reoperations for stiffness: 2; deep infection: 1

[a]The values are given as the mean points, with the range in parentheses when data available.

stantial reduction in the surgical time; better elbow scores; and better early Disabilities of the Arm, Shoulder and Hand scores. There was a trend to better motion and fewer reoperations in the arthroplasty group, but it was not significant.

Hemiarthroplasty

Some authors have reported good results using a distal humeral hemiarthroplasty with column fixation for distal humeral fractures.[30-33] Distal humeral hemiarthroplasty eliminates the potential for complications associated with the presence of polyethylene or an ulnar component. However, it does not eliminate the need for healing of the columns and may be complicated by instability or symptomatic changes in the articular surfaces of the unresurfaced ulna and radial head.

Approach

This chapter's author prefers a surgical approach to the joint through either the lateral column or with an olecra-

non osteotomy. For supraintercondylar fractures, the fractured lateral fragments may be reflected distally with the common extensor muscle group and underlying lateral collateral ligament complex origin. For low shear fractures of the articular surface, an olecranon osteotomy provides excellent exposure; alternatively, the joint may be approached through a lateral epicondylar osteotomy.

Surgical Technique

Currently, a limited number of implants may be used as a distal humeral hemiarthroplasty. The humeral component of the Sorbie-Questor system (Wright Medical Technology, Arlington, TN) has an anatomic design and may be used as a hemiarthroplasty.[33] Some authors have reported cases of patients managed with the Kudo humeral component (Biomet, Warsaw, IN).[30] This chapter's author favors the Latitude hemiarthroplasty prosthesis (Tornier, Saint-Ismier, France), which can be converted to a reliable total el-

bow arthroplasty, if necessary, and facilitates suture fixation of bone and/or soft tissues through the implant (**Figure 8**). Size is estimated with preoperative templates and confirmed with intraoperative trials. Healing of the columns is required for elbow stability. Column fixation may be achieved with screws, plates, or sutures, depending on the nature of the fracture, the surgeon's preference, and the implant used.

Outcomes

There are a limited number of studies on the outcome of distal humeral hemiarthroplasty. Adolfsson and Hammer[30] reported on four Kudo humeral hemiarthroplasties performed for distal humeral fractures in elderly women; results were rated as excellent in three elbows and good in one elbow at a mean follow-up of 10 months. Malone et al[34] reported on 30 hemiarthroplasties performed for either an acute distal humeral fracture or the failure of fracture fixation. Implants

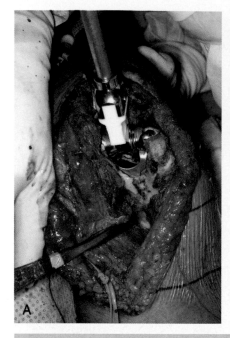
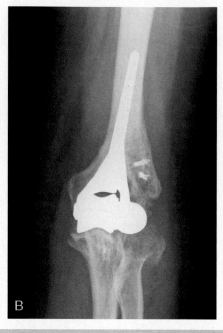
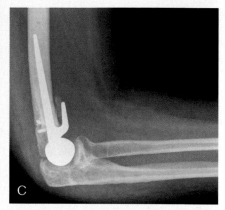

Figure 8　Distal humeral hemiarthroplasty is best suited for intra-articular fractures with severe destruction of the articular cartilage but with humeral column integrity. **A,** Intraoperative photograph made during a distal humeral hemiarthroplasty. **B,** Postoperative AP radiograph. **C,** Postoperative lateral radiograph.

used included the Sorbie component in 14 elbows and the Latitude component in 16 elbows. At a mean follow-up of 2 years, the mean range of motion included extension to 25° and flexion to 128°, and the mean Mayo elbow performance score was 77 points. Complications included periprosthetic fracture (one elbow), loosening (two elbows), symptomatic laxity (12%), and column nonunion (8%).

Shear Fractures of the Articular Surface

These injuries involve the articular surface of the distal end of the humerus without extension above the roof of the olecranon fossa.[2] Fractures of the capitellum represent the classic example of articular fractures of the distal end of the humerus, including the traditional descriptions of the Hahn-Steinthal fracture (a large fracture involving most of the capitellum) and the Köcher-Lorenz fracture (a small osteochondral fracture). Often, these fractures extend across the whole distal articular surface and may be associated with various amounts of impaction and comminution. The complexity of these fractures may be difficult to appreciate from radiographs, and CT scans with three-dimensional reconstructions are strongly recommended. Depending on the severity of articular cartilage damage, these fractures may require internal fixation or arthroplasty (**Figure 9**).

Internal Fixation

The surgical approach used for fixation of these fractures depends primarily on the presence of extension into the medial side of the joint. Fractures involving the capitellum and at most a very limited portion of the trochlea are approached through a lateral collateral ligament-preserving lateral approach. However, fractures affecting most of the anterior or posterior aspect of the trochlea, as well as those extending into the medial epicondyle, are best approached by mobilization of the extensor mechanism through an olecranon osteotomy or any of its alternatives. The simpler fracture patterns may be internally fixed with arthroscopically assisted techniques.

Thin osteochondral fractures are usually fixed with bioabsorbable pins, but excision of the fractured fragments may be done in elderly patients with low demands. Larger fractures require anatomic reduction and multiple articular screws, occasionally supplemented with bioabsorbable pins or threaded Kirschner wires. Plate fixation and/or bone grafting may be needed in elbows with extensive comminution and bone loss.

External fixation is sometimes considered to distract the elbow and neutralize the forces across the joint because articular fractures are placed at risk for fixation failure by shearing forces associated with elbow motion. This chapter's author prefers using a hinged elbow fixator for 3 to 6 weeks to allow early elbow motion. The successful use of such articulated fixators

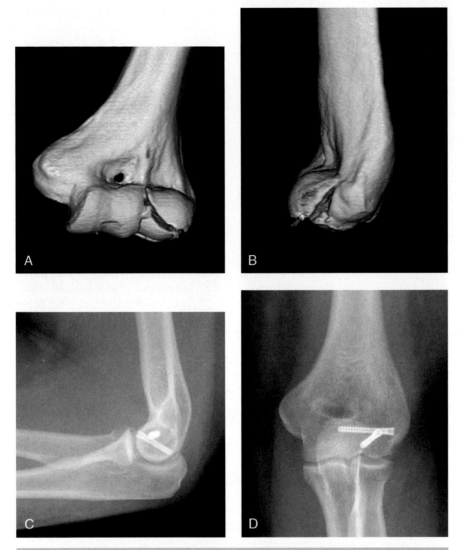

Figure 9   A simple fracture of the capitellum, as shown in this three-dimensional CT reconstruction of the distal end of the humerus, may be reliably fixed with articular screws through a lateral surgical approach. **A,** AP view. **B,** Lateral view. Lateral (**C**) and AP (**D**) radiographs made after fixation of the fracture with articular screws.

seven elbows. Mighell at al[36] reported on a selected group of 18 elbows with large coronal shear fractures of the capitellum and lateral aspect of the trochlea that were treated with open reduction and internal fixation with headless compression screws. At an average follow-up of 26 months, all but one patient had good or excellent results; three elbows showed radiographic evidence of osteonecrosis without clinical importance.

Arthroplasty

Total elbow arthroplasty and hemiarthroplasty may be indicated when the traumatic damage to the articular surface is severe. A distal humeral hemiarthroplasty may be ideal in these circumstances because there is integrity of the columns and collateral ligaments. Further studies are required to understand the role of both hemiarthroplasty and total elbow arthroplasty for articular distal humeral fractures.

Summary

The treatment of the distal end of the humerus continues to improve. Better imaging studies, sound internal fixation techniques and implants, and the selective use of elbow arthroplasty have all contributed to better overall management. However, some areas of controversy remain. Future advances will likely focus on less invasive surgical techniques and improved implants, as well as the prevention of complications that continue to compromise the final outcome of these injuries, such as wound problems, infection, ectopic bone formation, and persistent ulnar neuropathy.

References

1. Jupiter JB, Neff U, Holzach P, Allgöwer M: Intercondylar fractures of the humerus: An operative approach. *J Bone Joint Surg Am* 1985;67(2):226-239.

requires accurate reproduction of the axis of elbow flexion and extension.

The outcome of internal fixation for articular fractures of the distal end of the humerus has been reported by several authors. Ring et al[2] reported on 21 elbows followed for an average of 3.3 years. The mean arc of motion was from 27° of extension to 123° of flexion, and the overall results were graded as good or excellent in 76% of the elbows. Reoperations included contracture release in six elbows, ulnar nerve decompression in two elbows, early loss of fixation in one elbow, and implant removal in one elbow. Dubberley et al[35] reported on 28 elbows followed for a mean 4.6 years. Average motion ranged from 29° of extension to 138° of flexion, and results were considered satisfactory in 89% of the elbows. Reoperations included contracture release in seven elbows, revision internal fixation in two elbows, revision to an elbow arthroplasty in two elbows, and the removal of olecranon hardware in

2. Ring D, Jupiter JB, Gulotta L: Articular fractures of the distal part of the humerus. *J Bone Joint Surg Am* 2003;85-A(2):232-238.

3. Sanchez-Sotelo J, Torchia ME, O'Driscoll SW: Complex distal humeral fractures: Internal fixation with a principle-based parallel-plate technique. *J Bone Joint Surg Am* 2007;89(5): 961-969.

4. Cobb TK, Morrey BF: Total elbow arthroplasty as primary treatment for distal humeral fractures in elderly patients. *J Bone Joint Surg Am* 1997;79(6):826-832.

5. Sanchez-Sotelo J, Ramsey ML, King GJ, Morrey BF: Elbow arthroplasty: Lessons learned from the past and directions for the future. *Instr Course Lect* 2011;60: 157-169.

6. Nowak TE, Burkhart KJ, Mueller LP, et al: New intramedullary locking nail for olecranon fracture fixation: An in vitro biomechanical comparison with tension band wiring. *J Trauma* 2010;69(5): E56-E61.

7. Bryan RS, Morrey BF: Extensive posterior exposure of the elbow: A triceps-sparing approach. *Clin Orthop Relat Res* 1982;166: 188-192.

8. O'Driscoll SW: The triceps-reflecting anconeus pedicle (TRAP) approach for distal humeral fractures and nonunions. *Orthop Clin North Am* 2000; 31(1):91-101.

9. Chen RC, Harris DJ, Leduc S, Borrelli JJ Jr, Tornetta P III, Ricci WM: Is ulnar nerve transposition beneficial during open reduction internal fixation of distal humerus fractures? *J Orthop Trauma* 2010; 24(7):391-394.

10. Vazquez O, Rutgers M, Ring DC, Walsh M, Egol KA: Fate of the ulnar nerve after operative fixation of distal humerus fractures. *J Orthop Trauma* 2010;24(7): 395-399.

11. Schemitsch EH, Tencer AF, Henley MB: Biomechanical evaluation of methods of internal fixation of the distal humerus. *J Orthop Trauma* 1994;8(6):468-475.

12. O'Driscoll SW, Sanchez-Sotelo J, Torchia ME: Management of the smashed distal humerus. *Orthop Clin North Am* 2002;33(1): 19-33, vii.

13. Hughes RE, Schneeberger AG, An KN, Morrey BF, O'Driscoll SW: Reduction of triceps muscle force after shortening of the distal humerus: A computational model. *J Shoulder Elbow Surg* 1997;6(5): 444-448.

14. O'Driscoll SW, Giori NJ: Continuous passive motion (CPM): Theory and principles of clinical application. *J Rehabil Res Dev* 2000; 37(2):179-188.

15. Doornberg JN, van Duijn PJ, Linzel D, et al: Surgical treatment of intra-articular fractures of the distal part of the humerus: Functional outcome after twelve to thirty years. *J Bone Joint Surg Am* 2007;89(7):1524-1532.

16. Huang TL, Chiu FY, Chuang TY, Chen TH: The results of open reduction and internal fixation in elderly patients with severe fractures of the distal humerus: A critical analysis of the results. *J Trauma* 2005;58(1):62-69.

17. McKee MD, Kim J, Kebaish K, Stephen DJ, Kreder HJ, Schemitsch EH: Functional outcome after open supracondylar fractures of the humerus: The effect of the surgical approach. *J Bone Joint Surg Br* 2000;82(5): 646-651.

18. McKee MD, Wilson TL, Winston L, Schemitsch EH, Richards RR: Functional outcome following surgical treatment of intra-articular distal humeral fractures through a posterior approach. *J Bone Joint Surg Am* 2000; 82-A(12):1701-1707.

19. Ring D, Jupiter JB: Complex fractures of the distal humerus and their complications. *J Shoulder Elbow Surg* 1999;8(1):85-97.

20. Soon JL, Chan BK, Low CO: Surgical fixation of intra-articular fractures of the distal humerus in adults. *Injury* 2004;35(1):44-54.

21. Athwal GS, Hoxie SC, Rispoli DM, Steinmann SP: Precontoured parallel plate fixation of AO/OTA type C distal humerus fractures. *J Orthop Trauma* 2009;23(8): 575-580.

22. Shin SJ, Sohn HS, Do NH: A clinical comparison of two different double plating methods for intraarticular distal humerus fractures. *J Shoulder Elbow Surg* 2010; 19(1):2-9.

23. Kamineni S, Morrey BF: Distal humeral fractures treated with noncustom total elbow replacement. *J Bone Joint Surg Am* 2004; 86-A(5):940-947.

24. Gambirasio R, Riand N, Stern R, Hoffmeyer P: Total elbow replacement for complex fractures of the distal humerus: An option for the elderly patient. *J Bone Joint Surg Br* 2001;83(7):974-978.

25. Garcia JA, Mykula R, Stanley D: Complex fractures of the distal humerus in the elderly: The role of total elbow replacement as primary treatment. *J Bone Joint Surg Br* 2002;84(6):812-816.

26. Ray PS, Kakarlapudi K, Rajsekhar C, Bhamra MS: Total elbow arthroplasty as primary treatment for distal humeral fractures in elderly patients. *Injury* 2000; 31(9):687-692.

27. McKee MD, Pugh DM, Richards RR, Pedersen E, Jones C, Schemitsch EH: Effect of humeral condylar resection on strength and functional outcome after semiconstrained total elbow arthroplasty. *J Bone Joint Surg Am* 2003; 85-A(5):802-807.

28. Frankle MA, Herscovici D Jr, DiPasquale TG, Vasey MB, Sand-

ers RW: A comparison of open reduction and internal fixation and primary total elbow arthroplasty in the treatment of intraarticular distal humerus fractures in women older than age 65. *J Orthop Trauma* 2003;17(7): 473-480.

29. McKee MD, Veillette CJ, Hall JA, et al: A multicenter, prospective, randomized, controlled trial of open reduction: Internal fixation versus total elbow arthroplasty for displaced intra-articular distal humeral fractures in elderly patients. *J Shoulder Elbow Surg* 2009;18(1):3-12.

30. Adolfsson L, Hammer R: Elbow hemiarthroplasty for acute reconstruction of intraarticular distal humerus fractures: A preliminary report involving 4 patients. *Acta Orthop* 2006;77(5):785-787.

31. Athwal GS, Goetz TJ, Pollock JW, Faber KJ: Prosthetic replacement for distal humerus fractures. *Orthop Clin North Am* 2008; 39(2):201-212, vi.

32. Parsons M, O'Brien RJ, Hughes JS: Elbow hemiarthroplasty for acute and salvage reconstruction of intra-articular distal humerus fractures. *Tech Shoulder Elbow Surg* 2005;6:87-97.

33. Sorbie C: Hemiarthroplasty in the treatment of distal humeral fractures. *AO Dialogue* 2006;2:32-34.

34. Malone AA, Zarkadas P, Jansen S, Hughes JS: Elbow hemiarthroplasty for intra-articular distal humeral fracture. *J Bone Joint Surg Br* 2009;91(Suppl II):256.

35. Dubberley JH, Faber KJ, Macdermid JC, Patterson SD, King GJ: Outcome after open reduction and internal fixation of capitellar and trochlear fractures. *J Bone Joint Surg Am* 2006;88(1):46-54.

36. Mighell M, Virani NA, Shannon R, Echols EL Jr, Badman BL, Keating CJ: Large coronal shear fractures of the capitellum and trochlea treated with headless compression screws. *J Shoulder Elbow Surg* 2010;19(1):38-45.

Ligament Injury and the Use of Hinged External Fixators at the Elbow

Bernard F. Morrey, MD

Abstract

The indications and techniques for managing collateral ligament deficiencies after traumatic elbow injuries are continuing to evolve. Essentially, the lateral collateral ligament must be repaired, whereas the medial collateral ligament will heal in some instances. The repair of the medial collateral ligament is needed only in competitive athletes who place high valgus stress on the elbow joint. An understanding of the role of external fixators is also evolving. External fixation is effective in managing acute elbow trauma that results in an unstable elbow and reconstructive procedures in which the collateral ligaments or articular surface require protection in circumstances requiring movement of the elbow joint. Using half pins and a laterally placed external fixator provides the mechanical stability required in most traumatic settings.

Instr Course Lect 2012;61:215-225.

Ligament Injuries

The clinical circumstances and implications of injury to the medial collateral ligament (MCL) are markedly different than those of injury to the lateral ulnar collateral ligament (LUCL) complex.

MCL Injury

The vulnerability of throwing athletes to MCL injuries is well recognized, as is the mechanism of injury and its treatment.[1] Although the etiology of MCL injuries is beyond the scope of this chapter, an understanding of the causes of MCL injuries will provide valuable insight into the techniques of repair and reconstruction in patients with nonthrowing, traumatic MCL injuries.

Diagnosis

The diagnosis of insufficiency of the MCL is based on the patient's history and injury symptoms. MCL injury occurs in all elbow dislocations and is an essential component of terrible triad injuries involving a collateral tear and coronoid and radial head fracture.[2]

For reasons that have not been clarified, the MCL usually heals and is not generally believed to require formal repair in most acute injuries.[3,4] In chronic MCL injuries, insufficiency may be subtle and can present as pain, and the patient may not be aware of the instability.

Examination

The examination of the patient with an unstable elbow is usually relatively simple. MCL insufficiency is perceived as pain with valgus stress. If the diagnosis is subtle, a fluoroscopic image can be obtained. Lateral collateral ligament insufficiency is usually more problematic to diagnose. The instability may not be expressed as varus instability in the anteroposterior plane. The most subtle expression of collateral ligament deficiency is posterolateral rotatory instability. This form of instability is seen on a drawer test in which the elbow is placed at 90° with the biceps and triceps relaxed. The radial head is observed to subluxate on the capitellum with anterior and posterior directed pressure.

Imaging

In a patient with a chronic injury, plain AP and lateral radiographs are the first step in the imaging process. If the diagnosis is uncertain, this

Dr. Morrey or an immediate family member has received royalties from SBI and serves as a paid consultant to Zimmer.

chapter's author prefers an in-office fluoroscopic examination (**Figure 1**). MRI is rarely required in the non-throwing patient.

Management

It is well documented that there is no need to repair the MCL after a simple elbow dislocation.[3] However, the MCL is essential for elbow stability if the radial head has been removed.[5] The major dilemma facing a surgeon is whether or when to repair an acute MCL injury. In a terrible triad injury, the radial head and the coronoid fractures should be addressed, and the LUCL should be repaired. If the elbow remains unstable, the next step is either repair of the MCL or applying an external fixator.[4]

This chapter's author prefers the application of a hinged external fixator because the device is valuable in managing each component of the injury, and it renders the formal repair of the MCL unnecessary. If a medial exposure is used in treating the injury and the torn MCL is in the operative field, then it should be repaired. A running, locked No. 5-0 suture is preferred for the repair. The use of an external fixator is predicated on the stability of the elbow after all injured tissues have been addressed. If doubt exists, this chapter's author favors the application of an external fixator.

If an MCL deficiency is encountered in a chronic setting, reconstruction is performed unless the deficiency is an avulsion from the humerus and can be reliably reattached.

Technique

The original technique for MCL reconstruction in athletes as described by

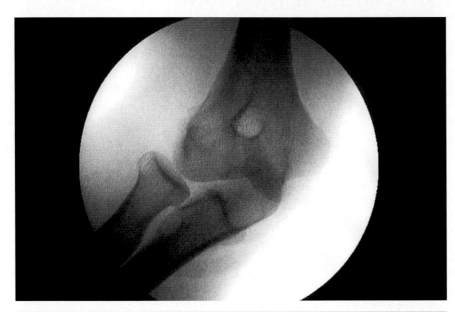

Figure 1 Fluoroscopic imaging of the elbow is helpful in the diagnosis of a chronic injury if the diagnosis is uncertain based on AP and lateral radiographs.

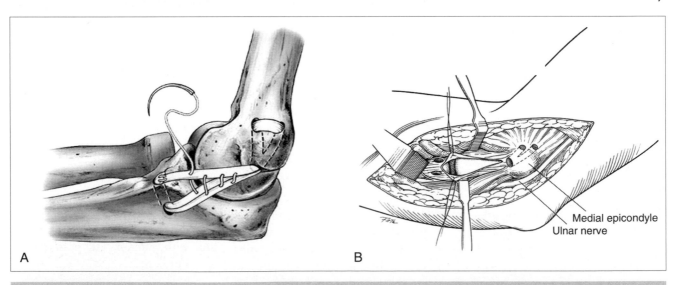

A   B

Figure 2 **A,** In the classic MCL reconstruction described by Jobe, a figure-of-8–type graft originated from the anatomic origin crossing the sublime tubercle and back to the anatomic origin. **B,** In the modified Jobe technique, the graft emerges anteriorly, and the ulnar nerve is not irritated. (Reproduced with permission from El Attrache NS, Ahmad CS: Diagnosis and treatment of ulnar collateral ligament injuries in athletes, in Morrey BF, ed: *The Elbow and Its Disorders*, ed 4. Philadelphia, PA, Saunders Elsevier, 2011, pp 660-700.)

Jobe et al[6] is still useful (**Figure 2**, *A*); however, most surgeons now prefer to modify the procedure by "docking" the proximal elements of the reconstruction in the medial epicondyle at the isometric point (**Figure 2**, *B*). To verify that stability is provided by the graft in the essential position when it is in or near full extension, two maneuvers are performed: (1) The humeral origin is placed just anterior and proximal to the true isometric point (**Figure 3**), and (2) the graft is tightened with the elbow flexed 30°. This chapter's author prefers a plantaris allograft, which is doubled on itself before it is passed through the ulnar tunnel placed under the sublime tubercle. This technique provides a four-ply graft to pass across and stabilize the joint (**Figure 4**). It is debated if the ulnar nerve should be moved or left in its grove. If the docking sutures are placed anteriorly, the nerve need not be moved.

Lateral Ulnar Collateral Ligament

It is now recognized that the LUCL is the key to symptomatic clinical elbow instability.[7] The ligament is compromised after a traumatic injury (usually following a simple or complicated dislocation). The second major source of LUCL inadequacy occurs after surgical intervention such as débridement for lateral epicondylitis or following surgery on the radial head. From a practical perspective, as is the case with the MCL, the LUCL does not require acute surgical treatment after a dislocation. However, recurrent instability may occur in this setting, especially in patients younger than 21 years. In contrast, the ligament must be formally repaired in all instances in which surgery is being performed because of a terrible triad injury or if it has been torn and there is also a radial head fracture.[2,8]

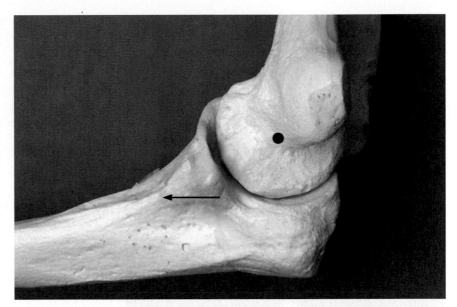

Figure 3 To avoid instability toward extension, moving the anatomic origin (black dot) of the ligament just proximal and posterior (arrow) improves the tension on the graft in extension but allows it to relax somewhat in flexion.

Diagnosis

Unlike the MCL, the patient history is not as helpful in diagnosing an LUCL problem. Some patients may sense an unstable elbow. In some instances, the insufficiency is perceived as pain rather than instability. The key elements of the patient history are a past injury suggesting a dislocation or a surgical intervention in this anatomic area. The classic diagnosis is made by demonstrating a positive posterior lateral rotatory insufficiency (PLRI) test, which is analogous to the pivot-shift test.[7] The examiner introduces a valgus, external rotatory force on the elbow as it is brought from 100° of flexion to full extension. Because of pain and apprehension, this test is sometimes difficult to perform in the physician's office; therefore, this chapter's author considers patient apprehension during the test as indicating a positive result. The initial description of the clinical consequences of LUCL deficiency is PLRI insufficiency. Regan and Lapner[9] made a significant contribution to diagnosing LUCL insufficiency with the observation that when the LUCL is compromised, a patient cannot perform a push-up or even rise from an arm chair using the affected extremity.

Imaging

When the diagnosis of LUCL deficiency is not obvious, this chapter's author routinely uses fluoroscopy to confirm a suspected diagnosis. A lateral projection is useful to show posterior subluxation of the radial head in supination and reduction in pronation (**Figure 5**). A varus stress test is also performed in the AP projection. MRI is not needed to make this diagnosis.

Management

The LUCL is formally addressed in all acute elbow disruptions that require an open surgical procedure. In patients in whom LUCL symptoms occur at a subsequent date, spontaneous healing does not appear to occur. Therefore, the injured ligament should be repaired if there is an acute tear. If a patient has PLRI after an injury, surgery should be offered as soon as the diagnosis is made.[8,10]

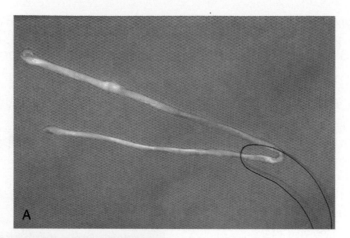

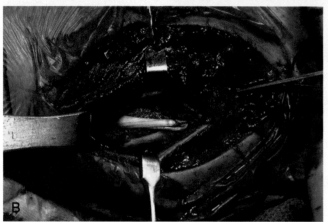

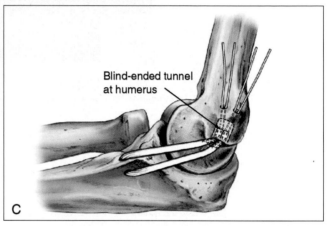

Figure 4 The graft material (a plantaris allograft is favored by this chapter's author) is folded on itself (**A**) and is brought through the sublime tubercle and "docked" in the medial epicondyle (**B** and **C**). (Panel B reproduced from Ahmad CS, El Attrache NS: Elbow valgus instability in the throwing athlete. *Instr Course Lect* 2006;14:693-700. Panel C reproduced with permission from El Attrache NS, Ahmad CS: Diagnosis and treatment of ulnar collateral ligament injuries in athletes, in Morrey BF, ed: *The Elbow and Its Disorders*, ed 4. Philadelphia, PA, Saunders Elsevier, 2011, pp 660-700.)

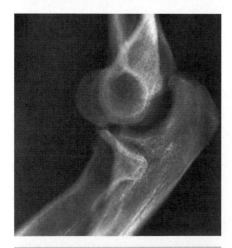

Figure 5 A lateral projection is useful to show posterior subluxation of the radial head.

Surgical Techniques

For an acute LUCL repair, this chapter's author uses a running, locked No. 5 nonabsorbable suture. It is driven through the tuft of the LUCL origin or through a bone tunnel at this site (**Figure 6**). The suture proceeds distally to the tubercle, at which point it passes under the insertion of the ligament at the tubercle. It then proceeds proximally with a running locked pattern and again penetrates the ligament origin. The forearm is pronated, and the elbow is flexed to 30° at closure.

For reconstructive procedures, a Kocher interval is used between the anconeus posteriorly and the extensor carpi radialis brevis anteriorly. The anconeus is detached from its bed to the point that the surgeon can identify the tubercle of the supinator crest, with sufficient exposure to fashion a tunnel at this site (**Figure 7**). A high-speed burr is used to create the tunnel. A suture is then passed through this tunnel and the isometric point in the vicinity of the humeral epicondyle is identified. Because the symptoms of instability occur with the elbow near full extension, the actual docking tunnel is made slightly anterior and proximal to the true isometric point. This chapter's author prefers a plantaris allograft tendon for the reconstruction. It is dou-

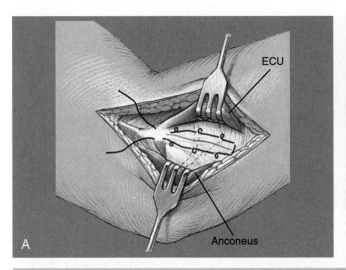
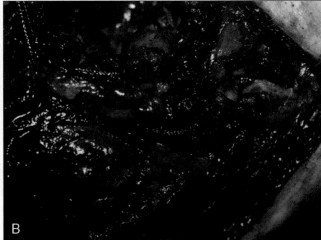

Figure 6 The anatomic origin of the lateral collateral ligament is at the lateral tubercle. Illustration (**A**) and intraoperative photograph (**B**) of the running locked stitch that originates from the origin, crosses the joint, and stabilizes the ligament at the sublime tubercle. The suture is brought proximally and again passed through bone holes stabilizing the reconstruction. ECU = extensor carpi ulnaris. (Reproduced with permission from Morrey BF: Radial head fractures, in Morrey BF, ed: *The Elbow and Its Disorders.* Philadelphia, PA, WB Saunders, 2008, pp 359-400.)

bled onto itself, and a four-ply graft is brought across the joint and docked into the humerus (**Figure 8**).

Results of Ligament Repair

Overall, surgical treatment to stabilize the elbow has been successful. For the MCL, the success rate in athletes is approximately 80%, and the success rate in nonathletes is approximately 90%.[1] Lateral ligament reconstruction to treat PLRI has a success rate of approximately 90%.[8,10]

Hinged External Fixation

Rationale

Hinged external fixation is valuable in protecting ligaments and providing early motion, protecting the articular surface and providing early motion, and a combination of both situations. With a properly constructed device, the ulna may be separated or distracted from the humerus yet still allow physiologic flexion and extension.

Concept

The mechanics and anatomic landmarks for the application of hinged fixator devices have been well defined. The axis of rotation of the distal humerus passes through the tubercle of origin of the lateral collateral ligament and through the anteroinferior aspect of the medial epicondyle[11] (**Figure 9**).

Indications

A properly applied hinged fixator maintains reduction and balance of the ulnohumeral joint during motion, thereby protecting repaired or reconstructed collateral ligaments. In traumatic injuries, fixators may be used to protect the surgical fixation of unstable fractures, protect ligament repairs, and manage long-standing elbow dislocation or recurrent instability.[12-18]

In elbow reconstruction, hinged fixators can be used in the treatment of instability, after ligamentous repair or with interposition arthroplasty.[19]

In most traumatic injuries, the goal is to neutralize the forces across the joint while maintaining elbow motion. The fixator can be applied acutely as an adjunct to surgical repair or as a secondary measure in failed reductions. The specific indications for dynamic external

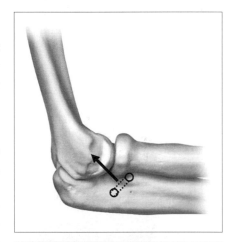

Figure 7 Tunnels (dotted lines) for lateral collateral ligament reconstruction are placed at the supinator crest and posteriorly at a distance of approximately 1 cm. The line of the reconstruction (arrow) is directed just proximal and posterior to the anatomic origin.

fixators to treat acute elbow trauma include instability, articular injury, and residual or recurrent subluxation.

Instability

Dynamic external fixation can be used to treat elbow dislocation with exten-

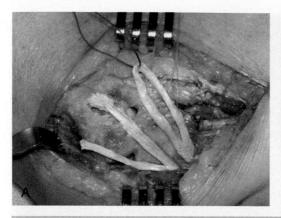
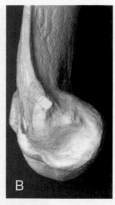
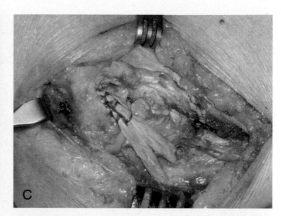

Figure 8   **A,** For lateral collateral ligament reconstruction, a plantaris allograft that has been folded on itself (see Figure 4A) is threaded through the tunnel placed in the crista of the supinator. **B,** A docking-type procedure is currently preferred. **C,** The graft is appropriately trimmed and brought into the docking tunnel and secured with the elbow in 60° of flexion and full pronation.

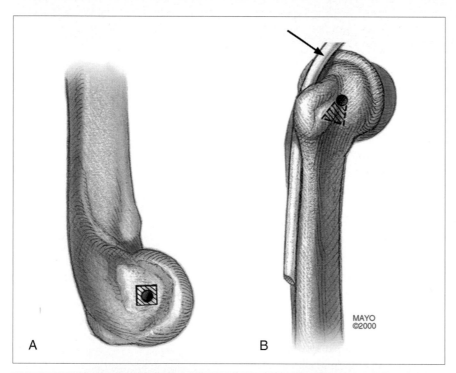

Figure 9   **A,** For external fixators, the axis is identified at the projected center of the capitellum and just anterior to the medial epicondyle, which is the projected center of the coronoid. **B,** The ulnar nerve (arrow) is protected by the medial epicondyle. (Reproduced with permission from the Mayo Foundation for Medical Education and Research, Rochester, MN.)

Articular Injury (Fracture-Dislocation)

Hinged external fixation is indicated for instability in fractures of the radial head, some olecranon fractures (Mayo type III), and Regan-Morrey type II and III coronoid fractures. The use of a hinged fixator for complex, unstable distal humerus fractures has been described.[12,20] Open fixation is the primary treatment modality. When gross instability persists or when fixation is deemed vulnerable, an external fixator can be added to allow immediate postoperative motion and neutralization or unloading of the stresses placed on the fracture fixation. Evidence of the efficacy of this adjunct has been reported experimentally and clinically.[12,17,21]

Residual or Recurrent Subluxation

Residual or recurrent subluxation may occur after simple or complex fracture-dislocations.[16] In this setting, the application of a percutaneous fixator can assist in reducing a subluxated joint without the need for an open procedure. Continued use of the device allows for early motion, with minimal risk of frank redislocation or continued subluxation. The added stability facilitates proper healing of the capsule and soft-tissue restraints.

sive soft-tissue injury that results in gross instability, even after surgical reduction or repair of the involved structures.[12,20] Adjunctive management of late untreated elbow dislocations involves the use an external fixator. The application of half-pin fixators has been shown to be adequate to stabilize both medial and lateral ligament insufficiency[14] (**Figure 10**).

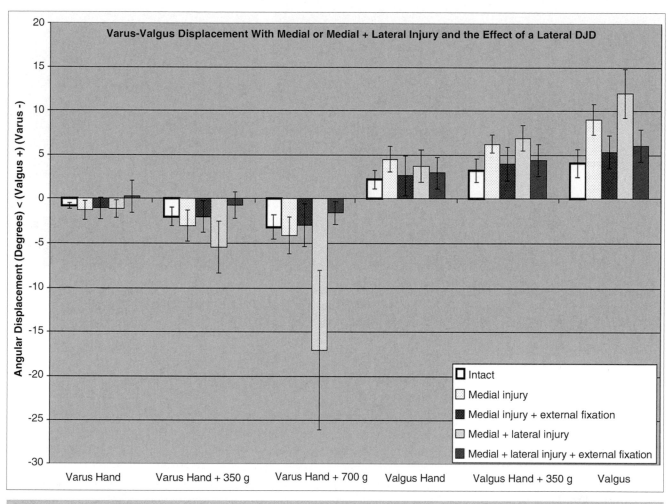

Figure 10 Experimental data demonstrate that lateral half-pin fixators can virtually restore normal stability to the elbow both in varus and in valgus. (Reproduced with permission from Kamineni S, Hirahara H, Neale P, et al: Effectiveness of the lateral unilateral dynamic external fixator after elbow ligament injury. *J Bone Joint Surg Am* 2007;89(8): 1802-1809.)

Relative Contraindications

There are several relative contraindications for using a hinged external fixator. (1) The presence of local sepsis at the desired site of pin insertion may preclude the use of an external fixator. In trauma cases, pins are ideally placed outside the zone of injury and should be located away from areas of anticipated hardware or prosthesis placement. (2) In situations in which there is uncertainty regarding the anatomic location of the neurovascular structures because of posttraumatic or postoperative disturbance of the anatomy,

a careful dissection with protection of the vulnerable nerves (usually the ulnar and radial) must be made when fixator placement is necessary. (3) The presence of fracture fixation devices in the humerus or proximal ulna can make pin placement impossible. However, there is some flexibility for pin placement, and the presence of internal fixation does not absolutely preclude its use. (4) Some surgeons may not have sufficient experience to use external fixation devices. (5) Some patients may be unable to comply with pin-site care or the rehabilitation program.

Fixator Configuration

Over the past few years several experiments have been conducted to better understand the optimal fixator configuration. Of particular importance is a study by Kamineni et al[22] that demonstrated that after release of both the MCL and the LUCL both varus and valgus stability was restored with the half-pin lateral configuration. Based on these findings, the current practice of this chapter's author is to use the lateral half-pin application of the Dynamic Joint Distractor (DJD) II (Stryker, Rutherford, NJ) in virtually

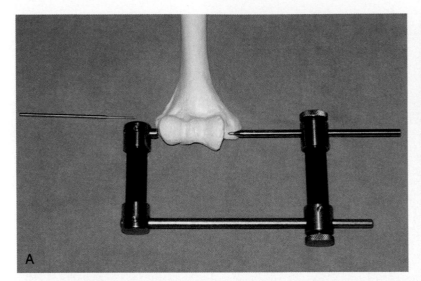
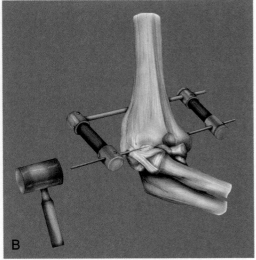

Figure 11 **A,** By using a sharp pointed stylus, the axis of the external fixator may be defined and stabilized without interfering with ligament repair or reconstruction. **B,** The stylus is tapped into place with a mallet. (Stryker Orthopaedics, Mahwah, NJ.)

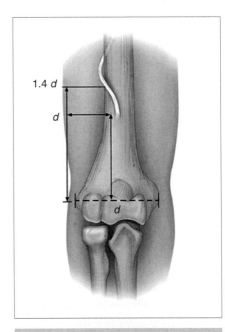

Figure 12 The closest the ulnar nerve comes to the axis of rotation is 1.4 times the epicondylar distance. Placing the most proximal pin at a distance (*d*) equal to the epicondylar distance is a safe location for this pin. (Stryker Orthopaedics, Mahwah, NJ.)

all clinical settings in which a fixator is believed to be necessary.

Technique: Dynamic Joint Distractor II
Patient Positioning
The patient is placed in the position required for proper treatment of the primary pathologic condition. In most cases of elbow trauma or reconstruction, a posterior skin incision is used, and the elbow joint is exposed either medially or laterally according to the pathologic condition being treated. After treatment of the pathologic condition, the lateral half-pin fixator is applied.

Axis Identification
The essential landmarks of the flexion axis are identified. On the lateral aspect of the joint, a tubercle, which represents the geometric center of curvature of the capitellum, is present at the origin of the lateral collateral ligament. On the medial aspect of the distal humerus, the axis of rotation lies just anterior and inferior to the medial epicondyle. This corresponds to the center of curvature of the medial contour of the trochlea.

Axis Stylus
A target device is used to identify the axis according to the previously described landmarks. A stylus pin is then driven across the lateral aspect of the humerus in a manner that does not interfere with the ligament repair or reconstruction but replicates the line of the flexion axis (**Figure 11**).

Humeral Pin Insertion
The maximum proximal placement of the humeral pin should not exceed the epicondylar dimension (**Figure 12**). This places the pin well below the radial nerve.[22] A self-tapping, 4-mm pin (or 3-mm pin for small bones) is advanced through a tissue sleeve into the lateral cortex and penetrates the medial cortex of the humerus. The proximal pin is fixed to the humeral rod, and a second pin is placed in a similar fashion. The axis of the fixator is now defined, and the stylus pin is removed.

Ulnar Pin Insertion
Two ulnar pins, usually 3 mm in diameter, are similarly placed in the proxi-

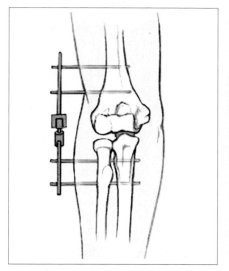

Figure 13 The half-pin configuration has been shown to be effective for most indications of ligamentous insufficiency. (Stryker Orthopaedics, Mahwah, NJ.)

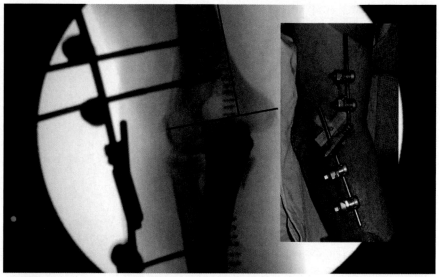

Figure 14 Fluoroscopic image of the elbow of a patient with a fracture-dislocation involving ligamentous instability that was stabilized by an external fixator placed in a percutaneous manner. Notice the accurate reduction of the elbow on the clinical photograph (inset). (Stryker Orthopaedics, Mahwah, NJ.)

Table 1

Articulated External Fixation: Dynamic Joint Distractor (DJD) II and Compass

Complications	Mayo Experience (100 patients)					
	DJD II No. Pins = 320	DJD II No. Patients = 80	Compass No. Pins = 113	Compass No. Patients = 20	P Value Compass > DJD II	P Value Compass > DJD II
Major complications	Per pin	Per patient	Per pin	Per patient	By pin	By patient
Purulent drainage/deep infection	2 (0.6%)	1 (1.3%)	12 (10%)	3 (15%)	> 0.05	
Loosening of pins; removal/ revision of pin placement	11 (3.4%)	4 (5%)	0	0		
Major complications, total	17 (5.3%)	7 (8.9%)	12 (10%)	3 (15%)	> 0.05	> 0.05

Reproduced from Cheung EV, Morrey BF, O'Driscoll SW: Abstract: Complications of hinged external fixators of the elbow. *74th Annual Meeting Proceedings.* Rosemont, IL, American Academy of Orthopaedic Surgeons, 2007, p 580.

mal ulna, distal to the surgical field. This completes the application of the device (**Figure 13**).

Distraction

If distraction is desired, typically 2 to 3 mm is sufficient to accomplish the goals of the procedure.

Fixator Removal

The fixator is removed at 3 weeks for soft-tissue injuries and ligament reconstruction and at 4 to 6 weeks when osseous protection is involved. In all instances, the fixator is removed with the patient under general anesthesia, and the elbow is examined for stability, smoothness of the articulation, and firmness of the end points of the flexion arc.[23] These end points are modified based on the intraoperative data.

Results

Hinged external fixators allow the surgeon to manage elbow trauma and its sequelae. Originally, these devices were successfully used as an adjunct for posttraumatic ankylosis surgery.[19] The value of external fixators in the management of acute trauma has been demonstrated both experimentally and clinically[12,24,25] (**Figure 14**). When used in conjunction with other procedures for the management of complex instability, an approximate 80% patient satisfaction rate has been reported.[12,15,16] However, in a challenging patient population with chronic joint subluxation and coronoid deficiency, Papandrea et al[2] were not able to demonstrate the value of the external fixator in the complex management of this injury treated at the Mayo Clinic.

It is important to remember that when treating patients with complex elbow disorders and instability, the outcome should not be directly attributed to the fixator; the outcome is influenced by the complexity of the injury and the totality of management. This is particularly true in the treatment of patients with subluxated or unstable joints. The use of an external fixator is not a principal treatment modality, but is an adjunct to stabilize the joint to protect the articulation, and allow early elbow motion.

Complications

Complications observed in the Mayo experience with 100 consecutive applications of 80 DJD II devices and 20 Compass fixators (Smith & Nephew, Memphis, TN) are shown in **Table 1**. Complications included superficial or deep infection, skin irritation, nerve injury, pin loosening, fracture, and pin breakage. There were statistically significant differences in the complication rate, which was greater when using the more complicated Compass device.[26] Differences in the frequency of these complications relate to several factors, including the indications for application and (possibly) technical difficulties encountered. No reoperations were required in any patient for pain-related problems.

Summary

Recognition of and the appropriate management of collateral ligament injuries is emerging, but additional study is needed. Specialized imaging should not replace the history and physical findings in diagnosing the problem. As a treatment adjunct, the external fixator is an important tool in the elbow surgeon's armamentarium for treating MCL and LUCL disorders. The protective effect and ability of these devices to replicate elbow kinematics has been experimentally verified. Although a low rate of significant pin-site complications has been reported, meticulous technique and appropriate monitoring of the pin sites are essential to achieving safe, successful results when using external elbow fixators.

References

1. Jobe FW, ElAttrache NS: Treatment of ulnar collateral ligament injuries in athletes, in Morrey BF (ed): *Master Techniques in Orthopaedic Surgery: The Elbow*. New York, NY, Raven Press, 1994.

2. Papandrea RF, Morrey BF, O'Driscoll SW: Reconstruction for persistent instability of the elbow after coronoid fracture-dislocation. *J Shoulder Elbow Surg* 2007;16(1):68-77.

3. Josefsson PO, Gentz CF, Johnell O, Wendeberg B: Surgical versus non-surgical treatment of ligamentous injuries following dislocation of the elbow joint: A prospective randomized study. *J Bone Joint Surg Am* 1987;69(4):605-608.

4. Morrey BF: Complex instability of the elbow. *Instr Course Lect* 1998;47:157-164.

5. Morrey BF, Tanaka S, An KN: Valgus stability of the elbow: A definition of primary and secondary constraints. *Clin Orthop Relat Res* 1991;265:187-195.

6. Jobe FW, Stark H, Lombardo SJ: Reconstruction of the ulnar collateral ligament in athletes. *J Bone Joint Surg Am* 1986;68(8):1158-1163.

7. O'Driscoll SW, Bell DF, Morrey BF: Posterolateral rotatory instability of the elbow. *J Bone Joint Surg Am* 1991;73(3):440-446.

8. Sanchez-Sotelo J, Morrey BF, O'Driscoll SW: Ligamentous repair and reconstruction for posterolateral rotatory instability of the elbow. *J Bone Joint Surg Br* 2005;87(1):54-61.

9. Regan W, Lapner PC: Prospective evaluation of two diagnostic apprehension signs for posterolateral instability of the elbow. *J Shoulder Elbow Surg* 2006;15(3):344-346.

10. Nestor BJ, O'Driscoll SW, Morrey BF: Ligamentous reconstruction for posterolateral rotatory instability of the elbow. *J Bone Joint Surg Am* 1992;74(8):1235-1241.

11. Kasparyan NG, Hotchkiss RN: Dynamic skeletal fixation in the upper extremity. *Hand Clin* 1997;13(4):643-663.

12. Cobb TK, Morrey BF: Use of distraction arthroplasty in unstable fracture dislocations of the elbow. *Clin Orthop Relat Res* 1995;312:201-210.

13. Hall J, Schemitsch EH, McKee MD: Use of a hinged external fixator for elbow instability after severe distal humeral fracture. *J Orthop Trauma* 2000;14(6):442-445.

14. Jupiter JB, Ring D: Treatment of unreduced elbow dislocations with hinged external fixation. *J Bone Joint Surg Am* 2002;84-A(9):1630-1635.

15. McKee MD, Bowden SH, King GJ, et al: Management of recurrent, complex instability of the elbow with a hinged external fixator. *J Bone Joint Surg Br* 1998;80(6):1031-1036.

16. Ring D, Hannouche D, Jupiter JB: Surgical treatment of persistent dislocation or subluxation of the ulnohumeral joint after fracture-dislocation of the elbow. *J Hand Surg Am* 2004;29(3):470-480.

17. Shin HD, Rhee KJ, Kim KC, Hong CH, Joo YB: Treatment of periarticular fracture of the elbow with a hinged external fixator. *J Korean Fracture Society* 2005;18:299-303.

18. Tan V, Daluiski A, Capo J, Hotchkiss R: Hinged elbow external fixators: Indications and uses. *J Am Acad Orthop Surg* 2005; 13(8):503-514.

19. Morrey BF: Post-traumatic contracture of the elbow: Operative treatment, including distraction arthroplasty. *J Bone Joint Surg Am* 1990;72(4):601-618.

20. Koslowsky TC, Mader K, Siedek M, Pennig D: Treatment of bilateral elbow dislocation using external fixation with motion capacity: A report of 2 cases. *J Orthop Trauma* 2006;20(7):499-502.

21. Deuel CR, Wolinsky P, Shepherd E, Hazelwood SJ: The use of hinged external fixation to provide additional stabilization for frac-tures of the distal humerus. *J Orthop Trauma* 2007;21(5):323-329.

22. Kamineni S, Ankem H, Patten DK: Anatomic relationship of the radial nerve to the elbow joint: Clinical implications of safe pin placement. *Clin Anat* 2009;22:684-688.

23. Araghi A, Celli A, Adams R, Morrey BF: The outcome of examination (manipulation) under anesthesia on the stiff elbow after surgical contracture release. *J Shoulder Elbow Surg* 2010; 19(2):202-208.

24. Kamineni S, Hirahara H, Neale P, O'Driscoll SW, An K-N, Morrey BF: Effectiveness of the lateral unilateral dynamic external fixator after elbow ligament injury. *J Bone Joint Surg Am* 2007;89(8):1802-1809.

25. Sekiya H, Neale PG, O'Driscoll SW, An KN, Morrey BF: An in vitro biomechanical study of a hinged external fixator applied to an unstable elbow. *J Shoulder Elbow Surg* 2005;14(4):429-432.

26. Cheung EV, Morrey BF, O'Driscoll SW: Abstract: Complications of hinged external fixators of the elbow. *74th Annual Meeting Proceedings*. Rosemont, IL, American Academy of Orthopedic Surgeons, 2007, p 580.

18

Complex Fractures of the Proximal Ulna: The Critical Importance of the Coronoid Fragment

Robbin C. McKee
Michael D. McKee, MD, FRCS(C)

Abstract

Complex fractures of the proximal ulna with associated elbow instability represent challenging disorders with a high incidence of complications, including malunion, arthrosis, stiffness, and recurrent instability. If a significant coronoid fragment is present, there is an increased risk of a poor outcome. Proper management of this coronoid fragment can be critical to a successful outcome. Information on identifying, reducing, and fixing the coronoid fragment in complex proximal ulnar fractures will help the treating orthopaedic surgeon maximize results with this difficult injury pattern.

Instr Course Lect 2012;61:227-233.

Elbow fracture-dislocations are complex injuries that are difficult to treat and generally have a high incidence of poor results.[1-3] Although simple elbow dislocations are relatively common, and when treated with early mobilization are associated with good results,[4] complex dislocations paired with intra-articular fractures greatly increase the probability of recurrent and persistent elbow instability, poor outcomes,

and the need for revision surgery[3,5,6] (**Figure 1**).

Multiple studies have shown that the coronoid process of the ulna plays a key role in elbow stability because its position on the distal side of the greater sigmoid notch prevents posterior dislocation of the ulna.[7,8] It also has been found that Monteggia-type fractures with an associated coronoid fragment have a significantly higher

rate of unsatisfactory outcomes.[9] Proper reduction and fixation of the coronoid process is an important but difficult surgical task that must be addressed in elbow fracture-dislocations.

There is considerable research on the terrible triad elbow injury, which is an elbow dislocation with radial head and coronoid fractures.[10,11] However, there is little specific information on elbow fracture-dislocations with complex proximal ulnar fractures that include a coronoid fragment. As such, outcomes of these injuries are difficult to determine and must be extracted from cases within larger clinical studies.

This chapter discusses clinical and radiographic outcomes of complex proximal ulnar fractures that include a significant coronoid fragment and presents a surgical strategy for reliable fixation to prevent recurrent elbow dislocation and subluxation and optimize functional outcomes.

Clinical Results

In a study focusing on fractures of the coronoid process, Regan and Morrey[12] classified coronoid fragments as type I, an avulsion of the tip; type II, a fragment of 50% or less of the whole

Ms. McKee or an immediate family member has received royalties from Stryker; is a member of a speakers' bureau or has made paid presentations on behalf of Synthes and Zimmer; serves as a paid consultant to Synthes and Zimmer; has received research or institutional support from Wright Medical Technology and Zimmer; and serves as a board member, owner, officer, or committee member of American Shoulder and Elbow Surgeons, the Orthopaedic Trauma Association, and the Canadian Orthopaedic Association. Dr. McKee or an immediate family member has received royalties from Stryker; is a member of a speakers' bureau or has made paid presentations on behalf of Synthes and Zimmer; serves as a paid consultant to Synthes and Zimmer; has received research or institutional support from Wright Medical Technology and Zimmer; and serves as a board member, owner, officer, or committee member of American Shoulder and Elbow Surgeons, the Orthopaedic Trauma Association, and the Canadian Orthopaedic Association.

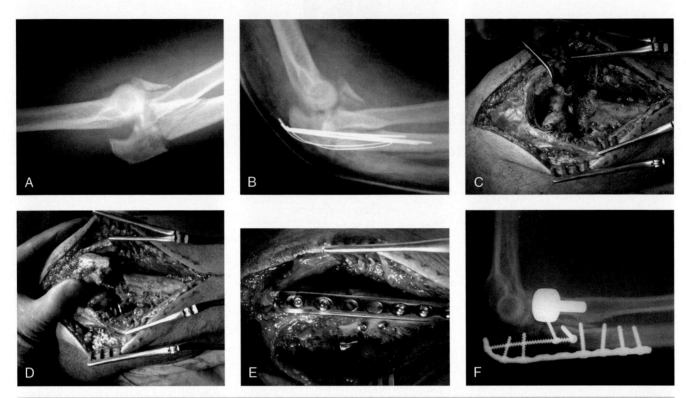

Figure 1 **A,** Lateral radiograph of a complex proximal ulnar fracture with a large coronoid fragment, probable radial head injury, and posterior dislocation of the ulnotrochlear joint. **B,** Lateral radiograph taken following fixation with a tension band wiring technique. The coronoid fragment was not reduced or fixed, the radial head injury was not addressed, and there was rapid redislocation of the ulnotrochlear joint. Tension band wiring is contraindicated in complex fractures of this type, especially if associated with ulnotrochlear instability. **C,** Intraoperative photograph taken from a posterior view after removal of the wiring. The olecranon fragment is retracted with the reduction forceps, revealing the main proximal ulnar fracture line. The coronoid fragment can be seen with difficulty in the depth of this fracture, opposed to the distal humeral joint surface. **D,** Intraoperative photograph after replacement of the damaged radial head. The coronoid fragment has been fixed with two lag screws, which typically are placed from posterolateral to anteromedial because the coronoid is primarily a medial structure. **E,** The main fracture line is reduced and secured with a contoured compression plate. **F,** Postoperative lateral radiograph shows reduction of the coronoid fragment and the primary proximal ulnar fracture line, replacement of the radial head with a metal modular prosthesis, and concentric reduction of the ulnohumeral joint. The eventual clinical result was good but prolonged rehabilitation was required, and there was significant residual stiffness in terms of flexion-extension and forearm rotation; these are typical sequelae following failed primary surgery. These problems could have been avoided and a better clinical result obtained by closer attention to surgical technique in the primary repair of this fracture.

coronoid process; and type III, a fragment larger than 50% of the coronoid process. Although this study focused on coronoid fractures, several patients had associated dislocations and fractures, including fractures of the proximal ulna. Three patients with type III coronoid fragments had concomitant proximal ulnar fractures, and all had radiographic evidence of a displaced coronoid fragment with posterior subluxation. When the three patients with type III coronoid fractures were grouped with one other patient with an associated fracture (not of the proximal ulna), the average Mayo Elbow Performance score was 60, which is considered a poor result. The authors compared simple coronoid fractures (with no associated dislocation or fracture) with more complex injuries (with associated dislocations and fractures) and reported that the simple injuries had a greater arc of flexion ($P < 0.001$), pronation ($P < 0.05$), less pain ($P < 0.01$), and a higher elbow score ($P < 0.001$).[12]

In a study by Doornberg et al,[13] which evaluated fracture-dislocations of the olecranon, there were 10 anterior and 16 posterior dislocations with proximal ulna fractures. Of the anterior dislocations, five had associated coronoid fractures, and four of the five coronoid fractures were fixed with a screw. A malunion and the development of grade 3 arthrosis in the unfixed coronoid fractures contributed the only poor result within this group.

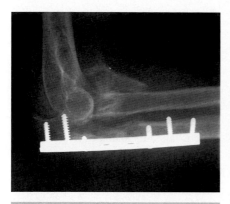

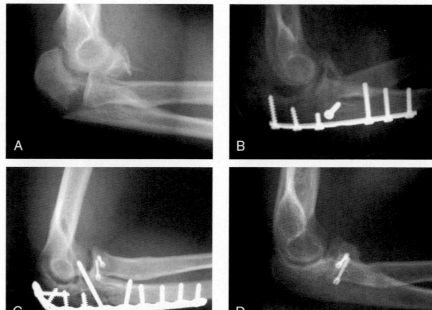

Figure 2 Postoperative lateral radiograph of a patient referred 3 months after injury for definitive care following the failed primary treatment of a complex proximal ulnar fracture with ulnotrochlear instability, similar to the patient in Figure 1. Deficiencies in technique of the primary treatment included failure to reduce and fix the large coronoid fragment, simple resection of the radial head without replacement, and failure to promptly recognize or treat the posterior subluxation/dislocation of the ulnohumeral joint. The large coronoid fragment and the corresponding bony defect in the proximal ulna can be clearly seen. Significant heterotopic ossification is evident posterior to the distal humerus. Reconstruction to salvage the joint will be technically difficult with an expected high complication rate (especially stiffness) and will produce a result significantly inferior to that which might have been achieved with proper primary surgical treatment. (Reproduced with permission from Saati AZ, McKee MD: Fracture-dislocation of the elbow. *Hand Clin* 2004;20:405-414.)

Figure 3 **A,** Lateral radiograph of a complex fracture-dislocation of the proximal ulna with an associated large coronoid fragment. **B,** Postoperative radiograph showing early redislocation caused by failure to adequately stabilize the coronoid fragment. A fracture of the radial head/neck also is evident. **C,** Lateral radiograph following revision stabilization with reduction and fixation of the coronoid and radial head fractures. This partial oblique view shows the screw inserted into the tip of the coronoid fragment. **D,** Lateral radiograph following removal of the ulnar plate because of local irritation. Anatomic healing of the coronoid fragment and concentric reduction of the ulnohumeral joint is evident.

All 16 patients in the group with a posterior dislocation and proximal ulna fracture had a corresponding coronoid fracture, 15 of which were fixed with a screw. Malalignment of the coronoid process that resulted in arthrosis developed in the patient with the unfixed coronoid fracture and one other patient. Proximal radioulnar synostosis developed in four patients in this group. The authors discussed the importance of proper restoration of the trochlear notch, and suggested that most preventable unsatisfactory results in their study were caused by improper treatment of the coronoid process, which led to an unstable trochlear notch with resultant stiffness and arthrosis (**Figures 2** and **3**). Doornberg et al[13] suggested a surgical technique for coronoid fixation that involves retraction of the olecranon fragment so the coronoid can be visualized, reduced, and fixed in proper anatomic position.

In a 1998 review of the AO experience with combined radius and ulna fractures at the elbow, Heim[14] reported on 120 total cases, 25 involving fractures of the coronoid process and the radial head. In these 120 cases, 11 patients were treated with primary radial head resection. Premature arthrosis developed in eight patients and

another eight had valgus instability. The author concluded that reduction of the coronoid fragment was critical to the restoration of elbow stability, and radial head resection is contraindicated if elbow instability is present.

In a study of Monteggia fractures, Ring et al[9] retrospectively reviewed 48 patients. Ten patients had a Bado type II (posterior or posterolateral) injury and associated fracture of the coronoid process, nine of which were fixed internally with screws. The authors found unsatisfactory results were significantly more common in patients with associated coronoid fractures than those without such fractures. Of the 10 patients with corresponding coronoid fractures, complications included persistent instability of the ulnohumeral joint, 2 patients with proximal radioulnar synostoses, and

3 patients with nonanatomically reduced coronoid fragments that led to elbow instability and painful posttraumatic osteoarthrosis. Radiographs were available for 19 patients 5 years after their original injury. The only signs of arthrosis were found in patients with malunited coronoid fractures. The authors concluded that large coronoid fragments must be anatomically reduced in Monteggia fractures.[9]

Rochet et al[15] studied the treatment of comminuted fractures of the proximal ulna with a double-plating technique. Of 18 patients, 11 had an associated coronoid fracture. These 11 patients had 3 complications (two nonunions and 1 elbow dislocation); the 7 patients without a coronoid fracture had no significant complications. The average flexion extension of the 11 elbows with coronoid fractures was 17° to 130°, and 85° to 65° for pronation-supination. The mean Morrey scores for the patients without coronoid fracture compared with those with coronoid fracture were 87 and 78, respectively. The authors discuss the importance of proper osteosynthesis of the coronoid fragment to improve overall results. The presence of a coronoid fracture results in lower subjective outcome scores, and the size of the coronoid fragment is important. Patients without a coronoid fracture and type I fragments had better results compared with patients with type II or III coronoid fragments.

In a more recent study, Ring et al[16] examined reconstruction of posterior Monteggia fractures that were malaligned after failed original surgery. Nine of 17 patients were identified as having a fracture of the coronoid process with the original injury. One patient was treated with suture fixation, one with wire fixation, three with screw fixation in a malaligned position, and four with no fixation. Revi-

sion surgery was needed in all nine patients because of ulnohumeral subluxation, pain, and stiffness. These findings clearly demonstrate the importance of accurate fixation of the coronoid fragment.

Surgical Technique

General surgical principles are to reduce and stabilize the fracture fragments of the proximal ulna sequentially (from deep to superficial) and identify and repair associated injuries, such as radial head fractures and collateral ligament tears. A general or regional anesthetic is administered, and the patient is placed in the lateral decubitus position with the affected side facing up. The arm is placed over a bolster, a tourniquet is applied, and the arm is draped free. This position allows excellent access to the proximal ulna, the radial head, the joint, and collateral ligaments. The pull of gravity provides a distally directed force that helps reduce the typically posteriorly and proximally displaced ulnar fracture or elbow subluxation. Alternatively, if the patient cannot be placed in the lateral decubitus position (for example, because of a concomitant severe chest injury), a supine position can be used with the arm draped free across the chest; however, this positioning typically requires an assistant to provide traction and support from the opposite side of the table. A portable imaging machine is positioned on the ipsilateral side of the patient for later use in radiographically evaluating the fracture reduction and fixation.

A direct posterior approach is used, and the proximal ulnar fracture site is identified. The incision can be extended to just proximal of the olecranon tip, and distally as far as is required for adequate fixation of the ulnar fracture; a minimum of three bicortical screws distal to the fracture site is recommended. It is not usually man-

datory to isolate and expose the ulnar nerve unless extensive surgery is anticipated on the medial side of the elbow. For example, a medial collateral ligament repair or a medial approach to a coronoid fragment would mandate isolation and protection of the nerve. Care is taken to manage any soft-tissue disruption created by the fracture with preservation of any intact soft-tissue structures.

Any associated radial head or neck fracture can then be evaluated. This can be done through the same posterior incision that exposes the ulna by retracting the extensor carpi radialis brevis laterally, then elevating the muscle attachment of the anconeus followed by the origin of the supinator from the lateral side of the proximal ulna. It is important to stay directly on the lateral bony surface of the ulna to minimize muscle damage and avoid the posterior interosseous nerve, especially distally. Dissection is carried down to the annular ligament, which can be incised or reflected to expose the radial head if required. The senior author (MDM) prefers this approach because the fractures can be well visualized and repaired through a single extensile incision. Often, much of the exposure has been created by soft-tissue disruption from the injury itself, most commonly in injuries involving posterior dislocation or subluxation. The disadvantage of the posterior exposure is that it increases the potential risk of loss of rotation from heterotopic ossification or synostosis, especially if extensive muscle damage occurs from the injury or the surgical approach. The alternative is to perform a separate skin incision with a standard lateral (Kocher) approach to the radial head and neck, thus reducing the risk of synostosis. Fracture fixation of the radial head is preferred when there are only one or two fracture fragments. If there is fracture

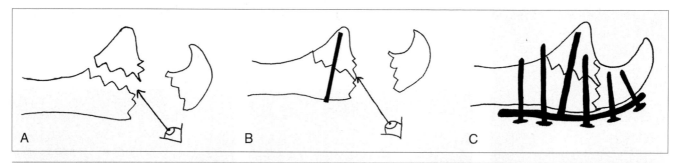

Figure 4   Illustration of the visualization and reduction technique for the coronoid fragment during a posterior approach to a complex proximal ulnar fracture. **A,** It is critical to visualize the coronoid fragment initially (before "closing the window") by reducing the principal proximal ulnar fracture line. It can then be reduced and stabilized to the shaft fragment either definitively or provisionally. **B,** Definitive lag screws can be placed distal laterally in the shaft fragment into the coronoid, which is proximal-medial. Alternatively, provisional fixation with Kirschner wires can be performed, followed by definitive fixation through the plate used to stabilize the primary ulnar fracture (**C**).

comminution, impaction, cartilage damage, or an associated radial neck fracture preventing a stable anatomic reduction, a radial head excision is performed. This enhances visualization of the coronoid fragment, allowing careful assessment of the size, location, and comminution of this fragment. Fixing the coronoid fragment at this point makes it difficult to subluxate the elbow sufficiently to insert the stem of the radial prosthesis without disrupting the fracture repair. Therefore, the radial stem and head prosthesis (a metal, modular prosthesis is preferred) is inserted first, and then the coronoid fracture is reduced and fixed to the ulnar shaft. One, or preferably two, partially threaded cancellous screws are inserted in a lag fashion, typically from distal-lateral on the shaft fragment to proximal-medial on the coronoid. Cannulated screws and image intensification facilitate the fixation. It is important to perform this fixation before reduction of the main proximal ulnar fracture line because the latter maneuver obscures the coronoid fragment (**Figure 4**). On occasion, a more direct approach to the coronoid may be required. This can be achieved through dissection on the medial surface on the ulna and reflecting the musculature. Alternatively, a direct approach, with a separate anteromedial incision while protecting the ulnar nerve and splitting the flexor-pronator mass, can be performed. This approach allows direct reduction of the fracture; a small buttress plate can be applied. After coronoid fixation has been performed, the main fracture line of the proximal ulna is reduced and can be fixed temporarily with Kirschner wires or, if the fracture pattern permits, definitive lag screws. The fracture is then stabilized by a plate placed directly on the posterior surface of the proximal ulna (**Figure 5**). Although compression plates contoured intraoperatively have traditionally been used, newer precontoured plates of equal strength but of lower profile are now readily available and are preferred. Screws inserted in a compression mode improve fracture healing, and a long screw inserted from the olecranon fragment down the intramedullary canal into the distal fragment will enhance fixation. Intraoperative imaging is performed to confirm fracture reduction and screw placement (no intra-articular hardware). Wounds are closed in layers followed by application of a sterile dressing. Drains are not routinely used.

Postoperative Management

A well-padded posterior plaster splint is applied with the elbow at 90° flexion, leaving the wrist free. Supervised motion can begin, directed by a physiotherapist, within 7 to 10 days of surgery when the sutures and splint are removed. Active-assisted range-of-motion exercises, including flexion, extension, and forearm rotation, are initiated at this time. Hinged splints or casts are not routinely used. Unrestricted shoulder and wrist motion is encouraged, as is the early discontinuation of splints. Bracing or splinting to improve motion is reserved for patients who do not show a progressive increase in motion with time.

Discussion

Elbow stability is dependent on both osseous integrity and soft-tissue constraint in equal proportions. The primary bony constraint is the coronoid process because of the buttress it offers against posterior translation of the ulna, whereas the medial collateral ligament inserts at the coronoid base and acts as a soft-tissue constraint.[8,17-19] The anatomic reduction and fixation of this fragment is of critical importance in the treatment of complex proximal ulnar injuries.[5,13,15] Although there is a paucity of literature dealing specifically with complex proximal ulnar fractures with associated el-

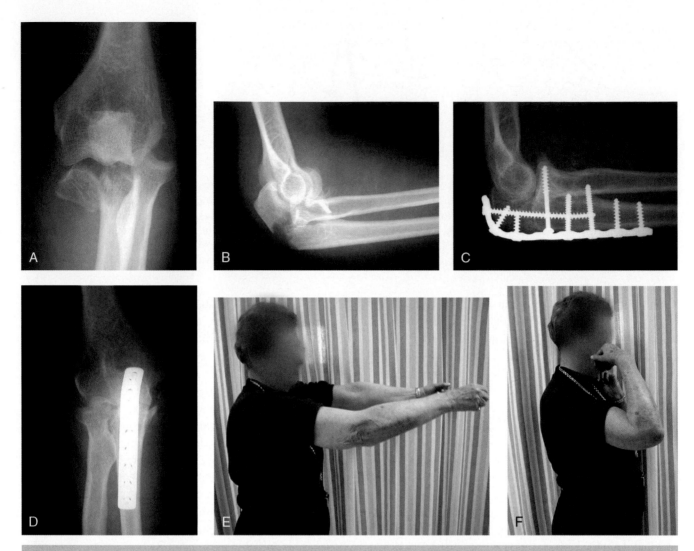

Figure 5   **A,** AP radiograph of a complex fracture-dislocation of the proximal ulna with a large coronoid fragment, which is displaced medially. **B,** Lateral radiograph showing posterior displacement of the shaft and radial head. **C,** Lateral radiograph after lag screw fixation of the coronoid fragment, plate fixation of the proximal ulna, and concentric reduction of both the ulnohumeral and radiocapitellar joints. **D,** AP radiograph shows concentric elbow reduction, some calcification of the medial collateral ligament (a sign of injury to this structure at the time of the fracture), and a small defect in the radial head. Although partial radial head excision is generally contraindicated, occasionally small fragments of less than 15% of the head in nonstrategic areas can be removed if examination reveals that elbow stability is not affected. **E** and **F,** The patient had an excellent clinical outcome with a range of elbow flexion-extension from 15° to 130°, full supination, and 50° of pronation. The results of successful primary fixation of this injury are, on average, significantly superior to the results of revision surgery, especially with regard to complications such as heterotopic ossification and stiffness.

bow instability, several facts are clear. Prolonged immobilization, in an attempt to maintain stability following a complex proximal ulnar fracture with elbow instability, is associated with a high incidence of stiffness, arthrosis, and poor results.[4,5,9,10,20] When the proximal ulnar fracture pattern includes a coronoid fragment, the occur-

rence of unsatisfactory outcome increases dramatically. This is primarily the result of recurrent posterior subluxation.[7,16,20,21] Coronoid fractures typically result from a shearing mechanism that occurs when the coronoid is driven against the distal humerus as the elbow subluxates and dislocates posteriorly. Proper surgical technique

that reduces and stabilizes the coronoid fragment(s) will dramatically improve the functional outcome of patients and avoid the need for revision surgery.

Summary

It is important to recognize the presence and significance of the coronoid fragment when treating complex fractures of the proximal ulna. In most patients, the coronoid fragment can be addressed and repaired through the main ulnar fracture line prior to definitive plate fixation. This technique optimizes elbow stability, facilitates early motion, and maximizes functional outcomes for patients.

References

1. Hotchkiss R, Green D: Fracture dislocation of the elbow, in Rockwood CA, Green DP, Bucholz RV, eds: *Rockwood and Green's Fractures in Adult*, ed 4. Philadelphia, PA, Lippincott Raven, 1996, pp 168-209.

2. Ring D, Jupiter JB: Fracture-dislocation of the elbow. *J Bone Joint Surg Am* 1998;80(4): 566-580.

3. Bruce HE, Harvey JP Jr, Wilson JC Jr: Monteggia fractures. *J Bone Joint Surg Am* 1974;56(8):1563-1576.

4. Mehlhoff TL, Noble PC, Bennett JB, Tullos HS: Simple dislocation of the elbow in the adult: Results after closed treatment. *J Bone Joint Surg Am* 1988;70(2):244-249.

5. Saati AZ, McKee MD: Fracture-dislocation of the elbow: Diagnosis, treatment, and prognosis. *Hand Clin* 2004;20(4):405-414.

6. Josefsson PO, Gentz CF, Johnell O, Wendeberg B: Dislocations of the elbow and intraarticular fractures. *Clin Orthop Relat Res* 1989; 246:126-130.

7. Papandrea RF, Morrey BF, O'Driscoll SW: Reconstruction for persistent instability of the elbow after coronoid fracture-dislocation. *J Shoulder Elbow Surg* 2007;16(1):68-77.

8. Closkey RF, Goode JR, Kirschenbaum D, Cody RP: The role of the coronoid process in elbow stability: A biomechanical analysis of axial loading. *J Bone Joint Surg Am* 2000;82-A(12):1749-1753.

9. Ring D, Jupiter JB, Simpson NS: Monteggia fractures in adults. *J Bone Joint Surg Am* 1998; 80(12):1733-1744.

10. Pugh DM, McKee MD: The "terrible triad" of the elbow. *Tech Hand Up Extrem Surg* 2002;6(1): 21-29.

11. Chemama B, Bonnevialle N, Peter O, Mansat P, Bonnevialle P: Terrible triad injury of the elbow: How to improve outcomes? *Orthop Traumatol Surg Res* 2010; 96(2):147-154.

12. Regan W, Morrey B: Fractures of the coronoid process of the ulna. *J Bone Joint Surg Am* 1989;71(9): 1348-1354.

13. Doornberg J, Ring D, Jupiter JB: Effective treatment of fracture-dislocations of the olecranon requires a stable trochlear notch. *Clin Orthop Relat Res* 2004;429: 292-300.

14. Heim U: Combined fractures of the radius and the ulna at the elbow level in the adult: Analysis of 120 cases after more than 1 year. *Rev Chir Orthop Reparatrice Appar Mot* 1998;84(2):142-153.

15. Rochet S, Obert L, Lepage D, Lemaire B, Leclerc G, Garbuio P: Ostéosynthèse des fractures comminutives de l'ulna proximal par deux plaques. *Rev Chir Orthop Reparatrice Appar Mot* 2010;96: 800-807.

16. Ring D, Tavakolian J, Kloen P, Helfet D, Jupiter JB: Loss of alignment after surgical treatment of posterior Monteggia fractures: Salvage with dorsal contoured plating. *J Hand Surg Am* 2004; 29(4):694-702.

17. Rosell P, Clasper J: Roles of the medial collateral ligament and the coronoid in elbow stability. *J Bone Joint Surg Am* 2003;85-A(3): 568-569.

18. Cage DJ, Abrams RA, Callahan JJ, Botte MJ: Soft tissue attachments of the ulnar coronoid process: An anatomic study with radiographic correlation. *Clin Orthop Relat Res* 1995;320: 154-158.

19. Morrey BF, Tanaka S, An KN: Valgus stability of the elbow: A definition of primary and secondary constraints. *Clin Orthop Relat Res* 1991;265:187-195.

20. Broberg MA, Morrey BF: Results of treatment of fracture-dislocations of the elbow. *Clin Orthop Relat Res* 1987;216: 109-119.

21. Ring D, Jupiter JB, Zilberfarb J: Posterior dislocation of the elbow with fractures of the radial head and coronoid. *J Bone Joint Surg Am* 2002;84-A(4):547-551.

MRI and Arthroscopy Correlations of the Elbow: A Case-Based Approach

Geoffrey D. Abrams, MD
David W. Stoller, MD
Marc R. Safran, MD

Abstract

The number of elbow arthroscopies and indications for the procedure have increased significantly since the advent of modern elbow arthroscopy in the 1980s. In addition to the patient history, physical examination, and plain radiography, MRI is an important tool for the clinician in diagnosing several pathologies within and around the elbow. Understanding the pathophysiology and clinical presentation and being familiar with the MRI characteristics of a variety of elbow conditions will assist the physician in making an accurate diagnosis and help guide appropriate treatment.

Instr Course Lect 2012;61:235-249.

The first successful arthroscopic evaluation of the elbow joint was reported in cadavers in 1932.[1] Modern elbow arthroscopy, however, did not begin until the mid 1980s when Andrews and Carson described the results of débridement and loose body removal for a small case series of patients with varied elbow pathologies.[2] Since that time, improved arthroscopic technology and a better understanding of the pathoanatomy of the elbow joint has led to an increase in the number of elbow arthroscopies being performed and has expanded the indications for the procedure. Despite these changes, less than 10% of arthroscopic procedures are performed for elbow pathology, and it remains the fourth or fifth most common joint undergoing arthroscopy. Improved MRI technology has allowed the clinician to more precisely identify elbow pathology and develop a treatment algorithm. This chapter will discuss the history, presentation, treatment, and correlations between MRI and subsequent arthroscopic findings for common pathologies within and around the elbow.

MRI Basics for the Elbow

MRI of the elbow can be both highly sensitive and specific when evaluating elbow pathology.[3-6] Standard sequences usually consist of T1-weighted, fat-suppressed T2-weighted, or proton density-weighted images. Additional pulse sequences, such as gradient echo sequences, can be used if either articular cartilage or ligament and tendon pathology is being investigated.[7,8] Imaging should extend from the distal humerus to the bicipital tuberosity of the radius. Axial images are used to create coronal oblique images prescribed along a line connecting the humeral epicondyles, whereas sagittal oblique images are prescribed perpendicular to the coronal axis. The use of a surface coil is essential to obtain adequate ligamentous detail.[8] The patient may be positioned either supine with the arm at the side or prone with the

Dr. Abrams or an immediate family member has stock or stock options held in Pfizer, Merck, Amgen, Johnson & Johnson, and MedCo. Neither Dr. Stoller nor any immediate family member has received anything of value from or owns stock in a commercial company or institution related directly or indirectly to the subject of this chapter. Dr. Safran or an immediate family member has received royalties from Stryker; serves as a paid consultant to Cool Systems, Cradle Medical, Arthrocare, and Biomimedica; has stock or stock options held in Cool Systems, Cradle Medical, and Biomimedica; has received research or institutional support from Ferring Pharmaceuticals; and serves as a board member, owner, officer, or committee member of American Shoulder and Elbow Surgeons; the American Orthopaedic Society for Sports Medicine; the International Society of Arthroscopy, Knee Surgery, and Orthopaedic Sports Medicine; and the Society for Tennis Medicine and Science.

arm overhead. The prone position allows the elbow to be placed in the center of the magnet, allowing for more uniform fat suppression, but is disadvantageous because it can cause patient discomfort and an increased risk for motion artifact. The flexed, abducted, and supinated position may be used for imaging distal biceps pathology.[9]

Direct magnetic resonance arthrography or the injection of intra-articular gadolinium or saline directly into the elbow can further increase detection of pathology, particularly articular cartilage lesions and subtle undersurface ligament tears.[10-12] Indirect magnetic resonance arthrography, which requires intravenous injection of gadolinium, is useful when evaluating arthropathies or synovial disorders.[13]

Osteochondritis Dissecans

Overview

The exact etiology of osteochondritis dissecans (OCD) of the capitellum is still unclear. It is usually seen in active children older than 12 years who have repetitive axial loading of the capitellum. The most widely accepted theory is that this repetitive trauma in genetically susceptible individuals causes a vascular insult to the capitellar subchondral bone, which lacks anastomoses and is subject to focal osteonecrosis when injured.[14] OCD may also occur in the radial head or trochlea. It is believed that the harder radial head compresses the softer capitellum, and the end arterioles within the capitellum are damaged.

Patients usually present with an insidious onset of dominant elbow pain and are usually involved in throwing sports, gymnastics, or weightlifting.[15] Tenderness may be elicited with palpation over the capitellum as the elbow is flexed and extended, and pronation and supination in extension may produce pain. A flexion contracture may also be present. The medial elbow

should be evaluated for concomitant pathology (ulnar collateral ligament [UCL] injury, ulnar neuropathy, and valgus extension overload). Imaging begins with plain radiography, which may show radiolucency within the capitellum. This is best done with the elbow in 45° of flexion because the OCD lesion is not directly distal in the capitellum.

MRI is most sensitive in evaluating the status of the articular cartilage and the extent of subchondral bone involvement, which is useful in classifying OCD lesions. MRI will occasionally show an OCD lesion before it is seen on plain radiographs. An unstable lesion will show fluid tracking between the lesion and the underlying bone on T2-weighted or proton density-weighted sequences. Bony edema may be seen within the capitellum. Although MRI can detect and help stage OCD, magnetic resonance arthrography is more accurate for staging the process, which ultimately is critical in the management of OCD. On T1-weighted images, there is a hypointense low signal zone of separation around the developing fragment and low signal within the fragment. Intermediate signal intensity synovial thickening and synovitis frequently are present. On fat-suppressed proton density-weighted fast spin-echo images, unstable lesions are characterized by fluid or contrast encircling the fragment and by variable signal within the fragment, depending on the degree of sclerosis and the chronicity of disease. Unstable lesions show an increased zone of separation from the capitellum. Short-tau inversion recovery protocols are also helpful in displaying the high signal rim of a loose fragment and the high signal within the fragment and in the deeper bone that indicate edema. Loose in situ lesions may also be identified by a cyst-like lesion beneath the OCD fragment. Intravenous

gadolinium will enhance the fluid within the joint and the granulation tissue in the defect, which is not as bright as joint fluid. The clinician must be knowledgeable regarding a pseudodefect of the capitellum, which is a normal variant, and not mistake this for true pathology.[16] This is found in the posterior portion of the capitellum, whereas OCD is usually anterior in the capitellum.

Difelice et al[17] developed a classification system based on the cartilage status and stability of the lesion. Based on this system, treatment options include nonsurgical treatment with rest from the offending activities, drilling the lesion, microfracture, fragment fixation, autologous osteochondral plug grafting, autologous chondrocyte implantation, and closing wedge osteotomy of the humerus.[14,18-22]

Generally, if the articular cartilage is intact, conservative management with relative rest is the initial treatment of choice. Some investigators recommend using an unloader brace to take pressure off the lateral elbow. Nonsurgical treatment is more often successful in skeletally immature patients than in those who have achieved skeletal maturity.[23] If symptoms persist or there is no radiographic evidence of healing by 6 months, then arthroscopic drilling, either anterograde or retrograde, is indicated. If the articular cartilage is violated but the lesion is in the bed, curettage—with or without microfracture of the base—and internal fixation of the fragment are often recommended. If the fragment is out of the bed and fragmented or overgrown, fragment removal may be indicated. In this situation, options include partial repair of the fragment, microfracture of the bed, or osteochondral plug grafting, which the senior author (MRS) prefers when the lateral column is affected. The senior author has no experience with autologous chondrocyte implantation or

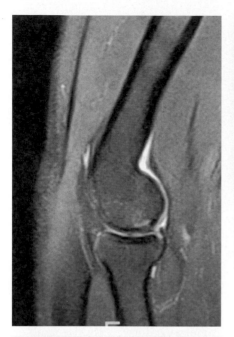

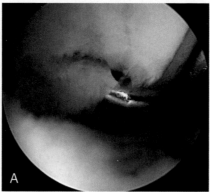

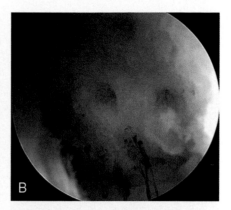

Figure 2 Arthroscopic image of the capitellum showing a large, full-thickness cartilage lesion before débridement (**A**) and following débridement and microfracture (**B**). (Courtesy of Marc R. Safran, MD, Redwood City, CA.)

Figure 1 Sagittal, proton density-weighted fat-saturated image of the left elbow showing increased signal within the capitellum and overlying cartilage irregularity. (Courtesy of Marc R. Safran, MD, Redwood City, CA.)

closing wedge osteotomy for this diagnosis.

Case Presentation

A 16-year-old cheerleader initially presented with persistent pain in her left elbow during activities of daily living. Her symptoms began approximately 3 years prior when she was competing in gymnastics. An MRI revealed OCD of the capitellum, and she was treated with chondroplasty and drilling of the lesion. The patient had initial improvement but symptoms returned. Imaging at that time showed subchondral edema within the capitellum and focal overlying cartilage irregularity without tracking of fluid beneath the lesion (**Figure 1**). The patient was subsequently treated with arthroscopic chondroplasty and microfracture of an osteochondral lesion measuring 8 mm in diameter × 3 mm deep (**Figure 2**).

Lateral Epicondylitis
Overview

Lateral epicondylitis, commonly called tennis elbow, has a prevalence of 3% in the general population.[24] This condition involves the more superior and deep fibers of the extensor carpi radialis brevis (ECRB) and is believed to be caused by overuse of wrist extensors.[25,26] The term epicondylitis is actually a misnomer because the classic histologic finding is angiofibroblastic tendinosis and not an inflammatory epicondylitis or tendinitis.[27] Lateral epicondylosis is probably a more appropriate term.

Patients typically report a history of pain over the lateral elbow, particularly with gripping or other repetitive wrist activities. There is usually tenderness to palpation over and just distal to the lateral epicondyle, which can be reproduced with resisted finger and wrist extension with the elbow in full extension. Other pathologies, including radiocapitellar arthritis, posterolateral plica, radial tunnel syndrome, and posterolateral rotatory instability, may cause pain over the lateral aspect of the elbow and should be excluded. Although lateral epicondylitis is usually a clinical diagnosis, plain radiography is required to evaluate the presence of other pathologies. Occasionally, calci-

fications may be seen near the lateral epicondyle. Ultrasound is increasingly being used in the diagnosis of this disorder and may reveal focal hypoechoic areas of the tendon or discrete tears.[28] MRI may reveal common extensor tendon degenerative changes, tendon thickening, and/or tearing. These changes include normal to increased tendon thickness with increased signal intensity on all pulse sequences. There may also be macroscopic tearing of the ECRB with or without tears of the extensor digitorum communis. Signal changes associated with steroid injections should be differentiated from those of tendinosis. Some physicians believe that MRI may be able to differentiate high-grade lesions that are less likely to be amenable to conservative treatment; however, more data are necessary to confirm this claim.

Initial treatment consists of rest, nonsteroidal anti-inflammatory drugs, and rehabilitation exercises focusing on strengthening and stretching of the wrist extensors. More than 90% of patients will respond to conservative measures.[29] If the condition does not improve with these initial measures, injection of corticosteroid is a common treatment, and blood and platelet-rich plasma treatment has shown promising early results.[30,31] Al-

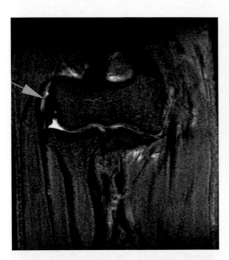

Figure 3 Coronal, T2-weighted fat-saturated image of the elbow showing increased signal within the common extensor tendons (arrow). (Courtesy of Marc R. Safran, MD, Redwood City, CA.)

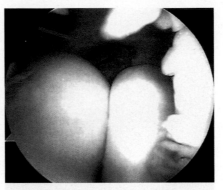

Figure 4 Arthroscopic view from the proximal anteromedial portal showing a lateral capsular rent (arrow), indicating tearing and degeneration of the ECRB tendon and underlying capsule. The radiocapitellar joint is seen in the foreground. (Courtesy of Marc R. Safran, MD, Redwood City, CA.)

though corticosteroids administered as an injection or via iontophoresis are beneficial in the short term, many physicians use corticosteroids as an adjunct to rehabilitation. Early reports suggest that platelet-rich plasma has a long-term advantage over corticosteroids, but further research is necessary. Both open and arthroscopic interventions for removal of abnormal tissue from the ECRB are also an option in severe cases that are recalcitrant to improvement after 6 months of proper rehabilitation and anti-inflammatory medications.

Case Presentation

A 54-year-old man who works as a computer software developer presented with right elbow pain that had persisted for 19 months. He actively worked out in the gym and was an avid motorcyclist. The pain started after performing biceps curls and progressed to the point that he now had pain when lifting a coffee cup and working on the computer (despite ergonomic changes to his workstation). The patient had four corticosteroid injec-

tions, which each resulted in temporary relief, and two courses of physical therapy. Examination revealed tenderness just distal to the lateral epicondyle, which was exacerbated by resisted wrist dorsiflexion with the elbow extended, as well as pain with passive palmar flexion of the wrist. The patient had full elbow range of motion, no tenderness over the arcade of Frohse, and an intact neurovascular status. Preoperative imaging demonstrated increased signal within the common extensor tendons just distal to the lateral epicondyle (**Figure 3**). Intraoperative arthroscopic images showed a lateral capsular rent, indicating tearing and degeneration of the ECRB tendon and underlying capsule (**Figure 4**).

Medial Instability

Overview

Common causes of UCL complex injury are acute valgus loading, elbow dislocation, and chronic attenuation in overhead athletes. It has been shown that 64 Nm valgus stress are placed on the UCL complex during the acceleration phase of throwing, whereas the ca-

daver strength of the UCL is only 33 Nm.[32-34] The primary restraint to valgus stress during throwing is the anterior oblique portion of the UCL complex.[35]

In patients with chronic attenuation, an insidious onset of medial elbow pain during the acceleration phase of throwing or during activities requiring valgus stress to the elbow is reported. A careful examination is required because medial elbow pain can result from other pathologies such as medial epicondylitis. In contrast with patients with medial epicondylitis, those having UCL complex pathology will show tenderness to palpation 2 cm distal to the medial epicondyle (over the UCL complex) and have a positive result on the milking maneuver, the valgus stress test, and/or the moving valgus stress test.[36-38] If UCL injury is suspected, a careful examination of the entire elbow should be performed because concomitant ulnar neuropathy and/or valgus extension overload may be present.

Plain radiography may show secondary findings of UCL insufficiency such as ossification of the ligament, loose bodies, or early arthritis.[39] MRI may reveal a complete or partial tear of the UCL. Acute injury to the UCL can be detected, localized, and graded with MRI. These injuries generally are midsubstance tears, especially in throwers. In younger athletes, however, the injuries may be avulsions, primarily from the humeral epicondyle. MRI findings consistent with a tear of the UCL include heterotopic ossification, indicated by increased fat signal of the bone marrow within the ligament, or hypointensity in sclerotic ossification; increased signal within the ligament on fat-suppressed proton density-weighted fast spin-echo images; a chronically thickened UCL that is hyperintense on T1-weighted or proton density-weighted images and hypointense on fat-suppressed proton density-weighted fast spin-echo images; and epicondylar avulsions. Other MRI findings consistent with a UCL tear include stress response or fracture at the humeral or ulnar attachments of the UCL; synovitis that is intermediate to hyperintense on fat-suppressed proton density-weighted fast spin-echo sequences; traction spurs that are hyperintense on T1-weighted and proton density-weighted images; possible edema within the lateral compartment or olecranon; possible discontinuity of the UCL fibers; possible hypertrophy of the sublime tubercle; hyperintense-associated strain of the flexor pronator mass or tear seen on fat-suppressed proton density-weighted fast spin-echo sequences; and extravasation of fluid when contrast is given intra-articularly. Partial tears of the UCL are indicated by a T-sign on magnetic resonance arthrography and represent undersurface tearing of the UCL distally off the sublime tubercle (**Figure 5**).

Both nonsurgical and surgical treatment options exist for UCL complex pathology. Nonsurgical treatment is successful in 42% of patients.[40] Surgery is usually reserved for high-level throwers and patients who had at least 3 months of nonsurgical rehabilitation without success. If surgical treatment is elected, reconstruction with ipsilateral palmaris tendon autograft is most often performed using a variety of reconstruction techniques; more than 90% of patients return to sports at their preinjury level.[41-45]

Case Presentation

A 20-year-old man who is a collegiate wrestler initially presented for treatment with a 3-month history of medial elbow pain in his dominant arm and swelling following acute valgus stress to his elbow that occurred while his hand was planted on the mat during a competition. Rest and other nonsurgical treatments failed to improve his

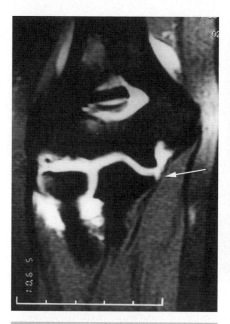

Figure 5   Coronal, fat-suppressed, gadolinium-enhanced T2-weighted MRI showing a partial tear of the anterior bundle of the UCL complex. The T-sign is shown by the arrow, with the inferior aspect of the T representing contrast tracking beneath the ligament and above its normal insertion on the sublime tubercle of the ulna. (Courtesy of Marc R. Safran, MD, Redwood City, CA.)

pain. Examination revealed maximal tenderness just distal to the medial epicondyle and a positive result on the modified milking maneuver, the valgus stress test, and the moving valgus stress test. MRI showed a near-complete tear of the UCL within its proximal midsubstance (**Figure 6**). Although the option of continued rest and nonsurgical treatment of the injury was discussed with the patient, he elected surgical treatment. Standard diagnostic arthroscopy was performed to evaluate concomitant intra-articular pathology. Laxity was confirmed with intraoperative stress testing, which demonstrated medial ulnohumeral gapping of 1 to 2 mm (**Figure 7**). A flexor carpi ulnar–splitting approach was used and the disrupted UCL was identified. Ipsilateral palmaris longus autograft was har-

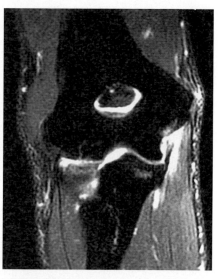

Figure 6   Coronal, oblique, T2-weighted fat-suppressed image showing increased signal intensity and the lack of fibers at the proximal aspect of the UCL, representing a near complete tear of the UCL. (Courtesy of Marc R. Safran, MD, Redwood City, CA.)

vested, and reconstruction was performed using a blind-end tunnel on the humeral side and a bone tunnel on the ulnar side (docking technique).[43] The ulnar nerve was not transposed.

Lateral Instability

Overview

Lateral elbow instability occurs when there is pathology within the lateral collateral ligament (LCL) complex. Although the most common cause is elbow dislocation, acute varus stress as well as iatrogenic injury may be implicated.[46] Lateral instability exists on a spectrum from posterolateral rotatory instability (subluxation of the radiocapitellar joint) to a perched elbow and culminates in frank dislocation. Investigations using serial sectioning of the LCL complex have shown that disruption of both the lateral ulnar collateral ligament (LUCL) and the radial collateral ligament are required to induce posterolateral rotatory instability.[47,48]

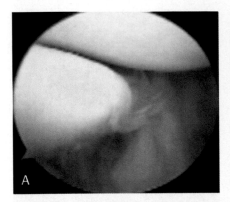
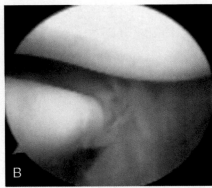

Figure 7 Intraoperative arthroscopic image of the trochlea (top) and the coronoid (bottom) showing normal congruity of the medial ulnohumeral joint (**A**) and a medial opening of 1 to 2 mm with valgus stress, indicating UCL incompetence (**B**). (Courtesy of Marc R. Safran, MD, Redwood City, CA.)

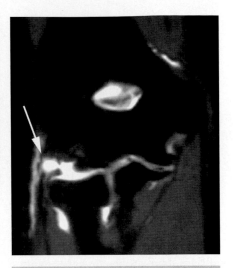

Figure 8 Coronal, T2-weighted fat-saturation sequence of the elbow showing a complete tear of the LUCL (arrow). (Courtesy of Marc R. Safran, MD, Redwood City, CA.)

Patients will often report previous trauma, surgery, or dislocation and laterally based elbow pain with giving way or catching. Clinical tests include the lateral pivot-shift test, the posterolateral drawer test, the chair sign, and the push up sign.[49,50] These tests usually elicit apprehension in the awake patient.

Plain radiographs are usually unremarkable unless there is an associated fracture. Stress radiographs may show the posterolateral rotatory motion (radial head posterior to the capitellum) and opening of the ulnohumeral joint, with a normal proximal radioulnar relationship. Posterolateral rotatory instability is a clinical diagnosis; however, MRI has been shown to be both sensitive and specific in detecting LCL complex pathology.[51] Radial head subluxation may be seen, as well as injury to the LCL itself, which is often seen as discontinuity of the ligament fibers surrounding hypointense edema or hemorrhage on T1-weighted images. LCL injury, especially when producing posterolateral rotatory instability, is usually an injury that occurs proximally at the level of the lateral epicondyle, and inspection of the MRI at this location is important (**Figure 8**).

Acute LCL complex injuries may be treated with a short period of immobilization followed by bracing in pronation.[52] Conservative treatment has no role in chronic LCL complex injuries with associated laxity. Direct repair and/or imbrication may be attempted; however, reconstruction with palmaris longus autograft is more commonly performed.

Case Presentation

A 20-year-old man who is an avid snowboarder fell on his outstretched left elbow when landing from a jump, eliciting immediate pain and deformity of the elbow. The elbow dislocation was reduced in the medical clinic at the ski slope, and he was referred for evaluation. An MRI was obtained and showed injury to the LCL complex. The patient was treated nonsurgically with a brace but had continued instability with activities of daily living. He reported difficulty when arising from the ground or pushing off when snowboarding, with his elbow giving way and popping. On examination, he had apprehension to the pivot-shift test and experienced discomfort during the chair-raise and push-up tests. Examination under anesthesia demonstrated a positive pivot shift maneuver. Arthroscopy showed radial head subluxation posterior to the capitellum, with supination near extension (**Figure 9**).

The patient was treated with LUCL reconstruction using a free palmaris longus graft (**Figure 10**).

Arthritis and Loose Bodies
Overview

Symptomatic elbow arthritis has been reported in 2% of the population that has not had elbow trauma, with a predisposition toward males and those engaged in heavy labor.[53] A study by Solia[54] found a 17% incidence of chondral damage in patients younger than 50 years and 29% in those older than 50 years. Common causes of elbow arthritis include trauma as well as excessive elbow torque, as found in athletes who participate in overhead sports.

Patients with elbow arthritis usually present with reports of medial or lateral pain and/or aching, especially in the mid ranges of motion; swelling; reduced range of motion; and/or decreased performance in athletic activities. If loose bodies are present, the patient may also report locking or catching. Examination may reveal effusion, pain with flexion/extension and pronation/supination, and popping or clicking if loose bodies are present.

Plain radiographs are required when evaluating for elbow arthritis and may show loose bodies, joint-space narrowing, and osteophytosis. MRI is the modality of choice for evaluating the status of the articular cartilage. In throwing athletes, articular cartilage changes occur in the postero-lateral area of the trochlear notch and the radiocapitellar joint. Older patients have cartilage loss at the radiohumeral articulation. With optimal MRI techniques, the thin articular cartilage of the elbow surfaces can be seen easily, particularly in the fat-suppressed sequences and with MR arthrography. In patients with more advanced arthritis, MRI also can be helpful in determining the size and location of loose bodies targeted for removal and in assessing ligament pathology and capsular contractures. The loose bodies are usually low signal structures, often round, with variable internal high signal equivalent to fat and adjacent moderate signal synovial thickening on T1-weighted images. There is usually high signal intensity, joint effusion with low signal loose bodies on fat-suppressed proton density-weighted, fast spin-echo scans. There often is increased signal within the loose bodies on short-tau inversion recovery images.

The management of elbow arthritis ranges from nonsurgical treatments (rest, nonsteroidal anti-inflammatory drugs, physical therapy, and activity modification) to injection with corticosteroids or viscosupplementation to surgical intervention. Arthroscopic surgical options for patients with global arthritis include débridement of chondral injuries and osteophytes, loose body removal, isolated capsulotomy, and the Outerbridge-Kawasaki procedure.[55-57] Open Outerbridge-Kawasaki procedures may also benefit

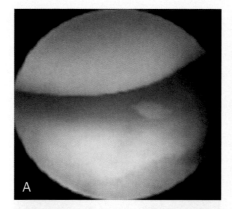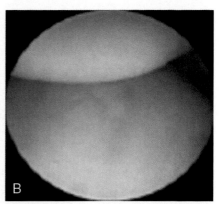

Figure 9   Arthroscopic images of the radial head in it reduced position within the radiocapitellar joint (**A**) and subluxating posterior to the capitellum with supination near extension, indicating posterolateral rotatory instability (**B**). (Courtesy of Marc R. Safran, MD, Redwood City, CA.)

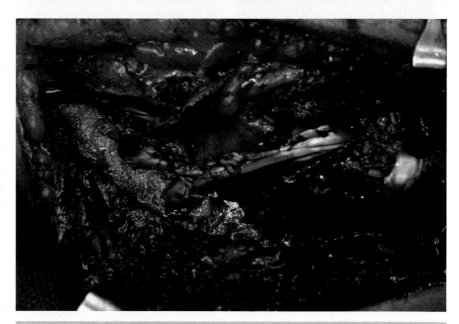

Figure 10   Intraoperative photograph of a LUCL reconstruction using a free palmaris longus graft. (Courtesy of Marc R. Safran, MD, Redwood City, CA.)

patients with degenerative arthritis of the elbow. Arthroplasty is usually reserved for patients with rheumatoid arthritis or lower-demand elderly patients with severe arthritis; it may also be an appropriate treatment for those with degenerative arthritis who are willing to accept postoperative lifestyle modifications.

Case Presentation

A 34-year-old man who is a former professional baseball pitcher presented

with a 6-month history of lateral elbow pain, even at rest, and intermittent locking of the elbow. He was unable to achieve full extension of the elbow and had some crepitus with flexion. No specific injury to the elbow was recalled by the patient, although he had been treated in past years with several cortisone injections into the elbow. Preoperative MRI showed evidence of loose bodies (**Figure 11**), which were confirmed during arthroscopic débridement (**Figure 12**).

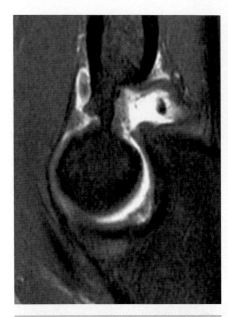

Figure 11   Sagittal, proton density-weighted image of the elbow showing loose bodies in the anterior and posterior capsular areas. (Courtesy of Marc R. Safran, MD, Redwood City, CA.)

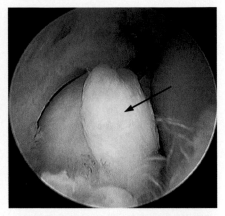

Figure 12   Arthroscopic view of the elbow from the proximal anteromedial portal showing a loose body within the anterior aspect of the joint. (Courtesy of Marc R. Safran, MD, Redwood City, CA.)

Valgus Extension Overload

Overview

Valgus extension overload predominantly exists in overhead athletes and involves posteromedial olecranon fossa osteophytes, posteromedial chondromalacia, and the risk of an olecranon stress fracture. The act of overhead throwing creates tension on the medial elbow (resisted primarily by the anterior oblique ligament of the UCL complex) and compression of the radiocapitellar joint laterally.[35] There is also shear of the proximal medial olecranon within the precisely fitting olecranon fossa. In the setting of an attenuated or disrupted UCL complex, medial tension and lateral compression are exacerbated and produce increased force at the posteromedial ulnohumeral articulation.[58] An uncontrolled deceleration phase of throwing will allow further impingement of the developing olecranon osteophytes within the olecranon fossa.[59]

Patients will typically report posterior elbow pain during both the acceleration and deceleration phases of throwing. Locking, catching, and/or an inability to fully extend the elbow may be reported. The valgus extension overload test is a useful diagnostic aid.[60] As valgus extension overload often occurs along with other elbow pathology, the UCL complex should be thoroughly evaluated.

Radiographs, including the elbow axillary view, may show the posteromedial osteophytes.[61] MRI is particularly useful because it can help to further define the posteromedial osteophytes as well as evaluate for loose bodies, the status of the UCL complex, and the presence of an olecranon stress fracture.

The initial treatment of a patient with valgus extension overload is rest, the administration of nonsteroidal anti-inflammatory drugs, and participation in a dedicated physical therapy program. Throwing mechanics should be addressed when the patient returns to activities.[62,63] If nonsurgical measures fail, arthroscopic débridement of the posteromedial osteophytes with or without UCL reconstruction may be

undertaken. Care should be taken to not remove an excessive amount of the posteromedial fossa because this may lead to increased stress on the UCL.[64]

Case Presentation

A 20-year-old man who plays collegiate baseball presented with posterior dominant elbow pain of 4 months' duration. He reported that the pain started after he increased the number of pitches thrown per game. The pain was located in the back of the elbow and began as soreness. It resolved with rest but returned when he tried to return to pitching, particularly after 30 throws. The pain started at ball release and follow-through during the pitching motion and was located along the posteromedial aspect of the elbow. He did not have any numbness, tingling, locking, or catching in the elbow. Examination showed that full extension of the affected elbow was 10° less than the contralateral elbow, but the patient was able to achieve full flexion. He had a slight elbow effusion and tenderness over the olecranon tip as well as posteromedially. The patient had no evidence of elbow laxity and no pain with resisted elbow or wrist maneuvers; his radiographs were unremarkable. A CT scan was obtained to better evaluate the bony anatomy. An MRI also could have shown the osteophyte, any bony edema from the impingement, and potentially a UCL injury. The axial CT scan demonstrated osteophyte formation off the medial olecranon (**Figure 13**).

Posterolateral Plica

Overview

Lateral or posterolateral elbow pain can have many etiologies. More commonly, lateral-sided pain may be caused by lateral epicondylitis, radiocapitellar arthritis, or loose bodies. In patients with refractory lateral-sided elbow pain and/or if mechanical symp-

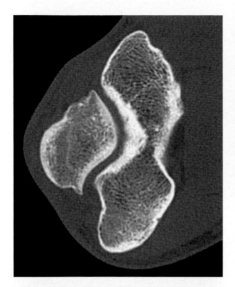

Figure 13 Axial CT scan showing the classic location of posteromedial osteophyte formation as seen in valgus extension overload. (Courtesy of Marc R. Safran, MD, Redwood City, CA.)

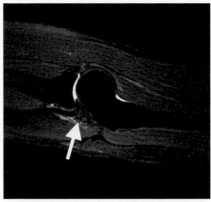

Figure 14 Sagittal, oblique, T2-weighted image of hypertrophic synovial impingement at the posterolateral aspect of the elbow (arrow). (Courtesy of Marc R. Safran, MD, Redwood City, CA.)

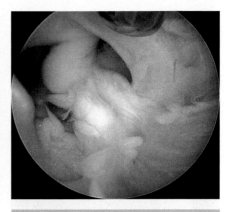

Figure 15 Arthroscopic view of the posterior aspect of the radiocapitellar joint shows multiple hypertrophic synovial plicae. (Courtesy of Marc R. Safran, MD, Redwood City, CA.)

toms such as snapping or catching are present, the clinician should evaluate for posterolateral plica. Plicae represent hypertrophic synovial folds that may become impinged with elbow range of motion.[65]

Patients with posterolateral plica are typically overhead athletes and report posterolateral elbow pain with associated mechanical symptoms.[66,67] They have often been unsuccessfully treated for lateral epicondylitis or other more common diagnoses of lateral elbow pain. Examination may reveal tenderness to palpation at the posterolateral aspect of the elbow behind the lateral epicondyle. The patient may be able to reproduce snapping of the elbow.

Plain radiography is usually unremarkable. MRI may reveal hypertrophic synovium or the synovial impingement itself, which is best seen on sagittal scans.[68] T2-weighted scans may show the edema within the synovium. Treatment may be nonsurgical, including rest, a rehabilitation program, and/or the administration of anti-inflammatory medications, including the injection of corticosteroids into the plica itself. Alternatively, the plica may be arthroscopically débrided.[65,67,69]

Case Presentation

A 20-year-old right-handed woman who is a collegiate volleyball player initially presented with posterior and lateral elbow pain associated with clicking and popping. The pain started after serving practice and progressed throughout the season, even with conservative therapy. Pain was most notable during serving and overhead smashing and was worse when the elbow was near full extension. MRI revealed a posterolateral synovial fold impinging within the posterolateral aspect of the elbow (**Figure 14**). Intraoperatively, two large posterolateral plicae were found adjacent to the distal humerus, with an additional plica band at the posterior radiocapitellar joint (**Figure 15**). The plicae were débrided, and the patient returned to full participation in sporting activities with complete resolution of symptoms.

Distal Biceps Tears

Overview

The short and long heads of the distal biceps brachii tendon insert on the radial tuberosity, giving the muscle its primary function as a forearm supinator and its secondary function as an elbow flexor. The short head inserts more distally, making it a more efficient elbow flexor, whereas the long head inserts more proximally and ulnarly onto the tuberosity, enhancing its function as a forearm supinator.[70,71] Although patients are generally asymptomatic before rupturing the biceps tendon, the end of the tendon usually shows chronic degenerative changes. Less commonly, partial tears of the distal biceps from the bicipital tuberosity and injuries to the musculotendinous junction may occur.

The patient with a distal biceps tendon rupture is often a middle-aged man; a pop and sudden pain in the antecubital fossa area is usually reported during eccentric supination or flexion activities. Muscle-tendon junction injuries also usually occur in males; however, the shoulder is usually in forward elevation or abduction and the elbow near extension at the time of injury.

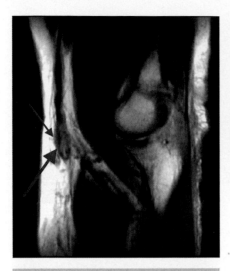

Figure 16 Sagittal T1-weighted MRI of the elbow showing proximal retraction of the distal biceps tendon, indicating a complete tear of the tendon (small arrow) as well as the lacertus fibrosus (large arrow). (Courtesy of Marc R. Safran, MD, Redwood City, CA.)

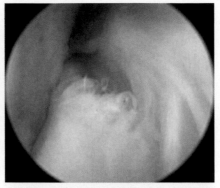

Figure 17 Tenoscopic view of the distal biceps tendon torn from the radial tuberosity. (Courtesy of Marc R. Safran, MD, Redwood City, CA.)

The examination may reveal swelling and ecchymosis extending proximally and distally from the antecubital fossa area as well as a Popeye sign indicating proximal retraction of the muscle belly in complete ruptures.[72] The examination is likely to show tenderness to palpation in the antecubital fossa, pain and/or loss of strength with supination, and a positive hook test (the examiner is unable to hook his or her finger under the biceps tendon because it has retracted proximally) in complete ruptures.

Because plain radiographs rarely show a bony avulsion from the radial tuberosity, ultrasound is used as an additional imaging modality, particularly in partial tears.[73,74] Although MRI is usually not needed to make the diagnosis of distal biceps tendon avulsions, it remains the imaging modality of choice for distal biceps pathology because it can help differentiate partial from complete tendon ruptures and distal tendon ruptures/avulsions from

musculotendinous junction pathology. MRI is also useful in determining the degree of tearing, the size of the gap, the location of the tear, and potentially the status of the lacertus fibrosus (when intact, a late primary repair is more feasible). The distal biceps tendon can be best visualized with a flexed, abducted, supinated view. The characteristic appearance of a distal biceps tendon avulsion includes fluid surrounding the tendon, which is thickened and usually retracted with a gap between the tendon end and the tuberosity; fraying and hyperintensity of the distal tendon if there is prior degeneration; hypertrophy of the radial tuberosity; a fluid-filled bicipital bursa; and blood adjacent to an acutely torn tendon. Fat-suppressed proton density-weighted fast spin-echo axial and sagittal scans are the most useful. Sagittal scans should include a field 10 cm proximal to the joint line to identify the tendon as it slingshots into the upper arm when the lacertus fibrosus is torn.

Treatment of distal biceps tendon pathology depends on the status of the tendon and the demands of the patient. Nonsurgical treatment is recommended for patients with less than 50% tendon disruption and/or low-

demand or medically unfit patients. The recommended nonsurgical treatment of partial tears is initial rest from supination and flexion activities followed by a rehabilitation program to regain strength. Surgical management is indicated for the active patient with a complete tendon rupture because up to 40% of supination strength and 30% of flexion strength may be lost with nonsurgical treatment of complete ruptures.[75,76] Surgical treatment may also be indicated in patients with partial tears if nonsurgical treatment has been unsuccessful. Endoscopy may be useful in determining the extent of partial tears of the distal biceps to help determine if acute repair is indicated. Partial tears may be treated by open or endoscopic débridement or tear completion and reattachment.[77-79] Full-thickness tears may be treated with a single- or dual-incision approach, with lower rates of lateral antebrachial cutaneous nerve palsies reported in the two-incision approach.[80-82] Fixation options include bone tunnels for the two-incision approach, and suture anchors, intraosseous screw fixation, and suspensory cortical buttons for the single-incision technique.[81,83-85] There also has been a report of endoscopically assisted fixation of distal biceps tears using a suspensory cortical button.[86]

Case Presentation

A 54-year-old, right-hand-dominant man who is an avid weight lifter reported left elbow weakness 6 weeks after a motocross racing crash. On examination, the patient had 5/5 elbow flexion strength without any pain and 4/5 supination strength associated with pain. The biceps muscle bulged in his upper arm. MRI showed a tear of the distal biceps tendon with proximal retraction (**Figure 16**), which was confirmed by tenoscopy (**Figure 17**).

Bursitis

Overview

Although there are several bursae surrounding the elbow, the olecranon bursa is the most common location of bursal pathology.[87] The olecranon bursa lies superficial to the olecranon and allows for reduced friction as the skin glides over the olecranon during elbow motion. Olecranon bursitis is an inflammation within the bursal space that can be caused by repetitive elbow motion or pressure on the bursa (chronic sterile bursitis), direct trauma with bleeding into the bursal space (hemorrhagic bursitis), or infection (septic bursitis). Chronic sterile bursitis is the most common form of olecranon bursitis and may be associated with several systemic diseases, including rheumatoid arthritis, gout, or other crystal deposition diseases.[88-91]

Patients will often report pain and swelling over the olecranon, occasionally as a result of trauma. The physical examination usually shows swelling and, occasionally, tenderness to palpation. If infection is present, fluctuation, erythema, and possibly skin abrasions or puncture wounds may be identified. Septic arthritis of the elbow should be ruled out.

Plain radiographs should be obtained to evaluate for the presence of foreign bodies or osteophytic changes of the olecranon. Because olecranon bursitis is mainly a clinical diagnosis, an MRI scan is usually not obtained; however, MRI may assist the clinician in distinguishing sterile from septic bursitis because the latter can reveal bursal loculation and increased soft-tissue signal intensity[92] and may help rule out osteomyelitis. The classic appearance of olecranon bursitis on MRI includes a high signal intensity fluid mass in the superficial soft tissues adjacent to the olecranon process and triceps insertion. Fat-suppressed proton

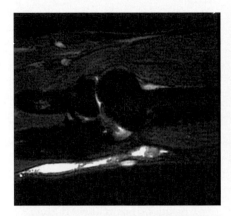

Figure 18 Sagittal T2-weighted MRI showing thickening of the olecranon fossa and fluid (light area at bottom of image) within the olecranon bursa. (Courtesy of Marc R. Safran, MD, Redwood City, CA.)

density-weighted spin-echo images will easily show the fluid, although chronic bursitis may be more difficult to delineate from other solid masses, including neoplasms, because there may be fibrosis, nodules, or granulomas. Aspiration and culture of bursal fluid may also assist in differentiating sterile from septic bursitis.

The initial treatment of chronic, sterile, olecranon bursitis should involve elbow rest, with or without splinting, and anti-inflammatory medications. Recalcitrant cases may be treated with corticosteroid injection.[93] Early septic olecranon bursitis may be treated with aspiration alone, oral or intravenous antibiotics, and close observation. Surgical treatment with bursectomy is reserved for recalcitrant cases of chronic, sterile, olecranon bursitis or septic bursitis. Open excision of the bursa may be performed, but there is a risk of wound healing complications.[94-96] Arthroscopic olecranon bursectomy may be used because it may reduce the risk of wound complications.

Case Presentation

A 21-year-old woman who plays collegiate basketball reported right elbow pain after falling on her elbow sev-

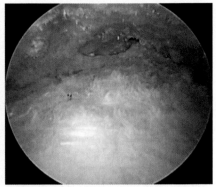

Figure 19 Arthroscopic view of the olecranon fossa of the elbow through the posterior portal following olecranon bursectomy. (Courtesy of Marc R. Safran, MD, Redwood City, CA.)

eral times during a game. She continued to experience pain and swelling with any elbow contact with the floor or an opposing player. Initial treatment consisted of nonsteroidal anti-inflammatory drugs, prednisone, and cortisone injections, as well as padding and rest from activity. Tenderness continued in the area over the olecranon, with periodic swelling of the bursa. On examination she had a palpable, slightly mobile, tender, 2-mm nodule consistent with a fibroma, but an otherwise normal elbow examination. Radiographs were normal; however, MRI showed thickening of the olecranon fossa and some fluid within the bursa (**Figure 18**). Four months after the injury, she was treated with arthroscopic bursectomy (**Figure 19**) and excision of the fibroma because of persistent tenderness and recurrent swelling.

Summary

MRI is a useful adjunct for evaluating the elbow. Arthroscopy can confirm MRI findings with a high degree of correlation. Preoperative planning that includes the use of MRI will help to decrease the likelihood of unexpected findings at the time of elbow arthroscopy.

References

1. Burman M: Arthroscopy of the elbow joint: A cadaver study. *J Bone Joint Surg* 1932;14:349-350.

2. Andrews JR, Carson WG: Arthroscopy of the elbow. *Arthroscopy* 1985;1(2):97-107.

3. Festa A, Mulieri PJ, Newman JS, Spitz DJ, Leslie BM: Effectiveness of magnetic resonance imaging in detecting partial and complete distal biceps tendon rupture. *J Hand Surg Am* 2010;35(1):77-83.

4. Dubberley JH, Faber KJ, Patterson SD, et al: The detection of loose bodies in the elbow: The value of MRI and CT arthrography. *J Bone Joint Surg Br* 2005;87(5):684-686.

5. Waldt S, Bruegel M, Ganter K, et al: Comparison of multislice CT arthrography and MR arthrography for the detection of articular cartilage lesions of the elbow. *Eur Radiol* 2005;15(4):784-791.

6. Thompson WH, Jobe FW, Yocum LA, Pink MM: Ulnar collateral ligament reconstruction in athletes: Muscle-splitting approach without transposition of the ulnar nerve. *J Shoulder Elbow Surg* 2001;10(2):152-157.

7. Stevens KJ: Magnetic resonance imaging of the elbow. *J Magn Reson Imaging* 2010;31(5):1036-1053.

8. Kaplan LJ, Potter HG: MR imaging of ligament injuries to the elbow. *Magn Reson Imaging Clin N Am* 2004;12(2):221-232, v-vi.

9. Giuffrè BM, Moss MJ: Optimal positioning for MRI of the distal biceps brachii tendon: Flexed abducted supinated view. *AJR Am J Roentgenol* 2004;182(4):944-946.

10. Nakanishi K, Masatomi T, Ochi T, et al: MR arthrography of elbow: Evaluation of the ulnar collateral ligament of elbow. *Skeletal Radiol* 1996;25(7):629-634.

11. Azar FM, Andrews JR, Wilk KE, Groh D: Operative treatment of ulnar collateral ligament injuries of the elbow in athletes. *Am J Sports Med* 2000;28(1):16-23.

12. Shahabpour M, Kichouh M, Laridon E, Gielen JL, De Mey J: The effectiveness of diagnostic imaging methods for the assessment of soft tissue and articular disorders of the shoulder and elbow. *Eur J Radiol* 2008;65(2):194-200.

13. Bergin D, Schweitzer ME: Indirect magnetic resonance arthrography. *Skeletal Radiol* 2003;32(10):551-558.

14. Baumgarten TE, Andrews JR, Satterwhite YE: The arthroscopic classification and treatment of osteochondritis dissecans of the capitellum. *Am J Sports Med* 1998;26(4):520-523.

15. Rudzki JR, Paletta GA Jr: Juvenile and adolescent elbow injuries in sports. *Clin Sports Med* 2004;23(4):581-608, ix.

16. Rosenberg ZS, Beltran J, Cheung YY: Pseudodefect of the capitellum: Potential MR imaging pitfall. *Radiology* 1994;191(3):821-823.

17. Difelice GS, Meunier MJ, Paletta GA Jr: Elbow injury in the adolescent athlete, in Altchek DW, Andrews JR, eds: *The Athlete's Elbow*. Philadelphia, PA, Lippincott Williams & Wilkins, 2001, pp 231-248.

18. Jones KJ, Wiesel BB, Sankar WN, Ganley TJ: Arthroscopic management of osteochondritis dissecans of the capitellum: Mid-term results in adolescent athletes. *J Pediatr Orthop* 2010;30(1):8-13.

19. Takeda H, Watarai K, Matsushita T, Saito T, Terashima Y: A surgical treatment for unstable osteochondritis dissecans lesions of the humeral capitellum in adolescent baseball players. *Am J Sports Med* 2002;30(5):713-717.

20. Iwasaki N, Kato H, Ishikawa J, Saitoh S, Minami A: Autologous osteochondral mosaicplasty for capitellar osteochondritis dissecans in teenaged patients. *Am J Sports Med* 2006;34(8):1233-1239.

21. Sato M, Ochi M, Uchio Y, Agung M, Baba H: Transplantation of tissue-engineered cartilage for excessive osteochondritis dissecans of the elbow. *J Shoulder Elbow Surg* 2004;13(2):221-225.

22. Kiyoshige Y, Takagi M, Yuasa K, Hamasaki M: Closed-wedge osteotomy for osteochondritis dissecans of the capitellum: A 7- to 12-year follow-up. *Am J Sports Med* 2000;28(4):534-537.

23. Takahara M, Mura N, Sasaki J, Harada M, Ogino T: Classification, treatment, and outcome of osteochondritis dissecans of the humeral capitellum. *J Bone Joint Surg Am* 2007;89(6):1205-1214.

24. Bot SD, van der Waal JM, Terwee CB, et al: Incidence and prevalence of complaints of the neck and upper extremity in general practice. *Ann Rheum Dis* 2005;64(1):118-123.

25. Nirschl RP, Ashman ES: Elbow tendinopathy: Tennis elbow. *Clin Sports Med* 2003;22(4):813-836.

26. Goldie I: Epicondylitis lateralis humeri (epicondylalgia or tennis elbow): A pathogenetical study. *Acta Chir Scand Suppl* 1964;57(suppl 339):339, 1.

27. Wittenberg RH, Schaal S, Muhr G: Surgical treatment of persistent elbow epicondylitis. *Clin Orthop Relat Res* 1992;278:73-80.

28. Levin D, Nazarian LN, Miller TT, et al: Lateral epicondylitis of the elbow: US findings. *Radiology* 2005;237(1):230-234.

29. Nirschl RP, Pettrone FA: Tennis elbow: The surgical treatment of lateral epicondylitis. *J Bone Joint Surg Am* 1979;61(6A):832-839.

30. Smidt N, van der Windt DA, Assendelft WJ, Devillé WL, Korthals-de Bos IB, Bouter LM: Corticosteroid injections, physio-

therapy, or a wait-and-see policy for lateral epicondylitis: A randomised controlled trial. *Lancet* 2002;359(9307):657-662.

31. Mishra A, Woodall J Jr, Vieira A: Treatment of tendon and muscle using platelet-rich plasma. *Clin Sports Med* 2009;28(1):113-125.

32. Fleisig GS, Andrews JR, Dillman CJ, Escamilla RF: Kinetics of baseball pitching with implications about injury mechanisms. *Am J Sports Med* 1995;23(2):233-239.

33. Werner SL, Fleisig GS, Dillman CJ, Andrews JR: Biomechanics of the elbow during baseball pitching. *J Orthop Sports Phys Ther* 1993;17(6):274-278.

34. Dillman CJ, Smutz P, Werner S: Valgus extension overload in baseball pitching. *Med Sci Sports Exerc* 1991;23(S4):S135.

35. Morrey BF, An KN: Articular and ligamentous contributions to the stability of the elbow joint. *Am J Sports Med* 1983;11(5):315-319.

36. Safran MR: Ulnar collateral ligament injury in the overhead athlete: Diagnosis and treatment. *Clin Sports Med* 2004;23(4):643-663, x.

37. Callaway GH, Field LD, Deng XH, et al: Biomechanical evaluation of the medial collateral ligament of the elbow. *J Bone Joint Surg Am* 1997;79(8):1223-1231.

38. O'Driscoll SW, Lawton RL, Smith AM: The "moving valgus stress test" for medial collateral ligament tears of the elbow. *Am J Sports Med* 2005;33(2):231-239.

39. Pappas AM: Elbow problems associated with baseball during childhood and adolescence. *Clin Orthop Relat Res* 1982;164:30-41.

40. Rettig AC, Sherrill C, Snead DS, Mendler JC, Mieling P: Nonoperative treatment of ulnar collateral ligament injuries in throwing athletes. *Am J Sports Med* 2001;29(1):15-17.

41. Jobe FW, Stark H, Lombardo SJ: Reconstruction of the ulnar collateral ligament in athletes. *J Bone Joint Surg Am* 1986;68(8):1158-1163.

42. Smith GR, Altchek DW, Pagnani MJ, Keeley JR: A muscle-splitting approach to the ulnar collateral ligament of the elbow: Neuroanatomy and operative technique. *Am J Sports Med* 1996;24(5):575-580.

43. Rohrbough JT, Altchek DW, Hyman J, Williams RJ III, Botts JD: Medial collateral ligament reconstruction of the elbow using the docking technique. *Am J Sports Med* 2002;30(4):541-548.

44. Ahmad CS, Lee TQ, ElAttrache NS: Biomechanical evaluation of a new ulnar collateral ligament reconstruction technique with interference screw fixation. *Am J Sports Med* 2003;31(3):332-337.

45. Dines JS, ElAttrache NS, Conway JE, Smith W, Ahmad CS: Clinical outcomes of the DANE TJ technique to treat ulnar collateral ligament insufficiency of the elbow. *Am J Sports Med* 2007;35(12):2039-2044.

46. Morrey BF: *The Elbow and Its Disorders*, ed 3. Philadelphia, PA, WB Saunders, 2000.

47. Dunning CE, Zarzour ZD, Patterson SD, Johnson JA, King GJ: Ligamentous stabilizers against posterolateral rotatory instability of the elbow. *J Bone Joint Surg Am* 2001;83A(12):1823-1828.

48. McAdams TR, Masters GW, Srivastava S: The effect of arthroscopic sectioning of the lateral ligament complex of the elbow on posterolateral rotatory stability. *J Shoulder Elbow Surg* 2005;14(3):298-301.

49. O'Driscoll SW, Bell DF, Morrey BF: Posterolateral rotatory instability of the elbow. *J Bone Joint Surg Am* 1991;73(3):440-446.

50. Regan W, Lapner PC: Prospective evaluation of two diagnostic ap-

prehension signs for posterolateral instability of the elbow. *J Shoulder Elbow Surg* 2006;15(3):344-346.

51. Potter HG, Weiland AJ, Schatz JA, Paletta GA, Hotchkiss RN: Posterolateral rotatory instability of the elbow: Usefulness of MR imaging in diagnosis. *Radiology* 1997;204(1):185-189.

52. Cheung EV: Chronic lateral elbow instability. *Orthop Clin North Am* 2008;39(2):221-228, vi-vii.

53. Stanley D: Prevalence and etiology of symptomatic elbow osteoarthritis. *J Shoulder Elbow Surg* 1994;3:386-389.

54. Solia P: Osteochonodrosis tables. *Acta Rheumatol Scand* 1960;6:151-160.

55. Kokkalis ZT, Schmidt CC, Sotereanos DG: Elbow arthritis: Current concepts. *J Hand Surg Am* 2009;34(4):761-768.

56. Adams JE, Wolff LH III, Merten SM, Steinmann SP: Osteoarthritis of the elbow: Results of arthroscopic osteophyte resection and capsulectomy. *J Shoulder Elbow Surg* 2008;17(1):126-131.

57. Krishnan SG, Harkins DC, Pennington SD, Harrison DK, Burkhead WZ: Arthroscopic ulnohumeral arthroplasty for degenerative arthritis of the elbow in patients under fifty years of age. *J Shoulder Elbow Surg* 2007;16(4):443-448.

58. Ahmad CS, Park MC, Elattrache NS: Elbow medial ulnar collateral ligament insufficiency alters posteromedial olecranon contact. *Am J Sports Med* 2004;32(7):1607-1612.

59. Ahmad CS, ElAttrache NS: Valgus extension overload syndrome and stress injury of the olecranon. *Clin Sports Med* 2004;23(4):665-676.

60. Andrews JR, Wilk KE, Satterwhite YE, Tedder JL: Physical examination of the thrower's elbow. *J Orthop Sports Phys Ther* 1993;17(6):296-304.

61. Wilson FD, Andrews JR, Blackburn TA, McCluskey G: Valgus extension overload in the pitching elbow. *Am J Sports Med* 1983;11(2):83-88.

62. Werner SL, Murray TA, Hawkins RJ, Gill TJ: Relationship between throwing mechanics and elbow valgus in professional baseball pitchers. *J Shoulder Elbow Surg* 2002;11(2):151-155.

63. Aguinaldo AL, Chambers H: Correlation of throwing mechanics with elbow valgus load in adult baseball pitchers. *Am J Sports Med* 2009;37(10):2043-2048.

64. Kamineni S, ElAttrache NS, O'driscoll SW, et al: Medial collateral ligament strain with partial posteromedial olecranon resection: A biomechanical study. *J Bone Joint Surg Am* 2004;86-A(11):2424-2430.

65. Clarke RP: Symptomatic, lateral synovial fringe (plica) of the elbow joint. *Arthroscopy* 1988;4(2):112-116.

66. Ruch DS, Papadonikolakis A, Campolattaro RM: The posterolateral plica: A cause of refractory lateral elbow pain. *J Shoulder Elbow Surg* 2006;15(3):367-370.

67. Kim DH, Gambardella RA, Elattrache NS, Yocum LA, Jobe FW: Arthroscopic treatment of posterolateral elbow impingement from lateral synovial plicae in throwing athletes and golfers. *Am J Sports Med* 2006;34(3):438-444.

68. Steinert AF, Goebel S, Rucker A, Barthel T: Snapping elbow caused by hypertrophic synovial plica in the radiohumeral joint: A report of three cases and review of literature. *Arch Orthop Trauma Surg* 2010;130(3):347-351.

69. Akagi M, Nakamura T: Snapping elbow caused by the synovial fold in the radiohumeral joint. *J Shoulder Elbow Surg* 1998;7(4):427-429.

70. Kulshreshtha R, Singh R, Sinha J, Hall S: Anatomy of the distal biceps brachii tendon and its clinical relevance. *Clin Orthop Relat Res* 2007;456:117-120.

71. Bain GI, Johnson LJ, Turner PC: Treatment of partial distal biceps tendon tears. *Sports Med Arthrosc* 2008;16(3):154-161.

72. Vidal AF, Drakos MC, Allen AA: Biceps tendon and triceps tendon injuries. *Clin Sports Med* 2004;23(4):707-722, xi.

73. Davis BM, Yassine Z: An etiologic factor in tear of the distal tendon of the biceps brachii. *J Bone Joint Surg Am* 1956;38A:1365-1368.

74. Tagliafico A, Michaud J, Capaccio E, Derchi LE, Martinoli C: Ultrasound demonstration of distal biceps tendon bifurcation: Normal and abnormal findings. *Eur Radiol* 2010;20(1):202-208.

75. Morrey BF, Askew LJ, An KN, Dobyns JH: Rupture of the distal tendon of the biceps brachii: A biomechanical study. *J Bone Joint Surg Am* 1985;67(3):418-421.

76. Baker BE, Bierwagen D: Rupture of the distal tendon of the biceps brachii: Operative versus nonoperative treatment. *J Bone Joint Surg Am* 1985;67(3):414-417.

77. Bourne MH, Morrey BF: Partial rupture of the distal biceps tendon. *Clin Orthop Relat Res* 1991;271:143-148.

78. Eames MH, Bain GI: Distal biceps tendon endoscopy and anterior elbow arthroscopy portal. *Tech Shoulder Elbow Surg* 2006;7:139-142.

79. Dellaero DT, Mallon WJ: Surgical treatment of partial biceps tendon ruptures at the elbow. *J Shoulder Elbow Surg* 2006;15(2):215-217.

80. Boyd HB, Anderson LD: A method for reinsertion of the distal biceps brachii tendon. *J Bone Joint Surg Am* 1961;43:1041-1043.

81. Kelly EW, Morrey BF, O'Driscoll SW: Complications of repair of the distal biceps tendon with the modified two-incision technique. *J Bone Joint Surg Am* 2000;82-A(11):1575-1581.

82. El-Hawary R, Macdermid JC, Faber KJ, Patterson SD, King GJ: Distal biceps tendon repair: Comparison of surgical techniques. *J Hand Surg Am* 2003;28(3):496-502.

83. John CK, Field LD, Weiss KS, Savoie FH III: Single-incision repair of acute distal biceps ruptures by use of suture anchors. *J Shoulder Elbow Surg* 2007;16(1):78-83.

84. Eardley WG, Odak S, Adesina TS, Jeavons RP, McVie JL: Bioabsorbable interference screw fixation of distal biceps ruptures through a single anterior incision: A single-surgeon case series and review of the literature. *Arch Orthop Trauma Surg* 2010;130(7):875-881.

85. Bain GI, Prem H, Heptinstall RJ, Verhellen R, Paix D: Repair of distal biceps tendon rupture: A new technique using the Endobutton. *J Shoulder Elbow Surg* 2000;9(2):120-126.

86. Sharma S, MacKay G: Endoscopic repair of distal biceps tendon using an EndoButton. *Arthroscopy* 2005;21(7):897.

87. Pien FD, Ching D, Kim E: Septic bursitis: Experience in a community practice. *Orthopedics* 1991;14(9):981-984.

88. Ho G Jr, Tice AD, Kaplan SR: Septic bursitis in the prepatellar and olecranon bursae: An analysis of 25 cases. *Ann Intern Med* 1978;89(1):21-27.

89. Fisher RH: Conservative treatment of distended patellar and olecranon bursae. *Clin Orthop Relat Res* 1977;123:98.

90. McCarty DJ Jr, Gatter RA: Recurrent acute inflammation associated with focal apatite crystal deposition. *Arthritis Rheum* 1966;9(6):804-819.

91. Macfarlane JD, van der Linden SJ: Leaking rheumatoid olecranon bursitis as a cause of forearm swelling. *Ann Rheum Dis* 1981; 40(3):309-311.

92. Floemer F, Morrison WB, Bongartz G, Ledermann HP: MRI characteristics of olecranon bursitis. *AJR Am J Roentgenol* 2004; 183(1):29-34.

93. Smith DL, McAfee JH, Lucas LM, Kumar KL, Romney DM: Treatment of nonseptic olecranon bursitis: A controlled, blinded prospective trial. *Arch Intern Med* 1989;149(11):2527-2530.

94. Stewart NJ, Manzanares JB, Morrey BF: Surgical treatment of aseptic olecranon bursitis. *J Shoulder Elbow Surg* 1997;6(1):49-54.

95. Kerr DR, Carpenter CW: Arthroscopic resection of olecranon and prepatellar bursae. *Arthroscopy* 1990;6(2):86-88.

96. Ogilvie-Harris DJ, Gilbart M: Endoscopic bursal resection: The olecranon bursa and prepatellar bursa. *Arthroscopy* 2000;16(3): 249-253.

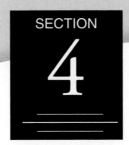
Adult Reconstruction: Hip

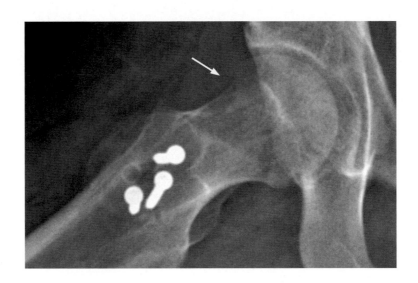

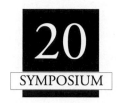

New Frontiers in Cartilage Imaging of the Hip

Paul E. Beaulé, MD, FRCSC
Young-Jo Kim, MD, PhD
Kawan S. Rakhra, MD, FRCPC
David Stelzeneder, MD
Thomas D. Brown, PhD

Abstract

High-resolution MRI for cartilage mapping is a rapidly evolving field that is contributing to a better understanding of osteoarthritis. The basic science of cartilage imaging uses different modalities (such as T1rho, T2 mapping, delayed gadolinium-enhanced MRI of cartilage) and has clinical applicability for treating hip disorders in the young adult. These imaging techniques rely on biomarkers to quantify early cartilage degeneration. The common biomarkers are proteoglycan concentration and collagen integrity. Imaging the hip presents unique challenges because of its sphericity, the close apposition of the two cartilage layers, and the limitations in using surface coils.

Instr Course Lect 2012;61:253-262.

Aberrant hip anatomy, such as developmental dysplasia or femoroacetabular impingement (FAI), is known to increase the risk of early osteoarthritis (OA).[1-3] The goal of surgical treatment is to correct these anatomic deformities before the onset of significant OA, providing pain relief and improved function for patients.[4] How-

ever, some patients continue to have significant pain, which is often associated with the progression of arthritis. Although the causes of surgical failure and/or arthritis progression are multifactorial, the relative health of the articular cartilage at the time of surgery is a strong predictor of outcomes.[4-7] Traditionally, clinicians have relied on

measuring the width of the joint space on conventional AP radiographs to assess the degree of OA. The Tönnis grade has been the most commonly used determinant for providing guidance on expected outcomes when surgically treating patients with hip dysplasia or FAI[5,6,8] (**Table 1**). However, because joint preservation surgery of the hip is mainly indicated for patients with no or only minor radiographic signs of OA, noninvasive quantification of cartilage quality before surgery is desirable to provide better counsel on the appropriateness and timing of surgical treatment before the occurrence of significant cartilage deterioration.[7]

Although current MRI techniques provide useful information regarding the macroscopic identification of cartilage defects and characterization of labral changes (hypertrophy with dysplasia), they do not provide prognostic information regarding the longevity of the hip joint.[9,10] Consequently, advanced MRI techniques are being applied to detect biochemical changes in the macromolecular matrix, which can alter the biomechanical properties of cartilage before gross morphologic

Dr. Beaulé or an immediate family member has received royalties from Wright Medical Technology; is a member of a speakers' bureau or has made paid presentations on behalf of Wright Medical Technology, Smith & Nephew, and MEDACTA; serves as a paid consultant to Corin USA, Smith & Nephew, Wright Medical Technology, and MEDACTA; owns stock or stock options held in Wright Medical Technology; and has received research or institutional support from Corin USA. Dr. Kim or an immediate family member serves as an unpaid consultant to Siemens Health Care; owns stock or stock options in Procter & Gamble; has received research or institutional support from Siemens Health Care; and has received nonincome support (such as equipment or services), commercially derived honoraria, or other non–research-related funding (such as paid travel) from Siemens Health Care. Dr. Brown or an immediate family member serves as a paid consultant to Smith & Nephew. Neither Dr. Rakhra and Dr. Stelzeneder nor any immediate family members have received anything of value from or own stock in a commercial company or institution related directly or indirectly to the subject of this chapter.

Table 1

Tönnis Classification System

Grade	Characteristics
0	No signs of osteoarthritis
1	Slight narrowing of joint space, slight lipping at the joint margin, and slight sclerosis of the femoral head or acetabulum
2	Small cysts in the femoral head or acetabulum, increasing narrowing of the joint space, and moderate loss of sphericity of the femoral head
3	Large cysts, severe narrowing or obliteration of the joint space, severe deformity of the femoral head, and osteonecrosis

cartilage damage occurs. These techniques have both diagnostic and prognostic value.[11] In developing better tools to assess cartilage health and deterioration, it is necessary to choose a surrogate (biomarker) to indicate the condition of the cartilage.[12] A biomarker is a characteristic that is objectively measured and evaluated as an indicator of normal biologic processes, pathogenic processes, or responses to a therapeutic intervention.[12] A biomarker that is predictive of clinical benefit or harm (or lack of benefit) is referred to as a surrogate end point. Biomarkers (including surrogate end points) require rigorous scientific validation. The process of developing a biomarker involves three phases: (1) face validity (Based on what is known, would the putative biomarker be generally viewed as relevant and useful?); (2) technical validity (Does the marker measure what it aims to measure?); and (3) pathophysiologic validity (Is the information provided by the marker of pathophysiologic or clinical use?).[12]

High-resolution MRI techniques, such as delayed gadolinium-enhanced MRI of cartilage (dGEMRIC), T2 mapping, and T1rho currently used in the knee[13] and more recently in the hip,[14] allow the quantification and characterization of the cartilage extracellular matrix (for example, proteoglycan content as well as orientation of type II collagen fibers) and provide

greater insight into the health of the articular cartilage. Characteristics of early cartilage breakdown include the loss of proteoglycans, changes in water content, and molecular-level changes in collagen.[15]

This chapter reviews the principles of cartilage imaging in terms of compositional assessment and reliable structural assessment (for example, geometric delineation of cartilage tissue boundaries). The physical basis and the respective advantages and disadvantages will be summarized for the three currently best-established techniques for MRI compositional assessments of cartilage: T2 mapping, dGEMRIC, and T1rho. Current clinical evidence of cartilage assessment in the hip and promising MRI techniques currently in the research stage will be considered.

Principles of Cartilage Imaging

The extensive experience with MRI of the knee provides a useful base of reference regarding the information potentially available to characterize the functional status of cartilage at the hip. Subjective or semiquantitative MRI structural assessments of knee joint cartilage are a mainstay of routine orthopaedic practice. All information present in MRI scans is necessarily indirect in that it merely reflects site-specific relative rates of relaxation/decay of magnet-induced perturba-

tions of the orientations of hydrogen nuclei in the tissue(s) being scanned.[16] Depending on the particulars of the transient magnetic pulses used to produce those nuclear orientation perturbations and on the particular aspect of the orientation change being monitored (information collectively designated as the MRI sequence), entirely different signal appearances result. Empirically, several sequences have emerged as especially useful for articular joints, including T1-weighted spoiled gradient echo and fast low-angle shot sequences, T2-weighted fast spin-echo and turbo spin-echo sequences, and fat-suppressed sequences.[17]

For purposes of MRI signal interpretation, it is important to remember that cartilage is richly heterogeneous at both the molecular and tissue levels.[18] The nuclear orientation relaxations that give rise to the MRI signals primarily arise from hydrogen present in the water of interstitial fluid, which comprises approximately 70% to 75% of the bulk weight of the tissues. The motility of these water molecules is influenced by the other extracellular matrix constituents, primarily the collagen (mainly type II) and the aggrecan. Of particular note, the chondroitin and keratan sulfate side units of proteoglycan macromolecules are negatively charged and are therefore hydrophilic, a property that can be exploited by MRI to detect the effective concentrations (fixed charge density) of those entities, and whose depletion is a key attribute of cartilage degeneration. At the tissue level, there are zonal (layer) differences in collagen architecture and in proteoglycan concentration that give rise to zonal differences in MRI signal intensity.

Structural Assessment

Delineation of cartilage boundaries (segmentation), a labor-intensive exercise (especially in three dimensions), is

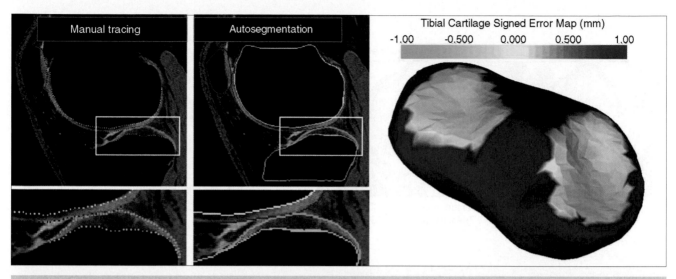

Figure 1 MRI scans on the left compare segmentations done manually versus automatically using the layered optimal graph image segmentation of multiple objects and surfaces (LOGISMOS) technique. The color image on the right shows the differences in thickness determined by these two techniques. It may be misleading to use the term "error," because that presumes that the manual technique is ground truth, which may not be the case. Submillimeter differences are indicated in the weight-bearing area. (Reproduced with permission from Yin Y, Zhang X, Williams R, et al: LOGISMOS-layered optimal graph image segmentation of multiple objects and surfaces: Cartilage segmentation in the knee joint. *IEEE Trans Med Imaging* 2010;29:2023-2037.)

approached at several levels of automation. Most commonly, segmentation is done manually by experienced observers identifying the visually apparent cartilage boundaries at many local sites, with continuous mathematical surfaces subsequently being fitted and various postprocessing operations then being performed (for example, measurement of cartilage thickness or volume).[19] Another broad class of segmentation assessments is semiautomated, wherein a human observer identifies one or more seed points at a cartilage boundary, after which computational edge-detection routines propagate the presumed boundary transverse to the direction of strongest magnetic resonance signal contrast.[20] Recently, fully automated segmentation techniques (**Figure 1**) have been introduced that require only a generic template of the expected anatomic features[21] (for example, distal femur, proximal tibia, and patella). The template is then morphed to match the individual patient's images, which in turn provide approximate starting points for definitive computational cartilage-edge detection. Another geometric challenge in cartilage MRI is image registration (identifying the same local anatomic site in images of a given patient collected at serial time points). Here, an attractive approach is to use landmarks that can be objectively identified at pixel or near pixel levels of precision.

Compositional Assessment
T2-Mapping

Although T2-weighted images have long been used for structural assessments, a change in T2-weighted signal intensity (change in T2 relaxation time) is influenced by changes in water-water and water-macromolecular interactions, which provide information about matrix alterations. Early-stage degeneration involves collagen disruption, which results in slower equilibration of magnet-perturbations of hydrogen nucleus orientation, and hence longer T2 times. Dunn et al[22] demonstrated that normalized T2 relaxation times differed from normal values for early-stage tibiofemoral arthritis, although further changes were not demonstrable between groups of patients with severe versus mild OA. In early degeneration, the spatial distribution of T2 times becomes more heterogeneous. Perhaps for that reason, Koff et al[23] was unable to document statistically significant changes in T2 signal of whole-thickness osteoarthritic patellofemoral cartilage despite clearly evident zone-dependent (depth-dependent) differences. When specific regions involving cartilage lesions are carefully segmented, degeneration-dependent T2 signal abnormalities emerge.[24] Another consideration limiting the use of T2 mapping is that the T2 signal is sensitive to collagen orientation (in the extreme, the signal disappears entirely for collagen oriented at the so-called magic angle to the main magnet field), thus making it difficult to establish site-independent relationships for T2 signal versus degeneration.

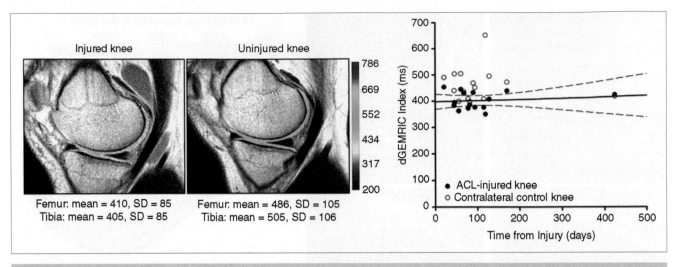

Injured knee

Femur: mean = 410, SD = 85
Tibia: mean = 405, SD = 85

Uninjured knee

Femur: mean = 486, SD = 105
Tibia: mean = 505, SD = 106

Figure 2   The two MRI scans on the left show dGEMRIC index spatial distributions in an anterior cruciate-injured knee versus the uninjured contralateral knee. The dGEMRIC index values are lower with injury because the cartilage presumably degenerates. The data graph on the right contrasts dGEMRIC index values for the injured versus uninjured knees for patients with anterior cruciate injuries whose MRI scans were obtained at various times after injury. (Reproduced with permission from Fleming BC, Oksendahl HL, Mehan WA, et al: Delayed Gadolinium-Enhanced MR Imaging of Cartilage (dGEMRIC) following ACL injury. *Osteoarthritis and Cartilage* 2010;18:662-667.)

Delayed Gadolinium-Enhanced MRI of Cartilage

Currently, the most widely used MRI technique for assessing cartilage composition is dGEMRIC. An intravenously injected, negatively charged contrast agent (gadopentetate^{2-}), upon equilibration, distributes within cartilage in an inverse relationship with the concentration of (negatively charged) glycosaminoglycan (GAG) fixed-charge density present in the cartilage matrix; this indirectly measures proteoglycan content within hyaline cartilage. A postcontrast T1 map can be obtained that provides quantitative information regarding the charge density of cartilage from which the amount of cartilage damage can be inferred. This technique requires the intravenous injection of gadolinium contrast, followed by a variable delay and/or exercise regimen. A very specific protocol must be followed in terms of exercise and time delay to reproducibly reach the equilibration stage,[25] and the injection of contrast medium is an invasive procedure. There also are some cautionary issues

in using dGEMRIC in patients with renal disorders, especially nephrogenic systemic fibrosis.

A large body of supporting evidence has documented a clear and direct relationship between GAG concentration assessed via dGEMRIC versus GAG concentration formally assayed biochemically.[26] Strong correlation has been demonstrated in cadavers between superficial-region tibial plateau stiffness versus dGEMRIC-assessed GAG concentration in the most superficial (600 μm) cartilage regions.[27] Reductions in dGEMRIC-apparent GAG concentrations have been documented in clinical situations involving early cartilage degeneration, both longitudinally in time and cross-sectionally[28,29] (**Figure 2**).

T1rho Mapping

A different MRI approach to cartilage compositional assessment is measuring spin-lattice relaxation time in a rotating reference frame, a technique known as T1rho mapping. This approach involves a specialty MRI pulse sequence, which is fully transparent to

the patient and has none of the logistic drawbacks associated with dGEMRIC. A trade-off, however, is that this sequence involves complex specialty programming and is not typically commercially available. Another consideration with T1rho is that radiofrequency energy transfer to the patient (specific absorption rate effect) tends to be higher than for most MRI sequences, which requires careful adherence to protocol guidelines. Like T2 relaxation, T1rho relaxation depends on a complex interaction between matrix water and the matrix macromolecules. Unlike dGEMRIC, T1rho has a substantial element of uncertainty regarding specifically what is being measured. Nevertheless, patients with reports of knee pain that plausibly involve early degeneration have exhibited readily detectable increases in T1rho relaxation time, substantially more vivid than those seen for T2 relaxation.[30] T1rho also has been shown to exhibit stronger and more consistent changes than T2 sequences in situations of relatively severe cartilage degeneration.[31] To date, relatively little work has been done to directly compare T1rho and dGEMRIC. In osteochondral specimens resected during total knee replacement surgery and from cadaver knees, regions of elevated dGEMRIC intensity were found to correspond to regions of reduced T1rho. However, formal correlations of the numerical values from these two respective imaging modalities failed to reach levels of statistical significance.[32]

Experience in structural and compositional assessment of cartilage at the knee provides motivational illustrations regarding the types of measurements that may be possible at the hip. However, the knee is substantially more amenable to MRI because of the generally greater thickness of the involved cartilage and especially because of the much more favorable anatomy for close-in circumferential positioning of receiver coils.

The Hip Joint

There are inherent challenges to biochemical imaging of hip cartilage compared with other joints such as the knee, which was the subject of much of the initial research on cartilage mapping. Hip hyaline cartilage is much thinner, especially in the periphery of the joint where the earliest chondral damage is known to occur.[33] The hip joint is grossly spherical, with resultant curvature of the joint space and articular surfaces, such that planar acquisition imaging slices can be susceptible to volume averaging artifacts. The articular surfaces of the acetabulum and femoral head are also closely opposed to one another, making it challenging to spatially separate the two surfaces.[34] For this reason, several studies on cartilage mapping in the hip performed the analysis on a combined bilayer, including both the acetabular and the femoral surfaces.[35,36] Several different biochemical imaging protocols, including dGEMRIC, T1rho, and T2 and T2-star (T2*) cartilage mapping, have

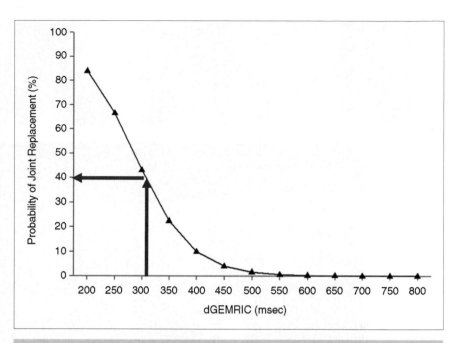

Figure 3 Graph showing probability of total hip replacement as a function of the dGEMRIC index. (Adapted from Cunnigham T, Jessel R, Zurakowski D, Millis MB, Kim YJ: Delayed gadolinium-enhanced magnetic resonance imaging of cartilage to predict early failure of Bernese periacetabular osteotomy for hip dysplasia. *J Bone Joint Surg Am* 2006;88(7):1540-1548.)

been conducted to varying degrees in normal and symptomatic hips.[35,37,38] To date, dGEMRIC has been the most widely studied imaging method used in the hip joint, mainly in the treatment of symptomatic hip dysplasia.[38-41] Jessel et al[7] studied 96 hips with acetabular dysplasia to evaluate risk factors of early OA as defined by dGEMRIC. Hips with a dGEMRIC index less than 390 ms (at 1.5 tesla) were defined as having early OA. These hips were significantly older, had significantly smaller lateral and anterior center-edge angles and joint space width, and had a significantly increased incidence of radiographic joint subluxation and labral tears. Using these data, a logistic regression model for the prediction of significant OA (dGEMRIC index < 390 ms) was calculated, showing the following odds ratios: age = 1.07/year; lateral center-edge angle = 0.94/degree; and the presence of labral tears = 3.28.[7] The

dGEMRIC index correlated with the Western Ontario and McMaster Universities Osteoarthritis Index score but not with joint space width measured with radiographs.[36] Cunningham et al[42] showed the value of the dGEMRIC index in predicting the clinical outcome of patients treated with a Bernese periacetabular osteotomy for hip dysplasia. In comparing the group in which the osteotomy failed (total hip arthroplasty was needed) with the group with a satisfactory outcome, radiographic joint subluxation, the Tönnis grade, joint space width, and the dGEMRIC index were significantly different.[42] The dGEMRIC index in the group with the failed osteotomy was 370 ± 88 ms compared with 498 ± 105 ms in the satisfactory group (*P* < 0.001). For a 100 ms increase in the dGEMRIC value, the likelihood of failure decreased by 77% (odds ratio 0.23; *P* = 0.002). The probability of total hip arthro-

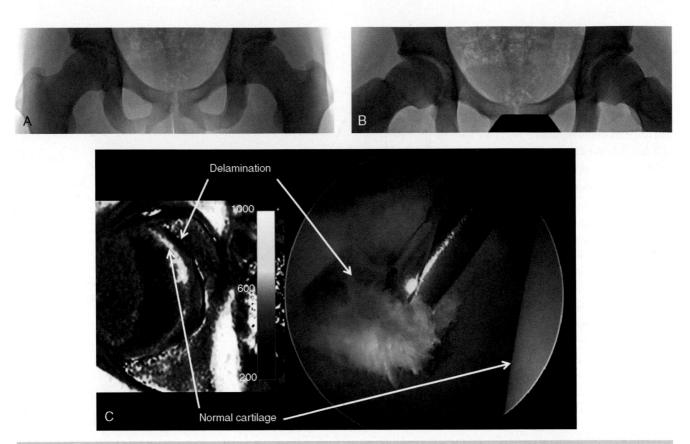

Figure 4 AP radiograph (**A**) and frog lateral radiograph (**B**) of the right hip of a 19-year-old man with FAI. No radiographic signs of OA are detectable. **C,** The low dGEMRIC index at the anterosuperior quadrant correlated with the intraoperative finding of cartilage delamination in this patient. (Courtesy of the Children's Orthopaedic Surgery Foundation, Boston, MA.)

plasty increased dramatically when the dGEMRIC index was less than 390 ms[42] (**Figure 3**).

A recent study evaluated the ability of dGEMRIC to detect cartilage damage preoperatively in FAI.[43] The average dGEMRIC index of hips with FAI was significantly lower compared with asymptomatic hips (464 ± 64 ms in hips with FAI). In the FAI hip, dGEMRIC has been shown to correlate with pain and the size of the cam deformity and demonstrate abnormal cartilage profiles even in asymptomatic individuals with FAI-predisposing joint morphology. The dGEMRIC index in morphologically normal hips averaged 570 ± 90 ms at 1.5 tesla. A dGEMRIC index of 390 ms is 2 SD below normal and can be used as a threshold value at 1.5 tesla.[7,36] The

use of 3.0 tesla magnetic resonance systems in clinical practice provides increased image resolution and/or reduced imaging time. However, absolute dGEMRIC index values must be interpreted differently on 1.5 and 3.0 tesla scans. Williams et al[44] reported 1.35-times average higher dGEMRIC index values at 3.0 compared with 1.5 tesla. The normal value of 570 ± 90 ms at 1.5 tesla would shift to 770 ms at 3.0 tesla, and the cutoff for OA would shift from 390 ms at 1.5 tesla to 527 ms at 3.0 tesla. These findings are consistent with the data of Pollard et al[38] who reported a dGEMRIC index of 720 to 790 ms for healthy asymptomatic individuals. A limitation to applying the dGEMRIC index in FAI is that only the weight-bearing area of the hip can be assessed with coronal

slices, whereas cartilage damage in cam-type impingement is often localized anteriorly; therefore, the areas of maximum damage may be missed in a two-dimensional scan. A recently developed three-dimensional sequence for dGEMRIC in the hip at 1.5 tesla was used for the preliminary assessment of 26 FAI patients and 10 healthy volunteers.[39,45] Additional spatial information on the pattern of cartilage damage was obtained (**Figure 4**). In this study, it was not possible to separate femoral and acetabular cartilages in the image analysis.

T1rho is another technique that provides information on the proteoglycan content of hyaline cartilage and does not require the administration of intravenous gadolinium contrast.[34,46-48] T1rho has been performed in the normal asymptomatic hip, in the OA hip, and recently in the FAI hip[37] (**Figure 5**). The technique can detect differences in the cartilage profiles of normal and diseased hips, although the number of published studies to date is small and further validation is required.

T2 cartilage mapping is a noncontrast-based technique that is sensitive to changes in collagen content and architecture as well as cartilage hydration but to date has not been performed in the FAI hip.[14,35] T2* mapping may provide similar information as T2 with regard to collagen status, although it is sensitive to other compositional changes, such as cartilage calcification.[14]

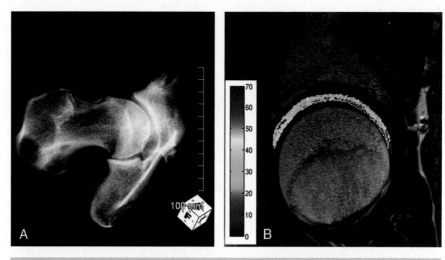

Figure 5 **A,** A 30-year-old man with a cam deformity of the hip as seen on a CT reconstruction of the Dunn view. **B,** The corresponding T1rho cartilage mapping shows loss of proteoglycans anterosuperiorly. The key represents the color map of the T1rho relaxation values.

Future Directions

Four lesser-known imaging techniques, which are currently in the research stage, have the potential to further improve cartilage compositional assessment. One promising pathway is to directly image magnet-induced orientation changes of sodium nuclei (a process conceptually analogous to conventional imaging of magnet-induced orientation changes of hydrogen nuclei). Like dGEMRIC, sodium imaging is attractive because it can directly quantify fixed charge density because the concentration of sodium in the cartilage matrix is compositionally in osmotic equilibrium with the water attracted to the (charged) chondroitin and keratan sulfate components of the GAG.[49] An important drawback of sodium imaging is that the signal-to-noise ratio is quite low, therefore requiring very high magnet field strength (7 tesla or more, whereas magnets in current clinical use are 1.5- or 3-tesla instruments). Also, specialty imaging equipment is required. These drawbacks potentially may be overcome by further technical developments.

Diffusion tensor imaging, in which differences in the direction of preferential motility of cartilage matrix water are transduced, is another promising technique in the research stage of development. This preferential water motility direction is predominantly influenced by the concentration and prevailing orientation of collagen fibers, which undergo change with early degeneration.[50] Diffusion tensor images specifically document the degree of local anisotropy of water motility and provide information on the status of the collagen fiber architecture. Very high magnet field strengths are needed to acquire usable images.

A third, lesser-developed technique is T2* imaging, which differs from conventional T2 imaging in terms of using a gradient-echo rather than a spin-echo pulse to perturb nuclear orientations. The resulting images appear to provide better discrimination of layerwise differences of cartilage compositional changes than those from T2 imaging and appear to offer better resolution at sites where cartilage is relatively thin.[51] However, like T2 imaging, T2* is relatively nonspecific re-

garding the specific compositional parameter(s) being imaged.

A fourth technique under development is magnetization transfer, which transduces the relative fraction of cartilage interstitial water, which is bound to matrix macromolecules. This reflects macromolecular integrity and concentration, which are altered in abnormal cartilage.[52]

Summary

Plain radiographs provide important information for defining bony abnormalities of the hip and determining the classic signs of arthritis; however, because of its two-dimensional nature, complete assessment of the health of the articular cartilage is limited from a structural standpoint. For these reasons, cartilage imaging in the hip provides a unique opportunity to study early degenerative changes and optimize the timing of interventions for joint preservation. The advent of high field scanners (3.0 tesla and higher), three-dimensional volume acquisitions, and continual advances in scanner hardware and surface coil technology will facilitate improved imaging with higher signal to noise ratios and shorter scan times. Future developments and increases in magnetic field strength will bring further improvements that will contribute to the understanding and treatment of early OA of the hip.

References

1. Murphy SB, Ganz R, Müller ME: The prognosis in untreated dysplasia of the hip: A study of radiographic factors that predict the outcome. *J Bone Joint Surg Am* 1995;77(7):985-989.

2. Cooperman DR, Wallensten R, Stulberg SD: Acetabular dysplasia in the adult. *Clin Orthop Relat Res* 1983;175:79-85.

3. Ganz R, Leunig M, Leunig-Ganz K, Harris WH: The etiology of osteoarthritis of the hip: An integrated mechanical concept. *Clin Orthop Relat Res* 2008; 466(2):264-272.

4. Beaulé PE, Allen DJ, Clohisy JC, Schoenecker PE, Leunig M: The young adult with hip impingement: Deciding on the optimal intervention. *J Bone Joint Surg Am* 2009;91(1):210-221.

5. Trousdale RT, Ekkernkamp A, Ganz R, Wallrichs SL: Periacetabular and intertrochanteric osteotomy for the treatment of osteoarthrosis in dysplastic hips. *J Bone Joint Surg Am* 1995;77(1): 73-85.

6. Ribas M, Ledesma R, Cardenas C, Marin-Peña O, Toro J, Caceres E: Clinical results after anterior mini-open approach for femoroacetabular impingement in early degenerative stage. *Hip Int* 2010; 20(S7, Suppl 7):36-42.

7. Jessel RH, Zurakowski D, Zilkens C, Burstein D, Gray ML, Kim YJ: Radiographic and patient factors associated with preradiographic osteoarthritis in hip dysplasia. *J Bone Joint Surg Am* 2009;91(5):1120-1129.

8. Tönnis D, Heinecke A: Acetabular and femoral anteversion: Relationship with osteoarthritis of the hip. *J Bone Joint Surg Am* 1999; 81(12):1747-1770.

9. Beaulé PE, Zaragoza EJ, Copelan N: Magnetic resonance imaging with gadolinium arthrography to assess acetabular cartilage delamination: A report of four cases. *J Bone Joint Surg Am* 2004; 86-A(10):2294-2298.

10. Leunig M, Podeszwa D, Beck M, Werlen S, Ganz R: Magnetic resonance arthrography of labral disorders in hips with dysplasia and impingement. *Clin Orthop Relat Res* 2004;418:74-80.

11. Burstein D, Gray M: New MRI techniques for imaging cartilage. *J Bone Joint Surg Am* 2003; 85-A(Suppl 2):70-77.

12. Gray ML: Toward imaging biomarkers for glycosaminoglycans. *J Bone Joint Surg Am* 2009; 91(Suppl 1):44-49.

13. Li X, Pai A, Blumenkrantz G, et al: Spatial distribution and relationship of T1rho and T2 relaxation times in knee cartilage with osteoarthritis. *Magn Reson Med* 2009;61(6):1310-1318.

14. Bittersohl B, Hosalkar HS, Hughes T, et al: Feasibility of T2* mapping for the evaluation of hip joint cartilage at 1.5T using a three-dimensional (3D), gradient-echo (GRE) sequence: A prospective study. *Magn Reson Med* 2009; 62(4):896-901.

15. Buckwalter JA, Mankin HJ, Grodzinsky AJ: Articular cartilage and osteoarthritis. *Instr Course Lect* 2005;54:465-480.

16. Peterfy CG, DiCarlo JC, Kathari M: Magnetic resonance imaging, in RW Moskowitz, Altman RD, Hochberg MC, Buckwalter JA, Goldberg VM, eds: *Osteoarthritis: Diagnosis and Medical/Surgical Management.* Philadelphia, PA, Lippincott, Williams & Wilkins, 2007, pp 167-192.

17. Gold GE, Hargreaves BA, Stevens KJ, Beaulieu CF: Advanced magnetic resonance imaging of articular cartilage. *Orthop Clin North Am* 2006;37(3): 331-347, vi.

18. Mow VC, Hou JS, Owens JM, Ratcliffe A: Biphasic and quasilinear viscoelastic theories for hydrated soft tissues, in Mow VC, Ratcliffe A, Woo LY, eds: *Biomechanics of Diarthrodial Joints.* New York, NY, Springer-Verlag, 1990, pp 215-260.

19. Wirth W, Larroque S, Davies RY, et al; OA Initiative Investigators Group: Comparison of 1-year vs 2-year change in regional cartilage thickness in osteoarthritis results from 346 participants from the Osteoarthritis Initiative. *Osteoarthritis Cartilage* 2011;19(1):74-83.

20. Koo S, Giori NJ, Gold GE, Dyrby CO, Andriacchi TP: Accuracy of 3D cartilage models generated from MR images is dependent on cartilage thickness: Laser scanner based validation of in vivo cartilage. *J Biomech Eng* 2009; 131(12):121004.

21. Yin Y, Zhang X, Williams R, Wu X, Anderson DD, Sonka M: LOGISMOS-layered optimal graph image segmentation of multiple objects and surfaces: Cartilage segmentation in the knee joint. *IEEE Trans Med Imaging* 2010;29(12):2023-2037.

22. Dunn TC, Lu Y, Jin H, Ries MD, Majumdar S: T2 relaxation time of cartilage at MR imaging: Comparison with severity of knee osteoarthritis. *Radiology* 2004; 232(2):592-598.

23. Koff MF, Amrami KK, Kaufman KR: Clinical evaluation of T2 values of patellar cartilage in patients with osteoarthritis. *Osteoarthritis Cartilage* 2007;15(2): 198-204.

24. Stehling C, Liebl H, Krug R, et al: Patellar cartilage: T2 values and morphologic abnormalities at 3.0-T MR imaging in relation to physical activity in asymptomatic subjects from the osteoarthritis initiative. *Radiology* 2010;254(2): 509-520.

25. Burstein D, Velyvis J, Scott KT, et al: Protocol issues for delayed Gd(DTPA)(2-)-enhanced MRI (dGEMRIC) for clinical evaluation of articular cartilage. *Magn Reson Med* 2001;45(1):36-41.

26. Gray ML, Burstein D, Kim YJ, Maroudas A: Magnetic resonance imaging of cartilage glycosaminoglycan: Basic principles, imaging technique, and clinical applications. *J Orthop Res* 2008;26(3): 281-291.

27. Baldassarri M, Goodwin JS, Farley ML, et al: Relationship between cartilage stiffness and dGEMRIC index: Correlation and prediction. *J Orthop Res* 2007;25(7):904-912.

28. Young AA, Stanwell P, Williams A, et al: Glycosaminoglycan content of knee cartilage following posterior cruciate ligament rupture demonstrated by delayed gadolinium-enhanced magnetic resonance imaging of cartilage (dGEMRIC): A case report. *J Bone Joint Surg Am* 2005; 87(12):2763-2767.

29. Fleming BC, Oksendahl HL, Mehan WA, et al: Delayed gadolinium-enhanced MR imaging of cartilage (dGEMRIC) following ACL injury. *Osteoarthritis Cartilage* 2010;18(5):662-667.

30. Duvvuri U, Charagundla SR, Kudchodkar SB, et al: Human knee: In vivo T1(rho)-weighted MR imaging at 1.5 T. Preliminary experience. *Radiology* 2001; 220(3):822-826.

31. Regatte RR, Akella SV, Lonner JH, Kneeland JB, Reddy R: T1rho relaxation mapping in human osteoarthritis (OA) cartilage: Comparison of T1rho with T2.

J Magn Reson Imaging 2006;23(4): 547-553.

32. Taylor C, Carballido-Gimio J, Majumdar S, Li X: Comparison of quantitative imaging of cartilage for osteoarthritis: T2, T1-rho, dGEMRIC and contrast-enhanced computed tomography. *Magn Reson Imaging* 2009;27(6):779-784.

33. Leunig M, Beck M, Woo A, Dora C, Kerboull M, Ganz R: Acetabular rim degeneration: A constant finding in the aged hip. *Clin Orthop Relat Res* 2003;413:201-207.

34. Carballido-Gamio J, Link TM, Li X, et al: Feasibility and reproducibility of relaxometry, morphometric, and geometrical measurements of the hip joint with magnetic resonance imaging at 3T. *J Magn Reson Imaging* 2008; 28(1):227-235.

35. Watanabe A, Boesch C, Siebenrock K, Obata T, Anderson SE: T2 mapping of hip articular cartilage in healthy volunteers at 3T: A study of topographic variation. *J Magn Reson Imaging* 2007;26(1): 165-171.

36. Kim YJ, Jaramillo D, Millis MB, Gray ML, Burstein D: Assessment of early osteoarthritis in hip dysplasia with delayed gadolinium-enhanced magnetic resonance imaging of cartilage. *J Bone Joint Surg Am* 2003;85-A(10):1987-1992.

37. Rakhra K, Lattanzio PJ, Cardenas-Blanco A, Cameron I, Beaule PE: 1.5T T1ñ MRI of acetabular cartilage in femoroacetabular impingement: Preliminary investigation. *Clin Orthop Relat Res* 2011, in press.

38. Pollard TC, McNally EG, Wilson DC, et al: Localized cartilage assessment with three-dimensional dGEMRIC in asymptomatic hips with normal morphology and cam deformity. *J Bone Joint Surg Am* 2010;92(15):2557-2569.

39. Bittersohl B, Steppacher S, Haamberg T, et al: Cartilage damage in

femoroacetabular impingement (FAI): Preliminary results on comparison of standard diagnostic vs delayed gadolinium-enhanced magnetic resonance imaging of cartilage (dGEMRIC). *Osteoarthritis Cartilage* 2009;17(10): 1297-1306.

40. Jessel RH, Zilkens C, Tiderius C, Dudda M, Mamisch TC, Kim YJ: Assessment of osteoarthritis in hips with femoroacetabular impingement using delayed gadolinium enhanced MRI of cartilage. *J Magn Reson Imaging* 2009;30(5): 1110-1115.

41. Tiderius CJ, Jessel R, Kim YJ, Burstein D: Hip dGEMRIC in asymptomatic volunteers and patients with early osteoarthritis: The influence of timing after contrast injection. *Magn Reson Med* 2007;57(4):803-805.

42. Cunningham T, Jessel R, Zurakowski D, Millis MB, Kim YJ: Delayed gadolinium-enhanced magnetic resonance imaging of cartilage to predict early failure of Bernese periacetabular osteotomy for hip dysplasia. *J Bone Joint Surg Am* 2006;88(7):1540-1548.

43. Burstein D, Bashir A, Gray ML: MRI techniques in early stages of cartilage disease. *Invest Radiol* 2000;35(10):622-638.

44. Williams A, Mikulis B, Krishnan N, Gray M, McKenzie C, Burstein D: Suitability of T(1Gd) as the dGEMRIC index at 1.5T and 3.0T. *Magn Reson Med* 2007; 58(4):830-834.

45. Mamisch TC, Dudda M, Hughes T, Burstein D, Kim YJ: Comparison of delayed gadolinium enhanced MRI of cartilage (dGEMRIC) using inversion recovery and fast T1 mapping sequences. *Magn Reson Med* 2008;60(4):768-773.

46. Vieira R, Regatte R, Cavalcanti C, Kubilay S, Schweitzer M: 3D-T1&[rho]-weighted MRI of the hip joint at 3T, in *Proceedings 14th Scientific Meeting International Society for Magnetic Reso-*

nance in Medicine, Berkely, CA, International Society for Magnetic Resonance in Medicine, 2006, p 3604.

47. Duvvuri U, Kudchodkar S, Reddy R, Leigh JS: T(1rho) relaxation can assess longitudinal proteoglycan loss from articular cartilage in vitro. *Osteoarthritis Cartilage* 2002;10(11):838-844.

48. Wheaton AJ, Dodge GR, Elliott DM, Nicoll SB, Reddy R: Quantification of cartilage biomechanical and biochemical properties via T1rho magnetic resonance imaging. *Magn Reson Med* 2005;54(5): 1087-1093.

49. Wheaton AJ, Borthakur A, Shapiro EM, et al: Proteoglycan loss in human knee cartilage: Quantitation with sodium MR imaging. Feasibility study. *Radiology* 2004; 231(3):900-905.

50. Crema MD, Roemer FW, Marra MD, et al: Articular cartilage in the knee: Current MR imaging techniques and applications in clinical practice and research. *Radiographics* 2011;31(1):37-61.

51. Krause FG, Klammer G, Benneker LM, Werlen S, Mamisch TC, Weber M: Biochemical T2* MR quantification of ankle arthrosis in pes cavovarus. *J Orthop Res* 2010;28(12):1562-1568.

52. Welsch GH, Trattnig S, Scheffler K, et al: Magnetization transfer contrast and T2 mapping in the evaluation of cartilage repair tissue with 3T MRI. *J Magn Reson Imaging* 2008;28(4):979-986.

Pathomorphology and Treatment of Femoroacetabular Impingement

Frank M. Klenke, MD, PhD
Klaus A. Siebenrock, MD

Abstract

Femoroacetabular impingement is recognized as a major cause of hip pain and early hip joint osteoarthritis in young adults. The dynamic conflict between the femoral neck and the acetabular rim has been shown to result in labral tears, cartilage lesions, and early osteoarthritis. To be successful, the treatment strategy should address the underlying pathomorphology at the femoral neck, the acetabulum, or both. An overview of the various pathomorphologies leading to femoroacetabular impingement and a treatment algorithm intended to preserve the native hip joint should be helpful to the orthopaedic surgeon treating patients with this condition.

Instr Course Lect 2012;61:263-272.

Femoroacetabular impingement (FAI) has been recognized as a major cause of hip pain and early hip joint osteoarthritis in young adults. The pathomechanics underlying FAI can be divided into those based on the dysmorphology of the acetabulum (pincer-type FAI) or the proximal femur (cam-type FAI). Both types of pathomorphology cause a conflict of the femoral neck with the acetabular rim, resulting in labral tears, cartilage lesions, and early osteoarthritis. The various pathomechanisms of FAI should be considered when planning surgery because the treatment should address the underly-ing pathomorphology. This chapter provides an overview of the various pathomorphologies of FAI that place the hip at risk for early osteoarthritis and provides a treatment algorithm for preserving the native hip joint.

Types of FAI

In principle, there are two types of FAI—the so-called cam and pincer types of impingement. The major pathomechanism of both types of FAI is a dynamic conflict of the femoral neck and the acetabular rim, which predominantly occurs with flexion–internal rotation of the hip joint (**Fig-**ure **1**) but may also occur with other hip movements such as circumferential acetabular overcoverage.[1] The disease entity of FAI describes the general pathomechanism, which may be caused by a variety of pathomorpho-logic conditions, including slipped capital femoral epiphysis (SCFE), Legg-Calvé-Perthes disease, and ac-etabular retroversion.

Normally, the anterosuperior femo-ral head-neck junction has a concave, spherical configuration. In cam-type FAI, the anterosuperior head-neck junc-tion is aspheric and may be either flat-tened or convex. During hip movement, the aspheric part immerges into the ac-etabulum and induces compression and shear forces at the junction between the labrum and the acetabular cartilage. These forces stretch the labrum and push it outward while the cartilage is compressed. The resulting articular damage is a separation between the labrum and the cartilage called an un-dersurface lesion; the labrum itself re-mains partially attached to the acetabu-lum and relatively deep cartilage lesion involving approximately one third of the total depth of the acetabulum. Those le-sions are usually restricted to the antero-superior quadrant of the acetabulum.

Dr. Klenke or an immediate family member has received research or institutional support from Amgen. Neither Dr. Siebenrock nor any immediate family member has received anything of value from or owns stock in a com-mercial company or institution related directly or indirectly to the subject of this chapter.

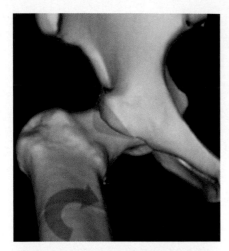

Figure 1 Schematic illustration of the anterosuperior impingement conflict between the femoral head-neck junction and the acetabular rim (red area). The curved arrow depicts the internal rotation of the femoral neck, causing impingement with the acetabular rim in 90° hip flexion.

Pincer-type FAI arises from a partially or globally overcovered acetabulum in which the femoral neck is leveraged on the front of the acetabulum. The linear contact between the acetabular rim and the femoral head-neck junction compresses the labrum between the acetabular rim and the femoral neck, resulting in anterior labral tears and cartilage lesions close to the acetabular rim. Often, cartilage lesions also occur posteriorly on the femoral head, reflecting a contrecoup lesion. Pincer impingement can be the result of excessive coverage by the acetabular rim or a massive, aspheric femoral head-neck junction in which the aspheric portion is too large to enter the joint. The excessive coverage by the acetabular rim can occur focally in one area of the joint or concentrically.

Cam impingement is usually caused by pathomorphology of the proximal femur and pincer impingement, usually arising from a malconfigured acetabulum. However, there are a few exceptions to this rule. FAI may also be classified based on the origin of the le-sions—those originating from the proximal femur or the acetabulum—because this distinction directly influences the therapeutic approach. Deformities leading to FAI are often idiopathic. Several other types of pathomorphology, such as SCFE and Legg-Calvé-Perthes disease, may cause secondary impingement.

Femoral Pathomorphology
Cam-Type Morphology
Cam-type morphologies include anterosuperior femoral head-neck deformities as seen in classic cam-type impingement caused by an extension of the epiphysis. In patients with SCFE, the inferior and posterior slip of the epiphysis relative to the metaphysis causes cam-type impingement because of the conflict of the prominent metaphysis and the anterosuperior acetabulum. On AP radiographs, the prominent metaphysis appears similar to a pistol grip (the so-called pistol-grip deformity), and it has been assumed that a silent slip is the predominant underlying pathology.[2-4] Even minor slips of less than 30° may result in cam-type impingement.[5] Deformities seen in malunited femoral neck fractures are similar to those found in SCFE; however, the cam morphology is more distal within the femoral neck. In most patients, the anterior portion of the distal head-neck junction is aspheric, causing cam-type impingement. More severe deformities show retroversion of the femoral neck and a coxa vara caused by the inferior-posterior tilt of the femoral head aggravating the conflict with the acetabular rim.

Malorientation of the Proximal Femur
The femoral offset may be normal in patients with coxa vara with femoral retrotorsion and coxa valga with femoral antetorsion. However, the femoral head-neck junction is closer to the acetabular rim, putting the hip at risk for cam impingement. The unfavorable position of the femoral neck in relation to the acetabulum results in an early conflict that can be provoked by certain movements of the hip joint. In coxa vara with femoral retrotorsion, an anterosuperior conflict is provoked by flexion and internal rotation (anterior impingement). In coxa valga with femoral antetorsion, a posteroinferior conflict arises in extension and external rotation (posterior impingement).

Acetabular Pathomorphology
Coxa Profunda/Protrusio Acetabuli
In coxa profunda/protrusio acetabuli, general overcoverage of the acetabulum causes classic pincer-type impingement.

Acetabular Retroversion
In patients with acetabular retroversion, the cranial portion of the acetabulum is oriented posteriorly, resulting in focal overcoverage of the anterior portion of the acetabulum. This configuration often occurs together with a deficient posterior wall. On AP radiographs, a positive crossover sign, a posterior wall sign, and an ischial spine sign indicate acetabular retroversion.[6,7]

Acetabular Anteversion
Posterior overcoverage is usually seen in patients with excessive acetabular anteversion and a simultaneous deficient anterior wall.

Combined Femoral and Acetabular Pathomorphology
In disorders with combined pathomorphology, such as Legg-Calvé-Perthes disease, the morphologic alterations affect the proximal femur as well as the acetabulum. On the femoral side, the dysmorphology consists of a grossly deformed femoral head, a high-riding

greater trochanter, functional coxa vara, and femoral retrotorsion. The acetabular pathomorphology includes a dysplastic hip with insufficient coverage, acetabular retroversion, and a steep acetabulum (acetabular index > 10°). Functionally, the morphologic abnormalities result in cam impingement (mild forms), head-induced pincer impingement (in severe forms, the grossly deformed femoral head is too large to enter the joint), and extra-articular impingement of the greater and lesser trochanter.[8-12]

Independent of the pathomorphologic changes, patients with general ligamentous hyperlaxity and/or excessive demands on the joint because of participation in high-impact sports (for example, hockey, soccer, or martial arts), especially those with extensive combined flexion–internal rotation movements, have an increased risk of developing symptoms of FAI.[13,14]

Preoperative Evaluation
Patient History
Patients with FAI often report groin pain with an insidious onset. Although groin pain is the most frequent symptom, patients may also report discomfort in the lateral hip, medial thigh, buttock, and knee regions. Pain is usually activity related. Initially, pain occurs after excessive activity. Over time, cartilage lesion pain may become severe and occur with activities of daily living.[15]

Clinical Evaluation
The clinical examination should assess the range of motion of the hip joint. Generally, patients with FAI have decreased range of motion, particularly for flexion and internal rotation. Typically, forced flexion and internal rotation (the anterior impingement test) is positive in patients with cam impingement and pincer impingement because of anterior overcoverage of the acetabulum.

Less commonly, excessive acetabular anteversion or global overcoverage will result in posterior impingement in forced flexion and external rotation (the posterior impingement test).

Radiographic Evaluation
The standard radiographic workup for diagnosing FAI and for decision making in joint-preserving hip surgery includes conventional radiographs and a specific magnetic resonance arthrogram (MRA).[16] Depending on the type of the pathomorphology, additional imaging studies such as CT may be necessary. The basic set of conventional radiographs includes an AP radiograph of the pelvis and a cross-table lateral radiograph of the hip. These views provide an overview of the major pathomorphology. To visualize the anterior coverage of the femoral head, a false-profile view can be obtained.[17] To obtain this view, the pelvis is rotated 65° from the plane of the radiographic table, with the axis of the ipsilateral foot parallel to the radiographic table. The specific MRA is obtained using a flexible surface coil and an intra-articular gadolinium contrast agent.[18] Besides the usual axial, coronal oblique, and sagittal oblique sequences, the specific technique also includes a radial proton–density-weighted sequence. These sections are placed orthogonal to the acetabular rim and labrum.

The diagnosis of FAI is based on symptoms, the clinical examination, suggestive conventional radiographs, and signs of chondrolabral degeneration on the radial MRA.[19] Asymptomatic patients with incidental findings on conventional radiographs do not require specific treatment and should be followed on a regular basis.

Surgical Treatment
Surgical treatment is indicated in symptomatic patients with correctable

pathomorphology with or without secondary changes such as labral tears and limited cartilage damage. In patients with established osteoarthritis (stage 2 or higher based on the Outerbridge classification system), surgical procedures aimed at correcting the pathomorphologic changes have a low probability of success. Nonsurgical treatment is recommended for these patients, including nonsteroidal anti-inflammatory drugs, intra-articular injections of anti-inflammatory drugs, and obturator nerve blocks to delay hip joint arthroplasty.

The goals of surgical treatment are to provide adequate and balanced femoral head coverage and impingement-free range of motion within physiologic limits. Generally, internal rotation should be 20° to 30° in 90° of hip flexion. Surgical hip dislocation is the standard treatment of FAI because this technique allows complete access to the acetabular rim and the femoral head and neck.[20] The following treatments can be performed via open surgical procedures: (1) trimming of the excessive acetabular rim and subsequent refixation of the labrum; (2) osteochondroplasty of the femoral head-neck junction to re-create a physiologic femoral head-neck offset; (3) relative neck-lengthening procedures; (4) transpositioning of the greater trochanter; and (5) reorientation osteotomies of the femoral head and neck in patients with deformities of the proximal femur, such as severe neck malrotation after a malunited femoral neck fracture, or a childhood disease, such as mild to severe SCFE or Legg-Calvé-Perthes disease.[9]

Hip arthroscopy is a valuable alternative to surgical hip dislocation. Pure cam-type deformities of the anterior portion of the femoral head-neck junction can be well treated with hip arthroscopy. However, arthroscopic treatment of pincer-type deformities is

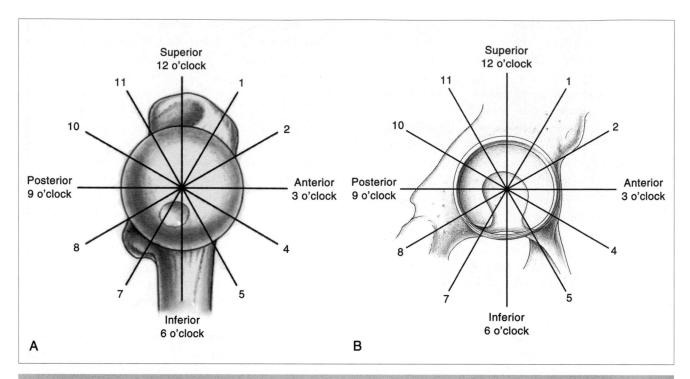

Figure 2   Schematic drawings showing the clockwise partitioning of the femoral head used to describe the exact location of impingement deformities with MRI. Partitioning of the left femur (**A**) and the right acetabulum (**B**) are illustrated.

technically demanding because of limited visualization and access to the acetabular rim and the difficulties associated with detachment and refixation of the labrum. In the experience of this chapter's authors, hip arthroscopy is most appropriate for remodeling the anterosuperior (12 o'clock to 6 o'clock) head-neck junction and the acetabular rim between the 10 o'clock and 4 o'clock positions (**Figure 2**). With the evolving progress of arthroscopic techniques and instruments, it is likely that the indications for hip arthroscopy in FAI will continue to broaden.

Independent of the surgical approach, the techniques applied in FAI treatment can be divided into remodeling and reorientation procedures. Remodeling procedures include all techniques that alter the shape of the acetabulum or proximal femur. Most often, they optimize the femoral neck waist (the so-called offset improvement) and trim either a segment or the

entire acetabular rim. Remodeling may also include relative lengthening of the femoral neck and distal transposition of the greater trochanter in patients with severely shortened femoral necks and varus morphology. In rare instances, remodeling procedures reduce the size of and reshape grossly deformed femoral heads, which are typically seen after Legg-Calvé-Perthes disease. The surgical technique must respect the blood supply to the femoral head via the terminal branches of the medial circumflex artery.[21,22]

Reorientation procedures include all osteotomies that change the spatial alignment or the position of either the proximal femur or the acetabulum. On the femoral side, intertrochanteric osteotomies may be required in patients with severe torsional deformities (retrotorsion and coxa vara or antetorsion and coxa valga). Femoral neck osteotomies are typically performed to correct secondary varus deformities after femoral neck fractures or SCFE. On the

acetabular side, reorientation procedures are performed for severe acetabular retroversion by means of a periacetabular osteotomy.[23,24]

Femoral Side

The most frequent pathologic finding is a nonspherical femoral head as indicated by α angles greater than 55°, resulting in insufficient offset of the femoral head-neck junction[25] (**Figure 3**). This pathomorphology can best be identified on a specific MRA with radial cuts and is predominantly seen anterosuperiorly.[26,27] However, the nonspherical segment of the head-neck junction will show considerable variation and may extend anteroinferiorly and posterosuperiorly, or even posteriorly to the superior retinaculum,[28] which contains the terminal branches of the medial circumflex artery that provides the blood supply to the femoral head.[21,22]

Pathomorphologies based on insufficient offset of the femoral head-neck

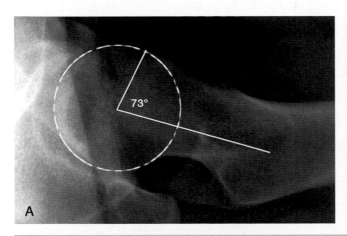
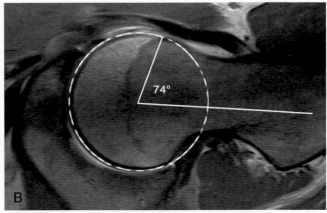

Figure 3 Cam impingement with an aspheric malformation of the femoral head-neck junction in a 20-year-old man. The malformation can be described using the α angle, which can be measured on a true lateral conventional radiograph (**A**) and on the axial planes of a hip MRA (**B**).

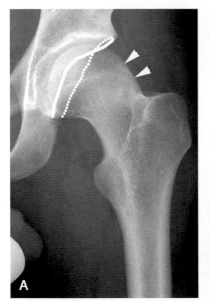
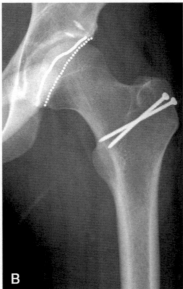
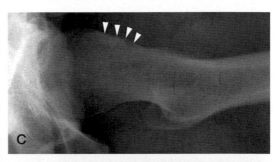
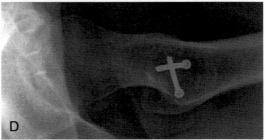

Figure 4 A through D, Radiographs of the femoroacetabular region in an 18-year-old man with combined cam and pincer impingement with a segmental overcoverage (solid line marking the anterior rim, dotted line marking the posterior rim) and nonsphericity of the femoral head-neck junction (marked by arrowheads). Preoperative AP (**A**) and lateral (**C**) radiographs of the deformity. Postoperative AP (**B**) and lateral (**D**) radiographs after a remodeling procedure consisting of osteochondroplasty of the nonspherical head-neck junction and trimming of the excessive acetabular rim with subsequent refixation of the labrum.

junction are usually treated with remodeling procedures to improve the offset. These remodeling procedures can be performed either arthroscopically or by means of open surgery via a surgical hip dislocation, depending on the location and the extent of the deformity.

Arthroscopic Surgery

Arthroscopic surgery can be used to treat cam impingement when the aspheric portion of the femoral head is confined to the anterior aspect of the head-neck junction (12 o'clock to 6 o'clock positions on a radial MRI) without relevant acetabular pathology.

Surgical Hip Dislocation

Cam impingement with the aspheric portion of the femoral head extending posterosuperiorly (9 o'clock to 12 o'clock positions on a radial MRI) and/or relevant acetabular pathology requires open surgery through surgical hip dislocation (**Figure 4**). Open sur-

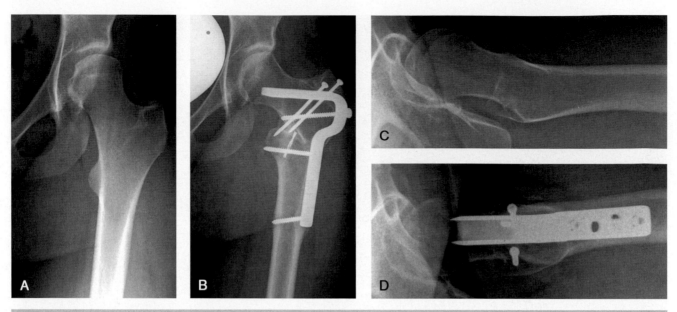

Figure 5   Preoperative AP (**A**) and axial (**C**) radiographs and postoperative AP (**B**) and axial (**D**) radiographs of the femoroacetabular region in a 19-year-old woman with dorsal impingement caused by coxa valga and femoral antetorsion. The patient was treated with an intertrochanteric osteotomy with a 20° correction of the femoral neck inclination and a 35° correction of the torsion deformity, along with transposition of the greater trochanter.

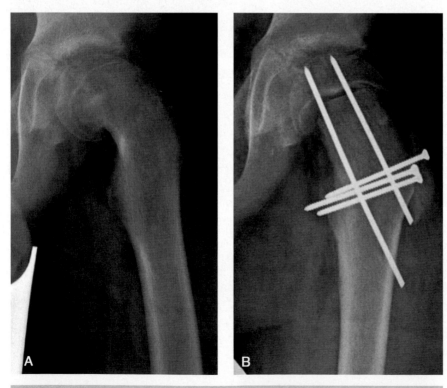

Figure 6   **A,** AP radiograph of the hip of a 16-year-old boy with a severe deformity of the left hip after chronic SCFE. The femoral neck had a posteroinferior deformation. **B,** Postoperative AP radiograph of the hip after treatment via a surgical hip dislocation with a retinacular flap. The femoral head was reoriented by trimming and relative neck lengthening, and the greater trochanter was transposed.

gery should be used to treat all pathologies requiring additional femoral head trimming and/or reorientation, femoral neck lengthening, correction of torsional deformities, and transpositioning of the greater trochanter. Open surgery is appropriate for three types of deformities. (1) Combined valgus and antetorsion deformities, as seen in congenital hip dysplasia, are treated with a femoral neck reorientation procedure by means of an intertrochanteric osteotomy (**Figure 5**). (2) Combined varus and retrotorsion deformities occurring after former SCFE and in malunited femoral neck fractures require reorientation procedures by means of intertrochanteric osteotomy or femoral neck osteotomy (**Figure 6**). (3) Complex deformities in Legg-Calvé-Perthes disease with head-induced pincer impingement, with or without functional retrotorsion, require a head reduction procedure, which is also performed via a surgical hip dislocation. Extra-articular impingement caused by a high-riding

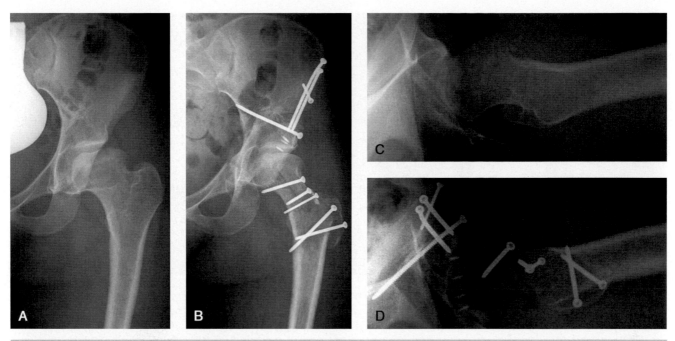

Figure 7   **A** through **D,** Radiographs of the left hip of a 22-year-old woman with severe pathomorphology of the left hip after Legg-Calvé-Perthes disease. Preoperative AP (**A**) and axial (**C**) radiographs show a grossly deformed femoral head, high-riding greater trochanter, functional coxa vara, and retrotorsion on the femoral side and a dysplastic hip with insufficient coverage, acetabular retroversion, and a steep acetabulum on the acetabular side. Postoperative AP (**B**) and axial (**D**) radiographs after surgical treatment of the femoral and acetabular pathomorphology with a combined remodeling and reorientation procedure. Treatment on the femoral side included a head reduction procedure, anterior osteochondroplasty with relative neck lengthening, and distalization of the greater trochanter. The acetabular deformity was corrected with a periacetabular osteotomy.

greater trochanter or, less commonly, by the lesser trochanter, can be treated by repositioning the greater and/or lesser trochanter (**Figure 7**). Mild deformities in which the aspheric portion of the femoral head enters the joint, resulting in cam impingement, are treated with anterior osteochondroplasty to optimize the shape of the head-neck junction and a relative lengthening of the femoral neck.

Acetabular Side

Understanding the definitive shape and orientation of the acetabulum is critical to making decisions on the treatment strategy. The most frequent acetabular pathology is segmental overcoverage, typically presenting as anterosuperior overcoverage or less frequently as severe retroversion with a positive posterior wall and an ischial spine sign on conventional radiographs[29] (**Figure 5**). Circumferential overcoverage, as seen in coxa profunda or protrusio acetabuli, may also lead to a predominant pincer-type impingement. Severe acetabular retroversion is seen more frequently in men, and circumferential overcoverage is more common in women.

Most patients with segmental and circumferential overcoverage can be treated with a remodeling procedure, including labrum detachment, trimming of the acetabular rim, and labrum refixation. When correcting circumferential or segmental overcoverage, care must be taken to prevent excessive trimming of the acetabular rim, which would create deficient acetabular coverage, resulting in secondary hip dysplasia. Reorientation procedures are required to correct acetabular retroversion and posterior wall deficiency.

Arthroscopic Surgery

Segmental overcoverage limited to the anterosuperior rim is usually accessible to allow reliable trimming of the rim and labral refixation by means of arthroscopy when performed meticulously and by an experienced surgeon.

Surgical Hip Dislocation

When segmental overcoverage is combined with extensive cam morphology, open surgery via surgical dislocation is recommended to most appropriately address the aspheric portion of the femoral head (**Figure 4**).

In FAI with circumferential overcoverage, surgical hip dislocation is generally recommended because the acetabular rim is not entirely accessible with hip arthroscopy.

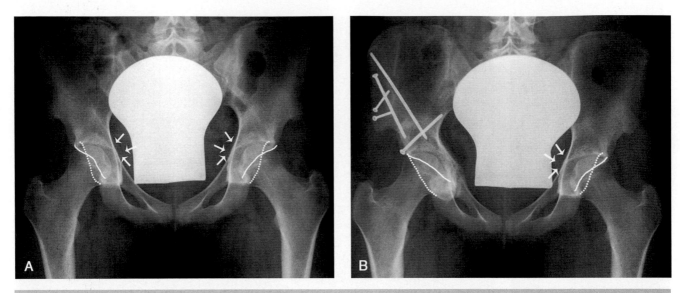

Figure 8 **A,** AP pelvic radiograph of an 18-year-old woman with pincer-type impingement caused by severe retroversion of the right and left acetabulum. The retroversion is demonstrated with the crossing sign (solid line marking the anterior rim, dotted line marking the posterior rim) and the prominent ischial spine (ischial spine sign) marked by arrows. **B,** Postoperative AP radiograph after the deformity was corrected with a reorientation procedure of the acetabulum on the right side through a periacetabular osteotomy.

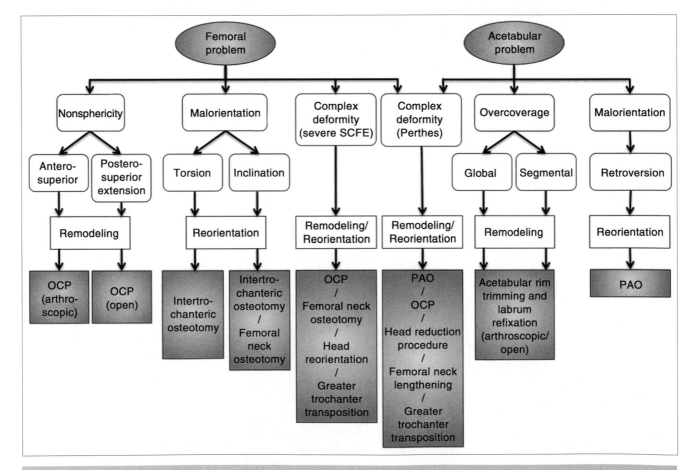

Figure 9 The Bernese treatment algorithm for FAI. OCP = osteochondroplasty, PAO = periacetabular osteotomy.

Video 21.1: Surgical Hip Dislocation for Femoroacetabular Impingement. Klaus A. Siebenrock, MD; Frank M. Klenke, MD (14 min)

Periacetabular Osteotomy

In FAI with significant acetabular retroversion (**Figure 8**), acetabular reorientation using periacetabular osteotomy is indicated if the following prerequisites are met: rim trimming would result in a center-edge angle less than 20°, there is a clear posterior wall deficiency, and the anterosuperior acetabular cartilage is largely intact.

In Legg-Calvé-Perthes disease with complex deformities, the femoral deformity is often combined with dysplastic hips showing insufficient coverage, acetabular retroversion, and a steep acetabulum requiring a periacetabular osteotomy to improve the hip joint containment (**Figure 7**).

Treatment Outcomes

Midterm outcomes after surgical treatment of FAI have not yet been published. However, encouraging short-term to midterm results are available for open surgical hip dislocation,[20,30] hip arthroscopy,[31,32] and periacetabular osteotomy.[23] Advanced degenerative osteoarthritis, age at the time of surgery, and overcorrection and undercorrection of both the acetabular and the femoral side seem to correlate with poor outcomes.[33] At a minimum follow-up of 5 years, preliminary results of a 2010 study of surgical hip dislocation for the treatment of FAI in 108 patients reported an improvement in the Merle d'Aubigné score in 95% of the patients, which was dependent on the individual joint alterations at the time of surgery.[34] Good to excellent results were obtained in 91% of all patients; the cumulative 5-year survivorship of the native hip joints was

91%. Despite these promising results, it is not yet proven that surgical treatment of FAI prevents or even delays osteoarthritis of the hip. The Bernese treatment algorithm for FAI is shown in **Figure 9**.

Summary

This chapter provides an overview of the various types of FAI pathomorphology, including classic cam- and pincer-type impingement, which place the hip at risk for early osteoarthritis. Although the field of diagnosing and treating of FAI is still young, midterm results of surgical treatment are encouraging. Studies providing long-term results and insights into the natural history of FAI will be needed to further improve treatment strategies and develop more sophisticated methods to detect and evaluate the pathomorphologies of the hip joint.

References

1. Ganz R, Parvizi J, Beck M, Leunig M, Nötzli H, Siebenrock KA: Femoroacetabular impingement: A cause for osteoarthritis of the hip. *Clin Orthop Relat Res* 2003; 417:112-120.

2. Goodman DA, Feighan JE, Smith AD, Latimer B, Buly RL, Cooperman DR: Subclinical slipped capital femoral epiphysis: Relationship to osteoarthrosis of the hip. *J Bone Joint Surg Am* 1997;79(10):1489-1497.

3. Harris WH: Etiology of osteoarthritis of the hip. *Clin Orthop Relat Res* 1986;213:20-33.

4. Stulberg SD, Cordell LD, Harris WH, Ramsey PL, MacEwen GD: Unrecognized childhood hip disease: A major cause of idiopathic osteoarthritis of the hip, in Mosby CV, ed: *Proceedings of the Third Open Scientific Meeting of the Hip Society*, St. Louis, MO, Hip Society, 1975, pp 212-228.

5. Loder RT, Aronsson DD, Weinstein SL, Breur GJ, Ganz R, Leunig M: Slipped capital femoral epiphysis. *Instr Course Lect* 2008; 57:473-498.

6. Kalberer F, Sierra RJ, Madan SS, Ganz R, Leunig M: Ischial spine projection into the pelvis: A new sign for acetabular retroversion. *Clin Orthop Relat Res* 2008; 466(3):677-683.

7. Werner CM, Copeland CE, Ruckstuhl T, et al: Radiographic markers of acetabular retroversion: Correlation of the cross-over sign, ischial spine sign and posterior wall sign. *Acta Orthop Belg* 2010; 76(2):166-173.

8. Eijer H, Podeszwa DA, Ganz R, Leunig M: Evaluation and treatment of young adults with femoro-acetabular impingement secondary to Perthes' disease. *Hip Int* 2006;16(4):273-280.

9. Ganz R, Huff TW, Leunig M: Extended retinacular soft-tissue flap for intra-articular hip surgery: Surgical technique, indications, and results of application. *Instr Course Lect* 2009;58:241-255.

10. Quain S, Catterall A: Hinge abduction of the hip: Diagnosis and treatment. *J Bone Joint Surg Br* 1986;68(1):61-64.

11. Snow SW, Keret D, Scarangella S, Bowen JR: Anterior impingement of the femoral head: A late phenomenon of Legg-Calvé-Perthes' disease. *J Pediatr Orthop* 1993; 13(3):286-289.

12. Wenger DR, Kishan S, Pring ME: Impingement and childhood hip disease. *J Pediatr Orthop B* 2006; 15(4):233-243.

13. Anderson SE, Siebenrock KA, Tannast M: Femoroacetabular impingement: Evidence of an established hip abnormality. *Radiology* 2010;257(1):8-13.

14. Beck M, Kalhor M, Leunig M, Ganz R: Hip morphology influences the pattern of damage to the acetabular cartilage: Femoroac-

etabular impingement as a cause of early osteoarthritis of the hip. *J Bone Joint Surg Br* 2005;87(7): 1012-1018.

15. Clohisy JC, Knaus ER, Hunt DM, Lesher JM, Harris-Hayes M, Prather H: Clinical presentation of patients with symptomatic anterior hip impingement. *Clin Orthop Relat Res* 2009;467(3): 638-644.

16. Tannast M, Siebenrock KA, Anderson SE: Femoroacetabular impingement: Radiographic diagnosis. What the radiologist should know. *AJR Am J Roentgenol* 2007; 188(6):1540-1552.

17. Lequesne M: The false profile view of the hip: Role, interest, economic considerations. *Joint Bone Spine* 2002;69(2): 109-113.

18. Leunig M, Werlen S, Ungersböck A, Ito K, Ganz R: Evaluation of the acetabular labrum by MR arthrography. *J Bone Joint Surg Br* 1997;79(2):230-234.

19. Tannast M, Siebenrock KA: Conventional radiographs to assess femoroacetabular impingement. *Instr Course Lect* 2009;58: 203-212.

20. Ganz R, Gill TJ, Gautier E, Ganz K, Krügel N, Berlemann U: Surgical dislocation of the adult hip: A technique with full access to the femoral head and acetabulum without the risk of avascular necrosis. *J Bone Joint Surg Br* 2001; 83(8):1119-1124.

21. Gautier E, Ganz K, Krügel N, Gill T, Ganz R: Anatomy of the medial femoral circumflex artery and its surgical implications.

J Bone Joint Surg Br 2000;82(5): 679-683.

22. Nötzli HP, Siebenrock KA, Hempfing A, Ramseier LE, Ganz R: Perfusion of the femoral head during surgical dislocation of the hip: Monitoring by laser Doppler flowmetry. *J Bone Joint Surg Br* 2002;84(2):300-304.

23. Siebenrock KA, Schoeniger R, Ganz R: Anterior femoroacetabular impingement due to acetabular retroversion: Treatment with periacetabular osteotomy. *J Bone Joint Surg Am* 2003; 85-A(2):278-286.

24. Steppacher SD, Tannast M, Ganz R, Siebenrock KA: Mean 20-year followup of Bernese periacetabular osteotomy. *Clin Orthop Relat Res* 2008;466(7):1633-1644.

25. Nötzli HP, Wyss TF, Stoecklin CH, Schmid MR, Treiber K, Hodler J: The contour of the femoral head-neck junction as a predictor for the risk of anterior impingement. *J Bone Joint Surg Br* 2002;84(4):556-560.

26. Mamisch TC, Zilkens C, Siebenrock KA, Bittersohl B, Kim YJ, Werlen S: MRI of hip osteoarthritis and implications for surgery. *Radiol Clin North Am* 2009;47(4): 713-722.

27. Siebenrock KA, Wahab KH, Werlen S, Kalhor M, Leunig M, Ganz R: Abnormal extension of the femoral head epiphysis as a cause of cam impingement. *Clin Orthop Relat Res* 2004;418:54-60.

28. Dudda M, Albers C, Mamisch TC, Werlen S, Beck M: Do normal radiographs exclude asphericity of the femoral head-neck junc-

tion? *Clin Orthop Relat Res* 2009; 467(3):651-659.

29. Reynolds D, Lucas J, Klaue K: Retroversion of the acetabulum: A cause of hip pain. *J Bone Joint Surg Br* 1999;81(2):281-288.

30. Murphy S, Tannast M, Kim YJ, Buly R, Millis MB: Debridement of the adult hip for femoroacetabular impingement: Indications and preliminary clinical results. *Clin Orthop Relat Res* 2004; 429:178-181.

31. Larson CM, Giveans MR: Arthroscopic management of femoroacetabular impingement: Early outcomes measures. *Arthroscopy* 2008;24(5):540-546.

32. Philippon MJ, Briggs KK, Yen YM, Kuppersmith DA: Outcomes following hip arthroscopy for femoroacetabular impingement with associated chondrolabral dysfunction: Minimum two-year follow-up. *J Bone Joint Surg Br* 2009;91(1):16-23.

33. Clohisy JC, St John LC, Schutz AL: Surgical treatment of femoroacetabular impingement: A systematic review of the literature. *Clin Orthop Relat Res* 2010; 468(2):555-564.

34. Tannast M, Siebenrock KA: Open therapy of femoroacetabular impingement. *Oper Orthop Traumatol* 2010;22(1):3-16.

Video Reference

21.1: Siebenrock KA, Klenke FM: Video. *Surgical Hip Dislocation for Femoroacetabular Impingement*. Bern, Switzerland, 2011.

Open Surgical Dislocation for the Treatment of Femoroacetabular Impingement: Past, Present, and Future

Christopher L. Peters, MD
Benjamin M. Stronach, MD
Christopher E. Pelt, MD
Jill A. Erickson, PA-C

Abstract

Femoroacetabular impingement results from a lack of clearance between the femoral neck and the acetabulum. This condition is most commonly seen in the young adult presenting with hip pain after activity. There have been rapid advancements in the understanding of femoroacetabular impingement to include diagnostic, imaging, and treatment options. An open surgical dislocation approach has been developed that offers a safe and effective method to dislocate the hip and allow direct visualization and full access to treat the often complex intra-articular pathologies of femoroacetabular impingement. The ultimate goal of treatment in carefully selected patients is relief of hip pain and preservation of the hip joint.[1-3]

Instr Course Lect 2012;61:273-286.

Femoroacetabular impingement (FAI) is a clinical condition in which abutment of the femoral head-neck junction and the acetabular rim produces acetabular chondrolabral injury and results in a painful hip. The characteristic structural abnormalities associated with FAI include decreased femoral head-neck offset and/or acetabular overcoverage, such as acetabular retroversion and coxa profunda.[1-3] If left untreated, FAI can lead to labrum and articular cartilage damage, resulting in early-onset osteoarthritis.[2,4-11] Decreased clearance in the hip joint appears to be responsible for the development of osteoarthritis early in life; these patients were once classified as having primary or idiopathic osteoarthritis.[12] FAI may be caused by cam impingement, pincer impingement, or a combination of both types (mixed impingement).[4,13] There has been a great deal of interest in this topic recently, resulting in rapid advancements in imaging, diagnosis, and treatment methodologies. More information on cam and pincer impingement is in chapter 21.

Historic Perspective

Many patients with end-stage osteoarthritis with no known underlying cause for the disease process were considered to have primary osteoarthritis until the 1960s. In 1965, Murray[14] performed a radiographic study to find an explanation for hip degeneration in patients with a previous diagnosis of primary arthritis and recognized a deformity in 65% of the hips. He identified a proximal femur abnormality that was termed femoral head tilt. In 1976, Solomon[15] used radiographs and anatomic specimens obtained at the time of surgery to elucidate the underlying pathology in these patients. He identified an underlying cause for joint degeneration in 300 of the 327 study patients (92%) and found femoral head tilt in 59 patients.[15] Stulberg et al[16] performed a radiographic review of the hips of 75 adults with osteoarthritis and found that 79% of patients had

Dr. Peters or an immediate family member has received royalties from Biomet; is a member of a speakers' bureau or has made paid presentations on behalf of Biomet; serves as a paid consultant to Biomet; and serves as a board member, owner, officer, or committee member of the American Academy of Orthopaedic Surgeons. None of the following authors or any immediate family member has received anything of value from or owns stock in a commercial company or institution related directly or indirectly to the subject of this chapter: Dr. Stronach, Dr. Pelt, and Ms. Erickson.

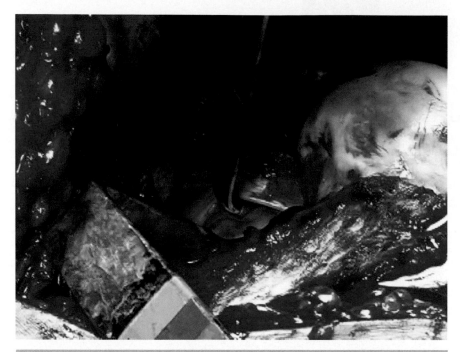

Figure 1 Image of the superior rim of the acetabulum with cartilage delamination lesion with hemostat inserted.

previously unidentified acetabular dysplasia or deformity of the femoral head and neck that was attributed to subtle Legg-Calvé-Perthes disease or slipped capital femoral epiphysis from childhood. This common finding in the proximal femur was termed a pistol grip deformity.[16] In each of these series, an underlying cause for some cases of osteoarthritis could not be found. It was hypothesized that these patients had a mechanical abnormality of the hip that could not be identified because of its subtle nature.[15-17]

Ganz et al[4] were able to identify subtle anatomic deformities that had not previously been described, likely providing an explanation for the small cohort of patients in previous investigations[15-17] with no identifiable mechanical abnormality. The authors noted continued anterior hip pain with decreased range of motion in a subset of their patients who had been treated with periacetabular osteotomy. On examination, the patients had a common finding of pain with flexion,

internal rotation, and adduction. Surgical exploration showed that these patients had obvious impingement of the anterior femoral neck on the anterior rim of the acetabulum. This condition was corrected by performing an osteoplasty of the anterior femoral neck and was the initial work describing open surgical dislocation for FAI.[18] The concept of impingement was then considered as a possible mechanical cause of the previously described idiopathic hip pain in young patients. Magnetic resonance arthrograms with radial sequencing of the femoral head and neck were obtained and provided a better appreciation for the anatomic variations seen in these patients. The patients were treated with open surgical dislocation; the resultant clinical improvement further validated the mechanical model proposed for impingement. Ganz et al[19] noted two distinct patterns of morphologic abnormalities causing impingement and coined the terms cam and pincer impingement. This work became the

foundation for the current understanding of FAI.[4,18]

Cam Impingement

Cam impingement results when an aspherical portion of the femoral head or the head-neck junction contacts the acetabulum during flexion and internal rotation of the hip, producing a shear force at the anterior chondrolabral junction, with subsequent labral and chondral injury. Decreased femoral head-neck offset had previously been described as a pistol grip deformity,[16] with more subtle variations now recognized as cam impingement.[2] Decreased femoral head-neck offset or a nonspherical head can result from multiple causes, including previous slipped capital femoral epiphysis, femoral neck fracture malunion, and decreased femoral anteversion.[20-22]

The pathomechanical shear stress on the anterosuperior chondrolabral junction resulting from cam impingement leads to acetabular cartilage damage, which typically presents as cartilage delamination from the underlying bone with a resultant chondral flap (**Figure 1**). Repetitive injury leads to failure of the articular margin of the labrum and progressive chondral damage. The capsular margin of the labrum is usually preserved until late in the disease process. The specific mechanism of damage to the acetabular cartilage is direct pressure from the aspherical femur during flexion and—to some degree—internal rotation. The process displaces the labrum from the acetabular margin, with resultant high tension and shear forces across this focused area. The rolling away of the labrum also exposes the osteochondral rim of the acetabulum to the impinging head-neck junction.[2,4,23]

Pincer Impingement

Pincer impingement is characterized by relative or absolute acetabular overcoverage of the femoral head. The result is premature abutment of the femoral head-neck junction against the acetabular rim, typically during flexion and internal rotation of the hip. Acetabular pathologic morphology associated with pincer impingement includes coxa profunda, coxa protrusio, acetabular retroversion, and calcified labra.[4,13,24,25] In pincer impingement, the femoral head-neck junction impinges against the prominent acetabular rim, which extends beyond the normal range of coverage. In contrast to cam impingement, the damage pattern in pincer impingement is characterized by direct labral compression, resulting in linear damage patterns to the labrum. There is evidence that the acetabular chondral surface is protected from damage with pincer impingement because the femur makes early contact with the acetabular rim and is prevented from entering the acetabulum.[23] Repeated labral compression leads to acetabular cartilage damage that is limited, with a mean of only 4 mm medial extension compared with 11 mm in cam impingement.[2] Ossification and cystic degeneration of the labrum can be pronounced in pincer impingement.[2,4,5] Secondary changes to the femoral head junction may be recognized as a so-called pincer groove or indentation.

Because most patients with FAI do not have isolated cam- or pincer-type impingement but have a combination of both impingement types,[2,26] the surgeon must have a thorough understanding of the specific hip pathomorphology to select the appropriate treatment for each patient. The available treatment options for FAI are evolving, and there is continued debate concerning which lesions are amenable to arthroscopic versus open procedures and which open procedure should be used in specific situations.

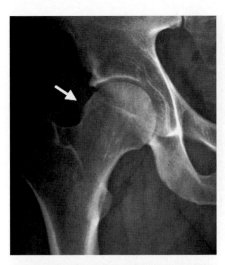

Figure 2   Preoperative AP radiograph of a right hip showing decreased femoral head-neck offset with a visible bump at the anterolateral femoral head-neck junction (arrow).

Presentation

Patients initially present for treatment because of pain and activity limitations. Most patients present with an insidious onset of hip pain that is frequently worsened with activity, but some patients present with an acute traumatic injury.[27,28] Specific activities that cause pain are associated with flexion, including rising from a sitting position, squatting, or sports that require high hip flexion, such as ballet, hockey, and soccer.[1,28] Pain is frequently localized to the groin but can also include regions proximal to the groin, such as the buttocks, the lateral hip, and the lower back.[28]

The physical examination includes an evaluation of gait for an antalgic or Trendelenburg gait pattern. Hip range of motion (adduction/abduction, flexion/extension, and internal/external rotation) should be documented. There is often decreased internal rotation of the affected hip(s) compared with patients with normal morphology.[27] The impingement test, which consists of flexing the hip to 90° with subsequent internal rotation and

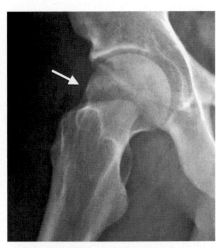

Figure 3   Preoperative frog-leg lateral radiograph of a right hip with decreased offset and visible anterolateral bump (arrow).

adduction, is useful in evaluating patients with suspected FAI.[4,7] One study reported a positive impingement test in all patients treated with open surgical dislocation,[1] and similar observations have been made in other patient populations.[29,30]

In some patients with hip pain, the source of the pain cannot be easily determined, and imaging is equivocal for intra-articular pathology. For these patients, this chapter's authors often use a fluoroscopically guided intra-articular hip injection with local anesthetic and corticosteroid as a diagnostic adjunct to determine if the pain generator is within the hip.

Imaging

Most FAI abnormalities can be detected on appropriately aligned AP pelvis and frog-leg lateral radiographs; however, the anterior bump seen in cam impingement can be missed on these views. Other views, such as the cross-table lateral, the false profile, and the Dunn view, may facilitate the diagnosis.[31] This chapter's authors obtain standing AP pelvis and hip (**Figure 2**), frog-leg lateral (**Figure 3**), and false profile lateral radiographs for all young

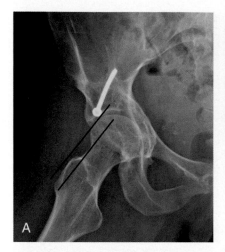

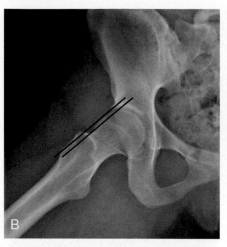

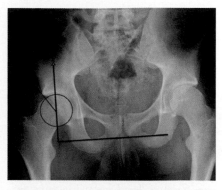

Figure 5 AP radiograph of the pelvis showing the lateral center-edge angle, which is determined by drawing a vertical line into the center of the femoral head with a connecting line from the femoral head center to the lateral rim of the acetabulum.

Figure 4 To determine the head-neck offset, the distance between a line drawn on a radiograph along the anteriormost portion of the femoral neck parallel to the neck axis and another line drawn parallel to this along the most anterior portion of the femoral head is measured. **A,** Radiograph of a hip with adequate head-neck offset. **B,** Radiograph of a hip with insufficient head-neck offset.

adult patients being evaluated for hip pain. Other views as necessary are used to augment the diagnosis.

Several measurements are used to help identify FAI on radiographs. The femoral anterior offset has been defined to help determine the presence of cam pathology on a lateral radiograph (**Figure 4**). This is accomplished by drawing a line along the anteriormost portion of the femoral neck parallel to the neck axis and drawing another line parallel to this along the most anterior portion of the femoral head. The distance between these two lines is measured. Tannast et al[32] recommend using a measurement of 10 mm or less to clinically identify cam pathology. The anterior offset can be divided by the diameter of the femoral head to determine the femoral head-neck offset ratio, with a value less than 0.17 highly suspicious for cam deformity.[33] The α angle is another useful measurement to identify cam impingement on a lateral radiograph. It is determined by drawing a line down the center of the femoral neck and connecting this with a line drawn from the head center to the

anterior point where the femoral head-neck contour becomes aspherical. An α angle greater than 50° is considered abnormal.[32,34] (See chapter 21, Figure 3 and chapter 27, Figure 15 for more information and an illustration of how the α angle is determined.)

Radiographic findings in pincer impingement reveal overcoverage of the femoral head. It is essential to obtain a true AP pelvis radiograph because pelvic tilt in an outlet or an inlet direction can give a false projection of overcoverage or undercoverage.[35,36] Coxa profunda (an acetabular fossa medial to the ilioischial line on an AP pelvis radiograph) and coxa protrusio (the femoral head is medial to the ilioischial line) result in a medialized femoral head with overcoverage.[32] The lateral center-edge angle is another measurement used for evaluating lateral acetabular coverage.[37] It is determined by drawing a vertical line into the center of the femoral head, with a connecting line from the femoral head center to the lateral rim of the acetabulum. A normal, lateral center-edge angle has been defined as 25° to 39°,

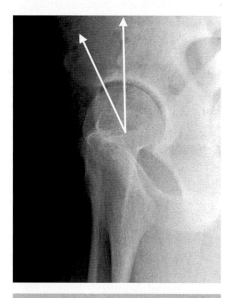

Figure 6 The lateral center-edge angle can be measured using a false-profile radiographic view of the hip.

with a value less than 25° defined as dysplasia[38] and a value greater than 39° indicative of overcoverage (**Figures 5** and **6**).[22]

Acetabular retroversion is a type of pincer impingement resulting in focal anterior overcoverage. The crossover sign (**Figure 7**) is used to identify retroversion on an AP pelvis radiograph by drawing a line along the lateral margin of anterior and posterior walls. In a normal, anteverted acetabulum, the posterior wall remains lateral to the anterior wall. In a retroverted acetabulum, the anterior wall crosses over the posterior wall, defining the crossover sign.[32,39] The posterior wall sign (**Figure** 7) is also useful in evaluating acetabular coverage. The posterior wall normally passes through the center of the femoral head. If the posterior wall is deficient, as is frequently seen in acetabular retroversion, the posterior wall is medial to the center of the femoral head. If the posterior wall crosses laterally to the femoral head, there is a prominent posterior wall with potential posterior overcoverage.[32]

MRI has become an important tool in the preoperative evaluation of FAI. It is useful in evaluating the hip for osteonecrosis, labral pathology, acetabular cartilage delamination lesions, and cam pathology. Magnetic resonance arthrography has become the gold standard for the detection of labral tears, with consistently good to excellent sensitivities (89% to 100%) and specificities (95% to 100%) in multiple studies.[40-44] Cartilage lesions can be difficult to detect with magnetic resonance arthrography because of the complex spherical shape of the hip and thinness of the cartilage.[44] MRI has shown fairly good sensitivities (47% to 93%) and specificities (66% to 89%) for detecting cartilage lesions[40,45-47] but is not yet effective enough to consistently detect acetabular delamination lesions (sensitivity, 22%).[23] MRI is currently the best noninvasive modality available for evaluating the cartilage despite these inherent shortcomings. Accuracy and detail in MRI continues to improve and helps the surgeon to fully appreciate the preoperative pathology and formulate a well-informed surgical plan.

CT arthrography is also a useful imaging modality in certain circumstances. A three-dimensional reconstruction of the joint can be obtained, which is helpful in understanding complex pathologic anatomy and is beneficial for surgical planning. This chapter's authors use CT arthrography on a select basis and do not believe this modality is necessary in evaluating all patients with FAI.

Treatment

A major challenge in treating FAI was finding a method to safely visualize the entire hip joint without damaging the cartilage or devascularizing the femoral head. A posterior approach to the hip risks damage to the medial femoral circumflex artery, which is the primary blood supply for the femoral head.[48,49] An anterior approach to the hip allows visualization of the anterior acetabular rim and the femoral head-neck junction but does not provide access to the superior femoral neck or the posterior acetabulum. This problem was solved by Ganz et al[19] when open surgical dislocation was first described. This procedure consisted of a lateral approach to the hip with a trochanteric flip osteotomy, which preserves the blood supply to the femoral head, followed by exposure of the anterior hip. An anterior capsulotomy and dislocation of the hip allows circumferential exposure of the acetabulum and most of the femoral head and neck.

The original procedure, which was described by Ganz et al[19] in 2001 has recently been updated with a comprehensive explanation of the surgery.[50] This chapter's authors use a similar exposure and surgical technique (**Figure** 8) with several minor modifications. After induction of anesthesia with complete relaxation, the patient is placed in the lateral decubitus position, and the pelvis is stabilized with an adjustable post system. After the patient is securely positioned and all

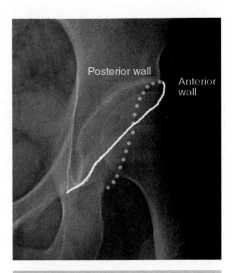

Figure 7 The posterior wall and crossover signs are shown on an AP pelvis radiograph.

nonsurgical regions are well padded, a wide surgical field from the ankle to the lower rib cage is prepared with an alcohol scrub, a chlorhexidine scrub, and an iodine-based sealant scrub. Sterile drapes are then placed to allow the operative leg to be manipulated, and a sterile pouch is positioned along the anterior portion of the patient. This allows the operative leg to remain sterile by placing it in the pouch during dislocation as it drops below the level of the surgical table.

The greater trochanter is fully palpated, and the incision is centered over this landmark in both the anterior-superior and the superior-inferior planes. Dissection is carried down through the subcutaneous fat to the level of the fascia overlying the gluteus maximus and the iliotibial band. At this point, the dissection is continued in a manner consistent with the initial portion of a posterior approach to the hip, which differs slightly from the Gibson approach used by Ganz et al[19] and Espinosa et al.[50] The midline of the femur is localized, the iliotibial band is incised, and dissection is performed superiorly through the anterior fibers of the gluteus maximus. A deep,

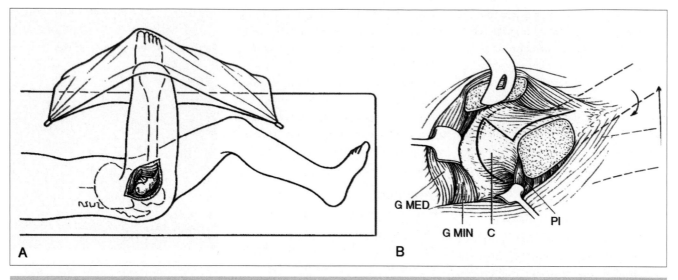

Figure 8 **A,** Illustration of patient positioning for surgical dislocation of the right hip. The patient is placed in the left lateral position with the right leg flexed and externally rotated until the hip dislocates anteriorly. The leg is then placed in a sterile anterior hip pouch. **B,** Illustration of the surgical approach as described by Ganz. G MED = gluteus medius, G MIN = gluteus minimus, C = capsule, PI = piriformis.

self-retaining retractor is placed, and the operative leg is then slightly internally rotated to visualize the posterior portion of the hip. It is critical at this point to understand the anatomic structures involved before proceeding to prevent injury to the blood supply to the femoral head. The posterior borders of the gluteus medius, greater trochanter, and vastus lateralis are identified. The fat overlying the external rotators is not disturbed, and no dissection should be performed in this specific region. The superior border of the piriformis is palpated, and the gluteus minimus is dissected from the capsule. No dissection is made inferiorly into the piriformis fossa, and the dissection always remains at or above the superior edge of the piriformis tendon. The joint capsule is now partially visualized, and a bent Hohmann retractor is placed in this interval deep to the gluteus minimus and superficial to the capsule. This chapter's authors have found that the definition of this interval before the trochanteric flip makes later dissection much easier and less traumatic to soft tissues. Attention

is then turned to the inferior border of the greater trochanter, where the posterior border of the vastus lateralis is identified and elevated from the femur. A retractor is placed onto the anterior femur in this interval, allowing retraction of the vastus lateralis. The posterior margin of the greater trochanter is well visualized, and the precise location of the trochanteric osteotomy can be determined.

The osteotomy starts superiorly at the posterior border of the gluteus medius and is carried inferiorly to the posterior margin of the vastus lateralis. The level of resection is parallel to the calf to ensure the osteotomy site is parallel to the alignment of the femur. After the osteotomy is completed, granular collagen/thrombin is placed on the osteotomy site to improve visualization and decrease blood loss for the remaining portion of the procedure. The wafer of bone is approximately 1.5 cm thick; however, this will vary slightly based on the patient's body habitus and osseous anatomy. If the osteotomy is performed correctly, the vastus lateralis, gluteus medius, and gluteus mini-

mus should be attached to the osteotomy fragment, allowing these structures to be retracted anteriorly. This is accomplished by placing a retractor onto the anterior border of the femur at the level of the remaining greater trochanter; the fragment is retracted anteriorly. The leg is then externally rotated gently to increase the exposure of the anterior capsule. The dissection is continued with electrocautery, releasing the adherent fibers of the rectus femoris and any remaining gluteus minimus. Once the capsule can be seen, the acetabular rim and the femoral head are palpated to ensure adequate exposure. The exposure is continued to include the anterior-inferior capsule and medially to the border of the iliopsoas tendon. After exposure of the capsule is complete, a Z-shaped capsulotomy is performed. The first incision is placed longitudinally down the anterior femoral neck. The second incision is started at the inferior margin of the first incision and carried anteriorly along the intertrochanteric line, releasing the inferior margin of the anterior capsule from

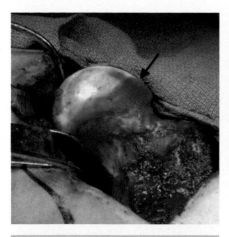

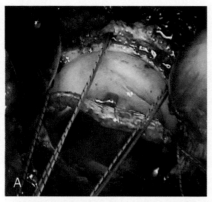

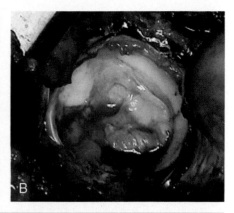

Figure 9   Photograph of the dislocated femoral head with decreased femoral head-neck offset and ecchymosis at the region of impingement against acetabulum (arrow).

Figure 10   Intraoperative photographs of the left hip labrum. **A,** Suture anchors have been placed in the acetabular rim. **B,** The labrum has been reconstructed with the suture anchors fixed back to the acetabular rim.

the inferior neck. Returning to the superior margin of the first incision, this capsulotomy is continued superiorly with visualization of the labrum to prevent injury. Once this incision is superior to the labrum, the third incision is made by releasing the capsule from the acetabulum in a posterior direction.

The hip can then be flexed and internally rotated to identify the area of impingement. Frequently, there is visible damage on the anterior femoral neck that includes periosteal blushing consistent with ecchymosis and osseous reaction (**Figure 9**). This area is delineated for femoral osteochondroplasty. The hip is then dislocated with gentle flexion and external rotation. The ligamentum teres often must be released to completely dislocate the femoral head. The foot is placed into the anterior drape bag during the dislocation maneuver. A retractor is placed anteriorly to the acetabulum on the ilium, staying deep to the iliopsoas to avoid damage to the femoral vessels. A second retractor is placed anteriorly to the femoral neck and onto the posterior column. This is used to retract the proximal femur posteriorly and al-

lows circumferential visualization of the acetabulum. The knee should be flexed during this portion of the procedure to decrease the tension on the sciatic nerve. The femoral head and acetabulum can be completely inspected for damage.

A labral takedown with subsequent repair is performed if required (**Figure 10**). This portion of the procedure is performed if there is a labral tear, cartilage damage on the acetabular rim, and/or a need for acetabuloplasty, which is often a necessary step to fully address the causative pathology. Acetabuloplasty is initiated with release of the labrum from the acetabular rim, usually from the anterior 4 o'clock position posteriorly to the 11 o'clock position. A high-speed burr is used for the acetabuloplasty, removing the amount of bone that was preoperatively templated. The amount of bone can be estimated by using the information provided by Philippon et al,[51] in which 1 mm of bone resection translates into a 2.4° decrease in the lateral center-edge angle, with each subsequent resected 1 mm of bone changing the center-edge angle by 0.6 mm. This translates into a bone resection of 5 mm, which decreases the center-edge angle by 5°.[51] This chapter's authors usually resect 3 to 5 mm of bone. If the

patient has acetabular dysplasia (lateral center-edge angle < 25°), acetabuloplasty is not recommended because of the potential risk for hip instability or iatrogenic dysplasia. After the work on the acetabulum has been completed, small suture anchors are placed 2 to 3 mm from the articular surface, and the labrum is repaired to the acetabular rim with horizontal mattress sutures. The sutures should be arranged so that the knots are on the outer surface of the labrum instead of the inner surface, which places the labrum as a barrier between the knots and the articulating surface of the hip joint. The sutures are spaced at approximately 2 cm and can involve two to five anchors based on the amount of labrum that requires reattachment. Repair of the labrum to the acetabular rim is recommended if possible,[52] but occasionally the labrum is too damaged or too hypotrophic to retain a suture. In these instances, the labrum is resected. A labral reconstruction can be performed in these patients with the use of the ligamentum teres[53] or a section of iliotibial band.[54,55]

Attention is then turned to the femoral neck, and the region of bone causing impingement is removed. An osteotome is initially used to define the superior border of the femoroplasty,

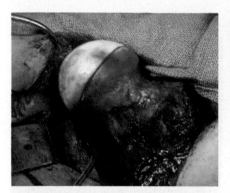

Figure 11 Image of a dislocated femoral head with the planned region of resection for femoroplasty delineated.

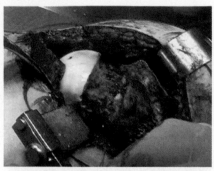

Figure 12 Image of a dislocated femoral head after completion of femoroplasty to restore femoral head-neck offset and remove the region of impingement.

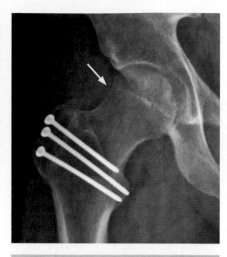

Figure 13 Postoperative AP radiograph of a right hip with trochanteric repair and the results of femoroplasty (arrow).

which is usually located proximal to the articular margin of the femoral head (**Figure 11**). The osteotome is directed distally and is used to remove periosteum with the assistance of a rongeur. The femoral osteochondroplasty is then completed with the use of a high-speed burr (**Figure 12**). The surgeon should strive to create a smooth transition from the articular surface of the femoral head to the femoral neck, with complete removal of the aspherical region. The final contour should be comparable to a ramp rather than a cliff to prevent the potential for a stress riser and allow for the restoration of a labral seal with normal fluid mechanics. Experience is needed to fully appreciate the amount of bone to remove; the amount may appear aggressive in a surgeon's initial experience. The assistant can now reduce the hip with gentle traction and internal rotation while the surgeon guides the head back into place. This chapter's authors have seen failure of the labral sutures on several occasions during this maneuver, requiring repeat dislocation and labral refixation. The number of dislocations should be minimized if possible. After the hip has been reduced, it can be taken through a range of motion to verify that no impingement occurs with flexion through an

arc of 0° to 90° and internal rotation through an arc of 0° to 20° if obtainable. Dynamic and static fluorographic images can be obtained to radiographically confirm impingement-free motion and visualize the extent of the bony débridement. If there is continued impingement, dislocation should be performed with revision of the femoral osteochondroplasty.

Once the range of motion is satisfactory with no residual impingement, the hip is irrigated thoroughly with normal saline, and the capsule is then repaired with absorbable sutures. It is advisable to leave laxity in the capsule if possible and not overtighten this closure because this can place the perforating branches of the medial circumflex femoral vessels at risk, with the potential for osteonecrosis of the femoral head. The greater trochanter is next reapproximated and repaired with the use of cortical screws under fluoroscopic guidance. A final fluorographic image is obtained to verify adequate screw position (angled toward the lesser trochanter with flush seating of the screw head against the greater trochanter) and proper reduction of the trochanteric fragment. A relative femoral neck lengthening can be performed during reattachment of the greater trochanter fragment. This

lengthening is performed in patients with coxa vara or a shortened neck as occurs in Legg-Calvé-Perthes disease, is accomplished by distalizing the fragment before reattachment, and results in increased tension on the hip abductors and thus improves mechanical function. The iliotibial band, subcutaneous layer, and skin are then closed with the suture material of choice. An intraoperative drain is not routinely placed. Postoperative radiographs can show the newly created contour on the femoral neck (**Figures 13** and **14**).

The average length of the patient's hospital stay is 3 days (range, 2 to 5 days).[1] This chapter's authors recommend compression stockings and mechanical foot compression pumps on the nonsurgical extremity during surgery and the placement of compression stockings and foot pumps bilaterally while the patient is in the hospital and in bed. All patients receive enoxaparin 30 mg subcutaneously twice a day while in the hospital unless contraindicated and are discharged on a regimen of 6 weeks of aspirin (325 mg once a day) to prevent deep venous thrombosis. Hip precautions for dislocation are not ordered for patients, but patients are required to observe 50% weight-bearing restrictions on the operated extremity for 6 weeks postoperatively to protect the trochanteric osteotomy site from excessive stress and prevent femoral neck fracture after femoral osteochondroplasty. Crutches are often sufficient ambulation aids in this young patient population. Radiographs are obtained at the 6-week postoperative visit, and weight bearing is progressed with the initiation of physical therapy at this time.

The described technique requires a thorough understanding of hip anatomy and is technically demanding. This procedure should not be used without proper preparation, which consists of spending time observing an experienced surgeon with a firm grasp of the technique and cadaveric study if possible.

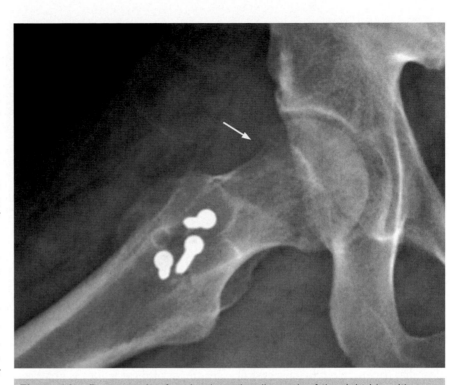

Figure 14   Postoperative frog-leg lateral radiograph of the right hip with restoration of the femoral head-neck offset (arrow).

Results

The treatment of FAI with open surgical dislocation has shown excellent functional outcomes and midterm survivorship in patients with no or minimal osteoarthritis[3,13,26,56] (**Table 1**). The first report of clinical results after surgical dislocation in 23 hips was encouraging, with 15 patients showing significant improvement in clinical outcomes at a minimum of 2 years postoperatively.[26] Similar findings were reported in 37 hips with an average follow-up of 3.1 years after surgical dislocation, with significant improvement in the average postoperative Western Ontario and McMaster Universities Osteoarthritis Index score compared with preoperative values.[56] A significant improvement in postoperative Harris hip scores in 96 hips with an average follow-up of 26 months was recently reported.[1]

In each of these studies, surgical failure, defined as no clinical improvement or conversion to hip arthroplasty, occurred in a small proportion of the patients. A common finding in these patients was moderate to severe arthritic changes at the time of surgery. In the first report documenting the results of open surgical dislocation, 15 of 23 patients had significant improvement with no further surgery, and 7 patients required conversion to total hip arthroplasty.[26] Five of those patients had significant preoperative arthritis, and the other two had residual, untreated acetabular dysplasia.[26] Beck et al[13] reported on 19 patients treated with open hip dislocation. In the five hips requiring total hip arthroplasty at a mean of 3.1 years, two of the patients had preoperative Tönnis grade 2 osteoarthritis, and the other three had Tönnis grade 1 or less preoperative arthritis; however, all were found to have severe arthritic changes intraoperatively, which were not always consistent with preoperative radiographs.[13] Two of this chapter's authors (CLP and JAE) initially reviewed 30 hips that had undergone open hip dislocation with an average follow-up of 32 months. There were four failures, with three patients requiring total hip arthroplasty.[3] This study was recently updated to include a total of 96 hips with an average follow-up of 26 months (range, 18 to 96 months). There were six failures defined as a decrease in the Harris hip score or conversion to arthroplasty. Four of the six patients were found to have severe acetabular cartilage damage (Outerbridge IV) at the time of surgery. Five of the 6 failures occurred in the initial 30 patients treated.[1] An improvement in the hip survival rate was seen when comparing the first group of 30 patients[3] treated with open surgical dislocation and the subsequent patients.[1] This improvement is attributed to the evolution in understanding the relationship of osteoarthritis and FAI and to greater patient selectivity in offering this surgical intervention. Philippon et al[57] also found a correlation between preexisting osteoarthritis and failure of

Table 1

Outcomes After Open Surgical Dislocation of the Hip for the Treatment of FAI

Study	No. of Patients	Average Age (Years)	Follow-up (Years)	Failures	Complications
Murphy et al[26]	23	35	2 to 12	7	0
Peters et al[3]	30	31	2.7	4	0
Beck et al[13]	19	36	4 to 5.2	5	0
Beaulé et al[56]	37	41	2.1 to 5	6	2
Peters et al[1]	96	28	2 to 9	6	2
Ganz et al[19]	213	34	2 to 7	NA	7

FAI = femoroacetabular impingement, NA = not available

arthroscopic femoroplasty. In the 10 procedures that failed, failure was directly correlated with intraoperative cartilage damage (6 with poor cartilage and 4 with moderate cartilage changes) and older patient age. It has become clear that patient selection has a critical effect on outcome results, especially in the presence of osteoarthritis. This has led to the development of improved preoperative imaging techniques to evaluate cartilage integrity and more selectivity in determining which patients should be offered the option of surgical dislocation.

Acetabular cartilage damage is frequently seen in patients with FAI.[13,23] These lesions are believed to be precursors to end-stage osteoarthritis that can eventually involve most of the hip joint. One important goal in the treatment of FAI is identifying these lesions early in the process and intervening in an attempt to halt the progression of joint degeneration. Cam impingement appears to be associated with a high prevalence of articular acetabular cartilage damage (specifically delamination). In a 2005 study, Beck et al[2] found acetabular cartilage damage in all 26 patients with a pure cam-type impingement pathology, with cartilage delamination in 10 of the patients. The acetabular lesions extended on average 11 mm medially toward the fovea. A study by Anderson et al[23] re-

ported similar findings with acetabular cartilage delamination, which was strongly associated with cam impingement pathology (odds ratio, 11.9), in 44% of all patients who underwent surgical dislocation. The appropriate treatment of these lesions is unknown and evolving. This chapter's authors currently recommend excising the delamination and then trimming the acetabular rim to a stable base for labral reattachment if the patient has adequate preoperative acetabular coverage (no dysplasia). The cartilage in the delaminated lesions is currently being evaluated to determine if it is alive and reparable. Fibrin glue has been used to reattach large delamination lesions in several patients, with mixed results. Another option is microfracture to stimulate the production of fibrocartilage.[58]

Damage to the acetabular labrum is a consistent finding in most patients treated with surgical dislocation for FAI. All of the 19 patients in a study by Beck et al[13] had labral tears, and 18 of 19 patients were found to have cartilage lesions in proximity to the labral tears. All of the labral lesions were located in the anterosuperior quadrant of the acetabulum, which is the region of abutment between the neck and the acetabulum. In a 2010 study, labral abnormalities were found in 82 of 96 hips during surgical dislocation, with 44 labral detachments, 15 tears,

9 degenerative labra, 10 calcified labra, and 4 absent labra secondary to previous surgery.[1] Graves and Mast[59] classified labral lesions in 48 hips. They found undersurface tears in 14 hips, base tears in 20 hips, ossification in 11 hips, and thickening in 4 hips. Espinosa et al[52] evaluated the options for the treatment of a labral tear by comparing the functional results of 20 patients who had labral resection and 32 patients in whom the labrum was repaired after acetabuloplasty. They found improved clinical outcomes in the patients with labral refixation compared with patients who had labral débridement.[52] It has become apparent that the labrum is frequently damaged in FAI, and it is an important component that should be addressed at the time of surgery to ensure a successful outcome. It is also important to address the underlying bony abnormality causing impingement that initially led to the labral damage.[2]

Complications

The treatment of FAI with open surgical dislocation is a technically demanding procedure with concern for specific complications, including osteonecrosis of the femoral head, sciatic neurapraxia, heterotopic ossification, femoral neck fracture, and nonunion of the greater trochanter. Multiple studies have shown a low complication rate despite these concerns. In their initial study of open surgical dislocation, Ganz et al[19] reported 2 cases of sciatic neurapraxia, which completely resolved; 3 failures of trochanteric fixation requiring reoperation; and heterotopic ossification in 79 hips. The authors found that the rate of heterotopic ossification decreased as they gained experience with the procedure.[19] This high rate of heterotopic ossification has not occurred in more recent series.[1,56,59]

The only reported complications in a recently published study of 96 hips were 2 failures of trochanteric fixation; no osteonecrosis, infection, femoral neck fracture, or sciatic neurapraxia were reported.[1] One patient subsequently experienced a sciatic neurapraxia, which has since resolved. That patient's hip was dislocated for an extended period of time (approximately 60 minutes) because of the need for extensive surgery on the acetabulum and the femoral neck. In the 37 hips reviewed by Beaulé et al,[56] failure of trochanteric fixation requiring reoperation occurred in 1 patient, heterotopic ossification requiring excision developed in 1 patient, and 9 hips required hardware removal for bursal irritation from trochanteric screws. Another series reported similar findings with minimal heterotopic ossification in nine hips, which required no further surgery, and two patients with symptomatic trochanteric irritation requiring screw removal.[59]

Trochanteric-related complications are a common thread in the reviewed studies. Patients should be counseled on the small risk of nonunion or the need for subsequent hardware removal. Femoral neck fracture is also a potential risk after femoral osteochondroplasty and has been reported in the arthroscopic literature[60] but not in the open dislocation series reviewed.[1,13,19,56,59] Mar-

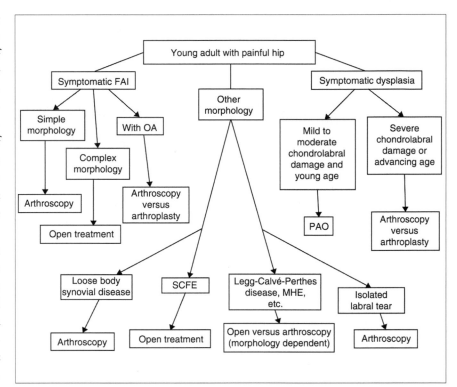

Figure 15 Treatment algorithm for the young patient with hip pain. OA = osteoarthritis, SCFE = slipped capital femoral epiphysis, PAO = periacetabular osteotomy, MHE = multiple hereditary exostoses.

dones et al[61] determined that up to 30% of the anterolateral neck could be removed before the proximal femur was at increased risk of fracture. This chapter's authors rarely remove an amount of bone approaching that limit and recommend against such an aggressive resection except in the most extreme circumstances. Postoperatively, patients are restricted to partial weight bearing for a period of 6 weeks as a precautionary measure to prevent femoral neck fracture.

Osteonecrosis of the femoral head remains a theoretic complication because it has not yet been reported in open surgical dislocation[1,13,19,56,59] or arthroscopic treatment of FAI.[62] This underscores the importance of meticulous surgical technique with protection of the medical circumflex femoral artery during the approach and the dislocation.

Discussion and Future Directions

FAI has received a great deal of attention recently, and the understanding of this condition has rapidly evolved. This renewed interest began with the development of a surgical procedure that allows safe access to the entire articular field without damaging the blood supply to the femoral head. The specific concepts of pincer and cam impingement came out of this initial work and provided the foundation for one current treatment algorithm for FAI (**Figure 15**). The arthroscopic treatment of FAI has correspondingly evolved, and the indications for this procedure continue to expand. The future direction for treating FAI will be finding the boundaries for arthroscopic versus open management, improving imaging modalities to detect pathology earlier in the process, and potentially using preoperative computer modeling to precisely reshape the acetabulum and the femoral neck to prevent impingement. There is a need to improve treatment options for cartilage lesions in an effort to improve the survival of hips after surgical treatment of FAI. Whether this takes the form of cartilage repair or advanced technologies, such as cartilage transplantation, remains to be determined.

Another controversial topic in FAI is when surgery should be performed. A course of nonsurgical management with physical therapy and nonsteroidal anti-inflammatory medication remains as the initial course of treatment for symptomatic patients. This chapter's authors have found that nonsurgical modalities are rarely successful in the midterm or the long-term treatment of symptomatic patients. There is currently no indication to surgically treat an asymptomatic patient with radiographic findings of FAI. There is interest in but no active program in place for screening at-risk populations and providing counseling for these individuals so they can seek treatment earlier if pain develops.

Summary

Rapid advancements in the understanding of FAI have resulted in changes in diagnostic and imaging techniques and treatment options. Regardless of the approach used, surgical intervention should be focused on correcting the underlying pathomorphology as well as the resultant chondrolabral tissue damage. The approach using open surgical dislocation offers a safe and effective method to dislocate the hip and allows direct visualization and full access to treat the often complex intra-articular pathologies that may be present.

References

1. Peters CL, Schabel K, Anderson L, Erickson J: Open treatment of femoroacetabular impingement is associated with clinical improvement and low complication rate at short-term followup. *Clin Orthop Relat Res* 2010;468(2):504-510.

2. Beck M, Kalhor M, Leunig M, Ganz R: Hip morphology influences the pattern of damage to the acetabular cartilage: Femoroacetabular impingement as a cause of early osteoarthritis of the hip. *J Bone Joint Surg Br* 2005;87(7):1012-1018.

3. Peters CL, Erickson JA: Treatment of femoro-acetabular impingement with surgical dislocation and débridement in young adults. *J Bone Joint Surg Am* 2006;88(8):1735-1741.

4. Ganz R, Parvizi J, Beck M, Leunig M, Nötzli H, Siebenrock KA: Femoroacetabular impingement: A cause for osteoarthritis of the hip. *Clin Orthop Relat Res* 2003;417:112-120.

5. Ito K, Leunig M, Ganz R: Histopathologic features of the acetabular labrum in femoroacetabular impingement. *Clin Orthop Relat Res* 2004;429:262-271.

6. Ito K, Minka MA II, Leunig M, Werlen S, Ganz R: Femoroacetabular impingement and the cam-effect: A MRI-based quantitative anatomical study of the femoral head-neck offset. *J Bone Joint Surg Br* 2001;83(2):171-176.

7. Wagner S, Hofstetter W, Chiquet M, et al: Early osteoarthritic changes of human femoral head cartilage subsequent to femoroacetabular impingement. *Osteoarthritis Cartilage* 2003;11(7):508-518.

8. Ecker TM, Tannast M, Puls M, Siebenrock KA, Murphy SB: Pathomorphologic alterations predict presence or absence of hip osteoarthrosis. *Clin Orthop Relat Res* 2007;465:46-52.

9. Leunig M, Beck M, Woo A, Dora C, Kerboull M, Ganz R: Acetabular rim degeneration: A constant finding in the aged hip. *Clin Orthop Relat Res* 2003;413:201-207.

10. Leunig M, Ganz R: Femoroacetabular impingement: A common cause of hip complaints leading to arthrosis. *Unfallchirurg* 2005;108(1):9-10, 12-17.

11. Tanzer M, Noiseux N: Osseous abnormalities and early osteoarthritis: The role of hip impingement. *Clin Orthop Relat Res* 2004;429:170-177.

12. Ganz R, Leunig M, Leunig-Ganz K, Harris WH: The etiology of osteoarthritis of the hip: An integrated mechanical concept. *Clin Orthop Relat Res* 2008;466(2):264-272.

13. Beck M, Leunig M, Parvizi J, Boutier V, Wyss D, Ganz R: Anterior femoroacetabular impingement: Part II. Midterm results of surgical treatment. *Clin Orthop Relat Res* 2004;418:67-73.

14. Murray RO: The aetiology of primary osteoarthritis of the hip. *Br J Radiol* 1965;38(455):810-824.

15. Solomon L: Patterns of osteoarthritis of the hip. *J Bone Joint Surg Br* 1976;58(2):176-183.

16. Stulberg SD, Cordell LD, Harris WH, Ramsey PL, MacEwen GD: Unrecognized childhood hip disease: A major cause of idiopathic osteoarthritis of the hip. *Proceedings of the Third Open Scientific Meeting of the Hip Society*. St. Louis, MO, CV Mosby, 1975, pp 2112-2228.

17. Harris WH: Etiology of osteoarthritis of the hip. *Clin Orthop Relat Res* 1986;213:20-33.

18. Myers SR, Eijer H, Ganz R: Anterior femoroacetabular impingement after periacetabular osteotomy. *Clin Orthop Relat Res* 1999;363:93-99.

19. Ganz R, Gill TJ, Gautier E, Ganz K, Krügel N, Berlemann U: Surgical dislocation of the adult hip a technique with full access to the

femoral head and acetabulum without the risk of avascular necrosis. *J Bone Joint Surg Br* 2001; 83(8):1119-1124.

20. Leunig M, Casillas MM, Hamlet M, et al: Slipped capital femoral epiphysis: Early mechanical damage to the acetabular cartilage by a prominent femoral metaphysis. *Acta Orthop Scand* 2000;71(4): 370-375.

21. Eijer H, Myers SR, Ganz R: Anterior femoroacetabular impingement after femoral neck fractures. *J Orthop Trauma* 2001;15(7): 475-481.

22. Tönnis D, Heinecke A: Acetabular and femoral anteversion: Relationship with osteoarthritis of the hip. *J Bone Joint Surg Am* 1999; 81(12):1747-1770.

23. Anderson LA, Peters CL, Park BB, Stoddard GJ, Erickson JA, Crim JR: Acetabular cartilage delamination in femoroacetabular impingement: Risk factors and magnetic resonance imaging diagnosis. *J Bone Joint Surg Am* 2009;91(2): 305-313.

24. Reynolds D, Lucas J, Klaue K: Retroversion of the acetabulum: A cause of hip pain. *J Bone Joint Surg Br* 1999;81(2):281-288.

25. Siebenrock KA, Schoeniger R, Ganz R: Anterior femoroacetabular impingement due to acetabular retroversion: Treatment with periacetabular osteotomy. *J Bone Joint Surg Am* 2003;85-A(2):278-286.

26. Murphy S, Tannast M, Kim YJ, Buly R, Millis MB: Debridement of the adult hip for femoroacetabular impingement: Indications and preliminary clinical results. *Clin Orthop Relat Res* 2004; 429:178-181.

27. Beaulé PE, Allen DJ, Clohisy JC, Schoenecker P, Leunig M: The young adult with hip impingement: Deciding on the optimal intervention. *J Bone Joint Surg Am* 2009;91(1):210-221.

28. Clohisy JC, Knaus ER, Hunt DM, Lesher JM, Harris-Hayes M, Prather H: Clinical presentation of patients with symptomatic anterior hip impingement. *Clin Orthop Relat Res* 2009;467(3): 638-644.

29. Philippon MJ, Maxwell RB, Johnston TL, Schenker M, Briggs KK: Clinical presentation of femoroacetabular impingement. *Knee Surg Sports Traumatol Arthrosc* 2007; 15(8):1041-1047.

30. Siebenrock KA, Wahab KH, Werlen S, Kalhor M, Leunig M, Ganz R: Abnormal extension of the femoral head epiphysis as a cause of cam impingement. *Clin Orthop Relat Res* 2004;418:54-60.

31. Meyer DC, Beck M, Ellis T, Ganz R, Leunig M: Comparison of six radiographic projections to assess femoral head/neck asphericity. *Clin Orthop Relat Res* 2006;445: 181-185.

32. Tannast M, Siebenrock KA, Anderson SE: Femoroacetabular impingement: Radiographic diagnosis. What the radiologist should know. *AJR Am J Roentgenol* 2007; 188(6):1540-1552.

33. Peelle MW, Della Rocca GJ, Maloncy WJ, Curry MC, Clohisy JC: Acetabular and femoral radiographic abnormalities associated with labral tears. *Clin Orthop Relat Res* 2005;441:327-333.

34. Nötzli HP, Wyss TF, Stoecklin CH, Schmid MR, Treiber K, Hodler J: The contour of the femoral head-neck junction as a predictor for the risk of anterior impingement. *J Bone Joint Surg Br* 2002;84(4):556-560.

35. Tannast M, Zheng G, Anderegg C, et al: Tilt and rotation correction of acetabular version on pelvic radiographs. *Clin Orthop Relat Res* 2005;438:182-190.

36. Siebenrock KA, Kalbermatten DF, Ganz R: Effect of pelvic tilt on acetabular retroversion: A study of pelves from cadavers.

Clin Orthop Relat Res 2003;407: 241-248.

37. Murphy SB, Kijewski PK, Millis MB, Harless A: Acetabular dysplasia in the adolescent and young adult. *Clin Orthop Relat Res* 1990; 261:214-223.

38. Murphy SB, Ganz R, Müller ME: The prognosis in untreated dysplasia of the hip: A study of radiographic factors that predict the outcome. *J Bone Joint Surg Am* 1995;77(7):985-989.

39. Clohisy JC, Carlisle JC, Beaulé PE, et al: A systematic approach to the plain radiographic evaluation of the young adult hip. *J Bone Joint Surg Am* 2008; 90(Suppl 4):47-66.

40. Neumann G, Mendicuti AD, Zou KH, et al: Prevalence of labral tears and cartilage loss in patients with mechanical symptoms of the hip: Evaluation using MR arthrography. *Osteoarthritis Cartilage* 2007;15(8):909-917.

41. Chan YS, Lien LC, Hsu HL, et al: Evaluating hip labral tears using magnetic resonance arthrography: A prospective study comparing hip arthroscopy and magnetic resonance arthrography diagnosis. *Arthroscopy* 2005;21(10):1250.

42. Freedman BA, Potter BK, Dinauer PA, Giuliani JR, Kuklo TR, Murphy KP: Prognostic value of magnetic resonance arthrography for Czerny stage II and III acetabular labral tears. *Arthroscopy* 2006;22(7):742-747.

43. Toomayan GA, Holman WR, Major NM, Kozlowicz SM, Vail TP: Sensitivity of MR arthrography in the evaluation of acetabular labral tears. *AJR Am J Roentgenol* 2006;186(2):449-453.

44. Fadul DA, Carrino JA: Imaging of femoroacetabular impingement. *J Bone Joint Surg Am* 2009; 91(Suppl 1):138-143.

45. Keeney JA, Peelle MW, Jackson J, Rubin D, Maloney WJ, Clohisy JC: Magnetic resonance arthrogra-

phy versus arthroscopy in the evaluation of articular hip pathology. *Clin Orthop Relat Res* 2004;429: 163-169.

46. Mintz DN, Hooper T, Connell D, Buly R, Padgett DE, Potter HG: Magnetic resonance imaging of the hip: Detection of labral and chondral abnormalities using non-contrast imaging. *Arthroscopy* 2005;21(4):385-393.

47. Schmid MR, Nötzli HP, Zanetti M, Wyss TF, Hodler J: Cartilage lesions in the hip: Diagnostic effectiveness of MR arthrography. *Radiology* 2003;226(2):382-386.

48. Gautier E, Ganz K, Krügel N, Gill T, Ganz R: Anatomy of the medial femoral circumflex artery and its surgical implications. *J Bone Joint Surg Br* 2000;82(5): 679-683.

49. Sevitt S, Thompson RG: The distribution and anastomoses of arteries supplying the head and neck of the femur. *J Bone Joint Surg Br* 1965;47:560-573.

50. Espinosa N, Beck M, Rothenfluh DA, Ganz R, Leunig M: Treatment of femoro-acetabular impingement: Preliminary results of labral refixation. Surgical technique. *J Bone Joint Surg Am* 2007; 89(Suppl 2 Pt.1):36-53.

51. Philippon MJ, Wolff AB, Briggs KK, Zehms CT, Kuppersmith DA: Acetabular rim reduction for the treatment of femoroacetabular impingement correlates with preoperative and postoperative center-edge angle. *Arthroscopy* 2010;26(6):757-761.

52. Espinosa N, Rothenfluh DA, Beck M, Ganz R, Leunig M: Treatment of femoro-acetabular impingement: Preliminary results of labral refixation. *J Bone Joint Surg Am* 2006;88(5):925-935.

53. Sierra RJ, Trousdale RT: Labral reconstruction using the ligamentum teres capitis: Report of a new technique. *Clin Orthop Relat Res* 2009;467(3):753-759.

54. Philippon MJ, Briggs KK, Hay CJ, Kuppersmith DA, Dewing CB, Huang MJ: Arthroscopic labral reconstruction in the hip using iliotibial band autograft: Technique and early outcomes. *Arthroscopy* 2010;26(6):750-756.

55. Philippon MJ, Schroder e Souza BG, Briggs KK: Labrum: Resection, repair and reconstruction sports medicine and arthroscopy review. *Sports Med Arthrosc* 2010; 18(2):76-82.

56. Beaulé PE, Le Duff MJ, Zaragoza E: Quality of life following femoral head-neck osteochondroplasty for femoroacetabular impingement. *J Bone Joint Surg Am* 2007; 89(4):773-779.

57. Philippon MJ, Briggs KK, Yen YM, Kuppersmith DA: Outcomes following hip arthroscopy for femoroacetabular impingement with associated chondrolabral dysfunction: Minimum two-year follow-up. *J Bone Joint Surg Br* 2009;91(1):16-23.

58. Philippon MJ, Schenker ML, Briggs KK, Maxwell RB: Can microfracture produce repair tissue in acetabular chondral defects? *Arthroscopy* 2008;24(1):46-50.

59. Graves ML, Mast JW: Femoroacetabular impingement: Do outcomes reliably improve with surgical dislocations? *Clin Orthop Relat Res* 2009;467(3):717-723.

60. Sampson TG: Complications of hip arthroscopy. *Clin Sports Med* 2001;20(4):831-835.

61. Mardones RM, Gonzalez C, Chen Q, Zobitz M, Kaufman KR, Trousdale RT: Surgical treatment of femoroacetabular impingement: Evaluation of the effect of the size of the resection. Surgical technique. *J Bone Joint Surg Am* 2006;88(Suppl 1 Pt 1):84-91.

62. Ilizaliturri VM Jr: Complications of arthroscopic femoroacetabular impingement treatment: A review. *Clin Orthop Relat Res* 2009; 467(3):760-768.

Arthroscopic Management of Hip Pathomorphology

Christopher M. Larson, MD

Abstract

The role for the arthroscopic correction of femoroacetabular impingement continues to evolve. As the understanding of hip pathomorphology improves and arthroscopic techniques for managing these disorders advance, the indications for arthroscopic femoroacetabular correction become clearer. Attention to detail with respect to diagnoses and surgical management is critical to optimize outcomes in this patient population. Studies have shown comparable outcomes for arthroscopic management and open surgical techniques. Further study is required to better define the role for arthroscopic versus open surgical management of selected pathomorphologies of the hip.

Instr Course Lect 2012;61:287-293.

The body of literature regarding the arthroscopic management of hip pathomorphology, particularly femoroacetabular impingement (FAI), continues to grow[1-22] (CM Larson, MD, et al, San Francisco, CA, unpublished data presented at the Arthroscopy Association of North America annual meeting, 2011). There is a long learning curve for treating FAI arthroscopically, and specific techniques and indications continue to evolve. It is critical to identify those patients who are appropriate candidates for arthroscopic FAI correction.

Indications and Contraindications

Indications and contraindications for the arthroscopic management of FAI are based on a physician's ability to treat the underlying pathomorphology. Arthroscopic indications include focal anterior acetabular overcoverage, mild to moderate degrees of acetabular retroversion, coxa profunda, associated rim fractures and os acetabuli, and anterolaterally based cam lesions.[23] Relative contraindications for arthroscopic treatment include associated significant structural instability, extra-

articular greater trochanteric impingement, posteriorly based cam lesions, and moderate to advanced degenerate arthritis.[23] More specifically, structural instability cannot be corrected with arthroscopy. Patients with center-edge angles less than 20°, evidence of femoral head lateralization, a break in the Shenton line, and more severe degrees of acetabular retroversion with a low volumetric acetabulum may be better treated with a corrective pelvic osteotomy. To more completely define instability in patients with milder degrees of structural instability, it is important to take into account other factors, such as acetabular inclination, the femoral neck-shaft angle, and femoral neck version. Although global rim resections can be performed for protrusio acetabuli, there are limitations associated with arthroscopic dynamic assessment. Ultimately, younger patients with more severe protrusio may be better treated with an open surgical dislocation.[23]

Surgical Technique Overview

When performing hip arthroscopy, the surgeon must be capable of treating a three-dimensional problem while viewing a two-dimensional image. Consequently, three-dimensional CT is valuable in better defining the pathology and correlating it with ar-

Dr. Larson or an immediate family member is a member of a speakers' bureau or has made paid presentations on behalf of Smith & Nephew; serves as a paid consultant to Smith & Nephew and A2 Surgical; owns stock or stock options in A2 Surgical; and has received research or institutional support from Smith & Nephew.

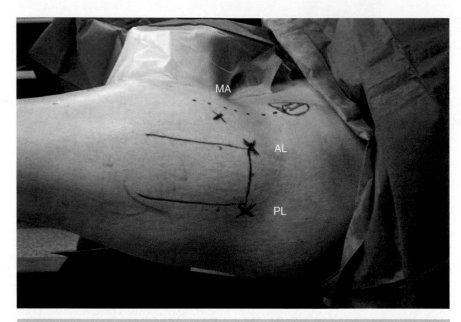

Figure 1   Typical portals used for hip arthroscopy (left hip shown) include the midanterior portal (MA), the anterolateral portal (AL), and the posterolateral portal (PL).

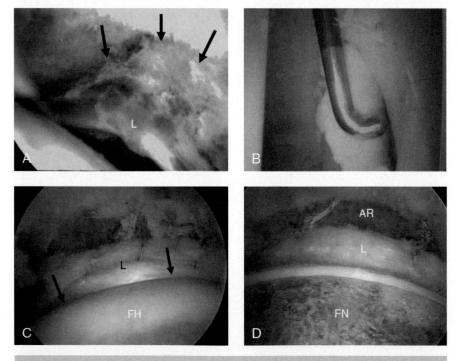

Figure 2   **A,** Arthroscopic image of the left hip shows labral bruising (L) and abnormal extension of the acetabular rim (arrows) beyond the labrochondral junction consistent with pincer-type impingement. **B,** Arthroscopic image of the left hip shows a chondral delamination with probing of the labrochondral junction. **C,** Arthroscopic image of the left hip after labral refixation (L) with mattress sutures shows maintenance of the labral seal (arrows) against the femoral head (FH). **D,** Arthroscopic image of the left hip after rim resection (AR), labral refixation (L), and femoral resection osteoplasty (FN) shows maintenance of the labral seal.

throscopic findings. Most procedures can be performed using a two-portal technique, with anterolateral and midanterior portals. A posterolateral portal can be used when posterior acetabular rim pathology is treated (**Figure 1**). Initially, central compartment arthroscopy is performed with traction. Generous capsulotomies from the midanterior to anterolateral or posterolateral portals are created to access most of the acetabular rim and the anterolateral femoral head-neck junction. Inspection of the labrum, labrochondral junction, acetabulum, and femur should confirm the suspected pathomorphology and guide specific procedures (**Figure 2**). Labral ecchymosis, calcification, ossification, extension of the acetabular rim well beyond the labrochondral junction, and difficulty visualizing or accessing the central compartment despite adequate distraction on fluoroscopy are all consistent with pincer-type FAI (**Figure 2, A**). Labrochondral disruptions, with varying degrees of acetabular chondral delaminations, are consistent with cam-type FAI (**Figure 2, B**). Many patients will have a combination of these findings because of the presence of both cam- and pincer-type FAI. All the described findings should be correlated with preoperative imaging studies and evaluated with intraoperative dynamic assessment.

Rim resections for pincer-type FAI are typically performed with the hip in traction, with or without labral takedown. The labrum can be taken down from the acetabular rim with an arthroscopic knife along the area of the pincer-type impingement. Rim resection is then performed with a motorized burr. Alternatively, more focal areas of pincer-type FAI with an intact labrum can be resected peripheral to the labrum without labral takedown. Intraoperative fluoroscopy can help guide and confirm appropriate resections if the pelvis is properly aligned to re-create a well-centered, preoperative anteroposterior pelvic radiograph[24] (**Figure 3**). This is primarily achieved by aligning the anterior superior iliac spines parallel to the floor and ceiling.[24] The extent and degree of rim resection is ultimately based on intraoperative findings, dynamic assessment, and preoperative imaging studies (**Figure 4**). The labrum is then refixed with suture anchors placed approximately 1 cm apart. A mattress and labral base refixation may be preferred to a loop-around refixation to preserve the sealing function of the labrum (**Figure 2**). Overresection of pincer-type pathology or resections in the setting of acetabular dysplasia should be avoided and can lead to iatrogenic postoperative instability.[25-27]

After treating the central compartment pathology, traction is released and the hip is flexed to approximately 40°. Portals can be maintained during traction release by withdrawing the arthroscope from the central compartment, which allows for visualization of the femoral head-neck junction. Dynamic assessment is then performed to evaluate for impingement secondary to cam-type FAI. Impingement is indicated by abnormal lifting of the acetabular labrum by the head-neck junction, levering of the femoral head out of the acetabulum, and/or limitations in hip range of motion with a firm end point during dynamic testing. The cam lesion is identified and correlated with preoperative imaging studies. Greater degrees of flexion and external rotation allow for visualization of the anteroinferior femoral head-neck junction and the medial synovial fold, whereas greater degrees of extension and internal rotation allow for visualization of the superoposterior femoral head-neck junction and the retinacular vessels.[5] A motorized burr is used to re-create a normal femoral-

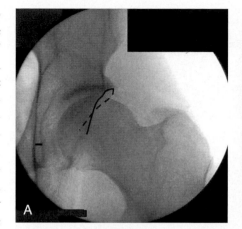
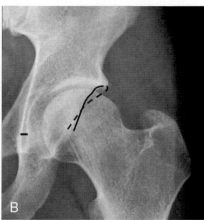

Figure 3   The intraoperative fluoroscopic image (**A**) of the left hip re-creates a well-centered preoperative AP pelvic radiograph (**B**) with respect to the relationship between the anterior (dashed line) and posterior acetabular walls (solid line), and between the ilioischial line and tear drop (horizontal line). (Reproduced with permission from Larson CM, Wulf CA: Intraoperative fluoroscopy for evaluation of bony resection during arthroscopic management of femoroacetabular impingement in the supine position. *Arthroscopy* 2009;25:1183-1192.)

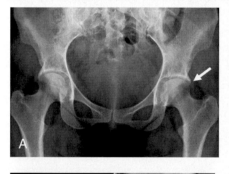
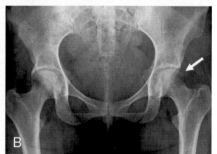
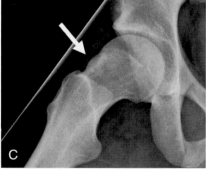
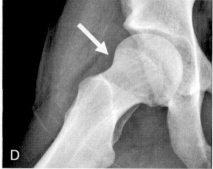

Figure 4   **A,** AP radiograph shows bilateral global acetabular overcoverage secondary to labral ossification (arrow). **B,** Postoperative radiograph after global anterior to posterior rim resection of the left hip (arrow). **C,** Lateral view of the right hip shows cam-type impingement (arrow). **D,** Postoperative radiograph of the right hip after femoral resection osteoplasty reveals improved head-neck offset.

head neck junction; a repetition of dynamic assessment and intraoperative fluoroscopy can confirm appropriate femoral resection (**Figure 4**). A broad-

er, more conservative resection is generally preferred over a more focal, aggressive resection because it may better maintain the labral seal. Resecting

Table 1
Clinical Outcomes After Arthroscopic Management of Femoroacetabular Impingement

Study	Hips	Mean Follow-up (Years)	Clinically Good or Excellent Outcomes
Brunner et al[12]	53	2.4	NA
Byrd et al[13]	200	1.6	95%
Byrd and Jones[1]	207	1.4	NA
Fabricant et al[18]	27	1.5	NA
Gedouin et al[14]	111	0.8	NA
Horisberger et al[15]	20	3.0	NA
Ilizaliturri et al[19]	14	2.5	NA
Ilizaliturri et al[2]	19	2.4	NA
Larson and Giveans[4]	75	1.6	DB, 66.7%; LR, 89.7%
Larson et al[20]	227	2.2	NA
Larson et al[a]	100	3.5	DB, 68%; LR, 92%
Nho et al[17]	47	2.2	93%
Philippon et al[7]	112	2.3	NA
Philippon et al[21]	28	2.0	NA
Schilders et al[22]	101	2.44	NA
Singh and O'Donnell[16]	27	1.8	NA

[a]CM Larson, MD, et al, San Francisco, CA, unpublished data presented at the Arthroscopy Association of North America annual meeting, 2011.
ADL = activities of daily living; DB = débridement (labral resection); HHS = Harris Hip score; HOS = Hip Outcome score; LR = labral refixation; MHHS = modified Harris Hip score; NAHS = Nonarthritic Hip score; NA = not available; OA = osteoarthritis; RTP = return to play; SF-12 = Medical Outcomes Study 12-Item Short Form; THA = total hip arthroplasty; VAS = visual analog pain scale, WOMAC = Western Ontario and McMaster Universities Osteoarthritis Index.
(Courtesy of Asheesh Bedi, MD, and Bryan Kelly, MD, New York, NY.)

greater than 30% of the femoral neck width is reported to significantly increase the risk for postoperative femoral neck fractures.[28] Impingement is a unique condition, with each case varying with respect to the region and extent of bony resections. At the completion of the procedure, a motorized shaver is used to meticulously remove all residual bony debris to minimize the risk for postoperative heterotopic ossification. Closure of the capsulotomy is controversial and should be considered in patients with capsular laxity, generalized hypermobility, and borderline dysplasia.

 Video 23.1: Arthroscopic Management of Pincer- and Cam-Type Femoroacetabular Impingement. Christopher M. Larson, MD; Rebecca M. Stone, ATC (8 min)

Postoperative Management
Early postoperative range of motion begins on the day of surgery with well-leg cycling or a continuous passive range-of-motion machine. Limits are placed on the extremes of external rotation for patients with capsular repairs. Foot-flat weight bearing is advised for 2 to 3 weeks until the patient is able to ambulate with a non-antalgic gait. Weight-bearing restrictions are maintained for 4 to 8 weeks if microfracture is performed or osteopenic bone is encountered during bony resections. Nonsteroidal anti-inflammatory drugs are taken for 2 to 3 weeks postoperatively to decrease

Table 1 *(continued)*

Clinical Outcomes After Arthroscopic Management of Femoroacetabular Impingement

Clinical Outcome Measure(s) and Mean Change in Hip Score (Points)	Failure Definition	Failure % (Number)
SF-12, 1.06; NAHS, 31.3; VAS, 4.1	NA	NA
MHHS, 21	Conversion to THA, inability to RTP	THA, 0.5%; professional RTP, 0.5%; intercollegiate RTP, 15%
MHHS, 20	NA	NA
HHS, 21; HOS, 16	NA	NA
WOMAC, 23	NA	NA
NAHS, 28; VAS, 4	Conversion to THA	THA, 8.6% (9)
WOMAC, 9.6	NA	0% (0)
WOMAC, 7	Advanced OA, recommended THA	5% (1)
DB: MHHS, 25; SF-12, 19; VAS, 5 LR: MHHA, 32; SF-12, 24; VAS, 5	MHHS less than 70, reconversion to THA, repeat débridement	DB, 11.1%; LR, 7.7%
No OA: MHHS, 22.8; SF-12, 20.9; VAS, 4.5 With OA: MHHS, 3.7; SF-12, 4.3; VAS, 2.6	No sustained improvement in MHHS	Failure rate, 12%; failure rate with mild joint-space narrowing, 33%; failure rate with OA, 82%
DB: MHHS, 20.2; SF-12, 18.4; VAS, 4.7 LR: MHHS, 26.1; SF-12, 28.1; VAS, 4.6	MHHS less than 70, reconversion to THA, repeat débridement	DB, 9.1%; LR, 8.0%
MHHS, 20; HOS, 13	Inability to RTP	7%
MHHS, 24; HOS-ADL, 17; HOS-Sport, 24; NAHS, 14	Conversion to THA	9% (10)
MHHS, 25	NA	NA
LR: HHS, 33; DB: HHS, 26	NA	NA
MHHS, 10; NAHS, 15	Continued hip pain or pain requiring surgical intervention	0% (0)

[a]CM Larson, MD, et al, San Francisco, CA, unpublished data presented at the Arthroscopy Association of North America annual meeting, 2011.

ADL = activities of daily living; DB = débridement (labral resection); HHS = Harris Hip score; HOS = Hip Outcome score; LR = labral refixation; MHHS = modified Harris Hip score; NAHS = Nonarthritic Hip score; NA = not available; OA = osteoarthritis; RTP = return to play; SF-12 = Medical Outcomes Study 12-Item Short Form; THA = total hip arthroplasty; VAS = visual analog pain scale, WOMAC = Western Ontario and McMaster Universities Osteoarthritis Index.

(Courtesy of Asheesh Bedi, MD, and Bryan Kelly, MD, New York, NY.)

the risk of heterotopic bone formation.

Arthroscopic Outcomes and Complications

Reports and systematic reviews evaluating arthroscopic management of FAI in properly selected patients have noted significant improvements in pain and functional scores[1-22] (CM Larson, MD, et al, San Francisco, CA, unpublished data presented at the Arthroscopy Association of North America annual meeting, 2011) (**Table 1**). To date, there has been only one review article comparing arthroscopic and open surgical treatment of FAI.[11] This report found substantial improvement in outcomes after both open and arthroscopic approaches, but neither treatment was found to be clearly superior. Cadaver studies have shown that arthroscopic femoral resections for anteriorly based cam-type FAI are comparable to anterior femoral resections performed with an open surgical approach.[29,30]

Complications have been reported after arthroscopic management of FAI.[5,25-28,31,32] Specifically, underresection of bony impingement has been reported as a primary reason for failure in arthroscopic hip procedures.[31] Iatrogenic hip instability and femoral neck fractures also have been reported after hip arthroscopy; this emphasizes the importance of appropriate diagnosis, surgical technique, and the avoidance of bony overresection.[25-28,31,32] Hip joint preservation procedures in the presence of substantial osteoarthritis will lead to higher failure rates regardless of the surgical approach.[20]

Summary

The understanding of FAI is evolving, and new patterns of impingement are being identified. With appropriate patient selection, indications, and surgical technique, hip arthroscopy has been shown to be effective in treating these disorders. Published outcomes and systematic reviews support a role for hip arthroscopy in patients with FAI; however, further studies are required to better define the most appropriate surgical approach when treating the varying patterns of FAI.

References

1. Byrd JW, Jones KS: Arthroscopic femoroplasty in the management of cam-type femoroacetabular impingement. *Clin Orthop Relat Res* 2009;467(3):739-746.

2. Ilizaliturri VM Jr, Orozco-Rodriguez L, Acosta-Rodríguez E, Camacho-Galindo J: Arthroscopic treatment of cam-type femoroacetabular impingement: Preliminary report at 2 years minimum follow-up. *J Arthroplasty* 2008; 23(2):226-234.

3. Larson CM, Giveans MR: Arthroscopic management of femoroacetabular impingement: Early outcomes measures. *Arthroscopy* 2008;24(5):540-546.

4. Larson CM, Giveans MR: Arthroscopic debridement versus refixation of the acetabular labrum associated with femoroacetabular impingement. *Arthroscopy* 2009;25(4):369-376.

5. Larson CM, Guanche CA, Kelly BT, Clohisy JC, Ranawat AS: Advanced techniques in hip arthroscopy. *Instr Course Lect* 2009; 58:423-436.

6. Ng VY, Arora N, Best TM, Pan X, Ellis TJ: Efficacy of surgery for femoroacetabular impingement: A systematic review. *Am J Sports Med* 2010;38(11):2337-2345.

7. Philippon MJ, Briggs KK, Yen YM, Kuppersmith DA: Outcomes following hip arthroscopy for femoroacetabular impingement with associated chondrolabral dysfunction: Minimum two-year follow-up. *J Bone Joint Surg Br* 2009;91(1):16-23.

8. Stevens MS, Legay DA, Glazebrook MA, Amirault D: The evidence for hip arthroscopy: Grading the current indications. *Arthroscopy* 2010;26(10):1370-1383.

9. Clohisy JC, St John LC, Schutz AL: Surgical treatment of femoroacetabular impingement: A systematic review of the literature. *Clin Orthop Relat Res* 2010; 468(2):555-564.

10. Lodhia P, Slobogean GP, Noonan VK, Gilbart MK: Patient-reported outcome instruments for femoroacetabular impingement and hip labral pathology: A systematic review of the clinimetric evidence. *Arthroscopy* 2011;27(2):279-286.

11. Botser IB, Smith TW Jr, Nasser R, Domb BG: Open surgical dislocation versus arthroscopy for femoroacetabular impingement: A comparison of clinical outcomes. *Arthroscopy* 2011;27(2):270-278.

12. Brunner A, Horisberger M, Herzog RF: Sports and recreation activity of patients with femoroacetabular impingement before and after arthroscopic osteoplasty. *Am J Sports Med* 2009;37(5):917-922.

13. Byrd JW, Jones KS: Arthroscopic management of femoroacetabular impingement in athletes. *Am J Sports Med* 2011;39(Suppl): 7S-13S.

14. Gedouin JE, May O, Bonin N, et al; French Arthroscopy Society: Assessment of arthroscopic management of femoroacetabular impingement: A prospective multicenter study. *Orthop Traumatol Surg Res* 2010;96(8, Suppl): S59-S67.

15. Horisberger M, Brunner A, Herzog RF: Arthroscopic treatment of femoral acetabular impingement in patients with preoperative generalized degenerative changes. *Arthroscopy* 2010;26(5):623-629.

16. Singh PJ, O'Donnell JM: The outcome of hip arthroscopy in Australian football league players:

A review of 27 hips. *Arthroscopy* 2010;26(6):743-749.

17. Nho SJ, Magennis EM, Singh CK, Kelly BT: Outcomes after the arthroscopic treatment of femoroacetabular impingement in a mixed group of high-level athletes. *Am J Sports Med* 2011;39(Suppl): 14S-19S.

18. Fabricant PD, Heyworth BE, Kelly BT: Hip arthroscopy improves symptoms associated with FAI in selected adolescent athletes. *Clin Orthop Relat Res* 2007. http://www. springerlink.com/content/r475m171023133r0/fulltext.html. August 11, 2011. Accessed October 4, 2011.

19. Ilizaliturri VM Jr, Nossa-Barrera JM, Acosta-Rodriguez E, Camacho-Galindo J: Arthroscopic treatment of femoroacetabular impingement secondary to paediatric hip disorders. *J Bone Joint Surg Br* 2007;89(8):1025-1030.

20. Larson CM, Giveans MR, Taylor M: Does arthroscopic FAI correction improve function with radiographic arthritis? *Clin Orthop Relat Res* 2011;469(6):1667-1676.

21. Philippon MJ, Weiss DR, Kuppersmith DA, Briggs KK, Hay CJ: Arthroscopic labral repair and treatment of femoroacetabular impingement in professional hockey players. *Am J Sports Med* 2010;38(1):99-104.

22. Schilders E, Dimitrakopoulou A, Bismil Q, Marchant P, Cooke C: Arthroscopic treatment of labral tears in femoroacetabular impingement: A comparative study of refixation and resection with a minimum two-year follow-up. *J Bone Joint Surg Br* 2011;93(8): 1027-1032.

23. Larson CM: Arthroscopic management of pincer-type impingement. *Sports Med Arthrosc* 2010; 18(2):100-107.

24. Larson CM, Wulf CA: Intraoperative fluoroscopy for evaluation of bony resection during ar-

throscopic management of femoroacetabular impingement in the supine position. *Arthroscopy* 2009; 25(10):1183-1192.

25. Matsuda DK: Acute iatrogenic dislocation following hip impingement arthroscopic surgery. *Arthroscopy* 2009;25(4):400-404.

26. Ranawat AS, McClincy M, Sekiya JK: Anterior dislocation of the hip after arthroscopy in a patient with capsular laxity of the hip: A case report. *J Bone Joint Surg Am* 2009;91(1):192-197.

27. Benali Y, Katthagen BD: Hip subluxation as a complication of arthroscopic debridement. *Arthroscopy* 2009;25(4):405-407.

28. Mardones RM, Gonzalez C, Chen Q, Zobitz M, Kaufman KR, Trousdale RT: Surgical treatment of femoroacetabular impingement: Evaluation of the effect of the size of the resection. Surgical technique. *J Bone Joint Surg Am* 2006;88(Suppl 1 Pt 1):84-91.

29. Mardones R, Lara J, Donndorff A, et al: Surgical correction of "cam-type" femoroacetabular impingement: A cadaveric comparison of open versus arthroscopic debridement. *Arthroscopy* 2009; 25(2):175-182.

30. Sussmann PS, Ranawat AS, Lipman J, Lorich DG, Padgett DE, Kelly BT: Arthroscopic versus open osteoplasty of the head-neck junction: A cadaveric investigation. *Arthroscopy* 2007;23(12): 1257-1264.

31. Heyworth BE, Shindle MK, Voos JE, Rudzki JR, Kelly BT: Radiologic and intraoperative findings in revision hip arthroscopy. *Arthroscopy* 2007;23(12):1295-1302.

32. Aveni OR, Bedi A, Lorich DG, Kelly BT: Femoral neck fracture after arthroscopic management of femoroacetabular impingement: A case report. *J Bone Joint Surg Am* 2010;93(9):e47.

Video Reference

23.1: Larson CM, Stone RM: Video. *Arthroscopic Management of Pincer- and Cam-Type Femoroacetabular Impingement.* Edina, MN, 2011.

Approaches for Revision Total Hip Replacement

William Jiranek, MD, FACS

Abstract

Choosing the approach for revision total hip replacement is an essential part of surgical planning and should be done well before the patient enters the operating room. Planning includes selecting patient positioning, the location of the incision, techniques for managing previous incisions, the needed exposure equipment, and the steps needed to extend the exposure. More extensive exposure on both the acetabular and femoral sides is often required in revision surgery.

Instr Course Lect 2012;61:295-302.

Considering options for the surgical approach is an essential part of planning for revision total hip replacement. Three basic questions should be asked: (1) Which components are being revised? (2) What defects are present? (3) What approaches were used previously?

In general, it is sensible to honor previous incisions and approaches, with the exception of extensive acetabular work when using the direct lateral approach or extensive femoral work when using the anterior approach. The surgeon also should determine the primary location of the surgery: Is it predominantly acetabular, predominantly femoral, or both?[1]

The chosen approach is influenced by the work that needs to be done. For example, if bulk allografts or buttress augments are required, greater than normal exposure of the ilium will be necessary; posterior plating of a pelvic discontinuity would be difficult to achieve through anterior or anterolateral approaches; and placing a cage or triflange cup is much easier to accomplish through a transtrochanteric approach. For planning purposes, the surgery may use an extensile acetabular exposure, an extensile femoral exposure, or both. An extensile acetabular exposure is needed for managing severe osteolytic lesions, placing bulk allografts, buttress augmentation, posterior column plating for discontinuity, or placing a cage or a triflange cup. An extensile femoral approach is needed for difficult stem or cement extraction, plac-

ing a modular stem, managing severe bone loss (type IIIB or IV defects), treating broken femoral stems, or managing a periprosthetic fracture.[2]

Patient Positioning

Because many revision situations require extension of the incision, the surgeon should choose the patient position that provides maximum flexibility. Many surgeons prefer the floppy lateral position because it allows access to both the front and the back of the hip. In this position, the patient is rolled approximately halfway between the supine and lateral decubitus positions, and a beanbag is used to allow some motion forward and backward. The supine position can be used if the surgeon is comfortable with it, but access to posterior structures is difficult. Regardless of the position chosen, there should be clear access to the top of the ilium without impingement by bars or pads that would prevent extension of the incision. Similarly, the positioning should allow a full range of motion of the involved extremity without limitation by the positioning equipment. Numerous positioning guides are available, but the most adjustable may be a beanbag, which allows control of the torso and contralateral limb without restricting the motion of the operated leg.

Dr. Jiranek or an immediate family member has received royalties from DePuy; serves as a paid consultant to DePuy; has received research or institutional support from Stryker; and serves as a board member, owner, officer, or committee member of the American Academy of Orthopaedic Surgeons, the American Association of Hip and Knee Surgeons, and the Knee Society.

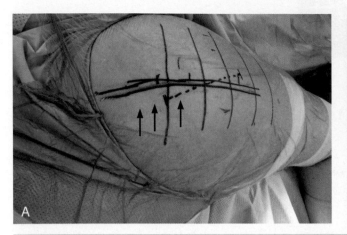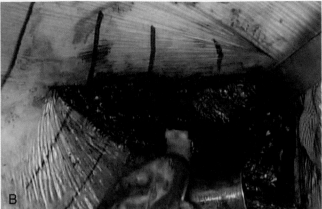

Figure 1 **A,** In managing multiple previous incisions, leaving a small area of potentially devascularized skin (arrows) should be avoided. **B,** Aspirating a hip joint of a failed metal-on-metal total hip replacement before capsulotomy.

Incisions

Rather than making a new incision in a better position, prior incisions should be used wherever possible and extended when necessary. Vascularity in the skin over the hip is considerably better than vascularity in the skin over the knee; however, care must be taken to avoid violating the 1:1 rule of flaps. This rule suggests that in any potential flap created by an old incision and a new incision, the length should be equal to the width (avoiding a strip of potentially devascularized skin) (**Figure 1,** *A*). In the situation where there are multiple prior incisions, the incision that is closest to the planned work should be used, and narrow flaps should be avoided. Attempts should be made to excise the previous incision, rather than merely incising it. This allows the surgeon to excise the dermal scar, which allows better apposition of the flaps on closure and avoids the unsightly appearance of multiple incisions. As with any incision, the surgeon should avoid the creation of large areas of dead space and should mobilize flaps only enough to access the joint and allow adequate closure.

If possible, the deep fascial incision should stay in the interval between the tensor fascia lata and gluteus maximus for both a lateral and a posterior approach. In revision approaches, it is often possible to reflect the posterior pseudocapsule and preserve it for later repair. It can be tagged in much the same manner as is done in a primary arthroplasty. The same is true for a revision performed through an anterolateral approach. Prior to incising the pseudocapsule, the synovial fluid should be aspirated for a cell count, differential, and culture (**Figure 1,** *B*). Findings from the cell count and differential can later help the surgeon differentiate a true positive bacterial culture from a contaminant.[3]

Exposure Equipment

The proper instruments facilitate accomplishing the exposure. Numerous retractors have been developed for revision surgery, including retractors that maintain the greater amounts of exposure required in revision surgery, as well as self-retaining retractors that provide exposure with less assistance. Longer cobra retractors can be used when an osteotomy fragment requires more anterior retraction. High-speed burrs and sharp osteotomes are helpful for creating osteotomies.

Extension of the Exposure

Soft-tissue releases and osteotomies can improve the mobilization of the hip joint. The soft-tissue releases are the anterior capsulectomy (versus capsulotomy), the gluteus maximus tendon release, the rectus strip, and the abductor strip (**Table 1**). Osteotomies include the traditional trochanteric osteotomy, the trochanteric slide, and the extended trochanteric osteotomy (**Table 2**).

Anterior Capsulectomy

The formal anterior capsulectomy is particularly valuable in acetabular revision surgeries performed through a posterior approach in which the femoral component is left in situ. Using this technique, the surgeon can safely differentiate the anterior pseudocapsule from the anterior neurovascular structures. Sufficient anterior capsule can be excised to create a pocket where the femoral trunnion or, in the case of monoblock femoral components, the femoral head can be safely retracted anterior to the anterior rim of the acetabulum. Prior to performing this maneuver, the surgeon should reflect the posterior pseudocapsule in a trapdoor fashion, tagging the capsule for later repair (**Figure 2**). An anterior capsulectomy is facilitated by leaving the prosthetic joint located, which allows the anterior capsule to be placed on tension. This technique is initiated by flexing and externally rotating the affected limb (**Figure 3,** *A*). The anterior border of the gluteus medius muscle belly is delineated, and a Cushing elevator is worked under the gluteus medius and the minimus muscle bellies from anterior to posterior (**Figure 3,** *B*). A long cobra retractor is inserted under the psoas tendon on top of the anterior hip pseudocapsule, with the tip resting over the iliopectineal eminence. The anterior border of the vastus lateralis muscle belly is mobilized, and a rake retractor is used to retract the muscle posteriorly. This provides good exposure of the anterior capsule. The first (superior) triangle is created by releasing the capsule along the vastus lateralis from distal to proximal to the level of the Cushing retractor (**Figure 4**). The release is then turned 90° along the anterior rim of the acetabulum toward the tip of the cobra retractor. The base of the triangle is then excised between these two limbs. The inferior triangle of capsule can be excised under direct vision so that any bleeding can be controlled. Following this excision, the surgeon should be able to place his or her fingers from the front and back of the femur and touch them anteriorly to posteriorly. The hip can then be dislocated, and the femoral head removed if it is modular. The tip of a long cobra retractor can be placed underneath the trunnion of the femoral component and then over the anterior superior rim of the acetabulum. With anterior retraction, the femoral component will slide anteriorly, thus affording wide exposure of the acetabulum.

Gluteus Maximus Tendon Release
The gluteus maximus tendon release aids in anterior mobilization of the femur and will decrease pressure on the sciatic nerve, which can occur with anterior mobilization. Some surgeons will

initiate the release by placing a tonsil clamp beneath the tendon to protect the sciatic nerve (**Figure 5**). The tendon can be tagged with suture before release to facilitate later repair. The tendon should be divided with a scalpel or an electrocautery device approximately 1 cm lat-

---

Table 1
Soft-Tissue Releases

Anterior Capsulectomy

Very helpful in acetabular revisions in which femoral component is left in situ and needs to be moved anterior to acetabulum.

Place leg in flexion and external rotation.

Place cobra retractor under iliopsoas and over anterior rim of pelvis.

Place Cushing elevator under abductors.

Remove lateral triangle medial to vastus lateralis and transverse across top of acetabulum.

Remove medial triangle inferior to medial aspect of acetabulum.

Gluteus Maximus Tendon Release

Helpful to mobilize femur anteriorly and takes pressure off sciatic nerve.

Sciatic nerve can be identified beneath gluteus maximus tendon.

Protect nerve by placing a tonsil clamp beneath tendon.

Divide tendon 1 cm lateral to the bony insertion.

Two relatively large vessels run in the deep section of tendon and should be coagulated.

Rectus Strip

Helps mobilize the femur anteriorly.

Place cobra retractor underneath the direct and reflected heads of the rectus femoris at the superomedial corner of the acetabulum.

Release the tendon origin from bone with electrocautery to allow the tendon to slide anteriorly.

Abductor Strip

Helps mobilize scarred abductors.

Identify superior margin of acetabulum.

Use curved 0.75-inch osteotome to slide up the iliac wing.

Avoid diving posteriorly into the sciatic notch.

Table 2
Osteotomies

Trochanteric

Use when wide exposure to the ilium is needed and the trochanter needs to be mobilized distally to improve abductor tension.

Trochanteric Slide

Use when wide exposure to the ilium is needed and the trochanter will be repaired in the same position.

Takes advantage of the tenodesis effect of the vastus lateralis attachment to prevent migration.

Place Cushing elevator beneath abductors.

Divide the posterior aspect of vastus lateralis and place Bennett retractor under vastus lateralis and over the femur.

Use oscillating saw to divide trochanter from beneath abductor insertion to beneath vastus tubercle.

Mobilize trochanter anteriorly.

Extended Trochanteric

Use when increased exposure of the femur is needed to remove implants or when femur is remodeled into varus.

Template the needed length to ensure that sufficient distal access is created.

Make posterior limb first; score femur 1 cm anterior to the linea aspera.

Make distal limb transversely; a pencil tip burr can be used to round corners.

Start anterior limb from distal to proximal; make drill holes along the line of the fragment parallel to the posterior limb; try to keep muscle attachments intact to fragment.

Distal to proximally, saw approximately one third the distance of the fragment.

Use an osteotome to complete osteotomy in line with the saw cut.

Make sure the distal corners are complete.

Use the two-osteotomes technique to mobilize the fragment from posterior to anterior.

Use particular care when mobilizing the trochanteric junction with the cortical fragment distal to the vastus tubercle.

The osteotomy weakens the femur approximately 60%, so the femur should be carefully mobilized.

Femoral Univalve

Occasionally indicated when a retained femoral stem for extraction needs to be torsionally mobilized for extraction.

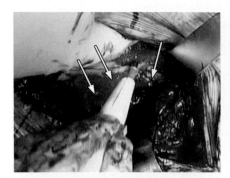

Figure 2   Tagging the posterior pseudocapsule (arrows) facilitates repair and protects the sciatic nerve posteriorly.

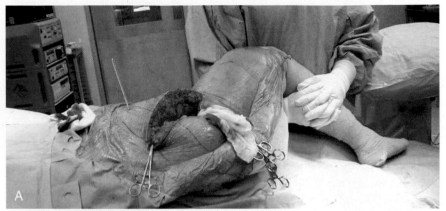

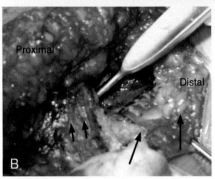

Figure 3   **A,** The capsule is placed on tension by leaving the hip located and flexing and externally rotating the limb. **B,** The anterior capsule is exposed by placing a retractor over the iliopectineal eminence, using a second retractor under the abductor tendons (short arrows), and using a third retractor to pull back the vastus lateralis tendon laterally (long arrows).

eral to the femur. This will facilitate easier repair and also allow control of the two relatively large blood vessels that run in the posterior aspect of the tendon. If exploration of the sciatic nerve is planned proximally, the nerve is located beneath the gluteus tendon.

The Rectus Strip

The rectus strip is used for exposing the superior acetabulum and anterior ilium to facilitate the removal of the acetabular components and the management of anterior bony defects. It allows placement of anterior retractors more medially on the anterior column and protects the anterior rim, which is often weakened and at risk for fracture. It involves releasing the direct head of the rectus femoris in a sliding fashion from anteromedially to posterolaterally. A cobra retractor is placed under the proximal femur and on the ilium superior and anterior to the socket (**Figure 6,** *A*). This placement puts the direct head of the rectus femoris under tension and will allow a window to slide a scalpel or electrocautery under the tendon and release it in a sliding fashion directly off its origin. Once the tendon is released, the surgeon can place the cobra retractor under the tendon in the iliac bone at the superior aspect of the acetabulum.

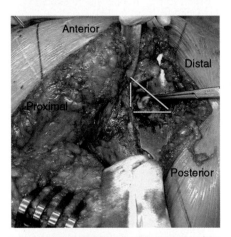

Figure 4   The first triangle of the anterior capsulotomy is excised. The margin of the inferior limb is just anterior to the vastus lateralis muscle belly, and the cephalad limb divides the capsule along the anterior rim of the socket.

The Abductor Strip

The abductor strip is used to expose the ilium for grafting or hardware placement or mobilize a proximally migrated hip or trochanteric fragment. It releases the muscle belly from its un-

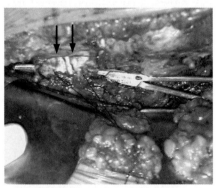

Figure 5   The gluteus maximus tendon (arrows) is isolated by placing a tonsil clamp beneath it; the sciatic nerve is protected inferiorly.

dersurface because the innervation of the muscle belly comes from the other side. The muscle belly may be released all the way to its origin on the iliac crest. The release starts just above the acetabulum, using a 0.75-inch curved osteotome or broad Cobb elevator beneath the muscle, directed in an anterosuperior fashion (**Figure 6,** *B*). Care should be taken to prevent the instrument from sliding into the sciatic

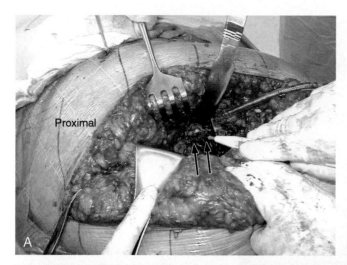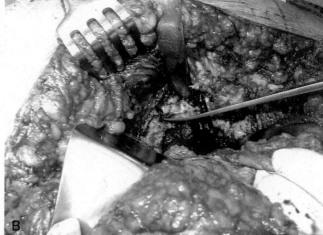

Figure 6 **A,** Sliding a retractor anterior and superior to the socket will place the anterior capsule and the direct head of the rectus femoris under tension (arrows) and allow them to be released in a sliding fashion. **B,** After a space is made between the superior edge of the socket and the rectus tendon, a curved osteotome can slide on bone to the top of the ilium. Caution is needed to prevent the osteotome from sliding posteriorly into the sciatic notch.

notch, which should be palpated before beginning the release. If a trochanteric fragment is present, it can be grasped with a bone-holding clamp, and distal traction can be placed on the fragment to aid in the release. In the case of extreme contracture, if this maneuver does not provide sufficient release, the abductor enthesis may be released from the iliac crest, and the entire muscle belly can be allowed to slide distally.

Osteotomies

A trochanteric osteotomy allows excellent exposure of the hip and femur; however, a trochanteric osteotomy should be used only when it provides clear advantages over soft-tissue releases alone (**Table 3**). The most common osteotomies are the traditional trochanteric osteotomy, the trochanteric slide, and the extended trochanteric osteotomy.[4] Less commonly used but occasionally helpful are the femoral univalve and the femoral window osteotomies.

Traditional Trochanteric

The traditional trochanteric osteotomy detaches the greater trochanter

from its distal attachments (the origin of the vastus lateralis muscle belly). It helps provide wide exposure to the acetabulum and also exposes the lateral side of the femoral endosteum to facilitate component exposure. This osteotomy is particularly suited for situations in which the trochanter must be advanced distally. Because of the orientation of the abductor muscles inserting into the proximal greater trochanter, the osteotomized fragment should be reflected proximally and anteriorly. The femur can usually be retracted either anteriorly or posteriorly. The osteotomy is started by templating the obliquity of the cut; a more transverse cut is used if the plan is to advance the trochanter, and a more vertical and superficial cut is used if the fragment is to be placed back onto the bed. The proximal aspect of the trochanter and the inserting abductor tendons should be differentiated from adjacent scar tissue. A Cushing retractor can be placed from anterior to posterior underneath the abductor tendons to delineate the proximal aspect of the osteotomy and protect the tendons from the saw. Distally, the vastus lateralis should be de-

Table 3
Indications for Osteotomy[a]

Remove solidly ingrown femoral component.

Remove solid cement mantle.

Bypass femoral deformity.

Need to retract abductors for wide exposure to the ilium.

Need to tighten abductor tension.

---

[a]Because osteotomy adds surgical time and puts the femur at risk for injury, it should be done only for sound indications.

tached from the vastus tubercle. The distal aspect of the osteotomy should come through the tubercle after the muscle is retracted. The osteotomy is repaired by using a four-wire technique (two vertical and two horizontal wires), by horizontal wires or cables, or by using a trochanteric claw device. The healing rate of traditional trochanteric osteotomies in older series was approximately 90% the first time it was repaired, but the rate decreased significantly (to 50% or less) on subsequent attempts at repair.[5]

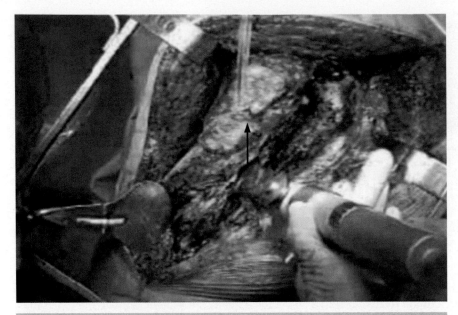

Figure 7 A Bennett retractor is placed beneath the vastus lateralis (arrow) to protect it as the posterior limb of the osteotomy is made through the femur with an oscillating saw. (Courtesy of C. Andrew Engh Jr, MD, Alexandria, VA.)

Trochanteric Slide

The trochanteric slide osteotomy was devised to preserve the distal attachment of the vastus lateralis, which likely improves the blood supply to the fragment and helps function as a tether to prevent proximal migration of the trochanter.[6-8] The only modification from the traditional osteotomy is that the posterior aspect of the vastus lateralis is mobilized just anterior to the intramuscular septum, and a Bennett retractor is used to retract the proximal portion of the muscle anteriorly, which protects the muscle as the osteotomy is made (**Figure 7**). This osteotomy is more appropriate when the trochanter will be repaired in situ and not advanced. Fixation is usually performed with horizontal wires or cables.

Extended Trochanteric

The extended trochanteric osteotomy was popularized by Paprosky in the 1990s to improve access to the femur for removing femoral components and providing more predictable healing of the trochanteric fragment.[9] Because

this type of osteotomy weakens the femur to torsional stress by up to 70%, it should be used only with clear indications.[10] The extended trochanteric osteotomy is indicated to allow access to extensively ingrown femoral components or the removal of distal cement, or when varus remodeling of the proximal femur makes placement of a new femoral component very difficult or impossible.

Because the femur is often encased in scar tissue during a revision surgery, the scar tissue should be released and the hip dislocated before starting the osteotomy. If this is not done, there is risk that the remaining femur will fracture as the limb is manipulated to dislocate the hip after the osteotomy. The osteotomy can be planned to include the lateral one third of the femoral circumference or as a more anterior (Wagner type) osteotomy. The Wagner osteotomy is performed 90° more anterior than the traditional extended trochanteric osteotomy and is easier to accomplish when using a Hardinge approach. Because the average femur has

a circumference of 6 to 8 cm, an osteotomy width of 2 to 2.5 cm provides sufficient access to the femur without markedly weakening it. The osteotomy can be templated with a 2-mm drill bit. It generally starts just anterior to the posterior intermuscular septum and progresses proximally to the posterior aspect of the greater trochanter and distally to the point that the surgeon determines will provide adequate access to the femoral component for extraction. The osteotomy is then turned 90° anteriorly for a distance of 2 to 2.5 cm and then turned 90° proximal and directed to the anterior aspect of the greater trochanter. Because the fibers of the vastus lateralis originate from this fragment (and presumably carry some of the blood supply), they should be preserved if possible. Consequently, once the anterior limb of the osteotomy has been started for a distance of 4 cm, a straight osteotome can be placed in the osteotomy track underneath the vastus lateralis fibers and impacted toward the anterior aspect of the trochanter (**Figure 8**). After the cortex is divided, the surgeon should ensure that the corners are mobilized. Then, using two wide osteotomes (one proximal and one distal) placed into the posterior limb of the osteotomy, the fragment should be slowly and carefully elevated. If there is extensive bony attachment to the undersurface of the fragment, a curved osteotome is used to gently disrupt the attachment to the underlying cement or prosthesis. The fragment can then be mobilized anteriorly, which provides wide exposure to the acetabulum.

Repair of the osteotomy is usually accomplished with three cables or wires. The proximal wire can be threaded through drill holes in the greater trochanter and passed inferior to the lesser trochanter. The other two wires are evenly spaced between the

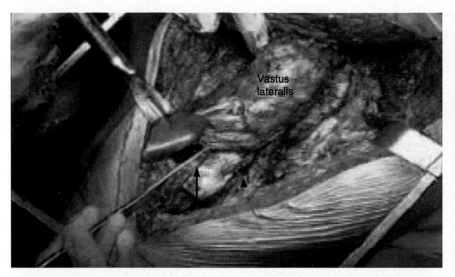

Figure 8 A straight osteotome is placed in the anterior limb (arrow) of the osteotomy from distal to proximal to complete the osteotomy without damaging the overlying muscle fibers. The posterior limb is indicated by the arrowhead. (Courtesy of C. Andrew Engh Jr, MD, Alexandria, VA.)

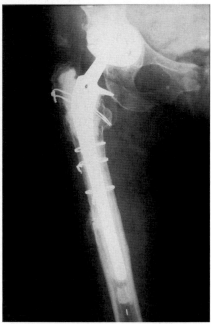

Figure 9 The wire location for repair of the osteotomy is shown. Three or four 18-gauge stainless steel wires or cables are equally spaced. The proximal wire must go under the lesser trochanter and through drill holes in the greater trochanter.

vastus tubercle and the end of the osteotomy fragment (**Figure 9**).

Femoral Univalve

The femoral univalve osteotomy is accomplished by first making the posterior cut of an extended trochanteric osteotomy. If the femoral component is somewhat loose or has fibrous ingrowth, this osteotomy often allows the surgeon to rotate the stem within the canal. The length of the single femoral cut should be close in length to the femoral component that will be removed. The femoral component can then be tapped out in a retrograde fashion. If the univalve is not sufficient to mobilize the femoral component, the remainder of the extended trochanteric osteotomy can be completed.

Femoral Window

The femoral window osteotomy can be an effective procedure for removing a well-fixed cement plug, a distal modular component of a femoral stem, or a broken portion of a femoral component.[11] It also can be helpful in revision surgery to monitor the preparation of the femoral canal. The size of the window should be templated preoperatively; several biomechanical studies have suggested that the anterior third of the femoral cortex causes the least amount of femoral weakening.[11,12]

Summary

Because each revision total hip replacement is unique, the surgeon must consider the previous approaches used, which components require revision, and what defects need to be addressed. Despite the best preparation, unplanned events can occur. The surgeon should be prepared to enhance the surgical exposure with a combination of bony and soft-tissue procedures.

References

1. Masterson EL, Masri BA, Duncan CP: Surgical approaches in revision hip replacement. *J Am Acad Orthop Surg* 1998;6(2):84-92.

2. Taylor JW, Rorabeck CH: Hip revision arthroplasty: Approach to the femoral side. *Clin Orthop Relat Res* 1999;369:208-222.

3. Spangehl MJ, Masri BA, O'Connell JX, Duncan CP: Prospective analysis of preoperative and intraoperative investigations for the diagnosis of infection at the sites of two hundred and two revision total hip arthroplasties. *J Bone Joint Surg Am* 1999;81(5): 672-683.

4. Masri BA, Campbell DG, Garbuz DS, Duncan CP: Seven specialized exposures for revision hip and knee replacement. *Orthop Clin North Am* 1998;29(2):229-240.

5. Glassman AH: Complications of trochanteric osteotomy. *Orthop Clin North Am* 1992;23(2): 321-333.

6. Engh CA Jr, McAuley JP, Engh CS Sr: Surgical approaches for revision total hip replacement surgery: The anterior trochanteric

slide and the extended conventional osteotomy. *Instr Course Lect* 1999;48:3-8.

7. Glassman AH, Engh CA, Bobyn JD: Proximal femoral osteotomy as an adjunct in cementless revision total hip arthroplasty. *J Arthroplasty* 1987;2(1):47-63.

8. Glassman AH, Engh CA, Bobyn JD: A technique of extensile exposure for total hip arthroplasty. *J Arthroplasty* 1987;2(1):11-21.

9. Miner TM, Momberger NG, Chong D, Paprosky WL: The extended trochanteric osteotomy in revision hip arthroplasty: A critical review of 166 cases at mean 3-year, 9-month follow-up. *J Arthroplasty*. 2001;16(8, Suppl 1):188-194.

10. Noble AR, Branham DB, Willis MC, et al: Mechanical effects of the extended trochanteric osteotomy. *J Bone Joint Surg Am* 2005;87(3):521-529.

11. Kerry RM, Masri BA, Garbuz DS, Duncan CP: The vascularized scaphoid window for access to the femoral canal in revision total hip arthroplasty. *Instr Course Lect* 1999;48:9-11.

12. Klein AH, Rubash HE: Femoral windows in revision total hip arthroplasty. *Clin Orthop Relat Res* 1993;291:164-170.

How to Do a Revision Total Hip Arthroplasty: Revision of the Acetabulum

Scott M. Sporer, MD

Abstract

The need for revision total hip arthroplasty continues to increase as the indications for total hip replacement broaden and the average life expectancy of patients and their demands for activity increase. To achieve a successful long-term outcome after revision acetabular surgery, the surgical reconstruction must provide a mechanically stable construct that will minimize micromotion, allow bone ingrowth, and restore appropriate hip biomechanics. Achieving these goals during revision acetabular surgery can be challenging because of periacetabular bone loss and a compromised biologic environment. Acetabular classifications can help to preoperatively predict areas of bone loss to guide treatment options. Most acetabular defects can be managed with a hemispheric or elliptic porous acetabular component; however, large areas of segmental or cavitary bone loss may require alternative treatments such as custom implants, metal/allograft augmentation, or an acetabular cage reconstruction.

Instr Course Lect 2012;61:303-311.

The most common indications for acetabular revision include instability, infection, polyethylene wear, and aseptic loosening.[1] The prevalence of these conditions remains essentially unchanged despite improved prosthetic component designs and enhanced surgical techniques. A successful acetabular revision must provide intimate contact between the acetabular implant and the host bone, a stable mechanical construct minimizing micromotion to allow bone ingrowth into a cementless acetabular component, and a mechanical construct that distributes the physiologic stresses to the surrounding acetabular bone. Additionally, the acetabular reconstruction must allow appropriate component orientation to minimize the risk of dislocation and reestablish the anatomic hip center to improve the overall joint kinematics. Biologic methods of acetabular reconstruction are advised except in cases of severe bone loss or prior radiation treatment in the hip region because nonbiologic revisions eventually fail.[2] Periacetabular bone loss can compromise component fixation, resulting in early loosening of the revised acetabulum. The amount of bone loss undoubtedly influences the ability to obtain initial optimal fixation. The location of remaining supportive bone, however, has a more important role in providing durable fixation than does the quantity of bone loss.

Defect Classification Systems

Acetabular defect classification systems can be used to predict the extent of bone loss seen intraoperatively and guide subsequent reconstructive options. The three most common classification systems for acetabular defects are the American Academy of Orthopaedic Surgeons (AAOS) classification system described by D'Antonio et al[3] (**Table 1**), the Gross classification system described by Saleh et al[4] (**Table 2**), and the Paprosky classification system[5] (**Table 3**). The AAOS classification system identifies the pattern of acetabular bone loss but does not quantify the size or location of the defect. Despite being the most commonly cited system, the AAOS defect classification system does not guide the

Dr. Sporer or an immediate family member serves as a paid consultant to Smith & Nephew and Zimmer and has received research or institutional support from Coolsystems.

identification of reconstructive options. The system described by Saleh et al[4] is based on the degree of bone loss seen on preoperative standard AP and lateral radiographs of the hip. A bone defect is considered uncontained if morcellized bone graft cannot be used to fill the defect. The Paprosky classification system is based on four radiographic criteria from an AP pelvic radiograph: (1) superior migration of the hip center, (2) ischial osteolysis, (3) acetabular teardrop osteolysis, and (4) position of the implant relative to the Kohler line[5] (**Figure 1**). Superior migration of the hip center represents bone loss of the acetabular dome involving the anterior and posterior columns. Ischial osteolysis indicates bone loss from the posterior column including the posterior wall, whereas teardrop osteolysis and migration beyond the Kohler line represent medial acetabular bone loss. Type III defects require structural support from bulk allograft, metallic augmentation, an acetabular cage, or a custom acetabular component. The Paprosky classification system is often used clinically, because it not only predicts bone loss encountered intraoperatively but also assists in determining reconstructive options.

Component Removal

Successful acetabular reconstruction begins with a meticulous surgical technique to remove a well-fixed acetabular component. The use of acetabular "explant osteotomes" (**Figure 2**) facilitates the safe removal of well-fixed components. An osteotome blade, which is the outer diameter of the acetabular component, is used with a so-called femoral head that matches the diameter of the bearing surface. The osteotome is rotated around the periphery of the socket, disrupting the interface between the implant and the host bone. Areas of the pelvis that are crucial for subsequent reconstruction are the anterosuperior and posteroinferior aspects of the acetabulum. Monoblock

Table 1

AAOS Classification System for Acetabular Defects

Type	Description
I	Segmental defect
II	Cavitary defect
III	Combined segmental and cavitary defect
IV	Pelvic discontinuity
IVa	Discontinuity with mild segmental or cavitary bone loss
IVb	Discontinuity with moderate to severe segmental or cavitary bone loss
IVc	Discontinuity with prior pelvic irradiation
V	Hip arthrodesis

AAOS = American Academy of Orthopaedic Surgeons

Table 2

Gross Classification System for Acetabular Defects

Type	Description
I	No substantial loss of bone stock
II	Contained loss of bone stock (columns and/or rim intact)
III	Uncontained loss of bone stock (< 50% acetabulum)
IV	Uncontained loss of bone stock (> 50% acetabulum)
V	Contained loss of bone stock with pelvic discontinuity

Table 3

Paprosky Classification System for Acetabular Defects

Type	Femoral Head Center Migration	Ischial Osteolysis	Kohler Line	Teardrop
I	Minimal (< 3 cm)	None	Intact	Intact
IIA	Mild (< 3 cm)	Mild	Intact	Intact
IIB	Moderate (< 3 cm)	Mild	Intact	Intact
IIC	Mild (< 3 cm)	Mild	Disrupted	Moderate lysis
IIIA	Severe (> 3 cm)	Moderate	Intact	Moderate lysis
IIIB	Severe (> 3 cm)	Severe	Disrupted	Severe lysis

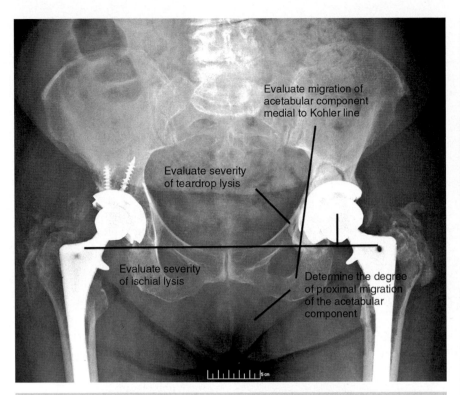

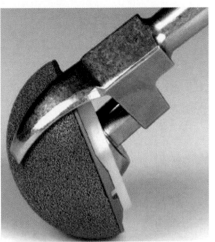

Figure 1   Components of the radiographic criteria in the Paprosky classification system for acetabular defects.

Figure 2   Acetabular component extraction tool. A bipolar femoral head may be used to remove a monoblock cobalt-chromium acetabular component. (Reproduced with permission from Taylor PR, Stoffel KK, Dunlop DG, Yates PJ. Removal of the well-fixed hip resurfacing acetabular component: A simple, bone preserving technique. *J Arthroplasty* 2009;24:484-486.)

acetabular components are removed with the use of a so-called bipolar articulation with a curved osteotome blade matching the outer diameter of the acetabular component. Alternatively, manual instruments such as curved chisels and motorized burrs can be used to disrupt the prosthesis-bone interface or section the cup. Forceful manipulation of the component during removal should be avoided because severe bone loss and associated pelvic discontinuity may occur. A preoperative angiogram and/or vascular surgery consultation should be obtained if the acetabular component has migrated medially past the Kohler line (**Figure 3**).

Treatment Algorithm

The treatment of acetabular defects depends on the degree and location of bone loss in addition to the potential for biologic fixation. Prior irradiation of the pelvis can result in periacetabu-

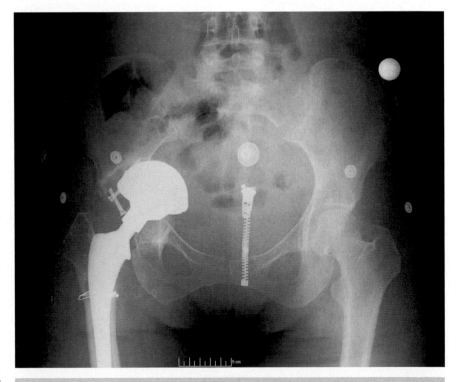

Figure 3   Intrapelvic migration of the acetabular component, a Paprosky type IIIB defect. A preoperative angiogram or vascular surgery consultation should be considered to minimize the risk of injury to the iliac vessel during revision arthroplasty.

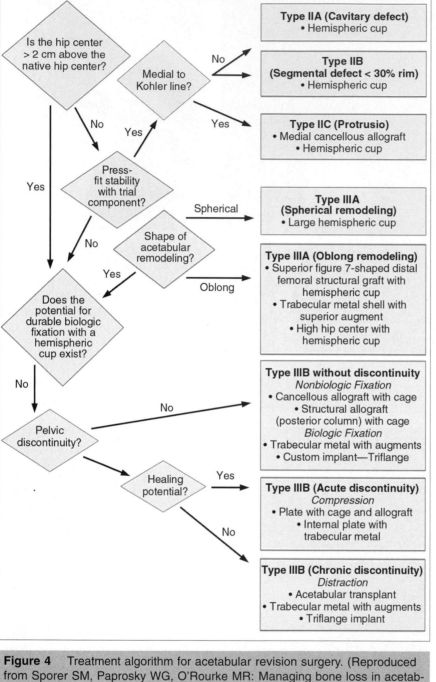

Figure 4   Treatment algorithm for acetabular revision surgery. (Reproduced from Sporer SM, Paprosky WG, O'Rourke MR: Managing bone loss in acetabular revision. *Instr Course Lect* 2006;55:287-298.)

lar osteonecrosis with limited ingrowth potential.[2] In these situations, nonbiologic fixation options, such as acetabular cages, custom implants, and fixed-angle devices, which offload the host bone, should be considered. Fortunately, most acetabular revisions can be managed successfully with a hemispheric component alone.[6-9] The goals of revision surgery are to obtain stable fixation on the remaining host bone and restore the hip center with the acetabular component near the Kohler line and the inferomedial aspect of the acetabular component near the inferior portion of the acetabular teardrop.

An algorithmic approach to acetabular defects helps preoperative planning as well as surgical decision making (**Figure 4**).

Acetabular Reconstruction

Hemispheric or Elliptic Component

An acetabular component with a hemispheric or elliptic design can be used in patients when the hip center of rotation has not migrated more than 3 cm proximally (Paprosky types I, IIA, IIB, and IIC).[10,11] After acetabular component removal, the remaining host bone should be exposed, and all granulation tissue should be thoroughly débrided. Pelvic discontinuity is assessed by looking for motion between the superior and the inferior hemipelvis when applying a caudal stress to the ischium with a Cobb elevator.

A retractor is placed in the obturator foramen to determine the level of the true acetabulum, which is the level of the inferior border of the acetabulum. Sequentially larger hemispheric acetabular reamers are used to determine the size of the acetabulum until the anterior and posterior columns are engaged by the reamer. To minimize the likelihood of creating pelvic discontinuity while reaming, in general, anterior acetabular bone should be sacrificed before posterior column bone. Trial acetabular components are used to assess the stability of the acetabular socket along with the degree of component coverage. Most acetabular defects have 5% to 20% of the acetabular component uncovered posterosuperiorly if the trial cup is placed in 40° of vertical inclination and 15° of anteversion. The temptation to place the component more vertically to improve coverage should be avoided because this can increase the risk of dislocation and wear. Cavitary bone defects are packed with either local autograft or allograft with the use of a reamer 2 mm smaller

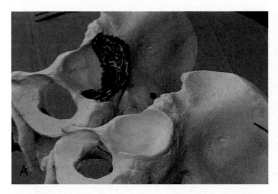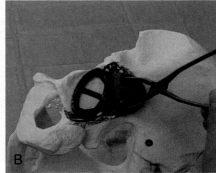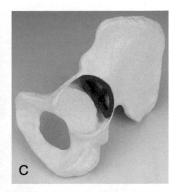

Figure 5   **A,** Type IIIA acetabular defect with superior and posterior bone loss. **B,** Acetabular augment used as a buttress to provide additional superior coverage. **C,** Augment used as a cavitary graft to fill cavitary bone defect and lower hip center.

than the last reaming in reverse. An acetabular component that is 2 mm larger at the periphery than the last reamer is used in most patients to obtain a so-called press-fit and initial fixation. Supplemental fixation with multiple screws is advised in all revisions to minimize micromotion and promote bone ingrowth. Screws should be placed not only posterosuperiorly into the dome of the acetabulum but also inferiorly into the ischium.

Surgical Treatment of Type IIIA Defects

Proximal and lateral migration of the acetabular component of more than 3 cm results in an acetabular dome deficiency that does not provide enough stability for a hemispheric acetabular component alone. Treatment options for patients with superior segmental bone loss include the use of structural bulk allograft, dual-geometry monoblock components, hemispheric components with metallic superior augmentation, or the placement of an implant with a high hip center. A high hip center places the hip abductor muscles at a mechanical disadvantage and necessitates the use of a small acetabular component. It can be challenging to obtain stable fixation and appropriate component orientation with use of a

monoblock dual-geometry acetabular component.[12,13] This chapter's author prefers to use a hemispheric acetabular component placed at the level of the true acetabulum and to create superior cup coverage with the use of metallic augmentation.

Hemispheric Component With Metallic Augmentation

The surgical treatment of a superior segmental bone defect with a hemispheric shell and augment begins by identifying the location of the true acetabulum with a retractor placed into the obturator foramen. Hemispheric reamers are then used to ream in the anatomic position until the anterior and posterior columns are engaged, which results in partial stability of a trial acetabular component. A superior augment is used either as a buttress in patients with primarily segmental bone loss or as a superior graft in patients with primarily oblong cavitary bone loss (**Figure 5**). It is crucial that the position of the augment not influence the ultimate position of the acetabular component. With the trial component in place, the augment is secured to the host bone with screws. The augment is then packed with bone graft, leaving the portion facing the cup exposed. Polymethyl methacrylate cement is placed directly on the porous

revision cup only in the areas mating with the augment. The acetabular component is firmly impacted to achieve a press-fit against the host bone. In severe bone loss, the polyethylene liner can be cemented into the acetabular shell to place screws at a fixed angle. Multiple screws are used in different planes to maximize stability and minimize the likelihood of component loosening.[14]

 Video 25.1: Type IIIA Acetabular Defect: Trabecular Metal Augment. Scott M. Sporer, MD; Wayne G. Paprosky, MD (11 min)

Hemispheric Component With Distal Femoral Allograft

The use of bulk allograft has been largely abandoned except in young patients because of the increased surgical time, the need for more soft-tissue exposure, and the concern for graft resorption.[15] Similar to metallic augmentation, the first step in the acetabular reconstruction with bulk allograft is to identify the location of the desired hip center and use acetabular reamers to size and shape the anteroposterior dimensions of the acetabulum to accept a hemispheric cementless implant. The distal femoral

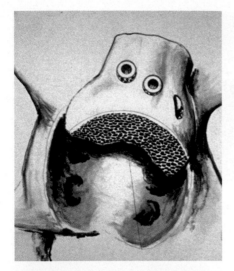

Figure 6 Distal femoral structural allograft used to reconstruct the superior dome of the acetabulum. (Reproduced with permission from Sporer SM, O'Rourke M, Chong P, Paprosky WG: The use of structural distal femoral allografts for acetabular reconstruction: Average ten-year follow-up. *J Bone Joint Surg Am* 2005;87:760-765.)

allograft is prepared to accommodate the segmental dome defect once it has been determined that there is inadequate coverage of a hemispheric component. The cortex of the distal femoral allograft shaft in the coronal plane relative to the condyles is removed. The posterior aspect of the condyles is then shaped to correspond with the superior acetabular defect with the use of a female reamer measuring 2 mm larger than the last reamer used to size the defect. The anterior to posterior aspect of the distal femoral allograft should correspond to the medial to lateral depth of the defect. The superior cortical limb of the graft should be approximately 4 to 5 cm to allow adequate fixation to the lateral aspect of the ilium. The contoured graft is impacted into the superior defect, obtaining a press-fit. The allograft is secured with three or four parallel 6.5-mm cancellous screws with washers. The screws are oriented obliquely into the ilium in

the direction of loading to provide compression of the graft against the remaining ilium. The acetabular cavity is reamed to contour the portion of the graft that will contact the hemispheric component[16] (**Figure 6**).

Surgical Treatment of Type IIIB Defects

Proximal and medial migration of the acetabular component of more than 3 cm results in an acetabular dome deficiency as well as a medial wall deficiency that does not provide enough intrinsic stability for a hemispheric acetabular component alone. Treatment options for patients with superomedial segmental bone loss include structural bulk allograft, custom implants spanning the iliac wing to the ischium, hemispheric components with multiple metal augments, or an acetabular cage. Pelvic discontinuity frequently occurs in patients with severe proximal medial migration of the acetabular component.

Acetabular Transplant With Cage

Acetabular reamers are used to size the acetabular cavity and identify the location of remaining bone along the superior aspect of the ilium that will abut the allograft. The acetabulum of the hemipelvic allograft is reamed on the back table to accept the cage. A curvilinear osteotomy is made in the allograft from the greater sciatic notch to the anterior-superior iliac spine. The pubic and ischial portions of the allograft are removed distal to the confluence of the acetabulum with enough length to accommodate any inferior defects. Leaving excessive inferior bone on the allograft that may prevent optimal medialization of the graft should be avoided because this leads to subsequent vertical cup placement and lateralization of the hip center. A female reamer, 1 to 2 mm larger than the

acetabular reamer used to size the acetabulum, should be used to mark and shape the medial aspect of the graft to fit the defect. A groove is made in the superior aspect of the ilium of the allograft to correspond to the ledge of bone along the superior aspect of the native acetabulum. This tongue-and-groove junction provides a stable buttress between the host and the allograft. A burr is used to debulk the inner table of the allograft ilium, while a shelf that will fill the defect of the acetabulum is maintained distally. The graft is secured with Steinmann pins provisionally until four 6.5-mm partially threaded screws are placed obliquely into the ilium from both the intra-articular and lateral aspects of the ilium of the graft. A pelvic reconstruction plate contoured to the posterior column with three screws in the native ilium and ischium is used for fixation. A cage is recommended to protect all transplants, and, if possible, the inferior flange of a cage is inserted into a slot in the ischium for fixation. A metal shell or a polyethylene liner is cemented into the cage-allograft composite, with care taken to avoid the tendency to place the acetabular component in a vertical and retroverted position.

Video 25.2: Type IIIB Acetabular Defect: Acetabular Transplant with Cage. Scott M. Sporer, MD; Wayne G. Paprosky, MD (3 min)

Type IIIB Defect: Modular Metal Augmentation

The acetabulum is reamed in the anatomic location and direction (anterior to posterior, anterior-inferior to posterior-inferior, or posterior-superior to anterior-inferior) for the eventual reconstruction until two

Table 4

Tips and Pearls for Acetabular Revision

Paprosky Classification of Defect	Tips and Pearls
Type IIB	Ream until the anterior and posterior columns are engaged to allow intrinsic stability of the trial component Ream slightly superiorly to improve coverage. Avoid attempts to provide coverage of the superior dome; the superior portion of the acetabular component may remain uncovered. Reverse ream with a reamer that is 1 to 2 mm undersized to pack cavitary defects. Use a cup with multiple holes. Avoid a spiked cup.
Type IIC	Ream until the anterior and posterior columns are engaged to allow intrinsic stability of trial cup along the acetabular rim. Medial bone graft is added until the reverse reamer, which is 1 to 2 mm undersized, disengages from the drive shaft. Use an acetabular component that is 2 mm larger than the last reamer to achieve press-fit fixation. Use a cup with multiple holes.
Type IIIA—distal femoral allograft	Verify that the surgical site is free of infection before opening the distal femoral allograft. Culture the femoral allograft. Avoid the use of femoral head allograft. Elevate abductor musculature with use of a Taylor retractor to allow adequate visualization of the iliac wing. Cut a figure 7-shaped portion of allograft at slightly less than 90° to allow intrinsic stability. Use 6.5-mm cancellous screws and always use with a washer. Tap screws in the allograft to avoid fracture. Avoid the tendency to place the component in excessive abduction and retroversion (the cup may remain uncovered). Place screws through cup-allograft-host bone if possible.
Type IIIA—hemispheric component with metal augment	Progressively ream in the anatomic position to engage the anterior and posterior columns to allow intrinsic stability to the acetabular trial component. Place the superior augment with the trial component in place (with appropriate version and abduction); the augment can be placed in any position or orientation to allow improved initial stability; leave 1 to 2 mm between the cup and the augment for the placement of cement. Use a motorized burr along the superior dome to fit the host bone to the augment to improve intrinsic stability and maximize bone contact. Pack the augment with bone graft, leaving the metal of the augment that faces the cup exposed. Place cement directly onto the porous revision cup only in areas mating with the augment. Insert the cup with cement in the doughy phase to improve interdigitation between the cup and the augment Consider the use of cement with antibiotics. Before the cement hardens, attempt to place a screw in the revision cup to eliminate motion during the final seating of the screws. Place bone wax in the end of the screws to facilitate cup removal.
Type IIIB—hemispheric component with metal augment and no discontinuity	Use augments to reconstruct the pelvis with nonbiologic material. Expose all margins of the acetabular defect. Progressively ream (anterior-posterior, anterior-inferior, and posterior-inferior) until two points of fixation are achieved. Loss of inferior bone stock (ischium) is often involved. Intrinsic stability will not be obtained with the trial component. Use augments to decrease acetabular volume and facilitate press-fit between the cup and the augment (attempt to place the augment in direct contact with the revision cup). Secure the augment first. Reverse ream with the augment in place to pack the bone graft. Clear bone graft from the exposed host bone (maximize the contact area between the host bone and the revision porous cup). Attempt to place screws inferiorly into the ischium to avoid cup pullout.
Type IIIB—pelvic discontinuity distraction	Use a porous acetabular component to reconstruct the pelvis with biologic material as an internal fixation device. Expose all margins of the acetabular defect and discontinuity thoroughly. Progressively ream (anterior to posterior, anterior-inferior to posterior-inferior, or posterior-superior to anterior-inferior) until two points of fixation are achieved. Intrinsic stability will not be obtained. Use augments to decrease acetabular volume and facilitate press-fit between the cup and the augment (attempt to place the augment in direct contact with the revision cup). Bridge the discontinuity with the augment and place screws cephalad and caudal to the discontinuity. Remove fibrous tissue in the discontinuity and place the bone graft. Reverse ream with the augment in place to pack the bone graft. Clear bone graft from exposed host bone (maximize contact area between the host bone and the revision cup).

points of fixation are achieved, because this determines the size of the acetabular defect. Acetabular augments are used to decrease the acetabular volume and restore a rim to support a revision cup. The location and orientation of augments depends on the pattern of bone loss. Augments are frequently placed along the medial aspect of the ilium or are stacked together to reconstruct the superomedial defect. It is more common to use augments with the wide base placed laterally and the apex medially, which is the opposite of how the augments are often used in the type IIIA defect. The revision acetabular cup directly contacts the augments, and the augments are necessary to achieve a press-fit of the acetabular component. Similar to the treatment of a type IIIA defect, augments for a type IIIB defect are initially secured to the host bone with the use of multiple screws. Portions of the augments are removed with a burr or a reamer as needed to optimize the surface area contact between the revision shell and the augments. Particulate bone graft is placed into any remaining cavities before the hemispheric revision shell is impacted in place. Similar to the treatment of a type IIIA defect, the interface between the revision shell and the augment is cemented to minimize micromotion and subsequent fretting. Multiple screws into both the ilium and ischium are used for fixation.

 Video 25.3: Type IIIB Acetabular Defect: Trabecular Metal Augment. Scott M. Sporer, MD; Wayne G. Paprosky, MD (6 min)

Pelvic Discontinuity

A hemispheric acetabular component alone does not provide adequate implant stability in patients with a pelvic discontinuity. Treatment options for a pelvic discontinuity include compression plating of the posterior column with use of a hemispheric component, placement of an acetabular cage, use of a custom implant that spans the discontinuity, or use of metal acetabular augments to "distract" across the pelvic discontinuity.[17] In patients with a chronic pelvic discontinuity, the amount of bone loss along the posterior column is often too severe to provide direct bone apposition during compression plating.

Modular Metal Augmentation With Distraction for Pelvic Discontinuity

The goal of the distraction technique for a pelvic discontinuity is to use ligamentotaxis secondary to the lengthening across the discontinuity to provide initial component stability. The location and severity of bone loss determine the type and position of the acetabular augments used to enhance initial component stability. Acetabular augments are frequently used to reconstruct portions of the anterosuperior aspect of the acetabulum as well as the posteroinferior aspect of the acetabulum to provide two secure points of fixation for the acetabular component both cephalad and caudal to the discontinuity. A porous acetabular component, which is 6 to 8 mm larger than the hemispheric reamer that engaged the anterior and posterior columns, is used to distract the superior hemipelvis from the inferior hemipelvis. Multiple screws are placed into the remaining ilium and ischium through the acetabular shell, and the augments are secured to the cup with polymethyl methacrylate. A polyethylene liner is cemented into the acetabular component, allowing screws to be placed at a fixed angle. A successful reconstruction of a pelvic discontinuity requires ingrowth of the host bone into both the superior and inferior portions of

the acetabular component to bridge the discontinuity. Consequently, as much contact as possible should be obtained between the host bone and the porous augments and acetabular component.

Tips and Pearls for Acetabular Revision

Tips and pearls for the acetabular revision of various types of Paprosky defects are listed in **Table 4**.

References

1. Bozic KJ, Kurtz SM, Lau E, Ong K, Vail TP, Berry DJ: The epidemiology of revision total hip arthroplasty in the United States. *J Bone Joint Surg Am* 2009;91(1): 128-133.

2. Jacobs JJ, Kull LR, Frey GA, et al: Early failure of acetabular components inserted without cement after previous pelvic irradiation. *J Bone Joint Surg Am* 1995; 77(12):1829-1835.

3. D'Antonio JA, Capello WN, Borden LS, et al: Classification and management of acetabular abnormalities in total hip arthroplasty. *Clin Orthop Relat Res* 1989;243: 126-137.

4. Saleh KJ, Holtzman J, Gafni ASaleh L, et al: Development, test reliability and validation of a classification for revision hip arthroplasty. *J Orthop Res* 2001;19(1): 50-56.

5. Paprosky WG, Perona PG, Lawrence JM: Acetabular defect classification and surgical reconstruction in revision arthroplasty: A 6-year follow-up evaluation. *J Arthroplasty* 1994;9(1):33-44.

6. Della Valle CJ, Berger RA, Rosenberg AG, Galante JO: Cementless acetabular reconstruction in revision total hip arthroplasty. *Clin Orthop Relat Res* 2004;420: 96-100.

7. Gaffey JL, Callaghan JJ, Pedersen DR, Goetz DD, Sullivan PM, Johnston RC: Cementless acetabular fixation at fifteen years: A comparison with the same surgeon's results following acetabular fixation with cement. *J Bone Joint Surg Am* 2004;86-A(2):257-261.

8. Hallstrom BR, Golladay GJ, Vittetoe DA, Harris WH: Cementless acetabular revision with the Harris-Galante porous prosthesis: Results after a minimum of ten years of follow-up. *J Bone Joint Surg Am* 2004;86-A(5):1007-1011.

9. Templeton JE, Callaghan JJ, Goetz DD, Sullivan PM, Johnston RC: Revision of a cemented acetabular component to a cementless acetabular component: A ten to fourteen-year follow-up study. *J Bone Joint Surg Am* 2001; 83-A(11):1706-1711.

10. Leopold SS, Rosenberg AG, Bhatt RD, Sheinkop MB, Quigley LR, Galante JO: Cementless acetabular revision: Evaluation at an average of 10.5 years. *Clin Orthop Relat Res* 1999;369:179-186.

11. Silverton CD, Rosenberg AG, Sheinkop MB, Kull LR, Galante JO: Revision total hip arthroplasty using a cementless acetabular component: Technique and results. *Clin Orthop Relat Res* 1995; 319:201-208.

12. Chen WM, Engh CA Jr, Hopper RH Jr, McAuley JP, Engh CA: Acetabular revision with use of a bilobed component inserted without cement in patients who have acetabular bone-stock deficiency. *J Bone Joint Surg Am* 2000;82(2): 197-206.

13. Schutzer SF, Harris WH: High placement of porous-coated acetabular components in complex total hip arthroplasty. *J Arthroplasty* 1994;9(4):359-367.

14. Sporer SM, Paprosky WG: The use of a trabecular metal acetabular component and trabecular metal augment for severe acetabular defects. *J Arthroplasty* 2006; 21(6, Suppl 2):83-86.

15. Sporer SM, O'Rourke M, Chong P, Paprosky WG: The use of structural distal femoral allografts for acetabular reconstruction: Average ten-year follow-up. *J Bone Joint Surg Am* 2005;87(4): 760-765.

16. Sporer SM, O'Rourke M, Chong P, Paprosky WG: The use of structural distal femoral allografts for acetabular reconstruction: Surgical technique. *J Bone Joint Surg Am* 2006;88(Suppl 1 Pt 1): 92-99.

17. Paprosky WG, O'Rourke M, Sporer SM: The treatment of acetabular bone defects with an associated pelvic discontinuity. *Clin Orthop Relat Res* 2005;441: 216-220.

Video References

25.1: Sporer SM, Paprosky WG: Video. *Type IIIA Acetabular Defect: Trabecular Metal Augment.* Winfield, IL, 2006.

25.2: Sporer SM, Paprosky WG: Video. *Type IIIB Acetabular Defect: Acetabular Transplant With Cage.* Winfield, IL, 2006.

25.3: Sporer SM, Paprosky WG: Video. *Type IIIB Acetabular Defect: Trabecular Metal Augment.* Winfield, IL, 2006.

Femoral Fixation in Revision Total Hip Arthroplasty

Curtis W. Hartman, MD
Kevin L. Garvin, MD

Abstract

Management of the femur during revision total hip arthroplasty can be challenging. Strategies for femoral reconstruction are based on understanding the degree of femoral bone loss. Numerous options exist for femoral reconstruction depending on the quantity and quality of the remaining femoral bone stock, including cemented fixation, cementless fixation using proximally porous-coated implants, cylindrical extensively porous-coated implants, modular and nonmodular tapered fluted stems, impaction bone grafting, allograft-prosthetic composites, and proximal femoral replacements (megaprostheses). An understanding of the results of various methods of femoral reconstruction is helpful in guiding the revision surgeon faced with a challenging femoral revision.

Instr Course Lect 2012;61:313-325.

Recent data project the number of total hip arthroplasty revisions to grow by 137% between 2005 and 2030.[1] Surgeons who manage the failed total hip replacement will find an ever-increasing workload and must have an understanding of the outcomes and treatment options for the failed femoral implant.

Management strategies for femoral implant revision are based on the femoral defect and the quality and quantity of the remaining femoral bone stock. Numerous options are available for femoral reconstruction, including cemented fixation, cementless fixation with the use of proximally porous-coated implants, cylindrical extensively porous-coated implants, modular and nonmodular tapered fluted stems, impaction bone grafting, allograft-prosthetic composites, and proximal femoral replacements (megaprostheses).

Preoperative Planning

Careful preoperative planning is a necessary step before any revision arthroplasty. An attempt should be made to identify the implants being revised. The implant manufacturer should be contacted for implant removal devices that may be specific to the implant being revised. Even when an isolated femoral revision is planned, it is beneficial to identify the acetabular implant because a modular polyethylene exchange may be possible.

The standard evaluation for preoperative planning includes four radiographic views: an AP view of the pelvis, an AP view of the affected hip, a frog-lateral view, and a shoot-through lateral view of the affected hip.[2] The radiograph should be examined for areas of osteolysis, stress shielding, femoral deformity, a cortical deficiency, and to detect the amount and location of cement. The radiographs provide substantial information as to the difficulty of implant removal and subsequent reconstruction. The degree and pattern of bone loss influence the revision implant choice. The bone stock distal to the implant should be visualized and evaluated because the diaphyseal bone may be essential to obtaining fixation during revision. Additionally, the radiographs should be of sufficient length to determine if a distal implant is present and if it will complicate the proximal reconstruction.

Serial radiographs help to determine whether the femoral stem to be revised is loose or well fixed. Cemented implants that have migrated or subsided, or have a fractured cement

Dr. Hartman or an immediate family member has received research or institutional support from Smith & Nephew. Dr. Garvin or an immediate family member serves as a board member, owner, officer, or committee member of the American Academy of Orthopaedic Surgeons and the American Orthopaedic Association and has received royalties from Biomet.

Table 1

Paprosky Classification System for Femoral Defects

Type	Description
I	Minimal metaphyseal bone loss
II	Extensive metaphyseal bone loss and an intact diaphysis
IIIA	Extensive metadiaphyseal bone loss and a minimum of 4 cm of intact cortical bone in the diaphysis
IIIB	Extensive metadiaphyseal bone loss and < 4 cm of intact cortical bone in the diaphysis
IV	Extensive metadiaphyseal bone loss and a nonsupportive diaphysis

Table 2

AAOS Classification System for Femoral Defects

Type	Description
I	Segmental defect involving loss of cortical osseous support[a]
II	Cavitary defect involving loss of cancellous or endosteal bone with an intact cortical shell
III	Combined segmental and cavitary defects
IV	Femoral malalignment in rotational or angular plane
V	Femoral stenosis with partial or complete occlusion of the intramedullary canal
VI	Femoral discontinuity usually due to fracture nonunion

[a]Type I defects are further specified as level I, indicating bone loss is proximal to the lower edge of the lesser trochanter; level II, loss is within 10 cm of the lower edge of the lesser trochanter; and level III, loss is distal to 10 cm below the lower edge of the lesser trochanter.

Table 3

Mallory Classification System for Femoral Defects

Type	Description
I	Cortex intact with cancellous bone present
II	Cortex intact with cancellous bone absent
IIIA	Cortical deficiency proximal to the lesser trochanter
IIIB	Cortical deficiency between the lesser trochanter and the isthmus
IIIC	Cortical deficiency involving the isthmus and distally

mantle, or implants that have fractured are definitely loose.[3,4] A continuous radiolucent line at the cement-bone interface indicates probable loosening, and a noncircumferential radiolucent line indicates possible loosening.[3,4] Cementless implants that demonstrate progressive subsidence, migration, or divergent radiolucent lines are considered unstable.[5] These femora typically demonstrate a distal pedestal and proximal cortical hyper-

trophy. An implant with parallel radiolucent lines and without progressive migration is likely to have stable fibrous ingrowth.[5] These femora usually do not have focal proximal cortical hypertrophy. A well-ingrown cementless implant does not have reactive lines or evidence of component migration.[5] These femora typically have proximal stress shielding.

Clear template overlays or digital templates are used to assess the length

and the diameter of the proposed revision implant. Templating also helps to determine whether proximal femoral remodeling has occurred. Loose femoral implants are often associated with femoral remodeling into varus alignment and retroversion.[6] If proximal femoral remodeling has occurred, it may be necessary to perform an extended trochanteric osteotomy to reduce the risks of cortical perforation during reaming, fracture during implant insertion, or undersizing the implant because of varus malpositioning.

Classification of Femoral Bone Loss

Multiple authors have proposed systems to characterize femoral bone loss in the setting of revision hip surgery.[7-10] Weeden and Paprosky[10] described a system based on the quantity of metaphyseal and diaphyseal bone stock (**Table 1**). This system uses a simple algorithm for femoral reconstruction based on the severity of the defect. D'Antonio et al[7] reported the classification system developed by the American Academy of Orthopaedic Surgeons (AAOS) (**Table 2**). Although this system is highly descriptive in detailing osseous abnormalities of the femur, it does not provide a guide for reconstructive options based on the femoral defect. Mallory[8] developed a system with three basic categories based on the presence or absence of cancellous bone and the extent of femoral cortical deficiency (**Table 3**). Although this system is simpler and more useful than that of the AAOS for determining the method of femoral reconstruction, as noted by Della Valle and Paprosky,[6] it fails to address several critical determinants of reconstruction. Saleh et al[9,11] also developed a system for classifying femoral bone loss, which is both reliable and valid (**Table 4**).

Paprosky Classification System

The classification system devised by Paprosky is based on the principle that as proximal bone becomes weak and unsupportive, the relatively spared diaphyseal bone can be successfully used to provide reliable, long-term fixation.[10,12-14] The system assigns the femur to one of four categories on the basis of the extent and the location of bone loss (**Figure 1**).

Table 4
Gross Classification System for Femoral Defects

Type	Description
I	No notable loss of bone stock
II	Contained loss of bone stock with cortical thinning
III	Uncontained loss of bone stock involving the calcar and the lesser trochanter
IV	Uncontained circumferential loss of bone stock > 5 cm in length that extends into the diaphysis
V	Periprosthetic fracture with circumferential loss of bone stock proximal to the fracture

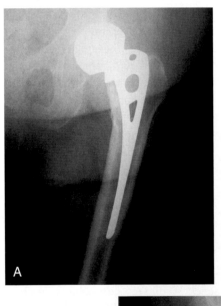

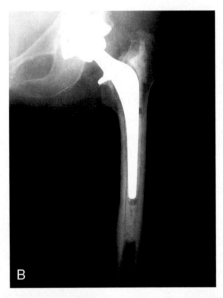

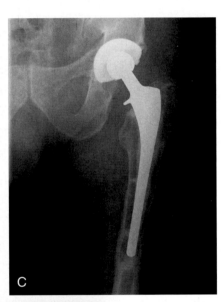

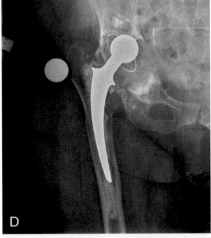

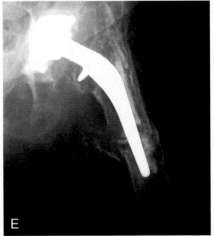

Figure 1   Radiographs showing femoral defects classified according to the Paprosky system. **A,** Type I femoral defect. **B,** Type II femoral defect. **C,** Type IIIA femoral defect. **D,** Type IIIB femoral defect. **E,** Type IV femoral defect. (Panels A, B, and E reprinted with permission from Della Valle CJ, Paprosky WG: Classification and an algorithmic approach to the reconstruction of femoral deficiency in revision total hip arthroplasty. *J Bone Joint Surg Am* 2003;85(Suppl 4):1-6.)

Type I

The femur with a type I defect has minimal loss of metaphyseal cancellous bone and an intact diaphysis (**Figure 1, A**).[10] This pattern of bone loss is uncommon in the revision setting and is more common with a failed resurfacing arthroplasty implant or an undersized, non–porous-coated cementless implant.[6]

Type II

The femur with a type II defect has extensive metaphyseal cancellous bone loss and minimal diaphyseal loss (**Figure 1, B**).[10] This is a common finding, particularly in the early stages of aseptic loosening.[6]

Types IIIA and IIIB

The femur with a type IIIA defect has extensive metaphyseal bone loss, leaving it unsupportive. The diaphysis is also involved, but a minimum of 4 cm of cortical bone is available at the isthmus to obtain a scratch fit (**Figure 1, C**).[10] This is probably the most frequently encountered defect in femoral revision surgery.[10]

The femur with a type IIIB defect has an unsupportive metaphysis secondary to extensive bone loss. Additionally, the diaphysis is more severely damaged, and less than 4 cm of scratch fit can be obtained at the isthmus (**Figure 1, D**).[10] This defect seems to be increasing in frequency with improved cementing techniques and the use of longer cementless stems.[6]

Type IV

The femur with a type IV defect has extensive metadiaphyseal bone loss. The femoral canal has expanded, and the isthmic cortical bone cannot provide reliable fixation (**Figure 1, E**). Although this pattern of bone loss is rare, its frequency is increasing.[6,10,15]

Results of Reconstruction

Based on the knowledge of this chapter's authors, Iorio et al[16] performed

the only randomized, prospective trial of femoral component fixation in revision total hip arthroplasty to date. In that study, femoral component fixation with the use of third-generation cementing techniques was compared with modular metaphyseal cementless fixation in Paprosky type I and type II femora. With a mean follow-up of 8 years, there was no difference in validated outcome measures or 5-year survivorship between the two groups. The relative paucity of comparative trials in revision arthroplasty makes interpretation of the results of revision arthroplasty difficult. Because of these shortcomings, it is most beneficial to evaluate the outcomes of different techniques on an individual basis.[17]

Cemented Fixation

The early results of cemented femoral implant revision had high failure rates. Pellicci et al[18] followed 99 hips for a mean 8.1 years after revision total hip arthroplasty and reported a 19% rate of rerevision and a 29% rate of femoral loosening. Similarly, Kavanagh et al[19] followed 166 hips for a mean 4.5 years and reported a 6% rate of rerevision but a 44% rate of radiographic femoral loosening.

These dismal results were credited to early cementing techniques, and revisions performed with more modern techniques (distal plug, medullary lavage, retrograde cement delivery, and pressurization) have higher rates of success. Callaghan et al[20] reported a 4.3% rate of rerevision in a cohort of 139 hips followed for a mean 3.6 years, with 16% showing definite mechanical loosening and 29% showing progressive radiolucencies. Rubash and Harris,[21] in a study of 43 hips followed for a mean 6.2 years after revision hip arthroplasty with cement, reported a 2% failure rate caused by aseptic loosening, whereas 11% demonstrated radiographic evidence of femoral com-

ponent loosening. Estok and Harris[22] described the long-term results for this cohort, which included 38 hips that were available for review at a mean follow-up of 11.7 years. They noted a 10.5% rerevision rate for aseptic failure and an additional 10.5% with radiographic evidence of loosening. In a third review of this cohort, Mulroy and Harris[23] reported a 26% rate of femoral component loosening at a mean follow-up of 15.1 years.

The so-called third-generation cementing technique that used pressurized, vacuum-mixed cement did little to improve the results of previous studies. Eisler et al[24] followed 83 consecutive hips after the first revision of the total hip replacement for 1.5 to 6.3 years. At a median follow-up of 3.6 years, the femoral failure rate was 39%.

These generally disappointing failure rates have led to further study in the laboratory in an attempt to understand the failure mechanisms more fully. Biomechanical tests evaluating the shear strength of the cement-bone interface found that a simulated revision setting reduces the interface shear strength to 20.6% of primary strength, and a second revision reduces the shear strength to 6.8% of primary strength.[25]

Impaction Grafting

Femoral impaction grafting was first reported by Simon et al[26] as a technique for femoral revision. The technique is relatively straightforward in concept but is time consuming and technically demanding.[27,28] The premise is that a damaged and ectatic femoral canal can be packed with cancellous allograft, creating a neomedullary canal. A highly polished, collarless, double-tapered stem is cemented into the graft bed with the use of contemporary cementing techniques. The graft is then vascularized and gradually incorporated with subsequent reconstitution of the deficient femoral bone stock (**Figure 2**). Full-thickness cortical defects can be reconstructed with mesh or cortical strut allografts to contain the morcellized cancellous graft.

Although some authors have reported worrisome results with impaction grafting,[29-33] numerous authors have reported short- and long-term success with this technique.[34-38] Meding et al[32] evaluated the results of 34 hips followed for a mean 30 months after femoral impaction grafting. The authors reported a 38% subsidence rate, with a mean subsidence of 10.1 mm and a 12% intraoperative femoral fracture rate. Similarly, Eldridge et al[29] reported massive subsidence (> 10 mm) in 11% of 79 hips followed for a mean 12.6 months. Ornstein et al[27] reported 39 femoral fractures within the first year after 108 femoral component revisions. Sierra et al[39] reviewed a subgroup of femoral revisions with use of stems of 220 mm or more in length, with the hypothesis that the longer stems would decrease the incidence of postoperative femoral fractures. The authors found 6 of the 42 hips reviewed required a reoperation. Survival analysis revealed a survival rate of 90% at 5 and 10 years with revision of the stem as the end point. However, with any femoral reoperation as the end point, the survival rate was 82% at both 5 and 10 years.

Similar to other procedures with a steep learning curve, the results of impaction grafting have improved as surgeons have become more comfortable with the procedure. Ornstein et al[34] reported the long-term results of a large cohort of femoral revisions in Sweden. They followed 1,305 femoral revisions for 5 to 18 years, identifying 70 repeat revisions. Survivorship for all causes of failure was 94% for women and 94.7% for men at 15 years. Survivorship at 15 years was 99.1% with aseptic loosening as the end point, 98.6% with infection as the end point, 99.0% with subsidence as the end point, and 98.7% with fracture as the end point. Wraighte and Howard[38] reported the results for 75 consecutive hips that had revision total hip replacement with a mean follow-up of 10.5 years. Survivorship with any further femoral operation as the end point was 92% at 10.5 years. They also found that subsidence correlated with the preoperative Endo-Klinik bone loss score, and the degree of subsidence at 1 year had a strong association with long-term subsidence. Halliday et al[36] reported that the survival of 226 hip replacements at 10 to 11 years was 90.5%, with any femoral operation as the end point. Mahoney et al[37] reviewed the results of 44 hips followed for a mean 4.7 years. With reoperation as the end point, the survivorship was 97%. These data support the use of impaction femoral bone grafting in select patients with substantial proximal femoral bone loss.

Cementless Fixation

The initial poor outcomes for cemented stems in revision arthroplasty led some to question their utility and search for other options. As a result, the use of cementless stems gained popularity. Multiple design philosophies have been used in cementless femoral fixation and have had important effects on the durability of the revision.

Proximally Porous-Coated Stems

The results of femoral implant revision with proximally porous-coated stems have been inferior compared with more modern techniques.[8,40-43] The primary reason for failure is the inability to obtain stable fixation of the stem in the deficient metaphysis. The results of proximally porous-coated stems in

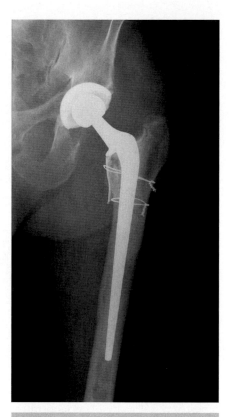

Figure 2 Radiograph of the femur after treatment of extensive osteolysis with impaction bone grafting. The patient had a cemented femoral stem and required revision because of extensive osteolysis. See Figure 1C for a radiograph of the femur before revision.

revision surgery can be summarized by the work of Berry et al.[44] The authors reviewed a series of 375 total hip arthroplasty revisions performed without cement and with the use of at least six different proximally porous-coated femoral components. A survivorship analysis at 8 years found that the survival rate, with revision for aseptic femoral failure as the end point, was 58%. The survival rate with aseptic femoral loosening (revision for aseptic loosening or radiographic loosening) as the end point was only 20%. In this series, greater preoperative bone loss correlated with worse survivorship. The authors concluded that the damaged and weakened proximal part of the femur does not provide an optimal

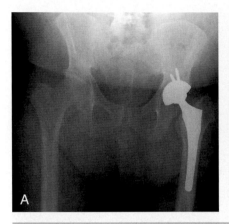
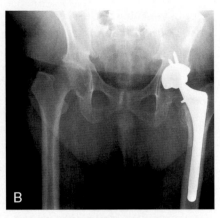

Figure 3 **A,** Radiograph of a hip with a loose, proximally porous-coated femoral stem before revision. **B,** Radiograph of the hip made after revision with an extensively porous-coated femoral stem.

environment for initial or long-term biologic fixation.

Fracture of the proximal part of the femur is a frequent complication in revisions with the use of proximally porous-coated implants. Berry et al[44] reported a 26% rate of intraoperative fracture. Malkani et al[45] reported a 45.9% incidence of intraoperative femoral fracture. The authors reported an overall 5-year survivorship free of moderate pain or revision of 82%; however, the fracture subgroup had survivorship of only 58% at 4 years. The difference in the survivorship between the groups was significant. Mulliken et al[46] reported a 40% intraoperative fracture rate. The authors did not report the failure rates in the fracture group but did find that the deficient proximal part of the femur was more likely to fracture, and most of the failures were in femora with severe proximal bone loss.

Proximally Porous-Coated Modular Stems

Proximally porous-coated modular femoral stems have appeal for cementless femoral revision because of their ability to obtain independent metaphyseal sizing and fixation relative to the diaphyseal portion of the implant. The goal of this technique is to reduce

stress shielding by attaining stable implant fixation in the proximal part of the femur.[47] This stem type has performed well for revisions with minimal bone loss (Paprosky types I and II);[47-49] however, for more difficult cases with more extensive bone loss, the results have been inferior. For example, McCarthy and Lee,[50] in a retrospective review of the results of revision hip replacement in 67 hips with a mean follow-up of 14 years, reported that 78% of the femora had Paprosky type III or IV defects. With revision as the end point, 14-year survival was 60%. All aseptic failures were in Paprosky type IIIB or IV femora. There were no long-term failures in femora classified as Paprosky type II or IIIA. Bolognesi et al[51] performed a randomized, prospective trial comparing hydroxyapatite-coated metaphyseal sleeves and porous-coated metaphyseal sleeves with use of the S-ROM prosthesis (DePuy, Warsaw, IN) in 53 patients followed for a mean of 4 years. The authors found that, with Paprosky type III defects, the hydroxyapatite-coated sleeve was 2.6 times more likely to achieve osseous ingrowth than the porous-coated sleeve. The authors also reported that regardless of which sleeve was used, the Harris hip scores were

significantly worse with worsening bone loss. For the entire cohort, the probability of femoral stem survival, with revision as the end point, was 95% at 3.9 years.

Cylindrical, Extensively Porous-Coated Stems

The use of extensively porous-coated femoral stems in revision arthroplasty is based on the principle that bypassing the damaged proximal part of the femur and engaging the diaphysis can reliably provide an ingrown and stable reconstruction (**Figure 3**). Despite concerns over proximal stress shielding, this technique is popular among surgeons who perform revisions because of the high rate of success and relative ease of technique. The results of revision with cylindrical, extensively porous-coated stems have been excellent[10,12,52-55] and are summarized in **Table 5**.

Several authors have reported the difficulty of using cylindrical, extensively porous-coated implants for femoral revision in the face of extensive bone loss.[10,52,56,57] Weeden and Paprosky[10] found that patients with type II or IIIA defects had a 5% failure rate, whereas patients with type IIIB defects had a 21% failure rate. Engh et al[57] identified 26 hips with bone loss extending 10 cm or more distal to the lesser trochanter that were followed for a mean of 13.3 years. The authors reported a 15% rate of mechanical loosening and a 10-year survivorship of 89%, with femoral revision as the end point. In another study by Engh et al,[52] the survival of femoral stems was significantly less if the preoperative bone loss extended more than 10 cm distal to the lesser trochanter. Sporer and Paprosky[56] investigated the failure rates of 51 patients with Paprosky type IIIA, IIIB, or IV femoral defects and reported no failures in 17 patients with type IIIA de-

Table 5
Results of Revision With Extensively Porous-Coated Femoral Stems

Study (Year)	Number of Hips	Implant Type[a]	Mean Patient Age (Years)	Mean (Range) of Follow-up (Years)	Results
Engh et al[52] (2004)	777	AML and Solution	NA	20[b]	Survival with revision for any reason as end point: 97.7% at 5 years, 95.8% at 10 years, and 95.8% at 15 years
Weeden and Paprosky[10] (2002)	170	AML and Solution	61.2	14.2	4.1% mechanical failure rate
Moreland and Moreno[55] (2001)	137	AML and Solution	63.0	9.3 (5-16)	4% revision rate for aseptic femoral loosening
Krishnamurthy el al[12] (1997)	297	AML	59.6	8.3 (5-14)	2.4% mechanical failure rate
Moreland and Bernstein[54] (1995)	175	AML and Solution	62.4	5 (2-10)	4% mechanical failure rate
Lawrence et al[53] (1994)	81	AML and Solution	57.0	9 (5-13)	11% mechanical failure rate

[a]AML = Anatomic Medullary Locking total hip replacement (DePuy, Warsaw, IN); Solution System (DePuy). [b]Twenty-year experience. NA = not available.

fects. They also found no failures in 15 patients with type IIIB femora if the endosteal canal was less than 19 mm; however, in the 11 patients with type IIIB femora and an endosteal canal diameter greater than 19 mm, the mechanical failure rate was 18%. Three of the eight patients with type IV femoral defects had mechanical failure. The authors noted that an additional 13 patients with type IV femora were treated with either impaction bone grafting or modular tapered fluted stems; patients treated with these techniques had no failures at the time of publication.

Tapered Fluted Stems

The concerns over proximal stress shielding and the difficulty of reconstructing femora with advanced bone loss with use of the cylindrical, extensively porous-coated stems have led to the development of other designs. Several authors have reported a generally favorable experience using the Wagner SL Revision stem (Zimmer, Warsaw, IN).[58-60] Although fixation with the Wagner SL Revision stem was reasonably good, most authors have also reported a relatively high rate of subsi-

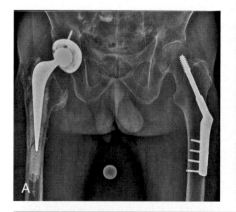
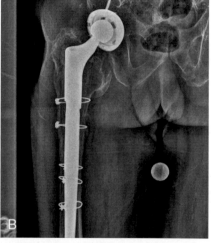

Figure 4   **A,** Radiograph of a hip with a periprosthetic femoral fracture and a loose cemented femoral stem before revision. **B,** Radiograph of the hip made after revision with a modular tapered fluted stem.

dence,[59,61] leading to the development of modular, fluted, tapered stems[62] (**Figure 4**). The results with modular, fluted, tapered stems have been excellent, with midterm survival rates of greater than 95% in several series.[63-70] The results of revision with modular, fluted, tapered stems are summarized in **Table 6**.

Richards et al[15] compared outcomes of femoral revisions with the use of either a tapered, fluted, modular titanium stem (ZMR Hip System; Zimmer) or a cylindrical, nonmodular cobalt-chromium implant (Solution System; DePuy). Despite the fact that patients in the tapered stem group had substantially worse osseous defects (65% had Paprosky type IIIB and IV defects), the cohort had better Western Ontario and McMaster Universities Osteoarthritis Index, Oxford-12, and

Table 6
Results of Revision With Tapered Fluted Stems

Study (Year)	Number of Hips	Implant Type[a]	Mean Duration of Follow-up (Months)	Stem Rerevision (%)	Any Rerevision (%)	Intraoperative Fractures (%)	Subsidence[c] (mm)
Wirtz et al[70] (2000)	142	MRP-Titan	28	1.4	4.9	NR	6 stems with > 5
Kwong et al[63] (2003)	143	Link MP	40	2.8	NR	2.1	2.1 (0-11.3)
Schuh et al[67] (2004)	79	MRP-Titan	48	3.8	NR	5.1	1 stem with > 2
Murphy and Rodriguez[65] (2004)	54	Link MP	42.6	2.9	16.3	NR	0
McInnis et al[64] (2006)	70	PFM	47	2.9	8.6	18.6	10 (0-52)
Park et al[66] (2007)	62	Lima-Lto	50	1.6	4.8	12.9	1 (0-25)
Rodriguez et al[87] (2009)	97	Link MP	39	5	NR	NR	5 stems with ≤ 2
Ovesen et al[69] (2010)	125	ZMR	50	3.2	6.4	3.2	2 (0-20)
Weiss et al[68] (2011)	90	Link MP	50[b]	2.0	10.0	1.0	2.7 (0-30)

[a]MRP-Titan (Peter Brehm Chirurgie Mechanik, Weisendorf, Germany); Link MP (Waldemar Link, Hamburg, Germany); PFM (Sulzer Orthopaedics, Baar, Switzerland); Lima-Lto (Lima Corporate, Udine, Italy); ZMR prosthesis (Zimmer, Warsaw, IN). [b]Median follow-up. [c]The values are given as the mean, with the range in parentheses, unless otherwise indicated. NR = not reported.

satisfaction scores. The authors also found that patients with a tapered stem had fewer fractures and more proximal osseous restoration.

Several authors have reported femoral stem fractures distal to the proximal modular junction.[15,69] Richards et al[15] reported four stem fractures in a cohort of 105 patients but noted that all the fractures occurred at the modular junction of an older design that is no longer in use. Although Berry[62] warned of the engineering challenges, given the location of this modular junction in a high-stress area, Postak and Greenwald[71] found the structural characteristics of the Link MP hip stem (Waldemar Link, Hamburg, Germany) are such that it offers the prospect of in vivo longevity.

Allograft-Prosthetic Composites

Proximal femoral allograft replacement

has been used successfully for the reconstruction of massive proximal femoral bone loss in the setting of multiple revision arthroplasties or oncologic resection. The obvious advantages to proximal femoral allograft are the ability to restore bone stock, particularly in younger patients, the provision of a biologic anchor for the abductor complex, and the ability to precisely adjust limb length.[72] The risks associated with proximal femoral allografts are the risk of disease transmission, graft resorption, and nonunion. Several authors have reported encouraging results of this technique with variable lengths of follow-up. Safir et al[73] reviewed the cases of 50 patients with a mean follow-up of 16.2 years who had been managed with a proximal femoral allograft. Survival at 15 years was 82.2%, with revision femoral surgery as the end point. Five patients required bone grafting and plate fixation for

symptomatic nonunion of the graft-host junction. The authors reported minor resorption of the graft in 58% of the patients, but only one patient in whom resorption led to failure of the construct. Graham and Stockley[74] reviewed the results of 25 allografts in 24 patients with a mean follow-up of 53 months. Two allografts required revision: one for aseptic failure and one for late infection. Another patient required augmentation of the graft-host junction for symptomatic nonunion. Babis et al[75] reported the results for 56 patients managed with an allograft-prosthetic composite. Survivorship of the reconstruction was 69% at 10 years with 26 hips remaining at risk. The authors reported the causes of failure were aseptic loosening in four, allograft resorption in three, allograft nonunion in two, allograft fracture in four, fracture of the femoral stem in one, and deep infection in five.

The authors also evaluated survival on the basis of the femoral defect and the number of previous revisions. Survival of the reconstructions was significantly worse for hips with Paprosky type IV defects than for those with type IIIB defects, and three or more previous femoral revisions significantly affected survival compared with one previous revision.

These results suggest that the use of proximal femoral allografts for massive segmental bone loss in revision total hip arthroplasty can provide durable long-term results, although the survival seems to be adversely affected by the amount of bone loss and the number of previous revisions.

Proximal Femoral Replacement

Proximal femoral replacements have been used extensively in the management of proximal femoral bone loss secondary to neoplastic disease.[76-82] There are few reports regarding the use of these prostheses in nonneoplastic conditions.[83-86] Parvizi and Sim[84] cautioned that these prostheses should be reserved for elderly or sedentary patients with massive proximal bone loss that cannot be reconstructed by other means.

Sim and Chao[83] reported encouraging results in a cohort of 21 patients who had been followed for 25 to 92 months after proximal femoral replacement. Two femoral components were revised: one because of recurrent instability and one because of acetabular loosening with substantial bone loss; the patient elected to have the well-fixed prosthesis removed. The authors cautioned that the results were preliminary, and longer term follow-up might change the results. In a follow-up report, Malkani et al[86] reviewed the 11.1-year results of 50 proximal femoral replacements. They reported that four femoral and seven acetabular components had been revised because of aseptic loosening. With any revision as the end point, survivorship was predicted to be 64% at 12 years following proximal femoral replacement. They also found that 11 of 50 hips had dislocated. Parvizi et al[85] reviewed the cases of 43 patients who had a proximal femoral replacement for a nonneoplastic condition at a mean of 36.5 months. With revision used as the end point, 37 of 43 implants had survived at 1 year and 31 of 43 implants at 5 years. Eight patients had hip instability, and six required revision for recurrent dislocation. Although the use of proximal femoral replacements can provide functional long-term results, the prostheses should be reserved for salvage situations in which massive proximal femoral bone loss cannot be reconstructed with other techniques.

Summary

Revision of a femoral implant is a challenging endeavor when there is substantial proximal bone loss. Numerous reconstructive options have been studied, and surgeons considering revision of a failed femoral prosthesis should be familiar with them. Careful preoperative planning is central to a successful outcome. Part of the preoperative plan will include a critical review of the radiographs in an effort to assess the degree of anticipated bone loss. Although several authors have proposed classification schemes for femoral bone loss, the Paprosky classification system provides a useful guide to femoral reconstruction based on the degree of bone loss. The rare type I defects can be treated with essentially any implant used in primary arthroplasty. The type II and IIIA defects can be reliably reconstructed with a cylindrical, extensively porous-coated implant. The type IIIB defect can usually be treated with a tapered, fluted, modular stem.

The complex type IV defect has been treated successfully with impaction grafting, modular tapered stems, allograft-prosthetic composites, and proximal femoral replacements. As technology and techniques have evolved, the success of femoral reconstruction in the face of extensive bone loss has improved. Continued follow-up and further evolution in technique and technology will continue to guide the management of femoral revision.

References

1. Kurtz S, Ong K, Lau E, Mowat F, Halpern M: Projections of primary and revision hip and knee arthroplasty in the United States from 2005 to 2030. *J Bone Joint Surg Am* 2007;89(4):780-785.

2. Agarwal S, Freiberg AA, Rubash HE: Preoperative planning for revision hip arthroplasty, in Callaghan JJ, Rosenberg AG, Rubash HE, eds: *The Adult Hip*, ed 2. Philadelphia, PA, Lippincott Williams & Wilkins, 2007, p 1313.

3. Harris WH, McCarthy JC Jr, O'Neill DA: Femoral component loosening using contemporary techniques of femoral cement fixation. *J Bone Joint Surg Am* 1982;64(7):1063-1067.

4. O'Neill DA, Harris WH: Failed total hip replacement: Assessment by plain radiographs, arthrograms, and aspiration of the hip joint. *J Bone Joint Surg Am* 1984;66(4): 540-546.

5. Engh CA, Bobyn JD, Glassman AH: Porous-coated hip replacement: The factors governing bone ingrowth, stress shielding, and clinical results. *J Bone Joint Surg Br* 1987;69(1):45-55.

6. Della Valle CJ, Paprosky WG: The femur in revision total hip arthroplasty evaluation and classification. *Clin Orthop Relat Res* 2004;420:55-62.

7. D'Antonio J, McCarthy JC, Bargar WL, et al: Classification of femoral abnormalities in total hip arthroplasty. *Clin Orthop Relat Res* 1993;296:133-139.

8. Mallory TH: Preparation of the proximal femur in cementless total hip revision. *Clin Orthop Relat Res* 1988;235:47-60.

9. Saleh KJ, Holtzman J, Gafni A, et al: Reliability and intraoperative validity of preoperative assessment of standardized plain radiographs in predicting bone loss at revision hip surgery. *J Bone Joint Surg Am* 2001;83-A(7):1040-1046.

10. Weeden SH, Paprosky WG: Minimal 11-year follow-up of extensively porous-coated stems in femoral revision total hip arthroplasty. *J Arthroplasty* 2002;17(4, Suppl 1):134-137.

11. Saleh KJ, Holtzman J, Gafni A, et al: Development, test reliability and validation of a classification for revision hip arthroplasty. *J Orthop Res* 2001;19(1): 50-56.

12. Krishnamurthy AB, MacDonald SJ, Paprosky WG: 5- to 13-year follow-up study on cementless femoral components in revision surgery. *J Arthroplasty* 1997;12(8): 839-847.

13. Lawrence JM, Engh CA, Macalino GE: Revision total hip arthroplasty: Long-term results without cement. *Orthop Clin North Am* 1993;24(4):635-644.

14. Della Valle CJ, Paprosky WG: Classification and an algorithmic approach to the reconstruction of femoral deficiency in revision total hip arthroplasty. *J Bone Joint Surg Am* 2003;85-A(Suppl 4):1-6.

15. Richards CJ, Duncan CP, Masri BA, Garbuz DS: Femoral revision hip arthroplasty: A comparison of two stem designs. *Clin Orthop Relat Res* 2010;468(2):491-496.

16. Iorio R, Healy WL, Presutti AH: A prospective outcomes analysis of femoral component fixation in revision total hip arthroplasty. *J Arthroplasty* 2008;23(5): 662-669.

17. Barrack RL, Folgueras AJ: Revision total hip arthroplasty: The femoral component. *J Am Acad Orthop Surg* 1995;3(2):79-85.

18. Pellicci PM, Wilson PD Jr, Sledge CB, et al: Long-term results of revision total hip replacement: A follow-up report. *J Bone Joint Surg Am* 1985;67(4):513-516.

19. Kavanagh BF, Ilstrup DM, Fitzgerald RH Jr: Revision total hip arthroplasty. *J Bone Joint Surg Am* 1985;67(4):517-526.

20. Callaghan JJ, Salvati EA, Pellicci PM, Wilson PD Jr, Ranawat CS: Results of revision for mechanical failure after cemented total hip replacement, 1979 to 1982: A two to five-year follow-up. *J Bone Joint Surg Am* 1985;67(7):1074-1085.

21. Rubash HE, Harris WH: Revision of nonseptic, loose, cemented femoral components using modern cementing techniques. *J Arthroplasty* 1988;3(3):241-248.

22. Estok DM II, Harris WH: Long-term results of cemented femoral revision surgery using second-generation techniques: An average 11.7-year follow-up evaluation. *Clin Orthop Relat Res* 1994;299: 190-202.

23. Mulroy WF, Harris WH: Revision total hip arthroplasty with use of so-called second-generation cementing techniques for aseptic loosening of the femoral component: A fifteen-year-average follow-up study. *J Bone Joint Surg Am* 1996;78(3):325-330.

24. Eisler T, Svensson O, Iyer V, et al: Revision total hip arthroplasty using third-generation cementing technique. *J Arthroplasty* 2000; 15(8):974-981.

25. Dohmae Y, Bechtold JE, Sherman RE, Puno RM, Gustilo RB: Reduction in cement-bone interface shear strength between primary and revision arthroplasty. *Clin Orthop Relat Res* 1988;236: 214-220.

26. Simon JP, Fowler JL, Gie GA, Ling RS, Timperley AJ: Impaction cancellous grafting of the femur in cemented total hip revision arthroplasty. *J Bone Joint Surg Br* 1991;73(Suppl 1):73.

27. Ornstein E, Atroshi I, Franzén H, Johnsson R, Sandquist P, Sundberg M: Early complications after one hundred and forty-four consecutive hip revisions with impacted morselized allograft bone and cement. *J Bone Joint Surg Am* 2002;84-A(8):1323-1328.

28. Oakes DA, Cabanela ME: Impaction bone grafting for revision hip arthroplasty: Biology and clinical applications. *J Am Acad Orthop Surg* 2006;14(11):620-628.

29. Eldridge JD, Smith EJ, Hubble MJ, Whitehouse SL, Learmonth ID: Massive early subsidence following femoral impaction grafting. *J Arthroplasty* 1997;12(5): 535-540.

30. Jazrawi LM, Della Valle CJ, Kummer FJ, Adler EM, Di Cesare PE: Catastrophic failure of a cemented, collarless, polished, tapered cobalt-chromium femoral stem used with impaction bone-grafting: A report of two cases. *J Bone Joint Surg Am* 1999;81(6): 844-847.

31. Masterson EL, Masri BA, Duncan CP: The cement mantle in the Exeter impaction allografting technique: A cause for concern. *J Arthroplasty* 1997;12(7): 759-764.

32. Meding JB, Ritter MA, Keating EM, Faris PM: Impaction bone-grafting before insertion of a femoral stem with cement in revision total hip arthroplasty: A minimum two-year follow-up study. *J Bone Joint Surg Am* 1997; 79(12):1834-1841.

33. Pekkarinen J, Alho A, Lepistö J, Ylikoski M, Ylinen P, Paavilainen T: Impaction bone grafting in

revision hip surgery: A high incidence of complications. *J Bone Joint Surg Br* 2000;82(1): 103-107.

34. Ornstein E, Linder L, Ranstam J, Lewold S, Eisler T, Torper M: Femoral impaction bone grafting with the Exeter stem: The Swedish experience. Survivorship analysis of 1305 revisions performed between 1989 and 2002. *J Bone Joint Surg Br* 2009;91(4): 441-446.

35. Edwards SA, Pandit HG, Grover ML, Clarke HJ: Impaction bone grafting in revision hip surgery. *J Arthroplasty* 2003;18(7): 852-859.

36. Halliday BR, English HW, Timperley AJ, Gie GA, Ling RS: Femoral impaction grafting with cement in revision total hip replacement: Evolution of the technique and results. *J Bone Joint Surg Br* 2003;85(6):809-817.

37. Mahoney CR, Fehringer EV, Kopjar B, Garvin KL: Femoral revision with impaction grafting and a collarless, polished, tapered stem. *Clin Orthop Relat Res* 2005; 432:181-187.

38. Wraighte PJ, Howard PW: Femoral impaction bone allografting with an Exeter cemented collarless, polished, tapered stem in revision hip replacement: A mean follow-up of 10.5 years. *J Bone Joint Surg Br* 2008;90(8):1000-1004.

39. Sierra RJ, Charity J, Tsiridis E, Timperley JA, Gie GA: The use of long cemented stems for femoral impaction grafting in revision total hip arthroplasty. *J Bone Joint Surg Am* 2008;90(6):1330-1336.

40. Gustilo RB, Pasternak HS: Revision total hip arthroplasty with titanium ingrowth prosthesis and bone grafting for failed cemented femoral component loosening. *Clin Orthop Relat Res* 1988;235: 111-119.

41. Harris WH, Krushell RJ, Galante JO: Results of cementless revisions of total hip arthroplasties using the Harris-Galante prosthesis. *Clin Orthop Relat Res* 1988;235: 120-126.

42. Hedley AK, Gruen TA, Ruoff DP: Revision of failed total hip arthroplasties with uncemented porous-coated anatomic components. *Clin Orthop Relat Res* 1988;235: 75-90.

43. Woolson ST, Delaney TJ: Failure of a proximally porous-coated femoral prosthesis in revision total hip arthroplasty. *J Arthroplasty* 1995;10(Suppl):S22-S28.

44. Berry DJ, Harmsen WS, Ilstrup D, Lewallen DG, Cabanela ME: Survivorship of uncemented proximally porous-coated femoral components. *Clin Orthop Relat Res* 1995;319:168-177.

45. Malkani AL, Lewallen DG, Cabanela ME, Wallrichs SL: Femoral component revision using an uncemented, proximally coated, long-stem prosthesis. *J Arthroplasty* 1996;11(4):411-418.

46. Mulliken BD, Rorabeck CH, Bourne RB: Uncemented revision total hip arthroplasty: A 4-to-6-year review. *Clin Orthop Relat Res* 1996;325:156-162.

47. Christie MJ, DeBoer DK, Tingstad EM, Capps M, Brinson MF, Trick LW: Clinical experience with a modular noncemented femoral component in revision total hip arthroplasty: 4- to 7-year results. *J Arthroplasty* 2000;15(7): 840-848.

48. Cameron HU: The long-term success of modular proximal fixation stems in revision total hip arthroplasty. *J Arthroplasty* 2002; 17(4, Suppl 1):138-141.

49. Smith JA, Dunn HK, Manaster BJ: Cementless femoral revision arthroplasty: 2- to 5-year results with a modular titanium alloy stem. *J Arthroplasty* 1997;12(2): 194-201.

50. McCarthy JC, Lee JA: Complex revision total hip arthroplasty with modular stems at a mean of 14 years. *Clin Orthop Relat Res* 2007;465:166-169.

51. Bolognesi MP, Pietrobon R, Clifford PE, Vail TP: Comparison of a hydroxyapatite-coated sleeve and a porous-coated sleeve with a modular revision hip stem: A prospective, randomized study. *J Bone Joint Surg Am* 2004;86-A(12): 2720-2725.

52. Engh CA Jr, Hopper RH Jr, Engh CA Sr: Distal ingrowth components. *Clin Orthop Relat Res* 2004; 420:135-141.

53. Lawrence JM, Engh CA, Macalino GE, Lauro GR: Outcome of revision hip arthroplasty done without cement. *J Bone Joint Surg Am* 1994;76(7):965-973.

54. Moreland JR, Bernstein ML: Femoral revision hip arthroplasty with uncemented, porous-coated stems. *Clin Orthop Relat Res* 1995; 319:141-150.

55. Moreland JR, Moreno MA: Cementless femoral revision arthroplasty of the hip: minimum 5 years followup. *Clin Orthop Relat Res* 2001;393:194-201.

56. Sporer SM, Paprosky WG: Revision total hip arthroplasty: The limits of fully coated stems. *Clin Orthop Relat Res* 2003;417: 203-209.

57. Engh CA Jr, Ellis TJ, Koralewicz LM, McAuley JP, Engh CA Sr: Extensively porous-coated femoral revision for severe femoral bone loss: Minimum 10-year follow-up. *J Arthroplasty* 2002;17(8): 955-960.

58. Böhm P, Bischel O: Femoral revision with the Wagner SL revision stem: Evaluation of one hundred and twenty-nine revisions followed for a mean of 4.8 years. *J Bone Joint Surg Am* 2001; 83-A(7):1023-1031.

59. Kolstad K, Adalberth G, Mallmin H, Milbrink J, Sahlstedt B: The

Wagner revision stem for severe osteolysis: 31 hips followed for 1.5-5 years. *Acta Orthop Scand* 1996;67(6):541-544.

60. Suominen S, Santavirta S: Revision total hip arthroplasty in deficient proximal femur using a distal load-bearing prosthesis. *Ann Chir Gynaecol* 1996;85(3):253-262.

61. Grünig R, Morscher E, Ochsner PE: Three- to 7-year results with the uncemented SL femoral revision prosthesis. *Arch Orthop Trauma Surg* 1997;116(4):187-197.

62. Berry DJ: Femoral revision: Distal fixation with fluted, tapered grit-blasted stems. *J Arthroplasty* 2002;17(4, Suppl 1):142-146.

63. Kwong LM, Miller AJ, Lubinus P: A modular distal fixation option for proximal bone loss in revision total hip arthroplasty: A 2- to 6-year follow-up study. *J Arthroplasty* 2003;18(3, Suppl 1):94-97.

64. McInnis DP, Horne G, Devane PA: Femoral revision with a fluted, tapered, modular stem seventy patients followed for a mean of 3.9 years. *J Arthroplasty* 2006;21(3):372-380.

65. Murphy SB, Rodriguez J: Revision total hip arthroplasty with proximal bone loss. *J Arthroplasty* 2004;19(4, Suppl 1):115-119.

66. Park YS, Moon YW, Lim SJ: Revision total hip arthroplasty using a fluted and tapered modular distal fixation stem with and without extended trochanteric osteotomy. *J Arthroplasty* 2007;22(7):993-999.

67. Schuh A, Werber S, Holzwarth U, Zeiler G: Cementless modular hip revision arthroplasty using the MRP Titan Revision Stem: Outcome of 79 hips after an average of 4 years' follow-up. *Arch Orthop Trauma Surg* 2004;124(5):306-309.

68. Weiss RJ, Beckman MO, Enocson A, Schmalholz A, Stark A: Mini-

mum 5-year follow-up of a cementless, modular, tapered stem in hip revision arthroplasty. *J Arthroplasty* 2011;26(1):16-23.

69. Ovesen O, Emmeluth C, Hofbauer C, Overgaard S: Revision total hip arthroplasty using a modular tapered stem with distal fixation: Good short-term results in 125 revisions. *J Arthroplasty* 2010;25(3):348-354.

70. Wirtz DC, Heller KD, Holzwarth U, et al: A modular femoral implant for uncemented stem revision in THR. *Int Orthop* 2000;24(3):134-138.

71. Postak PD, Greenwald AS: *The Influence of Modularity on the Endurance Performance of the LINK MP Hip Stem.* Cleveland, OH, Orthopaedic Research Laboratories, 2001.

72. Lee SH, Ahn YJ, Chung SJ, Kim BK, Hwang JH: The use of allograft prosthesis composite for extensive proximal femoral bone deficiencies: A 2- to 9.8-year follow-up study. *J Arthroplasty* 2009;24(8):1241-1248.

73. Safir O, Kellett CF, Flint M, Backstein D, Gross AE: Revision of the deficient proximal femur with a proximal femoral allograft. *Clin Orthop Relat Res* 2009;467(1):206-212.

74. Graham NM, Stockley I: The use of structural proximal femoral allografts in complex revision hip arthroplasty. *J Bone Joint Surg Br* 2004;86(3):337-343.

75. Babis GC, Sakellariou VI, O'Connor MI, Hanssen AD, Sim FH: Proximal femoral allograft-prosthesis composites in revision hip replacement: A 12-year follow-up study. *J Bone Joint Surg Br* 2010;92(3):349-355.

76. Bosquet M, Burssens A, Mulier JC: Long term follow-up results of a femoral megaprosthesis: A review of thirteen patients. *Arch Orthop Trauma Surg* 1980;97(4):299-304.

77. Donati D, Zavatta M, Gozzi E, Giacomini S, Campanacci L, Mercuri M: Modular prosthetic replacement of the proximal femur after resection of a bone tumour a long-term follow-up. *J Bone Joint Surg Br* 2001;83(8):1156-1160.

78. Kawai A, Backus SI, Otis JC, Inoue H, Healey JH: Gait characteristics of patients after proximal femoral replacement for malignant bone tumour. *J Bone Joint Surg Br* 2000;82(5):666-669.

79. Johnsson R, Carlsson A, Kisch K, Moritz U, Zetterström R, Persson BM: Function following mega total hip arthroplasty compared with conventional total hip arthroplasty and healthy matched controls. *Clin Orthop Relat Res* 1985;192:159-167.

80. Morris HG, Capanna R, Del Ben M, Campanacci D: Prosthetic reconstruction of the proximal femur after resection for bone tumors. *J Arthroplasty* 1995;10(3):293-299.

81. Ogilvie CM, Wunder JS, Ferguson PC, Griffin AM, Bell RS: Functional outcome of endoprosthetic proximal femoral replacement. *Clin Orthop Relat Res* 2004;426:44-48.

82. Zehr RJ, Enneking WF, Scarborough MT: Allograft-prosthesis composite versus megaprosthesis in proximal femoral reconstruction. *Clin Orthop Relat Res* 1996;322:207-223.

83. Sim FH, Chao EY: Hip salvage by proximal femoral replacement. *J Bone Joint Surg Am* 1981;63(8):1228-1239.

84. Parvizi J, Sim FH: Proximal femoral replacements with megaprostheses. *Clin Orthop Relat Res* 2004;420:169-175.

85. Parvizi J, Tarity TD, Slenker N, et al: Proximal femoral replacement in patients with non-neoplastic conditions. *J Bone Joint Surg Am* 2007;89(5):1036-1043.

86. Malkani AL, Settecerri JJ, Sim FH, Chao EY, Wallrichs SL: Long-term results of proximal femoral replacement for non-neoplastic disorders. *J Bone Joint Surg Br* 1995;77(3):351-356.

87. Rodriguez JA, Fada R, Murphy SB, Rasquinha VJ, Ranawat CS: Two-year to five-year follow-up of femoral defects in femoral revision treated with the link MP modular stem. *J Arthroplasty* 2009;24(5): 751-758.

MRI and Arthroscopy Correlations of the Hip: A Case-Based Approach

David A. McCall, MD

Marc R. Safran, MD

Abstract

Disorders of the hip joint can be physically disabling for the patient and a diagnostic challenge for the physician. Advances in imaging the hip with MRI can help the physician determine a more specific diagnosis for patients with acute or chronic hip pain. MRI and particularly magnetic resonance arthrography have helped raised awareness of nonarthritic hip problems and have made the diagnosis of hip problems much easier. Intra-articular and extra-articular processes can be evaluated with MRI; multiple sequences are available to increase the sensitivity and specificity for detecting specific pathology around the hip. Because the hip is a deep joint within a large soft-tissue envelope, MRI more precisely delineates the sources of hip pain by evaluating the soft tissues and ligamentous structures around the hip. It is helpful to understand the role of MRI in evaluating common pathologic conditions within the hip joint, including labral tears, chondral lesions, loose bodies, tears of the ligamentum teres, femoral acetabular impingement, developmental dysplasia of the hip, and pigmented villonodular synovitis.

Hip arthroscopy, a less invasive technique for treating hip problems, has also contributed to the rapid growth of interest in this area of orthopaedic surgery. Hip arthroscopy can be used to evaluate disorders in the intra-articular region (central and peripheral compartments) and periarticular region (iliopsoas bursa and tendon disorders) as well as those in the peritrochanteric region.

Instr Course Lect 2012;61:327-344.

The hip joint is designed to support the entire body weight and shifting mechanical loads during ambulation and activity. During ambulation, loads equal to four to seven times body weight are transmitted through the hip; these loads are even higher when performing activities like running and jumping. The hip joint has the unique structure of a ball-and-socket joint or enarthrodial joint.[1] The slightly aspheric femoral head can rotate freely and translate within the acetabulum, but it is also tightly opposed to the acetabulum for stability. Most biomechanists describe the hip joint as a gimbal joint (a pivoted support that allows the rotation of an object about an axis) rather than a true ball-and-socket joint. The stability of the hip joint is augmented by the bony anatomy and static and dynamic stabilizers of the joint, which include the surrounding capsule, ligaments, the acetabular labrum, and muscles.[2,3] These surrounding structures can be subsequently damaged by a myriad of pathologic conditions. Advances in MRI and hip arthroscopy have increased interest in the diagnosis and treatment of the nonarthritic painful hip joint and have improved understanding of the normal and pathologic mechanics of the hip.

Neither Dr. McCall nor any immediate family member has received anything of value from or owns stock in a commercial company or institution related directly or indirectly to the subject of this chapter. Dr. Safran or an immediate family member has received royalties from Stryker; serves as a paid consultant to Cool Systems and Arthrocare; serves as an unpaid consultant to Cool Systems, Cradle Medical, Ferring Pharmaceuticals, and Biomimedica; owns stock or stock options in Cool Systems, Cradle Medical, and Biomimedica; has received research or institutional support from Ferring Pharmaceuticals; and serves as a board member, owner, officer, or committee member of the American Shoulder and Elbow Surgeons; the American Orthopaedic Society for Sports Medicine; the International Society of Arthroscopy, Knee Surgery, and Orthopaedic Sports Medicine; and the Society for Tennis Medicine and Science.

Improved imaging is no substitute for a complete history and physical examination. The patient's gait, range of motion, and muscle strength should be evaluated and compared for side-to-side differences, including limb-length discrepancies. The clinician must be able to determine the frequency, severity, location, inciting factors, and radiation of painful symptoms. Mechanical symptoms such as clicking and locking occur with many types of hip pathology and may cause synovial irritation, which can present as pain in the hip or groin. Determining the factors that exacerbate or relieve symptoms and whether symptoms are chronic or acute can aid in the diagnosis. Intra-articular hip pain usually presents as groin pain and may radiate to the anterior thigh, although patients may describe pain on the lateral thigh or buttocks, oftentimes placing cupped hands over the greater trochanter (the C sign).[4] Evaluation and examination of the lumbar spine, genitourinary tract, and abdomen should be performed to rule out other sources of pathology as the cause of symptoms.[5]

Plain radiographs of the hip and pelvis are used to determine the presence of bony structural abnormalities of the hip, including dysplasia, femoral acetabular impingement, acetabular retroversion, and the presence of degenerative changes.[6] As with other joints, MRI should be used to help confirm the diagnosis of a hip disorder rather than make the diagnosis. Currently, the preoperative patient history and physical and MRI evaluation of the hip is still in need of refinement. Martin et al[7] reported that even experts in hip arthroscopy have difficulty making an accurate diagnosis of hip pain, although determining an intra-articular or extra-articular source of pain can be done reliably. MRI sensitivity for most hip pathologies is quite good. MRI is particularly helpful in di-

agnosing the source of intra-articular or periarticular hip pain.

Because the hip is a deep joint within an envelope of soft tissues, MRI helps provide a more precise delineation of the sources of hip pain by evaluating the soft tissues and ligamentous structures around the hip. Although MRI with a small field of view and particularly magnetic resonance arthrography are useful for detecting labral pathology, these modalities are not accurate in identifying chondral lesions.[8] With the addition of saline or gadolinium to distend the hip capsule, MRI has increased sensitivity for identifying intra-articular pathology such as acetabular labral tears, osteochondral injury, ligamentum teres tears, and loose bodies.[9-11] Studies comparing magnetic resonance arthrography to hip arthroscopy for the detection of labral and cartilage lesions show better sensitivity for labral pathology over articular defects.[10-12] Hip arthroscopy has become increasingly popular over the past several years as indications for its use have shifted from a diagnostic to a therapeutic role. This chapter will discuss some common pathologic conditions of the hip joint that are amenable to treatment with hip arthroscopy and correlate those conditions with magnetic resonance findings and imaging. There is a role for MRI in common pathologic conditions of the hip joint, including labral tears, chondral lesions and loose bodies, tears of the ligamentum teres, femoral acetabular impingement, developmental dysplasia, and pigmented villonodular synovitis (PVNS).

MRI Basics

When evaluating the pelvis, it is helpful to begin with a large field of view that includes both hips. Typical sequences include axial images obtained from the top of the iliac crest to below the lesser trochanters. A side-to-side

comparison may be performed with a coronal or an axial sequence of the entire pelvis. If the patient reports specific hip symptoms, additional sequences with smaller fields of view showing only the symptomatic side should be obtained. Dedicated hip imaging should include a T1-weighted sequence, a short tau inversion recovery sequence in the coronal plane, an oblique axial proton density-weighted sequence, and a sagittal T2-weighted sequence with fat saturation.[3] The T1-weighted sequence aids in evaluating the anatomy, including the bony anatomy. The short tau inversion recovery sequence in the coronal plane has sensitivity to fluids and uniform fat suppression and aids in the evaluation of the superior and inferior labrum, cartilage, and bone marrow edema. The oblique axial proton density-weighted sequence is performed to evaluate the anterior and posterior labrum and bone marrow edema and measure the alpha angle. The sagittal T2-weighted sequence with fat saturation is performed to evaluate the anterior and posterior labrum and the superior cartilage. This sequence can be particularly useful for identifying extra-articular fluid collections, such as paralabral cysts and subtle bone marrow edema.[13]

On MRI, the normal acetabular labrum appears as a triangular structure with sharp margins and low signal intensity. There is often a recess between the outer margin of the labrum and the joint capsule (**Figure 1**). If intra-articular pathology is suspected, it is helpful to use magnetic resonance arthrography to improve the visualization of the detailed articular structures, such as the labrum and the articular surface. With degeneration of the labrum, there is increased signal on T2-weighted fast spin-echo images. Frank tears of the labrum usually present as a fluid-filled cleft at the base of the labrum adjacent to the acetabular cartilage. Complete detachment of the labrum can be seen in advanced tears. The use of magnetic resonance arthrography has been shown to increase the sensitivity of detecting labral lesions, which can be a helpful in directing treatment.[10,14-16] Local anesthetic may be mixed with gadolinium injections during magnetic resonance arthrography for diagnostic purposes.[16] A greater than 50% reduction in pain within the first hour after the injection helps to confirm that the hip joint is the source of the pain.

Labral Tears

The acetabular labrum is a fibrocartilaginous structure that outlines the acetabular socket. Labral attachment occurs at the periphery and is anchored anteriorly and posteriorly at the transverse acetabular ligament. The labrum is predominantly type 1 collagen that extends 7 to 10 mm from the acetabular rim, contributing 22% of the articulating surface and 33% of the volume of the acetabulum.[17] The thickness of the labrum and its morphology may vary slightly, but it is usually approximately 2 to 3 mm thick and extends 2 to 3 mm past the acetabular socket.[18] The labrum is a structure that was initially believed to have no real function, although recent research has suggested that the labrum actually has several important hip functions.[2] The intact labrum has been shown to have a sealant effect on the hip joint that maintains fluid for articular cartilage nutrition, maintains articular cartilage stiffness to reduce consolidation by maintaining the fluid within the articular cartilage, and serves as a barrier to extrusion of fluid from the joint to provide a smoother gliding surface.[19-21] The periphery of the labrum has a limited blood supply; therefore, there is a decreased healing potential for detached labral tears with ar-

throscopic labral repair.[22] The labrum provides secondary stability to the bony constrained hip joint by deepening the joint, by maintaining negative intra-articular pressure, and through proprioceptive mechanisms. The free margin articulates with the articular surface and has been shown to have neuroreceptors, which may provide proprioception to the hip joint.[23]

Clinically, patients with labral tears of the acetabulum may present with nonspecific hip or groin pain because the labrum is innervated with free nerve endings. The acetabular labrum is abnormal in many hip disorders; however, less than 50% of patients with labral tears have a history of associated trauma.[24] Occasionally, the tear can be associated with painful snapping and clicking within the hip joint. The pain frequently occurs as the hip is actively extended from a flexed position. There are many etiologies for labral tears, including traumatic and degenerative causes; nearly 90% of atraumatic causes of hip pain are associated with radiographic structural abnormalities.[25] Structural abnormalities range from femoroacetabular impingement (cam- and pincer-type lesions) to developmental dysplasia of the hip, prior slipped capital femoral epiphysis, and Legg-Calvé-Perthes disease. Traumatic tears can occur from an isolated event or, more commonly, from repetitive trauma, which is believed to be associated with hip hyperextension (with or without external rotation) and hip hyperflexion, which often occurs in patients who play golf or football, respectively. Traumatic hip dislocations and acetabular fractures also have been associated with labral tears.[26] Degenerative labral tears can be the result of repetitive microtrauma and may be associated with degenerative changes to the hip joint. These types of tears often cause mechanical symptoms, leading to abnormal loading and irritation

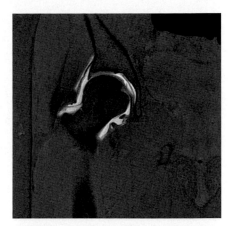

Figure 1 Coronal T2-weighted magnetic resonance arthrogram of a normal triangular-shaped labrum. Note that the capsule inserts directly onto the acetabulum, with a cleft between the labrum and the capsule. This is the normal appearance of the cleft and the labrum. (Courtesy of Marc R. Safran, MD, Redwood City, CA.)

to the hip and adjacent structures. Tears of the acetabular labrum may result in mechanical symptoms that can limit the ability to participate in daily activities or athletic events. The history and physical findings may suggest other etiologies, such as osteoarthritis, synovitis, juxta-articular soft-tissue abnormalities, osteonecrosis, and stress fracture. The clinical evaluation of patients with labral tears includes the labral stress test (pain and/or clicking as the hip is moved into extension, adduction, and internal rotation from a position of flexion-abduction and external rotation), the impingement test (pain with internal rotation of the hip flexed to 90° and adducted), and the McCarthy test (pain with extension of the flexed hip while supine with the contralateral hip held flexed; this test also can be performed in internal and external rotation). The clinician must consider that labral tears, labral fraying, and cartilage lesions all increase in prevalence with increasing age and may not always be symptomatic.

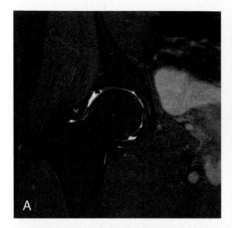

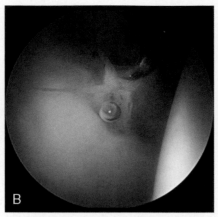

Figure 2   **A,** MRI scan of the hip of a 19-year-old patient who is a synchronized swimmer shows arthrographic contrast between the labrum and the acetabulum; this is consistent with a labral-chondral separation. **B,** Arthroscopic view of the anterior labral-chondral separation. (Courtesy of Marc R. Safran, MD, Redwood City, CA.)

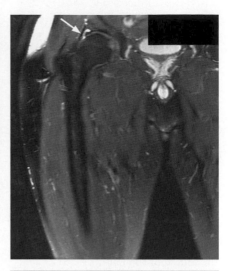

Figure 4   MRI scan of a perilabral cyst (arrow). The presence of the cyst is indicative of a labral tear. (Courtesy of Marc R. Safran, MD, Redwood City, CA.)

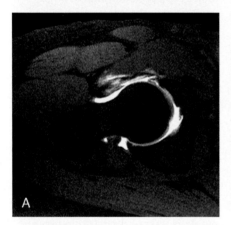

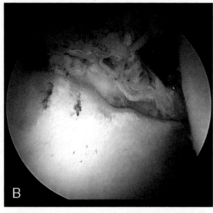

Figure 3   **A,** Magnetic resonance arthrogram of a 38-year-old patient who is a marathon runner shows intrasubstance labral tearing and degeneration. **B,** Arthroscopic appearance of the torn labrum. (Courtesy of Marc R. Safran, MD, Redwood City, CA.)

In patients with atraumatic labral tears, plain radiographs may show bony changes, such as those that occur in hip dysplasia, Legg-Calvé-Perthes disease, and femoroacetabular impingement, or evidence of prior slipped capital femoral epiphysis. Conventional MRI is limited for evaluating the labrum because of the lack of joint distention.[27] With magnetic resonance arthrography, the hip is injected with fluid before an MRI scan is performed. By distending the capsule, the labrum is outlined with contrast,

and tears are more readily identified.[10,16] The capsule does not insert on the labrum of the hip but instead inserts onto the acetabulum above the labrum; therefore, with magnetic resonance arthrography, a cleft may be seen between the capsule and the capsular side of the labrum (**Figure 1**). This cleft is occasionally misdiagnosed as a labral tear. Another pitfall in assessing the labrum occurs from a failure to recognize that the acetabular articular cartilage is in continuity with the labrum. Contrast fluid should not

be seen tracking perpendicular to the articular cartilage at the labral-chondral junction (**Figure 2**). A labral tear is usually identified by a bright line within the dark labrum (**Figure 3**) or at the labral-chondral junction on magnetic resonance arthrography. A perilabral cyst may also indicate that a labral tear is present (**Figure 4**).

Tears are often found at the anterior and anterosuperior aspects of the acetabular rim and can be characterized by their location and morphology. Labral tears have been classified morphologically as radial flap, radial fibrillated, longitudinal peripheral, and unstable.[28] Radial flap and radial fibrillated tears occur within the substance of the labrum. Longitudinal peripheral tears occur at the labral base and likely represent labral detachments. The unstable tear is identified by subluxing labral fragments.[29]

Labral tears also have been classified based on the histologic analysis of cadaver specimens. A type 1 labral tear is a detached labrum with displacement from the fibrocartilaginous labral-chondral junction. A type 2 labral tear

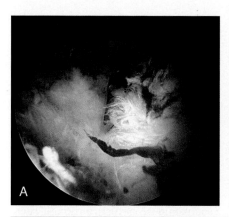
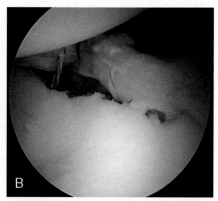

Figure 5 Arthroscopic views of a partial labrectomy of a complex degenerative labral tear using a meniscal biter (**A**) and labral repair with sutures in place before tying down the labrum (**B**). (Courtesy of Marc R. Safran, MD, Redwood City, CA.)

involves intrasubstance tears with variable depths.[17] McCarthy et al[30,31] described two types of labral pathology: fraying at the labral-chondral junction and tearing of the labrum with separation from the articular cartilage (chondrolabral separation). They referred to this chondrolabral separation as the watershed lesion. In addition to labral tears, magnetic resonance arthrography readily depicts articular cartilage, allowing for the diagnosis of early cartilage degenerative changes. Because classification systems are useful only if they predict outcomes or guide treatments, the simplest classification of whether the tear is at the watershed location of the labral-chondral junction (**Figure 2**) or is an intrasubstance tear (**Figure 3**) serves current treatment guidelines.

Treatment is based on the correlation of symptoms and clinical examination and imaging findings. The senior author (MRS) finds it useful to use intra-articular anesthetic as an adjunct in assessing the patient. If short-term pain relief (within 1 hour) can be achieved with a long-acting intra-articular anesthetic, the diagnosis of intra-articular pathology as the source of the pain can be confirmed. Pain relief may not be achieved with the in-

jection if (1) the injection is traumatic, (2) the injection is not made into the joint, (3) too little anesthetic is injected (7 cc preferred), and (4) the pain is not originating from inside the joint. On rare occasions, magnetic resonance arthrography with the addition of local anesthetic does not relieve pain; however, when a repeat intra-articular injection is given without gadolinium, there is a positive benefit. The reason for this is unclear because the amount of gadolinium is quite small in comparison with the amount of injected fluid.

If symptoms continue for more than 4 weeks, the clinical examination and imaging confirm that the pain is originating from inside the joint, and a labral tear can be seen, the patient may be a candidate for hip arthroscopy. Treatment options include a partial labrectomy (**Figure 5,** *A*) and labral repair (**Figure 5,** *B*). If the labrum is torn from the labral-chondral junction, these tears can be repaired because blood from the acetabular bone can heal the labrum to the acetabular rim. If there is an intrasubstance tear, a partial labrectomy to remove only the torn tissue is often recommended. However, treating only the labral pathology and not its underlying cause

may not result in the desired outcome. Arthroscopically débriding a labral tear when osteoarthritis is present has a poor outcome, and treating labral tears in patients with hip dysplasia or femoroacetabular impingement without treating the underlying bony problem has unacceptably high failure rates. The role of labral reconstruction is considered experimental.

Chondral Injury and Loose Bodies

Isolated cartilaginous lesions of the hip are infrequent injuries that are often related to acute shearing forces across the hip and often occur with a fall with direct landing onto the lateral hip.[32] More often, acetabular cartilaginous injuries are seen in tandem with labral pathology; both require treatment at the time of surgery. Cartilaginous lesions are also a frequent finding in femoral acetabular impingement. A magnetic resonance arthrogram is the imaging modality of choice for detailed evaluation of the articular cartilage and assessment of important data, including the size, location, stability, joint surface congruity, and viability of the fragments. Today, however, MRI has only moderate sensitivity for detecting cartilage lesions, in part because of the thin articular cartilage lining the hip and the signal-to-noise ratio of a deep structure such as the hip (**Figure 6**).

Loose bodies can originate from traumatic injury, degenerative changes, or other disease processes, such as spondyloepiphyseal dysplasia, Legg-Calvé-Perthes disease, osteochondritis dissecans, osteonecrosis, synovial chondromatosis, and osteoarthritis.[33] Osteochondritis dissecans, an osseous lesion with a mechanical or traumatic etiology, is uncommon in the hip, and its true pathophysiology is debatable. Cartilage flaps are particularly difficult to identify preoperatively because they

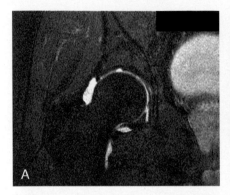
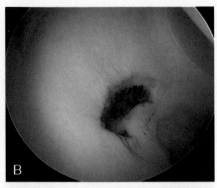

Figure 6 A 14-year-old boy had hip pain 1.5 years after an acetabular fracture that healed with nonsurgical management. **A,** MRI scan shows a filling defect of the weight-bearing portion of the acetabulum that is consistent with a full-thickness chondral injury. **B,** Arthroscopic view of the lesion after débridement. (Courtesy of Marc R. Safran, MD, Redwood City, CA.)

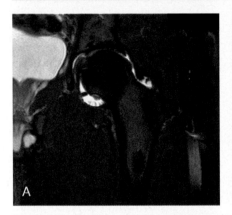
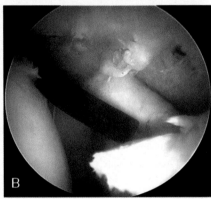

Figure 7 A 22-year-old patient who is a collegiate football player presented with a 2-year history of increasing hip pain. **A,** T2-weighted coronal MRI scan shows a labral tear with fluid tracking under the articular cartilage of the superolateral acetabulum. **B,** Arthroscopic view of the full-thickness flap of articular cartilage. This lesion was treated with débridement and microfracture. (Courtesy of Marc R. Safran, MD, Redwood City, CA.)

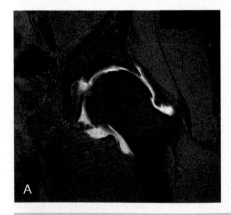
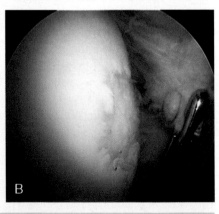

Figure 8 **A,** MRI scan of the hip of a 40-year-old patient who was a football player and a triathlete shows articular cartilage damage of the lateral acetabulum and superior femoral head. **B,** Arthroscopic view of the femoral head lesion. (Courtesy of Marc R. Safran, MD, Redwood City, CA.)

often lay within their bed against the subchondral bone (**Figure 7**). Cartilaginous abnormalities predominate on the acetabular articular surface, especially anterosuperiorly, with fewer lesions on the femoral head.[34] The clinical presentation of anterior groin pain, episodes of locking, painful clicking, buckling, giving way, or persistent pain within the hip during activity can be associated with intra-articular loose bodies, although there are no specific findings in patients with isolated chondral injury or loose bodies.[35,36] Although no definitive evidence exists, it appears chondral lesions of the femoral head (**Figure 8**) have a poorer prognosis than acetabular lesions.

The treatment of chondral injuries includes treatment of the underlying cause, débridement, and, in selected situations, microfracture (**Figure 9**). There have been some reports of chondral repair, although such treatment is experimental.[33,37] Chondrocyte viability in full-thickness cartilage flaps is poor.

Loose bodies can be ossified or nonossified and are classified as osteocartilaginous, cartilaginous, fibrous, and foreign. Ossified loose bodies, composed of bone and cartilage, are the most commonly identified loose body associated with the hip and may be detectable on plain radiographs. The classic disease process that results in ossified bodies is synovial osteochondromatosis. Cartilaginous loose bodies are radiolucent and usually originate from the articular surfaces of the femoral head and the acetabulum, although they also can occur in association with synovial chondromatosis or chronic synovial inflammation. Cartilaginous loose bodies are often detected with MRI, particularly with magnetic resonance arthrography (**Figures 10** and **11**). Loose bodies are commonly found in the cotyloid fossa or the posterior aspect of the central compartment (**Figure 10,** *B*) or in the peripheral compartment (**Figure 11,** *B*), especially in the posterior and medial femoral neck regions. The presence of a loose body within the articulating surfaces of any joint theoretically can result in destruction of the hyaline cartilage and ultimately result in degenerative arthritis. Loose bodies that gravitate into the posterior, medial, or inferior capsular recesses may be difficult to reach but generally are accessible arthroscopically.[38] If a fragment is visible posteriorly but not reachable, a mini-posterior arthrotomy has been advocated because it can be done easily and safely when the lateral position is used.[39]

The treatment of symptomatic loose bodies within the hip or in the pericapsular region is the most widely reported and accepted application for hip arthroscopy.[40] Although arthrotomy remains the gold standard for direct observation and removal of intra-articular and extra-articular objects or loose bodies, there is some morbidity associated with this procedure. The minimally invasive nature and low morbidity associated with hip arthroscopy make the procedure ideal for establishing an early preventive strategy to treat symptomatic patients with loose bodies in the hip. However, in some situations, particularly with larger loose bodies (> 6 mm) or when there are numerous loose bodies, arthroscopic removal of all the loose bodies may be long and tedious.

Ligamentum Teres Pathology

The ligamentum teres is a triangular structure located in the hip joint; its function is unclear. It has a broad origin, blending with the transverse ligament of the acetabulum and attached to the ischial and pubic sides of the acetabular notch by separate bands or bundles.[41] The length of the ligamen-

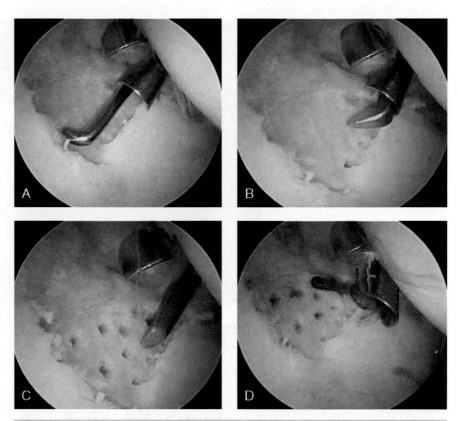

Figure 9 A 21-year-old patient with hip pain who is a collegiate water polo player was treated with débridement of an acetabular chondral lesion. Arthroscopic views showing measurement of the lesion (**A**), microfracture (**B**), fatty globules from the microfractured lesion (**C**), and blood coming from the microfractures (**D**). (Courtesy of Marc R. Safran, MD, Redwood City, CA.)

tum teres is typically between 30 mm and 35 mm on arthroscopic examination, but variations have been noted. It arises from the posteroinferior portion of the cotyloid fossa and inserts into the femoral head filling the fovea capitis femoris, which is an area of the femoral head devoid of cartilage lying slightly posterior and inferior to its center.[42] The ligamentum teres contains the anterior branch of the posterior division of the obturator artery, which supplies an area of the juvenile femoral head; the vessel remains patent in some adults, but its contribution to the vascularity of the femoral head is minimal after skeletal maturity. The fovea of the femoral head is connected to the posteroinferior portion of the acetabular fossa via the ligamentum teres, which becomes taut in hip flexion,

adduction, and external rotation, providing some stability to the hip. Any uncontrolled movement in the direction of maximal tension may cause injury to the ligament, such as hip dislocation or subluxation. Mechanical symptoms can occur with a ruptured ligamentum teres, including painful clicking and giving way.[43] Clinical examination may show a reduced and painful range of movement of the hip joint, either in extension or in combined flexion and internal rotation. Tears of the ligamentum teres have been classified into three types: type I (complete), type II (partial), and type III (degenerative) as seen in osteoarthritis.[44] Radiographs are usually unremarkable.

MRI remains the imaging modality of choice in evaluating suspected liga-

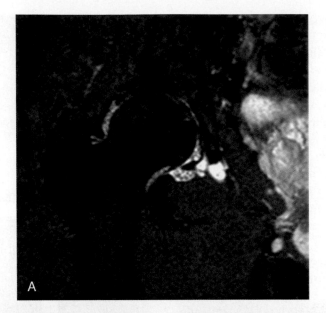

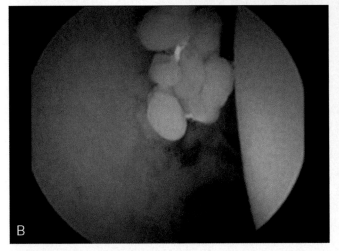

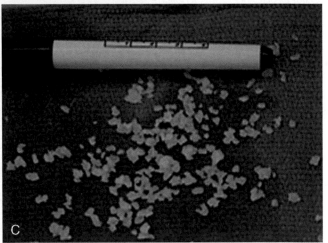

Figure 10   A 36-year-old man presented with hip pain. **A,** MRI scan revealed multiple small loose bodies in the peripheral compartment. **B,** Arthroscopic view of the multiple, small, loose bodies in the central compartment. **C,** Photograph of some of the small, chondral loose bodies after removal. (Courtesy of Marc R. Safran, MD, Redwood City, CA.)

mentum teres pathology. However, normal MRI dimensions of the ligamentum teres have not been defined, and MRI staging of ligamentum teres pathology is lacking. The normal ligamentum teres appears as a homogeneous structure with a low-intensity (dark) signal on T1- and T2-weighted sequences, much like other ligaments in the body. Magnetic resonance arthrography may also be used in the evaluation of the ligamentum teres when findings from contrast imaging are inconclusive (**Figure 12**).

Arthroscopy remains the most reliable diagnostic tool for assessing ligamentum teres pathology.[45,46] Tears of the ligamentum teres are usually treated with arthroscopic débridement to remove the innervated stump that may be intermittently caught within the joint and cause mechanical symptoms (**Figure 12**). There have been isolated reports of ligamentum teres reconstructions, although more research is needed.[47]

Femoroacetabular Impingement

Femoroacetabular impingement of the hip joint is a relatively new diagnosis that is increasingly being recognized as a common cause of hip pain and restriction of hip motion in young adults.[48] Physial stresses during development and genetic factors represent potential sources for the development of proximal femoral abnormalities. Posttraumatic acetabular dysplasia, femoral retrotorsion, and iatrogenic deformities of the hip are all factors

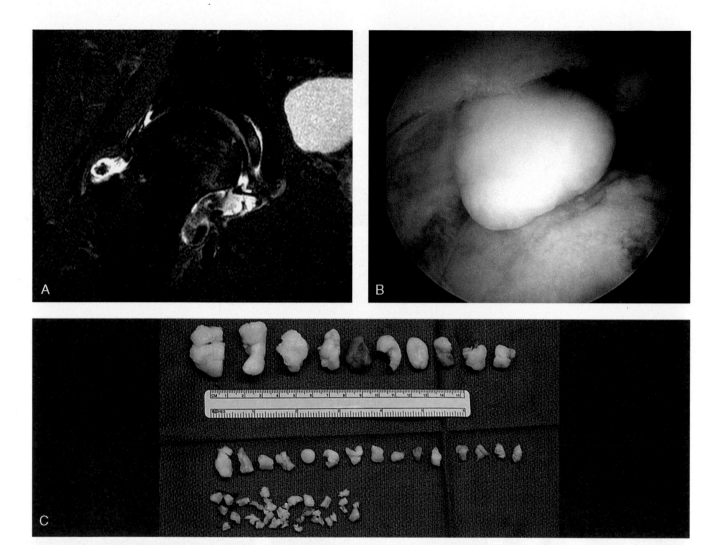

Figure 11 A 42-year-old man who works as a truck driver presented with hip pain and limited motion. **A,** MRI scan shows several large loose bodies in the peripheral compartment. **B,** Arthroscopic view showing one of the large loose bodies. **C,** Photograph of several of the loose bodies after removal. (Courtesy of Marc R. Safran, MD, Redwood City, CA.)

that can lead to femoroacetabular impingement (with acetabular deficiency or retroversion; concomitant coxa magna, which can cause impingement, is often present). Impingement has also been associated with childhood diseases such as Legg-Calvé-Perthes disease, slipped capital femoral epiphysis, hip dysplasia, and bladder exstrophy; however, the etiologies of most abnormalities causing femoroacetabular impingement have not been identified.[49] Morphologic features on the femoral and acetabular sides of the joint lead to impingement, which can be attributable to femoral causes (cam impingement) or acetabular causes (pincer impingement). Cam impingement is caused by abutment of an aspheric femoral head against the acetabulum during hip motion. Pincer impingement is the result of abnormal contact between the acetabular rim and the femoral neck as a result of acetabular abnormalities, such as acetabular retroversion (global or cranial) or overcoverage of the femoral head by the acetabulum, as in coxa profunda or protrusio.[50,51] These bony abnormalities lead to repetitive microtrauma associated with mechanical wear of the labrum and the articular cartilage and, if left untreated, cause pain, labral tears, and chondral injuries. The pathophysiology of cam-type impingement results in the initial sparing of the labrum, resulting in labral-chondral separation, whereas abutment against the acetabular rim results in deep (several millimeters from the acetabular rim) chondral injuries at the anterolateral acetabulum.[52] Conversely, pincer impingement results in crushing of the labrum between the acetabulum and the femoral neck, result-

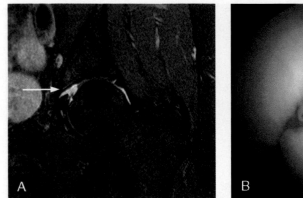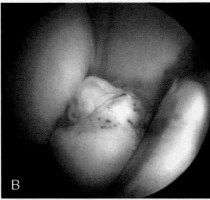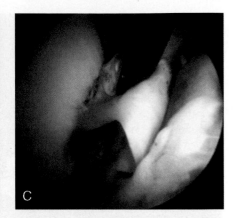

Figure 12 A 38-year-old patient who is a triathlete had pain in the left hip for 9 months. **A,** Coronal MRI scan shows the ligamentum teres pulled from the fovea (arrow). **B** and **C,** Arthroscopic images show the torn ligamentum teres with exposed bone at the fovea where the ligamentum teres was previously attached. (Courtesy of Marc R. Safran, MD, Redwood City, CA.)

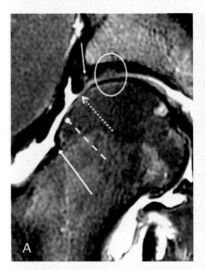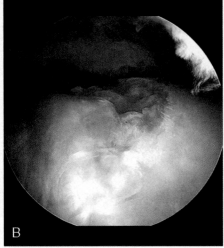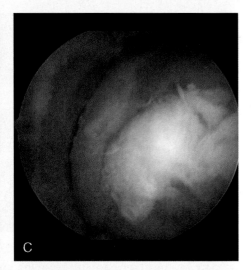

Figure 13 **A,** Coronal MRI scan showing changes of combined cam- and pincer-type femoroacetabular impingement. The circle highlights the changes in the articular cartilage. The short solid arrow points to the labral-chondral separation, and the dotted arrow points to a rounded labrum, suggestive of a labral tear. The dashed line ending in a circle demonstrates the femoral head-neck region with loss of offset (straight), and the long solid arrow points to the notching in the femoral neck, consistent with pincer impingement. **B,** Arthroscopic view of the peripheral compartment of a hip with notching of the femoral head caused by pincer impingement. The femoral head also has loss of offset of the head-neck region. **C,** Arthroscopic image shows bumpy bony changes of the femoral neck, resulting in symptomatic impingement of the hip. (Courtesy of Marc R. Safran, MD, Redwood City, CA.)

ing in intrasubstance labral damage. Chondral injuries associated with pincer impingement tend to be shallow (only 2 to 4 mm from the acetabular rim) but more global, involving more of the circumference of the acetabular rim. Further, posterior femoral head chondral damage may be seen with pincer impingement. Some authors believe that most patients have a com-

bination of cam and pincer impingement. Femoroacetabular impingement of the hip joint is often painful and is being increasingly acknowledged as a cause of early primary osteoarthritis of the hip.[53]

Radiography, CT, and MRI are useful for correlating the imaging findings, with history and clinical findings suggestive of femoroacetabular im-

pingement to confirm the diagnosis. Radiographs and MRI are currently considered the preferred combination of imaging modalities.[54] MRI can show labral tears, chondral damage, synovitis, asphericity of the femoral head-neck region, and occasionally periacetabular calcifications (os acetabuli, labral calcification and ossification) (**Figure 13**). As a result of the

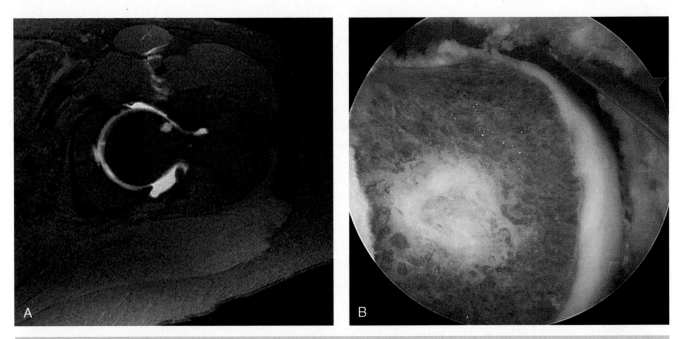

Figure 14   **A,** T2-weighted axial MRI scan showing a cyst or pit at the femoral head-neck junction, suggestive of femoroacetabular impingement. **B,** Arthroscopic appearance of the cyst after cheilectomy/osteoplasty and removal of lining in the peripheral compartment of the cyst. (Courtesy of Marc R. Safran, MD, Redwood City, CA.)

impingement of the acetabulum against the femoral neck, notching of the femoral neck may be seen. Cysts of the femoral head-neck region, often called Pitt's pits, are often seen in femoroacetabular impingement and may result from the impingement (**Figure 14**).[55] Nötzli et al[56] described an objective measure of cam-type femoroacetabular impingement using the alpha angle (**Figure 15**). This angle is a measure of loss of sphericity on radial axial MRI views. Recently its value has been called into question because of interobserver measurement variability and a lack of correlation with outcomes.[57,58]

Patients with femoroacetabular impingement often report groin pain, although they may also have pain laterally over the trochanter or in the buttock. These patients often have symptoms similar to those with labral tears because the bony anatomy puts the soft tissues, such as the labrum and the articular cartilage, at risk for breakdown and pain. The clinical examina-

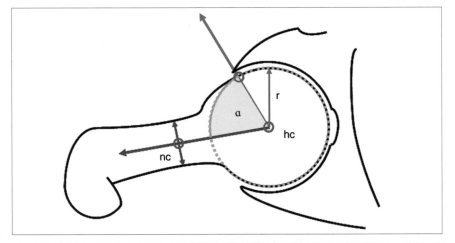

Figure 15   Schematic drawing of the alpha (α) angle. The angle is the result of two lines drawn on a radial axial MRI scan. One line (long magenta line) is drawn between the center of the femoral head (green circle) and the midway point of the narrowest part of the femoral neck. The second line (long blue line) is drawn between the center of the femoral head and the point where the distance from the center of the femoral head exceeds the radius (r; short blue line) of the subchondral surface of the femoral head. hc = femoral head center, nc = center of the narrowest part of the femoral neck. (Courtesy of Marc R. Safran, MD, Redwood City, CA.)

tion also has significant overlap with that performed for assessing the labrum. However, there frequently is a loss of internal rotation of the hip as examined in 90° of flexion, particularly in patients with large cam lesions.

Physiotherapy and anti-inflammatory medication remain the first line of treatment of musculoskeletal injuries; however, their benefits in femoroacetabular impingement are questionable. Attempting to gain motion may actually exacerbate the impingement, forcing the femur into the acetabulum and further damaging the soft tissues. Prolonged delay in the surgical correction of symptomatic bony abnormalities may lead to disease progression to the point where joint preservation is no longer indicated.[59]

Surgical treatment options for femoroacetabular impingement include open surgery with femoral head dislocation, arthroscopic surgery, or a combination of both. Open surgical dislocation is preferred by some surgeons because it allows 360° visibility of the femoral head and acetabulum. The open technique also allows femoral osteotomies at the level of the head and neck, the base of the neck, or the intertrochanteric region when these procedures are appropriate. Severe acetabular retroversion with intact cartilage may require acetabular reorientation, a decision that should be based on the position of the posterior wall in relationship to the center of rotation of the femoral head and on the quality of the cartilage in the superomedial area of the acetabulum.[60] When performed by an experienced surgeon, surgical dislocation is a safe and established technique with few complications. The most frequent complications are minor ectopic soft-tissue ossification and nonunion of the greater trochanter and painful hardware from fixation of the trochanteric osteotomy.

With an improved appreciation of the morphologies that cause femoroacetabular impingement, less invasive approaches, such as arthroscopy, have emerged as alternatives to open surgery in many clinical situations. The key to managing femoroacetabular impingement is to treat the bony abnormality and the associated labral or chondral lesions. Some chondral lesions are softening or delamination injuries that are amenable to less invasive techniques, such as débridement, abrasion arthroplasty, or microfracture. More advanced chondral lesions are often associated with joint space narrowing and represent a later stage of femoroacetabular impingement, which is usually less responsive to surgery.[34] Most, if not all, labral abnormalities occur in the presence of structural deformities. Treating physicians must not neglect the underlying bony pathology because this is a major cause of treatment failures.[61] After the bone has been addressed, refixation of the labrum should be done to allow the labrum to regain its physiologic function of dynamic stabilization and pressure distribution in the hip. There are several advantages of arthroscopic management over open surgical dislocation. The arthroscopic procedure is usually performed as an outpatient procedure, and there is less blood loss. The open technique requires the patient to use crutches to protect the trochanteric osteotomy, and nonunion may occur. However, the arthroscopic technique has a very steep learning curve.

Hip Dysplasia

Hip dysplasia refers to a developmental anomaly of the hip relating to the femoral head, the acetabulum, or both. Generally, the term is used to describe developmental dysplasia of the hip, a condition with undercoverage of the femoral head by a deficient acetabulum. There are multiple etiologies for the dysplasia, including neuromuscular diseases, particularly cerebral palsy, slipped capital femoral epiphysis, Legg-Calvé-Perthes disease, proximal focal femoral deficiency, traumatic injury, epiphyseal dysplasia, and developmental dysplasia of the hip. Normal development of the hip requires normal growth of the acetabulum and of the proximal femur as well as normal physiologic mechanical interaction. Dysplastic hips have some characteristic anatomic abnormalities. On the pelvic side, the true acetabulum is typically shallow, lateralized, anteverted, and deficient of bone anteriorly and superiorly. There often is a hypertrophied acetabular labrum, believed to exist to compensate for the bony deficiency of the acetabular roof (**Figure 16, A**). On the femoral side, the femoral head is small, oblong, with excessive anteversion on a short neck, although in some situations the head may be large (coxa magna). There is also an increased neck-shaft angle, with the greater trochanter displaced posteriorly, and a narrow femoral canal.[62] These abnormalities lead to a markedly decreased contact area between the femoral head and acetabulum and to lateralization of the center of hip rotation, which increases the body-weight lever arm. As a result, high forces are transmitted through a limited surface area. The increased contact pressures in the hip are the preliminary stages of a process that eventually leads to degenerative changes and the development of secondary osteoarthritis of this joint.[63] Longstanding hip dysplasia often results in groin pain that increases with activity and premature osteoarthritis in early adulthood.[64] This pain is often secondary to subluxation of the femoral head and can often be reproduced with hyperextension and external rotation of the hip. In less severe cases, patients may present for treatment later in life with pain in the hip, as the stability provided by the labrum is lost as the labrum degenerates, tears, or separates from the acetabular rim, with symptoms of labral tearing.[65] Additionally, there is associated articular cartilage injury from the increased loading of the shallow acetabular rim (**Figure 16, B**).

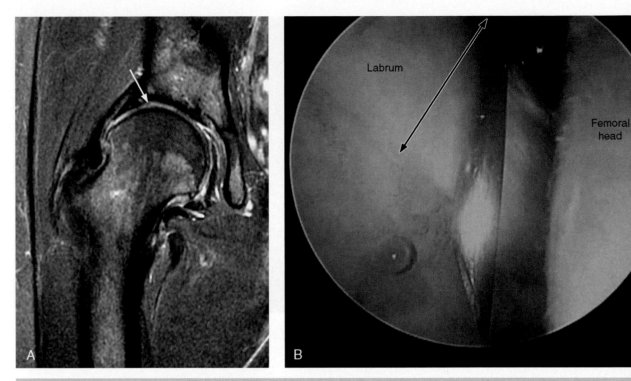

Figure 16   A, Coronal MRI scan of the hip of a 46-year-old patient (who was a ballet dancer) with developmental dysplasia of the hip. Note the very large labrum and some suggestion of chondral damage at the acetabular rim (arrow). **B,** Arthroscopic view shows the large labrum and chondral wear of the acetabular rim. (Courtesy of Marc R. Safran, MD, Redwood City, CA.)

Evaluation of hip dysplasia begins with an AP standing view of the pelvis, a false profile view, and a cross-table lateral radiograph of the hip. The AP radiograph may show degenerative changes and permit measurement of the center-edge angle of Wiberg, which suggests acetabular dysplasia if the measurement is less than 25°.[6] The false profile view of Lequesne and de Seze[66] is used to measure the anterior center-edge angle, and the cross-table lateral radiograph is used to measure the anterior femoral head-neck offset.[67] Other imaging modalities such as CT and MRI are also used in the evaluation of hip dysplasia and associated abnormalities. CT is used to evaluate the bony anatomy, and MRI is helpful for detecting labral and chondral abnormalities in patients with hip dysplasia. Magnetic resonance arthrography and arthroscopy also have been used for further evalua-

tion of pathology within the acetabular labrum and in the adjacent acetabular hyaline articular cartilage.[12,65] MRI typically shows an abnormally large and elongated labrum, with marginal irregularity and high signal intrasubstance change. There are often associated changes at the labral-chondral transitional zone, with thinning, fraying, fissuring, or full-thickness cartilage loss apparent.[68] These changes in the acetabular labrum may be secondary to chronic stress and abnormal loading through the labrum rather than through the bone.[48]

Patients with radiographic evidence of dysplasia and minimal symptoms should be treated nonsurgically. The natural history of dysplasia should be discussed with the patient, and radiographs should be taken at regular intervals to evaluate for the development of arthritis. Nonsteroidal anti-inflammatory agents, physical therapy,

lifestyle modifications, and avoidance of high-impact activities are the mainstays of conservative management. Surgical treatments are reserved for patients with persistent symptoms and limitations of daily activities. Options include arthroscopic surgery, pelvic osteotomy, femoral osteotomy, arthrodesis, reconstructive arthroplasty, and resection arthroplasty. The main goals of these procedures are to decrease pain, preserve hip function, and slow the progression of degenerative changes to the hip joint. Care must be taken if proceeding with hip arthroscopy for dysplasia. Because the underlying disorder is bony deficiency of the acetabular weight-bearing region, arthroscopy at this time cannot correct the underlying problem. Labral tears associated with acetabular dysplasia usually signify decompensation of the hip. Débridement of the labrum will not stop this deterioration and may poten-

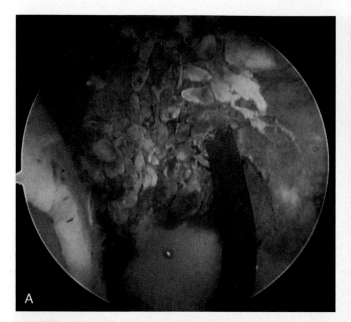 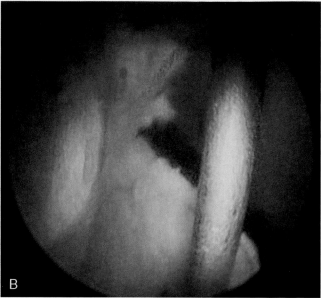

Figure 17 A 23-year-old patient who is a ballet dancer had a 5-year history of hip pain. MRI scans showed a large effusion of unclear etiology. **A,** Arthroscopic view of the PVNS. **B,** Arthroscopic view showing delamination of the articular cartilage of the femoral head. Biopsy confirmed the diagnosis of PVNS. (Courtesy of Marc R. Safran, MD, Redwood City, CA.)

tially accelerate it. There is often associated chondral wear at the acetabular rim from overloading of the acetabular bony rim. If symptomatic, consideration should be given to bony procedures to help with containment of the femoral head within the acetabulum, provided there are not too many degenerative changes. These procedures include periacetabular osteotomies and proximal femoral osteotomies. Arthroscopic or open labral repair should be considered in conjunction with these procedures. Labral tears associated with mild dysplasia, especially in older, less active patients, may be approached arthroscopically, but caution should be exercised in more advanced cases.

Pigmented Villonodular Synovitis

PVNS is a localized, nonneoplastic proliferative disorder that can affect any synovial-lined structure, including bursa, tendons, and joints. It is characterized by a proliferation of synovial fibroblasts and histiocytes that often cause pain, swelling, and a limp.[69] PVNS is most commonly reported in the knee, but the hip is the second most common site affected.[70] It usually presents in adults in the third or fourth decades of life with no sex bias and should be considered in the differential diagnosis for all young patients presenting with clinical or radiographic features suggestive of early hip degeneration.[70,71] The clinical examination of these patients is nonspecific and varies based on degree of associated pathology. The lesion typically presents in a monoarticular distribution with either a focal nodular or diffuse pattern characterized by multinucleated giant cells with pigmentation caused by intracellular and extracellular hemosiderin deposition.[72] PNVS may be locally invasive, resulting in periarticular cysts and occasionally delamination of the articular cartilage of the joint, eventually resulting in degenerative arthritis (**Figure 17**). The etiology and pathogenesis of PVNS are poorly understood. The most widely accepted theories are related to either a chronic inflammatory response or a benign but locally aggressive condition of fibrohistiocytic origin.[71,72]

On MRI, PVNS has a characteristic appearance with a focus of low signal intensity on T1- and T2-weighted imaging sequences related to the hemosiderin deposition (**Figure 18**). The use of MRI has improved the ability to diagnose and perform follow-up surveillance in these patients. Hip arthroscopy is a useful tool in both the diagnosis and treatment of PVNS because it can provide tissue for pathologic identification and allows partial synovectomy[73] (**Figure 17**).

Treatment options for patients with PVNS of the hip range from open and arthroscopic synovectomy to chemical or radionuclear synoviorthesis and/or total hip arthroplasty.[74] Synovectomy only is effective as a means of treatment when articular cartilage has been preserved. Patients with localized or focal disease in the hip have been

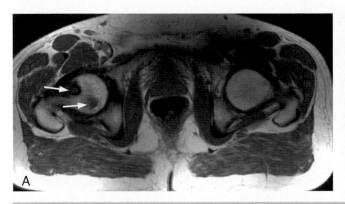
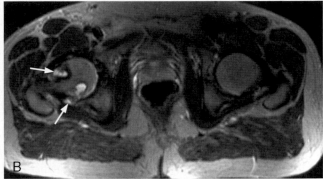

Figure 18 Axial T1-weighted (**A**) and T2-weighted (**B**) MRI scans showing PVNS of the hip joint, with cysts in the femoral head (arrows). (Reproduced with permission from Kenneth Buckwalter, MD, Indianapolis, IN.)

treated successfully with open and arthroscopic synovectomy. Considering the age of the patient population affected, hip arthroscopy is a viable alternative to formal open treatment of focal PVNS because it is less invasive and allows faster recovery and return to function.[75,76] The diffuse form is more difficult to treat and has a high likelihood of recurrence when a complete synovectomy is not done. Complete synovectomy of the hip is challenging if not impossible to achieve using arthroscopic techniques; it can be attempted at the time of the initial biopsy and followed with adjuvant therapy, such as radiation or yttrium therapy. Arthroscopy may allow the removal of loose bodies because chondral delamination may occur. There are reports of using a combined arthroscopic and open technique to perform a complete synovectomy without dislocation of the femoral head.[77] Diffuse recurrent PVNS eventually results in advanced joint degeneration, which is most predictably treated with total hip arthroplasty.[74]

Summary

MRI and magnetic resonance arthrography have helped raise awareness of nonarthritic hip disorders and have made the diagnosis of hip problems easier. Hip arthroscopy has proved useful in detecting and treating many nonarthritic hip disorders. As experience with hip arthroscopy expands, the ability to recognize and treat various injury patterns to the hip will also expand. An increasing understanding of the pathologic processes affecting the hip joint may improve the ability of physicians to intervene when appropriate and limit the progression of these disorders to frank osteoarthritis.

References

1. Arthrology: The joints of the lower limb the hip (coxal) joint, in Williams PL, Warwick R, eds: *Gray's Anatomy,* ed 36. Philadelphia, PA, WB Saunders, 1980, pp 477-482.

2. Safran MR: The acetabular labrum: Anatomic and functional characteristics and rationale for surgical intervention. *J Am Acad Orthop Surg* 2010;18(6):338-345.

3. Chatha DS, Arora R: MR imaging of the normal hip. *Magn Reson Imaging Clin N Am* 2005;13(4): 605-615.

4. Byrd JW: Hip arthroscopy: Patient assessment and indications. *Instr Course Lect* 2003;52:711-719.

5. Tibor LM, Sekiya JK: Differential diagnosis of pain around the hip joint. *Arthroscopy* 2008;24(12): 1407-1421.

6. Wiberg G: Studies on dysplastic acetabula and congenital subluxation of the hip joint. *Acta Chir Scand* 1939;83(suppl 58):5-135.

7. Martin RL, Kelly BT, Leunig M, et al: Reliability of clinical diagnosis in intra-articular hip diseases. *Knee Surg Sports Traumatol Arthrosc* 2010;18(5):685-690.

8. Mintz DN, Hooper T, Connell D, Buly R, Padgett DE, Potter HG: Magnetic resonance imaging of the hip: Detection of labral and chondral abnormalities using noncontrast imaging. *Arthroscopy* 2005;21(4):385-393.

9. Czerny C, Hofmann S, Neuhold A, et al: Lesions of the acetabular labrum: Accuracy of MR imaging and MR arthrography in detection and staging. *Radiology* 1996; 200(1):225-230.

10. Smith TO, Hilton G, Toms AP, Donell ST, Hing CB: The diagnostic accuracy of acetabular labral tears using magnetic resonance imaging and magnetic resonance arthrography: A meta-analysis. *Eur Radiol* 2011;21(4): 863-874.

11. James SL, Ali K, Malara F, Young D, O'Donnell J, Connell DA: MRI findings of femoroacetabular impingement. *AJR Am J Roentgenol* 2006;187(6):1412-1419.

12. Keeney JA, Peelle MW, Jackson J, Rubin D, Maloney WJ, Clohisy JC: Magnetic resonance arthro-

graphy versus arthroscopy in the evaluation of articular hip pathology. *Clin Orthop Relat Res* 2004; 429:163-169.

13. Steinbach LS, Palmer WE, Schweitzer ME: Special focus session: MR arthrography. *Radiographics* 2002;22(5):1223-1246.

14. Petersilge CA, Haque MA, Petersilge WJ, Lewin JS, Lieberman JM, Buly R: Acetabular labral tears: Evaluation with MR arthrography. *Radiology* 1996; 200(1):231-235.

15. Toomayan GA, Holman WR, Major NM, Kozlowicz SM, Vail TP: Sensitivity of MR arthrography in the evaluation of acetabular labral tears. *AJR Am J Roentgenol* 2006;186(2):449-453.

16. Byrd JW, Jones KS: Diagnostic accuracy of clinical assessment, magnetic resonance imaging, magnetic resonance arthrography, and intra-articular injection in hip arthroscopy patients. *Am J Sports Med* 2004;32(7):1668-1674.

17. Seldes RM, Tan V, Hunt J, Katz M, Winiarsky R, Fitzgerald RH Jr: Anatomy, histologic features, and vascularity of the adult acetabular labrum. *Clin Orthop Relat Res* 2001;382:232-240.

18. Bharam S: Labral tears, extra-articular injuries, and hip arthroscopy in the athlete. *Clin Sports Med* 2006;25(2):279-292, ix.

19. Ferguson SJ, Bryant JT, Ganz R, Ito K: The acetabular labrum seal: A poroelastic finite element model. *Clin Biomech (Bristol, Avon)* 2000;15(6):463-468.

20. Ferguson SJ, Bryant JT, Ganz R, Ito K: The influence of the acetabular labrum on hip joint cartilage consolidation: A poroelastic finite element model. *J Biomech* 2000;33(8):953-960.

21. Ferguson SJ, Bryant JT, Ganz R, Ito K: An in vitro investigation of the acetabular labral seal in hip joint mechanics. *J Biomech* 2003; 36(2):171-178.

22. Kelly BT, Shapiro GS, Digiovanni CW, Buly RL, Potter HG, Hannafin JA: Vascularity of the hip labrum: A cadaveric investigation. *Arthroscopy* 2005;21(1):3-11.

23. Kim YT, Azuma H: The nerve endings of the acetabular labrum. *Clin Orthop Relat Res* 1995;320: 176-181.

24. Burnett RS, Della Rocca GJ, Prather H, Curry M, Maloney WJ, Clohisy JC: Clinical presentation of patients with tears of the acetabular labrum. *J Bone Joint Surg Am* 2006;88(7):1448-1457.

25. Wenger DE, Kendell KR, Miner MR, Trousdale RT: Acetabular labral tears rarely occur in the absence of bony abnormalities. *Clin Orthop Relat Res* 2004;426: 145-150.

26. Philippon MJ: Arthroscopy of the hip in the management of the athlete, in McGinty JB, ed: *Operative Arthroscopy,* ed 3. Philadelphia, PA, Lippincott-Raven, 2003, pp 879-883.

27. Palmer WE: MR arthrography of the hip. *Semin Musculoskelet Radiol* 1998;2(4):349-362.

28. Lage LA, Patel JV, Villar RN: The acetabular labral tear: An arthroscopic classification. *Arthroscopy* 1996;12(3):269-272.

29. Petersilge C: Imaging of the acetabular labrum. *Magn Reson Imaging Clin N Am* 2005;13(4):641-652, vi.

30. McCarthy JC, Noble PC, Schuck MR, Wright J, Lee J: The Otto E. Aufranc Award: The role of labral lesions to development of early degenerative hip disease. *Clin Orthop Relat Res* 2001;393:25-37.

31. McCarthy J, Noble P, Aluisio FV, Schuck M, Wright J, Lee JA: Anatomy, pathologic features, and treatment of acetabular labral tears. *Clin Orthop Relat Res* 2003; 406:38-47.

32. Byrd JW: Lateral impact injury: A source of occult hip pathology. *Clin Sports Med* 2001;20(4): 801-815.

33. Yen YM, Kocher MS: Chondral lesions of the hip: Microfracture and chondroplasty. *Sports Med Arthrosc* 2010;18(2):83-89.

34. Schmid MR, Nötzli HP, Zanetti M, Wyss TF, Hodler J: Cartilage lesions in the hip: Diagnostic effectiveness of MR arthrography. *Radiology* 2003;226(2):382-386.

35. McCarthy JC: Hip arthroscopy: Applications and technique. *J Am Acad Orthop Surg* 1995;3(3): 115-122.

36. McCarthy JC, Busconi B: The role of hip arthroscopy in the diagnosis and treatment of hip disease. *Orthopedics* 1995;18(8): 753-756.

37. Sekiya JK, Martin RL, Lesniak BP: Arthroscopic repair of delaminated acetabular cartilage in femoroacetabular impingement. *Orthopedics* 2009;32(9):692.

38. Keene GS, Villar RN: Arthroscopic loose body retrieval following traumatic hip dislocation. *Injury* 1994;25(8):507-510.

39. Gondolph-Zink B, Puhl W, Noack W: Semiarthroscopic synovectomy of the hip. *Int Orthop* 1988; 12(1):31-35.

40. Byrd JW: Hip arthroscopy for posttraumatic loose fragments in the young active adult: Three case reports. *Clin J Sport Med* 1996; 6(2):129-133.

41. Brewster SF: The development of the ligament of the head of the femur. *Clin Anat* 1991;4(4): 245-255.

42. Keene GS, Villar RN: Arthroscopic anatomy of the hip: An in vivo study. *Arthroscopy* 1994; 10(4):392-399.

43. Rao J, Zhou YX, Villar RN: Injury to the ligamentum teres: Mechanism, findings, and results of treatment. *Clin Sports Med* 2001;20(4):791-799, vii.

44. Gray AJ, Villar RN: The ligamentum teres of the hip: An arthroscopic classification of its pathology. *Arthroscopy* 1997;13(5): 575-578.

45. Byrd JW, Jones KS: Traumatic rupture of the ligamentum teres as a source of hip pain. *Arthroscopy* 2004;20(4):385-391.

46. Kelly BT, Williams RJ III, Philippon MJ: Hip arthroscopy: Current indications, treatment options, and management issues. *Am J Sports Med* 2003;31(6):1020-1037.

47. Simpson JM, Field RE, Villar RN: Arthroscopic reconstruction of the ligamentum teres. *Arthroscopy* 2011;27(3):436-441.

48. Klaue K, Durnin CW, Ganz R: The acetabular rim syndrome: A clinical presentation of dysplasia of the hip. *J Bone Joint Surg Br* 1991;73(3):423-429.

49. Ganz R, Leunig M, Leunig-Ganz K, Harris WH: The etiology of osteoarthritis of the hip: An integrated mechanical concept. *Clin Orthop Relat Res* 2008;466(2): 264-272.

50. Pfirrmann CW, Mengiardi B, Dora C, Kalberer F, Zanetti M, Hodler J: Cam and pincer femoroacetabular impingement: Characteristic MR arthrographic findings in 50 patients. *Radiology* 2006;240(3):778-785.

51. Tannast M, Kubiak-Langer M, Langlotz F, Puls M, Murphy SB, Siebenrock KA: Noninvasive three-dimensional assessment of femoroacetabular impingement. *J Orthop Res* 2007;25(1):122-131.

52. Beck M, Kalhor M, Leunig M, Ganz R: Hip morphology influences the pattern of damage to the acetabular cartilage: Femoroacetabular impingement as a cause of early osteoarthritis of the hip. *J Bone Joint Surg Br* 2005;87(7): 1012-1018.

53. Ganz R, Parvizi J, Beck M, Leunig M, Nötzli H, Siebenrock KA:

Femoroacetabular impingement: A cause for osteoarthritis of the hip. *Clin Orthop Relat Res* 2003; 417:112-120.

54. Bredella MA, Stoller DW: MR imaging of femoroacetabular impingement. *Magn Reson Imaging Clin N Am* 2005;13(4):653-664.

55. Leunig M, Beck M, Kalhor M, Kim YJ, Werlen S, Ganz R: Fibrocystic changes at anterosuperior femoral neck: Prevalence in hips with femoroacetabular impingement. *Radiology* 2005;236(1): 237-246.

56. Nötzli HP, Wyss TF, Stoecklin CH, Schmid MR, Treiber K, Hodler J: The contour of the femoral head-neck junction as a predictor for the risk of anterior impingement. *J Bone Joint Surg Br* 2002; 84(4):556-560.

57. Lohan DG, Seeger LL, Motamedi K, Hame S, Sayre J: Cam-type femoral-acetabular impingement: Is the alpha angle the best MR arthrography has to offer? *Skeletal Radiol* 2009;38(9):855-862.

58. Brunner A, Horisberger M, Herzog RF: Evaluation of a computed tomography-based navigation system prototype for hip arthroscopy in the treatment of femoroacetabular cam impingement. *Arthroscopy* 2009;25(4):382-391.

59. Leunig M, Beaulé PE, Ganz R: The concept of femoroacetabular impingement: Current status and future perspectives. *Clin Orthop Relat Res* 2009;467(3):616-622.

60. Giori NJ, Trousdale RT: Acetabular retroversion is associated with osteoarthritis of the hip. *Clin Orthop Relat Res* 2003;417:263-269.

61. Heyworth BE, Shindle MK, Voos JE, Rudzki JR, Kelly BT: Radiologic and intraoperative findings in revision hip arthroscopy. *Arthroscopy* 2007;23(12):1295-1302.

62. Sanchez-Sotelo J, Trousdale RT, Berry DJ, Cabanela ME: Surgical treatment of developmental dysplasia of the hip in adults: I. Non-

arthroplasty options. *J Am Acad Orthop Surg* 2002;10(5):321-333.

63. Murphy SB, Ganz R, Müller ME: The prognosis in untreated dysplasia of the hip: A study of radiographic factors that predict the outcome. *J Bone Joint Surg Am* 1995;77(7):985-989.

64. Harris WH: Etiology of osteoarthritis of the hip. *Clin Orthop Relat Res* 1986;213:20-33.

65. Langlais F, Lambotte J-C, Lannou R, et al: Hip pain from impingement and dysplasia in patients aged 20-50 years: Workup and role for reconstruction. *Joint Bone Spine* 2006;73(6):614-623.

66. Lequesne M, de Sezes S: False profile of the pelvis: A new radiographic incidence for the study of the hip. Its use in dysplasias and different coxopathies. *Rev Rhum Mal Osteoartic* 1961;28:643-652.

67. Eijer H, Leunig M, Mahomed MN, Ganz R: Anterior femoral head-neck off-set: A method of measurement. *Hip Int* 2001;11: 37-41.

68. Horii M, Kubo T, Inoue S, Kim WC: Coverage of the femoral head by the acetabular labrum in dysplastic hips: Quantitative analysis with radial MR imaging. *Acta Orthop Scand* 2003;74(3): 287-292.

69. Newberg AH, Newman JS: Imaging the painful hip. *Clin Orthop Relat Res* 2003;406:19-28.

70. Cotten A, Flipo RM, Chastanet P, Desvigne-Noulet MC, Duquesnoy B, Delcambre B: Pigmented villonodular synovitis of the hip: Review of radiographic features in 58 patients. *Skeletal Radiol* 1995;24(1):1-6.

71. Goldman AB, DiCarlo EF: Pigmented villonodular synovitis: Diagnosis and differential diagnosis. *Radiol Clin North Am* 1988; 26(6):1327-1347.

72. Granowitz SP, D'Antonio J, Mankin HL: The pathogenesis and long-term end results of pig-

mented villonodular synovitis. *Clin Orthop Relat Res* 1976;114: 335-351.

73. Janssens X, Van Meirhaeghe J, Verdonk R, Verjans P, Cuvelier C, Veys EM: Diagnostic arthroscopy of the hip joint in pigmented villonodular synovitis. *Arthroscopy* 1987;3(4):283-287.

74. Gitelis S, Heligman D, Morton T: The treatment of pigmented vil-

lonodular synovitis of the hip: A case report and literature review. *Clin Orthop Relat Res* 1989;239: 154-160.

75. Rydholm U: Pigmented villonodular synovitis of the hip joint. *Int Orthop* 1987;11(4):307-310.

76. Krebs VE: The role of hip arthroscopy in the treatment of synovial

disorders and loose bodies. *Clin Orthop Relat Res* 2003;406:48-59.

77. Sekiya JK, Wojtys EM, Loder RT, Hensinger RN: Hip arthroscopy using a limited anterior exposure: An alternative approach for arthroscopic access. *Arthroscopy* 2000;16(1):16-20.

Adult Reconstruction: Knee

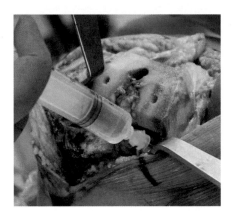

(Also see chapter 41 in Section 8)

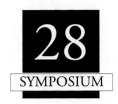

28

SYMPOSIUM

Current Controversies in Partial Knee Arthroplasty

Adolph V. Lombardi Jr, MD, FACS
Keith R. Berend, MD
Michael E. Berend, MD
Craig J. Della Valle, MD
Gerard A. Engh, MD
Wolfgang Fitz, MD
Jason M. Hurst, MD
Riyaz H. Jinnah, MD, FRCS
Jess H. Lonner, MD
William B. Macaulay, MD
John A. Repicci, DDS, MD
Giles R. Scuderi, MD

Abstract

Partial knee arthroplasty has enjoyed renewed interest during the past decade. It is helpful to be familiar with the classic and current indications, contraindications, and technical aspects of partial knee arthroplasty, including patellofemoral, medial unicompartmental, and lateral unicompartmental knee arthroplasty. Various implant choices for partial knee arthroplasty can be compared and evaluated based on patient characteristics, design qualities, and reported outcomes. It is also helpful to review the indications and techniques for performing medial or lateral unicompartmental knee arthroplasty in combination with arthroscopically assisted reconstruction of the anterior cruciate ligament.

Instr Course Lect 2012;61:347-381.

Partial knee arthroplasty has enjoyed renewed interest in the past decade. Isolated medial, lateral, and patellofemoral arthroplasties (PFAs) clearly have a role in the treatment of monocompartmental disease. This chapter reviews the classic and current indications, contraindications, and technical aspects of partial knee arthroplasty, including patellofemoral, medial unicompartmental, and lateral unicompartmental knee arthroplasty (UKA).

Implant choices for partial knee arthroplasty based on patient characteristics, design qualities, and reported outcomes will be compared and evaluated. Surgical tips and the perils of performing partial knee arthroplasty also are discussed.

The Patellofemoral Compartment

It has been reported that the prevalence of isolated patellofemoral arthritis in patients older than 55 years presenting with symptomatic osteoarthritis of the knee is 11% in men and 24% in women.[1] A review of the literature on PFA shows that 75% to 85% of the patients are female.[2-14] The overall higher prevalence of PFA in females is related to patellofemoral malalignment and dysplasia, conditions that are more common in females than males.[15-17] A history of adolescent anterior knee pain, trochlear dysplasia, patella alta, and recurrent patellofemoral instability are important contributing factors in patellofemoral arthrosis.

The clinical presentation of patellofemoral arthritis is anterior knee pain exacerbated by activities such as ascending or descending stairs, squatting, sitting with the knee flexed, rising from a seated position, and ambulating on uneven terrain. Patients may also report grinding and cracking localized to the patellofemoral articulation with range of motion. On physical examination, retropatellar crepitus with range of motion or effusion may be noted. Peripatellar facet tenderness and pain generally occurs with patellofemoral compression in patients with instability. A positive apprehension sign may be noted, and considerable quadriceps atrophy may be present. Symptoms are generally reproducible with provocative maneuvers such as squatting, stair stepping, or rising from a chair. Patellar tracking should be evaluated from 90° of flexion to extension. Malalignment or muscle imbalance can be detected by the J sign, which is the visible lateral subluxation of the patella as the knee proceeds from flexion into the terminal 20° of extension.[18] The quadriceps (Q) angle should also be measured.[18] A Q angle greater than 20° in females or greater than 15° in males may require treatment with an anterior medialization tibial tubercle osteotomy, known as a Fulkerson osteotomy.[19-21] Standing AP and PA flexed radiographs should be evaluated to determine the degree of degenerative disease involving the

tibial femoral articulation. Varus and valgus stress views may also be helpful in determining the extent of tibial femoral arthrosis. Lateral radiographs are useful for identifying patella alta or patella baja; often, patellofemoral osteophytes and joint-space narrowing are noted. Axial radiographs are examined for trochlear dysplasia, patellar tilt or subluxation, and the extent of patellofemoral arthrosis. Axial CT may have a role in accessing patellofemoral tracking in rare circumstances. MRI evaluation can further assess the status of the cartilage of the entire knee.

The initial treatment of patellofemoral arthritis should focus on nonsurgical measures such as weight loss, physiotherapy focused on quadriceps strengthening, nonsteroidal anti-inflammatory medications, and injection therapy of corticosteroids and/or viscosupplementation.[22] Arthroscopic débridement, microfracture articulation restoration, lateral retinacular release, soft-tissue realignment of the extensor mechanism, anterior medialization tibial tubercle osteotomy, mosaicplasty/autologous chondrocyte implantation, lateral patella partial fac-

etectomy, patellectomy, PFA, and total knee arthroplasty (TKA) are possible surgical options for treating patellofemoral arthrosis.[23]

There is a limited role for the nonarthroplasty options of arthroscopy, lateral retinacular release, and facetectomy.[24,25] Biologic articular restoration for PFA is limited by the inherent hostile force-load environment, distortions of joint congruency, and limitations of healing in avascular tissue. Currently, patellectomy is seldom used and has very limited applications in the active patient.[26] Anterior medialization tibial tubercle osteotomy is the most popular osteotomy. It is best suited for use in younger patients with combined lateral arthrosis and concomitant instability. In that combined setting, anterior medialization coupled with autologous chondrocyte implantation has shown more promising results than either procedure alone.[26,27]

The indications for PFA are isolated advanced patellofemoral osteoarthritis; posttraumatic arthritis; advanced chondromalacia of the patella, trochlea, or both; trochlear/patellar dysplasia; tibial femoral Ahlbäck scores of 1

Dr. Lombardi or an immediate family member has received royalties from Biomet and Innomed; is a member of a speakers' bureau or has made paid presentations on behalf of Biomet; serves as a paid consultant to Biomet; has received research or institutional support from Biomet; and serves as a board member, owner, officer, or committee member of the Hip Society, the Knee Society, and the New Albany Surgical Hospital Foundation. Dr. Keith R. Berend or an immediate family member has received royalties from Biomet; serves as a paid consultant to Biomet and Salient Surgical; has received research or institutional support from Biomet and Salient Surgical; and serves as a board member, owner, officer, or committee member of the American Association of Hip and Knee Surgeons. Dr. Michael E. Berend or an immediate family member has received royalties from Biomet; is a member of a speakers' bureau or has made paid presentations on behalf of Biomet; serves as a paid consultant to Angiotech; has received research or institutional support from Biomet and ERMI; and serves as a board member, owner, officer, or committee member of Piedmont Ortho. Dr. Della Valle or an immediate family member serves as a paid consultant to Angiotech, Biomet, Kinamed, and Smith & Nephew; has received research or institutional support from Pacira and Zimmer; and serves as a board member, owner, officer, or committee member of the American Association of Hip and Knee Surgeons and the Arthritis Foundation. Dr. Engh or an immediate family member has received royalties from DePuy; is a member of a speakers' bureau or has made paid presentations on behalf of Smith & Nephew; serves as a paid consultant to DePuy and Smith & Nephew; serves as an unpaid consultant to Alexandria Research Technologies; owns stock or stock options in Alexandria Research Technologies and TGS Knee Innovations; and has received research or institutional support from DePuy, Smith & Nephew, US Army Medical Research and Material Command and the Telemedicine and Advanced Technology Research Center, Medtronic, and Inova Health Systems. Dr. Fitz or an immediate family member has received royalties from Conformis; serves as a paid consultant to Conformis; owns stock or stock options in Conformis; and has received research or institutional support from Oped and IGB.com. Dr. Hurst or an immediate family member serves as a paid consultant to Biomet and Angiotech. Dr. Jinnah or an immediate family member has received royalties from Wright Medical Technology; is a member of a speakers' bureau or has made paid presentations on behalf of Wright Medical Technology and Mako Surgical; serves as a paid consultant to Wright Medical Technology and Mako Surgical; and has received research or institutional support from Smith & Nephew, Wright Medical Technology, and Mako Surgical. Dr. Lonner or an immediate family member has received royalties from Zimmer; is a member of a speakers' bureau or has made paid presentations on behalf of Zimmer and Mako Surgical; serves as a paid consultant to Zimmer and Mako Surgical; owns stock or stock options in Mako Surgical; and serves as a board member, owner, officer, or committee member of the Knee Society and the Philadelphia Orthopaedic Society. Dr. Macaulay or an immediate family member has received nonincome support (such as equipment or services), commercially derived honoraria, or other non–research-related funding (such as paid travel) from Pfizer and Wright Medical Technology. Dr. Repicci or an immediate family member has received royalties from Biomet and serves as an unpaid consultant to Biomet. Dr. Scuderi or an immediate family member has received royalties from Zimmer and Salient Surgical; is a member of a speakers' bureau or has made paid presentations on behalf of Zimmer and Salient Surgical; serves as a paid consultant to Zimmer and Salient Surgical; and serves as a board member, owner, officer, or committee member of the Knee Society and the International Congress for Joint Reconstruction.

or less, severe symptoms affecting daily activities that are referable to patellofemoral joint degeneration and unresponsive to physical therapy and nonsurgical treatments; anterior knee pain (retropatellar and peripatellar) with stair descent and sitting; and no medial or lateral joint line pain, tenderness, or wear. Some authors suggest that there are no age restrictions for patients treated with PFA, whereas others reserve PFA for their middle-age and/or elderly patients.

Video 28.1: Patellofemoral Arthroplasty. Jess H. Lonner, MD (17 min)

The contraindications to PFA are more than minimal tibiofemoral arthritis; advanced grade III to IV tibiofemoral chondromalacia; substantial chondrocalcinosis; active systemic inflammatory arthritis; significant coronal plane deformities, flexion contracture, or limited range of motion; uncorrected patellar maltracking or malalignment (Q angle); and the presence of complex regional pain syndrome or infection. Slight tilt and mild subluxation are acceptable if corrected. A Q angle greater than 20° in females and greater than 15° in males should be corrected with an anterior medialization tibial tubercle osteotomy before PFA.

The keys to successful PFA, whether using custom or off-the-shelf implants, are proper patient selection and meticulous attention to detail, especially with respect to patellofemoral tracking.

Onlay Versus Inlay Designs for PFA

The clinical results of PFA appear to be affected by several variables, including trochlear prosthesis design features, patient selection, surgical indica-

tions, trochlear and patellar prosthesis alignment and position, soft-tissue balance, and the duration of follow-up.[28] For clinical success, the patellar prosthesis must track well in the trochlear prosthesis. A poorly tracking patellar prosthesis (other than slight tilt and mild subluxation) will be evident within 6 months after surgery and will compromise function and outcome. If the patella tracks well, the primary mechanism of failure will be later progressive tibiofemoral arthritis (hence the reason that longer follow-up will affect clinical results). Aseptic loosening and patellar prosthesis wear are uncommon.

Several trochlear design features can affect patellar tracking, including the sagittal radius of curvature, proximal extension, width, thickness, tracking angle, asymmetry, constraint, and—perhaps most importantly—whether it is an inlay- or onlay-style prosthesis.[28-30] Inlay trochlear designs sit flush with the surrounding trochlear and condylar cartilage. Rotational alignment parallels trochlear inclination. Inlay trochlear components typically are shorter and narrower than onlay designs, ending at the proximal edge of the cartilage. Inlay-style prostheses may be off-the-shelf or custommade designs, including the Lubinus (Waldemar Link, Hamburg, Germany), Blazina (formerly Richards, now Smith & Nephew, Memphis, TN), CFS (Wright Medical Technology, Arlington, TN), Autocentric (DePuy, Warsaw, IN), patellar mobile-bearing LCS (DePuy), custom Sigma (DePuy) and custom Kinematch (Kinamed, Camarillo, CA). Inlay components are attractive at first because very little trochlear bone removal is required, which provides a very conservative method of bone preparation. The trochlear bed is prepared with a curet or motorized burr, removing a small volume of bone that accommo-

dates the prosthesis, which is inlayed so that its edges are flush with the surrounding trochlear and condylar cartilage surfaces. With this method of bone preparation, regardless of whether the component is an off-the-shelf or custom design, the axial rotational alignment of the trochlear prosthesis parallels the patient's native trochlear inclination. The inlay component typically ends at the proximal cartilage edge of the native trochlea, does not extend further up the femur, and is relatively narrow so that its edges can be inset within the surrounding cartilage and do not extend to the edges of the trochlea (**Figure 1,** *A*). Although inlay trochlear designs are advantageous because they conserve bone, they present difficulty in matching the variability in trochlear morphology.[31] These designs often have a relatively poor fit with the native trochlea because of considerable morphologic variability, unless the prosthesis is customized. The position of the prosthesis and its rotational alignment depend on the shape of the patient's trochlear surfaces[10,28-30] (**Figure 1,** *B*). These design issues are addressed with custom inlay designs, which use advanced imaging and rapid prototyping technology to determine bone morphology, component position, and rotational alignment.

The alternative trochlear component is an onlay design, which as a generic class of implants tend to be wider, have more favorable sagittal radii of curvature, and extend more proximally up the femur than the inlay designs.[29] Proponents of onlay trochlear designs note the ability to perform an anterior resection coincident with the anterior femoral cortex.[31] Onlay-style designs include the Avon (Stryker, Mahwah, NJ), Vanguard (Biomet, Warsaw, IN), and Gender Solutions (Zimmer, Warsaw, IN). The preparation of the trochlea is perpendicular to the anteroposterior axis or

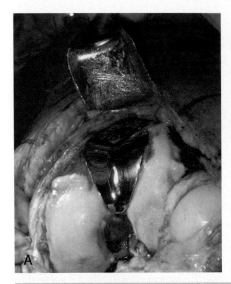
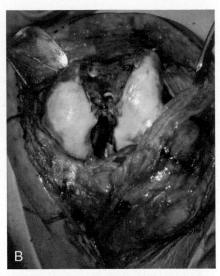

Figure 1 **A,** Intraoperative photograph of an inlay-style trochlear prosthesis. The component appears to be internally rotated. **B,** Bone preparation common with an inlay-style trochlear prosthesis demonstrating conservative removal of bone tangential to the articular surfaces. In this knee, a previous trochlear prosthesis was removed during revision to an onlay prosthesis.

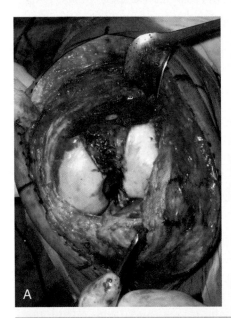
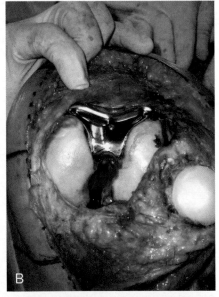

Figure 2 **A,** Intraoperative photograph showing the technique of anterior bone resection perpendicular to the anteroposterior axis (or parallel to the transepicondylar axis) for an onlay-style trochlear prosthesis. The resection was made during revision of an inlay- to an onlay-style trochlear prosthesis. **B,** Intraoperative photograph showing the position of an onlay trochlear prosthesis that is appropriately externally rotated relative to the anteroposterior axis of the femur.

the Whiteside line and parallel to the transepicondylar axis and flush with the anterior femoral cortex[32] (**Figure 2**). Design features and method of bone preparation may account for the better patellar tracking observed with onlay-style implants. A review of the literature suggests that secondary surgery to correct patellar maltracking and frank failures caused by patellar instability are substantially higher with inlay compared with onlay trochlear implants[2-14,23,28-49] (**Table 1**).

Superior results have been observed for cemented versus cementless fixation. Other factors affecting the clinical results include patient factors and adherence to surgical indications. Patient factors include patellofemoral alignment; tibiofemoral alignment (coronal plane); the presence of chondromalacia on weight-bearing condyles; and underlying diagnoses, such as dysplasia, primary osteoarthritis, or posttraumatic arthritis. Results also are influenced by the surgeon's technical proficiency, component alignment, and the duration of follow-up; tibiofemoral arthritis is found in approximately 20% of patients at 15-year follow-up. Patellar instability is the major source of failure with inlay-style trochlear components and is related to component malpositioning and extensor mechanism malalignment. The primary failure mode with onlay designs is tibiofemoral degeneration, which is more common in patients with osteoarthritis than posttraumatic arthritis. Loosening is rare after PFA, with studies observing no loosening at 5- to 11-year average follow-up and loosing in 2% at 13.3- to 20-year follow-ups;[3,5,11-13,41,44,48] however, the incidence is higher with cementless fixation.[39]

Variations in trochlear morphology have been described in several studies.[50-52] If the shape, morphology, and rotational alignment of the trochlear surfaces of the human knee are considered, it is clear why inlay designs may be predisposed to a higher incidence of patellar component maltracking and instability.[49] Lonner et al[50] studied 200 trochlear resection specimens (100 from women and 100 from men) at the time of TKA, and found

Table 1

Results of Patellofemoral Arthroplasty

Author(s)	Year	No. of Knees	Device (Manufacturer)	Follow-up (years)	Results
Blazina et al[33]	1979	57	Blazina I and II (Richards/ Smith & Nephew, Memphis, TN)	1-3.5	78% much improved
Lubinus[37]	1979	14	Lubinus (Waldemar Link, Hamburg, Germany)	0.5-2	All improved
Arciero and Toomey[38]	1988	25	Blazina II and CFS (Wright Medical, Arlington, TN)	3-9	72% good/excellent; 88% survival
Cartier et al[4]	1990	72	Blazina II and III	2-12	85% good/excellent; 8% mechanical complications
Argenson et al[39]	1995	66	Autocentric (DePuy, Warsaw, IN)	2-10	85% survival
Krajca-Radcliffe and Coker[6]	1996	16	Bechtol I and II (Richards/ Smith & Nephew)	2-18	88% good/excellent; 81% survival
de Winter et al[5]	2001	26	Blazina II	1-20	61% good/excellent; 81% survival
Tauro et al[13]	2001	62	Lubinus	5-10	45% satisfactory; 72% survival
Smith et al[40]	2002	45	Lubinus	0.5-7.5	64% good/excellent; 81% survival
Kooijman et al[41]	2003	45	Blazina II	15-21	62% survival
Board et al[34]	2004	17	Lubinus	1.6	53% satisfactory; 35% further surgery; 24% revised to TKA
Lonner[29]	2004	30	Lubinus	4	84% good/excellent; 17% maltracking
Lonner[29]	2004	25	Avon (Stryker, Mahwah, NJ)	0.5	96% good/excellent; 1% maltracking
Merchant[42]	2004	15	LCS (DePuy)	2.2-5.5	93% good/excellent on activities of daily living scale
Ackroyd and Chir[2]	2005	306	Avon	2-5	87% survival, complication free
Argenson et al[43]	2005	66	Autocentric	12-20	56% survival
Cartier et al[44]	2005	79	Blazina II and III	10	75% survival
Merchant et al[8]	2005	16	LCS	2.8-6.3	94% good/excellent
Sisto and Sarin[10]	2006	25	Kinematch (Kinamed, Camarillo, CA)	2.7-9.9	100% good/excellent; 100% survival
Ackroyd et al[3]	2007	109	Avon	5	96% survival; 28% progression; 80% success; 1% maltracking
Sisto and Sarin[11,12]	2007, 2008	25	Kinematch	6.1	100% survival; 72% excellent; 28% good
Mohammed et al[9]	2008	46 30 25	Lubinus FPV (Wright Medical) Avon	4	28% further surgeries; 4% revised to TKA
Minas[45]	2008	9 8 27	LCS Avon Sigma (DePuy)	5	78% survival; poor tracking and instability with LCS; 3/8 Avon and 3/27 Sigma revised due to tibiofemoral progression
Butler and Shannon[46]	2009	22	Custom Performa (Biomet, Warsaw, IN)	5	95% survival; 14% further surgery; 1 revised to TKA

TKA = total knee arthroplasty

Table 1 *(Continued)*

Results of Patellofemoral Arthroplasty

Author(s)	Year	No. of Knees	Device (Manufacturer)	Follow-up (years)	Results
Leadbetter et al[7]	2009	79	Avon	3	84% good/excellent; 16% clinical failures; 1.2% maltracking
van Wagenberg et al[14]	2009	24	Autocentric II (DePuy)	4.8	88% further surgery; 29% revised to TKA
Odumenya et al[47]	2010	50	Avon	5.3	94% survival; 22% progression
van Jonbergen et al[48]	2010	185	Blazina II	13.3	84% survival at 10 years; 69% survival at 20 years
AV Lombardi and KR Berend (unpublished data)	2011	22 9 2	Vanguard (Biomet) Gender Solution (Zimmer, Warsaw, IN) Kinematch	0.1-2.0	97% survival
Lonner[49]	2011	116	Gender Solution	0.25-3.0	< 1% patellar instability

TKA = total knee arthroplasty

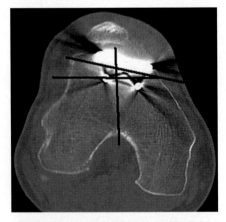

Figure 3 Axial CT scan of an inlay-style trochlear component implanted tangentially to the anterior trochlear surfaces, which results in component internal rotation and predisposes the knee to lateral patellar subluxation.

that the mean lateral and medial trochlear flange heights in women and men were 10.47 mm (range, 2.0 to 19.0 mm) and 6.95 mm (range, 2.0 to 18.0 mm), respectively. In men, the mean lateral and medial trochlear flange heights were 11.95 mm (range, 6.5 to 20.5 mm) and 7.71 mm (range, 1.0 to 18.0 mm), respectively. The differences in the mean heights between the lateral and medial trochlear

flanges, approximately 3.5 to 4 mm for both men and women, have implications for trochlear implant positioning when using inlay-style designs. These data were corroborated by Biedert et al[51] who reported that in a nondysplastic trochlea, the most anterior aspect of the lateral trochlear condyle is higher than the anterior aspect of the medial trochlear condyle.

The differences in the anterior heights of the lateral and medial trochlear peaks typically result in internal rotation of the anterior trochlear surface relative to the Whiteside axis or the transepicondylar axis, even in cases of trochlear dysplasia (**Figures 1** and **3**). In an unpublished study, (A. Kamath, MD, et al, San Diego, CA, 2011) MRIs of more than 300 patients were reviewed to evaluate a variety of random pathologic conditions in knees. The investigators found that the anterior trochlear inclination angle (angle from the lateral to the medial peaks of trochlear articular cartilage relative to the anteroposterior axis of femur) is internally rotated a mean of 11.3°, with no significant differences in the angles between women and men. Even in patients with trochlear

dysplasia, the mean trochlear inclination angle was 8.2°. Using 33 cadaver specimens, Shih et al[52] reported on the anterior femoral condylar angle, which is the equivalent of the anterior trochlear inclination angle. The authors reported that when using the articular cartilage surface as the point of measurement, the mean anterior condylar angle was 2.7° ± 6.2° (range, −11° to 10°), suggesting that most anterior trochlear surfaces are internally rotated relative to the transepicondylar axis, although some are externally rotated.

Based on these studies, it is clear that the more prominent lateral trochlear flange most often leads to internal rotation of inlay-style trochlear designs, except in rare cases of severe lateral trochlear dysplasia. Like malrotated femoral components in TKA, which have been implanted in internal rotation relative to the transepicondylar or Whiteside axes, internal rotation of the trochlear component in PFA effectively medializes the trochlear groove, increases the Q angle, and places tension on the lateral retinaculum, each of which predispose to patellar maltracking and instability[53] (**Figure 3**). These complications can be minimized with onlay-style trochlear designs, which are more likely to be implanted perpendicular to the anteroposterior axis of the femur (or parallel to the transepicondylar axis[30-32] (**Figure 4**).

An analysis of PFA results has shown a disparity in the early term and midterm failures that occur as a result of patellar instability and maltracking, depending on whether an inlay- or an onlay-style component is used.[2,3,5,10,13,23,28-36] If patella tracking is satisfactory after PFA, the primary mode of failure will be progressive tibiofemoral arthritis, irrespective of the type of trochlear prosthesis used. However, inlay-style components have a higher tendency than onlay designs for patellar maltracking, and more often require early secondary surgeries, including extensor mechanism realignment, revision PFA, or conversion to TKA.

In a study of 85 inlay trochlear components, Blazina et al[33] reported that extensor mechanism realignment was done in 37 knees to improve patellar tracking. Other studies reviewing the results of inlay-style implants have reported a 17% to 36% prevalence of patellar maltracking.[5,13,29,34] One series reviewing the results of a custom inlay trochlear component reported 100% good and excellent results.[10] The intraoperative photographs and postoperative radiographs published with that study depict a trochlear component that appears anteriorized and internally rotated; however, customization via rapid prototyping technology has corrected for internal rotation on the articulating surface of the implant.[11]

Most reports of onlay-style trochlear designs in PFA have found a low prevalence (typically less than 1%) of patellar maltracking.[2,23,29] Patellar tracking predictably improves when a maltracking inlay component is revised to an onlay component with im-

proved rotational positioning.[31,36] Hendrix et al[36] reported on 8 of 14 inlay trochlear components (57%) revised to an onlay design to treat iatrogenic patellar subluxation and instability. The authors found that at a mean follow-up of 5 years, Bristol knee scores improved significantly ($P < 0.001$), and patellar subluxation and instability were successfully treated in all the knees.

Custom PFA Designs

Advantages and Disadvantages

When considering PFA, the surgeon can choose between custom (patient-specific) designs and off-the-shelf designs. The disadvantages of off-the-shelf inlay and onlay designs are that they cannot be customized to match the patient, and specifically with onlay designs, require more aggressive bone resection. The advantages of custom PFA implants are that they do not require femoral bone resection.[10-12] Rapid prototyping technology based on CT modeling can be used to build a custom implant for the patient's femoral anatomy. More normal kinematics is achieved by reestablishing the alignment and depth of the trochlear groove. The overall thickness of the PFA implant and the patella component are designed to reestablish normal anatomy. The distal margin of the implant rests 3 to 5 mm from the apex of the femoral intercondylar notch. The implant has a thickened lateral border to compensate for the usual lateral bony deficiency of the trochlear groove.

The major disadvantage of custom PFA designs is the associated cost, which includes the preoperative CT scan, the implant cost, and the time required for manufacturing the implant. Critics of custom PFA implants also note the difficulty in orienting the component parallel to the anteroposterior axis and perpendicular to the

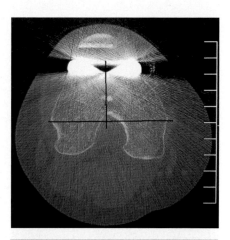

Figure 4 Axial CT scan of an onlay-style trochlear component shows improved positioning parallel to the transepicondylar axis and improved patellar tracking.

transepicondylar axis. However, these challenges can be addressed with careful preoperative planning. The surgeon reviews the three-dimensional model generated from the CT scan, and adjustments can be made to correctly position the component.

Because the surgical technique for PFA with a custom implant involves the procurement of a CT scan in accordance with the requirements of the implant manufacturer, the facility must be precertified by the manufacturer. Using rapid prototyping technology, a three-dimensional model of the distal femur is created for the surgeon to review. The surgeon can then modify the implant to specifically address orientation and component placement. The model is returned to the manufacturer for definitive component creation. The overall manufacturing time from the delivery of the CT scan to the manufacturer is approximately 4 weeks.

Surgical Technique

An incision is made over the medial third of the patella, generally commencing two finger-breadths proximal to the patella and extending one

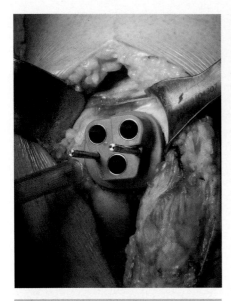

Figure 5   A custom PFA is performed using a custom drill guide developed based on preoperative imaging of the patient's anatomy.

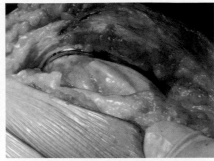

Figure 6   After cementation of the patellar component and a custom trochlear component based on preoperative imaging of the patient's anatomy, followed by tourniquet release and hemostasis, patellofemoral tracking is assessed using the "no thumbs" technique.

finger-breadth below the patella. A standard medial parapatellar arthrotomy is performed, taking care to avoid injury to the medial meniscus. The patella is displaced laterally. The tibialfemoral articulation is evaluated to determine if it is acceptable to proceed with PFA versus TKA. Proper fit of the custom drill guide is achieved by removing articular cartilage. The custom drill guide is used to assess the fit of the implant onto the trochlear groove. The position is then outlined with methylene blue, and a scalpel is used to dissect through and remove the cartilage. Curets are helpful in removing the articular cartilage within the outlined area and exposing the subchondral bone. The custom drill guide is then placed on the exposed bone, and the appropriate position is achieved (**Figure 5**). With the drill guide correctly positioned, three holes are drilled through the guide with an 8-mm stop drill. Small drill holes can be placed in the subchondral bone of the trochlear groove to enhance cement indigitation. The patella is then prepared in a

standard fashion. The thickness of the patella is noted before the resection and re-created with the patellar implant. The custom implant and patellar components are then cemented in place, and the cement is allowed to cure. The tourniquet is then released, hemostasis is accomplished, and patellofemoral tracking is assessed using the "no thumbs" technique (**Figure 6**). If there is any suggestion of less than satisfactory tracking of the patella, a lateral retinacular release is performed. Postoperatively, patients are allowed full weight bearing, and physiotherapy begins within hours of the surgical procedure to enhance range of motion.

Pitfalls
The major pitfalls to be avoided in PFA with a custom implant are a lack of adherence to the preoperative CT scanning protocol of the manufacturer, a lack of communication with the manufacturer regarding any planned osteophyte removal, and surgery for inappropriate indications. Other major pitfalls include aggressive removal of femoral trochlear cartilage with a burr, causing unintentional removal of the subchondral bone under the custom patellofemoral implant, under-

resection of the patella leading to over-stuffing of the patellofemoral articulation, and failure to correct patellar alignment and tracking intraoperatively.

Sisto and Sarin[10-12] reported the longest follow-up on PFA of the knee with a custom inlay design in which the trochlear component featured a lateral buildup and was anteriorized to enhance quadriceps function and provide a mechanical advantage. The cohort included 22 patients (25 knees) with a mean follow-up of 11.3 years (range, 7.8 to 14.9 years). All 25 PFAs were in place, and all patients reported satisfaction with the procedure. There were no reports of weakness, instability, or additional surgery. All 22 patients reported that they would undergo custom PFA again.

The Medial Compartment
The medial tibiofemoral compartment is the most common of the three compartments of the knee to be affected by degenerative joint disease.[1] Medial osteoarthritis is an extension gap disease. Varus is a highly destructive force. Greater than 2° of varus mechanical alignment provides a threefold greater risk for osteoarthritis progression in the knee. In a study of 2,958 knees without osteoarthritis at baseline, Sharma et al[54] found that varus but not valgus alignment increased the risk of incident tibiofemoral arthritis.

UKA had a resurgence as a treatment for end-stage disease of the medial compartment, reaching a peak in 2007 and 2008 and plateauing thereafter. Studies show that UKA provides better range of motion, a higher level of activity, and increased patient satisfaction.[55-60] Among the many controversies concerning UKA is the question of which design concept provides the most simple, reproducible surgical techniques combined with optimal long-term results. Specific controversies include onlay versus inlay designs, fixed-bearing versus mobile-bearing designs, the use of robotics and customization, and whether TKA represents a better treatment solution.

Fixed-Bearing Inlay Medial UKA

A fixed-bearing inlay design for UKA represents an option that conserves bone and is amenable to minimally invasive surgical techniques. Adding bone-sparing surface enhancement to an outpatient arthroscopic knee surgical procedure using a minimally invasive surgical approach through a 3-inch incision is an appealing concept to many elderly patients.[61-65] A bone-sparing technique allows a wider range of UKA indications and is of significant interest to elderly patients to relieve pain and prevent or delay the need for TKA. However, proper surgeon training, meticulous surgical technique, and the precise positioning of components are all necessary regardless of the implant choice.

The concept of minimally invasive surgery for joint arthroplasty began in the 1990s in conjunction with UKAs and was first reported by Repicci and Eberle.[61] They advocated arthroscopic confirmation of an intact lateral compartment to reduce early failures because lateral meniscal function cannot be adequately visualized via the flexion gap used in an open procedure. The incision length was reduced to 3 inches from the earlier standard of 8 inches, and eversion of the patella was avoided. A multimodal pain management strategy also was used, including soft-tissue injection with a combination of bupivacaine and epinephrine to enhance postoperative pain relief and hemostasis, a practice that has expanded to widespread use.[61,65] Patients were out of bed and ambulating independently 2 hours after the surgical procedure, which was performed as

outpatient surgery in 80% of the cases. Pharmacologic prophylaxis for deep venous thrombosis was unnecessary, probably because of the shorter incision, minimal soft-tissue trauma, reduced bleeding, and early ambulation. The need for formal, outpatient physical therapy was significantly reduced, and recovery time was considerably faster, with 90% of the patients achieving independent function at 2 weeks postoperatively.[61]

The use of a resurfacing UKA design with an inlay all-polyethylene tibial component requires minimal bone resection and preserves the medial buttress.[62,65] Five millimeters of bone are resected from the posterior femoral condyle with a sagittal saw to allow application of a joint distractor and improve visualization of the tibial plateau. Tibial bone and osteophytes are resected using a high-speed burr to a depth of 4 to 5 mm, creating a bed for the all-polyethylene tibial component within the layer of sclerotic bone. Stability is afforded by a 2- to 3-mm rim of bone preserved circumferentially. The high-speed burr is also used to complete preparation of the femoral condyle, removing 2 to 3 mm of bone and osteophytes. Preparation with the burr not only conserves bone but also reduces the need for an expanded exposure to place bulky jigs.[63]

In a study of 136 medial UKAs performed in 126 patients with a fixed-bearing, resurfacing inlay device (Repicci II; Biomet) and a minimally invasive surgical protocol, Romanowski and Repicci[62] reported 92.6% survival at 8-year follow-up. There were 10 revisions overall: 5 in 116 knees (4%) that were Ahlback stage II or III preoperatively and 5 in 20 knees (25%) that were Ahlback stage IV preoperatively. Five revisions (50%) were related to progression of disease in the remaining compartments at an average

of 66 months. Primary TKA components were used for all revisions.

Minimally invasive UKA using a fixed-bearing, resurfacing inlay component combined with a structured pain management program and early mobilization may be safely performed on an outpatient basis.[65] The bone-conserving nature of the device does not limit future treatment options, with subsequent revision to TKA being relatively straightforward. The rapid rehabilitation and return to function is favorable to patients who desire minimal lifestyle disruption. The procedure has high rates of patient satisfaction and a good implant survival rate at midterm follow-up.

Fixed-Bearing Onlay Medial UKA

Fixed-bearing onlay UKA has a long history that extends back nearly as far as the first tricompartmental designs. Because of the success of TKA and the initial erratic results of fixed-bearing onlay UKAs, many surgeons lost interest in this concept. However, with a better understanding of patient selection, appropriate design parameters, and surgical techniques, more consistent and favorable results have been reported with implant survivorship that rivals that of TKA[62,66-124] (**Table 2**). Despite the recent popularity of mobile-bearing UKA, there are several compelling reasons to select a fixed-bearing, onlay design.

Among the primary advantages of a fixed-bearing onlay UKA design with a metal-backed tibial component is that the surgical technique is straightforward and familiar to surgeons who regularly perform TKA. Intramedullary alignment can be used for the distal femoral cut with a measured, straightforward, resection technique. The tibial cut uses an extramedullary guide, which most surgeons find easier to use than a burr (as is necessary for an inlay

Table 2
Results of Medial Fixed-Bearing UKA

Author(s)	Year	No. of Knees	Type of Implant (Manufacturer)	Follow-up (range) years	Survivorship (No. of Revisions)
Scott and Santore[69]	1981	88	Brigham I and II (Stryker, Mahwah, NJ); cemented, all-polyethylene tibia	3.5 (2-6)	98.9% at 3.5 years (1)
Bae et al[70]	1983	72	Marmor all-polyethylene, Richards Mod II metal backed (both Smith & Nephew, Memphis, TN)	4 (minimum 2)	98.6% at 4 years (1)
Mallory and Danyi[71]	1983	38	Polycentric (Stryker) and Marmor; both cemented, all-polyethylene tibia	5.6 (5.1-8.1)	71% at 5.6 years (11)
Bernasek et al[72]	1988	28	PCA (Stryker); cementless, metal backed	2	78.6% at 2 years (6)
Mackinnon et al[73]	1988	115	St. Georg Sled (Waldemar Link, Hamburg, Germany); cemented, all-polyethylene tibia	4.8 (2-12)	94% at 4.8 years (7)
Marmor[74]	1988	53	Marmor; cemented, all-polyethylene tibia	11 (10-13)	70% at 10 years (20)
Kozinn et al[75]	1989	44	Brigham Mod (DePuy, Warsaw, IN); cemented, metal backed	5.5 (4.5-6)	100% at 5.5 years (0)
Magnussen and Bartlett[76]	1990	42	PCA; cementless, metal backed	(2-3.3)	92.9% at 2 years (3)
Christensen[77]	1991	524	St. Georg Sled; cemented, all-polyethylene tibia	3.9 (1-9)	98.4% at 3.9 years (NA)
Laurencin et al[78]	1991	23	19 Brigham, 4 Unicondylar (both DePuy)	6.8 (3.2-12.8)	95.6% at 6.8 years (1)
Rougraff et al[79]	1991	106	Compartmental I and II (Zimmer, Warsaw, IN); cemented, all-polyethylene	6.5 (0.7-13.5)	95.3% at 6.5 years (4)
Scott et al[80]	1991	88	Brigham I and II (Stryker); cemented, all-polyethylene tibia	(8-12)	87.5% at 9 years (11)
Stockelman and Pohl[81]	1991	63	Compartmental I and II; cemented, all-polyethylene	7.5 (5.5-12)	93.7% at 7.5 years (4)
Capra and Fehring[82]	1992	15	Marmor	11.1 (8-14)	66.7% at 11.1 years (5)
		25	Compartmental II	6.3 (4-11)	96% at 6.3 years (1)
Heck et al[83]	1993	255	Marmor and Compartmental I and II	6 (maximum 14.8)	94.1% at 6 years (15)
Sisto et al[84]	1993	61	Brigham; cemented, metal backed	4.3 (2-5.8)	95.1% at 4.3 years (3)
Swank et al[85]	1993	75	27 Fibermesh (Zimmer); 48 Microloc (DePuy); cementless and cemented	5.5 (4-8)	87.8% at 5.5 years (NA)
Weale and Newman[86]	1994	42	St. Georg Sled; cemented, all-polyethylene tibia	(12-17)	88% at 12-17 years (5)
Lewold et al[87]	1995	2181	Marmor; cemented, all-polyethylene tibia	6 (1-10)	96.3% at 10 years (87)
Cartier et al[88]	1996	60	Marmor; cemented, all-polyethylene tibia	12 (10-18)	93% at 10 years (7)
Ansari et al[89]	1997	461	St. Georg Sled; cemented, all-polyethylene tibia	4 (1-17)	95.7% at 4 years (20)

NA = not available

Table 2 *(Continued)*

Results of Medial Fixed-Bearing UKA

Author(s)	Year	No. of Knees	Type of Implant (Manufacturer)	Follow-up (range) years	Survivorship (No. of Revisions)
Bert[90]	1998	100	Performance (Biomet, Warsaw, IN); metal backed, 10% cementless, 85% cemented	10	87.4% at 10 years (12)
Schai et al[91]	1998	28	PFC (DePuy); age < 60 years, 20 all-polyethylene, 8 metal backed	3.3 (2-6)	92.8% at 3.3 years (2)
Tabor and Tabor[92]	1998	61	Marmor-style, cemented, all-polyethylene tibia	9.7 (5-20)	85.2% at 9.7 years (9)
Berger et al[93]	1999	62	Miller-Galante (Zimmer); cemented, metal backed	7.5 (6-10)	96.8% at 7.5 years (2)
Squire et al[94]	1999	48	Marmor; cemented, all-polyethylene tibia	18 (15.8-21.8)	84% at 22 years (5)
Argenson et al[67]	2002	145	Miller-Galante; cemented, metal backed	5.5 (3-9.33)	94% at 10 years (5)
Ackroyd et al[95]	2002	408	St. Georg Sled; cemented, all-polyethylene tibia	6.4 (4.2-21)	87.5% at 10 years (25)
Perkins and Gunckle[96]	2002	40	Miller-Galante II (Zimmer); cemented, metal backed (60%), all polyethylene (40%)	6 (3-10)	74% at 10 years (6)
Emerson et al[97]	2002	51	Brigham; cemented, metal backed	7.7 (2-13.2)	84.3% at 7.7 years (8)
Romanowski and Repicci[62]	2002	136	Repicci (Biomet) cemented, all-polyethylene	8	92.6% at 8 years (10)
Gioe et al[98]	2003	474	Nine different designs	NA	88.6% at 10 years (36)
Pennington et al[68]	2003	46	Miller-Galante; cemented, metal backed	11	92% at 11 years (3)
Confalonieri et al[99]	2004	20	Allegretto (Zimmer); cemented, metal backed	5.7	95% at 5.7 years (1)
Emerson and Higgins[100]	2004	164	Repicci; cemented, all-polyethylene tibia	1.3 (0.5-3) (first 30)	97% at 1.3 years (1)
Gleeson et al[101]	2004	57	St. Georg Sled; cemented, all-polyethylene tibia	2	93% at 2 years (4)
Kankovský et al[102]	2004	20	St. Georg Sled; cemented, all-polyethylene tibia	(10-16)	95% at 10-16 years (1)
Khan et al[103]	2004	50	St. Georg Sled; cemented, all-polyethylene tibia	10	96% at 10 years (2)
Naudie et al[104]	2004	113	Miller-Galante; cemented, metal backed	10 (2-14)	86% at 10 years (11)
Berend et al[105]	2005	79	48 EIUS (Stryker), 31 Repicci II; cemented, all-polyethylene	3.4 (2-5.8)	78% at 3 years (16)
Berger et al.[66]	2005	62	Miller-Galante; cemented, metal backed	12 (10-13)	95.7% at 13 years (2)
O'Rourke et al[106]	2005	122	Marmor; cemented, all-polyethylene tibia	24 (17-28)	72% at 25 years (17)
Tabor et al[107]	2005	100	Marmor-style; cemented, all-polyethylene tibia	12.2 (0.25-25.6)	86% at 12.2 years (14)
Eickmann et al[108]	2006	411	12 different designs	9 (0.1-19.3)	80% at 9 years (96)
Li et al[109]	2006	28	Miller-Galante; cemented, metal backed	2	100% at 1 years (0)

NA = not available

Table 2 *(Continued)*

Results of Medial Fixed-Bearing UKA

Author(s)	Year	No. of Knees	Type of Implant (Manufacturer)	Follow-up (range) years	Survivorship (No. of Revisions)
Steele et al[110]	2006	203	St. Georg Sled; cemented, all-polyethylene tibia	14.8 (10-29.4)	85.9% at 20 years; 80% at 25 years
Cartier et al[111]	2007	131	< age 60 years, Genesis (Smith & Nephew); 20% cementless, 43% all-polyethylene	(5-14)	94% at 10 years; 92% at 11 years; 88% at 12 years
Mariani et al[112]	2007	39	Preservation (DePuy); cemented, all-polyethylene tibia	(0.75-1.0)	61.5% at 1 year (15)
Koskinen et al[113]	2007	330 196 146	Miller-Galante II Duracon (Stryker) PCA	10 10 10	79% at 10 years 78% at 10 years 53% at 10 years
Newman et al[114]	2009	51	St. Georg Sled; cemented, all-polyethylene tibia	15	89.8% at 15 years (4)
Koskinen et al[115]	2009	46	Miller-Galante II; cemented, metal backed	7.2 (2.7-13.1)	86.6% at 7 years (5)
Lustig et al[116]	2009	84	HLS Evolution (Tornier, Edina, MN); cemented, all-polyethylene tibia	5.2 (2.1-13.3)	93.6% at 5 years; 90.4% at 10 years
Parratte et al[117]	2009	35	≤ age 50 years, Miller-Galante; metal backed	9.7 (5-16)	82.9% at 9.7 years (6)
Seyler et al[118]	2009	80	Miller-Galante II; cemented, metal backed	5 (2-14)	92% at 5 years; 84% at 10 years (9)
Biswal and Brighton[119]	2010	128	Allegretto (Zimmer); cemented, metal backed	5.7 (3-8)	93% at 5.7 years (9)
Saenz et al[120]	2010	144	EIUS; cemented, all-polyethylene tibia	3 (2-4.5)	89% at 3 years (16)
O'Donnell and Neil[121]	2010	114	Repicci II; cemented, all-polyethylene tibia	7.4 (5.2-9)	78% at 9 years (22)
John et al[122]	2010	85	Miller-Galante; cemented, metal backed	10.8 (2-16)	94% at 10 years, 87% at 15 years
Bruni et al[123]	2010	83	Preservation; cemented, all-polyethylene tibia	5	100% at 5 years (0)
Whittaker et al[124]	2010	150	Miller-Galante; cemented, metal backed	8.1 (1-17.8)	96% at 5 years (22)

design). The balance of the femoral sizing and preparation is simple, with most systems using a posterior referencing technique that ensures an appropriately sized flexion gap. The use of a modular, metal-backed tibial component eases the need to clear retained cement,[125] and in most series has proved more durable than all-polyethylene components.[120]

With a mobile-bearing design, there is a risk of bearing dislocation unless the flexion and extension gaps are precisely balanced;[101,126] such a risk is not present with fixed-bearing UKA. Comparative studies of fixed- and mobile-bearing UKAs show that mobile-bearing UKAs have a higher rate of early complications (including reoperation) compared with the fixed-bearing design.[101,124] In an effort to avoid bearing dislocation, the surgeon may be tempted to use a thicker bearing, which can predispose the patient to contralateral compartment arthritis.[127] Current mobile-bearing designs

are not used on the lateral side of the knee because of an unacceptable risk of bearing dislocation.[128]

When a fixed-bearing design is used, several tenets must be followed to optimize results. (1) The tibial cut should be conservative to ensure that good-quality bone is available to support the component and facilitate a straightforward revision if required in the future. (2) It is imperative to avoid oversizing the femoral component, which can lead to patellar impingement.[129] (3) The femoral component must track centrally on the tibial component to avoid edge loading of the polyethylene, which will lead to rapid wear and failure. (4) There must be 2 to 3 mm of laxity in both full extension and 90° of flexion; this ensures a neutral to slight varus alignment, which protects against lateral compartment degeneration.

The theoretic advantages of a mobile-bearing design include lower wear and a lower risk of loosening secondary to decreased stress at the implant interfaces. Interestingly, most studies of fixed-bearing designs find that wear is a relatively uncommon cause of failure. That is the case despite the fact that the bearing thickness is less than 6 mm in the most commonly used designs.[66-68,104] When present, wear appears to be associated with younger patients and with polyethylene that was gamma irradiated in air.[130,131] When excessive wear occurs, it is often amenable to an isolated exchange of the bearing surface.[117] Because loosening is a commonly reported mode of failure of mobile-bearing designs,[101,124,126] the risk of late wear must be balanced against the risk of an earlier failure related to bearing dislocation.

Several studies from multiple centers have shown excellent results with metal-backed fixed-bearing UKAs, with survivorship exceeding 90% (and reaching 98% in one report) at more than 10 years after surgery.[66-68,104] Although equally good results have been reported for mobile-bearing designs at centers where these procedures are performed in high volumes, the few comparative studies and meta-analyses do not suggest superiority over a fixed-bearing design.[124,132-134]

Mobile-Bearing Medial UKA

Mobile-bearing UKA has been approved by the US Food and Drug Ad-

ministration since 2004, with educational training. A mobile-bearing device offers the hope of restoring knee kinematics, decreasing polymer wear through increased implant conformity, and lowering polyethylene stresses, which together may improve long-term implant performance. Although Kozinn and Scott[135] described the standard indications for mobile-bearing medial UKA more than 15 years ago, many surgeons continue to follow those indications, which exclude patients weighing more than 82 kg (180 lb), patients younger than 60 years, patients who have more than minimal erosive changes in the patellofemoral articulation, and patients with anterior knee pain believed to be a sign of significant patellofemoral involvement. Other exclusions include cumulative angular deformity less than 15°, patients who are physically active or performing heavy labor, those with a range of motion greater than 90°, flexion contracture less than 5°, minimal pain at rest, noninflammatory arthropathy, and an intact anterior cruciate ligament (ACL).[134] With these conservative indications, 2% to 15% of patients with osteoarthritic knees may be candidates for UKA. A more liberal set of physiologic criteria has been advocated for mobile-bearing medial UKA by the Nuffield Orthopaedic Care Centre.[136-138] These indications include full-thickness medial cartilage loss, anterior disease with preserved posterior bone, fully correctable full-thickness lateral cartilage, and an intact ACL. The indication for medial UKA is anteromedial osteoarthritis, which is a clinical condition originally described by White et al.[136] Anteromedial osteoarthritis is a distinct disease that defines the indications for medial UKA. This disease involves complete bone-on-bone arthrosis medially on a weight-bearing radiograph, functionally intact ligamentous stabi-

lizers (ACL and medial collateral ligament), and a correctible varus deformity. The ability to correct the deformity and maintain the lateral joint space is evaluated using a valgus stress radiograph in each candidate for UKA[136,139] (**Figure 7**). Pain location and pattern are generally worse in or confined to the medial aspect of the knee but may be present globally or in other areas, particularly the posterior aspect of the knee. Applying these more liberal indications, approximately 35% of patients with osteoarthritic knees may be candidates for UKA. Although there are few contraindications to mobile-bearing medial UKA, this procedure is not indicated in patients with active infection (as is true for all arthroplasty procedures); in those with inflammatory disease because of its global rather than monocompartmental nature; and in patients with ligamentous instability or an absent ACL, which renders a disease process other than anteromedial osteoarthritis. It is also not indicated in patients with medial collateral ligament contracture, which would prevent correction of the intra-articular deformity, and in those with a history of high tibial osteotomy, which causes extra-articular overcorrection of the deformity and leads to rapid progression in the lateral compartment. Obesity, young age, activity level, and the presence of patellofemoral disease or anterior knee pain are not contraindications[87,97,99-101,109,113,124,127,132,140-163] (**Table 3**).

Excellent results with a 98% implant survival rate at up to 6-year follow-up have been reported using the liberal indications for mobile-bearing partial knee replacement in more than 1,500 knees.[155] Price and Svard[132] reported longer-term results of 91% for all-cause revision cumulative survival at 16 years in 543 patients treated with 682 mobile-bearing

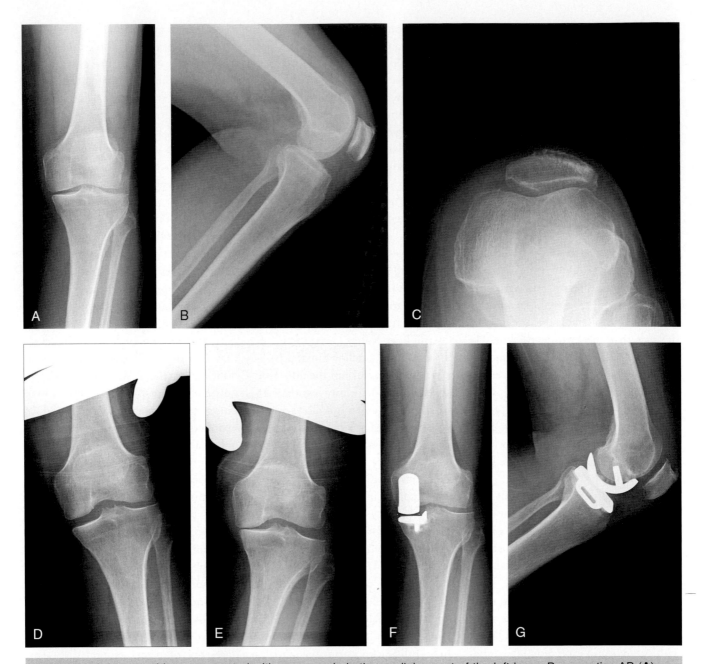

Figure 7   A 65-year-old man presented with severe pain in the medial aspect of the left knee. Preoperative AP (**A**), lateral (**B**), and axial patellar (**C**) radiographs revealed tibiofemoral alignment of 5° varus and severe narrowing of the joint space. **D,** A valgus stress view (technician applies stress with a protected hand) shows restoration of normal limb alignment without collapse of the lateral compartment and an intact medial collateral ligament. **E,** A varus stress view shows unsatisfactory restoration of normal limb alignment with collapse of the medial compartment. AP (**F**) and lateral (**G**) postoperative radiographs after medial UKA using a cemented, mobile-bearing device show that component position and alignment are satisfactory.

UKAs; the 91% survival rate was maintained at 20 years. In their series, all but seven knees (1%) fulfilled the expanded indications criteria, with four failures after high tibial osteotomy, two knees with an absent ACL, and one knee with inflammatory disease.

A recent report supported the practice of ignoring the radiographic status of the patellofemoral joint in patients selected for mobile-bearing UKA.[164] Standardized radiographs from 638 mobile-bearing medial UKAs, in which no patient was excluded based on the preoperative status of the patellofemoral joint, were graded by a blinded observer using a modified

Table 3
Results of Medial Mobile-Bearing UKA

Author(s)	Year	No. of Knees	Type of Implant (Manufacturer)	Follow-up (Range) Years	Survivorship (No. of Revisions)
Lewold et al[87]	1995	663	Oxford (Biomet, Warsaw, IN); cemented	6 (1-10)	63.2% at 6 years (45)
Murray et al[140]	1998	143	Oxford; cemented	7.6 (maximum 13.8)	98% at 10 years (5)
Kumar and Fiddian[141]	1999	100	Oxford; cemented	5.6 (1-11)	93% at 5.6 years (7)
Svärd and Price[142]	2001	124	Oxford; cemented	12.5 (10.1-15.6)	95% at 10 years (6)
Emerson et al[97]	2002	50	Oxford; cemented	6.8 (2-10.9)	86% at 6.8 years (7)
Keblish and Briard[143]	2004	156	LCS (DePuy, Warsaw, IN); cemented	11 (5-19)	81.4% at 11 years (29)
Saxler et al[144]	2004	315	AMC Uniglide (Corin, Gloucestershire, England); 72% cemented, 25% cementless, 3% hybrid	5.5 (2.3-12.5)	95% at 5.5 years (16)
Confalonieri et al[99]	2004	20	AMC (Alphanorm, Quiershied, Germany); cemented	5.7	100% at 5.7 years (0)
Emerson and Higgins[100]	2004	55	Oxford; cemented	10.2 (8.8-14.3)	87.3% at 14 years (7)
Gleeson et al[101]	2004	47	Oxford; cemented	2	85.1% at 2 years (7)
Jeer et al[145]	2004	66	LCS; cemented	5.9 (5.1-6.6)	90.9% at 5.9 years (6)
Keys et al[146]	2004	40	Oxford; cemented	7.5 (6-10)	100% at 7.5 years (0)
Rajasekhar et al[147]	2004	135	Oxford; cemented	5.8 (2-12)	94% at 10 years (5)
Skowroński et al[148]	2005	42	Oxford; cemented	11.2 (minimum 10)	86% at 11.2 years
Price et al[149]	2005	52	< age 60 years; Oxford	10	92.3% at 10 years (4)
		512	≥ age 60 years; Oxford	10	96.1% at 10 years (20)
Price et al[150]	2005	439	Oxford; cemented	15 (minimum 10)	93% at 15 years (19)
Li et al[109]	2006	28	Oxford; cemented	2	92.9% at 2 years (2)
Pandit et al[151]	2006	688	Oxford III; MIS, cemented	(1-8)	97.3% at 10 years (9)
Vorlat et al[152]	2006	149	Oxford; cemented	12.5	82% at 10 years (24)
Kort et al[153]	2007	154	Oxford III; cemented	(2-7)	89% at 2-7 years (17)
Koskinen et al[113]	2007	1145	Oxford	10	81% at 10 years
Emerson and Higgins[127]	2008	51	Oxford II; cemented	11.8 (8.8-14.3)	85% at 11.8 years (7)
Arastu et al[154]	2009	43	Preservation (DePuy); cemented	3.1 (0.8-4.4)	79% at 3.1 years (9)
Berend et al[155]	2009	257	Oxford III; cemented	3.8	96.1% at 3.8 years (10)
Heller et al[156]	2009	59	Oxford III; cemented	2.7 (2-5)	88% at 2.7 years (7)
Whittaker et al[124]	2010	79	Oxford; cemented	3.6 (1-11.3)	88% at 5 years (7)
Mercier et al[157]	2010	43	Oxford; cemented	14.8	90% at 5 years; 74.7% at 10 years; 70% at 15 years (13)
Parmaksizoğlu et al[158]	2010	38	Oxford III; cemented	2 (1.5-2.7)	100% at 2 years (0)
Sun and Jia[159]	2011	28	Oxford III; cemented	4.3 (3-6.7)	75% at 4.3 years (7)
Dervin et al[160]	2011	545	Oxford; cemented	3.8 (2.3-7.4)	94.1% at 3.8 years (32)
Lisowski et al[161]	2011	244	Oxford III; cemented	4.2 (1-10.4)	94.4% at 7 years (9)
Price and Svard[132]	2011	682	Oxford; cemented	5.9 (0.5-22)	91% at 20 years (29)
Pandit et al[162]	2011	1000	Oxford III; cemented	5.6 (1-11)	96% at 10 years (29)
White et al[163]	2011	100	Oxford Twin Peg, cemented	2	100% at 2 years (0)

Altman classification (0 to 3; normal to severe, erosive bone-on-bone disease). At 6 years, there were 17 revisions for an overall implant survival rate of 97.3%. Fourteen revisions (3.5%) occurred in the 396 knees (62%) graded as having a normal patellofemoral joint. Only 2 revisions (1.2%) occurred in the 168 grade 1 knees (26%), 1 revision (1.5%) in the 65 grade 2 knees (10%), and no revisions in the 9 grade 3 knees (1%). Many theories exist for this finding. Radiographic evaluation using standardized axial views has been shown to have poor sensitivity for detecting the severity of chondral changes. Correcting the varus malalignment with medial UKA may offload the medial facet of the patellofemoral joint and normalize joint forces. Preoperative radiographic changes in the patellofemoral joint can be safely ignored without compromising implant survivorship.

Another recent report studied the impact of body mass index (BMI) on the outcome of a consecutive, prospective series of 2,465 mobile-bearing UKAs at two high-volume centers in two countries with a maximum 12-year follow-up.[165] There were 380 patients (15%) with normal body weight (BMI < 25 kg/m²), 869 patients (35%) who were overweight (BMI 25 to < 30 kg/m²), 722 patients (29%) who were obese class I (BMI 30 to < 35 kg/m²), 290 patients (12%) who were obese class II (BMI 35 to < 40 kg/m²), and 204 (8%) who were morbidly obese (BMI > 40 kg/m²). The 7-year survival rates were not significantly different between the various groups: 97% in the normal group, 95% in the overweight group, 91% in the obese class I group, 94% in the obese class II group, and 98% in the morbidly obese group.

Metal backing of the tibial component may provide protection against the deleterious effects of a high BMI reported in previous studies with all-polyethylene bearings.[105,166] Small et al[167] investigated the influence of the metal backing on tibial loading throughout knee motion using in vitro photoelastic strain quantification methods. The authors found higher overall strains and more localized strain concentration in the posterior medial tibia with all-polyethylene implants compared with metal implant designs. This finding may partly explain the biomechanics behind tibial subsidence in patients with high BMI who are treated with all-polyethylene implants. The authors also studied the influence of bearing mobility on proximal tibial loading in UKA, simulating flexion and extension of the knee.[168] The greatest strains were reported in the anteromedial tibia and 2 cm distal to the joint line, which correlates with the area occasionally noted to have residual pain following UKA. Tibial overload may contribute to pain. These findings demonstrate the important role that bearing movement plays in load distribution throughout the tibia after UKA and may illuminate a biomechanical process of tibial remodeling that influences pain and implant loosening.

Polyethylene wear has been a concern in fixed-bearing metal-backed implants, with Collier et al[130] reporting severe polyethylene fatigue wear in 43 of 245 UKAs (17.6%) at a mean follow-up of 9 years in a cohort that included 7 fixed-bearing metal-backed designs. Knight et al[169] reported failure attributable to polyethylene wear in 6 of 43 UKAs (14%) with the Porous Coated Anatomic implant (PCA; Stryker, Mahwah, NJ), with a mean time to failure of 3.1 years. In a more recent study, Whittaker et al[124] reported on the Miller-Galante implant (Zimmer) and observed a 4.7% incidence of revision (7 of 150 UKAs) at a mean follow-up of 8.8 years. The limitations of polyethylene have been better understood with recognition of the adverse effects of oxidation with increased shelf life and sterilization in the presence of oxygen.[130,131] Polyethylene wear is an infrequent indication for revision of mobile-bearing implants. The wear rate on retrieved mobile bearings has been reported to be from 0.02 to 0.7 mm per year on penetration testing.[170-172] Bearing impingement has been shown to increase polyethylene wear in mobile-bearing devices and highlights the importance of surgical technique to ensure an impingement-free kinematic environment.[170]

Other risks unique to mobile-bearing UKAs are bearing dislocation, misinterpretation of postoperative tibial radiolucencies, and increased revision rates reported in registry data.[173,174] Dislocation of a medial mobile-bearing UKA requires simultaneous medial joint distraction and bearing spinning. Anatomic bearings have been designed to prevent 90° of bearing rotation on the tibial tray. The anterior portion of the bearing has a 5-mm lip, whereas the posterior aspect has a 3-mm lip. Bearing dislocation occurs when the bearing impinges on bone, cement, and retained osteophytes. Surgical technique is important to prevent bearing dislocation.

Radiolucencies have been reported under cemented metal-backed mobile-bearing UKA tibiae. The clinical significance of these radiolucencies has been investigated and does not correlate with pain or poor postoperative outcomes.[173] The importance of the correct radiographic interpretation of radiolucencies cannot be overemphasized. In the absence of implant migration, a cautious approach to revision should be used.

Registry data suggest higher revision rates for UKA than TKA.[174] Goodfellow et al[174] questioned the true meaning of these data, observing that UKAs had better clinical outcome scores than TKAs, and only 12% of TKAs with a poor outcome score (Oxford Knee Score < 20) are revised compared with 63% of UKAs with a similar score. It should be remembered that the threshold for some surgeons to revise a unsatisfactory UKA is much lower than the threshold to perform a revision for a painful TKA; therefore, the revision rate is not an objective measure and should not be used to compare these two procedures.

UKA has faster recovery with less perioperative morbidity compared with TKA.[55,175] In a study investigating the rate of transfusion, symptomatic thromboembolic events, and length of hospital stay in 1,000 consecutive UKAs managed with a rapid recovery protocol and multimodal venous thromboembolism prophylaxis, Berend et al[175] reported no deaths (0.0%), one deep venous thrombosis (0.1%), and one deep infection (0.1%). Five patients (0.5%) required a transfusion, and seven patients (0.7%) had a cardiac complication, including congestive heart failure, arrhythmia, or myocardial infarction. With the low rate of perioperative complications for UKA, surgeons may be overtreating patients with anteromedial knee osteoarthritis with TKA.

Robotics in Medial UKA

UKA is an excellent option for patients with a diseased tibiofemoral compartment. Minimally invasive UKA has many advantages over traditional TKA, including bone conservation, retention of normal knee kinematics, lower morbidity, shorter hospital stays, and increased patient satisfaction. Despite these advantages, UKA may be underutilized because the procedure is technically challenging, and accurate alignment may be difficult to obtain, even for experienced surgeons. Perhaps more importantly, early failures of

both tibial and femoral components have been well described.[105,112,176] It has been shown that proper implant positioning in UKA is important, and malalignment can lead to early failures. Improper component alignment has been shown to cause accelerated polyethylene wear, early implant loosening, fracture, and the progression of osteoarthritis in other compartments.[177,178] Excessive posterior slope is associated with injury to the ACL and component loosening.[179]

Robotically assisted UKA has been developed to improve implant positioning and potentially decrease component failure rates. With robotic assistance, bone resection and implant positioning can be performed with levels of precision and accuracy that are unmatched by manual surgery. Lonner et al[180] compared 27 UKAs performed using manual instrumentation with 31 robotically assisted arthroplasties. The root mean square error of the tibial slope was 3.1° manually compared with 1.9° robotically. The varus/valgus root mean square average error was 3.4° manually and 1.8° robotically. Cobb et al[181] described a series of 28 knees that were randomly allocated to have UKA performed manually or with robotic assistance. The primary outcome measurement was the angle of tibiofemoral alignment in the coronal plane. All the knees in the robotically assisted group had alignment within 2° of the planned position, whereas only 40% of the conventional group achieved this accuracy. It has been demonstrated that the average learning curve using robotic assistance for UKA is 16 cases (RH Jinnah, MD, et al, Big Island, Hawaii, unpublished data, 2009).

Haptic robotic technology consists of a robotic arm with a cutting burr at the end and is a passive system that prohibits the surgeon from resecting bone outside the planned area. The

system creates haptic boundaries based on the surgical plan. Although the surgeon actively controls the burr, the robot constrains the surgeon and does not allow bone resection outside the planned area. Any attempt to move the active burr outside the predefined area of resection will be met with firm resistance, keeping the burr within the zone of resection. The system essentially creates an artificial, three-dimensional cutting jig. In addition to tactile feedback, the surgeon also visually monitors progress. A three-dimensional bony model of the knee is displayed along with a virtual burr and highlighted areas of planned resection to create visual boundaries. Burr movements and bone removal are depicted in real time.

Haptic robotic technology can be coupled with excellent preoperative and intraoperative planning. A CT scan is taken preoperatively and is three-dimensionally reconstructed. Planning is then performed using three-dimensional, computer-aided design models of the implants. Any anatomic deformities or large cysts can be identified at this time. This comprehensive planning allows for evaluation of implant size and position, limb alignment, and implant tracking before the surgeon enters the operating room. Another benefit of this technology is the ability to adjust the plan intraoperatively to account for soft-tissue balancing. After the initial bone registration process, the knee is taken through its range of motion, and the tightness or looseness of the surgical compartment is measured at multiple angles. This information is then displayed in bar graph format, making it easy to determine imbalances between the flexion and extension gaps of the preoperative plan. The computer-derived, virtual implants can then be rotated or translated in any plane of motion on the three-dimensional model, and the corresponding planned changes to gap balancing are displayed.

Tibiofemoral tracking is adjusted in a similar manner. With multiple adjustments, it is not uncommon to have all gaps balanced to less than 1 mm throughout the range of motion, thus optimizing soft-tissue tensioning. Once the intraoperative plan is satisfactory, the plan is committed and the haptic robotic arm controls bone resection to execute the surgical plan. After resection, trial components are inserted and real-time, dynamic evaluation of the flexion and extension gaps and tibiofemoral tracking can be performed. An unpublished series of 44 patients showed that the actual gaps created at 0°, 30°, 60°, and 90° varied little from the gaps planned before resection (RH Jinnah, MD, unpublished data, 2011).

Robotically assisted UKA has several disadvantages. Additional time is required for setting up and calibrating the equipment. Two bicortical Schanz pins must be inserted into both the tibial and femoral diaphysis to provide rigid fixation for the navigation markers. In addition to increased morbidity, these sites could potentially act as stress risers. Extra time must also be allotted for computer registration of the tibia and femur. Any change in position of the navigation markers during surgery will alter the system's understanding of the femur and tibia in space. An inadvertent and unnoticed position change will lead to inaccurate bone resection.

Robotically assisted UKA has created a platform in which precise planning and execution of implant positioning can be accomplished in a minimally invasive fashion. Studies have shown that this emerging technology significantly improves implant positioning and limb alignment.[180-182] Whether improved implant alignment and soft-tissue balancing will prolong longevity or enable lower-volume surgeons to obtain excellent outcomes or will expand the indications for the procedure remains to be determined.

Patient-Specific Resurfacing Implants

Patient-specific, fixed-bearing resurfacing implants modeled from data obtained from preoperative CT scans can address many of the limitations of current off-the-shelf devices for the treatment of medial or lateral tibiofemoral compartment disease and bicompartmental disease involving the patellofemoral and one tibiofemoral compartment. The iUni and iDuo (Conformis, Burlington, MA) have been approved by the US Food and Drug Administration since 2007. Patient-specific disposable cutting jigs are provided with the custom implants, and the surgical technique is reduced to five simple steps.[183] Because the implants are derived from individual three-dimensional imaging data, they more accurately match the patient's anatomy than off-the-shelf devices, optimizing tibial plateau coverage, matching the J curve and coronal curvature of the femoral condyle, and accommodating anatomic differences between the medial and lateral compartments. Biomechanical and anatomic axes are factored into the preoperative plan, and custom jigs are generated that fit in a unique position on the condyle, achieving accurate cut planes, component position, and alignment without the use of navigation.

Based on the clinical examination, indications for the patient-specific unicompartmental iUni implant are range of motion greater than 90°, a correctable deformity of less than 10° varus, flexion contracture less than 10°, no evidence of inflammatory arthritis, an intact ACL, and osteoarthritis isolated to the medial or lateral compartment. Preoperative radiographs, including bilateral AP standing, Rosenberg standing, lateral standing, and skyline views, are obtained and assessed for the presence of monocompartmental, bicompartmental, or tricompartmental osteoarthritis. A CT arthrogram is useful to determine if the contralateral tibiofemoral compartment is intact and if the patellofemoral compartment is eburnated or intact. In the presence of arthritic changes in the patellofemoral joint, the bicompartmental iDuo may be used. The implants and instrumentation are derived from detailed, high-resolution CT scans of the knee, with additional slices of the ankle and hip to determine the mechanical axis for alignment. The surgeon receives a preoperative plan for modification or approval. After approval, implants and instruments are fabricated and delivered to the surgical facility in a single sterile box; two polyethylene inserts (6 and 8 mm) are included.

Surgical steps include removing all cartilage in the involved compartment off the femoral condyle inferior of the sulcus terminalis and off the tibial plateau. The knee is balanced at 10° to 30° using the individualized balancing chip supplied. The tibial cutting block is attached. The femoral cutting jig is placed, and pegs are drilled. The posterior femoral condyle is then cut, removing the planned amount of bone. For the bicompartmental device, an additional anterior cut is made. The anterior trench is prepared and a smooth transition to the posterior cut is fashioned using a 5-mm, high-speed burr. Trial implants are placed, and component positioning and balancing are verified. The femur and tibia are then prepared for cementation and implantation of the final components.

Koeck et al[184] conducted a radiographic analysis of 32 patient-specific medial UKAs performed in two German university centers between May 2008 and November 2009. The coronal femorotibial angle was corrected from a mean of 7° preoperatively to 1° postoperatively ($P < 0.001$), and the medial proximal tibial angle was corrected from a mean of 87° preoperatively to 89° postoperatively ($P < 0.001$). Patient-specific implants with personalized instrumentation were reliable in restoring the mechanical axis, obtaining a medial tibial angle of 90°, correctly positioning implants, and providing optimal tibial coverage.

Soft-Tissue–Guided Surgery for a Perfectly Balanced Knee

Knee arthroplasty procedures have changed little over the past 30 years. Traditional knee arthroplasty, including unicondylar arthroplasty, is performed by preparing the bone for the implant independent of the soft tissues. Intramedullary or extramedullary guides are used to align cutting blocks on both the femur and the tibia for the bone resections. In this process, the anatomy of both the distal femur and proximal tibia is altered. In most knees, the valgus alignment of the distal femur is reduced when variable amounts of bone are removed from each condyle. The varus alignment of the tibia is eliminated by making the bone resection perpendicular to the anatomic axis of the tibia.

Knee arthroplasty performed in the traditional manner does not take into account the individual differences in knee anatomy between patients. In most healthy knees, distal femoral valgus ranges from 5° to 12°. Varus in the proximal tibia ranges from 0° to 7°. The goal in knee arthroplasty is to place the mechanical axis of the extremity through the center of the knee by converting the variation in the patient's anatomy to an average of 6° valgus in the femur and neutral (0°) in the tibia. The amount of bone re-

moved from the distal femur is different on each condyle. The posterior condylar resections are made without consideration of the bone cuts from the distal end of the femur. Because these cuts are independent, the knee will have laxity in flexion if more bone is removed from the back of a condyle than the end of the condyle or will be too tight in flexion and result in limited knee motion if less bone is removed from the back of a condyle. Asymmetric or unequal bone resections create some degree of knee instability that results in altered knee kinematics and function. Often, ligament balancing is necessary to achieve acceptable knee function.

Altering the synergistic relationship between the capsular structures that provide stability to the knee and the underlying bone alters a patient's functional ability during higher-demand activities. Patients can sense imbalance caused by poor implant positioning and altered knee kinematics. Gait studies have confirmed changes in velocity, a decreased stride length, decreased midstance knee flexion (quad avoidance gait), decreased maximum knee flexion during stance and swing phases, and abnormal flexion-extension moments.[185-188] Studies by Andriacchi et al[188,189] have shown a decrease in knee motion during both ascent and descent of stairs, along with decreased velocity and knee motion during descent of stairs in knees with posterior-stabilized implants. The functional limitations that result from alterations in knee kinematics affect lateral movement, turning and cutting, carrying loads, leg strengthening, playing tennis, and gardening. Noble et al[190] has documented such limitations in 52% of patients after TKA compared with 22% of age-matched normal subjects. Sports activities following total hip arthroplasty increased from 36% to 52% but decreased from

42% to 34% following TKA.[191] In addition, 16% of patients continued to report some pain after knee arthroplasty compared to 9% of patients that reported pain after hip arthroplasty.

Kinematic changes that can be measured following TKA include femoral rollback and axial rotation. The patellar tendon angle, a simple but practical measure of anteroposterior knee stability, is reduced following traditional TKA. The reduction or absence of tension in the ACL allows the tibia to slide forward, thus disrupting the mechanical function of the extensor mechanism. Video fluoroscopy during activities such as deep knee bends can be used to evaluate both femoral rollback and axial rotation. Dennis and Komistek[192] demonstrated that the normal femoral rollback of 15 to 25 mm on the lateral side of the knee is essentially eliminated following cruciate-retaining or cruciate-substituting TKA. The normal axial rotation of 15° to 20° is reduced by almost two thirds with knee replacement surgery.

In tissue-guided surgery, bone cuts are performed only under the guidance of the soft-tissue envelope. This type of surgery is uniquely based on instrumentation that uses the patient's knee motion to guide bone preparation for the implants. This optimizes the implant position with the soft tissues spanning the knee. The surgeon places a cutting element inside the knee to machine the articular surface as the surgeon flexes and extends the knee. This process addresses two issues paramount to knee arthroplasty. (1) Traditional systems delay soft-tissue balancing until after the bone cuts are made and (2) soft-tissue balancing is considered to be one of the most challenging aspects of knee replacement. Frequently, some correction, either through ligament release or additional bone resection, is required to achieve knee stability. Tissue-guided surgery uses the patient's knee motion to balance the soft tissues as the bone cuts are made. Combining soft-tissue balancing with bone preparation removes the challenge of soft-tissue balancing from the procedure.

Tissue-guided surgery is based on the premise that changes to the hard tissue anatomy cannot be performed independent of the tension in the soft-tissue elements without creating a subclinical level of knee instability. With tissue-guided knee arthroplasty, a tibial cut is performed first to create space for the cutting element that will be mounted on a guide plate that is placed on the resected tibial plateau. A guide path aligns the femur precisely to the center of the resected tibia. Tension in the soft-tissue elements that guide motion and provide stability to the knee is integrated with the femoral bone preparation. The intra-articular cutting elements are mounted within the joint cavity and machine the femur a precise distance from the tibia, with the capsular structures distracted as the knee is moved throughout a full arc of knee motion.

Two steps are used to prepare the femoral condyle. First, the surgeon prepares a guide surface by placing a cutting element inside the knee and extending the leg. The cutting element is a side-cutting drill, which is mounted on a tibial guide plate that is placed on the resected tibial plateau. A guide plate that covers the resected tibial plateau is selected and used to center the cutting element that will remove bone from the femur. As the knee is extended, a groove is created in the center of the femoral condyle. This groove is oriented to the center of the tibial plateau, assuring precise component-to-component alignment. The primary cutter baseplate also provides tension on the joint space with a spring-loaded platform as the knee is articulated. The depth of the groove is

dictated by the patient's own soft-tissue envelope, which includes the collateral and cruciate ligaments. The second step is to use cutters that reference this guide surface to prepare an implant support surface. The secondary cutters have a fin that fits in the groove created with the first step. The fin holds and distracts the joint appropriately to keep the capsular envelope tensioned and guides the cutter to prepare the support surfaces for the femoral implant on either side of the central groove.

No planer cuts are made to prepare the femoral condyle. The implant used with tissue-guided surgery has a radius of 140°, with change in the sagittal radius of the implant of 2 mm between each size. The implant has the same curvature as the native condyle. The implant should precisely fit the condyle or can be off by only ± 1 mm.

Tissue-guided surgery is unique in that ligament balancing to restore optimum knee kinematics is integral to bone preparation. The technique provides the surgeon with an intuitive and reproducible procedure that achieves a perfectly balanced knee.

Combination ACL Reconstruction–Medial UKA in the ACL-Deficient Knee

Deficiency of the ACL is a common finding in end-stage osteoarthritis. Varus osteoarthritis in ACL-competent knees demonstrates the classic anteromedial osteoarthritic pattern that has been shown to be successfully treated with UKA. However, ACL-deficient knees have a unique pattern of osteoarthritis with a more posteromedial location.[193] Traditional indications for UKA have restricted the procedure to knees with normal ligaments and bone-on-bone medial compartmental arthrosis.[135] Previous studies have shown that UKA in knees without an intact ACL have decreased

survivorship.[85,139,194] With increasing interest in UKA, younger and more active patients are presenting with end-stage arthritis and concomitant ACL insufficiency.[195-197] In these patients with degenerative arthrosis and concomitant instability, cartilage restoration options are limited, and TKA is not the ideal treatment option considering the young age of the patients and their usual high level of activity. Less invasive arthroplasty options have been considered despite the relative contraindication of ACL deficiency. The indications and surgical technique for arthroscopically assisted simultaneous UKA and ACL were studied, and early outcomes of the procedure were noted (J Hurst, MD, et al, San Diego, CA, unpublished data, 2011). Between June 2007 and August 2010, arthroscopically assisted simultaneous UKA and ACL treatment was indicated and performed in 17 patients at Joint Implant Surgery (New Albany, OH), representing 1.6% of the medial UKAs during the study period. Indications for the procedure included ACL deficiency and medial joint arthrosis with a correctible deformity on valgus stress radiographs. Arthroscopic evaluation and confirmation of unicompartmental disease was performed, followed by arthroscopic establishment of the femoral and tibial tunnels using the all-inside technique. UKA was then performed via a limited arthrotomy; trial components were placed; then the graft was passed, tensioned, and fixed. Final cementation of the UKA components was performed.

The postoperative rehabilitation regimen was similar to typical UKA rehabilitation programs, with additional focus on proprioception, balanced hamstring/quadriceps strength, and graft protection until 9 months postoperatively. High-impact activities were discouraged, and participation in ACL-dependent sports was limited until 9 months after surgery. Two reoperations were needed in the 17 cases. One graft fixation failure required revision ACL, and one manipulation was needed. The average patient age was 50 years (range, 38 to 63 years). In patients with 1-year follow-up, the mean range of motion was 113° and the mean Knee Society pain score was 40. This group of young patients had a high success rate in terms of pain and range of motion.

Younger patients with significant medial arthrosis and concomitant ACL deficiency present a difficult clinical dilemma because TKA is not an ideal treatment option for young, active patients, and cartilage restoration is typically contraindicated. Even though ACL deficiency has been considered a contraindication to UKA, a less invasive arthroplasty option still remains attractive in this population because of the young age at which these patients present with severe medial disease. The combined ACL-UKA procedure may provide implant longevity considering the increased rate of implant failure in UKAs performed in patients with concomitant ACL deficiency. ACL-UKA treatment provides more normal kinematics and is a less invasive arthroplasty option compared with TKA. In addition, the combined ACL-UKA procedure in younger patients may delay arthritic progression.

When considering an ACL-UKA procedure, it is important to consider the etiology of the ACL deficiency. There are two main types of ACL deficiency: traumatic and attritional. In traumatic ACL deficiency, medial osteoarthritis is secondary to the ACL deficiency. In this type of deficiency, there is a classic isolated posteromedial pattern and limited contracture of the medial collateral ligament. The ACL-UKA combined procedure is a viable treatment option in patients with traumatic ACL deficiency because the varus deformity is still correctable. In attritional ACL deficiency, the ACL ruptures secondary to the degenerative process. In this type of disorder, the arthritic pattern starts anteromedially and progresses posteriorly as the ACL fails secondary to the degenerative process. There is often significant contracture of the medial collateral ligament with attritional ACL deficiency. When the varus deformity is uncorrectable, TKA is warranted.

The Lateral Compartment

Isolated unicompartmental arthritis occurs less frequently than tricompartmental arthritis. In isolated disease, the medial compartment is affected more commonly than the lateral compartment.[1] Isolated lateral compartment disease occurs at a rate of 5% to 10%.[198,199] Medial UKA is performed 10 times more often than lateral UKA, with lateral UKA representing approximately 1% of all arthroplasty procedures.[199] Lateral UKA is also considered more technically demanding than medial UKA or TKA because of the more complex lateral kinematic profile.[183,198-200]

The surgical technique begins with an abbreviated midline incision created from 2 cm proximal to the superior pole of the patella and extending to the proximal lateral aspect of the tibial tubercle. Via this skin incision, a lateral parapatellar approach is performed with careful dissection of the superficial fascia and preservation of the infrapatellar fat pad. Extramedullary tibial and femoral alignment guides are used. Instrumentation and implant technique proceeds according to the implant manufacturer's technique guidelines. A transpatellar tendon vertical resection of the tibia is used to allow appropriate internal rotation of the tibial baseplate and ensure that the femur articulates with the tibial polyethylene even through the screw-home mechanism. Balancing the lateral compartment is performed differently than is done in medial UKA or TKA. Laterally, in the knee with intact ligaments, the flexion gap is lax in comparison with the extension gap. This normal disparity in flexion and extension gap balance is re-created to avoid overcorrection. The surgeon should be familiar with a lateral approach for TKA in the event that intraoperative conversion is needed. Lateral UKA is a true resurfacing procedure in which the joint line should be reconstructed to anatomic level. This requires resection of the tibial plateau to the level at which the tibial trial can be inserted in extension, before making any bony resections to the distal femur. This procedure is very different from mobile-bearing medial UKA. It is currently recommended that a fixed-bearing device be used for lateral UKA because of the high range of motion, femoral posterior subluxation, the complexity of the screw-home mechanism perhaps leading to dislocation, and significant laxity of the lateral compartment in flexion.

The paucity of lateral UKAs performed since the inception of UKA approximately 40 years ago is puzzling. The original reports from that era concentrated primarily on experiences with medial UKA, with very few patients undergoing lateral UKA and available for study. However, the results of initial reports suggested that medial UKA was not a viable long-term option for treating unicompartmental femorotibial osteoarthritis, whereas lateral UKA seemed more promising.[69,201-203] Following refinements in patient selection criteria, surgical technique, and implant design, favorable results for medial and lateral UKAs were being published in the 1980s.[204] With enthusiasm for UKA growing, the procedure became more widespread, specifically regarding medial UKAs. Ten-year follow-up studies were reported showing survivorship that was slightly less than that reported for TKA but still acceptable considering the conservative nature of the surgery.[80,83,86]

Since that time, many studies have been published reporting survivorship of medial UKA ranging from 70% to 96% at a minimum 10-year follow-up among large patient cohorts (**Tables 2** and **3**). There have been fewer studies reporting the long-term results following lateral UKA[69,71,75-77,79,80,82, 83,85, 87,92,106,111,116,122,143,144,198,200,205-213] (**Table 4**). However, recent studies examining lateral UKA outcomes at midterm and long-term follow-up report survivorship rates of 100%.[197,208,213] Berend et al[213] recently reported on 109 knees (102 patients) with minimum 1-year follow-up (average follow-up, 30 months ± 16.5 months). The indications for lateral UKA were isolated lateral bone-on-bone arthrosis with maintenance of medial joint space confirmed radiographically, on a varus stress radiograph, or arthroscopically. Technically, a lateral parapatellar approach was used with the vertical tibial resection performed through the patellar tendon. Postoperatively, the average Knee Society clinical score improved significantly ($P < 0.001$) to a pain score of 46 (range, 10 to 50; SD = 9), a total score of 94 (range, 10 to 95; SD = 10.4), and a Knee Society function score of 89 (range, 40 to 100; SD = 16). Postoperative average range of motion also improved significantly ($P < 0.001$) to 124° (range, 95° to 145°; SD = 10.2°). There were 91% good or excellent results. Implant survivorship was 100% at up to the 5.8-year follow-up.

Pennington et al[208] reported excellent clinical results of lateral UKA in younger and more active patients with cemented, metal-backed, or all-polyethylene tibial components at an average follow-up of 12.4 years, with a survivorship of 100%. Argensen et al[210] reported survivorship of 92% at 10 years, and 84% at 16 years with lateral UKA. Sah and Scott[198] reported no revisions at 5.4 years in 49 patients treated with lateral UKA. Berend et al[213] used preoperative varus stress radiographs or diagnostic arthroscopy before lateral UKA, and in contradistinction to Sah and Scott,[198] there were no patients who required conversion to TKA intraoperatively using a less invasive lateral parapatellar approach (**Figure 8**). Pennington et al[208] and Berend et al[213] used a lateral parapatellar approach, whereas Sah and Scott[198] used a medial parapatellar approach, indicating the endurance of lateral UKA regardless of the surgical approach. These reports suggest that the outcomes of lateral UKA are at least comparable to, if not superior to, those of medial UKA.

The study by Argenson et al,[210] which analyzed outcomes of lateral UKA, reported a relatively disappointing survivorship rate of 84% at 16 years, with five revision surgeries necessary. However, the authors retrospectively reviewed all cases of lateral UKA between February 1982 and December 2004, and four of the five revisions occurred before 1989, whereas only one of five occurred after 1989 ($P = 0.007$). Prior to 1989, patient selection criteria were not as refined or as rigorous as current criteria. For example, the authors disclose that the absence of valgus deformity or full loss of cartilage in the opposite femorotibial compartments was not a reason for exclusion before 1989. Four of five revision surgeries were performed for painful progression of osteoarthritis to the adjacent femorotibial compartments. During the 1980s, surgical instrumentation was technically limited, and surgical cuts were handmade. The study authors believed that technical surgical errors were the reason for one of five revision surgeries for early tibial implant migration.[210] The use of the mobile-bearing Oxford unicompartmental prosthesis (Biomet, Bridgend, Wales) also may have contributed to the need for revision surgery. Gunther et al[206] reported a 21% failure rate and 10% rate of bearing dislocation in 53 lateral UKAs performed using the standard Oxford implant for medial UKA. Given the high range of motion, significant femoral rollback, and screw-home mechanism most noted laterally, a mobile bearing would be ideal.[206] Using a novel domed tibial plateau implant significantly reduced the rate of mobile bearing dislocation from 11% to 1.7%.[212] It is not yet known if a mobile-bearing design used laterally will yield the same long-term survivorship and low wear rate as that of medial mobile-bearing UKAs.[132,170]

Although the rates of revision surgery have recently decreased markedly, the prospect of the need for revision surgery following lateral UKA must be considered. Since 1990, reasons for revision reported in the literature include progression of arthritis in retained compartments, loosening of the femoral component, loosening of the tibial component, fracture of the femoral component, fracture of the tibial plateau, and valgus malalignment. A significant reason for revisions has been the progression of osteoarthritis in the retained medial and patellofemoral compartments. Walton et al[214] reported definite progression of osteoarthritis in 18% to 34% of lateral UKAs performed in a small cohort of 32 patients. Ashraf et al[200] revised 9 of 15 lateral UKAs for symptomatic progression of osteoarthritis, and Argenson et al[210] performed 4 of 5 revision surgeries for progression of osteoarthritis.

Three other reasons for revision (fracture of the femoral component,

Table 4

Published Results of Lateral UKA

Author(s)	Year	No. of Knees	Type of Implant (Manufacturer)	Follow-up (Range) Years	Survivorship (No. of Revisions)
Scott and Santore[69]	1981	12	Brigham I and II (DePuy, Warsaw, IN); cemented, all-polyethylene tibia	3.5 (2-6)	83.3% at 3.5 years (2)
Mallory and Danyi[71]	1983	4	Polycentric (Stryker, Mahwah, NJ), 17%; Marmor (Smith & Nephew, Memphis, TN), 83%; both cemented, all-polyethylene tibia	5.6 (5.1-8.1)	50% at 5.6 years (2)
Marmor[205]	1984	14	Marmor; cemented, all polyethylene tibia	7.4 (2.5-9.83)	85.7% at 7.4 years (2)
Kozinn et al[75]	1989	11	Brigham Mod; cemented, metal backed	5.5 (4.5-6)	100% at 5.5 years (0)
Magnussen and Bartlett[76]	1990	9	PCA (Stryker); cementless, metal backed	(2-3.3)	100% at 2 years (0)
Christensen[77]	1991	54	St. Georg Sled (Waldermar Link, Hamburg, Germany); cemented, all-polyethylene tibia	3.9 (1-9)	98.4% at 3.9 years (NA)
Rougraff et al[79]	1991	14	Compartmental I and II (Zimmer, Warsaw, IN); cemented, all-polyethylene	6.5 (0.7-13.5)	92.9% at 6.5 years (1)
Scott et al[80]	1991	12	Brigham I and II (Stryker); cemented, all-polyethylene tibia	(8-12)	83.3% at 9 years (2)
Capra and Fehring[82]	1992	4 8	Marmor Compartmental II	11.1 (8-14) 6.3 (4-11)	100% at 11.1 years (0) 100% at 6.3 years (0)
Heck et al[83]	1993	39	Marmor Compartmental I and II	6 (maximum 14.8)	97.4% at 6 years (1)
Swank et al[85]	1993	7	5 Fibermesh (Zimmer); 2 Microloc (DePuy); cementless and cemented	5.5 (4-8)	87.8% at 5.5 years (NA)
Lewold et al[87]	1995	36	Oxford (Biomet, Warsaw, IN); cemented, mobile bearing	6 (1-10)	86.1% at 6 years (5)
Gunther et al[206]	1996	53	Oxford; cemented, mobile bearing	5 (2.5-9.83)	82% at 5 years (11)
Tabor and Tabor[92]	1998	6	Marmor-style, cemented, all-polyethylene tibia	9.7 (5-20)	66.7% at 9.7 years (2)
Ohdera et al[207]	2001	18	Four different designs	8.25 (5-15.75)	NA (2)
Ashraf et al[200]	2002	83	St. Georg Sled; cemented all polyethylene tibia	9 (2-21)	74% at 15 years (15)
Keblish and Briard[143]	2004	19	LCS (DePuy), cemented, mobile bearing	11 (5-19)	84.2% at 11 years (3)
Saxler et al[144]	2004	46	AMC Uniglide (Corin, Gloucestershire, England); 72% cemented; 25% cementless; 3% hybrid, mobile bearing	5.5 (2.3-12.5)	89% at 5.5 years (5)
O'Rourke et al[106]	2005	14	Marmor; cemented all polyethylene tibia	24 (17-28)	72% at 25 years (2)
Pennington et al[208]	2006	29	Miller-Galante (Zimmer); cemented, metal backed (75%); all polyethylene tibia (25%)	12.4 (3.1-15.6)	100% at 12.4 years (0)
Cartier et al[111]	2007	30	< age 60, Genesis (Smith & Nephew); 20% cementless; 43% all-polyethylene	(5-14)	94% at 10 years 92% at 11 years 88% at 12 years

NA = not available

Table 4 *(Continued)*
Published Results of Lateral UKA

Author(s)	Year	No. of Knees	Type of Implant (Manufacturer)	Follow-up (Range) Years	Survivorship (No. of Revisions)
Forster et al[209]	2007	30	Preservation (DePuy); cemented, 13 mobile bearing, 17 all-polyethylene fixed	2	Mobile: 77% at 2 years (3); fixed: 100% at 2 years (0)
Sah and Scott[198]	2007	49	Four different designs	5.2 (2-14)	100% at 5.4 years (0)
Argenson et al[210]	2008	38	Four different designs	12.6 (3-23)	84% at 16 years (5)
Bertani et al[211]	2008	35	Four different designs	9 (2-22)	85.7% at 9 years (5)
Lustig et al[116]	2009	60	HLS Evolution (Tornier, Edina, MN); cemented, all-polyethylene tibia	5.2 (2.1-13.3)	98.3% at 5 years; 98.3% at 10 years (11/144)
John et al[122]	2010	9	Miller-Galante, cemented, metal backed, fixed bearing	10.8 (2-16)	97% at 5 years; 41% at 8 years
Pandit et al[212]	2010	53	Oxford I and II	5.2	82% at 4 years (11)
		65	Oxford III; flat tibia	4.7 (3-9)	91% at 4 years (9)
		101	Oxford III; domed tibia	2.3 (1-4)	98% at 4 years (1)
Berend et al[213]	2011	132	Vanguard M (Biomet); cemented, metal backed	2.4 (1-5.8)	100% at 2 years (0)

fracture of the tibial component, and valgus malalignment) were reported in the early but not the recent literature. Ashraf et al[200] reported performing 4 of 15 revision surgeries for the treatment of a fractured femoral component. The four revision surgeries were all performed before 1988, when the implant design was modified to incorporate a stronger femoral component. Argenson et al[210] reported one of five revision surgeries necessitated by a tibial plateau fracture. The authors attributed the fracture to a technical error secondary to the limitations of the available surgical instruments available in the late 1980s. Valgus malalignment as a reason for revision of a lateral UKA was originally reported by Scott and Santore[69] in 1981. At the same time, Cameron et al[215] reported that 9 of 20 lateral UKAs achieved poor results, likely resulting from difficulty in correcting the valgus malalignment. With refinement of patient selection criteria, uncorrectable valgus deformity is now considered a contraindication for lateral UKA.

The increase in survivorship and decrease in the revision rate of lateral UKA can be attributed to better-defined patient selection criteria, improvements in surgical technique and instrumentation, and modifications of implant design to better accommodate the lateral compartment. Current research is focusing on the development of customized patient-specific lateral implants, a spherical-dome design for mobile-bearing lateral UKAs to decrease polyethylene dislocation, and an oxidized zirconium countersurface on the femoral component to decrease polyethylene wear.[212,216]

Partial Knee Arthroplasty Versus TKA

Degenerative arthritis and posttraumatic arthritis in a young, active patient present a therapeutic dilemma. Nonsurgical management, such as nonsteroidal anti-inflammatory drugs, physiotherapy, and activity modification, should be exhausted before surgery is contemplated. Surgical options include arthroscopic débridement,

femoral or tibial osteotomy, unicondylar replacement, and TKA. Few patients are willing to accept the functional limitations of an arthrodesis. Arthroscopic débridement has achieved limited success but is not a predictable procedure, especially in patients with limb malalignment or chondrocalcinosis.[217] Proximal tibial or distal femoral osteotomy may be indicated for the young patient with limb malalignment and unicompartmental disease and in those who perform heavy labor or participate in sports. Although early results are good, the results deteriorate over time.[218-221] Previous osteotomy may not compromise the outcome of a subsequent TKA, but it does make the conversion to TKA more technically demanding. Unicondylar replacement offers an alternative, bone-sparing procedure, but often degenerative arthritis is not limited to one compartment of the knee.[222,223]

As the indications for TKA expand, the decision to proceed with this procedure in a young, active patient

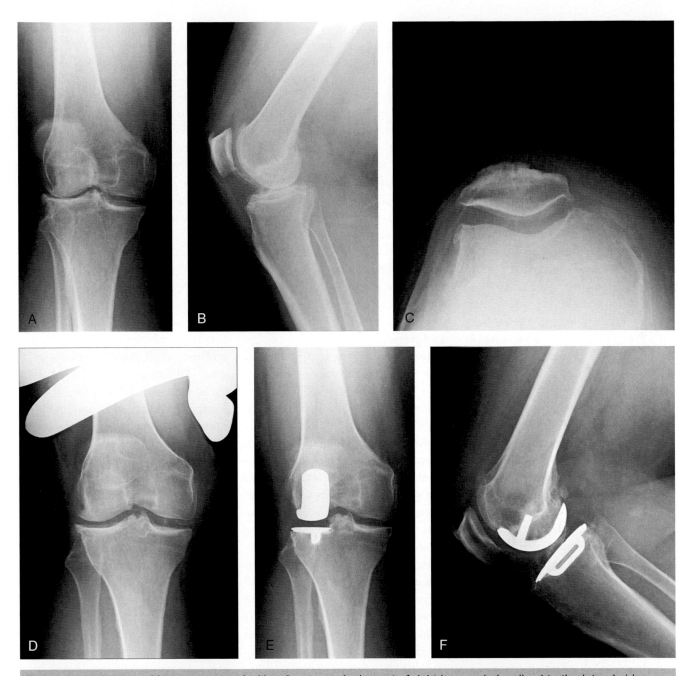

Figure 8 A 48-year-old man presented with a 3-year gradual onset of right knee pain localized to the lateral side. Preoperative AP (**A**), lateral (**B**), and axial patellar (**C**) radiographs revealed tibiofemoral alignment of 14° valgus, severe joint-space narrowing, sclerosis, and osteophyte formation. **D,** A varus stress test (technician applies stress with a protected hand) showed radiographic restoration of normal limb alignment without collapse of the medial compartment and an intact lateral collateral ligament. AP (**E**) and lateral (**F**) postoperative radiographs after treatment with a lateral UKA using a cemented, fixed-bearing device show that component position and alignment are satisfactory.

should be individualized and alternative treatments should be considered. TKA has been shown to be a durable and predictable procedure in elderly patients, providing pain relief, improving function, and correcting deformity.[224-228] Potential component loosening and the need for multiple revisions initially had discouraged the widespread use of TKA in young patients with degenerative arthritis. This concern arose from the poor results in young patients undergoing total hip replacement.[229-232] However, early results with TKA were encouraging and did not reflect the experience with total hip replacement.[233,234] Many of the initial studies included a large proportion of patients with rheumatoid arthritis or juvenile rheumatoid arthritis because there were no other treatment options available for these patients. Based on the initial success, the indications were then expanded to young patients with osteoarthritis.

Stuart and Rand[234] reviewed 44 cemented TKAs in patients with rheumatoid arthritis who were younger than 40 years. At an average follow-up of 5 years, 86% had an excellent or good result. Dalury et al[235] reported on 103 TKAs in patients younger than 45 years. Most of the patients (87%) had a diagnosis of rheumatoid arthritis. The average follow-up was 7 years. Although there were two patellar fractures and one infection, there were no revisions for component loosening. Boublik et al[236] reviewed 22 cementless TKAs in young patients with juvenile rheumatoid arthritis. At an average follow-up of 3.9 years, the average Hospital for Special Surgery knee score was 92. Ranawat et al[237] reported on 90 TKAs in patients younger than 55 years with rheumatoid arthritis and osteoarthritis. At an average follow-up of 6 years, the average Hospital for Special Surgery knee score was 87. In a study that reviewed only osteoarthritic knees, Stern et al[238] reported 55 excellent and 13 good results in patients age 55 years or younger at an average follow-up of 6 years.

These short-term and midterm results have withstood the test of time, even in more active patients with degenerative or posttraumatic arthritis. Duffy et al[239] reported on 74 consecutive TKAs in 54 patients who were 55 years or younger (average age, 43 years) at the time of the index procedure. All patients had a minimum follow-up of 10 years with an average follow-up of 13 years (range, 10 to 17 years). The preoperative diagnosis was rheumatoid arthritis in 47 patients; osteoarthritis in 12; posttraumatic ar-

thritis in 6; osteonecrosis in 3; hemophilia in 2; and 1 patient each with pigmented villonodular synovitis, tuberculosis, systemic lupus erythematosus, and achondroplasia. All knees had cemented condylar prostheses. The final functional score was 60 (range, 0 to 100 points) at latest follow-up. Two knees were revised: one at 3 years because of ligamentous laxity, and one at 13 years because of aseptic loosening of the tibial component. At last follow-up, there were no loose components. The authors concluded that the use of cemented TKAs in young patients is a reliable procedure, has achieved excellent results at 13-year follow-up, and has an estimated survivorship of 99% at 10 years.

Because most long-term studies include a larger percentage of older patients with a variety of diagnoses (including patients with rheumatoid arthritis and those with multiple joint involvement), it is important not to overinterpret these results and extrapolate them to younger, active patients with osteoarthritis. This subgroup of patients tends to be more active, and some may have employment requiring physical labor. Their activity requirements are greater and may put higher demands on the prosthetic surface and fixation. A study specifically evaluating this subset of patients was reported by Diduch et al.[240] The authors reviewed 108 knees in 84 patients with a diagnosis of either osteoarthritis or posttraumatic arthritis, with 58% having had prior knee surgery; all but 1 of these patients had a cemented posterior stabilized prosthesis (that patient had a total condylar prosthesis). One hundred three unrevised knees were available for clinical evaluation, with an average follow-up of 8 years (range, 3 to 18 years). Thirty-six knees were followed for more than 10 years. The average postoperative Hospital for Special Surgery knee score was 92, the

average Knee Society score was 94, and the functional score was 89. All knees were rated as either good or excellent. The average Tegner activity score improved from an average of 1.3 preoperatively to 3.5 postoperatively (range, 1 to 6). The level of activity improved in all but two patients, whereas 24% had an activity level greater than 5 points, indicating regular participation in activities such as tennis, skiing, cycling, or strenuous farm or construction work. There were two revisions for late infection, one for polyethylene wear, and one for flexion instability. In all the patients, the femoral and tibial components were well fixed. With failure defined as revision of either the femoral or tibial component, the cumulative survivorship was 94% at 18 years. There were an additional three knees that required revision of loose patellar components. These durable results support treatment of the osteoarthritic knee in a young, active patient with a cemented posterior-stabilized prosthesis when less invasive measures have failed.

Despite the good results experienced by several skilled surgeons and supported by clinical reports, common sense suggests that TKA should continue to be considered with caution for some young patients. Deferment of the definitive surgical procedure may be the best option until the symptoms warrant TKA. If total knee replacement is performed, young patients should be advised that activities involving high impact loads, such as running and jumping, should be avoided. Although some studies have reported good results at follow-ups as long as 18 years, these are incidental cases with specific implant designs and should not be construed as a guaranteed norm with all implants in all patients. Although there does not appear to be any evidence of catastrophic component loosening or failure, additional long-term data are needed before TKA is universally accepted in the treatment of osteoarthritis in young, active patients.

Acknowledgments

The authors would like to thank Joanne B. Adams, BFA, Joint Implant Surgeons, New Albany, OH; Ryan Bunch, DO, and Jason Lang, MD, Wake Forest University School of Medicine, Winston-Salem, NC; and Manish Noticewala, MS IV, New York Presbyterian Hospital, Columbia University, New York, NY, for their assistance in the preparation of this manuscript.

References

1. McAlindon TE, Snow S, Cooper C, Dieppe PA: Radiographic patterns of osteoarthritis of the knee joint in the community: The importance of the patellofemoral joint. *Ann Rheum Dis* 1992;51(7): 844-849.

2. Ackroyd CE, Chir B: Development and early results of a new patellofemoral arthroplasty. *Clin Orthop Relat Res* 2005;436:7-13.

3. Ackroyd CE, Newman JH, Evans R, Eldridge JD, Joslin CC: The Avon patellofemoral arthroplasty: Five-year survivorship and functional results. *J Bone Joint Surg Br* 2007;89(3):310-315.

4. Cartier P, Sanouiller JL, Grelsamer R: Patellofemoral arthroplasty. 2-12-year follow-up study. *J Arthroplasty* 1990;5(1):49-55.

5. de Winter WE, Feith R, van Loon CJ: The Richards type II patellofemoral arthroplasty: 26 cases followed for 1-20 years. *Acta Orthop Scand* 2001;72(5):487-490.

6. Krajca-Radcliffe JB, Coker TP: Patellofemoral arthroplasty: A 2- to 18-year followup study. *Clin Orthop Relat Res* 1996;330:143-151.

7. Leadbetter WB, Kolisek FR, Levitt RL, et al: Patellofemoral arthroplasty: A multi-centre study with minimum 2-year follow-up. *Int Orthop* 2009;33(6):1597-1601.

8. Merchant AC: A modular prosthesis for patellofemoral arthroplasty: Design and initial results. *Clin Orthop Relat Res* 2005;436: 40-46.

9. Mohammed R, Jimulia T, Durve K, Bansal M, Green M, Learmonth D: Medium-term results of patellofemoral joint arthroplasty. *Acta Orthop Belg* 2008;74(4): 472-477.

10. Sisto DJ, Sarin VK: Custom patellofemoral arthroplasty of the knee. *J Bone Joint Surg Am* 2006;88(7): 1475-1480.

11. Sisto DJ, Sarin VK: Custom patellofemoral arthroplasty of the knee: Surgical technique. *J Bone Joint Surg Am* 2007;89(Suppl 2 Pt. 2): 214-225.

12. Sisto DJ, Sarin VK: Patellofemoral arthroplasty with a customized trochlear prosthesis. *Orthop Clin North Am* 2008;39(3):355-362, vi-vii.

13. Tauro B, Ackroyd CE, Newman JH, Shah NA: The Lubinus patellofemoral arthroplasty: A five- to ten-year prospective study. *J Bone Joint Surg Br* 2001;83(5): 696-701.

14. van Wagenberg JM, Speigner B, Gosens T, de Waal Malefijt J: Midterm clinical results of the Autocentric II patellofemoral prosthesis. *Int Orthop* 2009;33(6): 1603-1608.

15. Arendt EA: Dimorphism and patellofemoral disorders. *Orthop Clin North Am* 2006;37(4): 593-599.

16. Csintalan RP, Schulz MM, Woo J, McMahon PJ, Lee TQ: Gender differences in patellofemoral joint biomechanics. *Clin Orthop Relat Res* 2002;402:260-269.

17. Varadarajan KM, Gill TJ, Freiberg AA, Rubash HE, Li G: Gender differences in trochlear groove orientation and rotational kinematics of human knees. *J Orthop Res* 2009;27(7):871-878.

18. Sheehan FT, Derasari A, Fine KM, Brindle TJ, Alter KE: Q-angle and J-sign: Indicative of maltracking subgroups in patellofemoral pain. *Clin Orthop Relat Res* 2010;468(1):266-275.

19. Fulkerson JP: Anteromedialization of the tibial tuberosity for patellofemoral malalignment. *Clin Orthop Relat Res* 1983;177:176-181.

20. Ebinger TP, Boezaart A, Albright JP: Modifications of the Fulkerson osteotomy: A pilot study assessment of a novel technique of dynamic intraoperative determination of the adequacy of tubercle transfer. *Iowa Orthop J* 2007;27: 61-64.

21. Lonner JH: Patellofemoral arthroplasty. *Instr Course Lect* 2010;59: 67-84.

22. Minkowitz RB, Bosco JA III: Patellofemoral arthritis. *Bull NYU Hosp Jt Dis* 2009;67(1):30-38.

23. Leadbetter WB: Patellofemoral arthroplasty in the treatment of patellofemoral arthritis: Rationale and outcomes in younger patients. *Orthop Clin North Am* 2008; 39(3):363-380, vii.

24. Becker R, Röpke M, Krull A, Musahl V, Nebelung W: Surgical treatment of isolated patellofemoral osteoarthritis. *Clin Orthop Relat Res* 2008;466(2):443-449.

25. Yercan HS, Ait Si Selmi T, Neyret P: The treatment of patellofemoral osteoarthritis with partial lateral facetectomy. *Clin Orthop Relat Res* 2005;436:14-19.

26. Fulkerson JP: Alternatives to patellofemoral arthroplasty. *Clin Orthop Relat Res* 2005;436:76-80.

27. Pascual-Garrido C, Slabaugh MA, L'Heureux DR, Friel NA, Cole BJ: Recommendations and treatment outcomes for patellofemoral

articular cartilage defects with autologous chondrocyte implantation: Prospective evaluation at average 4-year follow-up. *Am J Sports Med* 2009;37(Suppl 1): 33S-41S.

28. Lonner JH: Patellofemoral arthroplasty. *J Am Acad Orthop Surg* 2007;15(8):495-506.

29. Lonner JH: Patellofemoral arthroplasty: Pros, cons, and design considerations. *Clin Orthop Relat Res* 2004;428:158-165.

30. Lonner JH: Patellofemoral arthroplasty: The impact of design on outcomes. *Orthop Clin North Am* 2008;39(3):347-354, vi.

31. Lonner JH: Patellofemoral arthroplasty. *Orthopedics* 2010;33(9): 653.

32. Lonner JH: Patellofemoral arthroplasty, in Lotke PA, Lonner JH, eds: *Master Techniques in Orthopaedic Surgery: Knee Arthroplasty,* ed 3. Philadelphia, PA, Lippincott Williams and Wilkins, 2009.

33. Blazina ME, Fox JM, Del Pizzo W, Broukhim B, Ivey FM: Patellofemoral replacement. *Clin Orthop Relat Res* 1979;144:98-102.

34. Board TN, Mahmood A, Ryan WG, Banks AJ: The Lubinus patellofemoral arthroplasty: A series of 17 cases. *Arch Orthop Trauma Surg* 2004;124(5):285-287.

35. Lonner JH, Jasko JG, Booth RE Jr: Revision of a failed patellofemoral arthroplasty to a total knee arthroplasty. *J Bone Joint Surg Am* 2006;88(11):2337-2342.

36. Hendrix MR, Ackroyd CE, Lonner JH: Revision patellofemoral arthroplasty: Three- to seven-year follow-up. *J Arthroplasty* 2008; 23(7):977-983.

37. Lubinus HH: Patella glide bearing total replacement. *Orthopedics* 1979;2:119-127.

38. Arciero RA, Toomey HE: Patellofemoral arthroplasty: A three- to nine-year follow-up study. *Clin Orthop Relat Res* 1988;236:60-71.

39. Argenson JN, Guillaume JM, Aubaniac JM: Is there a place for patellofemoral arthroplasty? *Clin Orthop Relat Res* 1995;321:162-167.

40. Smith AM, Peckett WR, Butler-Manuel PA, Venu KM, d'Arcy JC: Treatment of patello-femoral arthritis using the Lubinus patellofemoral arthroplasty: A retrospective review. *Knee* 2002;9(1):27-30.

41. Kooijman HJ, Driessen AP, van Horn JR: Long-term results of patellofemoral arthroplasty: A report of 56 arthroplasties with 17 years of follow-up. *J Bone Joint Surg Br* 2003;85(6):836-840.

42. Merchant AC: Early results with a total patellofemoral joint replacement arthroplasty prosthesis. *J Arthroplasty* 2004;19(7):829-836.

43. Argenson JN, Flecher X, Parratte S, Aubaniac JM: Patellofemoral arthroplasty: An update. *Clin Orthop Relat Res* 2005;440:50-53.

44. Cartier P, Sanouiller JL, Khefacha A: Long-term results with the first patellofemoral prosthesis. *Clin Orthop Relat Res* 2005;436:47-54.

45. Minas T: Patellofemoral replacement: The third compartment. *Orthopedics* 2008;31(9):920-922.

46. Butler JE, Shannon R: Patellofemoral arthroplasty with a custom-fit femoral prosthesis. *Orthopedics* 2009;32(2):81.

47. Odumenya M, Costa ML, Parsons N, Achten J, Dhillon M, Krikler SJ: The Avon patellofemoral joint replacement: Five-year results from an independent centre. *J Bone Joint Surg Br* 2010; 92(1):56-60.

48. van Jonbergen HP, Werkman DM, Barnaart LF, van Kampen A: Long-term outcomes of patellofemoral arthroplasty. *J Arthroplasty* 2010;25(7):1066-1071.

49. Lonner JH: Symposium handout: Onlay trochlear designs in patellofemoral arthroplasty are most effective. *AAOS 2011 Annual Meeting Proceedings.* CD Rom, vol 12. Rosemont, IL, American Academy of Orthopaedic Surgeons, 2011, pp 145-146.

50. Lonner JH, Jasko JG, Thomas BS: Anthropomorphic differences between the distal femora of men and women. *Clin Orthop Relat Res* 2008;466(11):2724-2729.

51. Biedert R, Sigg A, Gal I, Gerber H: 3D representation of the surface topography of normal and dysplastic trochlea using MRI. *Knee* 2011;18(5):340-346.

52. Shih YF, Bull AM, Amis AA: The cartilaginous and osseous geometry of the femoral trochlear groove. *Knee Surg Sports Traumatol Arthrosc* 2004;12(4):300-306.

53. Berger RA, Crossett LS, Jacobs JJ, Rubash HE: Malrotation causing patellofemoral complications after total knee arthroplasty. *Clin Orthop Relat Res* 1998;356:144-153.

54. Sharma L, Song J, Dunlop D, et al: Varus and valgus alignment and incident and progressive knee osteoarthritis. *Ann Rheum Dis* 2010;69(11):1940-1945.

55. Lombardi AV Jr, Berend KR, Walter CA, Aziz-Jacobo J, Cheney NA: Is recovery faster for mobile-bearing unicompartmental than total knee arthroplasty? *Clin Orthop Relat Res* 2009;467(6):1450-1457.

56. Dalury DF, Fisher DA, Adams MJ, Gonzalez RA: Unicompartmental knee arthroplasty compares favorably to total knee arthroplasty in the same patient. *Orthopedics* 2009;32(4):pii.

57. Yang KY, Wang MC, Yeo SJ, Lo NN: Minimally invasive unicondylar versus total condylar knee arthroplasty: Early results of a matched-pair comparison. *Singapore Med J* 2003;44(11):559-562.

58. Walton NP, Jahromi I, Lewis PL, Dobson PJ, Angel KR, Campbell DG: Patient-perceived outcomes and return to sport and work:

TKA versus mini-incision unicompartmental knee arthroplasty. *J Knee Surg* 2006;19(2):112-116.

59. Manzotti A, Confalonieri N, Pullen C: Unicompartmental versus computer-assisted total knee replacement for medial compartment knee arthritis: A matched pair study. *Int Orthop* 2007;31(3): 315-319.

60. Hopper GP, Leach WJ: Participation in sporting activities following knee replacement: Total versus unicompartmental. *Knee Surg Sports Traumatol Arthrosc* 2008; 16(10):973-979.

61. Repicci JA, Eberle RW: Minimally invasive surgical technique for unicondylar knee arthroplasty. *J South Orthop Assoc* 1999;8(1): 20-27.

62. Romanowski MR, Repicci JA: Minimally invasive unicondylar arthroplasty: Eight-year follow-up. *J Knee Surg* 2002;15(1):17-22.

63. Romanowski MR, Repicci JA: Technical aspects of medial versus lateral minimally invasive unicondylar arthroplasty. *Orthopedics* 2003;26(3):289-293.

64. Repicci JA, Hartman JF: Minimally invasive unicondylar knee arthroplasty for the treatment of unicompartmental osteoarthritis: An outpatient arthritic bypass procedure. *Orthop Clin North Am* 2004;35(2):201-216.

65. Repicci JA, Hartman JF: MIS unicondylar arthroplasty: The bone-sparing technique, in Scuderi GR, Tria AJ, eds: *Minimally Invasive Surgery in Orthopedics.* New York, NY, Springer Science and Business Media, 2010, pp 229-238.

66. Berger RA, Meneghini RM, Jacobs JJ, et al: Results of unicompartmental knee arthroplasty at a minimum of ten years of follow-up. *J Bone Joint Surg Am* 2005; 87(5):999-1006.

67. Argenson JN, Chevrol-Benkeddache Y, Aubaniac JM: Modern unicompartmental knee arthroplasty with cement: A three to ten-year follow-up study. *J Bone Joint Surg Am* 2002;84-A(12): 2235-2239.

68. Pennington DW, Swienckowski JJ, Lutes WB, Drake GN: Unicompartmental knee arthroplasty in patients sixty years of age or younger. *J Bone Joint Surg Am* 2003;85-A(10):1968-1973.

69. Scott RD, Santore RF: Unicondylar unicompartmental replacement for osteoarthritis of the knee. *J Bone Joint Surg Am* 1981; 63(4):536-544.

70. Bae DK, Guhl JF, Keane SP: Unicompartmental knee arthroplasty for single compartment disease: Clinical experience with an average four-year follow-up study. *Clin Orthop Relat Res* 1983;176: 233-238.

71. Mallory TH, Danyi J: Unicompartmental total knee arthroplasty: A five- to nine-year follow-up study of 42 procedures. *Clin Orthop Relat Res* 1983;175: 135-138.

72. Bernasek TL, Rand JA, Bryan RS: Unicompartmental porous coated anatomic total knee arthroplasty. *Clin Orthop Relat Res* 1988;236: 52-59.

73. Mackinnon J, Young S, Baily RA: The St Georg sledge for unicompartmental replacement of the knee: A prospective study of 115 cases. *J Bone Joint Surg Br* 1988; 70(2):217-223.

74. Marmor L: Unicompartmental arthroplasty of the knee with a minimum ten-year follow-up period. *Clin Orthop Relat Res* 1988; 228:171-177.

75. Kozinn SC, Marx C, Scott RD: Unicompartmental knee arthroplasty: A 4.5 - 6-year follow-up study with a metal-backed tibial component. *J Arthroplasty* 1989; 4(Suppl):S1-S10.

76. Magnussen PA, Bartlett RJ: Cementless PCA unicompartmental joint arthroplasty for osteoarthritis of the knee: A prospective study of 51 cases. *J Arthroplasty* 1990; 5(2):151-158.

77. Christensen NO: Unicompartmental prosthesis for gonarthrosis: A nine-year series of 575 knees from a Swedish hospital. *Clin Orthop Relat Res* 1991;273: 165-169.

78. Laurencin CT, Zelicof SB, Scott RD, Ewald FC: Unicompartmental versus total knee arthroplasty in the same patient: A comparative study. *Clin Orthop Relat Res* 1991;273:151-156.

79. Rougraff BT, Heck DA, Gibson AE: A comparison of tricompartmental and unicompartmental arthroplasty for the treatment of gonarthrosis. *Clin Orthop Relat Res* 1991;273:157-164.

80. Scott RD, Cobb AG, McQueary FG, Thornhill TS: Unicompartmental knee arthroplasty: Eight- to 12-year follow-up evaluation with survivorship analysis. *Clin Orthop Relat Res* 1991;271: 96-100.

81. Stockelman RE, Pohl KP: The long-term efficacy of unicompartmental arthroplasty of the knee. *Clin Orthop Relat Res* 1991;271: 88-95.

82. Capra SW Jr, Fehring TK: Unicondylar arthroplasty: A survivorship analysis. *J Arthroplasty* 1992; 7(3):247-251.

83. Heck DA, Marmor L, Gibson A, Rougraff BT: Unicompartmental knee arthroplasty: A multicenter investigation with long-term follow-up evaluation. *Clin Orthop Relat Res* 1993;286:154-159.

84. Sisto DJ, Blazina ME, Heskiaoff D, Hirsh LC: Unicompartment arthroplasty for osteoarthrosis of the knee. *Clin Orthop Relat Res* 1993;286:149-153.

85. Swank M, Stulberg SD, Jiganti J, Machairas S: The natural history

of unicompartmental arthroplasty: An eight-year follow-up study with survivorship analysis. *Clin Orthop Relat Res* 1993;286: 130-142.

86. Weale AE, Newman JH: Unicompartmental arthroplasty and high tibial osteotomy for osteoarthrosis of the knee: A comparative study with a 12- to 17-year follow-up period. *Clin Orthop Relat Res* 1994;302:134-137.

87. Lewold S, Goodman S, Knutson K, Robertsson O, Lidgren L: Oxford meniscal bearing knee versus the Marmor knee in unicompartmental arthroplasty for arthrosis: A Swedish multicenter survival study. *J Arthroplasty* 1995;10(6): 722-731.

88. Cartier P, Sanouiller JL, Grelsamer RP: Unicompartmental knee arthroplasty surgery: 10-year minimum follow-up period. *J Arthroplasty* 1996;11(7):782-788.

89. Ansari S, Newman JH, Ackroyd CE: St. Georg sledge for medial compartment knee replacement: 461 arthroplasties followed for 4 (1-17) years. *Acta Orthop Scand* 1997;68(5):430-434.

90. Bert JM: 10-year survivorship of metal-backed, unicompartmental arthroplasty. *J Arthroplasty* 1998; 13(8):901-905.

91. Schai PA, Suh JT, Thornhill TS, Scott RD: Unicompartmental knee arthroplasty in middle-aged patients: A 2- to 6-year follow-up evaluation. *J Arthroplasty* 1998; 13(4):365-372.

92. Tabor OB Jr, Tabor OB: Unicompartmental arthroplasty: A long-term follow-up study. *J Arthroplasty* 1998;13(4):373-379.

93. Berger RA, Nedeff DD, Barden RM, et al: Unicompartmental knee arthroplasty: Clinical experience at 6- to 10-year followup. *Clin Orthop Relat Res* 1999;367: 50-60.

94. Squire MW, Callaghan JJ, Goetz DD, Sullivan PM, Johnston RC:

Unicompartmental knee replacement: A minimum 15 year followup study. *Clin Orthop Relat Res* 1999;367:61-72.

95. Ackroyd CE, Whitehouse SL, Newman JH, Joslin CC: A comparative study of the medial St Georg sled and kinematic total knee arthroplasties: Ten-year survivorship. *J Bone Joint Surg Br* 2002;84(5):667-672.

96. Perkins TR, Gunckle W: Unicompartmental knee arthroplasty: 3- to 10-year results in a community hospital setting. *J Arthroplasty* 2002;17(3):293-297.

97. Emerson RH Jr, Hansborough T, Reitman RD, Rosenfeldt W, Higgins LL: Comparison of a mobile with a fixed-bearing unicompartmental knee implant. *Clin Orthop Relat Res* 2002;404:62-70.

98. Gioe TJ, Killeen KK, Hoeffel DP, et al: Analysis of unicompartmental knee arthroplasty in a community-based implant registry. *Clin Orthop Relat Res* 2003; 416:111-119.

99. Confalonieri N, Manzotti A, Pullen C: Comparison of a mobile with a fixed tibial bearing unicompartmental knee prosthesis: A prospective randomized trial using a dedicated outcome score. *Knee* 2004;11(5):357-362.

100. Emerson RH Jr, Higgins LL: A comparison of highly instrumented and minimally instrumented unicompartmental knee prostheses. *Clin Orthop Relat Res* 2004;428:153-157.

101. Gleeson RE, Evans R, Ackroyd CE, Webb J, Newman JH: Fixed or mobile bearing unicompartmental knee replacement? A comparative cohort study. *Knee* 2004; 11(5):379-384.

102. Kankovský V, Ptácek Z, Kubát P: Long-term results of unicompartmental knee joint replacement. *Acta Chir Orthop Traumatol Cech* 2004;71(2):84-92.

103. Khan OH, Davies H, Newman JH, Weale AE: Radiological changes ten years after St. Georg Sled unicompartmental knee replacement. *Knee* 2004;11(5): 403-407.

104. Naudie D, Guerin J, Parker DA, Bourne RB, Rorabeck CH: Medial unicompartmental knee arthroplasty with the Miller-Galante prosthesis. *J Bone Joint Surg Am* 2004;86-A(9):1931-1935.

105. Berend KR, Lombardi AV Jr, Mallory TH, Adams JB, Groseth KL: Early failure of minimally invasive unicompartmental knee arthroplasty is associated with obesity. *Clin Orthop Relat Res* 2005;440:60-66.

106. O'Rourke MR, Gardner JJ, Callaghan JJ, et al: The John Insall Award: Unicompartmental knee replacement. A minimum twenty-one-year followup, end-result study. *Clin Orthop Relat Res* 2005; 440:27-37.

107. Tabor OB Jr, Tabor OB, Bernard M, Wan JY: Unicompartmental knee arthroplasty: Long-term success in middle-age and obese patients. *J Surg Orthop Adv* 2005; 14(2):59-63.

108. Eickmann TH, Collier MB, Sukezaki F, McAuley JP, Engh GA: Survival of medial unicondylar arthroplasties placed by one surgeon 1984-1998. *Clin Orthop Relat Res* 2006;452:143-149.

109. Li MG, Yao F, Joss B, Ioppolo J, Nivbrant B, Wood D: Mobile vs. fixed bearing unicondylar knee arthroplasty: A randomized study on short term clinical outcomes and knee kinematics. *Knee* 2006; 13(5):365-370.

110. Steele RG, Hutabarat S, Evans RL, Ackroyd CE, Newman JH: Survivorship of the St Georg Sled medial unicompartmental knee replacement beyond ten years. *J Bone Joint Surg Br* 2006;88(9): 1164-1168.

111. Cartier P, Khefacha A, Sanouiller JL, Frederick K: Unicondylar knee arthroplasty in middle-aged patients: A minimum 5-year follow-up. *Orthopedics* 2007;30 (8, Suppl):62-65.

112. Mariani EM, Bourne MH, Jackson RT, Jackson ST, Jones P: Early failure of unicompartmental knee arthroplasty. *J Arthroplasty* 2007;22(6, Suppl 2):81-84.

113. Koskinen E, Paavolainen P, Eskelinen A, Pulkkinen P, Remes V: Unicondylar knee replacement for primary osteoarthritis: A prospective follow-up study of 1,819 patients from the Finnish Arthroplasty Register. *Acta Orthop* 2007; 78(1):128-135.

114. Newman J, Pydisetty RV, Ackroyd C: Unicompartmental or total knee replacement: The 15-year results of a prospective randomised controlled trial. *J Bone Joint Surg Br* 2009;91(1):52-57.

115. Koskinen E, Paavolainen P, Eskelinen A, et al: Medial unicompartmental knee arthroplasty with Miller-Galante II prosthesis: midterm clinical and radiographic results. *Arch Orthop Trauma Surg* 2009;129(5):617-624.

116. Lustig S, Paillot JL, Servien E, Henry J, Ait Si Selmi T, Neyret P: Cemented all polyethylene tibial insert unicompartmental knee arthroplasty: A long term follow-up study. *Orthop Traumatol Surg Res* 2009;95(1):12-21.

117. Parratte S, Argenson JN, Pearce O, Pauly V, Auquier P, Aubaniac JM: Medial unicompartmental knee replacement in the under-50s. *J Bone Joint Surg Br* 2009; 91(3):351-356.

118. Seyler TM, Mont MA, Lai LP, et al: Mid-term results and factors affecting outcome of a metal-backed unicompartmental knee design: A case series. *J Orthop Surg Res* 2009;4:39.

119. Biswal S, Brighton RW: Results of unicompartmental knee arthroplasty with cemented, fixed-bearing prosthesis using minimally invasive surgery. *J Arthroplasty* 2010;25(5):721-727.

120. Saenz CL, McGrath MS, Marker DR, Seyler TM, Mont MA, Bonutti PM: Early failure of a unicompartmental knee arthroplasty design with an all-polyethylene tibial component. *Knee* 2010; 17(1): 53-56.

121. O'Donnell T, Neil MJ: The Repicci II® unicondylar knee arthroplasty: 9-year survivorship and function. *Clin Orthop Relat Res* 2010;468(11):3094-3102.

122. John J, Mauffrey C, May P: Unicompartmental knee replacements with Miller-Galante prosthesis: Two to 16-year follow-up of a single surgeon series. *Int Orthop* 2011;35(4):507-513.

123. Bruni D, Iacono F, Russo A, et al: Minimally invasive unicompartmental knee replacement: Retrospective clinical and radiographic evaluation of 83 patients. *Knee Surg Sports Traumatol Arthrosc* 2010;18(6):710-717.

124. Whittaker JP, Naudie DD, McAuley JP, McCalden RW, MacDonald SJ, Bourne RB: Does bearing design influence midterm survivorship of unicompartmental arthroplasty? *Clin Orthop Relat Res* 2010;468(1):73-81.

125. Howe DJ, Taunton OD Jr, Engh GA: Retained cement after unicondylar knee arthroplasty: A report of four cases. *J Bone Joint Surg Am* 2004;86-A(10):2283-2286.

126. Song MH, Kim BH, Ahn SJ, Yoo SH, Lee MS: Early complications after minimally invasive mobile-bearing medial unicompartmental knee arthroplasty. *J Arthroplasty* 2009;24(8):1281-1284.

127. Emerson RH Jr, Higgins LL: Unicompartmental knee arthroplasty with the oxford prosthesis in patients with medial compartment arthritis. *J Bone Joint Surg Am* 2008;90(1):118-122.

128. Robinson BJ, Rees JL, Price AJ, et al: Dislocation of the bearing of the Oxford lateral unicompartmental arthroplasty: A radiological assessment. *J Bone Joint Surg Br* 2002;84(5):653-657.

129. Hernigou P, Deschamps G: Patellar impingement following unicompartmental arthroplasty. *J Bone Joint Surg Am* 2002;84-A(7):1132-1137.

130. Collier MB, Eickmann TH, Sukezaki F, McAuley JP, Engh GA: Patient, implant, and alignment factors associated with revision of medial compartment unicondylar arthroplasty. *J Arthroplasty* 2006; 21(6, Suppl 2):108-115.

131. McGovern TF, Ammeen DJ, Collier JP, Currier BH, Engh GA: Rapid polyethylene failure of unicondylar tibial components sterilized with gamma irradiation in air and implanted after a long shelf life. *J Bone Joint Surg Am* 2002; 84-A(6):901-906.

132. Price AJ, Svard U: A second decade lifetable survival analysis of the Oxford unicompartmental knee arthroplasty. *Clin Orthop Relat Res* 2011;469(1):174-179.

133. Beard DJ, Pandit H, Gill HS, Hollinghurst D, Dodd CA, Murray DW: The influence of the presence and severity of preexisting patellofemoral degenerative changes on the outcome of the Oxford medial unicompartmental knee replacement. *J Bone Joint Surg Br* 2007;89(12):1597-1601.

134. Smith TO, Hing CB, Davies L, Donell ST: Fixed versus mobile bearing unicompartmental knee replacement: A meta-analysis. *Orthop Traumatol Surg Res* 2009; 95(8):599-605.

135. Kozinn SC, Scott R: Unicondylar knee arthroplasty. *J Bone Joint Surg Am* 1989;71(1):145-150.

136. White SH, Ludkowski PF, Good-fellow JW: Anteromedial osteoarthritis of the knee. *J Bone Joint Surg Br* 1991;73(4):582-586.

137. Berend KR, Lombardi AV Jr: Liberal indications for minimally invasive oxford unicondylar arthroplasty provide rapid functional recovery and pain relief. *Surg Technol Int* 2007;16:193-197.

138. Berend KR, Lombardi AV Jr, Adams JB: Obesity, young age, patellofemoral disease, and anterior knee pain: Identifying the unicondylar arthroplasty patient in the United States. *Orthopedics* 2007;30(5, Suppl):19-23.

139. Goodfellow JW, Kershaw CJ, Benson MK, O'Connor JJ: The Oxford Knee for unicompartmental osteoarthritis: The first 103 cases. *J Bone Joint Surg Br* 1988;70(5):692-701.

140. Murray DW, Goodfellow JW, O'Connor JJ: The Oxford medial unicompartmental arthroplasty: A ten-year survival study. *J Bone Joint Surg Br* 1998;80(6):983-989.

141. Kumar A, Fiddian NJ: Medial unicompartmental arthroplasty of the knee. *Knee* 1999;6(1):21-23.

142. Svärd UC, Price AJ: Oxford medial unicompartmental knee arthroplasty: A survival analysis of an independent series. *J Bone Joint Surg Br* 2001;83(2):191-194.

143. Keblish PA, Briard JL: Mobile-bearing unicompartmental knee arthroplasty: A 2-center study with an 11-year (mean) follow-up. *J Arthroplasty* 2004;19(7, Suppl 2): 87-94.

144. Saxler G, Temmen D, Bontemps G: Medium-term results of the AMC-unicompartmental knee arthroplasty. *Knee* 2004;11(5):349-355.

145. Jeer PJ, Keene GC, Gill P: Unicompartmental knee arthroplasty: An intermediate report of survivorship after the introduction of a new system with analysis of failures. *Knee* 2004;11(5):369-374.

146. Keys GW, Ul-Abiddin Z, Toh EM: Analysis of first forty Oxford medial unicompartmental knee replacement from a small district hospital in UK. *Knee* 2004;11(5):375-377.

147. Rajasekhar C, Das S, Smith A: Unicompartmental knee arthroplasty: 2- to 12-year results in a community hospital. *J Bone Joint Surg Br* 2004;86(7):983-985.

148. Skowroński J, Jatskewych J, Długosz J, Skowroński R, Bielecki M: The Oxford II medial unicompartmental knee replacement: A minimum 10-year follow-up study. *Ortop Traumatol Rehabil* 2005;7(6):620-625.

149. Price AJ, Dodd CA, Svard UG, Murray DW: Oxford medial unicompartmental knee arthroplasty in patients younger and older than 60 years of age. *J Bone Joint Surg Br* 2005;87(11):1488-1492.

150. Price AJ, Waite JC, Svard U: Long-term clinical results of the medial Oxford unicompartmental knee arthroplasty. *Clin Orthop Relat Res* 2005;435:171-180.

151. Pandit H, Jenkins C, Barker K, Dodd CA, Murray DW: The Oxford medial unicompartmental knee replacement using a minimally-invasive approach. *J Bone Joint Surg Br* 2006;88(1):54-60.

152. Vorlat P, Putzeys G, Cottenie D, et al: The Oxford unicompartmental knee prosthesis: An independent 10-year survival analysis. *Knee Surg Sports Traumatol Arthrosc* 2006;14(1):40-45.

153. Kort NP, van Raay JJ, Cheung J, Jolink C, Deutman R: Analysis of Oxford medial unicompartmental knee replacement using the minimally invasive technique in patients aged 60 and above: An independent prospective series. *Knee Surg Sports Traumatol Arthrosc* 2007;15(11):1331-1334.

154. Arastu MH, Vijayaraghavan J, Chissell H, Hull JB, Newman JH, Robinson JR: Early failure of a mobile-bearing unicompartmental knee replacement. *Knee Surg Sports Traumatol Arthrosc* 2009;17(10):1178-1183.

155. Berend KR, Lombardi AV Jr: The medial unicompartmental option: Mobile magic. *Semin Arthroplasty* 2009;20:11-14.

156. Heller S, Fenichel I, Salai M, Luria T, Velkes S: The Oxford unicompartmental knee prosthesis for the treatment of medial compartment knee disease: 2 to 5 year follow-up. *Isr Med Assoc J* 2009;11(5):266-268.

157. Mercier N, Wimsey S, Saragaglia D: Long-term clinical results of the Oxford medial unicompartmental knee arthroplasty. *Int Orthop* 2010;34(8):1137-1143.

158. Parmaksizoğlu AS, Kabukçuoğlu Y, Ozkaya U, Bilgili F, Aslan A: Short-term results of the Oxford phase 3 unicompartmental knee arthroplasty for medial arthritis. *Acta Orthop Traumatol Turc* 2010;44(2):135-142.

159. Sun PF, Jia YH: Mobile bearing UKA compared to fixed bearing TKA: A randomized prospective study. *Knee* 2011 Feb 21. Epub ahead of print.

160. Dervin GF, Carruthers C, Feibel RJ, Giachino AA, Kim PR, Thurston PR: Initial experience with the oxford unicompartmental knee arthroplasty. *J Arthroplasty* 2011;26(2):192-197.

161. Lisowski LA, van den Bekerom MP, Pilot P, van Dijk CN, Lisowski AE: Oxford Phase 3 unicompartmental knee arthroplasty: Medium-term results of a minimally invasive surgical procedure. *Knee Surg Sports Traumatol Arthrosc* 2011;19(2):277-284.

162. Pandit H, Jenkins C, Gill HS, Barker K, Dodd CA, Murray DW: Minimally invasive Oxford phase 3 unicompartmental knee

replacement: Results of 1000 cases. *J Bone Joint Surg Br* 2011; 93(2):198-204.

163. White SH, Roberts S, Jones PW: The Twin Peg Oxford partial knee replacement: The first 100 cases. *Knee* 2011 Jan 18. Epub ahead of print.

164. Berend KR, Lombardi AV Jr, Morris MJ, Hurst JM: Poster P204: Does preoperative patello-femoral joint state affect medial unicompartmental survival? *AAOS 2011 Annual Meeting Proceedings*. CD-Rom, vol 12. Rosemont, IL, American Academy of Orthopaedic Surgeons, 2011, p 572.

165. Murray DW, Pandit AJ, Price AJ, Lombardi AV Jr, Dodd CA, Berend KR: The impact of body mass index on the outcome of unicompartmental knee replacements. 2011 Specialty Day Meeting of the Knee Society. Final Scientific Program, p 20. http://www.kneesociety.org/web/2011%20SD%20Knee%20Final%20Program.pdf. Accessed April 18, 2011.

166. Aleto TJ, Berend ME, Ritter MA, Faris PM, Meneghini RM: Early failure of unicompartmental knee arthroplasty leading to revision. *J Arthroplasty* 2008;23(2):159-163.

167. Small SR, Berend ME, Ritter MA, Buckley CA, Rogge RD: Metal backing significantly decreases tibial strains in a medial unicompartmental knee arthroplasty model. *J Arthroplasty* 2010.

168. Small SR, Berend ME, Ritter MA, Buckley CA: Bearing mobility affects tibial strain in mobile-bearing unicompartmental knee arthroplasty. *Surg Technol Int* 2010;19:185-190.

169. Knight JL, Atwater RD, Guo J: Early failure of the porous coated anatomic cemented unicompartmental know arthroplasty: Aids to diagnosis and revision. *J Arthroplasty* 1997;12(1):11-20.

170. Kendrick BJ, Longino D, Pandit H, et al: Polyethylene wear in Oxford unicompartmental knee replacement: A retrieval study of 47 bearings. *J Bone Joint Surg Br* 2010;92(3):367-373.

171. Argenson JN, O'Connor JJ: Polyethylene wear in meniscal knee replacement: A one to nine-year retrieval analysis of the Oxford knee. *J Bone Joint Surg Br* 1992; 74(2):228-232.

172. Price AJ, Short A, Kellett C, et al: Ten-year in vivo wear measurement of a fully congruent mobile bearing unicompartmental knee arthroplasty. *J Bone Joint Surg Br* 2005;87(11):1493-1497.

173. Gulati A, Chau R, Pandit HG, et al: The incidence of physiological radiolucency following Oxford unicompartmental knee replacement and its relationship to outcome. *J Bone Joint Surg Br* 2009; 91(7):896-902.

174. Goodfellow JW, O'Connor JJ, Murray DW: A critique of revision rate as an outcome measure: Re-interpretation of knee joint registry data. *J Bone Joint Surg Br* 2010;92(12):1628-1631.

175. Berend KR, Morris MJ, Lombardi AV Jr : Unicompartmental knee arthroplasty: Incidence of transfusion and symptomatic thromboembolic disease. *Orthopedics* 2010; 33(9, Suppl):8-10.

176. Skyrme AD, Mencia MM, Skinner PW: Early failure of the porous-coated anatomic cemented unicompartmental knee arthroplasty: A 5- to 9-year follow-up study. *J Arthroplasty* 2002;17(2): 201-205.

177. Hernigou P, Deschamps G: Alignment influences wear in the knee after medial unicompartmental arthroplasty. *Clin Orthop Relat Res* 2004;423:161-165.

178. Ridgeway SR, McAuley JP, Ammeen DJ, Engh GA: The effect of alignment of the knee on the outcome of unicompartmental knee

replacement. *J Bone Joint Surg Br* 2002;84(3):351-355.

179. Hernigou P, Deschamps G: Posterior slope of the tibial implant and the outcome of unicompartmental knee arthroplasty. *J Bone Joint Surg Am* 2004;86-A(3):506-511.

180. Lonner JH, John TK, Conditt MA: Robotic arm-assisted UKA improves tibial component alignment: A pilot study. *Clin Orthop Relat Res* 2010;468(1):141-146.

181. Cobb J, Henckel J, Gomes P, et al: Hands-on robotic unicompartmental knee replacement: A prospective, randomised controlled study of the acrobot system. *J Bone Joint Surg Br* 2006;88(2): 188-197.

182. Pearl AD, O'Loughlin PF, Kendoff DO: Robot-assisted unicompartmental knee arthroplasty. *J Arthroplasty* 2010;25(2):230-237.

183. Fitz W: Unicompartmental knee arthroplasty with use of novel patient-specific resurfacing implants and personalized jigs. *J Bone Joint Surg Am* 2009; 91(Suppl 1):69-76.

184. Koeck FX, Beckmann J, Luring C, Rath B, Grifka J, Basad E: Evaluation of implant position and knee alignment after patient-specific unicompartmental knee arthroplasty. *Knee* 2011;18(5): 294-299.

185. Dorr LD, Ochsner JL, Gronley J, Perry J: Functional comparison of posterior cruciate-retained versus cruciate-sacrificed total knee arthroplasty. *Clin Orthop Relat Res* 1988;236:36-43.

186. Kramers-de Quervain IA, Stüssi E, Müller R, Drobny T, Munzinger U, Gschwend N: Quantitative gait analysis after bilateral total knee arthroplasty with two different systems within each subject. *J Arthroplasty* 1997;12(2): 168-179.

187. Kärrholm J, Saari T: Removal or retention: Will we ever know? The

posterior cruciate ligament in total knee replacement. *Acta Orthop* 2005;76(6):754-756.

188. Andriacchi TP, Galante JO, Fermier RW: The influence of total knee-replacement design on walking and stair-climbing. *J Bone Joint Surg Am* 1982;64(9):1328-1335.

189. Andriacchi TP, Galante JO: Retention of the posterior cruciate in total knee arthroplasty. *J Arthroplasty* 1988;3(Suppl):S13-S19.

190. Noble PC, Gordon MJ, Weiss JM, Reddix RN, Conditt MA, Mathis KB: Does total knee replacement restore normal knee function? *Clin Orthop Relat Res* 2005;431:157-165.

191. Huch K, Müller KA, Stürmer T, Brenner H, Puhl W, Günther KP: Sports activities 5 years after total knee or hip arthroplasty: The Ulm Osteoarthritis Study. *Ann Rheum Dis* 2005;64(12):1715-1720.

192. Dennis DA, Komistek RD: Kinematics of mobile-bearing total knee arthroplasty. *Instr Course Lect* 2005;54:207-220.

193. Ritter MA, Faris PM, Thong AE, Davis KE, Meding JB, Berend ME: Intra-operative findings in varus osteoarthritis of the knee: An analysis of pre-operative alignment in potential candidates for unicompartmental arthroplasty. *J Bone Joint Surg Br* 2004;86(1):43-47.

194. Deschamps G, Lapeyre B: Rupture of the anterior cruciate ligament: A frequently unrecognized cause of failure of unicompartmental knee prostheses. Apropos of a series of 79 Lotus prostheses with a follow-up of more than 5 years. *Rev Chir Orthop Reparatrice Appar Mot* 1987;73(7):544-551.

195. Lee GC, Cushner FD, Vigoritta V, Scuderi GR, Insall JN, Scott WN: Evaluation of the anterior cruciate ligament integrity and degenerative arthritic patterns in patients undergoing total knee

arthroplasty. *J Arthroplasty* 2005; 20(1):59-65.

196. Pandit H, Van Duren BH, Gallagher JA, et al: Combined anterior cruciate reconstruction and Oxford unicompartmental knee arthroplasty: In vivo kinematics. *Knee* 2008;15(2):101-106.

197. Pandit H, Beard DJ, Jenkins C, et al: Combined anterior cruciate reconstruction and Oxford unicompartmental knee arthroplasty. *J Bone Joint Surg Br* 2006;88(7):887-892.

198. Sah AP, Scott RD: Lateral unicompartmental knee arthroplasty through a medial approach: Study with an average five-year follow-up. *J Bone Joint Surg Am* 2007;89(9):1948-1954.

199. Scott RD: Lateral unicompartmental replacement: A road less traveled. *Orthopedics* 2005;28(9):983-984.

200. Ashraf T, Newman JH, Evans RL, Ackroyd CE: Lateral unicompartmental knee replacement survivorship and clinical experience over 21 years. *J Bone Joint Surg Br* 2002;84(8):1126-1130.

201. Insall J, Walker P: Unicondylar knee replacement. *Clin Orthop Relat Res* 1976;120:83-85.

202. Insall J, Aglietti P: A five to seven-year follow-up of unicondylar arthroplasty. *J Bone Joint Surg Am* 1980;62(8):1329-1337.

203. Laskin RS: Unicompartmental tibiofemoral resurfacing arthroplasty. *J Bone Joint Surg Am* 1978;60(2):182-185.

204. Deshmukh RV, Scott RD: Unicompartmental knee arthroplasty: Long-term results. *Clin Orthop Relat Res* 2001;392:272-278.

205. Marmor L: Lateral compartment arthroplasty of the knee. *Clin Orthop Relat Res* 1984;186:115-121.

206. Gunther T, Murray DW, Miller R: Lateral unicompartmental knee arthroplasty with Oxford meniscal knee. *Knee* 1996;3:33-39.

207. Ohdera T, Tokunaga J, Kobayashi A: Unicompartmental knee arthroplasty for lateral gonarthrosis: midterm results. *J Arthroplasty* 2001;16(2):196-200.

208. Pennington DW, Swienckowski JJ, Lutes WB, Drake GN: Lateral unicompartmental knee arthroplasty: Survivorship and technical considerations at an average follow-up of 12.4 years. *J Arthroplasty* 2006;21(1):13-17.

209. Forster MC, Bauze AJ, Keene GC: Lateral unicompartmental knee replacement: fixed or mobile bearing? *Knee Surg Sports Traumatol Arthrosc* 2007;15(9):1107-1111.

210. Argenson JN, Parratte S, Bertani A, Flecher X, Aubaniac JM: Long-term results with a lateral unicondylar replacement. *Clin Orthop Relat Res* 2008;466(11):2686-2693.

211. Bertani A, Flecher X, Parratte S, Aubaniac JM, Argenson JN: Unicompartmental-knee arthroplasty for treatment of lateral gonarthrosis: about 30 cases: Midterm results. *Rev Chir Orthop Reparatrice Appar Mot* 2008;94(8):763-770.

212. Pandit H, Jenkins C, Beard DJ, et al: Mobile bearing dislocation in lateral unicompartmental knee replacement. *Knee* 2010;17(6):392-397.

213. Berend KR, Kolczun MC II, George JW Jr, Lombardi AV Jr: Lateral unicompartmental knee arthroplasty vial a lateral parapatellar approach. *Clin Orthop Relat Res* 2011 Aug 6. Epub ahead of print.

214. Walton MJ, Weale AE, Newman JH: The progression of arthritis following lateral unicompartmental knee replacement. *Knee* 2006;13(5):374-377.

215. Cameron HU, Hunter GA, Welsh RP, Bailey WH: Unicompartmental knee replacement. *Clin Orthop Relat Res* 1981;160:109-113.

216. Heyse TJ, Tibesku CO: Lateral unicompartmental knee arthroplasty: A review. *Arch Orthop Trauma Surg* 2010;130(12):1539-1548.

217. Harwin SF: Arthroscopic debridement for osteoarthritis of the knee: Predictors of patient satisfaction. *Arthroscopy* 1999;15(2):142-146.

218. Coventry MB: Upper tibial osteotomy for gonarthrosis: The evolution of the operation in the last 18 years and long term results. *Orthop Clin North Am* 1979;10(1):191-210.

219. Insall JN, Joseph DM, Msika C: High tibial osteotomy for varus gonarthrosis: A long-term follow-up study. *J Bone Joint Surg Am* 1984;66(7):1040-1048.

220. McDermott AG, Finklestein JA, Farine I, Boynton EL, MacIntosh DL, Gross A: Distal femoral varus osteotomy for valgus deformity of the knee. *J Bone Joint Surg Am* 1988;70(1):110-116.

221. Ritter MA, Fechtman RA: Proximal tibial osteotomy: A survivorship analysis. *J Arthroplasty* 1988;3(4):309-311.

222. Katz MM, Hungerford DS, Krackow KA, Lennox DW: Results of total knee arthroplasty after failed proximal tibial osteotomy for osteoarthritis. *J Bone Joint Surg Am* 1987;69(2):225-233.

223. Windsor RE, Insall JN, Vince KG: Technical considerations of total knee arthroplasty after proximal tibial osteotomy. *J Bone Joint Surg Am* 1988;70(4):547-555.

224. Colizza WA, Insall JN, Scuderi GR: The posterior stabilized total knee prosthesis: Assessment of polyethylene damage and osteolysis after a ten-year-minimum follow-up. *J Bone Joint Surg Am* 1995;77(11):1713-1720.

225. Ewald FC, Jacobs MA, Miegel RE, Walker PS, Poss R, Sledge CB: Kinematic total knee replacement. *J Bone Joint Surg Am* 1984;66(7):1032-1040.

226. Insall JN, Kelly MA: The total condylar prosthesis. *Clin Orthop Relat Res* 1986;205:43-48.

227. Insall JN, Lachiewicz PF, Burstein AH: The posterior stabilized condylar prosthesis: A modification of the total condylar design. Two to four-year clinical experience. *J Bone Joint Surg Am* 1982;64(9):1317-1323.

228. Vince KG, Insall JN, Kelly MA: The total condylar prosthesis: 10- to 12-year results of a cemented knee replacement. *J Bone Joint Surg Br* 1989;71(5):793-797.

229. Dorr LD, Kane TJ III, Conaty JP: Long-term results of cemented total hip arthroplasty in patients 45 years old or younger: A 16-year follow-up study. *J Arthroplasty* 1994;9(5):453-456.

230. Joshi AB, Porter ML, Trail IA, Hunt LP, Murphy JC, Hardinge K: Long-term results of Charnley low-friction arthroplasty in young patients. *J Bone Joint Surg Br* 1993;75(4):616-623.

231. Solomon MI, Dall DM, Learmonth ID, Davenport JM: Survivorship of cemented total hip arthroplasty in patients 50 years of age or younger. *J Arthroplasty* 1992;7(Suppl):347-352.

232. Ewald F, Christie MJ: Results of cemented total knee replacements in young patients. *Orthop Trans* 1987;11:442.

233. Hungerford DS, Krackow KA, Kenna RV: Cementless total knee replacement in patients 50 years old and under. *Orthop Clin North Am* 1989;20(2):131-145.

234. Stuart MJ, Rand JA: Total knee arthroplasty in the young adult. *Orthop Trans* 1987;11:441-442.

235. Dalury DF, Ewald FC, Christie MJ, Scott RD: Total knee arthroplasty in a group of patients less than 45 years of age. *J Arthroplasty* 1995;10(5):598-602.

236. Boublik M, Tsahakis PJ, Scott RD: Cementless total knee arthroplasty in juvenile onset rheumatoid arthritis. *Clin Orthop Relat Res* 1993;286:88-93.

237. Ranawat CS, Padgett DE, Ohashi Y: Total knee arthroplasty for patients younger than 55 years. *Clin Orthop Relat Res* 1989;248:27-33.

238. Stern SH, Bowen MK, Insall JN, Scuderi GR: Cemented total knee arthroplasty for gonarthrosis in patients 55 years old or younger. *Clin Orthop Relat Res* 1990;260:124-129.

239. Duffy GP, Trousdale RT, Stuart MJ: Total knee arthroplasty in patients 55 years old or younger: 10- to 17-year results. *Clin Orthop Relat Res* 1998;356:22-27.

240. Diduch DR, Insall JN, Scott WN, Scuderi GR, Font-Rodriguez D: Total knee replacement in young, active patients: Long-term follow-up and functional outcome. *J Bone Joint Surg Am* 1997;79(4):575-582.

Video Reference

28.1: Lonner JH: Video. *Patellofemoral Arthroplasty.* Philadelphia, PA, 2011.

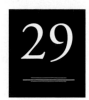

Current and Innovative Pain Management Techniques in Total Knee Arthroplasty

David F. Dalury, MD

Jay R. Lieberman, MD

Steven J. MacDonald, MD, FRCSC

Abstract

Pain management is a major concern for patients contemplating total knee replacement surgery and is one of the leading causes of dissatisfaction after knee replacement. Substantial progress has been made over the past several years in improving pain control after total knee replacement using multimodal pain control, preemptive analgesia, and periarticular injections.

Instr Course Lect 2012;61:383-388.

Pain is "an unpleasant sensory and emotional experience associated with actual or potential tissue damage."[1] It is of considerable concern to patients undergoing total knee replacement because the procedure has the reputation of being extremely painful, and fear of this pain is frequently cited as a reason for delaying the decision to undergo surgery.[2] Postoperative pain is intensified by movement and has a circadian rhythm with increasing pain at night.[3] Failure to adequately control pain after total knee replacement induces patho-physiologic responses, which increase postoperative morbidity, hinder physiotherapy, increase anxiety, disrupt sleep patterns, and, in general, decrease patient satisfaction and prolong recovery. Patients believe that physicians do not fully appreciate the need for perioperative pain management, and this adds to patient anxiety. Surgeons need to recognize the importance of managing pain. The Joint Commission has declared pain to be the "fifth vital sign" and stated that patients have a "right" to adequate pain management.[4]

Mechanism of Surgical Pain

The trauma of surgery activates the nociceptor system, including the nociceptors in peripheral nerves and in the central nervous system. There are two types of nociceptors that transmit information. A-delta fibers are myelinated nociceptors that are activated by mechanical and thermal stimulation and provide rapid information to the central nervous system. C fibers are unmyelinated nociceptors that are activated by mechanical, chemical, and cold stimulation and are involved in the inflammatory process.

Total knee arthroplasty produces a peripheral noxious stimulus. Action potentials are propagated from the nerve endings in the peripheral nerves to the spinal cord and then to the central nervous system, which generates a secondary inflammatory response. These signals induce prolonged changes in both the peripheral and central nervous systems that can amplify and prolong postoperative pain. The surgery also leads to cell injury and inflammation, which promote the release of various substances and cytokines including hydrogen and potassium, histamine, serotonin, prosta-

Dr. Dalury or an immediate family member has received royalties from DePuy; is a member of a speakers' bureau or has made paid presentations on behalf of DePuy; serves as a paid consultant to DePuy; and has received research or institutional support from DePuy. Dr. Lieberman or an immediate family member serves as a paid consultant to DePuy; has received research or institutional support from Amgen and Arthrex; and serves as a board member, owner, officer, or committee member of the American Academy of Orthopaedic Surgeons and American Association of Hip and Knee Surgeons. Dr. MacDonald or an immediate family member has received royalties from DePuy; serves as a paid consultant to DePuy; has received research or institutional support from DePuy, Smith & Nephew, and Stryker; and serves as a board member, owner, officer, or committee member of The Knee Society.

glandins, leukotrienes, thromboxane, and substance P. This leads to a reduction in the pain threshold of the nociceptor afferent terminals at the surgical site, a condition called primary hyperalgesia. The reduction in the pain threshold of the nociceptor afferent terminals in the surrounding noninjured tissue is called secondary hyperalgesia. Peripheral and central sensitization also leads to primary and secondary hyperalgesia. Peripheral sensitization occurs when there is inflammation of the site of the surgical trauma, which leads to a reduction in the threshold of nociceptors of afferent terminals. Central sensitization occurs when there is excitability of the spinal neurons secondary to persistent exposure to nociceptor afferent input from peripheral neurons. If the pain is prolonged, it may become chronic in nature.

To control surgery-associated pain, multimodal pain management can minimize these stimuli and limit activation of the central nervous system during and after a total knee arthroplasty.

Patient responses are variable, and there is not a direct correlation between noxious stimuli and perceived pain. Effective pain control takes this into consideration. Psychologic status influences a patient's perception of pain. Patients with higher depression and anxiety scores experience more pain, and patients with poor coping skills have increased pain perception. In 2010, Riddle et al[5] found that pain catastrophizing was a consistent predictor of poorer pain outcome after total knee replacement.

Racial and ethnic groups have different pain responses to noxious stimuli, concerns about drug addiction vary, and some patients prefer to rely on prayer to deal with their pain.[6-8] As a group, black Americans have more advanced disease and pain compared

with white Americans by the time they have surgery.[8]

Biologic differences explain some of the variability. Tseng et al[9] reported that 10% of whites do not have an enzyme needed to convert codeine to its active state, whereas only 0.5% of patients of African or Asian descent do not have the enzyme. The bioavailability of drugs is likely another biologic cause because of individual differences in drug metabolization.

Conventional Pain Management

The most common means of controlling pain associated with surgery is to start treating the pain by administering opioids postoperatively. Although parenteral opioids work quickly, there are more adverse side effects with parenterally administered pain medications compared with orally administered opioids.[10] Whether the medication is given orally or parenterally, the patient waits for the nurse to administer the pain medication, which reduces the effect of the pain medication.[11] Patient-controlled analgesia is an alternative method for the administration of pain medication that is attractive to patients because they are able to administer medications when and how they may need them. The sense of self-control is appealing; however, adverse reactions (excessive somnolence and sedation, respiratory depression, pruritus, nausea or vomiting, constipation, and urinary retention) associated with narcotic usage are common.[12]

New Approaches to Pain Management

Pain is probably easier to prevent than to eradicate and, on the basis of this concept, anesthesiologists originally termed this approach preemptive analgesia. The current understanding suggests that, when a noxious stimulus causes pain, there is a so-called recruit-

ment of adjacent neural pathways, which makes the pain worse and difficult to control. Prevention of the initial postoperative pain should make subsequent pain management simpler.[13,14]

The use of a variety of medications at relatively low doses is another new method, which is referred to as multimodal analgesia because it takes advantage of the multiple pain modulators. Using a variety of medications, which affect different steps along the pain pathway, results in lower narcotic use and fewer adverse side effects.

Multimodal pain management combined with preemptive analgesia results in optimal pain control. The preoperative phase includes patient education and preemptive analgesia. Preoperative education includes a frank discussion with the patient concerning issues related to pain management, including realistic goals in the perioperative period.

Intraoperatively, both the narcotic (or other primary mediators) and the anti-inflammatory agents are injected directly at the surgical site. Postoperatively, patients are administered oral pain medications and anti-inflammatory agents. Liberal use of antiemetics helps the patients to avoid nausea and minimizes or eliminates the use of patient-controlled analgesia and parenteral narcotics.

Preemptive analgesia limits the sensitization of the nervous system to painful stimuli and blocks the transmission of noxious efferent information from the peripheral nervous system to the spinal cord and brain. Analgesic agents must be given before the incision and must be of sufficient magnitude to limit sensitization of the nervous system. Opioids, nonsteroidal anti-inflammatory drugs (NSAIDs), acetaminophen, clonidine, and ketamine have all been shown to be effective agents in protocols designed to induce preemptive analgesia.

Table 1
Preoperative and Perioperative Medications

Medication	Dose	Administration	Frequency
Celecoxib[a]	400 mg	Oral	The day before surgery and then daily for 3 days postoperatively
Oxycodone controlled release	10 to 20 mg	Oral	Prior to surgery (10 mg if patient is older than 75 years or reports sensitivity to narcotics) and then every 12 hours for 24 hours postoperatively
Oxycodone	5 to 10 mg	Oral	Every 4 hours as needed
Acetaminophen	1,000 mg	Oral	Three times a day
Ketorolac	30 mg	Intramuscular	Every 8 hours as needed (3 doses maximum)
Tramadol	50 to 100 mg	Oral	Every 6 hours as needed
Gabapentin	300 mg	Oral	At bedtime
Ondansetron	4 mg	Oral	As needed for nausea

[a]If the patient has a sulfa allergy, substitute 15 mg of meloxicam for the celecoxib.

Prostaglandin E_2 (PGE_2) is upregulated in the central nervous system and peripheral tissue during and after surgery, and high levels of PGE_2 are associated with increased pain scores on a visual analog scale.[15-17] PGE_2 does not directly activate nociceptors but facilitates pain transmission by sensitizing nociceptors from mechanical and chemical stimuli, leading to central sensitization and lowering the pain threshold in the surrounding uninjured tissue. Patients with higher PGE_2 levels needed a longer time to achieve milestones in physical therapy, including the time to walk distances of 10 m and 25 m, the time needed to get out of bed, and the time needed to climb steps.[15] Perioperative multimodal analgesia can reduce the peripheral PGE_2 levels. A prostaglandin inhibitor (this chapter's authors prefer a cyclooxygenase-2 [COX-2] inhibitor) administered both preoperatively and postoperatively limits prostaglandin release, preventing the usual nervous system sensitization associated with surgical trauma. The authors of this chapter treat their patients with 400 mg of celecoxib (or 15 mg of meloxicam if the patient has a sulfa allergy) for 2 days before surgery and with 20 mg of oxycodone extended release (10 mg for a patient who is older than 75 years or has a narcotic sensitivity) 1 hour before surgery.

Buvanendran et al,[18] in 2003 performed a randomized placebo-controlled double-blind trial of treatment with or without oral rofecoxib in patients undergoing primary total knee arthroplasty with spinal and epidural anesthesia. Patients in the treatment arm were administered oral rofecoxib immediately before and for 13 days after the surgery. All patients were evaluated for pain, nausea, sleep disturbance, and knee range of motion. Patients who received the COX-2 inhibitor had less opioid consumption, pain, vomiting, and sleep disturbance and had improved knee range of motion at 1 month after surgery. Increased plasma levels of the COX-2 inhibitor at the beginning of the surgery were associated with decreased analgesic consumption postoperatively.

During the postoperative recovery, 400 mg of celecoxib are administered daily for 3 days; 10 to 20 mg of oxycodone controlled release (depending on age) for the first 24 hours after surgery; 5 to 10 mg of oxycodone every 4 hours, as needed; 1,000 mg of acetaminophen every 8 hours, as needed; 30 mg of ketorolac given intramuscularly every 8 hours (three doses maximum), 50 to 100 mg of tramadol every 6 hours, as needed; and ondansetron, as needed, for nausea (**Table 1**).

At discharge, the patient is advised to take 200 mg of celecoxib orally every day for 6 weeks and one or two 5/500-mg hydrocodone/acetaminophen tablets orally every 4 hours, as needed (**Table 2**). Elevated interleukin (IL)-6 and IL-8 levels are associated with an increased frequency of sleep disturbance. Gabapentin has been added because it has been shown to improve sleep disturbances associated with pain.[19,20]

All NSAIDs can induce cardiac toxicity. Therefore, COX-2-inhibitors should be avoided in high-risk patients who have a history of cardiac ischemia, stroke, congestive heart failure, or recent coronary artery bypass surgery.

Other Medications
Acetaminophen is often used in perioperative pain protocols. The mechanism of action of this drug is poorly un-

Table 2

Discharge Medications

Medication	Dose	Administration	Frequency
Celecoxib[a]	200 mg	Oral	Daily for 6 weeks
Hydrocodone	5/500 mg (1 to 2 tablets)	Oral	Every 4 hours as needed
Gabapentin	300 mg	Oral	At bedtime

[a]If the patient has a sulfa allergy, substitute 7.5 mg of meloxicam for the celecoxib.

derstood but leads to a decreased need for opioids.

Gabapentin was first developed as an anticonvulsant. When used preoperatively, it enhances the effect of morphine, NSAIDs, and COX-2 inhibitors. The adverse side effects of gabapentin include dizziness and somnolence with long-term use.

Clonidine is an α2-adrenergic agonist. Its mechanism of action of analgesia is unknown. Theoretically, it potentiates the effects of local anesthetics. It is administered intravenously or locally. Clonidine is presently used in some multimodal pain management protocols.

Ketamine is a general analgesic and a noncompetitive N-methyl-D-aspartate receptor and inhibitor. The N-methyl-D-aspartate receptors are associated with central sensitization. Ketamine has opioid-sparing effects but no reduction in opioid-related adverse effects. Intravenous ketamine can be used in conjunction with femoral nerve blocks or epidural analgesia after total knee arthroplasty. It can also be infiltrated into the wound.

Surgical Anesthesia Options

Overall pain relief is better with a regional anesthesia, blocks, and local injections than with general anesthesia.[21] Epidural anesthesia is a popular method of anesthesia for total knee replacement, and a meta-analysis of studies on epidural anesthesia has suggested that, regardless of the analgesic agent or location of the catheter, epidural analgesia provided superior postoperative analgesia compared with parenteral opioids.[22] Risks associated with this modality include motor block, numbness in the contralateral lower extremity, ileus, pressure phenomenon, pruritus, epidural hematoma, nausea and vomiting, technical issues, and limitations on anticoagulation choices, all of which can prolong hospitalization and delay rehabilitation.

Peripheral nerve blocks may be better. Barrington et al[23] compared femoral nerve block with epidural analgesia after total knee replacement and found equivalent pain scores, knee range of motion, and rehabilitation outcomes among the groups, but significantly less nausea and vomiting in the femoral nerve block group. On the other hand, a femoral nerve block may produce motor loss and a need for support (such as a knee immobilizer) or bed rest, is technically difficult, provides less predictable pain relief, and often needs to be combined with other blocks to achieve relief of posterior knee pain.

This chapter's authors prefer regional anesthesia. A spinal anesthetic, in general, is a more predictable regional anesthetic, should be used unless contraindicated, and is the preferred form of anesthesia for patients undergoing total knee replacement. In 2009, Macfarlane et al[24] performed a systematic review and found that, although a regional anesthetic did not decrease blood loss compared with general anesthesia, it did reduce postoperative pain and morphine consumption.

This chapter's authors use a direct intra-articular injection of a so-called cocktail of medications during surgery to improve immediate postoperative pain, and have studied four different combinations of medications to establish which medications should be included in the injection. Four groups of 12 patients undergoing total knee replacement with similar anesthetics and the identical orally administered pain management and physiotherapy protocols were evaluated. The pain score on a visual analog scale and pain assessments by the nursing staff were recorded every 4 hours for 3 days, and knee range of motion, pain scores, and walking distance were recorded by the physical therapists at each session. There was a trend for superior pain control in the group receiving all four medications, and their functional outcomes were significantly superior.[25] The most successful anesthetic cocktail contains 5 mg/mL of ropivacaine (49.25 mL), 30 mg/mL of ketorolac (1 mL), 1 mg/mL of epinephrine (0.5 mL), 0.1 mg/mL of clonidine (0.08 mg = 0.8 mL), and normal saline solution, which is added to the medications, for a total of 100 mL (**Table 3**). This mixture is prepared by the pharmacy and is stored for up to 24 hours. The placement of the injections is important, and the total volume should be divided into quarters, with one quarter injected into the posterior capsule, one quarter into the medial periosteum and medial capsule, one quarter into the lateral periosteum and lateral capsule, and one quarter into the soft tissues around the skin incision (**Figures 1** and **2**).

Table 3

Intraoperative Management

	Medication	Dose
1	Spinal anesthesia	
2	Pericapsular injection[a]	Total of 100 mL
	Ropivacaine	5 mg/mL (49.25 mL)
	Epinephrine	1 mg/mL (0.5 mL)
	Ketorolac	30 mg/mL (1 mL)
	Clonidine	0.1 mg/mL (0.08 mg = 0.8 mL)
	Normal saline solution	48.45 mL

[a]The combined medication is premixed by the pharmacy and remains stable for 24 hours. The injection is made behind the knee into posterior soft tissues (30 mL); into the medial and lateral gutters, which should include the periosteum of the femur (25 mL); and then into subcutaneous tissue (20 mL). The location of the injection is key.

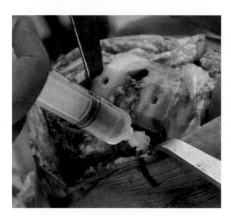

Figure 1 Injection into the posterior capsule of the knee.

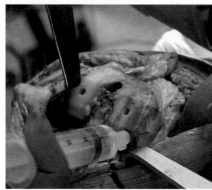

Figure 2 Injection into the periosteum and gutters of the femur.

Establishing a New Protocol for Total Knee Replacement Pain Management

Introducing a new pain management protocol requires the commitment of the surgeon; however, it also takes a team of committed anesthesiologists, pharmacists, physical therapists, and nursing staff to be successful. Education and patience are required to change from conventional methods of pain management after a total knee replacement. This chapter's authors have found that the effort is worthwhile, and believe that patients, staff, and surgeons can expect excellent perioperative and postoperative results.

References

1. Merskey H, Bogduk N, eds: *Classification of Chronic Pain*, ed 2. Seattle, WA, IASP Press, 1994, pp 209-214.

2. Trousdale RT, McGrory BJ, Berry DJ, Becker MW, Harmsen WS: Patients' concerns prior to undergoing total hip and total knee arthroplasty. *Mayo Clin Proc* 1999;74(10):978-982.

3. Ferrante FM, Orav EJ, Rocco AG, Gallo J: A statistical model for pain in patient-controlled analgesia and conventional intramuscular opioid regimens. *Anesth Analg* 1988;67(5):457-461.

4. American Pain Society: *Principles of Analgesic Use in the Treatment of Acute Pain and Cancer Pain*, ed 4. Glenview, IL, American Pain Society, 1999.

5. Riddle DL, Wade JB, Jiranek WA, Kong X: Preoperative pain catastrophizing predicts pain outcome after knee arthroplasty. *Clin Orthop Relat Res* 2010;468(3): 798-806.

6. Carragee EJ, Vittum D, Truong TP, Burton D: Pain control and cultural norms and expectations after closed femoral shaft fractures. *Am J Orthop (Belle Mead NJ)* 1999;28(2):97-102.

7. Anderson KO, Green CR, Payne R: Racial and ethnic disparities in pain: Causes and consequences of unequal care. *J Pain* 2009;10(12): 1187-1204.

8. Edwards RR, Doleys DM, Fillingim RB, Lowery D: Ethnic differences in pain tolerance: Clinical implications in a chronic pain population. *Psychosom Med* 2001;63(2):316-323.

9. Tseng CY, Wang SL, Lai MD, Lai ML, Huang JD: Formation of morphine from codeine in Chinese subjects of different CYP2D6 genotypes. *Clin Pharmacol Ther* 1996;60(2):177-182.

10. Wheeler M, Oderda GM, Ashburn MA, Lipman AG: Adverse events associated with postoperative opioid analgesia: A systematic review. *J Pain* 2002;3(3):159-180.

11. Sinatra RS, Torres J, Bustos AM: Pain management after major orthopaedic surgery: Current strategies and new concepts. *J Am Acad Orthop Surg* 2002;10(2): 117-129.

12. Macintyre PE: Safety and efficacy of patient-controlled analgesia. *Br J Anaesth* 2001;87(1):36-46.

13. Bridenbaugh PO: Preemptive analgesia: Is it clinically relevant? *Anesth Analg* 1994;78(2):203-204.

14. Katz J, Kavanagh BP, Sandler AN, et al: Preemptive analgesia: Clinical evidence of neuroplasticity contributing to postoperative pain. *Anesthesiology* 1992;77(3):439-446.

15. Buvanendran A, Kroin JS, Berger RA, et al: Upregulation of prostaglandin E2 and interleukins in the central nervous system and peripheral tissue during and after surgery in humans. *Anesthesiology* 2006;104(3):403-410.

16. Funk CD: Prostaglandins and leukotrienes: Advances in eicosanoid biology. *Science* 2001;294(5548):1871-1875.

17. Ebersberger A, Grubb BD, Willingale HL, Gardiner NJ, Nebe J, Schaible HG: The intraspinal release of prostaglandin E2 in a model of acute arthritis is accompanied by an up-regulation of cyclo-oxygenase-2 in the spinal cord. *Neuroscience* 1999;93(2):775-781.

18. Buvanendran A, Kroin JS, Tuman KJ, et al: Effects of perioperative administration of a selective cyclooxygenase 2 inhibitor on pain management and recovery of function after knee replacement: A randomized controlled trial. *JAMA* 2003;290(18):2411-2418.

19. Foldvary-Schaefer N, De Leon Sanchez I, Karafa M, Mascha E, Dinner D, Morris HH: Gabapentin increases slow-wave sleep in normal adults. *Epilepsia* 2002;43(12):1493-1497.

20. Takemura Y, Yamashita A, Horiuchi H, et al: Effects of gabapentin on brain hyperactivity related to pain and sleep disturbance under a neuropathic pain-like state using fMRI and brain wave analysis. *Synapse* 2011;65(7):668-676.

21. Busch CA, Shore BJ, Bhandari R, et al: Efficacy of periarticular multimodal drug injection in total knee arthroplasty: A randomized trial. *J Bone Joint Surg Am* 2006;88(5):959-963.

22. Block BM, Liu SS, Rowlingson AJ, Cowan AR, Cowan JA Jr, Wu CL: Efficacy of postoperative epidural analgesia: A meta-analysis. *JAMA* 2003;290(18):2455-2463.

23. Barrington MJ, Olive D, Low K, Scott DA, Brittain J, Choong P: Continuous femoral nerve blockade or epidural analgesia after total knee replacement: A prospective randomized controlled trial. *Anesth Analg* 2005;101(6):1824-1829.

24. Macfarlane AJ, Prasad GA, Chan VW, Brull R: Does regional anesthesia improve outcome after total knee arthroplasty? *Clin Orthop Relat Res* 2009;467(9):2379-2402.

25. Dalury DF, Kelley T, Adams MJ: Poster No. P142 Abstract: Efficacy of multimodal perioperative analgesia protocol with periarticular drug injection in total knee arthroplasty. A randomized, double blind study. *AAOS 2011 Annual Meeting Proceedings, Volume 12*. DVD. Rosemont, IL, American Academy of Orthopaedic Surgeons, 2011, p 551.

Multimodal Pain Management With Peripheral Nerve Blocks for Total Knee Arthroplasty

Michael R. Pagnotto, MD
Mark W. Pagnano, MD

Abstract

Multimodal pain management techniques using femoral and sciatic nerve blocks can dramatically improve a patient's experience after total knee arthroplasty. Nerve blocks reduce postoperative pain and the need for parenteral opioids and result in fewer medical complications associated with opioid use. Peripheral nerve blocks have traditionally been underutilized in lower extremity surgery; however, more modern techniques now allow for safe, efficient, and reliable femoral and sciatic blocks. Peripheral nerve blocks are now routinely used in both primary and revision total knee arthroplasty. Although it is difficult to isolate the added benefit of sciatic nerve blocks, there is a growing body of evidence for using femoral and/or sciatic nerve blocks as part of a multimodal approach to pain management. With many years of experience and published results on thousands of patients, it is clear that the risks of peripheral nerve blocks are minimal, whereas the benefits are substantial.

Instr Course Lect 2012;61:389-395.

Multimodal pain management techniques after total knee arthroplasty (TKA) have been shown to be reliable, reproducible, and safe in optimizing postoperative pain control and minimizing systemic opioid usage.[1-4] Peripheral nerve blocks, either single-injection or via a continuous-infusion catheter, provide excellent pain relief when used as part of a contemporary multimodal pain management regimen. When coupled with a comprehensive pain management approach, peripheral nerve blocks have dramatically decreased postoperative pain and markedly improved the overall patient experience after TKA.[1-4] Minimizing opioid use has helped to lower the rates of many opioid-induced complications (nausea, vomiting, excessive sedation, and disorientation) that were once accepted as an inevitable part of the postoperative course after TKA.

When compared with nerve blocks for upper extremity surgery, nerve blocks for lower extremity surgery have traditionally been underutilized.[5] That underutilization stems from at least two sources. First, it was previously believed that traditional anesthetic techniques provided adequate and appropriate pain control after TKA; however, it is now clear that, for many patients, traditional pain management techniques relying primarily on narcotics delivered via a patient-controlled analgesic device achieve suboptimal pain control and are associated with a substantial number of adverse side effects.[6] Second, lower extremity nerve blocks were historically more technically demanding to perform compared with upper extremity blocks.[3] Recent advances in high-quality, portable ultrasound technology (that allows real-time visualization of peripheral nerves), as well as nerve-stimulating needles and improved peripheral catheter systems, have made lower extremity nerve blocks reliable, reproducible, and safe for anesthesiologists to perform for a broader range of patients.[3,7]

Neither Dr. Pagnotto nor any immediate family member has received anything of value from or owns stock in a commercial company or institution related directly or indirectly to the subject of this chapter. Dr. Pagnano or an immediate family member has received royalties from DePuy and Mako; has received research or institutional support from Zimmer; and serves as a board member, owner, officer, or committee member of the Knee Society.

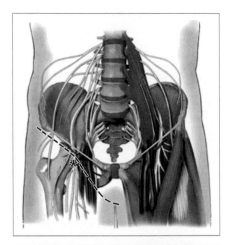

Figure 1 Illustration of the femoral nerve block. The needle is inserted 1 to 2 cm lateral to the femoral arterial pulsation at the level of the inguinal crease. A 5-cm needle is advanced until a quadriceps response is noted, and 20 mL of local anesthetic is incrementally injected. * = the femoral nerve, dashed line = the inguinal crease. (Reproduced with permission from the Mayo Foundation for Medical Education and Research, Rochester, MN.)

Indications

Peripheral nerve blocks are indicated in both primary and revision TKA. Nerve blocks can be used with minimally invasive techniques, and the benefits of improved pain control and decreased opiate consumption also are applicable to traditional surgical techniques. Although peripheral nerve blocks can be used to deliver complete lower extremity anesthesia, they are more commonly used to deliver postoperative analgesia in conjunction with either intraoperative general or spinal anesthesia. However, if placed preoperatively, the analgesic effects of peripheral nerve blocks frequently allow lighter general anesthesia or a shorter-acting spinal anesthesia than would be expected.

Contraindications

There are few absolute contraindications for lower extremity peripheral nerve blocks. For obvious reasons, nerve blocks should not be performed through areas of local infection. Relative contraindications are debatable. A severe coagulopathy may be considered a relative contraindication, but simply having an elevated international normalized ratio is not a contraindication for either a femoral or a sciatic block. Coagulopathy is more of a concern when performing a posterior lumbar plexus (psoas) block because of the risk of retroperitoneal hematoma or bleeding into the central nervous system. A history of peripheral nerve injury or a baseline neuropathy requires consideration but is not an absolute contraindication. In some medical practices, it is not uncommon to use a femoral nerve block and forego a sciatic block in a patient with a history of peripheral neuropathy. Similarly, some surgeons prefer not to use nerve blocks in particularly complex cases or cases in which there is a heightened concern for intraoperative nerve injury. For example, some surgeons prefer to avoid sciatic blocks in a patient with a fixed valgus deformity of the knee so that the peroneal nerve can be assessed immediately after surgery. One alternative in more complex cases is to perform the femoral nerve block preoperatively and then to proceed with a postoperative sciatic nerve block after normal peroneal function is documented by the postoperative neurologic examination. However, some experienced surgeons are comfortable using both sciatic and femoral blocks when treating a valgus deformity or performing a complex revision TKA.

Techniques

Femoral Nerve Blocks

Femoral nerve blocks can be achieved through psoas, femoral, or fascia iliaca approaches. Psoas blocks are not typically needed in TKA (but are quite useful after total hip arthroplasty) because a psoas block includes the femoral, obturator, and lateral femoral cutaneous nerves.[8] Because it is not clear that blocking the obturator nerve and the lateral femoral cutaneous nerves provides additional pain relief after TKA, many surgeons prefer to use a femoral or a fascial iliaca approach. Both approaches reliably block the femoral nerve but not the obturator or the lateral femoral cutaneous nerves.[8,9] For TKA, this chapter's authors prefer an indwelling femoral nerve catheter (**Figure 1**), with a fascia-iliaca perineural catheter as the secondary choice (**Figure 2**). The indwelling femoral nerve catheter technique used at the Mayo Clinic has been well described by Hebl et al.[1,2] The catheter is initially bolused with bupivacaine 0.5% (20 mL) and 1:200,000 epinephrine. In the postanesthesia care unit, the catheter is again bolused with 10 mL of 0.2% bupivacaine, and a continuous infusion of 0.2% bupivacaine is started at 10 mL/h. On the morning of postoperative day 1, the catheter infusion is changed to 0.1% bupivacaine at 12 mL/h for an additional 24 hours. The catheter is removed the morning of postoperative day 2.[1,2]

Sciatic Nerve Blocks

To achieve complete unilateral lower extremity anesthesia or maximize postoperative analgesia, the femoral nerve block must be combined with a sciatic block.[5] The need for some type of sciatic block in TKA has been described.[10,11] This chapter's authors prefer to augment the indwelling femoral or fascia iliaca continuous infusion block with a single-injection sciatic block (**Figure 3**). The sciatic block provides analgesic coverage of the entire posterior thigh and leg, with the exception of the saphenous nerve but including the posterior femoral cutaneous nerve.[12] The sciatic block markedly improves immediate postoperative pain control after TKA because patients commonly report early posterior knee pain.[12] For the sciatic nerve block, a single injection of 30 mL of 0.5% bupivacaine with 1:200,000 epinephrine is used.[1,2] If a sciatic block is not possible, a local intraoperative periarticular injection into the posterior capsule is recommended to improve postoperative posterior knee pain.

Results

Femoral Nerve Block

The benefits of femoral nerve blocks in TKA are well documented.[13-16] In a randomized controlled trial comparing a continuous femoral nerve block, patient-controlled intravenous analgesia, or epidural analgesia, the patients receiving the continuous femoral nerve block reported significantly lower pain scores, fewer adverse side effects, better knee flexion up to 6 weeks after surgery, faster ambulation, and a shorter hospital stay than those receiving patient-controlled analgesia.[16] In another study comparing a continuous femoral block with bupivacaine versus a continuous femoral block with placebo, the 0.2% bupivacaine group had reduced opioid requirements and improved range of motion.[15] Longer-term follow-up also has been assessed. In a study comparing a high-dose continuous femoral nerve block, a low-dose continuous femoral nerve block, and no femoral nerve block, the authors reported less pain, higher satisfaction, and lower morphine consumption in the immediate postoperative period in both groups receiving a femoral nerve block compared to those receiving no nerve block.[17] At 2 years, there was no significant difference between any of the groups in terms of functional outcome.

The authors of a recent meta-analysis analyzed 23 randomized controlled trials comparing a femoral nerve block with patient-controlled

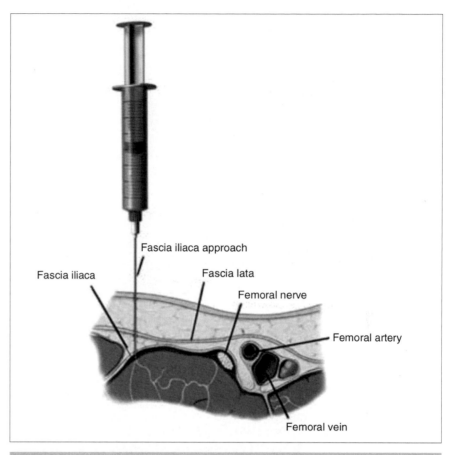

Figure 2   Illustration showing the fascia iliaca approach to a femoral nerve block. The inguinal ligament is identified, the junction of its lateral one third with its medial two thirds is determined, and a 17-gauge Tuohy needle is inserted 1 cm below this point. An initial loss of resistance is noted as the needle penetrates the fascia lata, and a second loss of resistance is felt as the needle penetrates the fascia iliaca; 30 mL of local anesthetic is incrementally injected. (Reproduced with permission from the Mayo Foundation for Medical Education and Research, Rochester, MN.)

analgesia or epidural analgesia.[18] Although the added benefits of continuous femoral nerve blocks were difficult to separate, the authors found clear evidence that single-shot femoral nerve blocks reduced patient-controlled morphine consumption at 24 and 48 hours after surgery, decreased activity-related pain scores at 24 and 48 hours, and reduced the incidence of postoperative nausea.[18] The authors concluded that the benefit of single-injection femoral nerve blocks was clear, and the potential benefit of continuous femoral nerve blocks and/or sciatic blocks warrants further study.

Sciatic Nerve Block

Multiple studies have demonstrated the benefit of combined sciatic and femoral nerve blocks when compared with no block.[19-21] However, unlike the proven benefits of femoral nerve blocks, the added benefits of using a sciatic nerve block are more controversial. In theory, a sciatic nerve block will help relieve pain in the popliteal space. In one prospective study, patients were randomized to receiving either a continuous femoral nerve block or continuous femoral and sciatic nerve blocks.[11] The group of patients who received both the femoral and sciatic

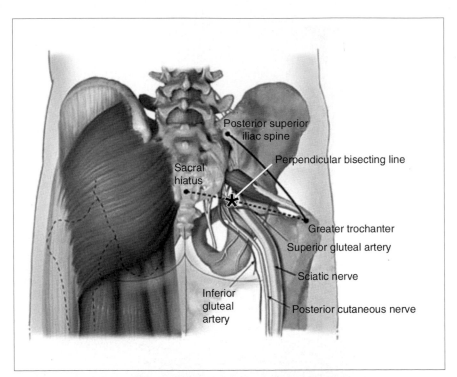

Figure 3   Illustration showing the classic posterior approach to the sciatic nerve. The needle insertion (*) is 5 cm along the perpendicular line (white line) that bisects a line connecting the greater trochanter and posterosuperior iliac spine (black line). The needle insertion is confirmed by the intersection of the perpendicular bisection line and a second line connecting the greater trochanter and sacral hiatus (black dashed line). A 10-cm stimulating needle is advanced until a tibial or peroneal motor response is elicited, then 20 to 30 mL of local anesthetic is incrementally injected. Light dashed lines = underlying osseous anatomy, light solid lines = gluteal fold. (Reproduced with permission from the Mayo Foundation for Medical Education and Research, Rochester, MN.)

blocks had an 81% decrease in morphine consumption and significantly less postoperative nausea and vomiting.[11] Another randomized trial compared three groups: femoral nerve block, femoral and sciatic nerve block, and psoas compartment block.[22] The femoral and sciatic nerve block group had reduced opiate consumption over the first 48 postoperative hours when compared with the other two groups.[22]

The potential additional benefit of a sciatic block with a femoral block was less clear when reviewed in the meta-analysis by Paul et al.[18] Although a single-shot femoral block, a single-shot femoral block with sciatic block, and a continuous femoral block all resulted in less morphine consumption when compared with patient-controlled analgesia alone at 24 and 48 hours postoperatively, there was no difference noted between a single-shot femoral nerve block compared with a single-shot femoral nerve block with an additional sciatic block. Because the additional benefits of sciatic nerve blocks may be small, some authors argue that the small benefit is not worth the theoretic risks.[23] The concern is that sciatic blocks may either potentiate an intraoperative nerve injury or mask a nerve injury in the postoperative period and therefore delay diagnosis and treatment.[23] Some surgeons prefer to use a femoral nerve block and inject the posterior capsule intraoperatively to help reduce pain in the popliteal space. Despite the largely theoretic risks, many institutions continue to use both femoral and sciatic blocks as the focal point of a comprehensive multimodal anesthesia protocol.[1-3] At the Mayo Clinic, a recent unpublished poll of orthopaedic anesthesiologists found widespread support for the contention that the addition of a sciatic block markedly improves pain relief after TKA, whereas orthopaedic surgeons remain divided on the relative merits of continuous femoral plus sciatic nerve blocks versus a continuous femoral block alone.

Complications

The two main types of potential complications associated with peripheral nerve blocks in TKA are the risk of direct nerve injury and the risk of complications that are secondary to the effects of well-functioning nerve blocks. The risk of direct nerve injury has been shown to be small.[24] A recent study examined all of the perioperative nerve injuries over a 20-year period at the Mayo Clinic.[24] The authors identified 97 cases of perioperative nerve injury in 12,329 patients treated with an elective TKA. Of the 12,329 TKA patients, 3,883 received peripheral nerve blocks for supplemental analgesia. The overall incidence of nerve injury was 0.79% in all patients, regardless of the type of nerve blockade. Perioperative nerve injury was not associated with peripheral nerve blocks. Young patients were less likely to sustain a nerve injury, whereas increased tourniquet time and bilateral procedures increased the risk of nerve injury. Interestingly, the authors found that patients who had peripheral nerve blocks and sustained a perioperative nerve injury were less likely to have full neurologic recovery.[24]

Although it is recognized that the risk of direct neurologic injury secondary to nerve blocks is low, some authors have reported complications that may be secondary to nerve blocks. Falls, knee dislocations, and heel ulcers have all been reported in association with peripheral nerve blocks after TKA.[25-28] A recent study attempted to quantify the risks of femoral nerve blocks in TKA.[26] The authors reviewed the complication rate in 709 single-shot femoral nerve blocks for TKA and found a 1.6% rate of falls and a 0.4% rate of reoperation secondary to falls.[26] The authors attributed the falls to decreased quadriceps function secondary to the blocks and recommended modified postoperative protocols for patients who receive a femoral nerve block. Although quadriceps weakness increases a patient's risk for falling, it is not clear that there is a higher rate of postoperative falls in patients who have nerve blocks. Certainly, some patients treated with TKA sustain falls even in the absence of nerve blocks. To minimize the risk of a fall, some institutions routinely place patients in a knee immobilizer while the block is in place (removing it during physical therapy for range-of-motion exercises), and other institutions use a comprehensive prehospital and in-hospital patient education program that emphasizes partial weight bearing until the nerve block has resolved.

Peripheral nerve blocks have the added benefit of decreasing some medical complications traditionally associated with postoperative opioid use. In a systematic review of adverse events associated with postoperative opioid analgesia, Wheeler et al[29] reported a 37% rate of adverse gastrointestinal effects, a 34% rate of cognitive adverse effects, urinary retention in 16% of patients, pruritus in 15%, and respiratory depression in 2%. A postoperative

pain regimen that minimizes opiate use can eliminate many complications that were once believed to be an inevitable part of TKA recovery. Data from the Mayo Clinic show a substantial decrease in the risks of postoperative ileus (1% versus 7%), urinary retention (31% versus 50%), and postoperative cognitive dysfunction (0% versus 15%) when comparing a multimodal anesthesia protocol (**Table 1**) to a matched historical control group, respectively, undergoing TKA and total hip arthroplasty.[1,2]

Summary

Multimodal pain regimens featuring peripheral nerve blocks have helped to dramatically improve the experiences of patients after TKA. With modern techniques, both femoral and sciatic blocks can be performed reliably, efficiently, and safely. The data are clear that femoral nerve blocks reduce pain and postoperative opiate consumption, and sciatic blocks may have an additional benefit. The risk of complications associated with nerve blocks using contemporary techniques is low,

---

Table 1

Mayo Clinic Multimodal Pain Management Regimen for TKA

Preemptive Analgesia (Given in Surgical Preparation Room)

Oxycodone controlled release 10 mg by mouth once if patient is age 15 to 59 years or 20 mg if patient is age 60 to 74 years

Gabapentin 600 mg by mouth

Celecoxib 400 mg by mouth

Nerve blocks

Femoral: indwelling catheter bolus with 20 mL of 0.5% bupivacaine and 1:200,000 epinephrine

Sciatic: single-shot 30 mL of 0.5% bupivacaine with 1:200,000 epinephrine

Intraoperative Anesthesia

Spinal anesthesia preferred

Postoperative Analgesia (Given in Postanesthesia Care Unit)

Femoral nerve catheter: bolus 10 mL of 0.2% bupivacaine; then continuous infusion 10 mL/h 0.2% bupivacaine

Oxycodone 5 mg and acetaminophen 500 mg by mouth as required for pain

Fentanyl 25 μg intravenously as needed for pain

Ketorolac 15 mg intravenously as needed for pain

Patient Care Unit

Femoral nerve catheter: Postoperative day 1 infusion reduced to 12 mL/h of 0.1% bupivacaine; removed morning of postoperative day 2

Acetaminophen 1,000 mg every 6 hours

Tramadol 50-100 mg as needed for pain every 6 hours

Oxycodone 5-10 mg as needed for breakthrough pain every 4 hours

Patient Mobilization

Sit in chair the evening of surgery

Patients are counseled on fall prevention

Ambulate with weight bearing as tolerated with assistance on postoperative day 1

Ambulate independently and climb stairs after femoral block is removed on postoperative day 2

Pain controlled with oral medication, and patient discharged from hospital on postoperative day 2 or 3

---

whereas the benefits of avoiding parenteral opioid medications are substantial.

References

1. Hebl JR, Dilger JA, Byer DE, et al: A pre-emptive multimodal pathway featuring peripheral nerve block improves perioperative outcomes after major orthopedic surgery. *Reg Anesth Pain Med* 2008;33(6):510-517.

2. Hebl JR, Kopp SL, Ali MH, et al: A comprehensive anesthesia protocol that emphasizes peripheral nerve blockade for total knee and total hip arthroplasty. *J Bone Joint Surg Am* 2005;87(Suppl 2):63-70.

3. Horlocker TT, Kopp SL, Pagnano MW, Hebl JR: Analgesia for total hip and knee arthroplasty: A multimodal pathway featuring peripheral nerve block. *J Am Acad Orthop Surg* 2006;14(3):126-135.

4. Vendittoli PA, Makinen P, Drolet P, et al: A multimodal analgesia protocol for total knee arthroplasty: A randomized, controlled study. *J Bone Joint Surg Am* 2006; 88(2):282-289.

5. Enneking FK, Chan V, Greger J, Hadzić A, Lang SA, Horlocker TT: Lower-extremity peripheral nerve blockade: Essentials of our current understanding. *Reg Anesth Pain Med* 2005;30(1): 4-35.

6. Filos KS, Lehmann KA: Current concepts and practice in postoperative pain management: Need for a change? *Eur Surg Res* 1999; 31(2):97-107.

7. Birnbaum J, Kip M, Spies CD, et al: The effect of stimulating versus nonstimulating catheters for continuous interscalene plexus blocks in short-term pain management. *J Clin Anesth* 2007;19(6): 434-439.

8. Awad IT, Duggan EM: Posterior lumbar plexus block: Anatomy, approaches, and techniques. *Reg Anesth Pain Med* 2005;30(2): 143-149.

9. Kardash K, Hickey D, Tessler MJ, Payne S, Zukor D, Velly AM: Obturator versus femoral nerve block for analgesia after total knee arthroplasty. *Anesth Analg* 2007; 105(3):853-858.

10. Ben-David B, Schmalenberger K, Chelly JE: Analgesia after total knee arthroplasty: Is continuous sciatic blockade needed in addition to continuous femoral blockade? *Anesth Analg* 2004;98(3): 747-749.

11. Pham Dang C, Gautheron E, Guilley J, et al: The value of adding sciatic block to continuous femoral block for analgesia after total knee replacement. *Reg Anesth Pain Med* 2005;30(2):128-133.

12. Krych AJ, Horlocker TT, Hebl JR, Pagnano MW: Contemporary pain management strategies for minimally invasive total knee arthroplasty. *Instr Course Lect* 2010; 59:99-109.

13. Capdevila X, Barthelet Y, Biboulet P, Ryckwaert Y, Rubenovitch J, d'Athis F: Effects of perioperative analgesic technique on the surgical outcome and duration of rehabilitation after major knee surgery. *Anesthesiology* 1999;91(1): 8-15.

14. Chelly JE, Greger J, Gebhard R, et al: Continuous femoral blocks improve recovery and outcome of patients undergoing total knee arthroplasty. *J Arthroplasty* 2001; 16(4):436-445.

15. Ganapathy S, Wasserman RA, Watson JT, et al: Modified continuous femoral three-in-one block for postoperative pain after total knee arthroplasty. *Anesth Analg* 1999;89(5):1197-1202.

16. Singelyn FJ, Deyaert M, Joris D, Pendeville E, Gouverneur JM: Effects of intravenous patient-controlled analgesia with morphine, continuous epidural analgesia, and continuous three-in-one block on postoperative pain and knee rehabilitation after unilateral total knee arthroplasty. *Anesth Analg* 1998;87(1):88-92.

17. Shum CF, Lo NN, Yeo SJ, Yang KY, Chong HC, Yeo SN: Continuous femoral nerve block in total knee arthroplasty: Immediate and two-year outcomes. *J Arthroplasty* 2009;24(2): 204-209.

18. Paul JE, Arya A, Hurlburt L, et al: Femoral nerve block improves analgesia outcomes after total knee arthroplasty: A meta-analysis of randomized controlled trials. *Anesthesiology* 2010;113(5): 1144-1162.

19. Hunt KJ, Bourne MH, Mariani EM: Single-injection femoral and sciatic nerve blocks for pain control after total knee arthroplasty. *J Arthroplasty* 2009;24(4): 533-538.

20. McNamee DA, Convery PN, Milligan KR: Total knee replacement: A comparison of ropivacaine and bupivacaine in combined femoral and sciatic block. *Acta Anaesthesiol Scand* 2001;45(4):477-481.

21. Zaric D, Boysen K, Christiansen C, Christiansen J, Stephensen S, Christensen B: A comparison of epidural analgesia with combined continuous femoral-sciatic nerve blocks after total knee replacement. *Anesth Analg* 2006;102(4):1240-1246.

22. Morin AM, Kratz CD, Eberhart LH, et al: Postoperative analgesia and functional recovery after total-knee replacement: Comparison of a continuous posterior lumbar plexus (psoas compartment) block, a continuous femoral nerve block, and the combination of a continuous femoral and sciatic nerve block. *Reg Anesth Pain Med* 2005;30(5):434-445.

23. Levesque S, Delbos A: Sciatic nerve block for total-knee replacement: Is it really necessary in all patients? *Reg Anesth Pain Med* 2005;30(4):410-411.

24. Jacob AK, Mantilla CB, Sviggum HP, Schroeder DR, Pagnano MW, Hebl JR: Perioperative nerve injury after total knee arthroplasty: Regional anesthesia risk during a 20-year cohort study. *Anesthesiology* 2011;114(2): 311-317.

25. Apsingi S, Dussa CU: Can peripheral nerve blocks contribute to heel ulcers following total knee replacement? *Acta Orthop Belg* 2004;70(5):502-504.

26. Sharma S, Iorio R, Specht LM, Davies-Lepie S, Healy WL: Complications of femoral nerve block for total knee arthroplasty. *Clin Orthop Relat Res* 2010;468(1): 135-140.

27. Sisak K, Lloyd J, Fiddian N: Multi-ligament instability after early dislocation of a primary total knee replacement: Case report. *Knee* 2011;18(1):59-61.

28. Todkar M: Sciatic nerve block causing heel ulcer after total knee replacement in 36 patients. *Acta Orthop Belg* 2005;71(6):724-725.

29. Wheeler M, Oderda GM, Ashburn MA, Lipman AG: Adverse events associated with postoperative opioid analgesia: A systematic review. *J Pain* 2002;3(3):159-180.

Complications After Total Knee Arthroplasty: How to Manage Patients With Osteolysis

Giles R. Scuderi, MD

Abstract

Total knee arthroplasty generally is a highly successful orthopaedic procedure, but mechanical failure sometimes occurs. Debris particles, especially from polyethylene, can affect the long-term durability of the implant. Revision total knee arthroplasty is complex, and preoperative planning must consider alignment, stability, fixation, and knee motion. The reason for failure must be identified before complex reconstruction in the presence of osteolysis, and the procedure must appropriately augment the defective bone and place a stable, well-fixed implant.

Instr Course Lect 2012;61:397-404.

Total knee arthroplasty is one of the most successful orthopaedic procedures. It improves quality of life and has high patient satisfaction and excellent longevity, with survivorship of more than 90% at 15 to 20 years. However, mechanical failure remains a complication. Debris particles, especially from polyethylene, affect the long-term durability of the implants.[1-3] Polyethylene debris incites a chemical and cellular inflammatory reaction, resulting in bone resorption and osteolysis. The extent of the osteolysis is dependent on the volume, size, and shape of the polyethylene debris. The main causative factor leading to osteolysis is small particulate debris, which stimu-lates an inflammatory foreign-body cellular response, resulting in bone resorption.[4] In contrast, the large polyethylene particles associated with delamination of the polyethylene and fatigue wear do not elicit the same cellular response.[2,3]

Wear is a motion-driven abrasive or adhesive process, and delamination is a stress-driven mechanical process. In total knee arthroplasty, polyethylene wear occurs from a combination of rolling, sliding, and rotational motions on the bearing surfaces. Polyethylene damage in total knee arthroplasty occurs on the articular surface as abrasive wear due to the sliding motion of the femoral component on the tibia. Pit-ting, delamination, and flaking are caused by the cyclic loading and oxidation of the polyethylene. Tibial post wear in posterior stabilized designs can be seen as delamination, deformation, or fracture. Tibial backside wear occurs as abrasive wear, pitting, flaking, or delamination. The magnitude and degree of polyethylene wear are multifactorial and depend on the material properties of the implant along with the alignment and stability of the prosthesis.

There are numerous causes of osteolysis, including the component design, quality of the polyethylene, manufacturing process, and sterilization techniques.[2,3,5-9] The impact of the component design depends on the conformity of the femoral component on the tibial polyethylene articular surface and the resultant contact stress. Articular surface designs with small contact areas between the femoral and tibial components distribute forces over a limited area and increase the stress on the tibial polyethylene. Some posterior cruciate-retaining prostheses have this design feature, resulting in increased contact stress on the polyethylene and predisposing it to wear and osteolysis, especially if there is condy-lar liftoff and edge loading of the femoral component on the flat tibial

Dr. Scuderi or an immediate family member has received royalties from Zimmer and Salient Surgical; is a member of a speakers' bureau or has made paid presentations on behalf of Zimmer and Salient Surgical; serves as a paid consultant to Zimmer and Salient Surgical; and serves as a board member, owner, officer, or committee member of the Knee Society and the International Congress for Joint Reconstruction.

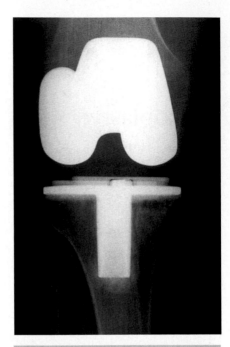

Figure 1 AP radiograph of a total knee replacement demonstrating a small area of osteolysis beneath the medial side of the tibial tray, which had subsided into mild varus alignment.

polyethylene surface. Furthermore, abnormal and erratic kinematics, such as paradoxical anterior femoral translation with flexion in some cruciate-retaining designs, potentially increases polyethylene wear.[10] Round-on-round designs are more conforming and lead to lower contact stresses and less polyethylene wear. These partially conforming designs improve anteroposterior stability and kinematics with a lower rate of polyethylene wear.[11] Retrieval studies have demonstrated that these more conforming designs have lower wear rates and fewer eccentric wear patterns than the less conforming designs.[5,12-14]

The introduction of modular tibial components resulted in new modes of failure of total knee replacement. Modular tibial baseplates with screw holes have been implicated as sources of polyethylene backside damage, and they create a portal for polyethylene

debris to enter the tibia. Some of the earliest reports on osteolysis implicated cementless designs with holes in the baseplate, tibial fixation screws, or discontinuous porous surfaces that served as conduits for debris, ultimately leading to osteolysis.[2,3] Later studies found that osteolysis also occurred in cemented designs with the invasion of the polyethylene debris through voids in the cement mantle.[7] Another design feature, introduced with the advent of tibial modularity, is the tibial polyethylene locking mechanism. Depending on the security of the locking mechanism, micromotion occurs between the tibial polyethylene and the baseplate, leading to backside wear of the tibial polyethylene component. Numerous studies have shown that micromotion between the tibial baseplate and polyethylene component occurs to a varying degree with most implant designs, and this motion progresses over time. The surface finish of the tibial baseplate also impacts the extent of backside wear. Manufacturers have attempted to reduce backside wear by improving the locking mechanism, improving mobile-bearing designs, and reintroducing monoblock tibial components.

Regarding the quality and manufacturing of the polyethylene, these factors vary among manufacturers.[15] The tibial polyethylene component is usually manufactured by either a net-shape molded technique or is machined from bar stock.[16] Machining of the polyethylene may predispose the polyethylene to surface and subsurface irregularities, which can lead to delamination and failure.[17] Compression-molded polyethylene has exhibited less wear than components machined from extruded bar stock. Finally, the method of sterilization impacts the mechanical properties and the durability of the tibial polyethylene component. Polyethylene sterilized by gamma

irradiation in air produces free radicals with oxidation of the polyethylene, which leads to premature mechanical failure, generation of polyethylene debris, and ultimately osteolysis. Current implants are sterilized in either ethylene oxide gas or gamma irradiation in an inert oxygen-free environment. The recent introduction of highly cross-linked polyethylene created a stronger three-dimensional structure of the polyethylene, resulting in improved wear-resistant polyethylene with less oxidation and a diminution of residual free radicals. Additional developments include the introduction of oxygen-quenching additives such as vitamin E (α-tocopherol) to further stabilize the polyethylene, improve the mechanical properties, and improve wear resistance.[18]

Osteolysis is a progressive condition that should be diagnosed early, and treatment should be initiated before a catastrophic failure, such as periprosthetic fracture or substantial bone loss that renders the revision arthroplasty more complicated.

Clinical Evaluation

Most patients who present with early osteolysis are asymptomatic, and osteolysis is an incidental radiographic finding. Osteolytic lesions are typically radiolucent lesions adjacent to the component. They may have a sclerotic border or thinning of the adjacent cortex (**Figure 1**). The implant may obscure the osteolysis, especially femoral osteolysis with posterior stabilized implants that have an intercondylar box. Oblique radiographs may help to visualize osteolysis in the posterior aspect of the femoral condyles, especially with a posterior stabilized prosthesis.[19] Radiographs tend to underestimate the extent of the osteolysis.[20] Multidetector CT is a useful imaging study to determine the extent of all lesions[21] (**Figure 2**). MRI with metal suppression has been recently used to evaluate the degree of osteolysis.[22]

Management of Osteolysis

Once an osteolytic lesion is identified, the goal is to intervene before component failure or periprosthetic fracture due to the bone loss. Management should address the reason for the osteolysis, restore the region of bone loss, and restore the appropriate component position and limb alignment with a stable implant.

Small areas of limited osteolysis are usually of little clinical importance, but these patients should be followed on an annual basis to determine whether the lesion is progressive or impacting the fixation of the prosthesis. Lesions that are asymptomatic, small, and nonprogressive usually require no treatment. Pharmacologic treatments, such as bisphosphonates and NSAIDs have been used to minimize the osteolytic process, but there are insufficient clinical data to support this course of treatment.[23]

Isolated osteolytic tibial lesions with well-fixed modular components, either cemented or cementless, with no malalignment, no malrotation, and no instability, may be treated with isolated tibial polyethylene exchange and impaction bone grafting of the lesion[24,25] (**Figure 3**). These lesions are usually incidental radiographic findings in asymptomatic patients but are concerning because of the size of the osteolytic lesion and the potential for later mechanical failure. It is important to determine the extent of the lesion, the integrity of the cortex, and the stability of the component fixation. Even when the above criteria are met, several other factors that must be considered include ensuring that the tibial locking mechanism is intact and functional, the new tibial polyethylene is of good quality and has not been on the shelf too long (an issue with older de-

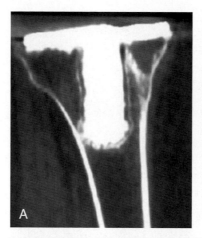
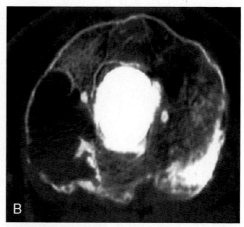

Figure 2 A coronal CT scan (**A**) showing a large area of osteolysis and an axial CT scan (**B**) showing large areas of osteolysis in the same area that was poorly visualized on the radiograph shown in Figure 1.

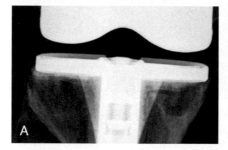
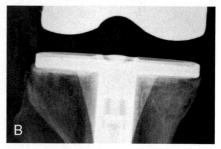

Figure 3 An osteolytic lesion in the medial aspect of the tibia beneath a well-fixed tibial component. **A**, AP radiograph made before revision. **B**, AP radiograph, made 5 years after tibial polyethylene exchange and impaction bone grafting, shows that the bone graft had incorporated and the tibial component had solid fixation.

signs), and there is no damage to the femoral surface or the tibial baseplate. If the femoral component surface is damaged, it should be exchanged because the irregular femoral surface will damage the new polyethylene tibial component.

Symptomatic patients with expanding osteolytic lesions or cortical disruption, loose components, instability, or periprosthetic fracture should have revision of the total knee replacement. This may involve either single-component revision or total revision. The amount of bone loss should be carefully assessed in planning the revision total knee arthroplasty.

Bone loss is common in revision total knee arthroplasty for osteolysis and can be compounded by subsidence of loose components, pathologic fracture, or removal of well-fixed components. The options available to treat the bone defects include the use of polymethyl methacrylate, autogenous bone graft, morcellized allogenic bone graft, structural bone allograft, modular augments, and megaprostheses.[26-37] The choice of augmentation is dependent on the degree of bone loss, patient age, and surgeon experience. Additional considerations include the need for implant stem extensions, the use of constrained prostheses, and the correction of anatomic deformity.[38]

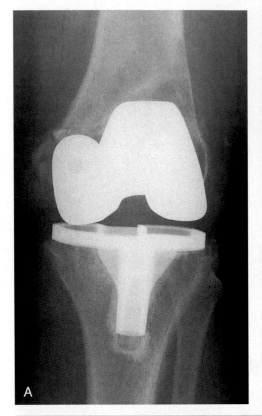
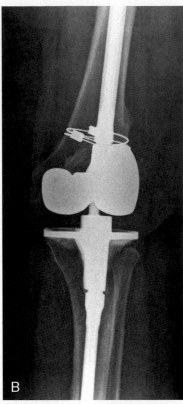

Figure 4 Medial tibial polyethylene wear, lateral joint-space widening, and a large osteolytic lesion in the lateral femoral condyle developed after a total knee replacement. **A,** AP radiograph made before revision. **B,** AP radiograph after revision total knee arthroplasty with the use of a long-stemmed constrained prosthesis with structural allograft of the distal end of the femur.

Preoperative assessment with radiographs is inadequate, but a CT scan will demonstrate the amount of bone loss. In a retrospective analysis of 31 patients with symptomatic total knee replacements who had osteolytic lesions, radiographs detected only 17% of the osteolytic lesions, whereas CT scans revealed lesions in all cases.[21] However, the intraoperative findings are often different from those predicted by imaging.[39] A useful classification system for bone loss is the Anderson Orthopaedic Research Institute (AORI) classification system, which grades the bone loss from the femur and the tibia independently as 1, 2, or 3.[8,10] The severity of bone loss and the proximity to the femoral epicondyles and the tibial tubercle determine the grade. Bone loss from the femoral condyles or tibial plateau is further subdivided into A or B, depending on whether one (A) or two sides (B) are involved. This classification system provides a useful guide for dealing with the degree of augmentation needed during revision arthroplasty.[32,40]

If the bone loss is minimal (AORI type 1) and the cortical rim is intact, the small cavitary defects can be augmented with bone cement or cancellous bone chips. In young patients, for whom bone preservation and restoration are important, impaction bone grafting of these bone defects has been valuable. For patients with greater bone loss (AORI type 2), structural allografts can provide a viable biologic option for restoration of the proximal part of the tibia or the distal part of the femur (**Figure 4**). Another easy option for AORI type 2 defects that is readily available in most revision systems is modular augmentation. These modular augments along with stem extensions—either press-fit or cemented—can be added to the femoral and tibial components and are useful in restoring the femoral and tibial components to their appropriate position. Modular augmentation helps to restore moderate-sized bone defects with biomechanically stable components to allow restoration of the proximal and distal femoral anatomy, assist in the creation of equal flexion and extension gaps during the revision procedure by restoring the joint line, and allow full weight bearing with functional motion. Severe bone loss (AORI type 3) results in a difficult revision arthroplasty and usually requires bulk structural allografts, tibial or femoral metaphyseal cones, or megaprostheses.

Modular revision implants with augmentation blocks or wedges facilitate the treatment of bone defects. These modular augments attach to the femoral and tibial components, are available in various shapes and sizes, and are fixed to the components with screws or cement. These augments are adaptable, allow intraoperative customization of the components, provide excellent biomechanical properties, and require minimal bone resection as the augments build off the residual bone. Femoral defects can be reconstructed, in most revision arthroplasty systems, with metal augments in increments of 5 mm. Because most bone loss is either from the distal end of the femur, the posterior condyles, or both, augments are fixed to the femoral component in an effort to restore the femoral anatomy, the posterior condylar offset, and the distal femoral joint line. Augmentation of the posterolateral part of the femur also assists with the rotational position of the

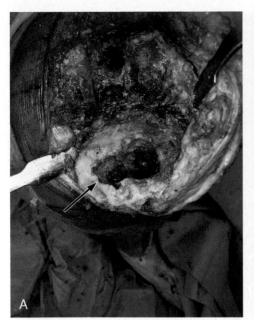
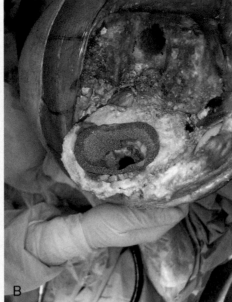
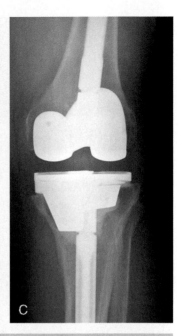

Figure 5   A knee with a large tibial osteolytic defect. **A,** Intraoperative photograph of the proximal part of the tibia showing a large area of osteolysis (arrow) in the central and medial aspects. **B,** Intraoperative photograph showing placement of a trabecular metal metaphyseal cone in the proximal end of the tibia. **C,** Postoperative AP radiograph of the trabecular metal cone filling the tibial osteolytic defect.

femoral component. The tibial modular augments are either wedges or blocks and assist in dealing with the bone defects and positioning the tibial component perpendicular to the mechanical axis. Modular wedges are useful when a loose tibial component subsides into a varus position with a resulting angular deformity, whereas tibial blocks are useful for revising a failed unicondylar knee replacement or a tibial defect that is more symmetric. With the use of modular augments in revision total knee arthroplasty, good or excellent results have been reported to range from 84% to 98%.[36,37]

The more challenging revision arthroplasties are those with substantial bone loss (AORI type 2B or 3). Reconstruction choices in these cases are modular augmentation, structural allograft, or megaprostheses. Trabecular metal cones and metaphyseal sleeves for the proximal part of the tibia and the distal end of the femur provide a modular alternative for metaphyseal augmentation

in patients with severe bone loss and provide a platform for the final components. Trabecular metal cones used in the proximal part of the tibia, implanted in a press-fit cementless manner, re-create the cortical rim and provide a stable platform for the final component. The variety of available shapes addresses both cancellous bone loss and cortical defects (**Figure 5**). The distal femoral cones help to reestablish the metaphyseal-diaphyseal junction and create a stable base for the femoral component. These modular constructs absorb compressive loads and provide both structural and mechanical support. The unique material properties of porous trabecular metal allow it to achieve rapid bone ingrowth and osseointegration with the potential for long-term biologic fixation and restoration of bone stock. Clinical studies with trabecular metal cones have demonstrated excellent short-term outcomes.[31,33] Further long-term studies are necessary to determine the durability of these new modular augments.

 Video 31.1: Trabecular Metal Tibial Cones for Proximal Tibial Bone Defects. Giles R. Scuderi, MD; Henrik B. Pedersen, MD (6 min)

With massive bone loss from osteolysis, it may be preferable, especially in younger patients, to attempt to restore the bone stock with structural allografts.[28,40] The advantage of this technique is that it is a biologic alternative with restoration of the distal end of the femur or the proximal part of the tibia. The disadvantages of structural allograft include nonunion, late collapse, and disease transmission or infection. Most clinical studies have noted clinical success when the allograft-prosthetic composite is rigidly fixed securely to the host bone.[41] Diaphyseal engaging implant stems are necessary to ensure stability and fixation. In the rare case of severe osteolysis in an older patient with a patho-

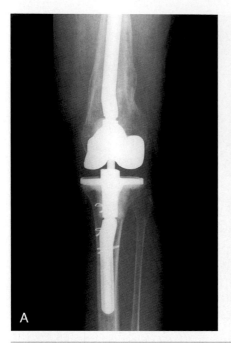 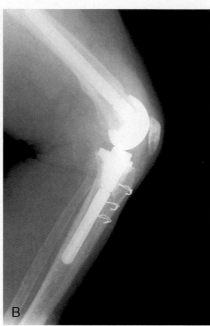

Figure 6 AP (**A**) and lateral (**B**) radiographs showing the utility of offset stems in both the femur and the tibia for achieving component position and fixation in revision total knee arthroplasty. The tibial tubercle osteotomy was used to improve surgical exposure, and wire fixation of the osteotomy was used.

Stem Fixation

In the presence of substantial osteolysis, fixation of the final components is important, and stem extensions are used to enhance the immediate stability of the implant in the residual bone. Methods of stem fixation are a controversial aspect of revision total knee arthroplasty. Some advocate the use of cemented stem fixation, whereas others advocate the use of cementless press-fit stem extensions. Each has its own advantages and disadvantages.[35,42] The length and diameter of the extensions should be determined on the basis of the integrity of the residual bone and the dimensions of the intramedullary canal.[36,43] Cemented stems allow for intraoperative adjustment with unusual anatomy and achieve fixation in large canals and osteopenic bone. It is recommended that short, narrow, non–canal-filling stem extensions be cemented. Longer diaphyseal stems should not be cemented. Cemented stems are difficult to remove if revision is necessary, and because they are not canal filling, they do not guarantee alignment.[44] Cementless press-fit stem extensions are easy to use and facilitate component alignment, and diaphyseal engaging stems ensure fixation. In revision total knee arthroplasty, the mechanical stability of the femoral and tibial components is increased by the addition of press-fit canal-filling stems, especially in the presence of poor metaphyseal bone quality or large bone defects.[43] Long modular stem extensions, which can be canal filling and diaphyseal engaging, can be used in a press-fit manner by cementing only the condylar and metaphyseal portions of the femoral prosthesis as well as the tibial surface and metaphysis of the tibial component. Whereas canal-filling stems are more predictable in guaranteeing alignment, anatomic variation may create the need for offset stems, especially in the tibia. In an anatomic study, Hicks et al[45] found that there was substantial variation in alignment between the center of the tibial plateau and the center of the tibial diaphyseal canal. Actual measurements of this difference ranged from 15 mm anterior to the center to 1.5 mm posterior to the center and 8 mm medial to the center to 4.5 mm lateral. Because of this variability, an offset tibial stem may be necessary in revision arthroplasty to ensure accurate alignment, secure fixation, and correct orientation of the tibial tray without overhang (**Figure 6**).

Summary

Revision total knee arthroplasty is a complex procedure that needs to address alignment, stability, fixation, and knee motion. For complex reconstruction in the presence of osteolysis, it is important to determine the reason for failure and then address the bone defects with appropriate augmentation of the bone loss and a stable well-fixed implant.

References

1. Engh GA, Ammeen DJ: Periprosthetic osteolysis with total knee arthroplasty. *Instr Course Lect* 2001;50:391-398.

2. Naudie DD, Ammeen DJ, Engh GA, Rorabeck CH: Wear and osteolysis around total knee arthroplasty. *J Am Acad Orthop Surg* 2007;15(1):53-64.

3. Naudie DD, Rorabeck CH: Sources of osteolysis around total knee arthroplasty: Wear of the bearing surface. *Instr Course Lect* 2004;53:251-259.

logic fracture, a megaprosthesis with either a distal femoral or a proximal tibial replacement may be an alternative.

4. Jacobs JJ, Roebuck KA, Archibeck M, Hallab NJ, Glant TT: Osteolysis: Basic science. *Clin Orthop Relat Res* 2001;393:71-77.

5. Fehring TK, Murphy JA, Hayes TD, Roberts DW, Pomeroy DL, Griffin WL: Factors influencing wear and osteolysis in press-fit condylar modular total knee replacements. *Clin Orthop Relat Res* 2004;428:40-50.

6. Huang CH, Ma HM, Liau JJ, Ho FY, Cheng CK: Osteolysis in failed total knee arthroplasty: A comparison of mobile-bearing and fixed-bearing knees. *J Bone Joint Surg Am* 2002;84(12): 2224-2229.

7. O'Rourke MR, Callaghan JJ, Goetz DD, Sullivan PM, Johnston RC: Osteolysis associated with a cemented modular posterior-cruciate-substituting total knee design: Five to eight-year follow-up. *J Bone Joint Surg Am* 2002; 84(8):1362-1371.

8. Tanner MG, Whiteside LA, White SE: Effect of polyethylene quality on wear in total knee arthroplasty. *Clin Orthop Relat Res* 1995;317:83-88.

9. Won CH, Rohatgi S, Kraay MJ, Goldberg VM, Rimnac CM: Effect of resin type and manufacturing method on wear of polyethylene tibial components. *Clin Orthop Relat Res* 2000;376: 161-171.

10. Dennis DA, Komistek RD, Colwell CE Jr, et al: In vivo anteroposterior femorotibial translation of total knee arthroplasty: A multicenter analysis. *Clin Orthop Relat Res* 1998;356:47-57.

11. Colizza WA, Insall JN, Scuderi GR: The posterior stabilized total knee prosthesis: Assessment of polyethylene damage and osteolysis after a ten-year-minimum follow-up. *J Bone Joint Surg Am* 1995;77(11):1713-1720.

12. Landy MM, Walker PS: Wear of ultra-high-molecular-weight polyethylene components of 90 retrieved knee prostheses. *J Arthroplasty* 1988;3(Suppl):S73-S85.

13. Bartel DL, Bicknell VL, Wright TM: The effect of conformity, thickness, and material on stresses in ultra-high molecular weight components for total joint replacement. *J Bone Joint Surg Am* 1986;68(7):1041-1051.

14. Li S, Scuderi G, Furman BD, Bhattacharyya S, Schmieg JJ, Insall JN: Assessment of backside wear from the analysis of 55 retrieved tibial inserts. *Clin Orthop Relat Res* 2002;404:75-82.

15. Lombardi AV Jr, Ellison BS, Berend KR: Polyethylene wear is influenced by manufacturing technique in modular TKA. *Clin Orthop Relat Res* 2008;466(11): 2798-2805.

16. Collier JP, Sutula LC, Currier BH, et al: Overview of polyethylene as a bearing material: Comparison of sterilization methods. *Clin Orthop Relat Res* 1996;333: 76-86.

17. Berzins A, Jacobs JJ, Berger R, et al: Surface damage in machined ram-extruded and net-shape molded retrieved polyethylene tibial inserts of total knee replacements. *J Bone Joint Surg Am* 2002; 84(9):1534-1540.

18. Oral E, Malhi AS, Wannomae KK, Muratoglu OK: Highly crosslinked ultrahigh molecular weight polyethylene with improved fatigue resistance for total joint arthroplasty. *J Arthroplasty* 2008; 23(7):1037-1044.

19. Miura H, Matsuda S, Okazaki K, Kawano T, Kawamura H, Iwamoto Y: Validity of an oblique posterior condylar radiographic view for revision total knee arthroplasty. *J Bone Joint Surg Br* 2005; 87(12):1643-1646.

20. Nadaud MC, Fehring TK, Fehring K: Underestimation of osteolysis in posterior stabilized total knee arthroplasty. *J Arthroplasty* 2004;19(1):110-115.

21. Reish TG, Clarke HD, Scuderi GR, Math KR, Scott WN: Use of multi-detector computed tomography for the detection of periprosthetic osteolysis in total knee arthroplasty. *J Knee Surg* 2006; 19(4):259-264.

22. Vessely MB, Frick MA, Oakes D, Wenger DE, Berry DJ: Magnetic resonance imaging with metal suppression for evaluation of periprosthetic osteolysis after total knee arthroplasty. *J Arthroplasty* 2006;21(6):826-831.

23. Talmo CT, Shanbhag AS, Rubash HE: Nonsurgical management of osteolysis: Challenges and opportunities. *Clin Orthop Relat Res* 2006;453:254-264.

24. Engh GA, Koralewicz LM, Pereles TR: Clinical results of modular polyethylene insert exchange with retention of total knee arthroplasty components. *J Bone Joint Surg Am* 2000;82(4):516-523.

25. Griffin WL, Scott RD, Dalury DF, Mahoney OM, Chiavetta JB, Odum SM: Modular insert exchange in knee arthroplasty for treatment of wear and osteolysis. *Clin Orthop Relat Res* 2007;464: 132-137.

26. Cuckler JM: Bone loss in total knee arthroplasty: Graft augment and options. *J Arthroplasty* 2004; 19(4, Suppl 1):56-58.

27. Dennis DA, Berry DJ, Engh G, et al: Revision total knee arthroplasty. *J Am Acad Orthop Surg* 2008;16(8):442-454.

28. Engh GA, Parks NL: The management of bone defects in revision total knee arthroplasty. *Instr Course Lect* 1997;46:227-236.

29. Haas SB, Insall JN, Montgomery W III, Windsor RE: Revision total knee arthroplasty with use of modular components with stems inserted without cement. *J Bone Joint Surg Am* 1995;77(11): 1700-1707.

30. Hockman DE, Ammeen D, Engh GA: Augments and al-

lografts in revision total knee arthroplasty: Usage and outcome using one modular revision prosthesis. *J Arthroplasty* 2005;20(1): 35-41.

31. Long WJ, Scuderi GR: Porous tantalum cones for large metaphyseal tibial defects in revision total knee arthroplasty: A minimum 2-year follow-up. *J Arthroplasty* 2009;24(7):1086-1092.

32. Lucey SD, Scuderi GR, Kelly MA, Insall JN: A practical approach to dealing with bone loss in revision total knee arthroplasty. *Orthopedics* 2000;23(10):1036-1041.

33. Meneghini RM, Lewallen DG, Hanssen AD: Use of porous tantalum metaphyseal cones for severe tibial bone loss during revision total knee replacement. *J Bone Joint Surg Am* 2008;90(1):78-84.

34. Nelson CL, Gioe TJ, Cheng EY, Thompson RC Jr: Implant selection in revision total knee arthroplasty. *J Bone Joint Surg Am* 2003; 85(Suppl 1):S43-S51.

35. Radnay CS, Scuderi GR: Management of bone loss: Augments, cones, offset stems. *Clin Orthop Relat Res* 2006;446:83-92.

36. Rand JA: Modular augments in revision total knee arthroplasty. *Orthop Clin North Am* 1998; 29(2):347-353.

37. Stulberg SD: Bone loss in revision total knee arthroplasty: Graft options and adjuncts. *J Arthroplasty* 2003;18(3, Suppl 1):48-50.

38. Scuderi GR: Revision total knee arthroplasty: How much constraint is enough? *Clin Orthop Relat Res* 2001;392:300-305.

39. Rand JA, Ries MD, Landis GH, Rosenberg AG, Haas S: Intraoperative assessment in revision total knee arthroplasty. *J Bone Joint Surg Am* 2003;85(Suppl 1): S26-S37.

40. Engh GA, Herzwurm PJ, Parks NL: Treatment of major defects of bone with bulk allografts and stemmed components during total knee arthroplasty. *J Bone Joint Surg Am* 1997;79(7):1030-1039.

41. Ghazavi MT, Stockley I, Yee G, Davis A, Gross AE: Reconstruction of massive bone defects with allograft in revision total knee arthroplasty. *J Bone Joint Surg Am* 1997;79(1):17-25.

42. Fehring TK, Odum S, Olekson C, Griffin WL, Mason JB, McCoy TH: Stem fixation in revision total knee arthroplasty: A comparative analysis. *Clin Orthop Relat Res* 2003;416:217-224.

43. Conditt MA, Parsley BS, Alexander JW, Doherty SD, Noble PC: The optimal strategy for stable tibial fixation in revision total knee arthroplasty. *J Arthroplasty* 2004;19(7, Suppl 2):113-118.

44. Parsley BS, Sugano N, Bertolusso R, Conditt MA: Mechanical alignment of tibial stems in revision total knee arthroplasty. *J Arthroplasty* 2003;18(7, Suppl 1): 33-36.

45. Hicks CA, Noble P, Tullos H: The anatomy of the tibial intramedullary canal. *Clin Orthop Relat Res* 1995;321:111-116.

Video Reference

31.1: Scuderi GR, Pedersen HB: Video. *Trabecular Metal Tibial Cones for Proximal Tibial Defects.* Insall Scott Kelly Institute for Orthopaedics and Sports Medicine, New York, NY, 2011.

Evaluation and Management of Complications of the Extensor Mechanism

Michael E. Berend, MD

Abstract

Extensor mechanism and patellofemoral joint complications occur infrequently following total knee arthroplasty but represent a high percentage of clinically significant problems. Accurately diagnosing and identifying specific complications of the underlying etiology are the keys to successful treatment. Patellofemoral joint complications may be broadly categorized into implant-related problems, tendinous and patellar bone integrity issues, and soft-tissue imbalance or instability of the patellofemoral joint. It is also important to be aware of issues surrounding implant selection, surgical technique, and the available treatment options for patellofemoral joint complications.

Instr Course Lect 2012;61:405-409.

Extensor mechanism and patellofemoral joint complications following total knee arthroplasty (TKA) may be broadly categorized into (1) implant-related problems, (2) tendinous and patellar bone integrity issues, and (3) soft-tissue imbalance or instability of the patellofemoral joint.

Patellofemoral Joint Implant-Related Issues

Patellar implant design plays a significant role in the long-term durability of the patellofemoral articulation after TKA. The patellar component of a TKA is subjected to high shear forces at the implant-bone interface. All-polyethylene implants appear to be more forgiving and have improved survivorship compared with metal-backed designs.[1-3] Importantly, complications with metal-backed implants usually require revision of the patellar component. The failure mechanism generally involves peripheral loading of the patellar implant in areas of relatively thin polyethylene; the end result from this process is severe polyethylene wear and the need for eventual revision because of metallosis (**Figure 1**). The incidence of metallosis appears be design sensi-

tive.[4] There is debate concerning the need for a corresponding femoral component revision in the setting of metal abrasion from a metal-backed patellar component.[5]

Metal-backed patellar implant failure and eventual revision represent an interesting contrast to complications that occur with cemented all-polyethylene patellar component designs (**Figure 2**). A 2001 study reported a 3.8% incidence of radiographic patellar loosening in a series of 3,152 TKAs; however, the loosening rarely led to revision (rate, 0.1%).[1] The natural history of patellar implant loosening has been reported to follow a predictable pathophysiologic pathway with (1) radiolucency, (2) increased osseous density, (3) subchondral collapse, (4) patellar fragmentation, and (5) lateral subluxation.[1] This cascade likely represents a complex biomechanical and biologic process. Numerous surgical variables, including resection depth and angle or tilt, implant positioning on the host bone, high body mass index, and male sex are known variables associated with a higher rate of patellar complications following TKA.[6]

Revision surgery for isolated patellar complications, such as excisional

Dr. Berend or an immediate family member has received royalties from Biomet; is a member of a speakers' bureau or has made paid presentations on behalf of Biomet; serves as a paid consultant to Angiotech; has received research or institutional support from Biomet and ERMI; and serves as a board member, owner, officer, or committee member of the Piedmont Orthopaedic Society.

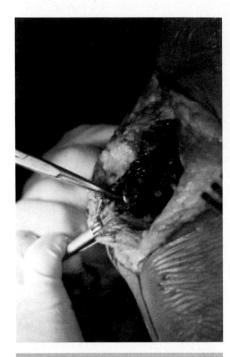

Figure 1   Intraoperative photograph of a failed TKA metal-backed patellar component with resulting metallosis. (Courtesy of Douglas A. Dennis, MD, Denver, CO.)

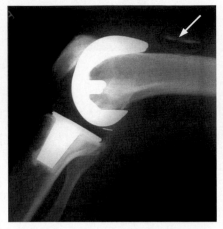

Figure 2   Lateral radiograph showing a loose all-polyethylene patellar component (arrow) displaced into the suprapatellar pouch.

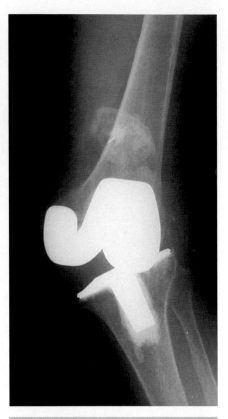

Figure 3   AP radiograph of an infrapatellar tendon disruption combined with rotational instability 7 years after a primary TKA.

arthroplasty, is a relatively straightforward and benign surgical procedure; however, multiple centers have reported that these procedures have a high complication rate.[7,8] Revision procedures should be performed with caution and be based on clinical symptoms rather than on radiographic findings alone.

All-polyethylene patellar component designs play a role in the durability and the mechanical stability of the implant. Design variables include inlay versus onlay and single versus a three-peg configuration. Biomechanically, inset designs offer 25% improvement in shear force resistance.[9] A large number of TKA revisions is needed to adequately power a study of the effects of patellar design. Because of the low overall revision rate, no clear advantage has been established for one- versus three-peg designs.[10] Femoral component design, such as posterior cruciate-retaining versus cruciate-substituting

designs, may also play a role in patellar implant survivorship.[1,10] It is important to recognize that, over the past 20 years, the influences of improved surgical technique, a better understanding of appropriate femoral component rotation, and measures to avoid osteonecrosis and reduce lateral retinacular release rates[11] have paralleled the improvement in patellar implant survival rates.

As is the case with many complications of the patellofemoral joint, implant failure may not be caused by an isolated component problem but may occur secondary to tibial or femoral component malpositioning. Excessive internal rotation of the femoral component places higher biomechanical shear forces on the patellar implant-bone fixation interface and precipitates higher loosening rates.

Increasing the composite thickness of the patella and the anterior position of the femoral component may result in what has been termed stuffing of the patellofemoral joint articulation. Relative retinacular tightness of the patellofemoral joint may result from a number of factors, including increasing patellar thickness, femoral component positioning in the sagittal plane, or a

combination of both factors. Rotational changes in the implant position may also increase retinacular tension and must be assessed within the context of the complete kinematics of the knee. Despite being widely discussed as a complication, limited evidence exists to support patellofemoral joint stuffing as a common or clinically relevant complication following TKA.[12] The theoretic risks associated with patellofemoral joint stuffing include decreased range of motion, arthrofibrosis, and pain.

Tendon and Bone Integrity

Quadriceps and patellar tendon disruption may lead to significant functional limitations and instability after TKA (**Figure 3**). Acute and chronic conditions require different surgical approaches. Acute injury with clinically significant functional limitations is amenable to acute repair with or without adjuvant soft-tissue reconstruction. This approach is indicated in knees with significant extensor lag and functional limitations. Repair with semitendinosus tendon autogenous graft supplementation was shown to enhance clinical outcomes in a small series of knees.[13] The semitendinosus graft serves as a source of supplemental collagen. The tendon graft can be passed through the quadriceps tendon or residual patellar bone. It can be attached from its trial insertion and used as a free tendon graft, or the distal tibial insertion can be left intact and the proximal end attached to the extensor mechanism. Each injury pattern and extensor mechanism deficiency will necessitate a unique use of the graft. The semitendinosus graft is secured to the extensor mechanism with absorbable sutures.

Chronic disruption of the extensor mechanism or failure of an acute repair requires a different surgical approach to change the biology of the articulation. One option is extensor mechanism allograft reconstruction. The surgical techniques have been well described by Nazarian and Booth.[14] The allograft bone block is fashioned to fit into the tibia in a reverse trapezoid shape, with the smaller end fitting proximally to prevent proximal migration. This is secured to the tibia with screws or cerclage wires. The host extensor mechanism tissue is opened longitudinally, and the proximal end of the graft is secured to the host tissue with nonabsorbable sutures with the knee in extension.

In their study of 40 patients (40 knees) with a chronic extensor mechanism disruption after TKA who were treated with extensor mechanism allograft placement to restore extensor function, Nazarian and Booth[14] reported satisfactory outcomes at mid-

term follow-up. At a mean follow-up of 3.6 years, the average range of motion in the 36 patients available for follow-up was 1.4° of extension and 98° of flexion. The average extensor lag was 13° in 15 of 36 patients. There were eight extensor allograft ruptures, which were treated by a repeat extensor allograft placement. Despite these initial ruptures, 34 of 36 patients (94%) had a successful clinical result. The average knee scores for function improved from 37 points preoperatively to 68 points postoperatively. The authors concluded that despite the complexity of the technique and the rehabilitation protocol, the results support extensor mechanism allograft placement for complete extensor mechanism loss after TKA when direct repair is unfavorable.

Implantation of the allograft requires careful surgical technique and postoperative rehabilitation. The rehabilitation regimen begins with bracing the extensor mechanism for 6 to 8 weeks, followed by progressive mobilization and physical therapy. Improved results were reported with tight fixation of the graft in full extension and delayed postoperative flexion.[15,16] Fixation of the tibial bone block can be achieved through stabilization with screws or cerclage wires.

Patellar osteonecrosis and fracture have been associated with lateral retinacular release and may represent the final pathophysiology of the disruption of the blood supply to the patella.[1,17] Patellar fracture was reported at long-term follow-up in 177 of 4,583 knees (3.8%) after TKA.[17] Patellar fracture treatment depends on fracture displacement, patellar component fixation, and the functional status of the extensor mechanism as determined by gait performance, the ability to climb stairs, and extensor lag. Individualized treatment with liberal host graft supplementation is the recom-

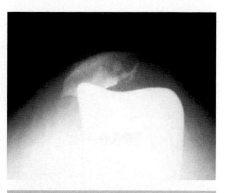

Figure 4   Sunrise radiographic view of patellar subluxation in a bicompartmental knee arthroplasty, which resulted from internal rotation of the femoral component.

mended treatment for surgically treated patients. Results from attempted open reduction and internal fixation are unpredictable and have included nonunion, infection, and hardware complications. Clinical success from the surgical treatment of displaced patellar fractures remains guarded, with 60% good results.[17]

Soft-Tissue Balance

Instability of the patellofemoral articulation is frequently related to factors outside the patella, notably femoral and tibial component internal rotation (**Figure 4**). When evaluating a patient with patellofemoral instability or stiffness, CT may help assess the role component rotational malpositioning plays in postoperative patellofemoral joint dysfunction.[18-20] Internal rotation of one or both of the implants has been reported.[18] It is critical to carefully consider and fully evaluate the patient prior to surgical intervention because a patellar-based solution often will not solve the pathologic effects of femoral or tibial rotational malrotation.

Femoral component internal rotational malpositioning has been associated with an increased rate of lateral retinacular release. Newbern et al[11] reported on the effects of a change from referencing the posterior condylar axis

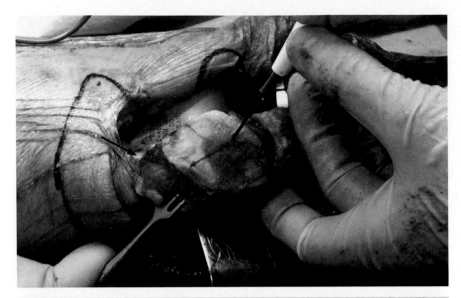

Figure 5 Intraoperative image of the soft-tissue synovium (arrow) that should be removed, especially with posterior stabilized and cam and post TKA implant designs.

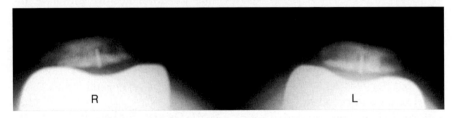

Figure 6 Sunrise radiograph showing lateral patellar contact in the patient's right knee but not in the left knee.

during TKA to a transepicondylar axis. The authors noted a reduction in the lateral retinacular release rate from 57% to 12% when referencing the epicondylar axis. Currently, with newer implant designs and an increased awareness of complications associated with lateral retinacular release, such as patellar osteonecrosis, fragmentation, and component loosening, the complication rate at St. Francis Hospital (Mooresville, IN) is less than 2%.[1]

Patellar clunk is another soft-tissue consideration that can complicate TKA. This complication has been reported most commonly with cam and post posterior stabilized implant designs and results from a fibrous nodule that forms superior to the patella (**Figure 5**). When symptomatic, the nod-ule can be removed with either an open or an arthroscopic procedure.[21] Increased early postoperative knee flexion has been associated with patellar clunk, whereas changes in femoral trochlear implant designs have been reported to lower the rate of patellofemoral joint complications.[22]

Pain and Failure

Anterior or so-called patellofemoral pain following TKA is poorly understood, and its causes are multifactorial. Anterior knee pain may be related to patellofemoral issues. Meding et al[6] reported that patients treated with TKA performed with a lateral release or those with a body mass index greater than 30 kg/m^2 were at the greatest risk of patellar loosening and fracture, re-spectively. Such complications are hypothesized to be associated with increase pain. Male sex, preoperative varus alignment of greater than 5°, and a large patellar component size also predicted a higher risk of patellar fracture. Medial patellar component position, tibial component thickness of greater than 12 mm, preoperative valgus alignment of 10° or greater, and preoperative flexion of 100° or greater are predictive of patellar loosening. Lateral patellar contact (**Figure 6**) of the remaining patellar bone with the femoral component has been hypothesized to result in postoperative pain in select patients. Ritter et al[23] evaluated the incidence of the radiographic finding of lateral patellar contact with the femoral component and correlated it with postoperative functional outcomes. The authors reported that in a review of 980 TKAs, 452 (46.1%) had lateral patellar contact, and it was not associated with increased postoperative pain or a compromise in the quality of postoperative outcomes.

Summary

Extensor mechanism and patellofemoral joint complications are infrequent complications of TKA but represent a high percentage of clinically significant problems. An accurate diagnosis and identification of the specific underlying etiology are the keys to successful treatment.

References

1. Berend ME, Ritter MA, Keating EM, Faris PM, Crites BM: The failure of all-polyethylene patellar components in total knee replacement. *Clin Orthop Relat Res* 2001; 388:105-111.

2. Rand JA, Trousdale RT, Ilstrup DM, Harmsen WS: Factors affecting the durability of primary total knee prostheses. *J Bone Joint Surg Am* 2003;85-A(2):259-265.

3. Crites BM, Berend ME: Metal-backed patellar components: A brief report on 10-year survival. *Clin Orthop Relat Res* 2001;388: 103-104.

4. Kraay MJ, Darr OJ, Salata MJ, Goldberg VM: Outcome of metal-backed cementless patellar components: The effect of implant design. *Clin Orthop Relat Res* 2001;392:239-244.

5. Garcia RM, Kraay MJ, Goldberg VM: Retention of superficially damaged femoral components after metal-backed patella component failure. *J Arthroplasty* 2008; 23(6):850-858.

6. Meding JB, Fish MD, Berend ME, Ritter MA, Keating EM: Predicting patellar failure after total knee arthroplasty. *Clin Orthop Relat Res* 2008;466(11): 2769-2774.

7. Berend ME, Harty LD, Ritter MA, Stonehouse DM II: Excisional arthroplasty for patellar loosening in total knee arthroplasty. *J Arthroplasty* 2003;18(5): 668-671.

8. Berry DJ, Rand JA: Isolated patellar component revision of total knee arthroplasty. *Clin Orthop Relat Res* 1993;286:110-115.

9. Rosenstein AD, Postak PD, Greenwald AS: Fixation strength comparison of onlay and inset patellar implants. *Knee* 2007; 14(3):194-197.

10. Larson CM, McDowell CM, Lachiewicz PF: One-peg versus three-peg patella component fixation in total knee arthroplasty. *Clin Orthop Relat Res* 2001;392: 94-100.

11. Newbern DG, Faris PM, Ritter MA, Keating EM, Meding JB, Berend ME: A clinical comparison of patellar tracking using the transepicondylar axis and the posterior condylar axis. *J Arthroplasty* 2006;21(8):1141-1146.

12. Pierson JL, Ritter MA, Keating EM, et al: The effect of stuffing the patellofemoral compartment on the outcome of total knee arthroplasty. *J Bone Joint Surg Am* 2007;89(10):2195-2203.

13. Cadambi A, Engh GA: Use of a semitendinosus tendon autogenous graft for rupture of the patellar ligament after total knee arthroplasty: A report of seven cases. *J Bone Joint Surg Am* 1992; 74(7):974-979.

14. Nazarian DG, Booth RE Jr: Extensor mechanism allografts in total knee arthroplasty. *Clin Orthop Relat Res* 1999;367:123-129.

15. Springer BD, Della Valle CJ: Extensor mechanism allograft reconstruction after total knee arthroplasty. *J Arthroplasty* 2008; 23(7, Suppl):35-38.

16. Burnett RS, Berger RA, Della Valle CJ, et al: Extensor mechanism allograft reconstruction after total knee arthroplasty. *J Bone Joint Surg Am* 2005;87(Pt 2, Suppl 1):175-194.

17. Keating EM, Haas G, Meding JB: Patella fracture after post total knee replacements. *Clin Orthop Relat Res* 2003;416:93-97.

18. Malo M, Vince KG: The unstable patella after total knee arthroplasty: Etiology, prevention, and management. *J Am Acad Orthop Surg* 2003;11(5):364-371.

19. Berger RA, Crossett LS, Jacobs JJ, Rubash HE: Malrotation causing patellofemoral complications after total knee arthroplasty. *Clin Orthop Relat Res* 1998;356:144-153.

20. Berger RA, Rubash HE: Rotational instability and malrotation after total knee arthroplasty. *Orthop Clin North Am* 2001;32(4): 639-647, ix.

21. Lucas TS, DeLuca PF, Nazarian DG, Bartolozzi AR, Booth RE Jr: Arthroscopic treatment of patellar clunk. *Clin Orthop Relat Res* 1999; 367:226-229.

22. Schroer WC, Diesfeld PJ, Reedy ME, LeMarr A: Association of increased knee flexion and patella clunk syndrome after mini-subvastus total knee arthroplasty. *J Arthroplasty* 2009;24(2): 281-287.

23. Ritter MA, Keating EM, Faris PM, Meding JB, Berend ME, Pierson JL: Lateral patellar contact after total knee arthroplasty: An analysis of the effects on postoperative pain and outcome. *J Arthroplasty* 2006;21(7):1017-1020.

Infection Following Total Knee Arthroplasty: Prevention and Management

Kevin L. Garvin, MD
Beau S. Konigsberg, MD

Abstract

Despite diligent efforts to prevent infection, prosthetic knee infection occurs in up to 2% of patients treated with total knee arthroplasty. Although the risk of infection is relatively low, the effects are considerable. The number of total knee arthroplasties is projected to increase by more than 600% by 2030, resulting in 3.48 million knee replacements, with a possible 70,000 prosthetic knee infections. Infection will be the most common indication for revision total knee arthroplasty.

Prophylactic antibiotics and minimizing patient risk factors are critical in preventing infections. Staphylococcus is the most common organism in infected total knee arthroplasties. Prompt diagnosis and treatment are crucial to the long-term outcomes of patients with prosthetic joint infections. The erythrocyte sedimentation rate, C-reactive protein level, and interleukin-6 serum level should be checked in all patients with clinical signs of infection or unexplained pain or stiffness. The surgical management of a prosthetic knee infection depends on several factors, but none is more important than the timing of infection in relationship to the index surgery. With a success rate of 80% to 90%, two-stage component exchange remains the treatment of choice for chronically infected total knee arthroplasties.

Instr Course Lect 2012;61:411-419.

Periprosthetic joint infection is one of the most formidable challenges for arthroplasty surgeons. Physicians and scientists have worked diligently to lower the incidence of infections around prosthetic joints, but the percentage of patients in whom an infection develops after primary total knee replacement remains in the range of 0.4% to 2%.[1-3] Medicare data indicate that the rate of periprosthetic infection within the first 2 years after knee arthroplasty is 1.55%. The infection rate in the following 2 to 10 years is an additional 0.46%.[4,5]

Although the percentage of prosthetic knees that are associated with infection is low, the numbers will increase with the growing number of total knee replacements. Kurtz et al[6] projected that the demand for primary knee arthroplasty will grow by 673%, from 450,000 in 2005 to 3.48 million in 2030. If infection develops in 2% of the 3.48 million patients within the first year after the knee arthroplasty, as many as 69,000 patients may be treated for periprosthetic knee infection each year. This group does not include patients in whom infection develops more than 1 year after the surgery or after a revision total knee arthroplasty. The burden and complexity are also increasing because of the number of resistant pathogens.

Staphylococcus aureus accounts for most periprosthetic joint infections. Infections caused by methicillin-resistant *S aureus* (MRSA) are especially difficult to treat.[7-9] The Staphylococcal infections may be acquired in the hospital, but some patients are known carriers of *S aureus* and infect themselves.[10,11] Patients who are

Dr. Garvin or an immediate family member has received royalties from Biomet; is a member of a speakers' bureau or has made paid presentations on behalf of ConvaTec; is an employee of Biomet; and serves as a board member, owner, officer, or committee member of the American Academy of Orthopaedic Surgeons and the American Orthopaedic Association. Neither Dr. Konigsberg nor any immediate family member has received anything of value from or owns stock in a commercial company or institution related directly or indirectly to the subject of this chapter.

Table 1

Risk Factors Associated With Periprosthetic Joint Infections of the Knee

Diabetes
Rheumatoid arthritis
Malnutrition
Smoking
Obesity
Steroids
Excessive anticoagulation
Chemotherapy
Cancer
Alcoholism
Urinary tract infection
Complex surgery
Revision surgery
Multiple blood transfusions

carriers can be screened and decolonization can be performed preoperatively, potentially lowering the risk of periprosthetic joint infection.

Prevention

A variety of interventions can reduce the incidence of infections. Prior to surgery, surgeons should identify and address host factors associated with an increased risk, carry out decolonization when a patient is a bacterial carrier, and use perioperative antibiotics. Prophylactic antibiotics are effective in preventing surgical site infections. The protocol should be to administer the antibiotics 1 hour before the surgical incision is made. Rosenberg et al[12] reported that, in a 3-month interval before the initiation of a protocol to ensure compliance with antibiotic dosing, only 26 of 40 patients (65%) received prophylactic antibiotics within 1 hour before the incision. After the protocol was started, the compliance increased to 180 of 186 patients (97%; $P < 0.0001$). The American Academy of Orthopaedic Surgeons (AAOS) has published guidelines for the most ap-

propriate antibiotics.[13-15] Cefazolin and cefuroxime are preferred, with clindamycin or vancomycin being recommended for patients with β-lactam allergies. Vancomycin may also be used for patients who are having surgery in an institution where the prevalence of MRSA or methicillin-resistant *Staphylococcus epidermidis* in the orthopaedic patients is greater than 25%.

Patients who are colonized with MRSA or who are so-called carriers of these resistant pathogens are also candidates for treatment with vancomycin. These patients also should receive additional treatment including chlorhexidine gluconate scrubs and nasal mupirocin. The decolonizing protocols have demonstrated the ability to reduce the rate of staphylococcal infections. Studies have also shown that a decolonizing protocol is effective in eradicating MRSA colonization of patients.[8,16-19]

Host Risk Factors

Periprosthetic joint infection has been associated with several host risk factors, including malnutrition, smoking, alcoholism, urinary tract infection, and obesity (**Table 1**). In a retrospective review that included 6,108 patients who had undergone a total of 8,494 hip or knee arthroplasties between 1991 and 2004, Malinzak et al[20] compared those in whom a deep infection developed with a noninfected control group. They found 43 deep infections (30 associated with total knee arthroplasty and 13 with total hip arthroplasty), for a prevalence of 0.51%. Obesity, younger age, and diabetes mellitus were identified as significant risk factors for infection. Morbidly obese patients (those with a body mass index [BMI] of >50 kg/m²) had an increased odds for the development of infection (odds ratio, 21.3). In the group treated with total knee arthroplasty, patients who had a BMI greater than 40 kg/m² but

less than 50 kg/m² had 3.3 times greater odds for the development of an infection compared with those with a BMI of less than 40 kg/m². The average age of the patients with an infected knee was 62.8 years, and the average age of those without an infected knee was 69.2 years. A deep infection was 3.1 times more likely to develop in patients with diabetes mellitus than in those without diabetes. Additional studies have shown a clinically relevant benefit to maintaining strict glycemic control in diabetic patients in the perioperative period.[21] Marchant et al[21] compared a group of patients with well-controlled diabetes with a group with poorly controlled diabetes when they underwent total knee arthroplasty and found the odds of a wound infection developing to be increased in the group with poorly controlled diabetes (odds ratio, 2.28). Bolognesi et al[22] reviewed the National Inpatient Sample (NIS) records of 751,340 primary and revision hip and knee replacements, including 64,239 in diabetic patients, and found no increase in infection in the diabetic population. However, this finding is likely due to the fact that the NIS was not designed to collect data on complications after the initial hospital stay and is not likely to include the great majority of periprosthetic joint infections.

Obesity is also a host risk factor for infection associated with wound-healing complications. Winiarsky et al[23] compared a group of morbidly obese patients who had a total of 50 total knee arthroplasties with a control group of nonmorbidly obese patients who had a total of 1,768 total knee arthroplasties. In the morbidly obese group, there was a 22% rate of wound complications (11 patients) and five deep infections. In contrast, the control group had a 2% rate of wound complications and a 0.6% rate of deep infections. The nutritional status of

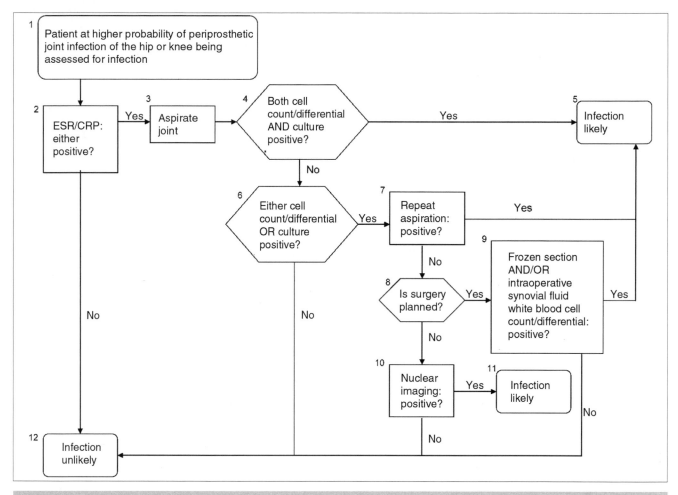

Figure 1   Algorithm for patients with a higher probability of having a hip or knee periprosthetic joint infection. (Reproduced from American Academy of Orthopaedic Surgeons: *Clinical Practice Guideline on the Diagnosis of Periprosthetic Joint Infections of the Hip and Knee.* Rosemont, IL, American Academy of Orthopaedic Surgeons, June 2010. http://www.aaos.org/Research/guidelines/PJIguideline.pdf.)

obese patients should be evaluated by obtaining serum albumin and transferrin levels as well as a total lymphocyte count. If their nutritional status is poor (a transferrin level of < 200 mg/dL, an albumin level of < 3.5 g/dL, or a total lymphocyte count of < 1,500 cells/mm³), obese patients should be referred to a primary care provider or nutritionist before total knee arthroplasty.

Patients at increased risk for infection because of obesity should be informed of that risk and counseled about ways to reduce it. If a morbidly obese patient has an adequate nutritional status, bariatric surgery may be recommended before arthroplasty.

Postoperative wound drainage and wound-healing complications are associated with an increased prevalence of infections. A study comparing 78 patients with a periprosthetic joint infection with a control population without an infection showed that hematoma formation, wound drainage, and a mean international normalized ratio (INR) greater than 1.5 had been more prevalent in the group with a periprosthetic joint infection.[24] Galat et al[25] reviewed the cases of 42 patients (42 knees) who had surgical evacuation of a postoperative hematoma within 30 days after a primary total knee arthroplasty. An additional group of 42 pa-

tients was matched to the group in an attempt to identify risk factors for the development of the hematoma. The 2-year probabilities of additional major surgery (component resection, muscle flap coverage, or amputation) and development of a deep infection were 12.3% and 10.5%, respectively, in the patients who had surgical evacuation of the hematoma. In the control group, the probabilities for the same complications were 0.6% and 0.8%. A history of a bleeding disorder had a significant association with the development of a hematoma requiring surgical evacuation ($P = 0.046$). Matar et al[26] reported several additional preop-

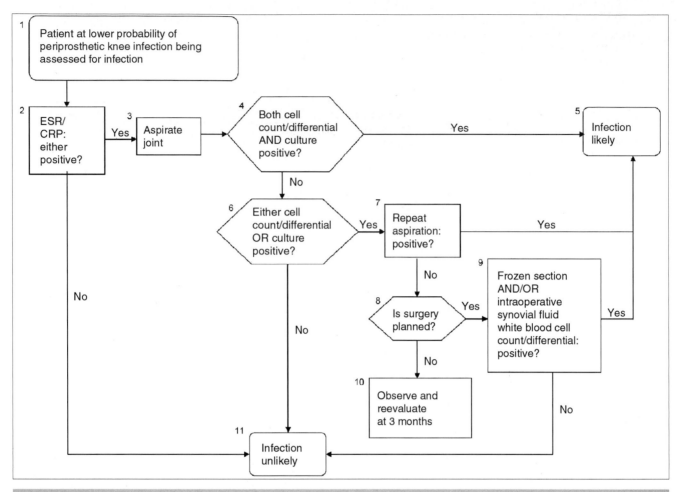

Figure 2 Algorithm for patients with a lower probability of having a periprosthetic knee infection. (Reproduced from American Academy of Orthopaedic Surgeons: *Clinical Practice Guideline on the Diagnosis of Periprosthetic Joint Infections of the Hip and Knee.* Rosemont, IL, American Academy of Orthopaedic Surgeons, June 2010. http://www.aaos.org/Research/guidelines/PJIguideline.pdf.)

erative, intraoperative, and postoperative factors that are associated with periprosthetic joint infection. These authors provide recommendations for addressing factors that may contribute to or increase the risk of infection.

Diagnosis

The evaluation of patients suspected of having a periprosthetic joint infection should follow a logical sequence. The AAOS developed a clinical practice guideline to help standardize this process (**Figures 1, 2,** and **3**). The patient's history and physical examination should initially raise suspicion that there is an infection. Typically, patients with a periprosthetic joint infec-

tion describe almost continuous pain and usually have stiffness or limited knee motion. Fever or malaise is strongly suggestive of infection, but they are not typical findings. If a draining sinus is present, the joint is considered to be infected until proven otherwise.

The next step in the evaluation of patients for whom there is a clinical suspicion of infection is the use of laboratory tests.[27] The erythrocyte sedimentation rate (ESR) and C-reactive protein (CRP) level should be measured whenever a patient is suspected of having an infection at the site of a total joint arthroplasty. The cutoff for normal and abnormal values for these

inflammatory markers was evaluated prospectively in a study of 151 knees in 145 patients who had presented for revision knee surgery.[27] This study suggests that an ESR greater than 22.5 mm/h (normal, 30 mm/h) and a CRP level greater than 13.5 mg/L (normal, 10 mg/L) were reliably suggestive of a periprosthetic joint infection.

The diagnostic accuracy of the interleukin-6 (IL-6) serum level was evaluated in a prospective study of 58 patients with a periprosthetic joint infection.[28] IL-6 is produced by stimulated macrophages, but the level returns to normal 48 to 72 hours after a procedure. The authors found that the IL-6 level was a more accurate marker

Higher probability of infection	One or more symptoms, AND at least one or more: 1) risk factor,[a] OR 2) physical exam finding; OR 3) early implant loosening/osteolysis (detected by radiography)
Lower probability of infection	Pain or joint stiffness only and none of the following: 1) risk factors;[a] OR 2) physical exam findings; OR 3) early implant loosening/osteolysis (as detected by radiography)

[a]risk factor supported by evidence or expert opinion

Factors for Risk Stratification

Symptoms	Risk Factors Supported by Evidence	Risk Factors Supported by Consensus	Physical Exam Findings	Other
1. Pain in the replaced joint 2. Stiffness in the replaced joint	1. Prior infection of the joint (knee) 2. Superficial surgical site infection (hip and knee) 3. Obesity (hip) 4. Extended operative time (> 2.5 hours, hip and knee) 5. Immunosuppression[a] (knee)	1. Any recent (< 1 yr) bacteremia or candidemia 2. Metachronous prosthetic joint infection 3. Skin disorders (psoriasis, chronic cellulitis, lymphedema, chronic venous stasis, skin ulcers) 4. IV drug use 5. Recent (< 3 yrs) MRSA infection or colonization 6. Active infection at other site	1. Warmth, effusion, redness, swelling 2. Sinus tract associated with the joint	1. Early (< 5 yrs) implant loosening or osteolysis (as detected by radiography)

Factors not supported as a risk by evidence
1. Smoking
2. Obesity (knee)
3. Use of drains
4. Hematoma or use of anticoagulation (INR > 2 or low molecular weight heparins)
5. Immunosuppression[b] (hip)

Figure 3 Factors for risk stratification. [b]In the systematic review, the following states were considered to be indicative of immunosuppression: HIV, diabetes, hepatitis, chemotherapy or other suppressive medication such as antimonoclonal antibodies (medications specified in search: prednisone, infliximab, adalimumab, methotrexate, and etanercept), autoimmune diseases (lupus, rheumatoid arthritis, ankylosing spondylitis, Reiter syndrome, and psoriatic arthropathy), inflammatory arthritis, renal disease (chronic renal failure and dialysis), liver failure, malnourishment, sickle cell disease, hemophilia, and solid organ transplant. IV = intravenous. (Reproduced from American Academy of Orthopaedic Surgeons: *Clinical Practice Guideline on the Diagnosis of Periprosthetic Joint Infections of the Hip and Knee.* Rosemont, IL, American Academy of Orthopaedic Surgeons, June 2010. http://www.aaos.org/Research/guidelines/PJIguideline.pdf.)

than either the ESR or the CRP level for the detection of periprosthetic infection. A meta-analysis of publications related to the diagnosis of infections around prosthetic joints included 30 eligible studies with data on a total of 3,909 hip and knee arthroplasties.[29]

The prevalence of periprosthetic joint infection was 32.5%. The best diagnostic accuracy was provided by the IL-6 level, followed by the CRP level, ESR, and white blood cell (WBC) count. One of the weaknesses of that meta-analysis was that it included only

one large study and two smaller studies measuring the usefulness of the IL-6 level, but 25 studies evaluating the usefulness of the ESR, 23 evaluating the usefulness of the CRP level, and 15 evaluating the usefulness of the WBC count. The cost of each of these tests was not evaluated.

The next step when suspicion of infection persists is aspiration at the site of the prosthetic joint and analysis of the periprosthetic fluid. The analysis of the aspirated fluid should include a cell count to determine the absolute number of leukocytes and the percentage of cells that are neutrophils. Somewhere between 1,100 and 3,000 leukocytes/μL indicates an infection.[30,31] The percentage of leukocytes that are neutrophils should be at least 60% for the joint to be considered infected.[32-34] Finally, specimens of the fluid should be cultured to identify bacteria and their sensitivity to available antibiotics. Gram staining of fluid specimens has a poor sensitivity and a poor predictive value, and the results do not generally alter the patient's treatment.[35]

In the early postoperative period, levels of inflammatory markers and the synovial WBC count may be elevated despite the joint not being infected. Bedair et al[36] evaluated the results of knee aspirations performed within 6 weeks after primary total knee arthroplasties and compared the ESR, CRP level, and WBC count and differential between patients with and those without a postoperative infection. The CRP level, synovial WBC count, and percentage of polymorphonuclear cells in the differential WBC count were found to be higher in the infected group, but the optimal cutoff for the synovial WBC count as a reliable marker of infection was much higher than the numbers previously given. This study showed a synovial WBC count of 27,800 cells/μL in the aspi-

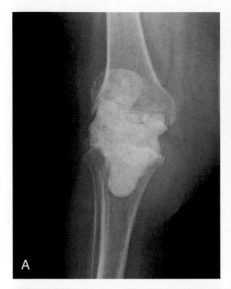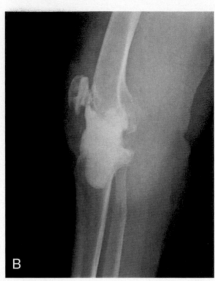

Figure 4 AP (**A**) and lateral (**B**) radiographs of a patient with a static spacer before placement of total knee arthroplasty implants after resolution of an infection.

rate from the site of a total knee arthroplasty in the acute postoperative period to be the best predictor of infection. With the use of this cutoff, there was a 94% positive predictive value and a 98% negative predictive value.

Aerobic, anaerobic, and fungal cultures are performed routinely, whereas molecular testing has the potential for routine use but currently is developmental. The challenges facing orthopaedic surgeons include both false-positive and false-negative cultures. False-positive fluid and tissue cultures are unfortunately common.[37] If the history, physical findings, levels of inflammatory markers, and cell count in the fluid are normal, then it is highly probable that a positive culture is false-positive. The corollary to this dilemma is when the history, physical findings, levels of inflammatory markers, and cell count in the fluid are elevated but the culture is negative. This problem of false-negative cultures is also common; it may occur 5% to 10% of the time.[38] Berbari et al[38] studied 897 cases of periprosthetic joint infection seen over a 10-year interval. Sixty (7%) of the infections were associated with

negative cultures, and in 32 of these 60 cases (53%), the patient had received prior antibiotics. Of the 60 infections, 34 (57%) were treated with a two-stage implant exchange; 12 (20%), with débridement and component retention; 8 (13%), with resection arthroplasty; 5 (8%), with one-stage exchange; and 1 (2%), with amputation. Patients were treated with parenteral antibiotics for an average of 28 days, with 49 of them (82%) receiving a cephalosporin. The 5-year estimate of implant survival without infection was 94% for the patients with a two-stage exchange and 71% for those treated with débridement and component retention. The study highlights the importance of treating these patients like patients with positive cultures. The protocol of parenteral antibiotics and a two-stage exchange can be expected to have a high rate of success for patients with a periprosthetic joint infection who have negative cultures.

Management

Segawa et al[39] suggested a clinically useful classification of deep periprosthetic infections. Type I infections are

those identified from routine cultures of specimens obtained at the time of an arthroplasty revision when an infection was not expected. The surgical revision used to treat this type of infection includes appropriate débridement and component exchange and therefore is comparable with a one-stage reimplantation. The treatment is completed by administering parenteral antibiotics for 4 to 6 weeks. Oral antibiotic therapy may be used after the completion of parenteral antibiotic therapy.

Type II infections are early postoperative infections, such as those discovered within the first month after surgery. A type II infection should be treated with surgical débridement and component retention followed by a 4- to 6-week course of parenteral antibiotics and possibly oral antibiotics for a defined interval. If the surgeon has assumed the care of a patient who had surgical revision elsewhere and notes that the culture of specimens obtained during the surgical procedure is positive, then it may be necessary to repeat the débridement. Several factors should be considered, including the type of bacteria and antibiotic sensitivity, the complexity of an anticipated resection and reimplantation at a later date, and the general health and immune status of the patient.

Type III infections occur years after implantation and are acute hematogenous infections from a remote source that is normally known. If the symptoms of infection have been present for 2 to 3 weeks or less, the implant is well fixed, and the patient is immunocompetent, then surgical débridement, component retention, and parenteral antibiotics may salvage the arthroplasty. Salvage has a success rate ranging from 30% to as high as 90%.[40-42] Azzam et al[43] recently studied the success of irrigation and débridement with component retention for treatment of type II and type III infections around prosthetic joints in 104 patients treated at a single institution and followed for an average of 5.7 years. With component resection or microbiologically proven infection as the end point, the success rate was 44%. The authors noted that patients with staphylococcal infection, higher American Society of Anesthesiologists scores, and purulence around the prosthesis had a higher failure rate. Patients who had been treated within 2 weeks after the onset of symptoms had the best results (a 60% rate of success).

Type IV infections are those that have been present for 1 month or more and are classified as chronic indolent infections. A one- or two-stage reimplantation including resection of the implant, thorough débridement of the joint, and parenteral antibiotic therapy for 4 to 6 weeks is recommended. When a two-stage procedure is done, antibiotic-impregnated polymethyl methacrylate in the form of either a static spacer or an articulating spacer is used to replace the removed implant, and the implant is replaced 6 weeks or more after it was removed (**Figures 4** and **5**). Initially, low doses (1 to 2 g per joint) of antibiotics in the polymethyl methacrylate were used, but larger doses have been found to be safe and more effective.[44] Springer et al[44] used 10.5 g of vancomycin and 12.5 g of gentamicin in 34 patients, 17 of whom had risk factors for infection. Only one patient had a transient 1-day rise in the serum creatinine level (1.7 mg/dL; normal, 0.6 to 1.3 mg/dL), and none had renal insufficiency, renal failure, or other adverse side effects. Others have reported complications with this high dose of local antibiotic delivery, so patients should be followed closely. If antibiotic-related side effects are identified, the spacer should be removed immediately.[45]

Jämsen et al[46] reported success rates of 73% to 100% for one-stage revi-

sions and 82% to 100% for two-stage revisions. Haleem et al[47] reported the survivorship after two-stage revisions to be 93.5% at 5 years and 85% at 10 years, with implant removal because of infection as the end point.

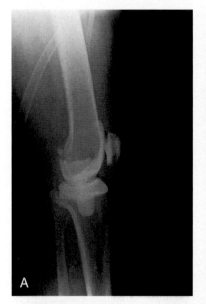
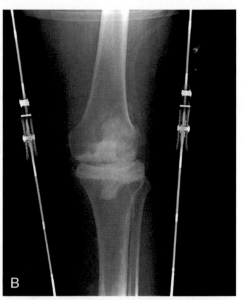
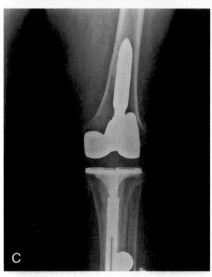
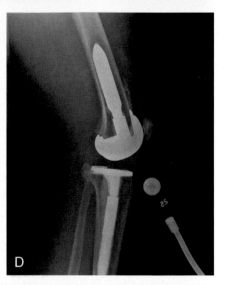

Figure 5   **A** and **B,** Radiographs of a 78-year-old man who presented with acute knee pain and swelling after dental manipulation. He had an infection at the site of a total knee arthroplasty 5 years postoperatively. The radiographs demonstrate an articulating spacer with high-dose antibiotic delivery for the treatment of a methicillin-resistant staphylococcal infection. AP (**C**) and lateral (**D**) knee radiographs demonstrating the results 2 years after a two-stage reimplantation of a total knee prosthesis was done because of a periprosthetic infection.

Summary

Infection after total knee arthroplasty is fortunately rare, but it is not likely that this complication will be eliminated. The surgeons' and patients' efforts should continue to focus on prevention by optimizing hospital and surgeon aseptic techniques and addressing patient-specific risk factors. Periprosthetic joint infection is a major complication that occurs after up to 2% of total knee arthroplasties. Once infection is suspected clinically, timely diagnosis and treatment are crucial. Any patient with a total knee prosthesis who has pain or stiffness without another identifiable cause should be evaluated for infection. When the diagnosis is made, prompt surgical treatment, usually a two-stage reimplantation in conjunction with antibiotic therapy, has a high rate of success and can provide good long-term results.

References

1. Mahomed NN, Barrett J, Katz JN, Baron JA, Wright J, Losina E: Epidemiology of total knee replacement in the United States Medicare population. *J Bone Joint Surg Am* 2005;87(6):1222-1228.

2. Wilson MG, Kelley K, Thornhill TS: Infection as a complication of total knee-replacement arthroplasty: Risk factors and treatment in sixty-seven cases. *J Bone Joint Surg Am* 1990;72(6):878-883.

3. Windsor RE, Bono JV: Infected total knee replacements. *J Am Acad Orthop Surg* 1994;2(1):44-53.

4. Bozic KJ, Kurtz SM, Lau E, et al: The epidemiology of revision total knee arthroplasty in the United States. *Clin Orthop Relat Res* 2010;468(1):45-51.

5. Kurtz SM, Ong KL, Lau E, Bozic KJ, Berry D, Parvizi J: Prosthetic joint infection risk after TKA in the Medicare population. *Clin Orthop Relat Res* 2010;468(1):52-56.

6. Kurtz SM, Lau E, Schmier J, Ong KL, Zhao K, Parvizi J: Infection burden for hip and knee arthroplasty in the United States. *J Arthroplasty* 2008;23(7):984-991.

7. Ayers DC, Dennis DA, Johanson NA, Pellegrini VD Jr: Common complications of total knee arthroplasty. *J Bone Joint Surg Am* 1997;79A:278-311.

8. Rao N, Cannella B, Crossett LS, Yates AJ Jr, McGough R III: A preoperative decolonization protocol for staphylococcus aureus prevents orthopaedic infections. *Clin Orthop Relat Res* 2008;466(6):1343-1348.

9. Fulkerson E, Valle CJ, Wise B, Walsh M, Preston C, Di Cesare PE: Antibiotic susceptibility of bacteria infecting total joint arthroplasty sites. *J Bone Joint Surg Am* 2006;88(6):1231-1237.

10. Price CS, Williams A, Philips G, Dayton M, Smith W, Morgan S: Staphylococcus aureus nasal colonization in preoperative orthopaedic outpatients. *Clin Orthop Relat Res* 2008;466(11):2842-2847.

11. Lindeque B, Rutigliano J, Williams A, McConnell J: Prevalence of methicillin-resistant Staphylococcus aureus among orthopedic patients at a large academic hospital. *Orthopedics* 2008;31(4):363.

12. Rosenberg AD, Wambold D, Kraemer L, et al: Ensuring appropriate timing of antimicrobial prophylaxis. *J Bone Joint Surg Am* 2008;90(2):226-232.

13. American Academy of Orthopaedic Surgeons. Recommendations for the use of intravenous antibiotic prophylaxis in primary total joint arthroplasty. 2004. http://www.aaos.org/about/papers/advistmt/1027.asp. Accessed June 1, 2011.

14. American Academy of Orthopaedic Surgeons. The use of prophylactic antibiotics in orthopaedic medicine and the emergence of vancomycin-resistant bacteria. 1998. Revised in 2002. http://www2.aaos.org/aaos/archives/bulletin/apr02/acdnws4.htm.

15. Finkelstein R, Rabino G, Mashiah T, et al: Vancomycin versus cefazolin prophylaxis for cardiac surgery in the setting of a high prevalence of methicillin-resistant staphylococcal infections. *J Thorac Cardiovasc Surg* 2002;123(2):326-332.

16. Hacek DM, Robb WJ, Paule SM, Kudrna JC, Stamos VP, Peterson LR: Staphylococcus aureus nasal decolonization in joint replacement surgery reduces infection. *Clin Orthop Relat Res* 2008;466(6):1349-1355.

17. Kalmeijer MD, Coertjens H, van Nieuwland-Bollen PM, et al: Surgical site infections in orthopedic surgery: The effect of mupirocin nasal ointment in a double-blind, randomized, placebo-controlled study. *Clin Infect Dis* 2002;35(4):353-358.

18. Kim DH, Spencer M, Davidson SM, et al: Institutional prescreening for detection and eradication of methicillin-resistant Staphylococcus aureus in patients undergoing elective orthopaedic surgery. *J Bone Joint Surg Am* 2010;92(9):1820-1826.

19. Simor AE, Phillips E, McGeer A, et al: Randomized controlled trial of chlorhexidine gluconate for washing, intranasal mupirocin, and rifampin and doxycycline versus no treatment for the eradication of methicillin-resistant Staphylococcus aureus colonization. *Clin Infect Dis* 2007;44(2):178-185.

20. Malinzak RA, Ritter MA, Berend ME, Meding JB, Olberding EM, Davis KE: Morbidly obese, diabetic, younger, and unilateral joint arthroplasty patients have elevated total joint arthroplasty infection rates. *J Arthroplasty* 2009;24(6, Suppl):84-88.

21. Marchant MH Jr, Viens NA, Cook C, Vail TP, Bolognesi MP: The impact of glycemic control and diabetes mellitus on perioperative outcomes after total joint arthroplasty. *J Bone Joint Surg Am* 2009;91(7):1621-1629.

22. Bolognesi MP, Marchant MH Jr, Viens NA, Cook C, Pietrobon R, Vail TP: The impact of diabetes on perioperative patient outcomes after total hip and total knee arthroplasty in the United States. *J Arthroplasty* 2008;23(6, Suppl 1): 92-98.

23. Winiarsky R, Barth P, Lotke P: Total knee arthroplasty in morbidly obese patients. *J Bone Joint Surg Am* 1998;80(12):1770-1774.

24. Parvizi J, Ghanem E, Joshi A, Sharkey PF, Hozack WJ, Rothman RH: Does "excessive" anticoagulation predispose to periprosthetic infection? *J Arthroplasty* 2007;22(6, Suppl 2):24-28.

25. Galat DD, McGovern SC, Larson DR, Harrington JR, Hanssen AD, Clarke HD: Surgical treatment of early wound complications following primary total knee arthroplasty. *J Bone Joint Surg Am* 2009; 91(1):48-54.

26. Matar WY, Jafari SM, Restrepo C, Austin M, Purtill JJ, Parvizi J: Preventing infection in total joint arthroplasty. *J Bone Joint Surg Am* 2010;92(Suppl 2):36-46.

27. Greidanus NV, Masri BA, Garbuz DS, et al: Use of erythrocyte sedimentation rate and C-reactive protein level to diagnose infection before revision total knee arthroplasty: A prospective evaluation. *J Bone Joint Surg Am* 2007;89(7): 1409-1416.

28. Di Cesare PE, Chang E, Preston CF, Liu CJ: Serum interleukin-6 as a marker of periprosthetic infection following total hip and knee arthroplasty. *J Bone Joint Surg Am* 2005;87(9):1921-1927.

29. Berbari E, Mabry T, Tsaras G, et al: Inflammatory blood laboratory levels as markers of prosthetic joint infection: A systematic review and meta-analysis. *J Bone Joint Surg Am* 2010;92(11):2102-2109.

30. Ghanem E, Parvizi J, Burnett RS, et al: Cell count and differential of aspirated fluid in the diagnosis of infection at the site of total knee arthroplasty. *J Bone Joint Surg Am* 2008;90(8):1637-1643.

31. Schinsky MF, Della Valle CJ, Sporer SM, Paprosky WG: Perioperative testing for joint infection in patients undergoing revision total hip arthroplasty. *J Bone Joint Surg Am* 2008;90(9):1869-1875.

32. Duff GP, Lachiewicz PF, Kelley SS: Aspiration of the knee joint before revision arthroplasty. *Clin Orthop Relat Res* 1996;331:132-139.

33. Mason JB, Fehring TK, Odum SM, Griffin WL, Nussman DS: The value of white blood cell counts before revision total knee arthroplasty. *J Arthroplasty* 2003; 18(8):1038-1043.

34. Kersey R, Benjamin J, Marson B: White blood cell counts and differential in synovial fluid of aseptically failed total knee arthroplasty. *J Arthroplasty* 2000;15(3): 301-304.

35. Morgan PM, Sharkey P, Ghanem E, et al: The value of intraoperative Gram stain in revision total knee arthroplasty. *J Bone Joint Surg Am* 2009;91(9):2124-2129.

36. Bedair H, Ting N, Jacovides C, et al: The Mark Coventry Award: Diagnosis of early postoperative TKA infection using synovial fluid analysis. *Clin Orthop Relat Res* 2011;469(1):34-40.

37. Bauer TW, Parvizi J, Kobayashi N, Krebs V: Diagnosis of periprosthetic infection. *J Bone Joint Surg Am* 2006;88(4): 869-882.

38. Berbari EF, Marculescu C, Sia I, et al: Culture-negative prosthetic joint infection. *Clin Infect Dis* 2007;45(9):1113-1119.

39. Segawa H, Tsukayama DT, Kyle RF, Becker DA, Gustilo RB: Infection after total knee arthroplasty: A retrospective study of the treatment of eighty-one infec-tions. *J Bone Joint Surg Am* 1999; 81(10):1434-1445.

40. Rand JA: Alternatives to reimplantation for salvage of the total knee arthroplasty complicated by infection. *J Bone Joint Surg Am* 1993;75(2):282-289.

41. Mont MA, Waldman B, Banerjee C, Pacheco IH, Hungerford DS: Multiple irrigation, debridement, and retention of components in infected total knee arthroplasty. *J Arthroplasty* 1997;12(4): 426-433.

42. Silva M, Tharani R, Schmalzried TP: Results of direct exchange or debridement of the infected total knee arthroplasty. *Clin Orthop Relat Res* 2002;404:125-131.

43. Azzam KA, Seeley M, Ghanem E, Austin MS, Purtill JJ, Parvizi J: Irrigation and debridement in the management of prosthetic joint infection: Traditional indications revisited. *J Arthroplasty* 2010; 25(7):1022-1027.

44. Springer BD, Lee GC, Osmon D, Haidukewych GJ, Hanssen AD, Jacofsky DJ: Systemic safety of high-dose antibiotic-loaded cement spacers after resection of an infected total knee arthroplasty. *Clin Orthop Relat Res* 2004;427: 47-51.

45. van Raaij TM, Visser LE, Vulto AG, Verhaar JA: Acute renal failure after local gentamicin treatment in an infected total knee arthroplasty. *J Arthroplasty* 2002; 17(7):948-950.

46. Jämsen E, Stogiannidis I, Malmivaara A, Pajamäki J, Puolakka T, Konttinen YT: Outcome of prosthesis exchange for infected knee arthroplasty: The effect of treatment approach. *Acta Orthop* 2009;80(1):67-77.

47. Haleem AA, Berry DJ, Hanssen AD: Mid-term to long-term followup of two-stage reimplantation for infected total knee arthroplasty. *Clin Orthop Relat Res* 2004; 428:35-39.

Foot and Ankle

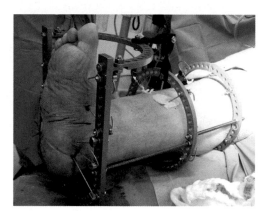

Charcot Foot: A Surgical Algorithm

Michael S. Pinzur, MD
Vincent James Sammarco, MD
Dane K. Wukich, MD

Abstract

The historic treatment of Charcot foot has entailed non–weight-bearing immobilization during the acute active phase, followed by longitudinal management with accommodative bracing. This treatment plan yields poor outcomes, even in cases classified as successful. An appreciation of poor outcomes convinced experts to attempt correction of the resultant deformities. Early attempts at surgical correction of the acquired deformities in patients with medical comorbidities were complicated by infection, wound failure, and mechanical loss of correction. New surgical techniques have been designed to obtain and maintain correction and minimize the risks for complications and poor outcomes in this complex patient population.

Instr Course Lect 2012;61:423-438.

The American Diabetes Association estimates that the number of individuals with diabetes in the United States is rapidly increasing, with a current estimate of more than 18 million. Improvements in the longitudinal management of diabetes and its associated comorbidities has allowed many patients to live longer and lead more active, productive lives. This heightened appreciation of diabetes and its associated comorbidities has encouraged many orthopaedic foot and ankle surgeons to attempt creative methods of deformity correction and stabilization, thus avoiding the need for cumbersome and expensive custom fabricated orthotic devices.

The historic treatment of Charcot foot arthropathy involves immobilization of the involved foot in a short leg, non–weight-bearing, total contact cast until the process resolves, followed by longitudinal management with accommodative bracing. This treatment regimen is based primary on expert opinion and the results of a few small retrospective case series. An observational study using the American Orthopaedic Foot and Ankle Society (AOFAS) diabetic foot questionnaire reported that Charcot foot results in a severe negative impact on health-related quality of life, which is not lessened even with successful treatment using methods based on the standard of care circa 2000.[1]

Several recent investigations have supported using a weight-bearing total contact cast only when the involved foot is both clinically and radiographically plantigrade.[2-5] The development of late ulceration overlying deformity and osteomyelitis is likely when the foot is not clinically or radiographically plantigrade.[4,5] These observations have led most experts to advise surgical correction when deformity is present.

Midfoot Arthrodesis With Internal Fixation

If untreated, neuroarthropathic dislocation of the foot often leaves the patient with a nonplantigrade foot and a bony prominence in the arch where the soft tissue is least equipped to deal with abnormally high pressures. One approach has been to protect the limb from weight bearing with a total con-

Dr. Pinzur or an immediate family member is a member of a speakers' bureau or has made paid presentations on behalf of Small Bone Innovations, Smith & Nephew, and Tornier; serves as a paid consultant to SBI; has received research or institutional support from Biomimetic; and serves as a board member, owner, officer, or committee member of the American Orthopaedic Foot and Ankle Society and the American Academy of Orthopaedic Surgeons. Dr. Sammarco or an immediate family member serves as a board member, owner, officer, or committee member of the American Academy of Orthopaedic Surgeons. Dr. Wukich or an immediate family member has received royalties from Arthrex and serves as a board member, owner, officer, or committee member of the American Academy of Orthopaedic Surgeons Membership Committee.

tact cast or other off-loading device and then excise the bony prominence after the acute Charcot phase has ended and the foot has consolidated into its final position.[6] Although this technique is often effective, a subset of patients never seems to achieve a stable foot position, and management of those patients with an orthosis can be exceedingly difficult and is often unsuccessful. Saltzmann et al[7] reviewed 115 patients who were treated with an intensive nonsurgical protocol, including close physician surveillance and bracing, to manage diabetic neuroarthropathy. The authors reported a 2.7% annual risk of amputation and a 49% rate of recurrent ulceration, suggesting that earlier surgical treatment may be more appropriate for some patients.

Early surgical studies focused on reconstruction of the Charcot dislocation with reduction and arthrodesis. Standard fixation techniques developed for fusion in nonneuropathic bone were used but often were inadequate to maintain reduction. Most surgeons recommended that the non–weight-bearing period be doubled or even tripled to account for poor bone healing and the inherent weakness of the underlying osseous structures.[8-11] Clinical experience shows that diabetic patients are often poorly compliant with postoperative protocols that demand non–weight-bearing periods. Often these patients are debilitated from multiple medical problems, including obesity, and overall poor physical conditioning that hinders their ability to ambulate while maintaining a non–weight-bearing status. Bohannon and Kelly[12] showed that a patient with neuropathy is unable to adequately modulate the amount of weight on his or her extremity, which the author believed was caused by a lack of feedback from the neuropathic limb. Early surgical series showed improvement in restoring a plantigrade foot and preventing recurrence of ulceration, although complications were frequent.[9,10,13,14] Often osseous nonunion, failure or cutout of hardware, and loss of initial correction were reported despite foot salvage.

Superconstruct Techniques

There are many problems associated with achieving a successful arthrodesis in a patient with neuroarthropathy. Often, the primary area of involvement in the foot undergoes bony dissolution, a process whereby increased vascularity combined with repetitive trauma causes fragmentation and resorption of bone. The Charcot process is mediated by not only repetitive trauma in an insensate foot but also sympathetic denervation, which leads to hypervascularity of the foot in the acute phase. Increased blood flow leads to a loss of calcium and osteoporosis in the involved bone and eventually to scarring and fibrosis of the bone itself. The combination of dissolution with gross instability is cumulative and leads to progressive bone loss and deformity. If the foot dislocates through the midfoot, the cuboid, the navicular, and/or the cuneiforms will become prominent in the mid-arch, and ulceration often ensues. The challenge for surgeons has been to develop fixation strategies that overcome the problems of poor bone quality, gross instability, poor patient compliance, and extended healing times. Early experience seemed to dictate a "more is better" philosophy in which more hardware was added without necessarily modifying the techniques or positioning of the implants; however, more hardware in osteopenic and avascular bone adds little to the quality of fixation. Surgeons eventually sought methods to improve the overall quality of the constructs used for fixation of the arthrodesis (**Figure 1**). Poor results, including nonunion, hardware failure, and recurrence of deformity have led to an evolution in fixation techniques. Over the past 10 years, surgeons have gradually increased the strength of the implants used and modified procedures so that fixation spans the area of dissolution, with the belief that better fixation can achieve successful arthrodesis.

The concept of a superconstruct has been introduced to summarize the principles that dictate reconstruction in these cases.[15] Superconstruct techniques abandon some of the normal principles of fusion surgery to maximize the stability of the fusion fixation. A superconstruct is defined by three techniques: fusion extended beyond the zone of injury, bone resection performed to allow reduction without significant tension on the soft-tissue envelope, and the use of the strongest device that can be tolerated by the soft-tissue envelope.

Fusion Beyond the Injury Zone

To improve fixation, fusion is extended beyond the zone of injury to include unaffected joints. This technique ignores the traditional principle of sparing unaffected joints to preserve motion segments in the foot. In the Charcot foot, single joint fusions are often not possible because of poor bone quality and fragmentation. By applying hardware that spans the area of dissolution and by including noninvolved joints, the risk of hardware cutout is diminished. Some authors prefer performing a formal arthrodesis with joint preparation of all involved segments that will be spanned by hardware.[16,17] Other authors have achieved successful results by formally preparing only the involved section for fusion and crossing hardware through some unprepared joints.[18-20] These authors argue that although crossing unfused joints increases the risk of hardware migration and long-term breakage, the technique allows the procedure to be done with less soft-tissue stripping and without removing the stronger subchondral bone of normal joints.

Bone Resection to Allow Reduction With Limited Tension on the Soft-Tissue Envelope

Bone resection is performed to allow reduction without significant tension on the soft-tissue envelope. The traditional principle of reestablishing length to reconstruct the shape of the foot must be abandoned to establish a tension-free reduction; otherwise there will be risks of redislocation and hardware cutout. Loss of the vascular supply of the forefoot may occur if the arterial supply is put under too much tension during the reduction because atherosclerosis may compromise the compliance of the vessels. Deforming forces include the strong pull of the Achilles tendon and contracted posterior calf musculature, which pulls the ankle and hindfoot into plantar flexion. In cases of midfoot dislocation, the tibialis anterior tendon and the digital extensors pull the forefoot dorsally; as instability progresses, the fore-

foot is pulled into abduction. When combined with midfoot instability, these opposing forces will lead to a bayonet apposition of the forefoot on the hindfoot, which allows the soft-

tissue envelope to further contract and become quite rigid (**Figure 2**). This rigid soft-tissue contracture cannot be stretched to allow for reduction of the foot, thus the osseous structures must

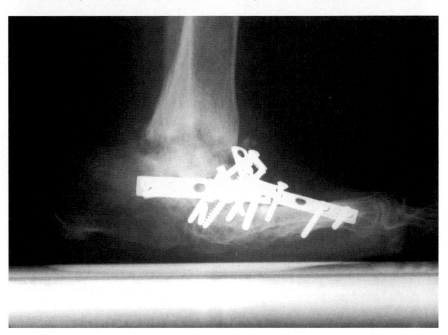

Figure 1   Lateral radiograph of the foot in a patient with diabetic foot neuroarthropathy showing nonunion, recurrent deformity, and broken hardware after an attempted midfoot fusion using a standard crossed screw and plate technique. (Reproduced with permission from Sammarco VJ: Superconstructs in the repair of Charcot midfoot dislocations. *Foot Ankle Clin* 2009;14(3):393-407. Http://www.sciencedirect.com/science/journal/10837515.)

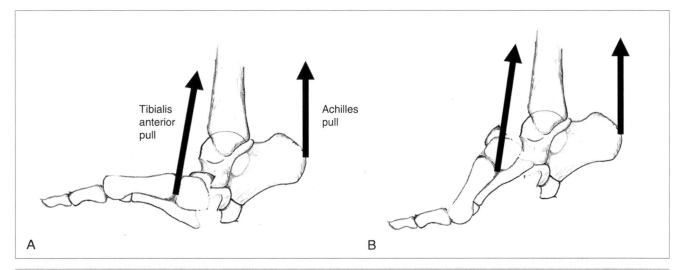

Figure 2   A, Illustration of deforming forces in the Charcot foot, including contracture of the Achilles tendon, which pulls the calcaneus and the ankle into plantar flexion, and the pull of the tibialis anterior and digital extensors, which cause a dorsal/lateral pull on the forefoot. **B,** Illustration showing the bayonet apposition of the forefoot on the hindfoot that occurs when the midfoot dislocates.

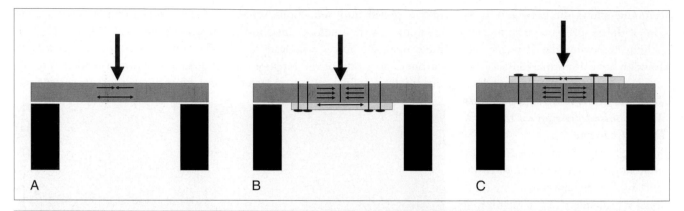

Figure 3 **A,** Illustration of force distribution in a beam bridge model with a three-point bending moment applied. Tension occurs dorsally and compression occurs plantarly. **B,** A plate applied plantarly will act as a load-sharing device as tension is generated through the plate and compression occurs through the fusion site. **C,** In a dorsally applied plate, the plate compresses, and distraction may occur at the fusion site as the plate deforms.

be shortened to allow a tension-free reduction.

Use of the Strongest Device Tolerated by the Soft-Tissue Envelope

The strongest device that can be tolerated by the soft-tissue envelope is used, and the device is applied in a manner that maximizes mechanical stability. Early attempts at fusing dislocated neuropathic feet were frustrated by nonunion and hardware failure. Fixation has evolved whereby the small diameter screws used in earlier series have been replaced by larger, more fatigue-resistant devices. Surgeons have also revised methods for applying the devices. Techniques have been developed to maximize the mechanical properties of the devices. Three fixation techniques have evolved to correct Charcot midfoot deformity: planter plating, locked plating, and axial screw fixation. Only limited data are available for evaluating the use of these techniques.

Plantar Plating and Locked Plating Techniques

Plating techniques for midfoot fusion are increasing in popularity because of a large influx of new plates and

procedure-specific devices. Plate fixation for fusion in reconstruction of the neuropathic foot offers many benefits. The plate can easily span the area of dissolution, affording fixation in more normal bone proximally and distally with multiple screws. Applying plates dorsally, medially, or laterally requires that the plate function as a load-bearing device. In neuroarthropathic feet, these plates may be at increased risk of fatigue failure because of extended healing times and incomplete healing. Schon (LC Schon, MD, Baltimore, MD, personal communication, 1998) noted that applying plates on the plantar aspect of the foot places the device under tension, allowing the plate to act as a load-sharing device (**Figure 3**). Deformation that occurs with weight bearing with the plate in a plantar position applies tension to the plate and forces compression at the fusion site. The plate itself is stronger under tension than compression. As weight is borne by the foot, the osseous structures are loaded along with the hardware to create a more stable construct.

Marks et al[21] tested this concept in a biomechanical model using cadavers. A midfoot fusion model was done in eight matched cadaver pairs, fixing the

fusion with either multiple crossed screws or a plantar plating construct at the tarsometatarsal joints. The models were loaded cyclically and also loaded to failure. The authors reported a much lower initial deformation and higher load to failure with the plantar plate technique and noted that this afforded a much sturdier preparation for arthrodesis. Campbell et al[22] studied the stability of metatarsal osteotomies fixed with crossed screws versus plantar plates and similarly found the plantar plate construct to be stronger and more resistant to deformation under cyclical loading. Schon et al[23] reported on the clinical results of patients treated with midfoot arthrodesis using the plantar plate technique. Thirty-four patients underwent reduction and midfoot fusion for treatment of neuroarthropathic midfoot dislocation. Fusions were fixed with plantar plates applied medially, laterally, or both. The authors reported successful deformity correction and adequate arthrodesis for all patients treated with the procedure. Poor results were noted in patients treated nonsurgically during the same period.

Plantar plating has enjoyed success anecdotally, although the study by Schon et al[23] is the only published re-

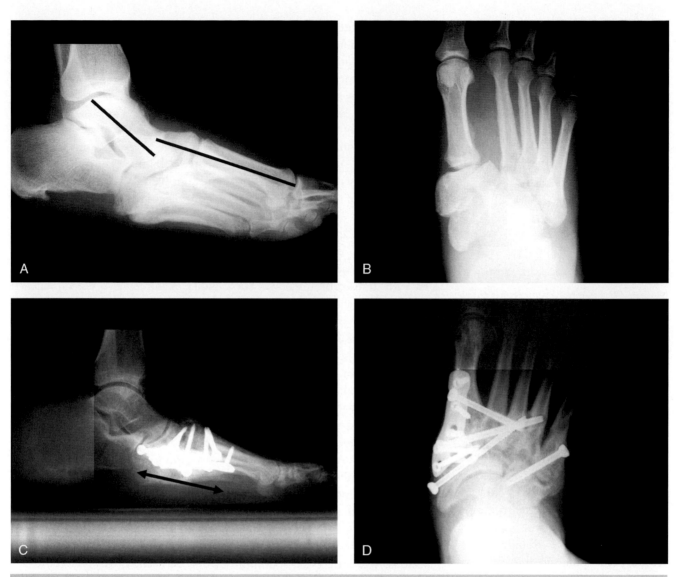

Figure 4   Radiographs of the foot of a 36-year-old man with diabetes with neuropathic dislocation through the midfoot. **A,** Lateral radiograph with lines indicating the midlateral axis of the talus (hindfoot) relative to the midlateral axis of the first metatarsal (forefoot). **B,** AP radiograph. Lateral (**C**) and AP (**D**) 2-year postoperative radiographs show solid fusion achieved with a plantar plating technique. Note that deformation of the plate caused compression of the fusion mass. The arrow in part C represents the tension band effect of the screw-plate construct. (Reproduced with permission from Sammarco VJ: Superconstructs in the repair of Charcot midfoot dislocations. *Foot Ankle Clin* 2009;14(3):393-407. Http://www.sciencedirect.com/science/journal/10837515.)

port to date of this technique. In the experience of this chapter's authors, that technique offers excellent fixation and deformity correction (**Figure 4**). Because the plantar tissues are thicker and more robust than dorsal and medial soft tissues, they allow the use of thicker, stronger implants. The technique works well when the dislocation involves the tarsometatarsal joints; however, in cases of navicular fragmen-

tation, the plates cannot be adequately positioned on the plantar aspect of the talar neck because of the proximity of the sustentaculum of the calcaneus. Technically, this is a demanding procedure that requires an extensive plantar exposure to allow application of the plates. There is concern that stripping of the entire soft-tissue envelope from the plantar aspect of the osseous structures may devascularize the arthrodesis

bed and, if deformity recurs or the screws back out, the hardware is more likely to be exposed directly in the event of a plantar ulceration.

Locked plating technology has mechanical advantages for fixation of bone in patients with neuropathy. Locked plating refers to devices in which the screws mechanically engage the plate to create a fixed-angle device.[24] This allows for the creation of a

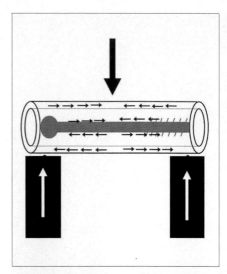

Figure 5 Illustration of an axial screw acting as reinforcement bar (rebar) in a beam model. The screw shares tension and compression with the bone when a three-point bend is applied to the beam. The large black arrow indicates the bending force. The white arrows represent the resting state of the biomechanical system.

much stronger construct than a conventional plate and allows rigid fixation of fragmented bone into the fusion site. Locked plates have been shown to have improved initial stability and screw pull-out strength in osteoporotic bone compared with their nonlocked counterparts.[25] These plates allow fixation on the dorsal and medial talar neck when navicular comminution is present and multiple fixed-angle fixations in the navicular when medial cuneiform comminution is present. Thicker, stronger plates are recommended with this technique because the plate will act as a load-bearing structure once weight bearing has been initiated, and the plate will be at risk for device failure because of cyclic loading. Although there are no published clinical series of reconstruction for neuropathic foot disease, successful long-term results have been reported in individual cases.[15,26]

Axial Screw Reconstruction

Axial screw fixation refers to the placement of screws within the intramedullary canal of the metatarsals distally and extension of those screws proximally to span the area of dissolution (**Figure 5**). The screws may be applied either antegrade through the calcaneus and talus or retrograde through the metatarsal heads. Axial screw fixation has several advantages of more traditional fixation methods. One advantage is that relatively large diameter screws can be applied without creating large stress risers in the metatarsal shafts, which occurs with transcortical screws. The technique also facilitates deformity reduction because if cannulated screws are used, the final alignment and hardware positioning can be checked and adjusted before the screws are actually placed. The technique allows preparation of the arthrodesis bed through a less extensile exposure because only the area of dislocation needs to be opened surgically. A more limited exposure limits stripping of the soft-tissue envelope and periosteal blood supply of the osseous structures, which in turn may improve the rate of fusion and decrease the chances of wound complications. The intraosseous positioning of the hardware also decreases the risk of direct hardware contamination in the event of postoperative wound complications or recurrent ulceration. Although the origin of the technique is unclear, this chapter's authors believe the first published account of the axial screw technique involved a large cannulated screw used to bridge the lateral column of a neuropathic dislocation from the calcaneus to the fourth metatarsal shaft during an arthrodesis.[27] Applying the screws retrograde through the metatarsophalangeal joints or antegrade through the talus is disadvantageous because the articular surfaces of these joints are disrupted.

During application, tightening the screws compresses the fusion mass and helps achieve good bony apposition of the fused segments. Mechanically, the screws function as load-sharing devices during weight bearing (**Figure 6**). Hansen suggested that the screw/fusion mass creates a structure similar to steel-reinforced concrete, in which the multiple axial screws function similar to rebar in the distribution of tensile and compressive forces (SV Hansen, MD, personal communication 2002). Two mechanical studies have been published evaluating this technique. Kann et al[28] tested matched pairs of cadavers for the stability of calcaneocuboid joint fusions fixed either with an obliquely applied screw or an axial screw applied across the joint. Initial stability and load to failure were higher in the axial screw model. A plantar plate/oblique screw construct was compared with multiple axial screw fixation in a matched-pair cadaver model in which the tarsometatarsal joint was disarticulated and fixed (KJ Mroczek, MD, et al, Washington, DC, unpublished data, 2010). There was no significant difference in initial stiffness or load to failure between the two groups, and none of the constructs failed during cyclic loading to 5,000 cycles.

Two clinical studies reported on the use of axial screws for the reconstruction of Charcot midfoot deformity. Sammarco et al[18] reported on 22 patients with severe deformity caused by neuropathic dislocation who were treated with midfoot arthrodesis fixed with multiple axial screws. Fusions were done in patients with continued gross instability and recurrent ulceration despite conservative management with a contact cast and accommodative bracing. Excellent deformity correction with normalization of radiographic parameters was reported at short- and long-term follow-up.

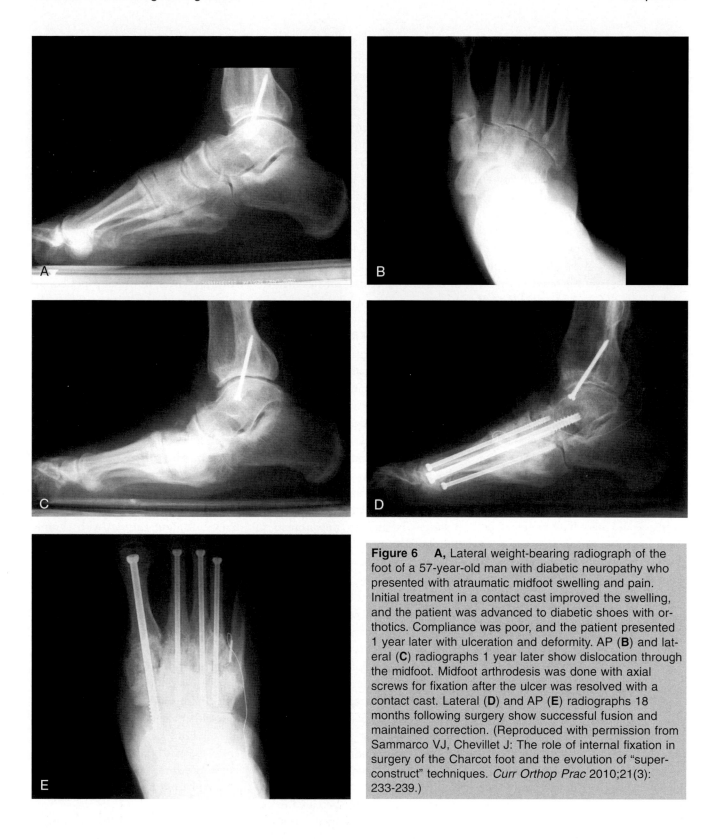

Figure 6 **A,** Lateral weight-bearing radiograph of the foot of a 57-year-old man with diabetic neuropathy who presented with atraumatic midfoot swelling and pain. Initial treatment in a contact cast improved the swelling, and the patient was advanced to diabetic shoes with orthotics. Compliance was poor, and the patient presented 1 year later with ulceration and deformity. AP (**B**) and lateral (**C**) radiographs 1 year later show dislocation through the midfoot. Midfoot arthrodesis was done with axial screws for fixation after the ulcer was resolved with a contact cast. Lateral (**D**) and AP (**E**) radiographs 18 months following surgery show successful fusion and maintained correction. (Reproduced with permission from Sammarco VJ, Chevillet J: The role of internal fixation in surgery of the Charcot foot and the evolution of "superconstruct" techniques. *Curr Orthop Prac* 2010;21(3): 233-239.)

Because complications were more common when the talonavicular joint was bridged with axial screws, the authors recommended using larger diameter screws in the medial column when the talonavicular joint was crossed. At a minimum 2-year follow-up, there were no amputations, and all patients were ambulatory and used standard diabetic shoe wear. Assal and Stern[17] reported on 15 patients treated with midfoot fusion for intractable ulceration caused by chronic Charcot midfoot deformity. A single, antegrade, longitudinal screw was used to fix the medial column, and the middle and lateral columns were fixed with a variety of techniques including plates and obliquely applied screws. Successful results were reported in all patients except one who required amputation because of persistent deep infection. The primary difference between these series is that Sammarco et al[18] do not recommend surgery in the presence of active ulceration, whereas Assal and Stern[17] consider intractable ulceration as an indication for surgery. Sammarco et al and Assal and Stern have presented detailed descriptions of techniques for performing reconstruction using axial screws.[19,20,29,30]

Video 34.1: Midtarsal Arthrodesis in the Treatment of Charcot Midfoot Arthropathy. V. James Sammarco, MD; G. James Sammarco, MD (28 min)

Future Direction

First-generation superconstruct techniques were developed because of inadequate results achieved with standard fixation methods in neuropathic bone. The previously described techniques were developed to improve internal fixation by improving the ability of standard orthopaedic trauma implants to hold together osteoporotic

and fibrotic bone for extended periods of time. The past 5 years have seen an explosion of procedure-specific implants, including screws designed for axial fixation and anatomically contoured locking plates designed specifically for foot arthrodesis. It is hoped that these devices will improve the ability of surgeons to achieve successful limb salvage in this challenging patient population. Similarly, biologic adjuvants such as recombinant bone morphogenetic proteins may improve the ability to achieve a successful arthrodesis by speeding the healing process.

Static Ring Fixation

Internal fixation methods are not appropriate for all patients. Surgery has generally been avoided in diabetic patients with Charcot arthropathy because of the high incidence of morbid obesity and the likelihood for wound infection or mechanical failure caused by poor quality bone.[31-35] The high incidence of postoperative wound infections in diabetic patients is well appreciated because of impairments in both humeral and cellular immunity.[36] The use of standard implants is further precluded in more than 50% of patients because of the presence of contaminated wounds overlying the deformity or, more likely, by complications from underlying osteomyelitis at the time of presentation.[37,38] Even if infection is avoided, the associated mechanically poor-quality bone often leads to mechanical failure of the surgical construct.[39]

These confounding variables have led several surgeons to modify the Ilizarov method to obtain and maintain correction of the acquired deformities with a minimal risk of complications.[37,38,40-43] This surgical technique obtains deformity correction through a limited surgical approach and maintains that correction

with a preassembled circular external fixator.

Surgical Technique

The first step in static ring fixation surgery is lengthening the gastrocnemius-soleus muscle unit by either percutaneous triple hemisection of the Achilles tendon or fractional lengthening at the musculotendinous junction. This step is performed to establish a muscle balance between the ankle plantar flexors and dorsiflexors. It is appreciated that diabetes-associated peripheral neuropathy, which is universally present in this patient population, affects the smaller muscles and nerves of the anterior leg. The resultant motor imbalance creates an equinus bending moment at the junction between the hindfoot and the forefoot during the midstance phase of gait.

The second step is excising all infected bone contiguous with any open wounds. The surgically obtained cultures are used to direct culture-specific parenteral antibiotic therapy that is used for all patients with evidence of bony infection. Patients with chronic wounds, negative cultures with microscopic demonstration of chronic infection (inflammatory granulation tissue with a large population of white blood cells), and a history of recurrent ulceration are also treated with a course of parenteral therapy with the antibiotic most likely appropriate to the clinical scenario. Many patients with no current clinical evidence of infection, who have either a history of an ulcer overlying the bony deformity or had apparently been successfully treated for bony infection, have positive cultures obtained from bony specimen at surgery.

The next step is deformity correction and creation of both a clinical and radiographically plantigrade foot. This is generally accomplished by excising a wedge of bone from the apex of the ac-

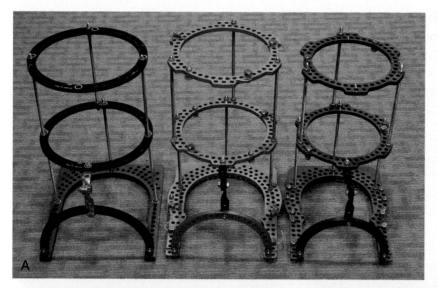

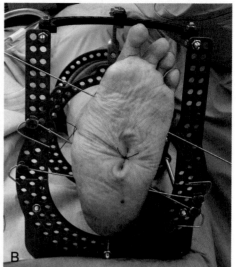

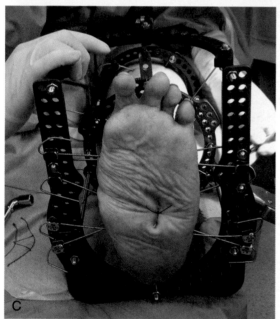

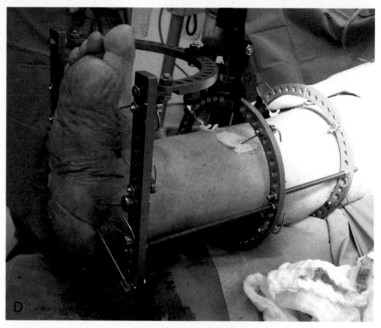

Figure 7   **A,** Circular frames can be prebuilt and available for use at surgery. **B,** Two olive wires are drilled through the calcaneus at 30° angles to each other, parallel to the weight-bearing surface of the heel. With the heel centered and oriented in the foot ring, these wires are pretensioned to 120 kg and attached to the foot ring, being careful to have no pressure on the skin. **C,** The forefoot is reduced to the hindfoot. Wires are drilled through the metatarsals, again at 30° angles to each other and parallel to the weight-bearing surface of the foot. To create compression fixation, the wires are arched. **D,** Two olive wires are then drilled through the tibia at approximately 60° angles to each other. The wires are drilled through the bone and then tapped through the soft tissues with a mallet to avoid neurovascular injury. With the tibia centered in the middle of the proximal ring, the wires are pretensioned to 120 kg and attached to the ring.

quired deformity. Standard principles of deformity correction osteotomy are used. The first osteotomy is made perpendicular with the axis of the hindfoot. The second osteotomy is made perpendicular to the axis of the forefoot. If done correctly, closing the wedge should create a clinical and a radiographic plantigrade foot.[37,38,44] Percutaneous smooth wires can be used to provide provisional fixation before application of the circular external fixator. Rarely, a corrective modified triple arthrodesis combined with bony resection, as historically used in patients with polio, can be used to correct the acquired deformity.

The final step is applying a preconstructed static external fixator to maintain the correction (**Figure 7,** *A*). With the foot positioned by hand in the center of a closed foot ring, two wires are drilled through the heel (**Figure 7**, *B*). The olive wires are placed at 30° angles to each other and parallel to the weight-bearing surface of the heel. These wires are pretensioned at 90 to 120 kg and attached to the foot ring. Two wires are then drilled through the metatarsals, again at 30° angles to each other and parallel to the weight-bearing surface of the forefoot. With the foot centered in the foot ring, the wires are again tensioned and attached to the foot ring (**Figure 7**, *C*). By placing the pin holders for the metatarsal wires in the hole just proximal to the resting position of the wire, the forefoot is compressed to the hindfoot. Two olive wires are then drilled through the tibia at the level of the proximal ring. With the tibia centered in the ring, the olive wires are pretensioned to 120 kg and attached to the ring. Olive or smooth wires can then be used at the level of the middle ring to achieve stability (**Figure 7**, *D*).

Postoperative Care

Dressings are removed on the second postoperative day. Pin care is performed daily with a mixture of chlorhexidine and hydrogen peroxide until the pin sites become dry. Patients are allowed to shower following discharge. A protective "frame shoe" is applied at the first postoperative visit to allow limited weight bearing during transfers. Pin tract infections are treated with broad-spectrum oral antibiotics and cutting of the skin to relieve tension from the wires. The frame is removed at 8 to 12 weeks after surgery, and the patient is transitioned to a weight-bearing total contact cast, which is used for 4 to 6 weeks. The patient is then transitioned into a removable fracture boot until volume is sufficiently stable to allow fitting of therapeutic footwear.

Midfoot Correction With Dynamic Circular Fixation

Jean-Francois Malgaigne introduced the concept of circular external fixation in 1840, when he fabricated an apparatus consisting of hemicircular arcs secured to point screws to reduce fracture fragments.[45-48] Modern external fixation dates back to the early 1900s when various forms of fixation were developed.[49-53] Anderson[54] developed the original pins-in-plaster concept, ultimately modifying this technique so that casting was not required. Another major improvement occurred when Stader[55] introduced compression and distraction across the fracture site. Despite the early success of external fixation, it remained unpopular in North America because of high complication rates associated with a lack of experience. These devices were banned by the US Army Surgeon General in most medical facilities during World War II.[56] Charnley[57,58] from England and Hoffman[59-61] from Switzerland furthered the understanding of external fixation after World War II. Hoffman[61] developed a unilateral fixator that incorporated universal joints at the pin fixator interface, allowing for the reduction of poorly aligned fracture fragments through a process termed osteotaxis. The Committee on Fractures and Traumatic Surgery of the American Academy of Orthopaedic Surgeons provided support for this technique in 1950, although this acceptance was granted with some reservation. They recommended that only experienced surgeons use this technique.

Ilizarov[62] developed an external ring fixator in Siberia in 1951, although it remained obscure for many years. The Ilizarov method incorporated Kirschner wires with circular rings for fracture stabilization and limb immobilization. Ilizarov discovered the concept of distraction osteogenesis when he noted that slow distraction of an osteotomy led to the formation of regenerate bone within the distracted osteotomy site.[63-65] Ilizarov expanded the indications for external ring fixation in the 1960s to include osseous lengthening, deformity correction, and soft-tissue contractures.[63-65] The methods of Ilizarov were essentially unknown outside the Soviet block until the early 1980s when Italian surgeons introduced the techniques.[66] The Ilizarov external fixation system provides an effective method for stabilizing and correcting osseous deformities while potentially minimizing surgical trauma with smaller incisions or percutaneous techniques. The ability to lengthen both osseous and soft-tissue structures has been invaluable in correcting severe deformities, nonunions, malunions, osteomyelitis, and soft-tissue contractures. Applications for the Ilizarov techniques have continued to evolve over time (**Figure 8**).

The components of circular fixation include rings, connecting rods, wires, and half-pins. Full rings are usually used in the leg; however, the anatomy of the foot and ankle often requires the use of partial rings and foot plates. Proper insertion techniques and tensioning of the fine wires is required to minimize pin tract problems. Tibial half pins are used more frequently in the United States and offer the ability to achieve orthogonal pin placement in difficult areas vulnerable to neurovascular injury. A thorough knowledge of cross-sectional anatomy is paramount to avoid injury to vital structures.

Advantages

External fixation was first used in the treatment of Charcot neuroarthropathy in the late 1990s.[8,67] There are several potential advantages of external fixation in patients with Charcot neu-

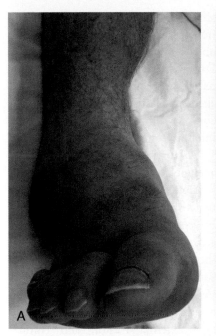

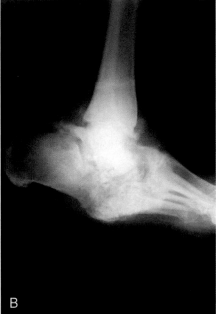

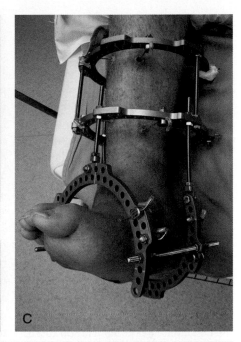

Figure 8   **A,** Photograph of a foot with a complex Charcot foot deformity. **B,** Lateral radiograph showing the deformity. **C,** Foot after applying a dynamic circular fixator.

roarthropathy, including the ability to perform acute or gradual correction during the postoperative period.[68-70] Because bone quality is often compromised in patients with neuropathic arthropathy as a result of regional osteopenia, the use of internal fixation may be compromised. Circular fixation provides the ability to obtain bone stability with multiple fine wires placed in multiple planes. Smaller bones, such as the tarsal and metatarsal bones, will not tolerate screw or plate fixation, and fine wires offer an advantage in these distal regions. Patients with diabetic neuropathy are often morbidly obese, and the increased stability provided by circular fixation can withstand some degree of weight bearing in these challenging patients. Traditional methods of internal fixation mandate the use of strong and bulky plates in neuropathic patients, typically requiring large incisions. Smaller incisions may be possible with external fixation, permitting realignment through less complicated soft-tissue flaps. A particularly difficult problem

to treat is the combination of Charcot neuroarthropathy and osteomyelitis. External fixation allows reconstruction to proceed concurrently with the treatment of infection. The ability to monitor wounds and soft-tissue envelopes during the postoperative periods is also a benefit of circular fixation The acceptance of external fixation in the treatment of Charcot arthropathy has increased greatly over the past 15 years despite Myerson's recommendation that external fixation should be used only in the presence of infection, large wounds, or gross ankle instability.[71]

Technique Evolution

Most of the literature describing the use of external fixation in the surgical management of Charcot neuroarthropathy consists of review articles and case reports.[37,69,72-74] Most commonly, external fixation has been used during the acute correction of deformities. Open realignment osteotomy and fusion are performed through a limited incision, followed by application of a static circular frame.[41,75]

Compression of the fusion site through arched wires can increase stability and improve healing.[69] The recent development of multiplane fixators allows the gradual correction of some of these deformities. Although gradual correction of Charcot deformities is possible with the Ilizarov-type frame, it is technically challenging and relies on the ability of the surgeon to places the wires and hinges in a very accurate manner. The introduction of the Taylor Spatial Frame (Smith & Nephew, Memphis, TN) simplifies correction with the use of a computer program that allows realignment in various planes. Multiaxial dynamic correction is used in concert with deformities that are mobile, either through intervention early in the Charcot process or through an osteotomy.[73,76,77] The frame permits gradual correction in the sagittal, coronal, and axial planes, thus restoring the appropriate anatomy. Elongating struts replace threaded rods and hinges, greatly simplifying the process. Once optimal alignment is obtained, internal fixation and arthrodesis through less invasive incisions can be performed to maintain the correction. Early results of this technique have been encouraging. Roukis and Zgonis[73] used the Taylor Spatial Frame to slowly compress and distract the osteotomy site, attempting to duplicate the Wolff law and promote healing. Once the frame is removed, stability is assessed; if any motion is detected, multiple screws are inserted to provide a rebar effect.

Challenging Patient Conditions and Study Results

Some patients with acute Charcot neuroarthropathy have compromised soft tissues; circular external fixation can be used in patients with severe deformity and less than optimal soft-tissue quality. Deformity about the ankle can cause ulceration over the malleoli, and acute correction may require large bone resections. Vascular embarrassment and further soft-tissue complications can arise with acute correction and significant bone shortening. By gradually correcting the deformity, neurovascular structures and skin can adapt over time, thus minimizing soft-tissue problems. Associated ulcers can be managed concurrently with gradual deformity correction. This technique has been used successfully in patients with posttraumatic equinovarus deformity.[77] The Charcot deformity is evaluated much like a long-bone fracture. The various parameters that are entered include the type of angulation, displacement, rotation, and length. The simplest method is to describe the characteristics of the deformity using a proximal reference that is normally analogous to a fracture. For example, a varus deformity of the ankle would be described as apex lateral angulation and medial displacement (translation) of the distal fragment. Virtually all Charcot deformities result in a short-

ened limb and require distraction as a part of the gradual realignment process. These parameters are entered into the computer program, and the computer generates a plan that allows correction over time. Once the soft tissues improve and ulcers heal, reconstructive options can include definitive arthrodesis with internal and/or external fixation.

In 2002, Cooper[68] reported the results of his experience in treating 100 patients with Charcot neuroarthropathy. Eighty-three of 100 patients (83%) were available for follow-up. More than 80% of the patients had a Wagner stage III ulcer, often with underlying osteomyelitis. The surgical technique included excision of any ulcers, correction of equinus deformity, biplanar osteotomy, and the application of circular external fixation. At an average follow-up of 22 months, limb salvage was accomplished in 96% of the patients. Complications included seven pin tract infections and two tibial fractures.

Saltzman[78] described his experience with multiplane external fixation in patients with Charcot neuroarthropathy. He applied 40 frames as a part of fusion treatment; the average duration of wearing the frame was 110 days. The postoperative protocol involved limited weight bearing on the involved side until the fusion was stable. After frame removal, a total contact cast was applied, and patients advanced to progressive weight bearing. The author reported that 31 of 40 patients had at least one complication, and several patients had more than one complication.

In 1998, Prokuski and Saltzman[67] reported on the use of an articulated monolateral external fixator in a patient with bilateral ankle Charcot arthropathy. Papa et al[8] described the use of external fixation in 4 of 29 patients who had diabetic neuropathic arthrop-

athy of the foot and ankle and mentioned the requirement of additional open surgery for salvage. Myerson and Edwards[79] discussed the use of an external ring fixation system in the management of an infected diabetic Charcot foot deformity as a supplement to internal fixation techniques.

Farber et al[41] reported the results of a single-stage correction with external fixation to treat ulcerated feet in patients with Charcot neuroarthropathy. Eleven patients with ulceration associated with midfoot Charcot arthropathy (10 diabetic patients and 1 patient with end-stage renal disease) were treated with débridement, corrective osteotomy, application of a Hoffman-type external fixator, and culture-directed antibiotic therapy. The duration of external fixation averaged 8 weeks and was followed by application of a total contact cast for an average of 19 weeks. Subsequently, therapeutic shoe wear and/or braces were prescribed. All patients remained ulcer free at an average follow-up of 24 months. Despite the fact that a bony union was achieved in only 4 of 11 feet (36%), the presence of a fibrous union did not appear to affect the final outcome, and all patients were satisfied with their result. This was the first study to describe a single-stage correction in a high-risk group.

The results of salvage ankle arthrodesis using circular fine-wire external fixation in a heterogeneous group of patients included 11 of 41 patients who were treated for Charcot arthropathy of the ankle.[80] The authors reported encouraging results with solid union in 10 of 11 patients (91%). Eight of the 11 patients (72%) experienced a complication during treatment, including 1 patient who required a transtibial amputation for infection.

A retrospective review of 28 patients with diabetic Charcot foot and ankle deformities reported that osseous consolidation was achieved at a mean of 3.1 months. In this series, patients were treated with hybrid ring fixation, percutaneous Achilles tendon lengthening, and external bone growth stimulators.[81] The authors reported that no further breakdown occurred, and there were minimal complications; however, no statistical conclusions were reported.

Fabrin et al[75] treated a high-risk group of patients with a Charnley-type external frame, including nine patients with ankle ulcers and six patients with foot ulcers. The frame was removed at 6 weeks, which was followed by an additional 6-week non–weight-bearing period in a total contact cast. Five patients were treated with tibiocalcaneal fusion and seven patients with tibiotalar fusion. Bony union was achieved in 6 of 12 extremities (50%), although the authors reported that the functional result of fibrous union was satisfactory in 5 of 6 patients in whom osseous union was not achieved. A transtibial amputation was required in one of the six nonunions because of recalcitrant infection and instability.

A recently published study reported on neutral ring fixation for high-risk, nonplantigrade Charcot midfoot deformity in obese patients (average body mass index of 38).[37] Twenty-six consecutive diabetic patients, 14 of whom had open wounds and osteomyelitis, were treated with Achilles tendon lengthening, excision of infected bone, deformity correction, and culture-specific antibiotic therapy. Patients were allowed to bear up to 30 lb of weight. The postoperative protocol included removal of the frame at 8 weeks followed by the use of a weight-bearing total contact cast for 4 to 6 weeks. Subsequent to this, a removable pneumatic fracture boot was used until the foot was stable to allow fitting for therapeutic shoes. Twenty-four of 26

patients were free of infection and ulcers at a minimum follow-up of 1 year. One patient died of unrelated causes, and the other patient underwent a transtibial amputation for persistent infection. Recurrent plantar ulceration, which resolved with exostectomy, developed in 4 of the remaining 24 patients (17%) whose limbs were successfully salvaged. Tibial stress fractures developed in 2 of the 24 patients (8%); 1 patient required surgical treatment and 1 patient healed with bracing. The average weight-bearing anteroposterior talar-first metatarsal angle improved from 14° to 3°, and the average lateral talar-first metatarsal angle improved from 17° to 10°.[37]

Complications are common when circular fixation is used in patients with Charcot neuroarthropathy. Patients with neuropathy often have chronic edema, the inability to sense how much weight is being applied, altered proprioception, and impaired vision. Consequently, pin tract complications are very common; however, most complications do not affect the final result.

Saltzman[78] reported that approximately 75% of patients had at least one postoperative complication and several had more than one complication during treatment with an external fixator. Twenty-eight patients had pin tract infections. Five of these required a 7- to 10-day course of an oral antibiotic, and 21 required more than one 7- to 10-day course of antibiotics. Thin wires were removed in two patients because of infection. A pin or wire broke in five other patients, the foot frame broke in one patient, and one patient had a pulmonary embolus with a negative venous Doppler leg examination.

In a small retrospective case series, Rogers et al[82] reported on 15 patients with 16 frame applications. Eighteen complications were reported (5 serious pin tract infections [31%], 4 minor

pin tract infections [25%], and 9 wound dehiscences [56%]). Ten of 16 frame applications (63%) had at least one pin tract complication. The authors stated that young age, higher elevations of preoperative glucose levels, and prolonged tourniquet times were significant predictors of complications.

A retrospective, controlled study by Wukich et al[36] compared circular fixation in 33 diabetic patients and a control group of 23 nondiabetic patients. Despite the fact that there were no significant differences with regard to age, body mass index, or duration of fixator application, the patients with diabetes experienced significantly more complications than patients without diabetes. Multivariate analysis demonstrated that males and patients with diabetes were at increased risk for complications. The overwhelming number of complications was related to pin tract problems, representing 93% of the complications in patients with diabetes and 100% of the complications in the nondiabetic patients. Other complications in diabetic patients included one tibial fracture, one deep venous thrombosis, and one death from cardiac arrest.

As experience with this technique increases, the use of circular fixation in the management of Charcot neuroarthropathy is becoming more popular. Thus far, the literature does not offer any studies that directly compare this method of fixation to the more traditional methods of internal fixation in the treatment of this disease. Published studies regarding the use of external fixation in the treatment of Charcot neuroarthropathy are level III, IV, or V (retrospective studies, case-control studies, case series, or expert opinion). Definitive recommendations regarding indications and outcomes will be forthcoming as the number of patients with Charcot neuroarthropathy who are treated with external fixation increases. The past 15 years have demonstrated that circular ring fixation clearly has a role in reconstructive surgery for patients with Charcot arthropathy.

Summary

Although there have been no comparative studies to date, the treatment of Charcot foot arthropathy has evolved from accommodative bracing to surgical correction of the deformity. Surgical stabilization has involved either internal fixation with augmented methods or modification of the Ilizarov method of external fixation with tensioned wires. It is likely that the next step in the treatment of Charcot foot arthropathy will be the refinement of these new methods of maintaining surgical stabilization.

References

1. Dhawan V, Spratt KF, Pinzur MS, Baumhauer J, Rudicel S, Saltzman CL: Reliability of AOFAS diabetic foot questionnaire in Charcot arthropathy: Stability, internal consistency, and measurable difference. *Foot Ankle Int* 2005;26(9):717-731.

2. Pinzur MS, Lio T, Posner M: Treatment of Eichenholtz stage I Charcot foot arthropathy with a weightbearing total contact cast. *Foot Ankle Int* 2006;27(5):324-329.

3. de Souza LJ: Charcot arthropathy and immobilization in a weightbearing total contact cast. *J Bone Joint Surg Am* 2008;90(4):754-759.

4. Bevan WP, Tomlinson MP: Radiographic measures as a predictor of ulcer formation in diabetic charcot midfoot. *Foot Ankle Int* 2008;29(6):568-573.

5. Pinzur MS: Surgical versus accommodative treatment for Charcot arthropathy of the midfoot. *Foot Ankle Int* 2004;25(8):545-549.

6. Brodsky JW, Rouse AM: Exostectomy for symptomatic bony prominences in diabetic charcot feet. *Clin Orthop Relat Res* 1993;296:21-26.

7. Saltzman CL, Hagy ML, Zimmerman B, Estin M, Cooper R: How effective is intensive nonoperative initial treatment of patients with diabetes and Charcot arthropathy of the feet? *Clin Orthop Relat Res* 2005;435:185-190.

8. Papa J, Myerson M, Girard P: Salvage, with arthrodesis, in intractable diabetic neuropathic arthropathy of the foot and ankle. *J Bone Joint Surg Am* 1993;75(7):1056-1066.

9. Myerson MS, Henderson MR, Saxby T, Short KW: Management of midfoot diabetic neuroarthropathy. *Foot Ankle Int* 1994;15(5):233-241.

10. Pakarinen TK, Laine HJ, Honkonen SE, Peltonen J, Oksala H, Lahtela J: Charcot arthropathy of the diabetic foot: Current concepts and review of 36 cases. *Scand J Surg* 2002;91(2):195-201.

11. Stone NC, Daniels TR: Midfoot and hindfoot arthrodeses in diabetic Charcot arthropathy. *Can J Surg* 2000;43(6):449-455.

12. Bohannon RW, Kelly CB: Accuracy of weightbearing at three target levels during bilateral upright stance in patients with neuropathic feet and control subjects. *Percept Mot Skills* 1991;72(1):19-24.

13. Early JS, Hansen ST: Surgical reconstruction of the diabetic foot: A salvage approach for midfoot collapse. *Foot Ankle Int* 1996;17(6):325-330.

14. Sammarco GJ, Conti SF: Surgical treatment of neuroarthropathic foot deformity. *Foot Ankle Int* 1998;19(2):102-109.

15. Sammarco VJ: Superconstructs in the treatment of charcot foot deformity: Plantar plating, locked plating, and axial screw fixation. *Foot Ankle Clin* 2009;14(3):393-407.

16. Schon LC, Marks RM: The management of neuroarthropathic fracture-dislocations in the diabetic patient. *Orthop Clin North Am* 1995;26(2):375-392.

17. Assal M, Stern R: Realignment and extended fusion with use of a medial column screw for midfoot deformities secondary to diabetic neuropathy. *J Bone Joint Surg Am* 2009;91(4):812-820.

18. Sammarco VJ, Sammarco GJ, Walker EW Jr, Guiao RP: Midtarsal arthrodesis in the treatment of Charcot midfoot arthropathy. *J Bone Joint Surg Am* 2009;91(1):80-91.

19. Sammarco VJ, Sammarco GJ: Axial screw technique for midfoot arthrodesis in Charcot foot deformity, in Wiesel SW, ed: *Operative Techniques in Orthopaedic Surgery*. Philadelphia, PA, Lippincott Williams & Wilkins, 2011, pp 3802-3808.

20. Sammarco VJ, Sammarco GJ, Walker EW Jr, Guiao RP: Midtarsal arthrodesis in the treatment of Charcot midfoot arthropathy: Surgical technique. *J Bone Joint Surg Am* 2010;92(Suppl 1, Pt 1):1-19.

21. Marks RM, Parks BG, Schon LC: Midfoot fusion technique for neuroarthropathic feet: Biomechanical analysis and rationale. *Foot Ankle Int* 1998;19(8):507-510.

22. Campbell JT, Schon LC, Parks BG, Wang Y, Berger BI: Mechanical comparison of biplanar proximal closing wedge osteotomy with plantar plate fixation versus crescentic osteotomy with screw fixation for the correction of metatarsus primus varus. *Foot Ankle Int* 1998;19(5):293-299.

23. Schon LC, Easley ME, Weinfeld SB: Charcot neuroarthropathy of the foot and ankle. *Clin Orthop Relat Res* 1998;349:116-131.

24. Haidukewych GJ, Ricci W: Locked plating in orthopaedic

trauma: A clinical update. *J Am Acad Orthop Surg* 2008;16(6): 347-355.

25. Zehnder S, Bledsoe JG, Puryear A: The effects of screw orientation in severely osteoporotic bone: A comparison with locked plating. *Clin Biomech (Bristol, Avon)* 2009; 24(7):589-594.

26. Sammarco V, Chevillet J: The role of internal fixation in surgery of the Charcot foot and the evolution of "super-construct" techniques. *Curr Orthop Pract* 2010; 21:233-239.

27. Sammarco GJ, ed: *The Foot in Diabetes*. Philadelphia, PA, Lea & Febiger, 1991.

28. Kann JN, Parks BG, Schon LC: Biomechanical evaluation of two different screw positions for fusion of the calcaneocuboid joint. *Foot Ankle Int* 1999;20(1):33-36.

29. Assal M, Ray A, Stern R: Realignment and extended fusion with use of a medial column screw for midfoot deformities secondary to diabetic neuropathy: Surgical technique. *J Bone Joint Surg Am* 2010;92(Suppl 1, Pt 1):20-31.

30. Sammarco VJ, Sammarco GJ: *Midtarsal Arthrodesis in the Treatment of Charcot Midfoot Arthropathy: Video Technique Guide* [DVD]. Rosemont, IL, American Academy of Orthopaedic Surgeons, 2010.

31. Stuck RM, Sohn MW, Budiman-Mak E, Lee TA, Weiss KB: Charcot arthropathy risk elevation in the obese diabetic population. *Am J Med* 2008;121(11):1008-1014.

32. Sohn MW, Stuck RM, Pinzur M, Lee TA, Budiman-Mak E: Lower-extremity amputation risk after charcot arthropathy and diabetic foot ulcer. *Diabetes Care* 2010; 33(1):98-100.

33. Pinzur MS, Freeland R, Juknelis D: The association between body mass index and foot disorders in diabetic patients. *Foot Ankle Int* 2005;26(5):375-377.

34. Reiber GE, Pecoraro RE, Koepsell TD: Risk factors for amputation in patients with diabetes mellitus: A case-control study. *Ann Intern Med* 1992;117(2):97-105.

35. Sohn MW, Lee TA, Stuck RM, Frykberg RG, Budiman-Mak E: Mortality risk of Charcot arthropathy compared with that of diabetic foot ulcer and diabetes alone. *Diabetes Care* 2009;32(5): 816-821.

36. Wukich DK, Belczyk RJ, Burns PR, Frykberg RG: Complications encountered with circular ring fixation in persons with diabetes mellitus. *Foot Ankle Int* 2008; 29(10):994-1000.

37. Pinzur MS: Neutral ring fixation for high-risk nonplantigrade Charcot midfoot deformity. *Foot Ankle Int* 2007;28(9):961-966.

38. Pinzur MS: Use of platelet-rich concentrate and bone marrow aspirate in high-risk patients with Charcot arthropathy of the foot. *Foot Ankle Int* 2009;30(2): 124-127.

39. Herbst SA, Jones KB, Saltzman CL: Pattern of diabetic neuro-pathic arthropathy associated with the peripheral bone mineral density. *J Bone Joint Surg Br* 2004; 86(3):378-383.

40. El-Gafary KA, Mostafa KM, Al-Adly WY: The management of Charcot joint disease affecting the ankle and foot by arthrodesis controlled by an Ilizarov frame: Early results. *J Bone Joint Surg Br* 2009; 91(10):1322-1325.

41. Farber DC, Juliano PJ, Cavanagh PR, Ulbrecht J, Caputo G: Single stage correction with external fixation of the ulcerated foot in individuals with Charcot neuroarthropathy. *Foot Ankle Int* 2002; 23(2):130-134.

42. Lamm BM, Paley D: Charcot neuroarthropathy of the foot and ankle, in Rozbruch SR, Ilizarov S, eds: *Limb Lengthening and Reconstructive Surgery*. New York, NY, Informa Healthcare, 2007, pp 221-232.

43. Kirienko A, Villa A, Calhoun JH: *Ilizarov Technique for Complex Foot and Ankle Deformities*. New York, NY, Marcel Dekker, 2004.

44. Pinzur MS: Static ring fixation for nonplantigrade Charcot midfoot deformity. *Oper Tech Orthop Surg* 2009;8:91-93.

45. Berenger-Feraud L: De l'emploi de la pointe de Malgaigne dans les fractures. *Rev Ther Med Chir* 1867;15:228.

46. Parkhill C: A new apparatus for the fixation of bones after resection and in fractures with a tendency to displacement. *Trans Am Surg Assoc* 1897;15:251.

47. Parkhill C: I. Further observations regarding the use of the bone-clamp in ununited fractures, fractures with malunion, and recent fractures, with a tendency to displacement. *Ann Surg* 1898;27(5): 553-570.

48. The classic: A new apparatus for the fixation of bones after resection and in fractures with a tendency to displacement, with report of cases. By Clayton Parkhill. 1897. *Clin Orthop Relat Res* 1983; 180:3-6.

49. Freeman L: XII. The treatment of oblique fractures of the tibia and other bones by means of external clamps inserted through small openings in the skin. *Ann Surg* 1911;54(3):381-389.

50. Freeman L: The application of extension to overlapping fractures, especially of the tibia, by means of bone screws and a turnbuckle, without open operation. *Ann Surg* 1919;70(2):231-235.

51. Lambotte A: L'intervention operatoire dans les fractures recent et anciennes, in Relter LF, ed: *Fractures*. Brussels, Belgium, Henri Lamertin, 1907, pp 59-60.

52. Lambotte A: The operative treatment of fractures: Report of fractures committee. *BMJ* 1912;2:1530.

53. Lambotte A: *Chirurgie operatoire des fractures*. Paris, France, Masson, 1913.

54. Anderson R: Castless ambulatory method of treating fractures. *J Int Coll Surg* 1942;5:45.

55. Stader O: A preliminary announcement of a new method of treating fractures. *N Am Vet* 1937;18:37.

56. Coates JB: *Orthopaedic Surgery in the European Theater of Operations*. Washington, DC, Office of the Surgeon General, Department of the Army, 1957.

57. Charnley J: Compression arthrodesis of the ankle and shoulder. *J Bone Joint Surg Br* 1951;33B(2):180-191.

58. Charnley J, Baker SL: Compression arthrodesis of the knee: A clinical and histological study. *J Bone Joint Surg Br* 1952;34-B(2):187-199.

59. Hoffman R: Rotules a os pour la reduction dirigee non sanglante, des fractures. *Congres Francais de Chirugie*. Paris, France, 1938, pp 601-610.

60. Hoffman R: Closed osteosynthesis with special reference to war surgery. *Acta Chir Scand* 1942;86:235.

61. Hoffman R: Osteotaxis: External osteosynthesis with pins and ball-and-socket joints. *Acta Chir Scand* 1954;107(1):72-88.

62. Ilizarov GA: A mode of uniting bones in fractures and an apparatus to implement this mode, USSR Authorship Certificate 98471, 1952.

63. Ilizarov GA: The tension-stress effect on the genesis and growth of tissues: Part I. The influence of stability of fixation and soft-tissue preservation. *Clin Orthop Relat Res* 1989;238:249-281.

64. Ilizarov GA: The tension-stress effect on the genesis and growth of tissues: Part II. The influence of the rate and frequency of distraction. *Clin Orthop Relat Res* 1989;239:263-285.

65. Ilizarov GA, Okulov GV: Compression arthrodesis of the ankle joint and adjacent foot joints. *Ortop Travmatol Protez* 1976;11:54-57.

66. Cattaneo R: Ilizarov from Kurgan to Lecco and to the world. *European Orthopaedic Bulletin of EFFORT*. 1997;(6):10-11.

67. Prokuski LJ, Saltzman CL: External fixation for the treatment of Charcot arthropathy of the ankle: A case report. *Foot Ankle Int* 1998;19(5):336-341.

68. Cooper PS: Application of external fixators for management of Charcot deformities of the foot and ankle. *Foot Ankle Clin* 2002;7(1):207-254.

69. Jolly GP, Zgonis T, Polyzois V: External fixation in the management of Charcot neuroarthropathy. *Clin Podiatr Med Surg* 2003;20(4):741-756.

70. Pinzur MS: Ring fixation in Charcot foot and ankle arthropathy. *Tech Foot Ankle Surg* 2006;5(2):68-73.

71. Myerson M: Diabetic neuroarthropathy, in Myerson M, ed: *Foot and Ankle Disorders*. Philadelphia, PA, WB Saunders, 2000, p 450.

72. Burns PR, Wukich DK: Surgical reconstruction of the Charcot rearfoot and ankle. *Clin Podiatr Med Surg* 2008;25(1):95-120, vii-viii.

73. Roukis TS, Zgonis T: The management of acute Charcot fracture-dislocations with the Taylor's spatial external fixation system. *Clin Podiatr Med Surg* 2006;23(2):467-483, viii.

74. Zgonis T, Roukis TS, Lamm BM: Charcot foot and ankle reconstruction: Current thinking and surgical approaches. *Clin Podiatr Med Surg* 2007;24(3):505-517, ix.

75. Fabrin J, Larsen K, Holstein PE: Arthrodesis with external fixation in the unstable or misaligned Charcot ankle in patients with diabetes mellitus. *Int J Low Extrem Wounds* 2007;6(2):102-107.

76. Belczyk R, Wukich D: Correction of rockerbottom deformity using the butt frame. *Oper Tech Orthop Surg* 2006;16(1):23-31.

77. Wukich D, Dial D: Equinovarus deformity correction with the Taylor spatial frame. *Oper Tech Orthop Surg* 2006;16(1):18-22.

78. Saltzman C: Ankle arthritis: Ankle neuroarthropathy, in Coughlin M, Mann R, Saltzman CL, eds: *Surgery of the Foot and Ankle*, ed 8. Philadelphia, PA, Mosby/Elsevier, 2007, pp 960-968.

79. Myerson MS, Edwards WH: Management of neuropathic fractures in the foot and ankle. *J Am Acad Orthop Surg* 1999;7(1):8-18.

80. Zarutsky E, Rush SM, Schuberth JM: The use of circular wire external fixation in the treatment of salvage ankle arthrodesis. *J Foot Ankle Surg* 2005;44(1):22-31.

81. Wang JC, Le AW, Tsukuda RK: A new technique for Charcot's foot reconstruction. *J Am Podiatr Med Assoc* 2002;92(8):429-436.

82. Rogers LC, Bevilacqua NJ, Frykberg RG, Armstrong DG: Predictors of postoperative complications of Ilizarov external ring fixators in the foot and ankle. *J Foot Ankle Surg* 2007;46(5):372-375.

Video Reference

34.1: Sammarco VJ, Sammarco GJ: Video. Excerpt. *Midtarsal Arthrodesis in the Treatment of Charcot Midfoot Arthropathy*. JBJS, DVD. Rosemont, IL, American Academy of Orthopaedic Surgeons, 2009.

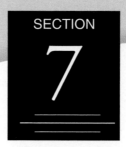

SECTION 7

Spine

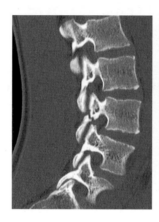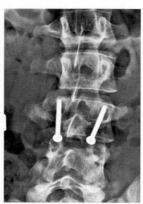

Advanced Techniques in Cervical Spine Surgery

Wellington K. Hsu, MD

Abstract

Many disorders of the cervical spine can be effectively treated through a posterior approach. Generally, posterior decompressions such as a laminectomies, laminoplasties, and/or foraminotomies result in fewer postoperative complications compared with anterior approaches for multilevel surgery. Complications can include dysphagia, dysphonia, and pseudarthrosis. Fusion is indicated in spinal conditions that involve cervical instability, subluxation, or severe sagittal imbalance. During the past decade, techniques have been developed for instrumentation of the upper and subaxial cervical spine. Several recent studies have led to a better understanding of the cervical spine anatomy, which has helped limit complications and facilitate surgical procedures.

Instr Course Lect 2012;61:441-450.

Disorders of the cervical spine can lead to compression of neural elements and cause myelopathy, radiculopathy, or a combination of these conditions. Spinal cord or nerve root compression can be caused by a soft herniated nucleus pulposus, osteophyte formation, facet joint hypertrophy, and/or congenital abnormalities of the cervical spine. If nonsurgical treatment fails, surgical treatment can often lead to excellent long-term clinical outcomes. The surgical treatment of these disorders depends on patient preference, clinical findings, and the evidence-based literature. In the properly selected patient, posterior cervical decompression for the treatment of radiculopathy pro-

vides potential advantages, including preservation of neck motion, the avoidance of complications from anterior surgery, and fewer postoperative restrictions.

A posterior fusion is indicated for conditions involving an unstable, kyphotic, or severely spondylotic cervical spine. Advances in the understanding of cervical spine anatomy have greatly enhanced the surgeon's options for osseous fixation to achieve fusion. Cadaver and imaging studies have demonstrated a high rate of anatomic variability and the importance of preoperative imaging and planning before surgery.[1-3] These studies have also established reliable guidelines for screw

placement to avoid critical vascular, neurologic, and visceral structures during cervical spine instrumentation. Awareness of these principles is essential to avoid complications and provide excellent outcomes.

Posterior Cervical Decompression

Foraminotomy

The foramina are bordered superiorly and inferiorly by the respective pedicles, anteriorly by the disk and uncovertebral joint, and posteriorly by the superior articular facet. The average dimensions of a cervical foramen are 9 to 12 mm in height and 4 to 6 mm in width.[4] These foramina are oriented at an angle of 45° from the midsagittal plane. Consequently, patients are more susceptible to foraminal narrowing in the anteroposterior plane.

Patients with radiculopathy from nerve root compression in the foramina can benefit from a foraminotomy, which decompresses the nerve root by removing a portion of the superior articular facet (**Figure 1**). This procedure allows the nerve root to be mobilized, increasing the space between it and the disk. In many patients with foraminal disk herniation, a partial pediculectomy and gentle retraction of the nerve root can aid in the

Dr. Hsu or an immediate family member is a member of a speakers' bureau or has made paid presentations on behalf of Stryker and has received research or institutional support from Baxter, Medtronic Sofamor Danek, and Pioneer Surgical.

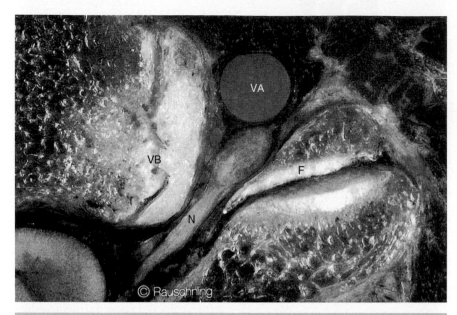

Figure 1 Axial cross-sectional view of a cadaver upper cervical spine with facet joint arthrosis (F) and uncovertebral hypertrophy (VB), causing encroachment on the exiting nerve root (N). VA = vertebral artery. (Reproduced with permission from Papadopoulos SM, ed: *Manual of Cervical Spine Internal Fixation*. Philadelphia, PA, Lippincott Williams & Wilkins, 2004.)

diskectomy, particularly when there is soft disk pathology rather than a disk-osteophyte complex, which is difficult to remove posteriorly. A preoperative CT scan is helpful in determining the etiology of the foraminal compression. Posterior foraminotomies are contraindicated for centrally located disk herniations, central spinal canal stenosis, and ossification of the posterior longitudinal ligament.

A posterior foraminotomy can be performed with the patient in either a sitting or a prone position. The sitting position decreases the incidence of intraoperative bleeding. It carries a theoretic risk of air embolism, but this position has been used in hundreds of cases without that complication.[5] When the prone position is used, Mayfield or Gardner-Wells tongs are used to stabilize the head. Both arthroscopic and microscopic techniques have been described to aid visualization during this procedure. After a preoperative localization radiograph identifies the cervical spine location, an incision is made

1.5 cm off the midline at the appropriate level. Sharp dissection is then performed through the fascia, with either a self-retaining McCullough retractor or a tube retractor docked onto the lateral mass and the facet joint. A localizing lateral radiograph is obtained to confirm the cervical spine level.

The medial third of the facet joint is identified, and the overlying inferior articular facet is then removed (at the C5 level for a C6 foraminotomy) with a high-speed oscillating burr (**Figure 2**). The superior articular facet is well visualized and is removed to unroof the foramen and expose the traversing nerve root. An oscillating burr, micro-Kerrison rongeurs, and angled curets are used to remove up to the medial 50% of the facet joint. To ensure adequate decompression once the nerve root is exposed, a nerve hook can be used to carefully palpate the caudad pedicle (at the C6 level for a C6 foraminotomy) (**Figure 2**, *D*). The procedure must be performed lateral to the pedicle to ensure a complete decompression.

When a soft disk herniation is present, a partial pediculectomy is done to minimize nerve root retraction. Once the medial third of the pedicle is removed with an oscillating burr, the traversing nerve root can be gently mobilized with a nerve hook to expose the disk fragment. Because this space is quite limited, an arthroscopic grabber or micropituitary rongeur from a tympanoplasty set can facilitate free disk fragment removal.

Posterior foraminotomies provide excellent clinical outcomes when used for the treatment of cervical radiculopathy.[5,6] Of 736 patients with a posterior-lateral foraminotomy, 91.5% were reported to have a good or excellent result at an average of 2.8 years postoperatively,[5] a finding that has been supported by other reports.[7,8] Factors that contribute to worsening sagittal alignment after posterior foraminotomy include age older than 60 years and preoperative cervical lordosis of less than 10°.[7]

A posterior cervical foraminotomy provides several advantages over anterior approaches in properly selected patients. Anterior surgical approaches for radiculopathy may be associated with complications, including recurrent laryngeal nerve palsy, dysphagia, dysphonia, and adjacent segment degeneration. The incidence of symptomatic adjacent segment degeneration after anterior cervical diskectomy and fusion is 2.9% per year (26% in a group of patients seen at 10 years postoperatively).[9] Posterior foraminotomy avoids the complications of anterior surgery and may also reduce the risk of adjacent segment degeneration postoperatively. In a study of 303 patients followed for an average of 7.2 years after a single-level posterior foraminotomy, symptomatic adjacent segment degeneration developed in 4.9% of the patients.[10] The 10-year rate of adjacent segment degeneration was calcu-

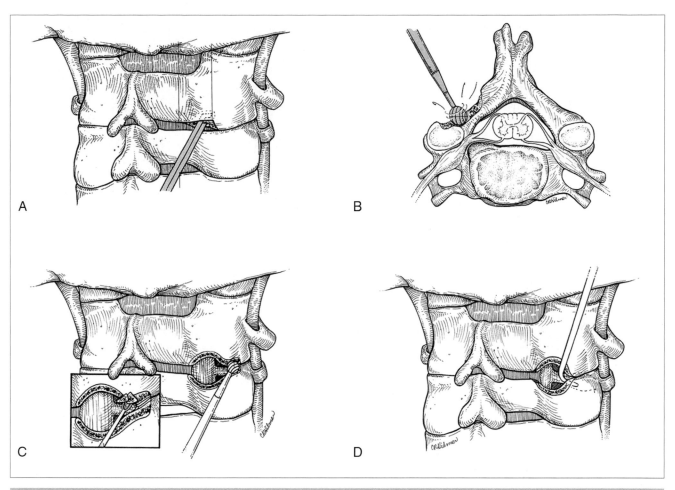

Figure 2 Illustrations showing the posterior foraminotomy procedure. After the medial third of the corresponding facet joint is identified, the inferior articular facet is removed with either micro-Kerrison rongeurs (**A**) or an oscillating burr (**B**) to expose the overlying superior facet. **C,** Decompression of the facet is continued to the level of the nerve root. **D,** A nerve hook can be used to palpate the pedicle inferiorly and ensure adequate lateral decompression. (Adapted with permission from An HS, Xu R: Posterior cervical spine procedure, in An HS, Riley LH III, eds: *An Atlas of Surgery of the Spine*. London, England, Martin Dunitz, 1998.)

lated to be 6.7%. Unlike anterior fusion, posterior decompression maintains cervical spine motion. In patients with multilevel pathologic involvement, a posterior approach can lead to outcomes that are comparable with those of the anterior approach without limiting neck motion.[6]

Some authors have suggested that a C5 foraminotomy with a decompressive procedure, such as a laminoplasty, would lead to a decreased incidence of C5 nerve root palsy. Patients with this complication can have severe deltoid weakness, preventing them from performing some activities of daily living.

Although the exact cause of C5 nerve root palsy is unclear, many authors have suggested an ischemic etiology from nerve root stretch after decompression. No treatment modalities have been successful in improving the outcome if iatrogenic C5 nerve root palsy occurs, but most patients regain functional deltoid strength within 6 to 9 months after surgery.[11] Even though a posterior foraminotomy would theoretically decrease nerve root tension after posterior drift of the spinal cord, it is unclear whether this would decrease the incidence of this difficult postoperative complication.

Laminectomy

Posterior cervical laminectomy has primarily been used to treat central cervical spine stenosis caused by spondylosis, neoplastic conditions, or ossification of the posterior longitudinal ligament. Preoperative positioning is similar to that for a foraminotomy, but a more extensive soft-tissue dissection is required to expose the posterior cervical spine.

Bilateral exposure of the lamina-lateral mass junction is required for a full laminectomy. One of several techniques that have been described is use of a high-speed oscillating burr to

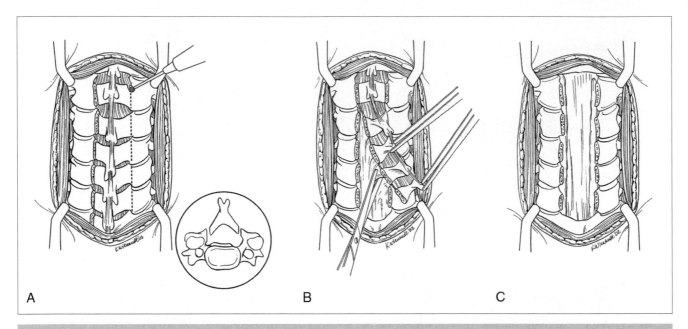

Figure 3   Illustrations showing a standard open posterior cervical laminectomy. **A,** After adequate soft-tissue exposure of the lamina-lateral mass junction bilaterally, a high-speed oscillating burr can be used to separate this junction. **B,** Once the inner cortical bone is adequately separated on each side, symmetric traction is necessary to safely remove the bone from the underlying cervical cord. **C,** Final inspection of the laminectomy site should show retention of the facet joint capsules and wide exposure of the cervical dura. (Reproduced with permission from Cooper PR, Ratliff JK: Cervical laminectomy, in Herkowitz HN, ed: *The Cervical Spine Surgery Atlas*, ed 2. Philadelphia, PA, Lippincott Williams & Wilkins, 2003.)

remove this osseous bridge bilaterally (**Figure 3**, *A*). After removal of the outer osseous cortex, the burr tip can be switched to an extra-rough diamond-tip drill bit to avoid catching soft tissue and dural tears. Excision of the ligamentum flavum is performed both cephalad and caudad to the laminectomy sites. Lamina removal is done with symmetric upward traction with the use of a towel clamp at both ends of the decompression (**Figure 3**, *B*). Care must be taken to avoid rotation of the fragments and subsequent impingement on the cervical cord. Remaining ligamentum flavum attachments to the lamina during this part of the procedure can be removed with a Kerrison rongeur.

Posterior Cervical Fusion

Posterior fusion is indicated for cervical spine instability resulting from traumatic, iatrogenic, or degenerative causes; pseudarthrosis after a prior ar-

throdesis; or multilevel anterior procedures requiring enhanced fixation. Surgeons can choose between wiring and screw fixation techniques. Recent studies have shown screw constructs to have greater rigidity and result in higher fusion rates than spinous process wiring.[12]

Subaxial Cervical Spine

Several techniques for subaxial screw fixation of the lateral mass have been described. First described in 1979, the Roy-Camille technique uses a starting point at the midpoint of the lateral mass.[13] With neutral alignment of the cervical spine (plumb line), the screw trajectory is perpendicular in the superior-inferior plane with a 10° lateral orientation (**Figure 4**). The primary risk with this technique is a breach of the facet joint in the area of both the vertebral artery and the nerve root (**Figure 5**). The Magerl (transarticular screw) technique[14] uses a start-

ing point just medial and superior to that used with the Roy-Camille procedure and orients the screw in a cephalad angle of 30° and a laterally directed angle of 25° (**Figure 4**). A broad or prominent spinous process can interfere with the screw trajectory with the Magerl technique, which may increase the risk of lateral screw cutout. There is a risk of nerve root injury with both techniques if they are not performed properly.

Anderson et al[15] modified the lateral-mass screw technique by using a starting point slightly medial to the midpoint of the lateral mass and a 35° to 40° superior and 10° lateral orientation. This chapter's author prefers the method in which a variable-length drill guide is used to optimize screw lengths at each cervical level. Advancement of drilling in 2-mm increments ensures the strongest bone purchase without violating the traversing nerve root. This screw trajectory

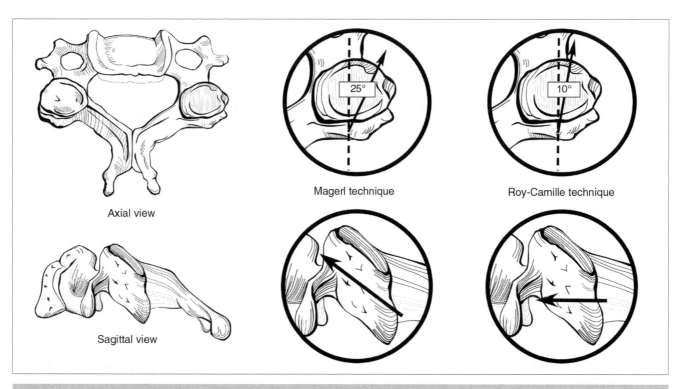

Axial view

Sagittal view

Magerl technique

Roy-Camille technique

Figure 4 Illustrations showing cervical lateral mass fixation with use of either a Magerl or a Roy-Camille technique. Although both techniques use a starting point at the midpoint of the lateral mass in both the cephalad-caudad and the medial-lateral plane, the Magerl screw is inserted in a 30° superior and 25° lateral orientation. The Roy-Camille screw takes a more perpendicular trajectory (0°) and 10° lateral approach. (Reproduced with permission from Stemper BD, Marawar SV, Yoganandan N, Shender BS, Rao RD: Quantitative anatomy of subaxial cervical lateral mass: An analysis of safe screw lengths for Roy-Camille and Magerl techniques. *Spine [Phila Pa 1976]* 2008;33[8]:893-897.)

appears to be the most reliable method for avoiding critical neurovascular structures.

Stemper et al[16] demonstrated the variations in the anatomy of the subaxial cervical lateral mass in an in vivo CT study of the cervical spine. Bicortical screw paths created with use of the Roy-Camille and Magerl techniques were drawn on sagittal CT images of 98 asymptomatic volunteers. Although there was a moderate amount of variation in screw lengths, no correlation was found between screw length and stature, body weight, or neck length. At C3-C6, Magerl screw trajectories were, on average, at least 2 mm longer than Roy-Camille screw trajectories. The screw lengths were the shortest (average, 9.8 mm in males and 8.5 mm in females) at the C7 lateral mass.

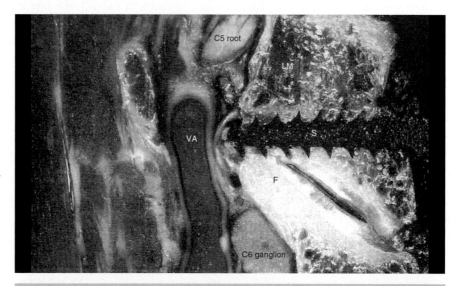

Figure 5 Sagittal cross section of a cadaver specimen of a lateral mass (LM) in a man treated with 3.5-mm cancellous screws when he was 72 years old. The lateral mass screw (S) is seen violating the inferior articular process of C5 with its tip just short of the vertebral artery (VA) in between the C5 nerve root and C6 ganglion. F = facet joint. (Reproduced with permission from Papadopoulos SM, ed: *Manual of Cervical Spine Internal Fixation.* Philadelphia, PA, Lippincott Williams & Wilkins, 2004.)

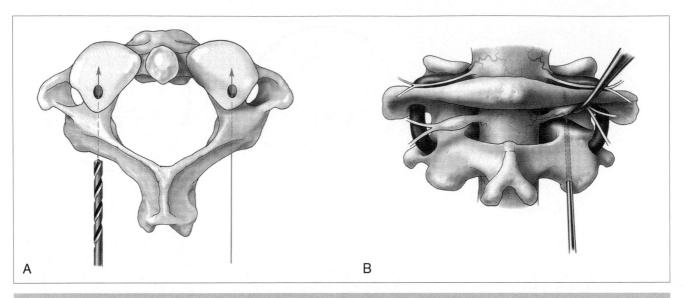

A   B

Figure 6   Illustrations showing transarticular screw fixation at C1-C2. **A,** The entry point for the transarticular screw is located in the inferomedial quadrant of the lateral mass with a neutral trajectory in the medial-lateral plane. **B,** Identification of the vertebral artery and the C2 nerve root can aid in the drilling of this screw. (Reproduced with permission from Feiz-Erfan I, Klopfenstein JD, Vougioukas VI, Dickman CA: Surgical therapy for fractures and dislocations of the craniocervical junction and upper cervical spine, in Kim DH, Henn JS, Vaccaro AR, Dickman CA, eds: *Surgical Anatomy and Techniques to the Spine.* New York, NY, Elsevier, 2006.)

Atlantoaxial Junction

Atlantoaxial fusions are indicated for patients showing more than 5 mm of instability on flexion-extension views; those with severe cervical cord compression; and those with traumatic injuries, such as a Jefferson fracture or an unstable hangman's fracture. Historically, the use of sublaminar wiring alone to stabilize this junction with the modified Gallie[17] or Brooks[18] technique has led to acceptable clinical outcomes, but the development of safe and efficient protocols with lateral mass and pedicle screw fixation in the upper cervical spine has increased fusion rates and often obviates the need for halo vest immobilization postoperatively. Patients with a concomitant subaxial cervical fracture or osteoporotic bone leading to poor bone purchase may require a halo postoperatively, but the potential for complications with halo use must be carefully considered, especially in elderly patients.[12]

The Magerl technique uses a cancellous screw that crosses the C1-C2 facet joint (**Figure 6**). Percutaneous starting points are made as caudad as T1 to obtain the proper angle for adequate fixation. Biplanar fluoroscopy is often required to identify the correct trajectory of 0° in the medial-lateral plane and 45° in the cephalad-caudad plane. With a starting point in the inferomedial quadrant of the C2 lateral mass, the trajectory is aimed toward the anterior tubercle of C1 on a lateral fluoroscopy view. Either cannulated or noncannulated screws can be used, but the placement and control of the initial Kirschner wire can be challenging. One advantage of this technique is that a standard set of fracture repair screws is sufficient for adequate fixation. A preoperative CT scan of the cervical spine is required to track the course of the vascular structures at this level. The presence of an anomalous vertebral artery precludes the use of this screw.

The Harms technique uses axial pedicle or pars interarticularis and atlas lateral mass screws.[19] Pedicle screws have been found to have a greater in-sertional torque and pullout strength than either laminar or pars interarticularis screws in cadaver spines.[20] The C2 pedicle screw is inserted with a starting point that is just superior and medial to the center of the lateral mass (**Figure 7**). A small laminotomy and palpation with a nerve hook can often assist with the medial-lateral orientation (10°), and lateral fluoroscopy can guide the cephalad-caudad direction (15°). The C1 entry point is identified at the junction of the lateral mass and the inferior aspect of the posterior arch (**Figure 7**). Often, the overhang of the C1 arch should be removed with an oscillating burr at the level of the lateral mass to identify the landmarks and provide room for the screw head. A Penfield retractor can be used to palpate the medial aspect of C1 to guide a 10° medial and 20° cephalad trajectory. The most commonly used titanium screw size is 3.5 × 28 mm. With this procedure, the surgeon should try not to violate the C2-C3 interspinous space and leave as many muscle attach-

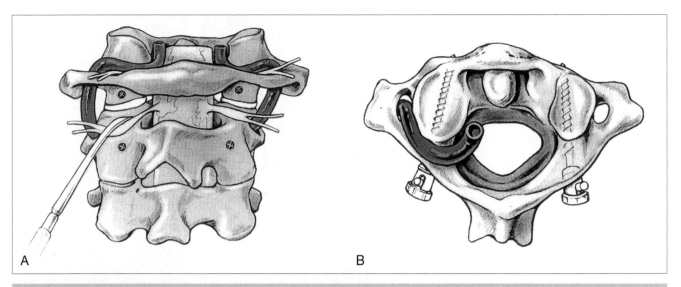

Figure 7   Illustrations showing C1-C2 fixation with use of the Harms technique. **A,** The entry point for the C2 pedicle screw is the superomedial quadrant of the lateral mass directed in a 15° cephalad and 10° medial trajectory. **B,** The C1 lateral mass screw is started in the midpoint of the lateral mass just below the arch and oriented in a 10° medial direction for bicortical purchase. (Reproduced with permission from Harms J, Melcher RP: Posterior C1-C2 fusion with polyaxial screw and rod fixation. *Spine [Phila Pa 1976]* 2001;26[22]:2467-2471.)

ments as possible to reduce postoperative pain and increase stability. Any bleeding from the venous plexus between C1 and C2 should be controlled with FloSeal Hemostatic Matrix (Baxter Healthcare, Fremont, CA); cottonoid; or a combination of microfibrillar collagen (Avitene; Devol, Warwick, RI), Gelfoam (Upjohn, Kalamazoo, Michigan), and thrombin.

Although the C1 lateral mass screw is ideally placed with bicortical purchase, anterior structures such as the internal carotid artery must be avoided. In a study of 149 CT reconstruction images of the cervical spine, Murakami et al[21] defined the variation of the anatomy of the internal carotid artery anterior to the C1 anterior arch. In 64% of the patients, the internal carotid artery was directly anterior to the middle of the C1 lateral mass, and in 55% of the patients, it was over the lateral third. The authors concluded that a 10° medial orientation of the C1 lateral mass screw with the proper entry point can avoid injury to the internal carotid artery. This ideal trajectory was confirmed with an anatomic study of

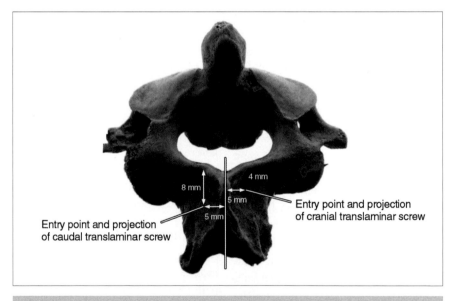

Figure 8   Entry points for C2 laminar screws. (Reproduced with permission from Ma XY, Yin QS, Wu ZH, Xia H, Riew KD, Liu JF: C2 anatomy and dimensions relative to translaminar screw placement in an Asian population. *Spine [Phila Pa 1976]* 2010;35[6]:704-708.)

atlas specimens that demonstrated less variability in C1 lateral mass measurements compared with those of other levels.[22]

When it is not possible to use C2 pedicle or pars interarticularis screws because of anatomic variations, lami-

nar fixation can be considered. With an entry point 5 mm lateral to the midline of the spinous process and 6 mm caudad to the cranial border of the lamina, a 3.5 × 26-mm screw can often be inserted[2] (**Figure 8**). In a biomechanical analysis of C1 lateral mass-

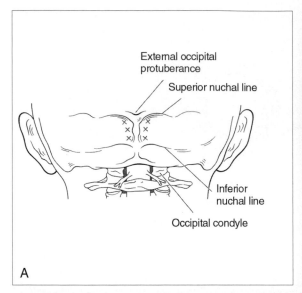
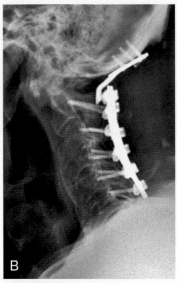
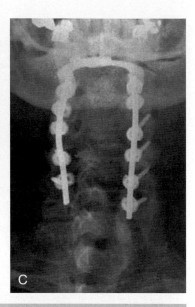

Figure 9 Occipital-cervical fixation. **A,** The identification of anatomic landmarks is essential to providing the optimum screw fixation in the occiput. (Reproduced with permission from Herkowitz HN, ed: *The Cervical Spine Surgery Atlas*, ed 2. Philadelphia, PA, Lippincott Williams & Wilkins, 2003.) **B** and **C,** Instrumentation systems should provide for screws in the midline of the occiput and a plate-rod interface that is secure and can be contoured to fit the skull.

C2 pedicle screw fixation, C1 lateral mass-C2 intralaminar screw fixation, and C1-C2 sublaminar wire fixation techniques, Elgafy et al[23] reported that all three instrumentation systems were equally stable in flexion-extension and lateral bending. Although both screw constructs were superior to the wiring technique in axial rotation, there were no significant differences between the lateral mass-intralaminar and lateral mass-pedicle constructs in flexion-extension. In an anatomic study of the axis in an Asian population, Ma et al[2] reported that 83% of the patients had anatomic parameters that allowed for a 3.5-mm screw, whereas only a unilateral screw was suitable in 12% of the patients. In 5% of the patients examined, the laminae were too thin to accommodate screws on either side. This and other studies highlight the importance of preoperative CT planning when either C2 pedicle or C2 laminar screws are considered.

Occipital-Cervical Junction

Posterior fixation for occipital-cervical fusion is required for clinical condi-

tions such as atlanto-occipital dissociation and/or instability or basilar invagination. Depending on the associated condition, a decompression of the opisthion (the hindmost point on the posterior margin of the foramen magnum) may be needed as well.

It is important to identify several landmarks before formal instrumentation. The external occipital protuberance is a palpable uprising that marks the thickest portion of the bone (**Figure 9**, *A*). The superior and inferior nuchal lines are ridges that extend in the medial-lateral direction from the external occipital protuberance. The path from the external occipital protuberance to the foramen magnum marks a sharp anterior trajectory that can make plate contouring a substantial challenge. All screw fixation should be caudad to the external occipital protuberance to ensure good bone quality and adequate soft-tissue coverage. At the external occipital protuberance, 12-mm to 18-mm-thick bone is expected. However, the identification of this point is important because a starting point just 1 cm lateral and inferior

to it provides only 5 to 7 mm of bone thickness. Although some authors have advocated bicortical screw purchase, unicortical screws at the external occipital protuberance provide adequate pullout strength as the inner table has only 10% of the overall thickness. A wide array of occipital-cervical plate-screw constructs that allow contouring and flexibility in this articulation are available. Regardless of the instrumentation system, the construct should allow adequate soft-tissue coverage, avoid hardware prominence, and provide a stable plate-to-screw interface to avoid postoperative complications (**Figure 9**).

Bone Graft

The choice of bone graft to be used in conjunction with posterior cervical fusion depends on several factors, including fusion rates, the volume required, complications, comorbidities, and cost. Historically, structural and cancellous autologous iliac crest bone grafting has been successfully used in Brooks and Gallie as well as subaxial fusion constructs. Because the posterior cervical spine is a more favorable biologic milieu for bone healing than is the posterior lumbar spine, iliac crest bone grafting can often be avoided. Just as important as the bone graft choice is the preparation of the fusion surfaces, which should include a subtotal facetectomy in the subaxial spine and thorough preparation of the lamina, facet joint, and occiput surfaces in the upper cervical spine. Local bone graft from a laminectomy site can provide an osteoinductive stimulus necessary for bone healing in this environment.[24] Bone graft extenders such as ceramic scaffolds, used in conjunction with local bone graft, also can increase osseous healing (the preferred method of this chapter's author). The use of bone morphogenetic protein has led to high fusion rates in the posterior cervical spine, but its use may lead to wound complications and local seroma formation.[25] At the present time, use of bone morphogenetic protein in this surgical setting has not been approved by the US Food and Drug Administration. The complications appear to be linked to the dose of growth factor used.

Summary

In properly selected patients, posterior cervical decompression and fusion can successfully treat cervical myelopathy and radiculopathy. The choice of a posterior approach versus an anterior approach depends on several factors, including sagittal alignment, the type and extent of the pathologic involvement, and patient preference. Recent advances in spine surgeons' understanding of anatomy and technique have increased their level of comfort with using instrumentation in the upper and subaxial cervical spine. The use of concomitant, minimally invasive techniques with these procedures leads to faster recovery times with equivalent outcomes. Awareness of the strengths and limitations of posterior cervical techniques can greatly enhance the surgeon's ability to achieve excellent clinical outcomes.

References

1. Liu J, Napolitano JT, Ebraheim NA: Systematic review of cervical pedicle dimensions and projections. *Spine (Phila Pa 1976)* 2010; 35(24):E1373-E1380.

2. Ma XY, Yin QS, Wu ZH, Xia H, Riew KD, Liu JF: C2 anatomy and dimensions relative to translaminar screw placement in an Asian population. *Spine (Phila Pa 1976)* 2010;35(6):704-708.

3. Yeom JS, Buchowski JM, Park KW, Chang BS, Lee CK, Riew KD: Undetected vertebral artery groove and foramen violations during C1 lateral mass and C2 pedicle screw placement. *Spine (Phila Pa 1976)* 2008;33(25): E942-E949.

4. Czervionke LF, Daniels DL, Ho PS, et al: Cervical neural foramina: Correlative anatomic and MR imaging study. *Radiology* 1988; 169(3):753-759.

5. Henderson CM, Hennessy RG, Shuey HM Jr , Shackelford EG: Posterior-lateral foraminotomy as an exclusive operative technique for cervical radiculopathy: A review of 846 consecutively operated cases. *Neurosurgery* 1983; 13(5):504-512.

6. Holly LT, Moftakhar P, Khoo LT, Wang JC, Shamie N: Minimally invasive 2-level posterior cervical foraminotomy: Preliminary clinical results. *J Spinal Disord Tech* 2007;20(1):20-24.

7. Jagannathan J, Sherman JH, Szabo T, Shaffrey CI, Jane JA: The posterior cervical foraminotomy in the treatment of cervical disc/osteophyte disease: A single-surgeon experience with a minimum of 5 years' clinical and radiographic follow-up. *J Neurosurg Spine* 2009;10(4):347-356.

8. Witzmann A, Hejazi N, Krasznai L: Posterior cervical foraminotomy. A follow-up study of 67 surgically treated patients with compressive radiculopathy. *Neurosurg Rev* 2000;23(4):213-217.

9. Hilibrand AS, Carlson GD, Palumbo MA, Jones PK, Bohlman HH: Radiculopathy and myelopathy at segments adjacent to the site of a previous anterior cervical arthrodesis. *J Bone Joint Surg Am* 1999;81(4):519-528.

10. Clarke MJ, Ecker RD, Krauss WE, McClelland RL, Dekutoski MB: Same-segment and adjacent-segment disease following posterior cervical foraminotomy. *J Neurosurg Spine* 2007;6(1):5-9.

11. Sakaura H, Hosono N, Mukai Y, Ishii T, Yoshikawa H: C5 palsy after decompression surgery for cervical myelopathy: Review of the literature. *Spine (Phila Pa 1976)* 2003;28(21):2447-2451.

12. Hsu WK, Anderson PA: Odontoid fractures: Update on management. *J Am Acad Orthop Surg* 2010;18(7):383-394.

13. Roy-Camille R, Gaillant G, Bertreaux D, Marie-Anne S: Early management of spinal injuries, in McKibbin B, ed: *Recent Advances in Orthopaedics*. Edinburgh, Scotland, Churchill-Livingstone, 1979, pp 57-87.

14. Jeanneret B, Magerl F, Ward EH, Ward JC: Posterior stabilization of the cervical spine with hook plates. *Spine (Phila Pa 1976)* 1991;16(3, Suppl):S56-S63.

15. Anderson PA, Henley MB, Grady MS, Montesano PX, Winn HR: Posterior cervical arthrodesis with AO reconstruction plates and bone graft. *Spine (Phila Pa 1976)* 1991;16(3, Suppl):S72-S79.

16. Stemper BD, Marawar SV, Yoganandan N, Shender BS, Rao RD: Quantitative anatomy of subaxial cervical lateral mass: An analysis of safe screw lengths for Roy-Camille and magerl tech-

niques. *Spine (Phila Pa 1976)* 2008;33(8):893-897.

17. Gallie WE: Skeletal traction in the treatment of fractures and dislocations of the cervical spine. *Ann Surg* 1937;106(4):770-776.

18. Brooks AL, Jenkins EB: Atlanto-axial arthrodesis by the wedge compression method. *J Bone Joint Surg Am* 1978;60(3):279-284.

19. Harms J, Melcher RP: Posterior C1-C2 fusion with polyaxial screw and rod fixation. *Spine (Phila Pa 1976)* 2001;26(22): 2467-2471.

20. Lehman RA Jr, Dmitriev AE, Helgeson MD, Sasso RC, Kuklo TR, Riew KD: Salvage of C2 pedicle and pars screws using the intralaminar technique: A biomechanical analysis. *Spine (Phila Pa 1976)* 2008;33(9):960-965.

21. Murakami S, Mizutani J, Fukuoka M, et al: Relationship between screw trajectory of C1 lateral mass screw and internal carotid artery. *Spine (Phila Pa 1976)* 2008; 33(24):2581-2585.

22. Seal C, Zarro C, Gelb D, Ludwig S: C1 lateral mass anatomy: Proper placement of lateral mass screws. *J Spinal Disord Tech* 2009; 22(7):516-523.

23. Elgafy H, Potluri T, Goel VK, Foster S, Faizan A, Kulkarni N: Biomechanical analysis comparing three C1-C2 transarticular screw salvaging fixation techniques. *Spine (Phila Pa 1976)* 2010;35(4): 378-385.

24. Huang RC, Girardi FP, Poynton AR, Cammisa FP Jr: Treatment of multilevel cervical spondylotic myeloradiculopathy with posterior decompression and fusion with lateral mass plate fixation and local bone graft. *J Spinal Disord Tech* 2003;16(2):123-129.

25. Crawford CH III, Carreon LY, McGinnis MD, Campbell MJ, Glassman SD: Perioperative complications of recombinant human bone morphogenetic protein-2 on an absorbable collagen sponge versus iliac crest bone graft for posterior cervical arthrodesis. *Spine (Phila Pa 1976)* 2009; 34(13):1390-1394.

Cervical Spine Surgery: Anterior Microsurgery

Alan Hilibrand, MD
Jeremy S. Smith, MD

Abstract

Anterior cervical decompression and fusion is one of the most commonly used procedures to treat myelopathy and radiculopathy. With the addition of the surgical microscope, enhanced visualization of the microanatomy has allowed the safe and efficient treatment of compressive pathology. It is important to understand the critical steps required to successfully treat cervical spine pathology from an anterior approach with the assistance of a surgical microscope, the factors involved in choosing a decompressive method, the technical considerations for intervertebral grafting, and the use of cervical plating. The knowledge of surgical pearls may optimize spinal cord and nerve root decompression, increase fusion rates, and give patients the best chance for a successful clinical outcome.

Instr Course Lect 2012;61:451-459.

The anterior approach is commonly used to treat compressive conditions of the cervical spine. Anterior cervical decompression and fusion represents one of the most common spinal procedures performed, with most clinical outcomes being quite favorable.[1,2] The surgical microscope is a tool used in anterior cervical spine microsurgery to enhance visualization of the microanatomy and improve the precision of surgical decompression. However, there is a learning curve for the surgeon to master the microscopic technique. This chapter will focus on current surgical techniques of anterior cervical microsurgery.

Indications and Results

Myelopathy

Cervical myelopathy is a common progressive spinal disorder seen in patients older than 55 years. Patients may report a constellation of symptoms, including a decrease in coordination or dexterity, poor balance, and difficulties with gait. When such symptoms are correlated with imaging studies showing spinal cord compression, a diagnosis of cervical myelopathy is indicated. Based on the natural history of the disease, a significant proportion of patients (up to 50%) have neurologic deterioration following conservative treatment.[3] In a study by Clarke and Robinson,[3] most of the patients (70%) displayed a stepwise decline in neurologic function, with stable intervals of variable length without deterioration. The remaining 30% of the patients had a gradual worsening of function, with 5% of the patients having rapid progression of their symptoms. Minor trauma in patients with compromised spinal cord function can result in a catastrophic neurologic injury.

The goals of anterior cervical surgery are to eliminate cord compression, protect the vulnerable spinal cord, and prevent further neurologic deterioration. Some patients may recover neurologic function. Emery et al[1] reviewed 108 patients with 2 to 17 years follow-up after anterior cervical decompression and arthrodesis for cervical spondylotic myelopathy. Eighty-seven percent of the patients had gait improvement, and 89% had motor function improvement.

Certain criteria must be met when considering an anterior cervical approach for the treatment of cervical

Dr. Hilibrand or an immediate family member has received royalties from Aesculap/B. Braun, Alphatec Spine, Amedica, Biomet, Stryker, and Zimmer; owns stock or stock options in Amedica, Benvenue Medical, Lifespine, Nexgen, Paradigm Spine, Pioneer Surgical, PSD, Spinal Ventures, Syndicom, and Vertiflex; and serves as a board member, owner, officer, or committee member of the American Academy of Orthopaedic Surgeons, the American Orthopaedic Association, the Cervical Spine Research Society, and the North American Spine Society. Neither Dr. Smith nor any immediate family member has received anything of value from or owns stock in a commercial company or institution related directly or indirectly to the subject of this chapter.

myelopathy.[4,5] The compressive spinal cord pathology must be anterior. For patients with myelopathy and concomitant radicular symptoms, this chapter's authors believe both pathologies are best treated with an anterior decompression. The ideal candidate for anterior decompression is a patient who presents with anterior compressive pathology involving one to three levels. If the cervical kyphosis involves more than three levels, an anterior approach may help decompress the pathology and realign the deformity.

Radiculopathy

Cervical radiculopathy typically results from nerve root compression and manifests as pain radiating in the sensory distribution of the involved nerve. Associated clinical findings may include motor weakness or reflex disturbances. Acute cervical radiculopathy should initially be treated conservatively with nonsteroidal anti-inflammatory drugs and physical therapy, with or without cervical traction and epidural steroid injections. Conservative treatment usually results in symptom resolution in 75% of patients.[6]

The anterior surgical approach can successfully treat various compressive pathologies that may cause cervical radiculopathy. Soft disk herniations may cause compression posterolaterally as the nerve exits or at the neural foramen more laterally. Hard disk nerve root impingement is caused by chronic degenerative disk disease, with or without calcification of the anulus in the posterolateral aspect of the vertebral body, with resulting nerve root compression. Degeneration of the intervertebral disk and the subsequent loss of disk height may result in cranial migration of the superior facet and subsequent foraminal narrowing. Facet hypertrophy also can cause nerve root impingement.[7]

The failure of nonsurgical treatments characterized by persistent radicular symptoms and ongoing functional limitations is an indication for surgical treatment. Patients presenting with substantial weakness that affects activities of daily living or occupational requirements may also be appropriate surgical candidates. Indications for an anterior approach include spondylosis, loss of disk height, disk herniation, and neck pain associated with arm pain. The goals of anterior cervical surgery are to adequately decompress the nerve roots and eliminate nerve root irritation. Neck pain may also be treated with the anterior approach.[8] Anterior decompression allows direct decompression of most lesions that cause cervical radiculopathy. Decompression can be achieved without placing traction on the nerve roots (as is necessary in many posterior decompressive procedures). The ability to place an intervertebral graft also allows indirect decompression of the neural foramen. A fusion at the diseased level will prevent recurrence of compressive pathology and potentially treat associated neck pain.

Outcomes following anterior cervical diskectomy and arthrodesis are good. Based on the surgeons' assessment of the patients' pain, Bohlman et al[2] reported no pain or mild pain in 113 of 122 patients in their study (93%) at follow-ups of more than 5 years. There was no deterioration over 5 to 6 years, although 10% of the patients required reoperation at another level secondary to adjacent level pathology.

Anterior Decompression and Fusion: Surgical Techniques

Operating Microscope

The operating microscope has been available to spine surgeons for more than 20 years and has been a useful tool in spinal surgery (**Figure 1**). Its first reported use in the spine was in the late 1970s for lumbar diskectomy.[9] The operating microscope is now commonly used for surgical procedures throughout the spine. Although the operating microscope offers many advantages that may make surgical decompressions faster, safer, and more accurate, many surgeons are reluctant to adopt this technology.

The operating microscope offers a detailed view of the microanatomy of the spine and allows for a more thorough decompression of the neural elements. Specifically, it allows detailed visualization of the posterior longitudinal ligament (PLL) and safer resection of its fibers. In addition, sequestered fragments of a herniated disk can be easily visualized and extracted. Dural tears are easily visualized and repaired through the microscope. In high-risk patients with ossification of the PLL, the operating microscope may reduce the risk of cerebrospinal fluid leakage during PLL resection.[10,11] When compared with loupe magnification, the microscope offers a range of magnifications; a superior light source, which remains perfectly aligned with the field of vision; and the ability for adequate visualization of the surgical field by an assistant. Three-dimensional visualization is maintained in a narrow field, optimizing the surgical view and coordination. Operating room staff and medical students may watch the procedure on a monitor (**Figure 1, A**).

The most commonly cited disadvantage of the operating microscope is the extra time required to set up and then maintain the proper orientation of the microscope throughout the procedure. This chapter's authors believe that the inexperienced surgeon may find it challenging to use the operating microscope; however, the learning curve is not steep, and the operating microscope permits more accurate and

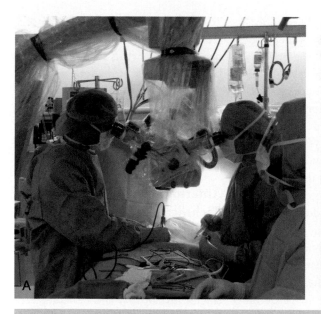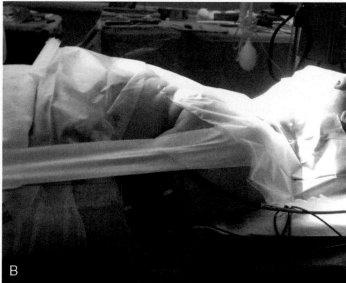

Figure 1   **A,** The setup of the operating microscope allows both the surgeon and an assistant to have the same view during surgery. **B,** The patient is placed in a slight reverse Trendelenburg position with the shoulders gently distracted.

safer spinal decompressions, which can be performed with minimal additional surgical time. As noted, the orientation of the microscope is crucial and must be maintained throughout the procedure. This is particularly important when performing a corpectomy. If the orientation is oblique or lost, there is a high risk of creating a trough that does not adequately decompress the spinal cord, potentially placing the vertebral arteries at risk for injury. When performing a diskectomy, it is important to maintain a sagittal orientation parallel to the disk space. Proper orientation requires adjustments at each disk level. If the orientation is not properly maintained, an unwanted end-plate resection may result. Under higher magnifications, epidural bleeding can appear quite dramatic, making a small amount of blood seem much larger.

Prepping and positioning the microscope requires some effort and experience; however, once the task is learned, it becomes routine and does not consume excessive time. Most surgeons perform the initial anterior cervical surgical exposure under loupe

magnification and introduce the microscope for spinal decompression. Some surgeons complete the reconstruction with bone grafting and plate application under the microscope using a lower magnification, whereas other surgeons remove the microscope to confirm proper alignment and orientation.

The microscope is sterilely draped by a member of the operating room staff. The entire microscope, including the objective and ocular lens, is wrapped with sterile plastic and then carefully brought into the field and appropriately positioned by the surgeon. Most modern microscopes have a base attached to a long, multijointed arm to avoid surgical field contamination. The eyepieces are adjusted to the appropriate refraction depending on the surgeon's visual acuity. The adjustment of the ocular lenses by the surgeon and assistant are best accomplished prior to the start of surgery.

When first attempting to incorporate the use of an operating microscope into any surgical procedure, the surgeon should realize that there will be a learning curve and only experience will

improve technique and time efficiency. Once a routine is developed and maintained, the benefits of a more detailed view of the microanatomy and the ability to more efficiently decompress the neural elements will be appreciated.

Instruments

Some of the instruments used in anterior cervical microsurgery require modification from those used with loupe magnification. Microcurets of various sizes and orientations (such as forward versus backward or angled versus straight) are essential to ensure adequate decompression while maintaining appropriate visualization. As with any anterior cervical procedure, a high-speed burr is absolutely necessary for adequate decompression of the anterior spinal cord, particularly with a corpectomy. This chapter's authors recommend using a burr with a high rotational speed, pedal controls, and a matchstick tip to protect the neural elements. Micro Kerrison rongeurs of various sizes are necessary to safely achieve a wide and thorough foraminotomy and efficiently resect the posterior anulus, PLL, and osteophyte complexes. To avoid compromising the field of view, a Kerrison rongeur with a rotating arm may be preferred depending on the desired angle of resection. Micro nerve hooks assist in developing a plane between the PLL and dura and can assist in determining the patency of the foraminotomy.

Surgical Approach

The Smith-Robinson approach is most commonly used to treat the anterior cervical spine.[12] The patient is positioned supine in a slight reverse Trendelenburg position. If a corpectomy is planned, Gardner-Wells tongs are placed, and gentle in-line traction is used intraoperatively to create the appropriate distraction (**Figure 1**, *B*).

A left-sided approach minimizes injury to the recurrent laryngeal nerve. It is important to understand the course of the laryngeal nerve and protect it, because damage will result in a permanent hoarseness. The left-sided recurrent laryngeal nerve courses around the arch of the aorta and is protected in the lower cervical spine within the tracheoesophageal groove. The right-sided nerve travels around the subclavian artery and is vulnerable to injury as it makes its way to the larynx. Anatomic landmarks used to guide the incision include the hyoid bone (overlying C3), the thyroid cartilage (overlying the C4-5 intervertebral disk space), and the cricoid ring (overlying C6). Depending on the number of levels treated in the procedure, a transverse or longitudinal incision is used. A transverse incision is made in line with a skin crease, just across the midline and extending just beyond the medial border of the sternocleidomastoid.

Following the skin incision, the skin and subcutaneous tissues are undermined slightly, and the platysma is divided with careful attention to avoid injury to the underlying external jugu-

lar venous structures. Dissection is continued to the medial border of the sternocleidomastoid. If the approach necessitates exposure of levels higher than C3-4, the appropriate interval is between the sternocleidomastoid laterally and the omohyoid medially. At lower levels, the interval is between the sternocleidomastoid and the omohyoid laterally and the strap muscles medially. The deep cervical fascia between the sternocleidomastoid and the strap muscles is carefully divided with a combination of blunt dissection and Metzenbaum scissors. If the omohyoid presents in the surgical field and multiple levels are to be decompressed, it may be divided. Dissection is continued superiorly and inferiorly. The thyroid vessels may be visualized (superior thyroid above C4 and inferior thyroid below C6). If these arteries are encountered, they should be protected if possible; if the arteries cannot be mobilized, they should be exposed and ligated. Blunt digital dissection through the pretracheal fascia between the carotid sheath laterally and the strap muscles with the esophagus medially is continued to the level of the prevertebral fascia on the anterior cervical spine. The finger is used to bluntly undermine the esophagus and expose the prevertebral fascia. The prevertebral fascia is then divided longitudinally, and a peanut is used to separate the fascia from the underlying structures. Using a protected tipped bovie electrocautery, the vertebral bodies are then exposed. A curved needle is carefully placed in the disk of interest. A lateral radiograph is obtained to confirm the level.

After confirming the level, the interval between the longus colli and the vertebral column is dissected using the bovie. Dissection proceeds laterally to expose the uncovertebral joints. Self-retaining retractors are placed under the developed bone-muscle interval.

To maintain the position of the self-retaining retractor, weights (2 lb) are tied to the retractors and hung off the bed on each side at the level of the patient's shoulders. Depending on the surgeon's preference, Caspar distractor pins may be placed into the superior and inferior vertebral bodies to provide distraction for the diskectomy.

Anterior Cervical Diskectomy: Technical Considerations

It is necessary to understand the pathoanatomy and appropriate level of resection required to relieve spinal cord and nerve root compression in the setting of myelopathy and radiculopathy. Identifying any retrovertebral spinal cord compression that may not be treated by a diskectomy is important in the preoperative analysis of CT and MRI studies. In such cases, hemicorpectomy or full corpectomy may be necessary. The surgeon should be aware of the anatomic limitations of the intervertebral approach to the spinal canal and the risks to the spinal cord associated with reaching behind the vertebral body to remove any retrovertebral compression.

Under loupe magnification, the anterior cervical spine is exposed as has previously been described. Once the appropriate level is identified, a No. 15 scalpel is used to incise the anterior anulus fibrosus, which is removed with a pituitary rongeur. A No. 0 curet is used to clear remaining anulus and nucleus material. A Kerrison rongeur is often required to remove the remaining lateral anulus fibrosus. Osteophytes from the anterior superior end plate are removed with a Kerrison rongeur to expose the entire disk space. If needed, a 4-mm, round, long burr may be used to further prepare the end plate. After the disk space has been mobilized with the help of a small Cobb elevator, Caspar pins may be placed in the cranial and caudal vertebral bodies. Gentle

Caspar pin distraction is then applied. The uncovertebral joints are identified and serve as the lateral margins of the exposure for the foraminotomy and aid as landmarks to help prevent vertebral artery injury. Using the curets, cartilaginous end-plate material is removed medially and laterally into the uncinate processes. The superior and inferior end plates and associated osteophytes are resected using a high-speed burr. A variable amount of the uncus may be removed to allow appropriate access for the foraminotomy. No more than two thirds of the uncovertebral joint should be resected to prevent instability. A 3-0 angled curet is useful for clearing behind the uncinate processes to clear a path for the foraminotomy. Next, 1- and 2-mm Kerrison rongeurs are used to complete the foraminotomy by removing the uncinates and any potential compressive bony pathology. A micro nerve hook may be used to gently observe the patency of the decompression and palpate behind the end plates for any remaining osteophytes. There is some question regarding the necessity to resect all of the uncinate osteophytes. It has been suggested that a well-positioned interbody graft may provide indirect decompression of the neural foramina.[2] However, this chapter's authors prefer using a combination of a high-speed burr, small curets, and a micro Kerrison rongeur to directly resect any end-plate osteophytes causing nerve root or spinal cord compression. This process is facilitated with the operating microscope.

Video 36.1: Advanced Techniques in Cervical Spine Surgery. Alan Hilibrand, MD; Jeremy S. Smith, MD (4 min)

The decision to resect the PLL depends on the characteristics of the compressive pathology. If the disk has herniated within or posterior to its fibers, the PLL should be resected. If the PLL is ossified, the entire PLL should be removed. Once all disk material is removed, the PLL is readily identified by its characteristic vertical striations. Under microscopic visualization, any posterior osteophytes are removed using a high-speed burr until there is a near-rectangular area of visualized disk space. Most commonly, the inferior vertebral end plate from the cranial vertebral body has prominent osteophytes that may require resection with a high-speed burr or a Kerrison rongeur. This resection ensures appropriate visualization and assists in preparing for graft placement. Once the osteophytes are removed and the PLL is fully visualized, a vertical plane is developed with a micro nerve hook or curet. This allows passage of a No. 1-0 or 2-0 Kerrison rongeur for resection of the PLL and any remaining disk or osteophytes. The operating microscope offers significant benefit over loupe magnification during this portion of the surgery. After the PLL is fully removed, a nerve hook is passed posterior to the vertebral bodies to check for any remaining disk material or compressive pathology. When the decompression is complete, the pedicle is palpated with a nerve hook to verify completion of the lateral decompression.

Anterior Cervical Corpectomy: Technical Considerations

Surgical indications for anterior cervical corpectomy depend on the pathoanatomy and degree of spinal cord compression. Corpectomy is generally reserved for patients with spondylotic myelopathy, burst fractures, and tumors. If there is significant retrovertebral compressive pathology, corpectomy is appropriate. If there is no

evidence of multilevel involvement, ossification of the PLL can usually be treated with a corpectomy.

In preparing for a corpectomy, Gardner-Wells tongs are placed in standard fashion to allow for intraoperative traction for stability and graft placement. After the standard Smith-Robinson exposure, a diskectomy is performed at the levels above and below the vertebra level of interest as previously described. This allows adequate visualization of the uncovertebral joints and posterior vertebral depth for safe lateral and anterior-posterior resection. Using a high-speed burr, troughs are burred in line within the uncovertebral joints delineating the lateral aspects of the corpectomy. A Leksell rongeur is then used to remove the anterior cortex and underlying cancellous bone. Hemostasis is maintained with pieces of gel foam or a thin layer of bone wax. With careful attention to maintaining orientation, the corpectomy is continued with a burr. The tendency is to resect more of the vertebral body that lies to the contralateral side of the surgeon. This can be prevented by periodically changing the view of the microscope to ensure a proper view and orientation. It is important that the width of corpectomy be 16 mm. The resection is continued with a combination of a rongeur and a high-speed burr to the posterior cortex of the vertebral body (**Figure 2,** *A*). Once the posterior cortex has been adequately thinned to a nearly transparent layer, microcurets and Kerrison rongeurs can be used to expose the underlying PLL. Preoperative imaging evaluation and intraoperative observation should be used to determine if the PLL should be resected. If the PLL is contributing to the compressive pathology (ossification of the PPL), it must be resected. Often, it is not contributing to the pathologic process and does not require resection. After the

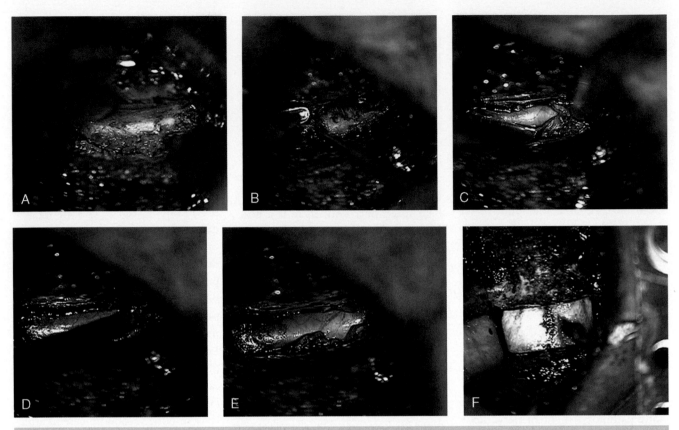

Figure 2 Anterior cervical diskectomy as viewed from the operating microscope. **A,** End-plate cartilage is burred, and posterior osteophytes are resected to the level of the PLL. **B,** A nerve hook placed between the longitudinal fibers of the PLL allows passage of a No. 1 or 2 Kerrison rongeur. **C,** Posterior vertebral bodies are undercut using a Kerrison rongeur. **D,** Foraminal decompression is performed with a Kerrison rongeur. Note that the exiting nerve root travels ventrally at an angle of approximately 30°. **E,** Completed decompression. **F,** The graft is gently inserted after final preparation of the end plates.

PLL is exposed, a small curet may by used to enter its fibers. In revision surgeries or in cases of ossification, the PLL may adhere to the dura. Once an adequate plane is achieved, careful resection with a small (No. 1 or 2) Kerrison rongeur can be performed (**Figure 2,** *B* and *C*). To ensure appropriate spinal cord decompression, an additional 1 to 2 mm should be undercut laterally. The resection should be sufficiently completed laterally to relieve compressive pathology (**Figure 2,** *D* through *F*). The higher concentration of epidural veins in this area may cause significant bleeding. A thrombin-soaked sponge or absorbable gelatin powder may be used to assist in hemostasis. It is important to treat end-plate osteophytes at the cranial

and caudal levels that may be contributing to the pathology.

Corpectomy Versus Multilevel Diskectomy

The choice of anterior decompressive procedure depends primarily on the pathoanatomic considerations and the area of spinal cord compression. If there is evidence of retrovertebral pathology, a corpectomy should be performed to adequately decompress the spinal cord. In patients with multilevel spondylosis in which there is no clear indication for wide bony decompression, the superiority of one technique over another is controversial. In a retrospective comparison study of 190 patients, Hilibrand et al[13] re-

ported a fusion rate of 93% in patients treated with corpectomy compared with a 66% arthrodesis rate in those treated with multilevel diskectomy and fusion, although these reconstructions were performed without the use of an anterior plate. Similar discrepancies in arthrodesis rates have been documented in the literature.[2,13-17] Fusion rates decrease as the number of grafted levels increases.[2,17-19] Evidence has suggested that there is no significant difference in fusion rates between two-level anterior diskectomy and single-level corpectomy.[20] When three or more levels are involved, corpectomy appears to be associated with higher fusion rates.[21] Anterior plating increases the fusion rate with either approach. The rationale behind the higher fusion rates with anterior cervical corpectomy is that there are only two bony surfaces to heal as opposed to two bony surfaces at each level in a multilevel diskectomy and fusion.[1] Although the rate of pseudarthrosis is higher following multilevel diskectomy and fusion, there is inconclusive data regarding the implications because the development of a pseudarthrosis may not have a significant impact on clinical outcome.[13,22,23] Other investigators have found a significant association between clinical outcome and fusion rates.[2,24,25] If the patient remains asymptomatic, the pseudarthrosis can be observed and does not require surgical intervention. Although the union rates are higher, complications associated with corpectomy and strut grafting should be taken into consideration when choosing a surgical approach. Extrusion of the graft and hardware failure are potential complications that occur more frequently with multilevel procedures.[26,27]

Patients with a variable pattern of disease process between segments can be treated with a hybrid construct using diskectomy and corpectomy. Evidence suggests that improved fusion rates, postoperative alignment, and reduced surgical times are a benefit of such reconstructions.[28]

Interbody Grafting: Technical Considerations

Prior to interbody grafting, end-plate preparation is pivotal in preventing graft dislodgment and improving fusion rates. The cartilage must be thoroughly denuded to create a healing environment. The subchondral end plates are perforated or drilled down to expose osteogenic factors. Distraction is performed with previously placed Caspar distraction or with Gardner-Wells traction for strut graft placement. The goal is to widen the space from 3 to 5 mm to adequately distract the neuroforamen.[2] The appropriate depth and width of the graft is measured, and the chosen graft is appropriately sized. Graft heights typically measure from 6 to 10 mm in height and 12 to 14 mm in depth. Lordosis can be built into the graft, particularly if deformity correction is a goal. The graft (the chapter's authors prefer a tricortical iliac crest allograft) is gently tamped into place and countersunk approximately 1 to 2 mm beyond the anterior edge of the vertebral body.

Some controversy exists regarding the use of an intervertebral graft following anterior cervical diskectomy for the treatment of degenerative disk conditions in the cervical spine. Limited data suggest the superiority of an intervertebral graft to diskectomy without graft placement. The rationale behind graft placement is to restore the prediscase disk height (indirectly decompressing the level by normalizing the foraminal diameter) and potentially address axial neck pain.[8]

Autograft Versus Allograft

The choice of the intervertebral graft is a widely debated topic. When choosing between autograft and allograft, factors such as donor site morbidity, fusion rate, and cost and time efficiency should be considered. With the advent of anterior cervical spine surgery, tricortical iliac crest autograft was initially considered the gold standard. Clinical studies have proven that graft integration and maintenance of disk height were superior to allograft. With the addition of cervical plate fixation, fusion rates have become comparable with those obtained with autograft.[29,30] Allograft reduces donor site morbidity and surgical time, has become more widely accepted, and is recognized as a cost-effective technique compared with autograft. In choosing a specific allograft, the integration and biomechanical graft integrity must be considered. Tricortical iliac crest allografts have better fusion rates compared with fibular allograft because of their greater osteoconductive potential.[31] Fibular allografts can maintain disk heights more effectively than iliac crest allografts, which can exhibit more than 50% graft collapse.[32]

With the advent of new technology, synthetic devices are now more widely used as interbody grafts in anterior cervical spine surgery. These devices have many advantages over human grafts, including no donor site morbidity, an unlimited supply of virtually any size, and no risk of disease transmission. However, synthetic grafts significantly increase cost, and there are limited data indicating comparable fusion rates.[33,34]

Cervical Plating

The use of anterior plate fixation in cervical fusions has substantially increased over the past 25 years. With the addition of plating, external bracing in the postoperative period is minimized. Plating improves fusion rates for long cervical fusions (two or more levels).[29,35] The benefit is less clear for single-level fusion.[36-38] Although fusion rates are improved with multilevel fusions, the pseudarthrosis rates remain high, and supplemental posterior fixation should be considered for fusions of more than three intervertebral levels. Plate design has evolved since its introduction in anterior cervical surgery, providing the surgeon with many hardware options. Screw fixation may be fixed (static) or variable angle. Plate designs range from static (round holes) to dynamic (slotted holes or moving platforms). Dynamic plating provides a load-sharing environment and aids in the reduction of stress shielding.[39] Although clinical and biomechanical results have suggested that dynamic plates may be an improvement over static plates, dynamic plates are not yet used routinely in anterior cervical surgery.[40,41] Complications of plate fixation include instrumentation failure (screw/plate breakage, screw backout), dysphagia, adjacent-level ossification, and esophageal injury, which appear to be more common with longer plated fusions.

Summary

Anterior cervical decompression allows the surgeon to directly treat pathology without manipulating the spinal cord. The addition of the surgical microscope allows better visualization of the neural elements and improves the precision and accuracy of decompression. The choice of diskectomy versus corpectomy depends on the pathoanatomic considerations and the area of compression. The decompression method used, the amount of decompression necessary, and the choice of graft and plate should be tailored to the individual patient.

References

1. Emery SE, Bohlman HH, Bolesta MJ, Jones PK: Anterior cervical decompression and arthrodesis for the treatment of cervical spondylotic myelopathy: Two to seventeen-year follow-up. *J Bone Joint Surg Am* 1998;80(7):941-951.

2. Bohlman HH, Emery SE, Goodfellow DB, Jones PK: Robinson anterior cervical discectomy and arthrodesis for cervical radiculopathy: Long-term follow-up of one hundred and twenty-two patients. *J Bone Joint Surg Am* 1993;75(9):1298-1307.

3. Clarke E, Robinson PK: Cervical myelopathy: A complication of cervical spondylosis. *Brain* 1956;79(3):483-510.

4. Rao RD, Gourab K, David KS: Operative treatment of cervical spondylotic myelopathy. *J Bone Joint Surg Am* 2006;88(7):1619-1640.

5. Witwer BP, Trost GR: Cervical spondylosis: Ventral or dorsal surgery. *Neurosurgery* 2007;60(1 Suppl 1):S130-S136.

6. Lees F, Turner JW: Natural history and prognosis of cervical spondylosis. *Br Med J* 1963;2(5373):1607-1610.

7. Ahlgren BD, Garfin SR: Cervical radiculopathy. *Orthop Clin North Am* 1996;27(2):253-263.

8. Garvey TA, Transfeldt EE, Malcolm JR, Kos P: Outcome of anterior cervical discectomy and fusion as perceived by patients treated for dominant axial-mechanical cervical spine pain. *Spine (Phila Pa 1976)* 2002;27(17):1887-1895, discussion 1895.

9. Williams RW: Microlumbar discectomy: A conservative surgical approach to the virgin herniated lumbar disc. *Spine (Phila Pa 1976)* 1978;3(2):175-182.

10. Hannallah D, Lee J, Khan M, Donaldson WF, Kang JD: Cerebrospinal fluid leaks following cervical spine surgery. *J Bone Joint Surg Am* 2008;90(5):1101-1105.

11. Smith MD, Bolesta MJ, Leventhal M, Bohlman HH: Postoperative cerebrospinal-fluid fistula associated with erosion of the dura: Findings after anterior resection of ossification of the posterior longitudinal ligament in the cervical spine. *J Bone Joint Surg Am* 1992;74(2):270-277.

12. Aronson N, Filtzer DL, Bagan M: Anterior cervical fusion by the Smith-Robinson approach. *J Neurosurg* 1968;29(4):396-404.

13. Hilibrand AS, Fye MA, Emery SE, Palumbo MA, Bohlman HH: Increased rate of arthrodesis with strut grafting after multilevel anterior cervical decompression. *Spine (Phila Pa 1976)* 2002;27(2):146-151.

14. Yonenobu K, Fuji T, Ono K, Okada K, Yamamoto T, Harada N: Choice of surgical treatment for multisegmental cervical spondylotic myelopathy. *Spine (Phila Pa 1976)* 1985;10(8):710-716.

15. Swank ML, Lowery GL, Bhat AL, McDonough RF: Anterior cervical allograft arthrodesis and instrumentation: Multilevel interbody grafting or strut graft reconstruction. *Eur Spine J* 1997;6(2):138-143.

16. Nirala AP, Husain M, Vatsal DK: A retrospective study of multiple interbody grafting and long segment strut grafting following multilevel anterior cervical decompression. *Br J Neurosurg* 2004;18(3):227-232.

17. Emery SE, Fisher JR, Bohlman HH: Three-level anterior cervical discectomy and fusion: Radiographic and clinical results. *Spine (Phila Pa 1976)* 1997;22(22):2622-2624, discussion 2625.

18. Emery SE, Bolesta MJ, Banks MA, Jones PK: Robinson anterior cervical fusion comparison of the standard and modified techniques. *Spine (Phila Pa 1976)* 1994;19(6):660-663.

19. Brodke DS, Zdeblick TA: Modified Smith-Robinson procedure for anterior cervical discectomy and fusion. *Spine (Phila Pa 1976)* 1992;17(10, Suppl):S427-S430.

20. Wang JC, McDonough PW, Endow KK, Delamarter RB: A comparison of fusion rates between single-level cervical corpectomy and two-level discectomy and fusion. *J Spinal Disord* 2001;14(3):222-225.

21. Fraser JF, Härtl R: Anterior approaches to fusion of the cervical spine: A metaanalysis of fusion rates. *J Neurosurg Spine* 2007;6(4):298-303.

22. White AA III, Southwick WO, Deponte RJ, Gainor JW, Hardy R: Relief of pain by anterior cervical-spine fusion for spondylo-

sis: A report of sixty-five patients. *J Bone Joint Surg Am* 1973;55(3): 525-534.

23. DePalma AF, Rothman RH, Lewinnek GE, Canale ST: Anterior interbody fusion for severe cervical disc degeneration. *Surg Gynecol Obstet* 1972;134(5): 755-758.

24. Phillips FM, Carlson G, Emery SE, Bohlman HH: Anterior cervical pseudarthrosis: Natural history and treatment. *Spine (Phila Pa 1976)* 1997;22(14):1585-1589.

25. Newman M: The outcome of pseudarthrosis after cervical anterior fusion. *Spine (Phila Pa 1976)* 1993;18(16):2380-2382.

26. Vaccaro AR, Falatyn SP, Scuderi GJ, et al: Early failure of long segment anterior cervical plate fixation. *J Spinal Disord* 1998; 11(5):410-415.

27. Wang JC, Hart RA, Emery SE, Bohlman HH: Graft migration or displacement after multilevel cervical corpectomy and strut grafting. *Spine (Phila Pa 1976)* 2003; 28(10):1016-1021, discussion 1021-1022.

28. Lian XF, Xu JG, Zeng BF, Zhou W, Kong WQ, Hou TS: Noncontiguous anterior decompression and fusion for multilevel cervical spondylotic myelopathy: A prospective randomized control clinical study. *Eur Spine J* 2010;19(5): 713-719.

29. Kaiser MG, Haid RW Jr, Subach BR, Barnes B, Rodts GE Jr: Anterior cervical plating enhances arthrodesis after discectomy and fusion with cortical allograft.

Neurosurgery 2002;50(2):229-236, discussion 236-238.

30. Samartzis D, Shen FH, Matthews DK, Yoon ST, Goldberg EJ, An HS: Comparison of allograft to autograft in multilevel anterior cervical discectomy and fusion with rigid plate fixation. *Spine J* 2003;3(6):451-459.

31. Martin GJ Jr, Haid RW Jr, MacMillan M, Rodts GE Jr, Berkman R: Anterior cervical discectomy with freeze-dried fibula allograft: Overview of 317 cases and literature review. *Spine (Phila Pa 1976)* 1999;24(9):852-858, discussion 858-859.

32. Young WF, Rosenwasser RH: An early comparative analysis of the use of fibular allograft versus autologous iliac crest graft for interbody fusion after anterior cervical discectomy. *Spine (Phila Pa 1976)* 1993;18(9):1123-1124.

33. Hacker RJ, Cauthen JC, Gilbert TJ, Griffith SL: A prospective randomized multicenter clinical evaluation of an anterior cervical fusion cage. *Spine* 2000;25(20): 2646-2654.

34. Park HW, Lee JK, Moon SJ, Seo SK, Lee JH, Kim SH: The efficacy of the synthetic interbody cage and Grafton for anterior cervical fusion. *Spine* 2009;34(17): E591-E595.

35. Wang JC, McDonough PW, Endow KK, Delamarter RB: Increased fusion rates with cervical plating for two-level anterior cervical discectomy and fusion. *Spine (Phila Pa 1976)* 2000;25(1): 41-45.

36. Wang JC, McDonough PW, Endow K, Kanim LE, Delamarter RB: The effect of cervical plating on single-level anterior cervical discectomy and fusion. *J Spinal Disord* 1999;12(6):467-471.

37. Nabhan A, Pape D, Pitzen T, et al: Radiographic analysis of fusion progression following one-level cervical fusion with or without plate fixation. *Zentralbl Neurochir* 2007;68(3):133-138.

38. Grob D, Peyer JV, Dvorak J: The use of plate fixation in anterior surgery of the degenerative cervical spine: A comparative prospective clinical study. *Eur Spine J* 2001;10(5):408-413.

39. Rhee JM, Riew KD: Dynamic anterior cervical plates. *J Am Acad Orthop Surg* 2007;15(11): 640-646.

40. Goldberg G, Albert TJ, Vaccaro AR, Hilibrand AS, Anderson DG, Wharton N: Short-term comparison of cervical fusion with static and dynamic plating using computerized motion analysis. *Spine* 2007;32(13):E371-E375.

41. Saphier PA, Arginteau MS, Moore FM, Steinberger AA, Camins MB: Stress-shielding compared with load-sharing anterior cervical plate fixation: A clinical and radiographic prospective analysis of 50 patients. *J Neurosurg Spine* 2007;6(5):391-397.

Video Reference

36.1 Hilibrand A, Smith JS: Video. *Advanced Techniques in Cervical Spine Surgery.* Philadelphia, PA, 2011.

Cervical Spine Surgery: Cervical Laminaplasty

Mark M. Mikhael, MD
Christopher F. Wolf, MD
Jeffrey C. Wang, MD

Abstract

Multilevel cervical spondylosis resulting in myelopathy is a complex condition to treat surgically. Several anterior and posterior procedures have been described. Cervical laminaplasty is a procedure that provides multilevel posterior cord decompression while attempting to eliminate the postoperative development of instability and kyphosis by retaining the posterior elements. Because laminaplasty does not involve arthrodesis, more postoperative motion is preserved and early range of motion is encouraged to avoid stiffness. Although laminaplasty is a relatively straightforward procedure, understanding several key points can help avoid common technical challenges and ensure the best possible outcomes for patients. A variety of fixation techniques, each with advantages and limitations, are available to keep the laminaplasty door open. The surgeon should be aware of the complications associated with cervical laminaplasty.

Instr Course Lect 2012;61:461-468.

Cervical myelopathy results from central canal impingement, possibly resulting from disk material or osteophyte formation, which causes cervical spinal cord compression. Multilevel central stenosis caused by advanced cervical spondylosis is more challenging to treat surgically than single-level disease (**Figure 1**). With multilevel disease, the surgeon must contend with issues regarding adequate decompression, stability, preserved motion, solid fixation, and complete fusion (when necessary). Multiple surgical strategies have been used to treat this complex condition. In general, these strategies can be categorized into anterior decompression procedures (including diskectomy and/or vertebral corpectomy and fusion) and posterior decompression procedures (including laminectomy alone, laminectomy and fusion, and cervical laminaplasty). The surgeon must be aware of the specific challenges, disadvantages, and complications associated with each procedure when planning a multilevel cervical decompression.

Cervical laminaplasty is used to achieve multilevel posterior cord decompression while attempting to eliminate the postoperative development of instability and kyphosis by retaining the posterior elements. Laminaplasty is associated with a 30% to 50% loss of cervical spine motion.[1,2] Because this procedure does not include arthrodesis, adjacent segment disease is less likely to occur following laminaplasty. These advantages suggest that patients treated with a laminaplasty procedure may have fewer postoperative limitations and a lower incidence of reoperation. There is also the possibility of preserving motion with a laminaplasty procedure as opposed to a fusion.

Although several techniques have been described for performing a laminaplasty, all are based on the concept of canal widening by opening the posterior elements in a "door-hinge"

Dr. Wang or an immediate family member has received royalties from Aesculap/B. Braun, Biomet, Medtronic Sofamor Danek, Stryker, Zimmer, Osprey, Alphatech, Seaspine, and Amedica; owns stock or stock options in Fziomed, Promethean Spine, Paradigm Spine, Benevenue, NexGen, K2 Medical, Pioneer, Amedica, Vertiflex, Electrocore, Surgitech, Invuity, Axiomed, Bone Biologics, VG Innovations, Corespine, Expanding Orthopaedics, Syndicom, Curative Biosciences, Facet Solutions, and Pearldiver; and serves as a board member, owner, officer, or committee member of the Cervical Spine Research Society, the North American Spine Society, and the Scoliosis Research Society. Neither of the following authors nor any immediate family member has received anything of value from or owns stock in a commercial company or institution related directly or indirectly to the subject of this chapter: Dr. Mikhael and Dr. Wolf.

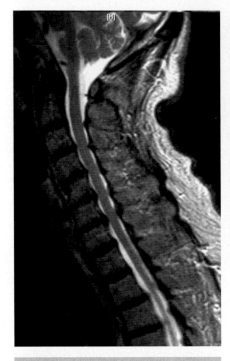

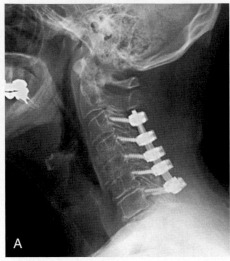

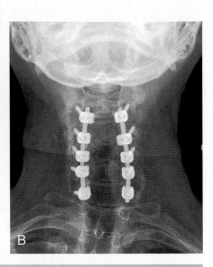

Figure 2 Lateral (**A**) and AP (**B**) radiographs of the cervical spine after laminectomy decompression and posterior instrumented fusion.

Figure 1 Sagittal MRI scan of the cervical spine showing multilevel cervical spondylosis with neutral alignment.

fashion without completely removing the posterior arch. Because compressive structures are generally located anteriorly (for example, disk material or osteophytes), this procedure allows indirect decompression of the spinal cord by expanding the central canal and allowing the spinal cord to drift dorsally. Laminaplasty is reported to provide long-term, stable neurologic improvement for patients with cervical myelopathy.[3-5]

Comparison of Procedures

Anterior decompression procedures can be fairly straightforward in patients with single-level disease involving a soft-disk herniation. These procedures become more complex in multilevel disease involving hard disks and central osteophyte formation. Rates of pseudarthrosis following anterior diskectomy and fusion can be low for single-level procedures but can range from 11% to 46% for multilevel

fusions involving multiple corpectomies and strut grafting.[6-8] The occurrence of graft dislodgement following multilevel corpectomy and strut grafting ranges from 6% to 20%.[9,10] Anterior plating has not been shown to prevent this complication because long-plated corpectomies have been shown to lose stability under fatigue loading, leading to failure.[11] Some complications involving the anterior approach to the cervical spine, such as speech and swallowing disturbance, esophageal injury, airway obstruction, and vertebral artery injury, are more likely after multilevel fusions or corpectomy procedures.[12,13] These complications can ultimately lead to pain, neurologic compromise, and reoperation. One study comparing outcomes from anterior corpectomy and fusion to laminaplasty reported similar clinical outcomes but a significant difference in the major complication rate between the groups, with a 29% rate in the group treated with anterior procedures compared with 7% in the laminaplasty group.[14]

Multilevel posterior laminectomy without fusion can be disadvantageous because of complications involving

neck pain, exposed dura, postlaminectomy kyphosis/instability, and recurrent myelopathy.[15,16] Rates of postoperative deformity and instability following multilevel posterior decompression without fusion can range from 25% to 95% and may require early reoperation.[17,18] Multilevel posterior laminectomy is generally combined with posterior instrumented fusion in an attempt to avoid the complications associated with decompression alone (**Figure 2**). One study comparing anterior corpectomy and fusion, laminectomy alone, and laminaplasty found statistically equivalent clinical outcomes in the groups treated with anterior corpectomy and fusion and those treated with laminaplasty; inferior outcomes were reported in the laminectomy group.[19] An independent matched cohort analysis of laminectomy and fusion versus laminaplasty showed better clinical outcomes and fewer complications, including myelopathy progression, nonunion, instrumentation failure, adjacent degeneration, infection, kyphotic deformity, and graft-site donor pain in the laminaplasty group.[20] However, no prospective, randomized trial has been done to directly compare laminaplasty with laminectomy and fusion.

Indications

The indications for a laminaplasty are similar to those for other decompression procedures, including evidence of multilevel (three or more levels) cervical canal compression causing myelopathy. Ideally, the curvature of the cervical spine should be lordotic or neutral without evidence of instability on flexion-extension radiographs.[21] Because one of the goals of the procedure is to maintain cervical motion, the patient should have little or no neck pain before surgery. Laminaplasty also can be used to treat patients with congenital spinal stenosis or ossification of the posterior longitudinal ligament.

Contraindications

The decompression achieved by performing a laminaplasty procedure relies on posterior drift of the spinal cord after the canal is hinged open (**Figure 3**). In patients with preoperative cervical kyphosis, the decompression may not be adequate because the kyphotic alignment does not allow the spinal cord to drift posteriorly. Because laminaplasty does not typically involve arthrodesis, patients with evidence of preoperative cervical instability must be identified. Flexion-extension radiographs of the cervical spine should not show evidence of increased angular motion or translation greater than 3 mm with motion. Patients with debilitating preoperative neck pain should be aware that the symptoms may not improve or may worsen because of surgical pain. Two studies investigating neck pain following laminaplasty found that the procedure did not affect the resolution or the development of those symptoms postoperatively.[22,23] The surgeon should be aware that these are all relative con-

traindications, yet laminaplasty can still be advantageous even in these settings. The appropriate surgical plan must be individualized to the specific needs and desires of the patient.

Procedure

Patient Positioning and Setup

Cervical spine precautions should be maintained during patient positioning, and fiberoptic intubation while the patient is awake is recommended. The patient is then positioned prone on a Jackson frame. The Mayfield headrest attachment with pinions is used to allow unrestricted access to the head and neck and for easy intraoperative alterations in positioning if needed. Care should be taken when positioning the head to ensure that both neck extension and flexion are avoided and there is minimal rotation through the cervical spine; this will aid with symmetric trough placement during the procedure. Ideally, the patient's head should be placed in a neutral position. Slight Trendelenburg positioning allows better visualization during the procedure. Some surgeons use intraoperative neurologic monitoring (electromyelography, motor-evoked and/or somatosensory-evoked potentials) and measure baseline potentials before, during, and immediately after the procedure. Intraoperative fluoroscopy can aid in proper placement of the skin incision, confirmation of the levels to be decompressed, and proper placement of instrumentation. When fluoroscopy is used, adequate space is needed for the sterile draped intensifier at the head of the table between the surgeon and anesthesiologist.

Exposure

A midline posterior incision is made at the desired levels after the location is confirmed with intraoperative imaging. The incision should be carried down through the ligamentum nuchae

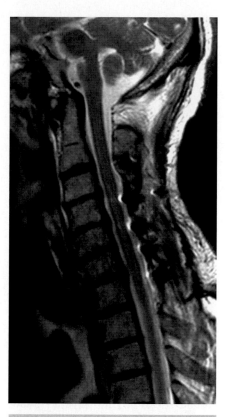

Figure 3 Postoperative MRI scan of the cervical spine after a laminaplasty procedure. Note that the canal is widened dorsally to allow for posterior drift of the spinal cord for decompression.

to the spinous process of each level. Preoperative imaging may help identify any bifid spinous process that may be incomplete in the midline, leaving unprotected dura at those levels; these processes will require added care to identify during the exposure (**Figure 4**). The muscular attachments to C2 should not be disrupted in an effort to increase stability and help preserve postoperative extension and motion. Each lamina should be exposed with subperiosteal dissection laterally to each facet capsule without violating the facet capsule. Typically, this procedure is performed anywhere from C3 to C7. If the posterior decompression needs to extend to C2, a burr and/or Kerrison punch may be used to remove the lower margin of the C2 arch

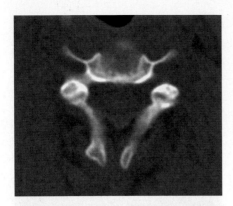

Figure 4 Axial CT scan of the cervical spine showing a completely bifid spinous process with a central defect allowing direct access to the central canal. Care must be taken during exposure to recognize these segments and avoid entering the dura centrally.

while preserving the muscular attachments superiorly. For levels below C2, a portion of the spinous processes should be excised immediately above and below the surgical levels to ensure unrestricted "opening of the door" at the end of the procedure. These resected fragments should be saved and used as local bone graft if needed. At this point in the procedure, some surgeons prefer to remove portions of the intraspinous and supraspinous ligaments for better visualization. Prior to starting the bone cuts, the ligamentum flavum should be exposed and identified immediately above and below the ends of the planned levels for decompression. The ligamentum flavum should then be released with a 1-mm Kerrison punch at the cranial and caudal ends of the planned procedure to assist in unrestricted mobilization and opening of the laminaplasty door. Some surgeons prefer to preserve the ligamentum flavum at these levels to add to the stability of the construct; however, this technique can be technically challenging and is discouraged when dural adhesions are present dorsally. Dorsal dural adhesions may inhibit opening of the laminaplasty.

Supplemental foraminotomies may be performed at any level with radiographic evidence of foraminal stenosis and associated radicular symptoms. Some authors recommend routine bilateral foraminotomies at C4-5 and at every level with radiographic foraminal stenosis to help decrease the incidence of postoperative neck pain, radiculopathy, and nerve root palsy caused by stretch injuries.[21] When performing a foraminotomy during a laminaplasty, care should be taken to avoid creating facet joint instability. No more than 50% of the inferior articular facet should be removed to gain access to the underlying superior articular facet. Resection of the superior facet lateral to the pedicle is unnecessary and will likely cause postoperative instability. Enough bone should be removed so that the lateral wall of the superior and inferior pedicles can be palpated.

Bone Trough Preparation

Several techniques have been described for performing a laminaplasty; the two most common are the French-door and the open-door techniques.[24,25] The French-door technique involves forming bilateral troughs in the laminae just medial to the pedicles, followed by a midline split of the spinous process to facilitate opening the posterior elements like a French door. This door is then held open with a plate, a ceramic spacer, or a bone spacer, which is placed just dorsal to the open canal. The open-door technique, which is preferred by this chapter's authors, is more commonly performed. In this technique, the laminae are hinged open on one side through a controlled greenstick-type fracture of the contralateral cortex, thus expanding the spinal canal.

When planning the location of the bone troughs, the surgeon must identify the junction of the lamina to the most medial portion of the lateral mass without disrupting the facet joints. The bone cuts are made just medial to the pedicles at each level. The operating microscope is helpful in making the troughs for the laminaplasty because the surgeon can see the transition from the cancellous to the deeper cortical bone. Typically, the complete (opening-side) osteotomy is made on the side that is either more stenotic or symptomatic because this side may be slightly more decompressed than the door-hinge side. If supplemental foraminotomies are made on one side (for example, to treat unilateral radicular symptoms), the opening side is typically made ipsilaterally. Ultimately, the unique features of the patient's disease and the surgeon's preference dictate the opening side. A 3- to 4-mm burr is used to score the cortex, marking the location of the bone troughs along the entire side for the complete osteotomy. Starting at the most cranial level, the osteotomy is performed using a burr and syringe irrigation to help prevent thermal injury. While viewing through the operating microscope, the surgeon can see when all cancellous bone within the trough has been removed and the deep cortical bone exposed. Hemostasis can be achieved between cuts with either a thin layer of bone wax or hemostatic thrombin foam and thrombin solution applied to the osteotomy site. The deep cortical bone is carefully removed with the burr or a 1-mm Kerrison punch until completion of the osteotomy is seen under magnification. This process is repeated at sequential caudal levels until the osteotomy is complete along the entire length. The surgeon must ensure that complete bone separation has occurred at every level before proceeding because it is critical in assessing the hinge stiffness in subsequent steps.

The surgeon then performs a partial osteotomy on the contralateral side to create the door hinge. The cortex is scored with the burr, marking the location of the bone trough at every level. It is especially important to ensure that this osteotomy is straight along the entire length of the decompression because this will assist with proper, uninhibited opening of the laminaplasty. Care also should be taken to ensure that the troughs are not made too medially or too deep because this could compromise the stiffness of the hinge. Starting at the most cranial level, the burr is used to deepen the bone troughs to the level of the cancellous bone. The stiffness of the hinge at each level is then checked to ensure that the lamina hinge opens slightly with moderate force. Generally, it is better to leave more cancellous bone than expected because additional bone can be removed if necessary. If the surgeon suspects that adequate bone has been removed but the hinge remains stiff, the osteotomy should be checked to make sure it is complete on the opening side. When there is adequate give with equal yielding stiffness at every level, opening the laminaplasty can begin.

Opening the Laminaplasty

Opening the laminaplasty is accomplished by creating a controlled greenstick-type fracture through the hinge-side osteotomy. Any structure that may inhibit a smooth, adequate, and controlled opening (such as facet capsule fibers, epidural veins, or residual ligamentum flavum at the cranial and caudal ends of the laminaplasty) should be addressed. The lamina is gently opened from one end to the other. Some surgeons prefer to place a small curet or other tool to assist in holding the door open and help prevent the lamina from springing back closed over the dura. As the door opens, an angled probe may be used to help separate any epidural veins or du-

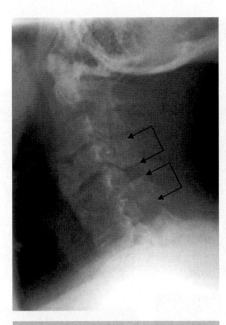

Figure 5 Lateral radiograph of the cervical spine after a laminaplasty procedure performed using a bone block spacer (bracket arrows) to hold the door open without plate fixation.

ral attachments from the underside of the lamina, which may inhibit proper opening. Once the laminaplasty is hinged open at every level, there should be enough residual stiffness at the hinge to hold the door in an open position before any fixation. The laminaplasty is typically opened from 8 mm to 18 mm to provide adequate decompression.

Fixation Strategies

Several techniques have been described to fix the laminaplasty door open. Typically, a bone block, suture fixation, or a plate and screws is placed. A bone block such as a spinous process remnant or allograft rib to hold the laminaplasty door open can allow healing of a new lamina and the hinge (**Figure 5**). Placing a bone block alone does not provide strong initial fixation; therefore, some surgeons are reluctant to start early range of motion before there is evidence of early healing. Suture fixation alone can be used to keep

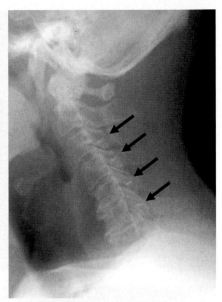

Figure 6 Lateral radiograph of the cervical spine showing a laminaplasty procedure performed using suture anchors (arrows) to hold the door open. The anchors are placed within the lateral masses on the hinge side while suture is looped through and around the spinous processes to keep them open.

the laminaplasty door open. Typically, a suture anchor is placed into the lateral mass on the hinge side, and the suture is driven through and looped around the spinous process, securing it in an open position (**Figure 6**). A disadvantage compared with placing a bone block is that there is no potential to re-create a new arch, and stability relies solely on healing of the hinge side. Probably the most secure and forgiving technique is plate fixation, which provides strong initial fixation and allows for early range of motion. Plate fixation can be combined with a bone graft to facilitate rigid fixation, increased union of the hinge side and graft, and formation of a new bony lamina (**Figure 7**). Laminaplasty plates can be fixed with two 3- to 5-mm screws in the lateral mass and a screw in the lamina. The graft can be secured to the plate through an oval hole to allow fine adjustments to the graft/plate

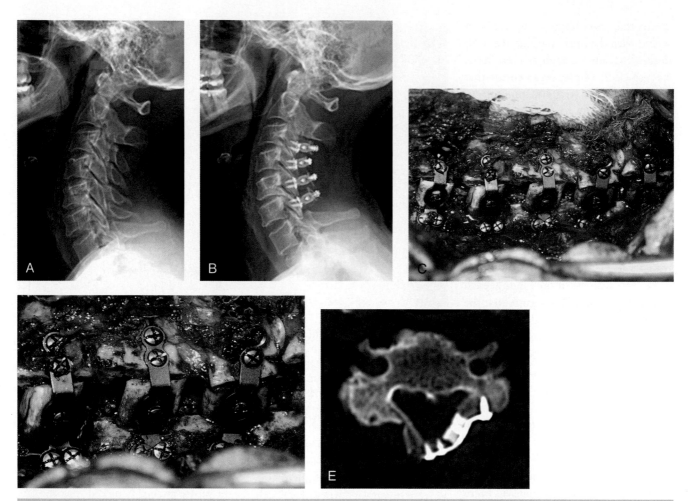

Figure 7 **A,** Preoperative lateral radiograph of a patient with multilevel cervical spondylosis with symptomatic myelopathy. Note that the lordotic sagittal alignment will facilitate posterior spinal cord drift postoperatively. **B,** Postoperative lateral radiograph after laminaplasty with plate and bone block fixation. Note the increased space available for the cord compared with the preoperative radiograph. **C,** Intraoperative photograph showing the placement of the plate and bone block construct at multiple levels. **D,** A closer view of the plate and bone block construct showing the fixation of the graft to the plate. The graft is secured with a screw through an oval hole in the plate allowing for minor adjustments of both graft and plate placement. **E,** Axial CT scan of the cervical spine showing the placement of the plate and bone block construct postoperatively. Note that the laminaplasty door is opened by hinging through the intact deep cortex on the hinge side.

positioning. Care must be taken when placing the screws in the lateral mass to avoid disrupting the facet joints. The surgeon should aim the screws slightly cranial in line with the slope of the facets.

Final Resection and Assessment

After the door is securely fixed open, the final step is removal of the spinous processes with a burr at the base of the lamina. This allows easier and symmetric closure of the muscles over the posterior neck. In addition, neck extension should be evaluated before closure to ensure that there is smooth motion without bony impingement. Areas of impingement should be carefully resected with the burr. Adequate hemostasis should be obtained before closure; bone bleeding can be controlled with a thin layer of bone wax or hemostatic thrombin foam and thrombin solution.

Postoperative Care

Because one of the advantages of performing a laminaplasty procedure is greater motion preservation compared with arthrodesis, postoperative immobilization with a cervical collar should be limited. A soft cervical collar is usually placed immediately postoperatively for comfort. No official cervical range-of-motion restrictions are given, and the patient is encouraged to discontinue the soft collar when the postoperative pain is adequately managed with oral analgesics. The patient should be encouraged to work on neck motion as tolerated immediately after discharge from the hospital. The wound should be inspected, and progress should be evaluated at 2 weeks after surgery. At that time, formal physical therapy can be initiated with gentle motion and strengthening exercises if needed. The next follow-up examination usually occurs at 6 to 8 weeks postoperatively; motion and symptom resolution are evaluated. Patients can usually return to normal activities at that time, including regular exercise. Some surgeons prefer to obtain cervical flexion-extension radiographs at the second follow-up visit to confirm the absence of any iatrogenic instability or fixation/graft failure.

Complications

The incidence of C5 nerve root palsy following laminaplasty has been reported as 1% to 3%.[2] Progressive recovery can be expected in most patients; however, some patients never have full recovery. At this time, it is unclear whether performing bilateral foraminotomies at the time of laminaplasty is helpful in preventing the occurrence of transient nerve palsies. The etiology of the palsies is believed to be a stretch injury caused by the relatively short length of the C5 nerve root and its typical location at the area of maximal cervical lordosis.

Failure of the graft or open-door fixation (such as plate or suture fixation) is also a potential complication after laminaplasty. Restenosis following hinge closure was the most common reason for failure before the use of more recent fixation techniques (**Figure 8**). If most fixation points are still intact, it is unusual for the door hinge to return to a closed position. The patient should be monitored for any evidence of neurologic compromise or progression. Patients with fixation failure in the setting of a stable neurologic examination can be safely observed with serial examination and imaging. Any evidence of neurologic deterioration or return of myelopathy necessitates reoperation.

Postoperative neck pain following laminaplasty has been studied by several authors.[22,23] Proper surgical indications, patient selection, and education are important to provide the patient with realistic postoperative expectations. Patients with debilitating preoperative neck pain who elect a laminaplasty procedure to treat multilevel cervical disease need to be aware that neck pain will not improve and may even worsen after surgery.

Summary

Cervical laminaplasty is a posterior decompressive procedure to surgically treat multilevel cervical spondylosis. Laminaplasty has some advantages over anterior and other posterior procedures used to treat this complex condition. Because the posterior elements are retained during the procedure, laminaplasty affords cervical stability without arthrodesis and allows the possibility for greater postoperative motion.

Several key technical points are important when performing a laminaplasty. The C2 muscular attachments should be maintained during exposure. The trough for the opening-side osteotomy should not be too deep or medial to avoid the creation of a loose hinge. All dural adhesions, residual ligamentum flavum, and epidural veins that may restrict uninhibited opening of the laminaplasty door should be recognized and resected. Multiple fixation techniques are available to keep the laminaplasty door open. A laminaplasty plate with bone graft allows for rigid initial fixation and improved healing of the hinge side with re-

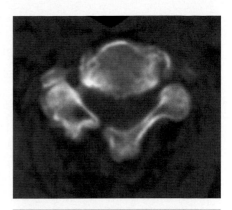

Figure 8 Postoperative axial CT scan of the cervical spine showing a laminaplasty that healed in the closed position after suture-anchor fixation failed to keep the door open.

creation of the lamina on the opening side. Postoperative range of motion can be started early. Complications following laminaplasty can include C5 nerve root palsy, fixation failure, and persistent or increased neck pain.

References

1. Edwards CC II, Heller JG, Silcox DH III: T-Saw laminoplasty for the management of cervical spondylotic myelopathy: Clinical and radiographic outcome. *Spine (Phila Pa 1976)* 2000;25(14): 1788-1794.

2. Satomi K, Nishu Y, Kohno T, Hirabayashi K: Long-term follow-up studies of open-door expansive laminoplasty for cervical stenotic myelopathy. *Spine (Phila Pa 1976)* 1994;19(5):507-510.

3. Shiraishi T, Fukuda K, Yato Y, Nakamura M, Ikegami T: Results of skip laminectomy: Minimum 2-year follow-up study compared with open-door laminoplasty. *Spine (Phila Pa 1976)* 2003; 28(24):2667-2672.

4. Kawaguchi Y, Kanamori M, Ishihara H, Ohmori K, Nakamura H, Kimura T: Minimum 10-year followup after en bloc cervical laminoplasty. *Clin Orthop Relat Res* 2003;411:129-139.

5. Seichi A, Takeshita K, Ohishi I, et al: Long-term results of double-door laminoplasty for cervical stenotic myelopathy. *Spine (Phila Pa 1976)* 2001;26(5):479-487.

6. Connolly ES, Seymour RJ, Adams JE: Clinical evaluation of anterior cervical fusion for degenerative cervical disc disease. *J Neurosurg* 1965;23(4):431-437.

7. Swank ML, Lowery GL, Bhat AL, McDonough RF: Anterior cervical allograft arthrodesis and instrumentation: Multilevel interbody grafting or strut graft reconstruction. *Eur Spine J* 1997;6(2):138-143.

8. Saunders RL, Pikus HJ, Ball P: Four-level cervical corpectomy. *Spine (Phila Pa 1976)* 1998;23(22):2455-2461.

9. Vaccaro AR, Falatyn SP, Scuderi GJ, et al: Early failure of long segment anterior cervical plate fixation. *J Spinal Disord* 1998;11(5):410-415.

10. Wang JC, Hart RA, Emery SE, Bohlman HH: Graft migration or displacement after multilevel cervical corpectomy and strut grafting. *Spine (Phila Pa 1976)* 2003;28(10):1016-1021, discussion 1021-1022.

11. Isomi T, Panjabi MM, Wang JL, Vaccaro AR, Garfin SR, Patel T: Stabilizing potential of anterior cervical plates in multilevel corpectomies. *Spine (Phila Pa 1976)* 1999;24(21):2219-2223.

12. Emery SE, Bohlman HH, Bolesta MJ, Jones PK: Anterior cervical decompression and arthrodesis for the treatment of cervical spondy-

lotic myelopathy: Two to seventeen-year follow-up. *J Bone Joint Surg Am* 1998;80(7):941-951.

13. Smith MD, Emery SE, Dudley A, Murray KJ, Leventhal M: Vertebral artery injury during anterior decompression of the cervical spine: A retrospective review of ten patients. *J Bone Joint Surg Br* 1993;75(3):410-415.

14. Yonenobu K, Hosono N, Iwasaki M, Asano M, Ono K: Laminoplasty versus subtotal corpectomy: A comparative study of results in multisegmental cervical spondylotic myelopathy. *Spine (Phila Pa 1976)* 1992;17(11):1281-1284.

15. Mikawa Y, Shikata J, Yamamuro T: Spinal deformity and instability after multilevel cervical laminectomy. *Spine (Phila Pa 1976)* 1987;12(1):6-11.

16. Kato Y, Iwasaki M, Fuji T, Yonenobu K, Ochi T: Long-term follow-up results of laminectomy for cervical myelopathy caused by ossification of the posterior longitudinal ligament. *J Neurosurg* 1998;89(2):217-223.

17. Albert TJ, Vacarro A: Postlaminectomy kyphosis. *Spine (Phila Pa 1976)* 1998;23(24):2738-2745.

18. Guigui P, Benoist M, Deburge A: Spinal deformity and instability after multilevel cervical laminectomy for spondylotic myelopathy. *Spine (Phila Pa 1976)* 1998;23(4):440-447.

19. Herkowitz HN: A comparison of anterior cervical fusion, cervical laminectomy, and cervical lamino-

plasty for the surgical management of multiple level spondylotic radiculopathy. *Spine (Phila Pa 1976)* 1988;13(7):774-780.

20. Heller JG, Edwards CC II, Murakami H, Rodts GE: Laminoplasty versus laminectomy and fusion for multilevel cervical myelopathy: An independent matched cohort analysis. *Spine (Phila Pa 1976)* 2001;26(12):1330-1336.

21. Lehman RA Jr, Taylor BA, Rhee JM, Riew KD: Cervical laminoplasty. *J Am Acad Orthop Surg* 2008;16(1):47-56.

22. Hosono N, Yonenobu K, Ono K: Neck and shoulder pain after laminoplasty: A noticeable complication. *Spine (Phila Pa 1976)* 1996;21(17):1969-1973.

23. Yoshida M, Tamaki T, Kawakami M, et al: Does reconstruction of posterior ligamentous complex with extensor musculature decrease axial symptoms after cervical laminoplasty? *Spine (Phila Pa 1976)* 2002;27(13):1414-1418.

24. Faccioli F, Buffatti P, Grosslercher JC, Bricolo A, Dalle Ore G: Open-door decompressive cervical laminotomy: Technic and initial experiences. *Neurochirurgie* 1987;33(1):38-43.

25. Hirabayashi K, Watanabe K, Wakano K, Suzuki N, Satomi K, Ishii Y: Expansive open-door laminoplasty for cervical spinal stenotic myelopathy. *Spine (Phila Pa 1976)* 1983;8(7):693-699.

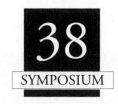

Patient Evaluation and Clinical Assessment of Adult Spinal Deformity

Adam L. Wollowick, MD
Steven D. Glassman, MD
Joseph H. Perra, MD
Frank J. Schwab, MD

Abstract

The clinical evaluation of adults with spinal deformity can be challenging for both general orthopaedic surgeons and spinal specialists. To properly treat these patients, the physician must be aware of the various types of adult spinal deformity and the basic principles of spinal misalignment. A complete patient assessment must include a thorough history and physical examination. Appropriate imaging studies can be used to characterize the extent of the deformity and determine the need for surgical intervention or referral to a spine specialist. The ultimate goal of the evaluation of an adult with spinal deformity is to determine the impact of the deformity on the patient's quality of life, including the ability to work and perform activities of daily living. For patients considering surgical treatment, additional factors must be included in the assessment because of the high rate of complications associated with adult deformity procedures.

Instr Course Lect 2012;61:469-479.

Because of the aging population and the increasing number of patients with spinal complaints, both general orthopaedic surgeons and spine specialists must frequently evaluate adults with spinal deformity. Although spinal deformity may not be the specific reason for the office visit and is sometimes not initially obvious, it may be discovered as part of a routine musculoskeletal examination and workup. The thorough evaluation of an adult with spinal deformity is a complex endeavor and requires diligence on the part of the examining physician. A complete history and physical examination and the appropriate use of imaging studies will ensure that urgent issues are not missed and can help define the source of the patient's symptoms. Although the assessment and management of adults with spinal deformity is challenging, this chapter will provide the treating physician with the information needed to assess and initiate care for these patients.

Basic Principles of Spinal Deformity

Spinal deformity is a misalignment of the spine, which can result from known or unknown causes. In many patients, spinal deformity is idiopathic in nature and has no clear etiology. Conversely, the deformity may be caused by a variety of congenital or

Dr. Wollowick or an immediate family member is a member of a speakers' bureau or has made paid presentations on behalf of DePuy; serves as a paid consultant to DePuy; has received research support from Stryker and DePuy; and serves as a board member, owner, officer, or committee member of the Scoliosis Research Society. Dr. Glassman or an immediate family member has received royalties from Medtronic Sofamor Danek; serves as a paid consultant to Medtronic Sofamor Danek; has received other non–research-related funding (such as paid travel) from Stryker; and serves as a board member, owner, officer, or committee member of the American Academy of Orthopaedic Surgeons, the North American Spine Society, and the Scoliosis Research Society. Dr. Perra or an immediate family member has received royalties from Medtronic; is a member of a speakers' bureau or has made paid presentations on behalf of Medtronic; serves as a paid consultant to Medtronic; owns stock or stock options in Medtronic; has received research support from DePuy; and serves as a board member, owner, officer, or committee member of the Scoliosis Research Society and Abbot Northwestern Hospital. Dr. Schwab or an immediate family member serves as a paid consultant to Medtronic Sofamor Danek and DePuy; owns stock or stock options in Nemaris; and has received research support from Medtronic Sofamor Danek and DePuy.

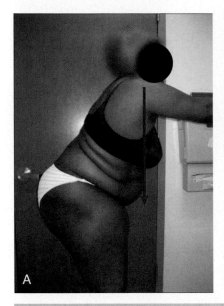
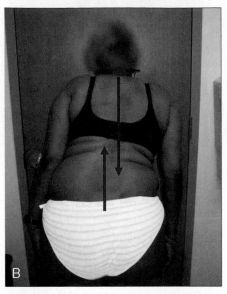

Figure 1   Clinical photographs of a 54-year-old woman with adult scoliosis. The images show both sagittal (**A**) and coronal (**B**) plane imbalance.

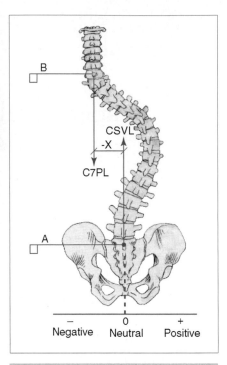

Figure 2   Coronal balance is measured by calculating the horizontal offset of the C7 plumb line (C7PL) from the center sacral vertical line (CSVL). (Adapted with permission from Medtronic Sofamor Danek, Memphis, TN.)

degenerative conditions as well as traumatic, infectious, or other medical processes such as tumors or inflammatory disorders. The alteration of various normal anatomic parameters can contribute to spinal deformity, including scoliosis, kyphosis, lordosis, and spondylolisthesis. Normally, the spine is straight in the coronal or frontal plane; however, curvature of more than 10° in the coronal plane is considered scoliosis. Although 10° has been a threshold for defining scoliosis in past literature, it is not a magnitude that necessarily implies clinical significance. The spine has natural contours in the sagittal plane, including cervical and lumbar lordosis and thoracic kyphosis. Normal thoracic kyphosis is typically between 10° and 40°, whereas normal lumbar lordosis ranges from 40° to 60°.[1-3] The sum of these sagittal contours typically results in a balanced overall posture. However, abnormal kyphosis or lordosis can develop and result in either a decrease or an increase in the magnitude of these parameters. Spondylolisthesis, which is the forward displacement of one vertebra on its ad-

jacent caudal vertebra, has a variety of causes.

Even in the presence of significant spinal deformity and abnormal spinal alignment, the patient may still maintain a balanced posture. The spine or the patient can compensate for the deformity through a variety of mechanisms such as the development of secondary curves or by hip or knee flexion. In some instances, the body is unable to compensate for the deformity and coronal or sagittal plane imbalance develops (**Figure 1**). Coronal balance exists when a plumb line drawn through the center of the C7 vertebral body is aligned with a line drawn through the center of the sacrum. When these lines do not meet, the patient has coronal plane decompensation (**Figure 2**). Normally, the C7 plumb line in the sagittal plane falls through the posterosuperior aspect of the S1 end plate. The sagittal vertical axis is the horizontal offset of the C7 plumb line from the posterosuperior aspect of S1 and is normally less than 5 cm. If the sagittal vertical axis is greater than 5 cm, the patient is be-

lieved to have sagittal plane imbalance (**Figure 3**). Recent studies have shown that sagittal plane decompensation is the most significant identified finding correlated to pain and disability in adults with spinal deformity.[4,5]

When considering a patient's overall balance, the spine cannot be evaluated in isolation. The spine works together with the pelvis, hips, and lower extremities to determine global alignment. Recent research has focused on the contribution of the pelvis to sagittal balance; several significant parameters have been identified, including pelvic incidence, pelvic tilt, sacral slope, and overhang (**Figure 4**). Pelvic incidence is defined as the angle between the perpendicular line to the sacral end plate at its midpoint and the line connecting this point to the axis of the femoral heads.[6] Pelvic incidence is

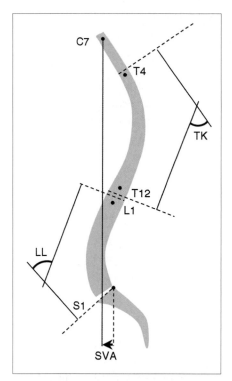

Figure 3 Sagittal spinal radiographic parameters. The magnitude of sagittal curvatures is measured using the Cobb method on the lateral radiograph. Thoracic kyphosis (TK) is measured from T4 to T12, and lumbar lordosis (LL) is measured from L1 to S1. The sagittal vertical axis (SVA) is the horizontal offset of the C7 plumb line from the posterosuperior aspect of the sacrum. (Adapted with permission from Schwab F, Lafage V, Boyce R, et al: Gravity line analysis in adult volunteers. *Spine* 2006;31: E959-E967.)

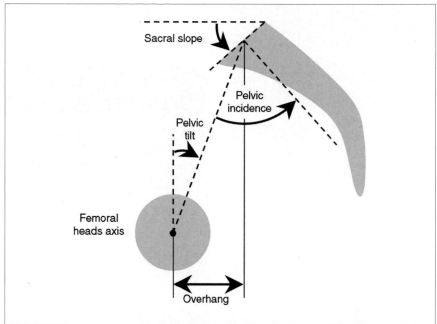

Figure 4 Illustration of the pelvic parameters (pelvic incidence, pelvic tilt, and sacral slope), which are critical to the assessment of patients with spinal deformity. See text for a description of these parameters. (Adapted with permission from Schwab F, Lafage V, Boyce R, et al: Gravity line analysis in adult volunteers. *Spine* 2006;31:E959-E967.)

unique to each patient and is independent of the position of the pelvis. Functionally, pelvic incidence is closely related to the optimal lumbar lordosis (lumbar lordosis = pelvic incidence ± 9°).[7] Pelvic tilt is a measure of pelvic rotation/version, and an increased pelvic tilt reflects compensation caused by spinal misalignment. As the spine falls forward because of loss of sagittal balance, the patient will rotate the pelvis backward around the hips to maintain an upright posture.

Importantly, pelvic tilt has been correlated with patient-reported quality-of-life measures.[8] Sacral slope is the angle between the horizontal and the sacral end plate. All three of these pelvic parameters are interrelated; pelvic incidence is equal to the sum of the pelvic tilt and the sacral slope. Overhang is defined as the horizontal offset between the midpoint of the sacral end plate and the femoral head axis.

Types of Adult Spinal Deformity

Adult spinal deformity can be classified into three general categories: spondylolisthesis, scoliosis, and sagittal plane deformity. Spondylolisthesis is one of the most common types of spinal deformity in adults. The Wiltse classification includes six types of spondylolisthesis, the most common of which is degenerative spondylolisthesis. Isthmic spondylolisthesis, which is caused by a defect in the pars

interarticularis, typically occurs during childhood or adolescence but may not become symptomatic until the patient is much older. The Meyerding grade is used to express the extent of slippage on a lateral radiograph as the percentage of forward displacement of the cephalad vertebra on the adjacent caudal vertebra. In the Meyerding system, the severity of the slippage is measured by the distance from the posterior aspect of the superior vertebra to the posterior aspect of the inferior vertebra. The distance is expressed as a percentage of the total superior vertebral body length. Adult scoliosis can be divided into two broad categories: idiopathic scoliosis in an adult and de novo scoliosis. Adolescent idiopathic scoliosis that is untreated may progress in adulthood or become symptomatic after the patient reaches skeletal maturity. Scoliosis may also develop in adults because of degeneration of the spine, fracture, tumor, or infection.

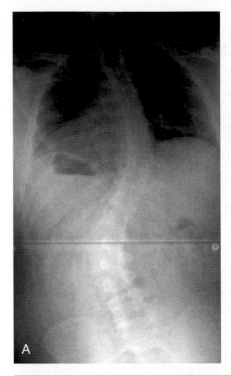

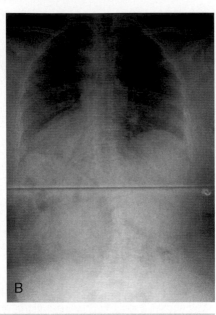

Figure 5 **A,** AP full-length spinal radiograph of a 38-year-old man with adolescent idiopathic scoliosis in an adult. **B,** AP full-length spinal radiograph of a 67-year-old woman with degenerative scoliosis.

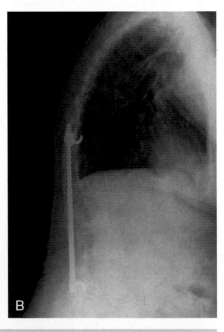

Figure 6 Lateral full-length spinal radiographs of two patients with sagittal plane deformity. **A,** Diffuse degenerative disk disease in a 72-year-old woman that led to decreased lumbar lordosis and a loss of sagittal balance. **B,** Harrington rod instrumentation placed at age 14 for the treatment of scoliosis in a now 44-year-old woman. A flat back deformity and proximal junctional kyphosis leading to sagittal plane decompensation subsequently developed.

Degenerative scoliosis primarily involves the lumbar spine (**Figure 5**).

Sagittal plane deformity can be quite disabling to a patient. There are many causes of sagittal misalignment, including degenerative disk disease; flat back deformity caused by a loss of lumbar lordosis; iatrogenic loss of normal contours; postlaminectomy kyphosis; or hyperkyphosis resulting from trauma, tumor, or infection (**Figure 6**). Historically, the most common cause of flat back deformity was the use of a Harrington rod or other distraction-based spinal instrumentation. However, a recent increase in the incidence of flat back deformity has been attributed to the increased number of multilevel, instrumented spinal fusion procedures being performed for degenerative conditions. Failure to restore or maintain normal lumbar lordosis in these patients can result in sagittal decompensation. Kyphosis and sagittal imbalance proximal to previously fused segments can develop postoperatively, especially at or near the thoracolumbar junction. With an aging population, osteoporosis is becoming more prevalent, and an increased number of compression fractures are being identified. Severe single-level or multilevel compression fractures can also lead to hyperkyphosis and spinal misalignment.

Patient History

A thorough patient assessment begins with a comprehensive history. Careful attention should be given to the chief complaint of the patient, which can be quite variable in adults with spinal deformity. For example, a patient who reports unilateral radiculopathy, even in the context of severe scoliosis, will be treated very differently from a patient with symptoms mainly caused by sagittal plane decompensation. The history begins with a full evaluation of the patient's complaints, including pain and neurologic symptoms. Although pain is the most frequent symptom in adults with spinal deformity, it is important to remember that all patients with a deformity do not have pain. Spinal deformity is frequently an incidental finding on imaging studies obtained for another reason, such as a chest or abdominal radiograph. When pain is present, a complete evaluation of the pain should include the location, onset, character, timing, and severity, as well as alleviating and exacerbating factors. It is important to determine if the pain is centered at the apex of a deformity or at a distant site. Special attention should be paid to distinguishing axial back pain from radiculopathy. Many patients present with pain caused by claudication, which can be neurogenic or vascular in nature. Claudication must be distinguished from muscle fatigue caused by coronal or sagittal imbalance.

Patients may also report neurologic symptoms, including numbness or tingling, and bowel and/or bladder dysfunction. The details of these findings should be thoroughly investigated. All patients should be questioned about symptoms of myelopathy or other upper motor neuron disease, which may include ataxia, fine-motor difficulty, or dropping objects. Ambulatory tolerance should be assessed in detail, with particular attention to any recent changes or a decline in overall function. The patient's ability to work and perform basic activities of daily living must be considered in detail because it is critical to understand the impact of the deformity on the patient's quality of life. Although some patients may tolerate seemingly large deformities without limitation, others may be significantly disabled by a disorder that appears to be minor on imaging studies. The impact of the deformity on the patient's appearance cannot be minimized. The cosmetic concerns of

the patient and his or her family must be considered.

The physician should also inquire about evidence of deformity progression. The patient may report a change in the fit of his or her clothing, such as a waistline alteration. The patient may notice a change in height or posture as well as an increase in the prominence of the abdomen, the rib cage, or a lumbar hump. When a change in the deformity is apparent, it is critical to understand the timing of any progression. The patient should be asked about constitutional symptoms, including weight loss, fever, chills, sweating, and night pain, which may suggest tumor or infection as the cause of the deformity.

A complete record includes the patient's past medical, surgical, and family history, medications and allergies, and previous treatments. The past medical history is critical to a full understanding of the source of the deformity and for preoperative planning. For example, medical conditions such as ankylosing spondylitis or Marfan syndrome may be the dominant cause of the deformity. A family history of spinal deformity, genetic disorders, or other syndromes should be elicited. Specific attention should be paid to cardiac and pulmonary issues, which may require further workup. The patient's nutritional status should be evaluated, including laboratory studies when appropriate. In some instances, the deformity can compromise the patient's ability to eat and may result in malnutrition. A history of osteopenia or osteoporosis should be determined. Compression fractures may be the cause of the deformity, and decreased bone mineral density can lead to intraoperative difficulty if surgery is needed.

Past surgical treatment, in particular prior spinal procedures, as well as previous musculoskeletal surgery, such as total joint arthroplasty, must be un-

derstood in relationship to the patient's deformity and overall status. Many adult deformities are the result of previous spinal surgeries, including the development of flat back deformity, postlaminectomy kyphosis, and proximal junctional kyphosis. A review of the patient's medications is also critical, particularly narcotic usage and drugs that increase the risk of bleeding during nonsurgical and surgical treatment. A patient who is dependent on narcotics can be especially challenging to treat regardless of whether surgery is being considered. Herbal supplements and alternative medications should be recorded. A complete review of previous treatments of the deformity should be discussed. The physician should inquire about medications, exercise, physical therapy, and chiropractic care. The patient should also be asked about bracing and interventional pain procedures, including epidural steroid injections, facet blocks, and alternative treatments such as acupuncture. A thorough history should provide the treating physician with a full understanding of the impact of the deformity on the patient's life and will aid in the decision to pursue imaging studies or make a referral to a spinal specialist.

Physical Examination
The physical examination of an adult patient with a known or suspected spinal deformity begins with an evaluation of the patient's gait and stance. The patient should be examined in a gown that is open to the back to allow full visualization of the entire spine. The patient should be viewed from the back and from the side to evaluate his or her overall coronal and sagittal balance. The physician should note if the patient stands with bent hips or knees or is pitched forward at rest or with walking. The patient should be asked to stand with the knees maximally extended to assess true sagittal balance. A

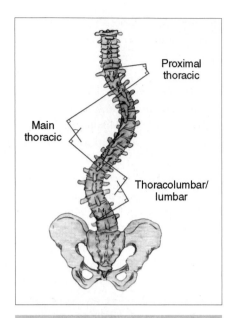

Figure 7 Illustration showing the Cobb angle measurement. See text for details. Measurement of all curves should be performed in every patient. (Courtesy of Medtronic Sofamor Danek, Memphis, TN.)

Labels in figure: Proximal thoracic; Main thoracic; Thoracolumbar/lumbar

full assessment of the patient's balance and coordination should be performed, including tandem gait (heel-to-toe walking), heel and toe walking, and the static Romberg test. During the static Romberg test, the patient is asked to stand with his or her arms outstretched and palms up. The patient is then asked to close his or her eyes. A loss of balance with the eyes closed suggests a proprioceptive deficit. The movement of the spine should be reviewed, including forward bending, extension, side bending, and rotation.

Attention should then be turned to inspecting the back itself. The position of the neck relative to the gluteal cleft should be noted, as should any shoulder asymmetry or scapular prominence. The patient may also have asymmetric skin folds or pelvic tilt as a result of an underlying deformity. In severe cases of lumbar or thoracolumbar scoliosis, the rib cage may abut the pelvis and may be a source of tremendous pain or can interfere with eating.

In this situation, the abdomen may become more protuberant, which may be the patient's initial complaint. Pelvic tilt, as manifested by asymmetric iliac crests, may be causing an apparent limb-length discrepancy. In some patients, scoliosis may be caused by a true limb-length inequality; treating the extremity may correct the spinal deformity. The skin of the back should be examined for the presence of abnormalities, such as café au lait spots, hairy tufts, dimples, sinuses, or midline defects, which may suggest underlying pathology. Patients with spondylolisthesis may have a palpable step-off, excessive lumbar lordosis, or heart-shaped buttocks. The Adams forward bend test can be performed to look for rib or lumbar humps. When asymmetry is noted in forward bending, the angle of trunk rotation may be assessed with a scoliometer. An angle of trunk rotation greater than 7° suggests scoliosis measuring at least 20°, thereby necessitating radiographic imaging to fully characterize the extent of the underlying spinal deformity.

A complete physical examination includes comprehensive testing of upper and lower extremity motor and sensory function and the assessment of deep tendon reflexes in the arms and legs. Hyperreflexia can be a sign of cervical myelopathy or other upper motor neuron diseases, whereas decreased reflexes can indicate radiculopathy caused by nerve root compression. Root tension signs, which suggest lumbar nerve irritation, such as the straight leg raise and the femoral stretch test should be elicited, as well as upper motor neuron signs of myelopathy, including clonus, the Hoffmann sign, the Babinski reflex, and the inverted radial response. The differential diagnosis of upper motor neuron disease includes cervical spondylotic myelopathy, multiple sclerosis, amyotrophic lateral sclerosis, syringomyelia, and vi-

tamin B_{12} deficiency. The hips and knees should be examined in all patients with spinal deformity for the presence of contractures or painful range of motion. When surgery is being considered, hip and knee disorders may need to be treated before proceeding with the spinal surgery. Tight hamstrings are frequently found in patients with spondylolisthesis and can be managed as needed.

Imaging Studies

The initial radiographic evaluation of an adult patient with a spinal deformity should consist of full-length (36-inch), standing, frontal and lateral radiographs of the entire spine. At a minimum, these radiographs should include visualization of C7 down to the pelvis and hips. The patient should stand with the hips and knees maximally extended to decrease compensatory mechanisms and allow assessment of sagittal plane imbalance. The feet should be positioned at shoulder width, and the hands should rest on the clavicles in a closed fist with the dorsum of the hands facing away from the body. This consistent patient position has been shown to be highly accurate and allows the surgeon to track deformity progression.[9,10]

The magnitude of spinal curves is determined by calculating the Cobb angle (**Figure 7**). The Cobb measurement is taken from the most tilted vertebra at the end of each curve. All curves should be measured on both the frontal and lateral views, including proximal thoracic, main thoracic, and thoracolumbar/lumbar scoliosis as well as thoracic kyphosis and lumbar lordosis. Additional radiographic views (supine, side-bending, fulcrum bending, traction, and push-prone views) of the entire spine can be helpful to assess the flexibility of the deformity and determine the potential for intraoperative correction[11,12] (**Figure 8**). If other abnormalities such as spondylolisthesis are detected on long cassette radiographs, selective imaging of specific regions can be performed.

CT can be useful to define bony anatomy and identify congenital spinal anomalies. Patients with a history of significant trauma and spinal deformity may benefit from a CT scan to fully characterize the extent of injury or any posttraumatic misalignment. However, CT carries the risk of radiation exposure to the patient. CT scans are sometimes used in preoperative planning, especially when considering the use of thoracic pedicle screws (**Figure 9**). Three-dimensional reconstructions are helpful to fully understand complex, multiplanar deformities. CT myelography can be performed if MRI cannot be used to assess the status of the neurologic elements. Myelography also can be used to assess the extent of stenosis related to the deformity with weight bearing. Myelography may be a more efficacious approach in the setting of complex spinal deformity than MRI, which may not provide appropriate cuts for complete assessment of neurologic compression. Lower-dose CT protocols are currently being investigated to decrease the patient's exposure to potentially hazardous ionizing radiation.

MRI can be used to detect herniated disks, spinal stenosis, and degenerative disk disease. MRI scans should be obtained in all patients with clinical evidence of persistent or significant radiculopathy, myelopathy, or claudication (**Figure 10**). Upright or dynamic MRI scans, including flexion-extension and side-bending sequences, can be obtained when stenosis is suspected but not seen on supine MRI studies. Although this technology can be helpful, it may not be readily available to all surgeons. Any patient with a suspected tumor or infection should be screened with MRI.

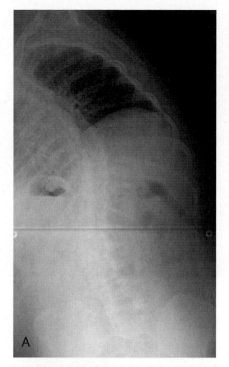
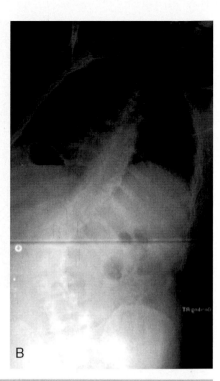

Figure 8   Side-bending radiographs of the patient described in Figure 5A. Bending to the left (**A**) does not correct the thoracolumbar curve, whereas bending to the right (**B**) corrects the main thoracic curve.

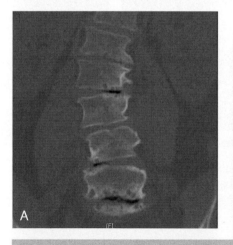
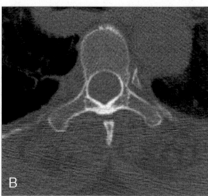

Figure 9   CT scans of a patient with adult degenerative scoliosis. **A,** The coronal reconstruction allows the surgeon to fully characterize the extent of the degenerative changes. **B,** The axial image shows significantly narrowed pedicles at T10. The presence of such dysplastic pedicles can lead to intraoperative difficulty with screw placement.

Imaging of adult patients with spondylolisthesis should include standing frontal and lateral radiographs of the lumbar spine. The lateral view should include visualization of the pelvis because consideration of pelvic parameters and sagittal balance are critical aspects of a thorough assessment of a patient with spondylolisthesis (**Figure 11**). Obtaining full-length radiographs to allow complete evaluation of the patient's entire spine and overall alignment should be considered. Flexion and extension views can

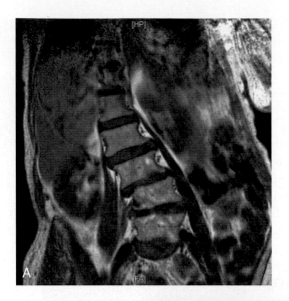

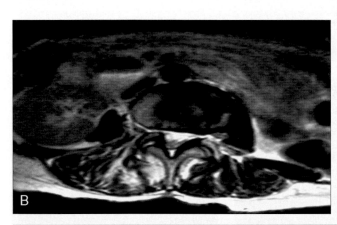

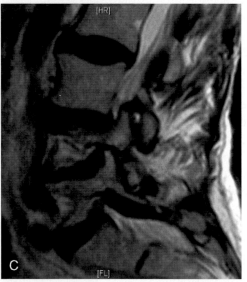

Figure 10   MRI scans of a patient with adult degenerative scoliosis. **A,** The coronal image shows the coronal plane deformity. **B,** The axial image shows moderate central stenosis caused by facet hypertrophy and ligamentum flavum buckling. **C,** The sagittal image shows severe L4-5 and L5-S1 foraminal stenosis, which caused significant radiculopathy.

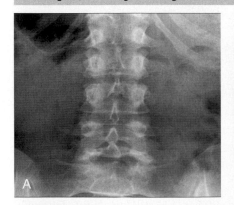

Figure 11   AP (**A**) and lateral (**B**) spinal radiographs of a 44-year-old woman with L5-S1 isthmic spondylolisthesis.

be used to identify significant spinal instability through the segment with spondylolisthesis (**Figure 12**). Oblique views can be used to identify a spondylolysis that is not seen on a lateral radiograph. When spondylolysis is suspected but not seen on radiographs, a CT scan can be obtained. MRI is used in patients with spondylolisthesis who have significant radiculopathy or neurogenic claudication (**Figure 13**). Single-photon emission computed tomography (SPECT) nuclear studies also can be used to identify spondylolysis. SPECT has been shown to be superior to standard bone scans for this purpose and can indicate the metabolic activity of the pars defect.[13] In younger adults, SPECT also can be used to monitor healing of the lysis as well as to determine if a patient is a candidate for pars repair. An MRI scan should be obtained in patients with spondylolisthesis and radiculopathy or claudication and in those with high-grade slips (grade III or higher).

Indications for Referral to a Spine Specialist

All adult patients with spinal deformity do not empirically need to be referred to a spine specialist, but there are many reasonable indications to do so (the most common reason is progressive pain and/or disability). There is no consensus about the magnitude of deformity that requires surgical management. The decision to proceed with surgery is often multifactorial and must be individualized to each patient's needs. In some cases, the patient's symptoms may be worsening or may be unresponsive to nonsurgical treatment. The nonsurgical management of patients with spinal deformity includes many treatment options (**Table 1**); the details of nonsurgical treatments are beyond the scope of this chapter. Patients with evidence of a significant neurologic deficit or myelopathy and those with deterioration in neurologic function or ambulatory status should be evaluated by a spine surgeon. A patient with a deformity of lesser magnitude but who requires decompression for stenosis or a herniated disk also may be referred to a spine specialist. In addition, adults with scoliosis that measures more than 50° are at risk for deformity progression and should be considered for a surgical consultation.[14,15] Patients with sagittal

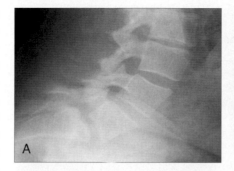
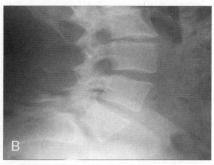

Figure 12   Lateral flexion (**A**) and extension (B) views of the patient in Figure 11 fail to demonstrate significant instability.

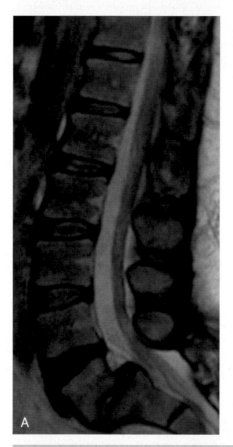
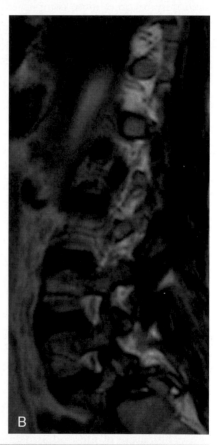

Figure 13   Sagittal MRI scans of the patient in Figure 11. **A,** No significant central stenosis is seen. **B,** Severe foraminal narrowing caused by the displacement of L5 on S1 as well as disk bulging into the neural foramen.

and/or coronal plane decompensation that is causing difficulty with activities of daily living, decreased quality of life, or debilitating pain should be referred to a spine specialist. It is never inappropriate to request consultation from a spine surgeon for any adult patient with a spinal deformity. Physician

comfort with the management of patients with challenging spine conditions will often determine the timing of the need for consultation with a spine specialist.

Preoperative Considerations

Evaluating adult patients with spinal

Table 1

Nonsurgical Treatment for Spinal Deformity

Medications	Anti-inflammatory drugs, analgesics, muscle relaxants, and neurologic agents (such as gabapentin or pregabalin)
Noninvasive interventions	Vigorous aerobic exercise, physical therapy, bracing, and aquatic therapy
Invasive procedures	Epidural steroid injections, nerve root blocks, facet joint blocks, and spondylolysis injections
Nontraditional interventions	Herbal supplements, acupuncture, chiropractic spinal manipulation, and yoga

deformity becomes more complicated when considering surgical intervention. Many studies have documented the high rate of perioperative complications associated with adult deformity surgery and the potential impact of these complications on outcomes.[16-18] As such, it is critical to fully inform the patient about potential perioperative and long-term adverse events, which will aid the patient in his or her decision making. The treating surgeon must fully assess the patient's fitness for surgery and perform thorough preoperative planning, including the consideration of various surgical techniques and potential complications. Several conditions that can lead to postoperative morbidity should be optimized before undertaking the surgical correction of an adult spinal deformity.

A complete preoperative pulmonary assessment is essential, including a possible evaluation by a pulmonologist. The nature of most adult deformity procedures, including long surgical times and the frequent need for blood transfusion, places patients at risk for pulmonary complications. Smokers and those with chronic respiratory illness are highly susceptible to these complications; patients should quit smoking before surgery, especially given the increased risk of pseudarthrosis. Patients with known cardiovascular disease, including coronary artery disease or prior stroke, should

have a preoperative cardiac workup, which may include a stress test, an echocardiogram, carotid duplex, and/or cardiac catheterization. Some patients may also benefit from the use of perioperative β-blockers to decrease morbidity. Patients with diabetes should have strict glycemic control in both the preoperative and postoperative periods. These patients should be counseled about the potential for increased surgical risks.

Adults undergoing deformity correction should be evaluated for nutritional deficiencies and osteoporosis because these conditions can have a significant impact on intraoperative management and postoperative healing. Malnutrition, which may result from chronic medical disorders, infection, spinal cord injury, or poor dietary intake, can lead to an increased number of complications.[19] Appropriate patients should be screened with laboratory studies such as albumin and prealbumin analyses. Preoperative dietary supplementation can be beneficial and may decrease postoperative morbidity.[20] Patients with osteoporosis should be treated preoperatively with antiresorptive agents or parathyroid hormone, which may increase bone mineral density before surgery. However, the surgeon should be prepared for adverse intraoperative events in patients with osteoporosis, including poor hardware fixation,

which may necessitate the need for multiple supplemental strategies to obtain adequate stability. Such strategies may include the use of bone cement, sublaminar wires, multiple points of fixation, and/or a circumferential approach.

Psychological factors also should be considered before surgery. Because many patients with adult spinal deformity have experienced pain for many years, narcotic dependence, depression, and anxiety are common. All of these factors should be addressed before electing surgical treatment. Consultation with a pain management specialist, psychiatrist, psychologist, or social worker may help the patient anticipate potential postoperative difficulties and make the recovery process smoother. Patients with ongoing significant psychosocial stress may not be good candidates for surgery. Spinal deformity correction in adults necessitates a strong support system for the patient. Patients with domestic or financial difficulties may not be appropriate candidates for reconstructive surgery. Consideration should be given to postponing surgery until stressors or personal issues have stabilized.

Summary

The evaluation of adult patients with spinal deformity is challenging, especially for surgeons without advanced training in spinal disorders. Many patients present with disabling symptoms and difficulty in performing the activities of daily living. The assessment should always include a thorough patient history and physical examination, which can identify significant underlying pathology that may require prompt investigation. The appropriate use of imaging studies can define the extent of the deformity and rule out abnormalities such as tumors, infection, fractures, or significant neurologic compression. The ultimate goal of the evaluation is to determine the impact of the deformity on the patient's quality of life and the need for referral to a spine specialist. If nonsurgical management has failed and the patient is interested in surgical treatment, the evaluation should include a thorough risk assessment. Meticulous preoperative planning is vital in adult spinal deformity correction. All spinal deformities are not the same, and treatment should be tailored to the individual patient.

References

1. Bernhardt M, Bridwell KH: Segmental analysis of the sagittal plane alignment of the normal thoracic and lumbar spines and thoracolumbar junction. *Spine (Phila Pa 1976)* 1989;14(7):717-721.

2. Berthonnaud E, Dimnet J, Roussouly P, Labelle H: Analysis of the sagittal balance of the spine and pelvis using shape and orientation parameters. *J Spinal Disord Tech* 2005;18(1):40-47.

3. Vialle R, Levassor N, Rillardon L, Templier A, Skalli W, Guigui P: Radiographic analysis of the sagittal alignment and balance of the spine in asymptomatic subjects. *J Bone Joint Surg Am* 2005;87(2):260-267.

4. Glassman SD, Berven S, Bridwell K, Horton W, Dimar JR: Correlation of radiographic parameters and clinical symptoms in adult scoliosis. *Spine (Phila Pa 1976)* 2005;30(6):682-688.

5. Glassman SD, Bridwell K, Dimar JR, Horton W, Berven S, Schwab F: The impact of positive sagittal balance in adult spinal deformity. *Spine (Phila Pa 1976)* 2005;30(18):2024-2029.

6. Legaye J, Duval-Beaupère G, Hecquet J, Marty C: Pelvic incidence: A fundamental pelvic parameter for three-dimensional regulation of spinal sagittal curves. *Eur Spine J* 1998;7(2):99-103.

7. Boulay C, Tardieu C, Hecquet J, et al: Sagittal alignment of spine and pelvis regulated by pelvic incidence: Standard values and prediction of lordosis. *Eur Spine J* 2006;15(4):415-422.

8. Lafage V, Schwab F, Patel A, Hawkinson N, Farcy JP: Pelvic tilt and truncal inclination: Two key radiographic parameters in the setting of adults with spinal deformity. *Spine (Phila Pa 1976)* 2009;34(17):E599-E606.

9. Horton WC, Brown CW, Bridwell KH, Glassman SD, Suk SI, Cha CW: Is there an optimal patient stance for obtaining a lateral 36″ radiograph? A critical comparison of three techniques. *Spine (Phila Pa 1976)* 2005;30(4):427-433.

10. Vedantam R, Lenke LG, Bridwell KH, Linville DL, Blanke K: The effect of variation in arm position on sagittal spinal alignment. *Spine (Phila Pa 1976)* 2000;25(17):2204-2209.

11. Klepps SJ, Lenke LG, Bridwell KH, Bassett GS, Whorton J: Prospective comparison of flexibility radiographs in adolescent idiopathic scoliosis. *Spine (Phila Pa 1976)* 2001;26(5):E74-E79.

12. Vedantam R, Lenke LG, Bridwell KH, Linville DL: Comparison of push-prone and lateral-bending radiographs for predicting postoperative coronal alignment in thoracolumbar and lumbar scoliotic curves. *Spine (Phila Pa 1976)* 2000;25(1):76-81.

13. Collier BD, Johnson RP, Carrera GF, et al: Painful spondylolysis or spondylolisthesis studied by radiography and single-photon emission computed tomography. *Radiology* 1985;154(1):207-211.

14. Weinstein SL: Idiopathic scoliosis: Natural history. *Spine (Phila Pa 1976)* 1986;11(8):780-783.

15. Lonstein JE, Carlson JM: The prediction of curve progression in untreated idiopathic scoliosis during growth. *J Bone Joint Surg Am* 1984;66(7):1061-1071.

16. Dickson JH, Mirkovic S, Noble PC, Nalty T, Erwin WD: Results of operative treatment of idiopathic scoliosis in adults. *J Bone Joint Surg Am* 1995;77(4):513-523.

17. Daubs MD, Lenke LG, Cheh G, Stobbs G, Bridwell KH: Adult spinal deformity surgery: Complications and outcomes in patients over age 60. *Spine (Phila Pa 1976)* 2007;32(20):2238-2244.

18. Glassman SD, Hamill CL, Bridwell KH, Schwab FJ, Dimar JR, Lowe TG: The impact of perioperative complications on clinical outcome in adult deformity surgery. *Spine (Phila Pa 1976)* 2007;32(24):2764-2770.

19. Klein JD, Hey LA, Yu CS, et al: Perioperative nutrition and postoperative complications in patients undergoing spinal surgery. *Spine (Phila Pa 1976)* 1996;21(22):2676-2682.

20. Mandelbaum BR, Tolo VT, McAfee PC, Burest P: Nutritional deficiencies after staged anterior and posterior spinal reconstructive surgery. *Clin Orthop Relat Res* 1988;234:5-11.

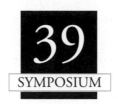

39

SYMPOSIUM

Pediatric Spinal Deformity: What Every Orthopaedic Surgeon Needs to Know

Paul D. Sponseller, MD
Behrooz A. Akbarnia, MD
Lawrence G. Lenke, MD
Adam L. Wollowick, MD

Abstract

Pediatric spinal deformity is an integral part of orthopaedic surgical practice. In a general or specialized practice, the well-versed orthopaedic surgeon should be aware of the diagnostic methods and the natural history from which practice standards are derived. It is important to be aware of the spectrum of spinal deformity in children (from early-onset scoliosis to adolescent idiopathic scoliosis, kyphosis, and spondylolisthesis) and current principles of growth and maturation as applied to the spine and the thorax. This information should be helpful in attaining the appropriate diagnosis, treatment, and/or referral for a pediatric patient with a spinal deformity.

Instr Course Lect 2012;61:481-497.

Early-Onset Scoliosis

Early-onset scoliosis (EOS), which is diagnosed between birth and 5 years of age, has a variety of causes. Although there has been substantial progress in understanding the natural history and management of patients with progressive EOS, treating a growing child with EOS remains challenging, primarily because of the presence of underlying conditions that often have a negative effect on patient outcomes and traditional treatment options that often require multiple procedures.

Idiopathic scoliosis has been classified into three groups that are based on the patient's age: infantile (birth to 3 years), juvenile (4 through 9 years), and adolescent (10 to 18 years). The term early-onset scoliosis was introduced by Dickson and Archer[1] for patients age 5 years or younger because of the unique characteristics of that age group. EOS is now a commonly used term and includes scoliosis from all causes, including infantile idiopathic scoliosis. The first 5 years of life include a period of accelerated growth similar to that in adolescent scoliosis and unlike that in juvenile scoliosis; if left untreated, EOS carries a high likelihood of cardiopulmonary complications. The causes of EOS include idiopathic, congenital, and neuromuscular disorders (such as cerebral palsy, myelodysplasia, and muscle diseases), and syndromes, such as Marfan and neurofibromatosis, which are not necessarily categorized in the other diagnostic groups.

Understanding the patterns of normal spinal and thorax growth helps orthopaedic surgeons appreciate the

Dr. Sponseller or an immediate family member has received royalties from Globus Medical and DePuy; serves as a paid consultant to DePuy; has received research or institutional support from DePuy; and serves as a board member, owner, officer, or committee member of the Pediatric Orthopaedic Society of North America and the Scoliosis Research Society. Dr. Akbarnia or an immediate family member has received royalties from DePuy Spine and Nuvasive; serves as a paid consultant to Nuvasive, K2M, Ellipse, K Spine, and DePuy; owns stock or stock options in Nuvasive, Ellipse, K Spine, and Nocimed; has received research or institutional support from K2M, DePuy Spine, Nuvasive, and Ellipse; and serves as a board member, owner, officer, or committee member of the Growing Spine Foundation, the Scoliosis Research Society, the Pediatric Orthopaedic Society, and the San Diego Spine Foundation. Dr. Lenke or an immediate family member has received royalties from Medtronic; serves as an unpaid consultant to Medtronic; has received research or institutional support from DePuy and Axial Biotech; and serves as a board member, owner, officer, or committee member of the Scoliosis Research Society. Dr. Wollowick or an immediate family member is a member of a speakers' bureau or has made paid presentations on behalf of DePuy; serves as a paid consultant to DePuy; has received research or institutional support from Stryker and DePuy; and serves as a board member, owner, officer, or committee member of the Scoliosis Research Society.

natural history of the disease and choose the most appropriate treatment for a growing child with progressive EOS. Human skeletal growth involves a change in proportions.[2-6] At birth, the ratio of the sitting height to the length of the lower limb is 70:30, but the ratio progressively approaches 50% at skeletal maturity. The average gain in sitting height and (subischial) leg length from birth to skeletal maturity is estimated to be 58 and 63 cm, respectively. Because spinal growth varies by age (approximately 2 cm per year from birth to 5 years, 1 cm per year from 5 to 10 years, and 2 cm per year from 10 to approximately 15 years), growth deficits can be predicted. For example, an anterior and posterior spinal fusion from T1 to S1 in a 5-year-old patient can result in a total deficit of 15 cm in sitting height (10 cm in the thoracic spine and 5 cm in the lumbar spine). DiMéglio et al[3] termed the thorax the "fourth dimension of the spine." The volumetric growth of the thorax increases from 6% of its final size in the newborn to 30% at 5 years, 50% at 10 years, and 100% at 15 years of age. As the lungs are developing, the lung tissues and pulmonary vascular tree develop relative to the size of the thorax, not to the patient's age. The number of alveoli increases from 20 million at birth to 250 million at 4 years of age and reaches adult levels at age 8 years. Campbell et al[7] described thoracic insufficiency syndrome as the inability of the thorax to support normal respiration or lung growth. Therefore, potentially life-threatening health risks can develop in children younger than 5 years who have clinically significant progressive scoliosis. These deformities affect the growth potential of the spine and the thorax and often lead to pulmonary complications.

If infantile and juvenile idiopathic scoliosis remain untreated, the mortality rate for patients can be significantly higher than what would be expected over time.[8] Early upper thoracic spinal fusion has deleterious effects on pulmonary function, as was shown by Canavese et al,[9] who performed posterior spinal fusions in a rabbit model. The T1 to T6 fusions decreased thoracic volume more than T7 to T12 spinal fusions, contributing to the hypothesis that the ribs between T1 and T6 articulate with the sternum, whereas the ribs at T7 to T12 do not.[9] Karol et al[10] studied the relationship of thoracic height to lung disease in 28 patients (average age, 14 years) who were treated with spinal fusion at a mean age of 3 years. Of the 16 patients with a thoracic spine height less than 18 cm, 10 (62%) had restrictive lung disease, which is defined as having less than 50% of normal vital capacity. None of the four patients with a thoracic spine height of more than 22 cm had restrictive lung disease. The authors concluded that restrictive lung disease is less likely when the thoracic spine is allowed to reach a minimum height of 22 cm.[10] Thoracic insufficiency syndrome substantially impairs the quality of life of pediatric patients and results in a quality of life that is as low as that of pediatric patients with asthma, juvenile rheumatoid arthritis, and heart transplants.[11]

Treatment

The goals of EOS treatment are deformity correction and prevention of curve progression and pulmonary disease while preserving normal spinal growth. Although there is some consensus regarding surgical indications (including curve magnitude, diagnosis, patient age, and "final" spinal fusion method), there is wide variation among surgeons regarding the type of treatment that should be used to treat a spinal and/or chest wall deformity.[12,13] Nonsurgical methods include orthosis, casting, and/or traction, all of which may be used as definitive treatment of small, idiopathic curves (**Figure 1**). Nonsurgical methods also are used to delay surgery for progressive deformities if surgery is contraindicated in a very young patient. Spinal fusion surgery typically involves posterior spinal fusion with instrumentation, which can lead to the crankshaft phenomenon of anterior column overgrowth in a young child.[14] However, if anterior and posterior spinal fusions are performed in an effort to prevent anterior overgrowth, the trunk is unlikely to reach full thoracic height. For focal spinal deformities, limited fusion of selected vertebrae (often including vertebral resections) may be indicated.

Growth-friendly surgical procedures have become increasingly popular over the past decade because they allow correction and control of the deformity while allowing spine and thorax growth. Sankar et al[15] classified various growth-friendly procedures into three unique treatment groups: (1) distraction-based devices, such as growing rods, the Vertically Expandable Prosthetic Titanium Rib (VEPTR, Synthes Spine, Paoli, PA), and remotely controlled distraction devices; (2) tension-based devices, such as intervertebral staples and spinal tethers; and (3) growth-guided procedures, such as hemiepiphysiodesis and the Shilla procedure.[16]

Nonsurgical Treatment

More effective casting methods, incorporating rotational correction, have been recently popularized by Mehta.[17] The author reported that all 94 patients (age range, 6 to 48 months; mean Cobb angle, 32°) experienced reversal of the deformity and resolution of scoliosis at an average age of 3.5 years, whereas 36% of older patients (age range, 11 to 48 months) with larger curves (mean Cobb angle,

52°) required spinal fusion. Sanders et al[18] reported on 55 patients who were treated with derotational casting and found that casting was most effective for patients younger than 20 months who had curves less than 60°. Cast treatment was less effective for patients with nonidiopathic scoliosis with larger curves.[18] In contrast, Lloyd-Roberts and Pilcher[19] reported that 92% of idiopathic scoliosis curves resolved spontaneously in the first year of life. Because of the possibility for some idiopathic curves to improve spontaneously, it is not yet known if Mehta casting with derotation will prove as revolutionary as the Ponseti technique. No prospective comparison studies have shown that casting is superior to observation. It is also well accepted that cast treatment is not beneficial for patients with congenital scoliosis.

Surgical Treatment

Early spinal fusion leads to a short trunk. Hemiepiphysiodesis is not effective at reversing the progression of early-onset deformity; however, if instrumentation is used, progression may be halted.[20] Early spinal fusion can control focal areas of progressive congenital deformity, but total spinal fusion (anterior and posterior) results in lung underdevelopment and a substantial decrease in pulmonary function in young children.[10]

Because none of the growth-friendly devices currently in use, except for VEPTR, is approved by the Food and Drug Administration, they are used as physician-directed or off-label implants. Tension-based treatment methods include staples and tethers, which are applied to the convexity of the curve to modulate growth in an attempt to prevent curve progression. Staples are metallic and more rigid than tethers, but clinical experi-

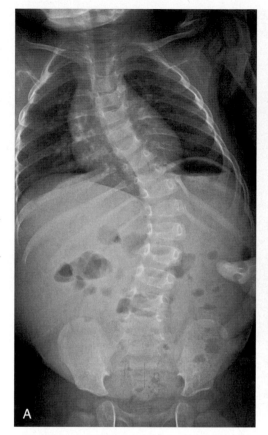
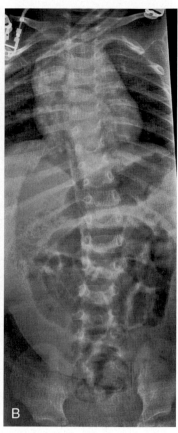

Figure 1   Radiographs of the spine of a patient with early-onset scoliosis. **A,** Upright PA radiograph before casting. **B,** Radiograph after casting in a derotational Mehta cast.

ence with them is limited, particularly in EOS applications.

Growth-guiding procedures, such as the Shilla technique, control the apex of the curve by creating a short apical fusion. Upper and lower foundations are placed using nonlocking pedicle screws so that bilateral rods can slide through the pedicle screws, guiding the spine to straight, vertical growth. The Shilla technique has been described in a preclinical study,[16] and follow-up data are currently being reviewed.

Distraction-based procedures typically use anchors in the spine and/or rib. The VEPTR has become a widely used rib-to-rib or rib-to-spine device that is indicated for thoracic insufficiency syndrome, primary or secondary thoracic dysplasia syndrome, and

volume depletion deformities of the thorax (**Figure 2**); it is intended to indirectly correct the spine or chest wall deformity and promote growth of the thorax. VEPTR has been successfully applied to a wide variety of deformities in the growing spine.[21,22]

Growing rods are most often used in patients with progressive EOS (**Figure 3**). The Harrington rod technique has a long history. Harrington recommended that, in an effort to optimize spinal growth, patients younger than 10 years should not undergo spinal fusion.[23] In 2002, the Growing Spine Study Group was established to evaluate growth-friendly procedures for patients with EOS. Historically, a single rod was used, with anchors placed at the cephalad and caudad ends of the spinal deformity.[24,25] More recently, a

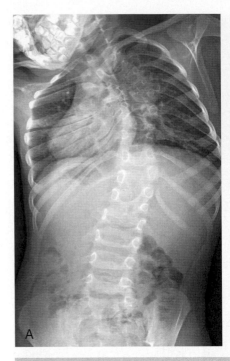

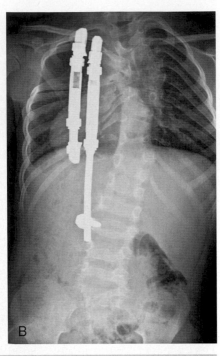

Figure 2 Radiographs of the spine of a patient with progressive congenital scoliosis and fused ribs. **A,** Preoperative AP radiograph of the patient at age 4 years. **B,** PA radiograph at age 7 years after expansion thoracoplasty and 3 years of distraction with a VEPTR device.

dual-rod technique was used for 23 patients with favorable results, including maintenance of curve correction, spinal height, and space available for the lungs.[25]

Video 39.1: Dual Growing Rod Surgery for the Surgical Treatment of Infantile Idiopathic Scoliosis. Behrooz A. Akbarnia, MD; Gregory M. Mundis Jr, MD; Burt Yaszay, MD (6 min)

Growing-rod surgery is associated with major complications. Bess et al[26] reported that the risk of complications increased by 24% for each additional surgical procedure performed but decreased 13% for each year of increased patient age at the initiation of treatment. To minimize complications, the authors suggested delaying the initial

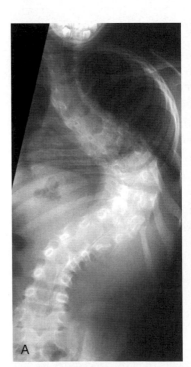
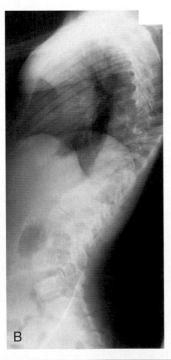
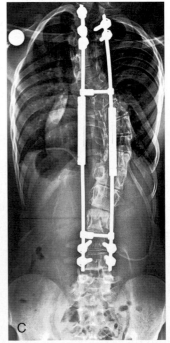
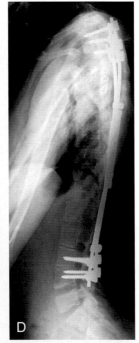

Figure 3 Radiographs showing the course of growing rod treatment of a male patient with early onset idiopathic scoliosis. Preoperative AP (**A**) and lateral (**B**) radiographs taken at age 7 years show a 95° curve. Postoperative AP (**C**) and lateral (**D**) radiographs taken at age 16 years after seven distractions. There was a gain of 10 cm in T1-S1 height until the patient was 13 years old. The spine has been stable for 3 years without surgical fusion.

growing-rod treatment, placing dual rods in a submuscular fashion, and limiting the number of lengthenings. It was also recently reported that syndromic patients with thoracic kyphosis of more than 40° should be closely monitored for complications after growing-rod surgery, particularly for implant failure.[27] Anchor fixation complications, brachial plexopathy, chest-wall scarring, fusion beneath the implants, and wound infection are possible complications associated with most distraction-based methods, including growing rods and VEPTR.

Avoiding Complications

It is important to choose the most appropriate surgical procedure for a particular patient, including the levels to be instrumented, the patient's sagittal alignment, the surgical technique of exposure, the method of tissue handling, and early planning to detect potential complications. Although complications are common, they can usually be overcome; the long-term goal of treatment should always be kept in mind.

To determine the best time to start surgical treatment, Sankar et al[28] evaluated the amount of T1-S1 gain versus the number of rod lengthenings and found a law of diminishing returns with regard to spinal height after approximately seven rod lengthenings. Myung et al[29] reported that in patients who were initially considered to have "failure to thrive" (less than or equal to the fifth percentile), 44% showed an increase in weight percentile after growing-rod surgery, a percentage similar to that reported for patients treated with VEPTR. However, patients younger than 4 years at the time of initial surgery did not experience gains in weight percentiles even at up to 4 years after surgery.[29] Both of these studies suggest there might be a benefit to delaying growing-rod surgery, but this possibility must be weighed against the risk of curve progression.

To improve on the traditional growing-rod technique, remotely controlled magnetic distraction devices have been introduced, first in France and now in the United States and other countries. The devices are implanted using surgical techniques similar to those currently used for growing-rod surgery, but the lengthenings are done remotely without the need for anesthesia and can be performed in an outpatient facility. These devices have not been approved by the US Food and Drug Administration, but initial results from an international study have been encouraging.[30]

Discussion

Curve progression in patients with EOS can be life threatening, and early spinal fusion leads to a short trunk and decreased thoracic volume, which may lead to pulmonary complications. Improvement in pulmonary function and quality of life should be the primary treatment goals. Growth-friendly procedures are promising but still carry a substantial risk of complications. In the future, new and effective treatment methods to avoid multiple surgeries can be expected. The assessment of the effectiveness of treatment methods on the quality of life of children with progressive spinal and chest abnormalities also must be improved by using a reliable outcomes tool. Future regulatory policies should allow necessary innovations and make them more readily available to patients and surgeons. A multicenter research effort with long-term follow-up is essential to answer many of the complex questions regarding this group of pediatric patients with EOS.

Adolescent Idiopathic Scoliosis

Idiopathic scoliosis is the most common spinal deformity in the pediatric population. Patients older than 18 years are considered to have adult idiopathic scoliosis. Of all pediatric spinal deformities, adolescent idiopathic scoliosis (AIS) is by far the most common type. The prevalence of AIS is 2% to 3% of all children 10 to 18 years old.[31] The female to male ratio is 3.6:1 overall, but it is nearly 1:1 for small curves (approximately 10°) and 9:1 for curves greater than 50° (Cobb measurement).[31] The prevalence of AIS declines with increasing curve magnitude: 0.5% for curves less than 20° and 0.1% for curves greater than 40°. As documented by several investigators, the natural history of AIS indicates that patients who present at a young age with low skeletal maturity (as measured by the Risser sign) and a large Cobb angle will have a markedly higher risk for progression than children who present at an older age.[32,33] It is hoped that future analysis of genetic markers will provide additional information on the risk of curve progression.

Evaluation

The cause of AIS is unknown, and it is a diagnosis of exclusion. The treating physician must exclude other causes of scoliosis, including congenital and neuromuscular reasons and syndromes such as Ehlers-Danlos, neurofibromatosis, and Marfan. Patients with atypical histories, physical examinations, and/or spinal radiographs also must be excluded from a diagnosis of AIS. Atypical features in the patient's history include substantial pain that may indicate a spinal tumor (such as an osteoid osteoma), a history of neurologic complaints (such as numbness or weakness), and bladder problems that may indicate spinal canal anomalies (such as a tethered spinal cord). On the physical examination, the clinician should search for anomalies, such as cavus feet, severe joint hyperlaxity, or

Table 1

Curve Types

Type	Proximal Thoracic	Main Thoracic	Thoracolumbar/Lumbar
1 Main thoracic	Nonstructural	Structural[a]	Nonstructural
2 Double thoracic	Structural	Structural[a]	Nonstructural
3 Double major	Nonstructural	Structural[a]	Structural
4 Triple major	Structural	Structural[a]	Structural[a]
5 Thoracolumbar/lumbar	Nonstructural	Nonstructural	Structural[a]
6 Thoracolumbar/lumbar–main thoracic	Nonstructural	Structural	Structural[a]

[a]Indicates major curve

weakness and/or long tract signs. The typical radiographic curve patterns associated with AIS (including right thoracic, right thoracic and/or left lumbar, and left thoracolumbar/ lumbar [TL/L]) are quite consistent. Therefore, atypical radiographic features include a left main thoracic (MT) curve, sharply angulated curves, curves with congenital bony anomalies, and very large curves, which may be indicative of a nonidiopathic diagnosis. MRI of the entire spine is indicated if these features are seen. Left thoracic curves have a known incidence of syringomyelia of 20% to 30%.[34] Recently, thoracic hyperkyphosis in combination with a thoracic scoliosis was found to indicate an increased incidence of spinal canal anomalies such as Arnold-Chiari malformations and syringomyelia.[31] Therefore, a thorough evaluation of the patient history, physical examination, and radiographs is needed to exclude other conditions and establish the diagnosis of AIS.

The clinical examination of a patient with AIS begins by evaluating the posterior trunk and torso with as much of the trunk, extremities, and feet visible as possible. Shoulder height is evaluated to determine if the patient has level shoulders or if one shoulder is higher than the other. Trunk shift is noted by asymmetry of the ribcage on the pelvis (distinct from decompensa-

tion), which is an overall alignment of C7 to the sacral plumb line in the coronal plane. When waistline asymmetry is noted, it usually indicates a major thoracolumbar or lumbar deformity. The examiner should inspect for various skin lesions such as café-au-lait spots or hairy dimples. A forward-bending examination is then performed to evaluate thoracic and lumbar asymmetries. A scoliometer (inclinometer), which is commonly used as an objective screening test for AIS, is used to measure the proximal thoracic (PT), thoracic, and TL/L regions. A scoliometer measurement of 7° or more has a sensitivity of 74% to 100% for AIS. The device also quantifies the relative rotation of each curve.

Classification

The system by Lenke et al[35] is the most commonly used classification system for AIS curves. This system combines the radiographic triad of the curve type, the coronal lumbar modifier, and the sagittal thoracic modifier (**Table 1**). Classification begins by evaluating upright coronal, sagittal, and side-bending radiographs. In the coronal plane, the PT, MT and TL/L curves are measured using the Cobb method. The major curve is defined as the largest Cobb measurement, and the other two minor curves then are evaluated on the appropriate side-bending radiograph for flexibility to

categorize the curves as less than 25° or greater than or equal to 25° of residual curve. On the sagittal radiograph, the T5-T12 region is measured, and the PT (T2-T5) and TL/L (T10-L2) regions are measured for the degree of kyphosis. Minor curve structural criteria include a residual side-bending Cobb measurement of 25° or more and/or PT or TL/L kyphosis of 20° or more. A template of six curve types can be created depending on the structural nature of the PT, MT, and TL/L curves. In curve types 1 through 4, the MT region is the major curve, whereas in curve types 5 and 6, the TL/L region is the major curve. A coronal lumbar spine modifier is then added based on the position of the lumbar TL/L apex to the center sacral vertical line, noting an A, B, or C modifier (**Figure 4**). The sagittal thoracic modifier (–, N, or +) is then added based on a T5-T12 hypokyphosis, normal kyphosis, or hyperkyphosis Cobb measurement, respectively. This triad classification system indicates regions of the spine that should be treated; that is, the major region and the structural minor curves (which should be treated with arthrodesis) and the nonstructural minor curve(s) (which should not be treated with arthrodesis). This system has been shown to be up to 90% predictive for indicating the regions of the spine that may be fused successfully[35] (**Table 2**).

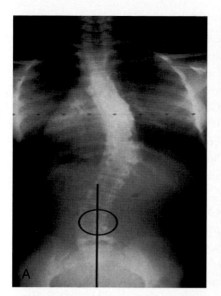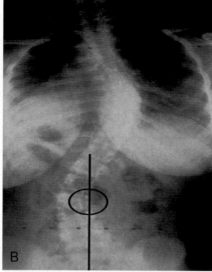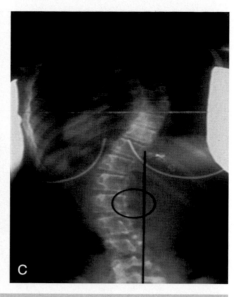

Figure 4   The three lumbar modifiers. **A,** This coronal lumbar modifier has the center sacral vertical line bisecting the apex of the curve between the pedicles. **B,** This coronal lumbar modifier has the center sacral vertical line touching the apical pedicles. **C,** This coronal lumbar modifier has the apical pedicles completely outside the center sacral vertical line.

Table 2
Treatment Approaches Based on the Lenke Classification System

Type	Regions Fused	Approach
1 Main thoracic	Main thoracic	Anterior or posterior spinal fusion
2 Double thoracic	Proximal thoracic and main thoracic	Posterior spinal fusion
3 Double major	Main thoracic and thoracolumbar/lumbar	Posterior spinal fusion
4 Triple major	Proximal thoracic, main thoracic, and thoracolumbar/lumbar	Posterior spinal fusion
5 Thoracolumbar/lumbar	Thoracolumbar/lumbar	Anterior or posterior spinal fusion
6 Thoracolumbar/lumbar–main thoracic	Main thoracic and thoracolumbar/lumbar	Posterior spinal fusion

The frequency of occurrence of these six curve patterns has recently been evaluated in a large multicenter study.[36] Of the 756 patients with AIS, 47% had type 1 MT curves, 22% had type 2 double thoracic curves, and 13% had type 5 TL/L curves; the remaining 18% had a mixture of the three types of curves. The most common posterior constructs were hybrid constructs (hooks, wires, pedicle screws; 56%); 40% had all pedicle-screw constructs, and only 4% had all hook constructs. Of the 756 patients, 91.1% had no complications from surgery through hospital discharge. Scoli-osis Research Society scores[36] improved significantly in the domains of appearance (3.3 to 4.2 points), satisfaction (3.7 to 4.4 points), and total score (3.9 to 4.3 points) (all $P < 0.05$) (**Figure 5**).

Most recently, acknowledgment that three-dimensional scoliotic deformities should be evaluated and classified using a three-dimensional perspective is gaining acceptance.[36] The Scoliosis Research Society has commissioned a committee to develop a clinically useful, three-dimensional classification system for AIS. Using the basic principle that the AIS curva-ture includes a deviation of the normal sagittal curvatures of thoracic kyphosis and lumbar lordosis from the midsagittal plane, a plane of maximum deformity is created and quantified by the Da Vinci representation,[37] which is a top-down vector representation of all major curves. Additional work is required to confirm the validity and reliability of this system; however, a dramatic change in the evaluation and classification of AIS using a three-dimensional method is expected in the next decade.[37,38]

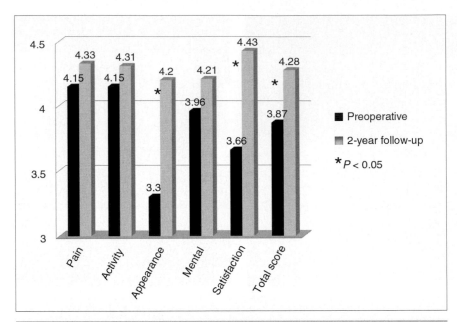

Figure 5   Bar graph of preoperative and 2-year postoperative Scoliosis Research Society scores after surgery to treat scoliosis show statistically significant improvement in the domains of appearance, overall satisfaction, and total score.

Treatment

There are four basic methods available for treating AIS: nonconventional, observational, bracing, and surgical.

Nonconventional

Nonconventional treatments include electrical stimulation, therapeutic exercises, chiropractic manipulation, and Rolfing. Although many of these methods have been popularized via the Internet, there is no demonstrated scientific validity in the ability of these treatments to limit progression in patients susceptible to curve progression.

Observational

Observation of AIS is the most common treatment used for patients with mild deformity (for example, a Cobb measurement of less than 25° in a skeletally immature or mature individual). Patients with mild deformities usually have acceptable alignment and cosmesis. Depending on the degree of skeletal maturity, patients are followed every 4 to 6 months, at least initially, to watch

for curve progression. If the skeletally immature patients (Risser 0 to 1) show progression with more than 25° of scoliosis, bracing may be indicated.

Bracing

Bracing is used for skeletally immature patients with AIS to try to limit curve progression and avoid spinal fusion surgery.[39] Rough guidelines for bracing of AIS curves include patients with a Cobb measurement of 25° to 40°, skeletally immature patients (Risser 0, 1, or 2), and those who will be compliant with brace wear. Compliance is an important component to brace wear. It has been shown (with in-brace devices such as heat thermoresisters) that the actual compliance of North American teenagers with brace wear averages approximately 60%.[40] In almost every scientifically validated brace study, the results were better for patients who wore the brace for long periods each day (ideally, 20 to 22 hours) than for patients with shorter brace-wear times.[40]

There are many types of braces; however, the most common brace for AIS is an underarm thoracolumbosacral orthosis or Boston-type brace. Also available are nighttime bending braces such as the Charleston brace (Charleston Bending Brace Foundation, Charleston, SC), the Providence orthosis (Providence Brace, Spinal Technologies, Providence, RI), and the Spinecor Dynamic Brace (Spine Corporation, Derbyshire, UK), but their efficacy is not as strongly researched for most curve patterns as that of the Boston brace.

Although the results of bracing are somewhat controversial, one of the best studies was performed by Nachemson et al.[41] In 1995, the authors published the results of their surgeon-randomized multicenter study of girls (Risser 0-2) with curves of 25° to 40° treated with Boston bracing or observation. The authors reported that bracing was 75% effective in preventing progression (defined by a greater than 5° increase in thoracic curves reviewed until skeletal maturity); these results were significantly better than those obtained with observation.[41] Although North American studies have been unable to reproduce these excellent results, a National Institutes of Health–funded study has recently completed enrollment, and follow-up is under way to ultimately provide more concrete information from this randomized prospective study of bracing in patients with AIS (S Weinstein, MD, unpublished data, 2011).

Surgical

Betz et al[42] and Cuddihy et al[43] recently promoted anterior thoracic and lumbar spinal stapling, which mimics the results of bracing. The authors reported on a series of 49 patients with idiopathic scoliosis, a Risser sign of 0 to 1 at first visit, curve sizes between 25° and 45°, and a minimum 2-year follow-up. The patients had mean preoperative curves of 32° in the thoracic spine and 31° in the lumbar spine. Stapling had a success rate of 80% in preventing progression of less than 10° in thoracic curves, with a similar success rate in the lumbar curve. Additional studies of this promising alternative surgical option for limiting the progression of moderate-size AIS curves in skeletally immature patients are needed to determine if such results can be replicated by other surgeons.

The surgical treatment of AIS follows the major tenets of deformity correction, with procurement of a solid spinal fusion and maintenance of correction over time. However, the methods of obtaining these two goals of correction and fusion have evolved in recent years. The current modality for most curve patterns of AIS is posterior treatment with segmental spinal fixation.

Overall, the trend during the past decade has been a decrease in the use of anterior-only and circumferential anteroposterior surgery and an increase in posterior-only surgery for patients with AIS. Major factors influencing that change have been the use of pedicle screw anchors for three-column purchase of the vertebrae, various forms of posterior spinal releases, osteotomies to increase curve flexibility, and interest in minimizing chest wall violation with its deleterious effect on pulmonary function by avoiding a formal anterior thoracotomy and/or thoracoabdominal approach or a posterior thoracoplasty.[44,45] Even large and stiff AIS curves (greater than 70° to 100° or more) can be managed with a posterior-only approach, including the rare use of a complete vertebrectomy or vertebral column resection approach for the largest and stiffest curves[46-48] (**Figure 6**).

Discussion

The evaluation and overall treatment of patients with AIS continues to evolve slowly and carefully. The diagnosis of AIS remains a diagnosis of exclusion. Performing a thorough history and physical examination, evaluating appropriate spinal radiographs, and obtaining a total spine MRI scan (when needed to rule out intraspinal anomalies) are the main tenets of the diagnostic assessment. Observation remains the most common treatment of small curves in all patients or moderate-size curves in skeletally mature pediatric patients. Bracing is still the main method for preventing the progression of mild or moderate curves in skeletally immature patients, but results are variable. Surgical management has evolved with the frequent use of a posterior approach with segmental fixation and now often includes pedicle screws with or without various spinal releases and osteotomies. However, the ultimate goal of AIS surgery is still the attainment of a stable spine fusion over the minimum number of spinal levels, centered over the pelvis in both planes, without complications.

Scheuermann Kyphosis

Scheuermann kyphosis is a focal developmental kyphosis that has been recognized for more than a century, although the causes are not understood. Characteristics include irregularity of the vertebral end plates (at times with Schmorl nodes) of at least three consecutive vertebrae, defects in maturation of their peripheral or ring apophyses, narrowing of the disk spaces, and wedging of the vertebral bodies. This disorder is best conceptualized as an osteochondrosis or growth disturbance secondary to abnormal loads or the inability of the growing spine to adapt to normal loading.

Natural History and Basic Principles

The normal range for thoracic kyphosis in adolescents is 20° to 45°, usually extending from T2 to T12. The vertebrae from T10 to L2 are typically parallel. Because Scheuermann kyphosis is often progressive, patients should be monitored. The condition is often—but not always—associated with pain in the area of the deformity. The condition is diagnosed in most patients around the time of puberty. After skeletal maturity, the risk and rate of progression are lower, but the kyphosis is likely to increase.[49] Untreated patients report increased back pain and are likely to elect lower activity levels as adults; however, most patients can remain employed, and pulmonary function is not diminished unless the curve exceeds 100°.

Signs and Symptoms

Increasing focal deformity with or without pain is noted by the patient and/or the family. The neurologic examination is typically normal. Hamstring tightness is common, but this characteristic is generally common in adolescents. A forward-bending test reveals the focal nature of the kyphosis and the fact that up to one third of cases are associated with a mild to moderate scoliosis.[49,50] The differential diagnosis includes healed compression fractures, type I osteogenesis imperfecta, spondyloepiphyseal dysplasia tarda, neurofibromatosis, and connective tissue disorders such as Marfan and Ehlers-Danlos syndromes.[51]

Treatment

Nonsurgical treatment of Scheuermann kyphosis includes physical therapy and orthotic management. Physical therapy (core strengthening and hamstring stretching) may alleviate pain, but it does not improve the deformity. Brace treatment has been shown to improve the angle of the kyphosis in appropriate settings, including kyphotic curves of 55° to 75° in patients who have substantial growth remaining. Milwaukee

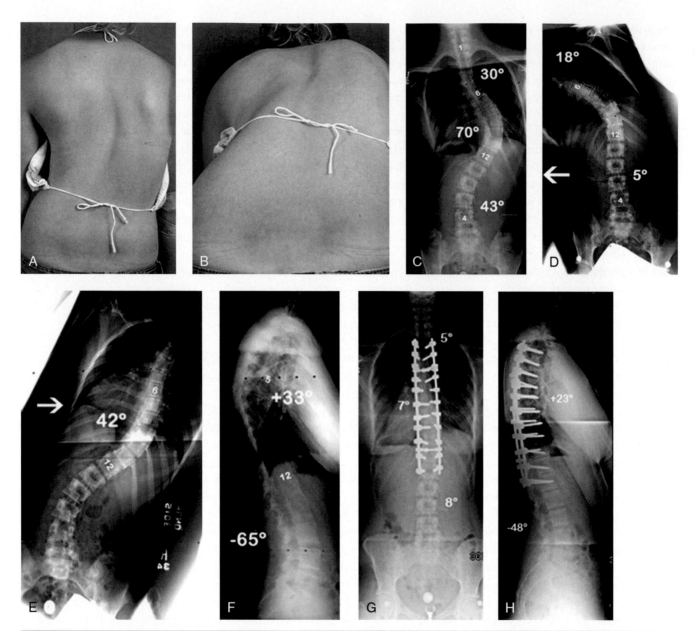

Figure 6 A 14.5-year-old adolescent girl had a progressive 70° right thoracic AIS deformity. **A,** Preoperative upright clinical photograph. **B,** Preoperative bending photograph. **C,** Preoperative upright AP radiograph. **D,** On the preoperative left-side bending radiograph, her PT curve was 18°, and her lumbar curve was 5°; both curves were nonstructural. The arrow shows the direction of the bend. **E,** The right-bending radiograph showed improvement in the main thoracic curve to 42°. The arrow shows the direction of the bend. **F,** On the preoperative lateral radiograph, the coronal lumbar coronal modifier is A, and the sagittal thoracic modifier was N because of the +33° T5 to T12 kyphosis. The complete classification was 1AN, the most common curve pattern seen. AP (**G**) and lateral (**H**) radiographs at 2 years after a posterior spinal fusion from T3-L1 with segmental pedicle screw fixation and a derotation maneuver. AP (**G**) and lateral (**H**) radiographs at 2 years after a posterior spinal fusion from T3-L1 with segmental pedicle screw fixation and a derotation maneuver. The patient had excellent coronal and sagittal spinal realignment.

and underarm orthoses have been shown to be beneficial, with the former likely being more effective.[50,52] With a properly indicated brace and wear compliance, correction of 10° to 20°

may occur by maturity.

Surgical treatment is an option for a curve larger than approximately 75° if it is associated with substantial pain or deformity. Many surgeons obtain preoper-

ative MRI to rule out stenosis, prominent disks, or other neuraxial findings. Posterior fusion, combined with appropriate posterior osteotomies and segmental fixation, can correct most

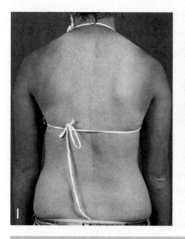
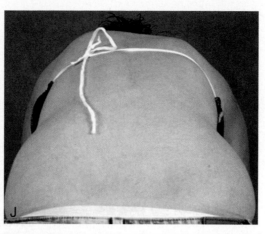

Figure 6 *(Continued)*   Postoperative standing (**I**) and bending (**J**) clinical photographs show truncal correction and improvement of the rib hump.

curves. Arthrodesis should encompass all vertebrae in the kyphotic region and extend distally into the sagittal stable zone, the first vertebra intersected by a line from the posterosuperior corner of the first sacral vertebra.[53] Complications in kyphosis surgery include failure of fixation, neurologic deficit, and superior mesenteric artery syndrome. Patient satisfaction is generally high because of the noticeable improvement in pain and deformity.

Discussion

Scheuermann kyphosis is a common disorder. Moderate deformities can be improved with bracing during growth, and symptoms may be ameliorated with physical methods. Surgical treatment, usually from a posterior approach, can be successful in correcting severe deformity.

Pediatric Spondylolysis and Spondylolisthesis

Spondylolysis and spondylolisthesis are among the most challenging spinal disorders to treat. Orthopaedic surgeons can use the knowledge of natural history and treatment outcomes to guide treatment decisions and optimize outcomes for pediatric patients with spondylolysis and spondylolisthesis.

Natural History and Basic Principles

Much of what is known about the natural history of spondylolysis and spondylolisthesis comes from the landmark population study of patients in Sayre, Pennsylvania more than 50 years ago.[54] A lateral lumbar radiograph was obtained for each of 500 children at birth and at ages 6, 8, 10, 15, and 18 years. The study showed that spondylolysis or spondylolisthesis was not evident at birth; however, the onset of the disorders appeared in 4.4% of the population by 5 years of age and 6% at adulthood (18 years of age). Most of the deformities occur early in life, presumably as children assume an upright posture. Other studies have identified special risk groups: high-performance athletes and patients with Scheuermann kyphosis, athetosis, or osseous fragility.[55-57] Even without advanced imaging, a familial tendency was identified. There was a positive family history in more than one third of the patients, and most patients had other posterior element defects, such as spina bifida occulta. The lytic defect led to spondylolisthesis in two thirds of the patients but never exceeded a 39% slip in the study population. The patients were followed for up to 45

years, and the results were striking. The patients' symptoms were rare and mild. The mean Medical Outcomes Study 36-Item Short Form scores were equal to that of the general population, and no patient reported a back disability. The mean slip was 18% (maximum slip, 39%). Only one patient from the study required spinal fusion.

Other studies have contributed additional information. Saraste[56] investigated the 20-year natural history in a large series of 255 patients with spondylolisthesis and found that progression was usually mild. That study showed the need for further investigation of the natural history of the much more rare high-grade slips. In 1987, Harris and Weinstein[55] examined patients with severe grade III or IV slips. At the 20-year follow-up, two thirds of the patients had symptoms, and 45% had neurologic findings. Patients with high-grade slips merit intervention. Identified factors that predict progression from the relatively common low-grade slip to the much rarer high-grade slip include female sex, a dysplastic slip, the presence of a grade II slip during the growing years, a high slip angle (kyphosis at the slip level), a family history of a substantial slip, and the presence of substantial laxity or a connective tissue disorder.[55,56]

Symptoms, Signs, and Imaging

Symptoms vary from person to person. It is important to remember that some patients with spondylolysis or spondylolisthesis are asymptomatic. Although approximately 6% of the population is affected by this condition, many individuals are unaware of it.[54] If symptoms develop, they most often appear during adolescence. The most common symptom is activity-related back pain that worsens with spinal extension and sports participation. Pain may extend to the buttocks and proximal thighs. Signs may include altered gait, most commonly described as a stiff-legged or a pelvic waddle; both result from compensations that limit hip flexion or hamstring excursion. Movement patterns include limited forward flexion. Patients with more severe degrees of slippage display prominent ilia as the pelvis is relatively extended. The slip itself is more subtle and may manifest as a palpable step-off of spinous processes. This step-off is one level above the vertebral body slip because the posterior elements remain contiguous with the caudal portion of the spine. Therefore, for a spondylolisthesis of L5-S1, the step-off of the spinous processes is between L4 and L5.

Imaging studies include conventional radiographs of the lumbar spine centered on the area of concern. Oblique films are often not definitive. Depending on clinical decision making, it may be reasonable to obtain more definitive imaging with CT or bone scanning. CT can provide more anatomic detail, such as the size and precise location of the defect. A bone scan provides an indication of osseous activity at the lesion, which some experts believe correlates with the pain level.[58-60] One of this chapter's authors (PDS) finds the information obtained from the CT study to be more useful than that obtained from a bone scan. MRI can show bony edema in patients with a recent fracture but often does not show the bony defect well. MRI is most helpful in defining the degree of disk protrusion and space for the nerve roots in patients with a severe slip who will require surgery.

Treatment of Spondylolysis
Nonsurgical Treatment
A brace or cast may be used for healing or symptom relief. Most clinicians use a lumbosacral orthosis for approximately 2 months. Although a biome-

chanical study has shown that a pantaloon brace is the most effective device,[61] it is also the least practical. The likelihood of true bony healing of the defect is rather low; a report in 2009 showed that radiographic healing occurred in approximately 5% of lesions.[62] However, the period of immobilization relieves symptoms in most patients. If satisfactory relief is obtained, the brace interval is followed by a supervised return to activity, which can be done under the guidance of a physical therapist or a trainer to reduce the chance of activity stresses resulting in symptom recurrence. This phase of treatment should focus on stretching, strengthening core muscles, and rebuilding endurance. If the symptoms are controlled, follow-up may be dictated by the degree of pain. Preadolescent patients or those with connective tissue laxity should be followed periodically throughout the growth period.

Surgical Treatment
Patients who have continued pain from a pars defect after a trial of nonsurgical treatment and who cannot return to their desired level of activity may be offered surgery. MRI to assess the adjacent disks and a radiographically guided injection of local anesthetic into the defect may be helpful in decision making if the cause of the pain is questionable. Surgical repair of the pars defect is an effective procedure for controlling pain without fusing motion segments. Indications for this procedure include persistent symptoms in a patient younger than 25 years, a slip of 5 mm or less, and no substantial disk degeneration. Repair of the defect is strongly indicated in levels above L5, but good results have been reported even at level L5.[63,64] Surgery involves cleaning the fibrous tissue from the laminar defect, stabilizing the defect, and inserting bone graft

across the defect with internal fixation of the pars fracture. Many forms of fixation have been successful, including figure-of-8 wires compressing the spinous process to the transverse process on either side, hook and pedicle screw combinations, and intraosseous screw fixation[64,65] (**Figure 7**). These devices are associated with a high success rate in relieving pain and returning athletes to sports participation.[63]

Treatment of Spondylolisthesis
Nonsurgical Treatment
Nonsurgical care is the mainstay of treatment for spondylolisthesis in most patients with grade 0 to 2 slips.[54,56,57] No restrictions are needed for asymptomatic patients with grade 1 or 2 slips. If back pain is severe, activity should be restricted during symptomatic periods. After symptoms improve, rehabilitation should begin with abdominal and extensor strengthening as well as hamstring stretching in a maintenance program. The use of a lumbosacral orthosis for acute or persistent symptoms is a treatment option. Periodic follow-up (every 1 to 2 years) should be continued during the patient's growth period.

Surgical Treatment
Arthrodesis is indicated for any patient with a slip greater than 50% or with persistent symptoms even with a smaller defect. In situ arthrodesis is a valid option. Instrumentation is not mandatory because many low-grade slips in young patients will fuse without it. However, uninstrumented arthrodesis will have poorer results in a patient with small transverse processes because the processes are the only available surface connected to the vertebral body (the lamina is detached at the pars interarticularis).[66] For severe slips, circumferential (anterior and posterior) arthrodesis has been shown to be slightly better than posterior-

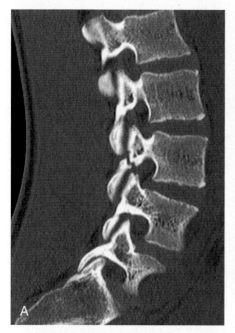
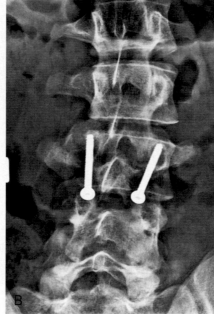
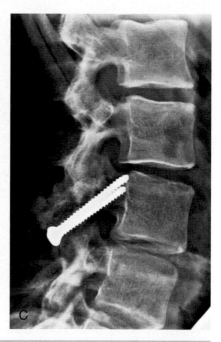

Figure 7   **A,** CT of the spine of a 17-year-old patient who plays soccer. The patient had painful L3 spondylolysis (with mild scoliosis) that persisted despite rest, bracing, and therapy. One-year postoperative AP (**B**) and lateral (**C**) radiographs showing screw fixation of the defect. The patient successfully returned to sports participation without fusion of a motion segment.

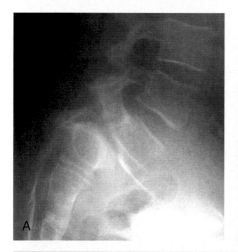
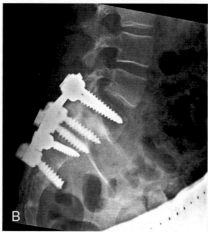
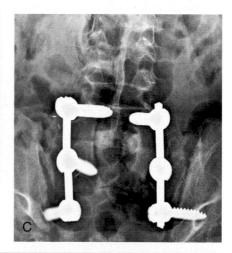

Figure 8   **A,** Radiograph of the spine of a 12-year-old child with an 80% slip with back and leg pain but no motor weakness. Lateral (**B**) and AP (**C**) radiographs after monosegmental reduction and circumferential fusion with fixation of L5-S2, which relieved the patient's pain.

only arthrodesis at long-term follow-up.[66,67] Patient appearance improves with a solid fusion, even in the absence of reduction.[68] Arthrodesis should include only the slip level if the degree of slip is mild (less than 50%) or can be successfully reduced (**Figure 8**). Arthrodesis should include two levels if the degree of slip is not reduced below approximately 50%. When considering reduction of the spondylolisthesis, the risks must be balanced against the benefits. The risk of palsy of the nerve root at the level of the slip should be discussed when counseling the patient. It is most likely that nerve root palsy occurs secondary to tension as the slipped vertebra is pulled posteriorly at the same time that the spinal column is slightly elongated. If the reduction can be achieved without complications, it can improve control of severe deformities and provide a more stable instrumented construct that is more likely to fuse and have good long-term results. Reduction of a grade 3 or 4 slip may decrease the arthrodesis level to a single segment because the vertebral alignment is more stable.

During surgery, the surgeon should be aware of laminar integrity and avoid midline exposure through bifid levels. If instrumentation is used, fixation of the slipped vertebra must be robust because of the forces that will be applied during reduction and maintenance of fixation. Serious consideration should be given to using alar screws in S2 to provide foundational purchase for reduction, especially in skeletally immature patients. Reduction begins with laminar excision, wide exposure and decompression, and stimulation of the nerve roots. Interbody grafting is an option, especially if there is substantial compression by the disk, the foramina are narrowed, or the patient is skeletally mature. A good posterolateral bone graft is a key component of the procedure. With rigid segmental fixation, postoperative bracing is not mandatory.

Another option for stabilizing severe slips is interbody dowel-type bone grafting with an allograft or autograft fibula. Although an anterior technique was first described by Jones et al,[69] Smith and Bohlman[70] reported excellent results with a posterior-only technique that is somewhat easier to perform. This technique does not require reduction and provides stabilization of both columns.

Spondylectomy and reduction is an option for severe, complete slips with substantial spinal shortening (high grade 4 or grade 5 slips). This modality avoids lengthening the abnormally foreshortened spinal column but requires a two- to three-stage procedure and involves the risk of neurologic deficit.[71]

Pitfalls and Controversies

Neurologic deficit has been reported in at least 3% to 5% of most spondylolisthesis series.[72] Deficits may arise from stretching the nerve roots at the affected levels, from compression at the foraminal or extraforaminal levels, or from compression by the deformed or bulging disk or across the dome of the sacrum. Regular monitoring is required in the first postoperative days because deficit onset may be delayed. Postoperative hyperalgesia in the absence of motor deficits may be observed. According to another review, there have been some reports of cauda equina syndrome in the absence of a reduction;[73] this complication most likely represents additional compromise of a barely compensated, stretched cauda equina while the patient is under anesthesia.

Adding-on or junctional kyphotic deformity of the spine may develop at the level above the fused level and is more likely if that level was temporarily instrumented or the slip was severe.[74]

Discussion

Spondylolysis and spondylolisthesis range from a defect with minimal deformity and symptoms to one with progressive pain and deformity. Grade 3 or greater slips are best treated surgically, and the risks of complications are proportionate to the treatment. Treatment at the early stages of deformity is preferable. Nevertheless, the improvement in pain, function, and deformity is gratifying after treatment of this challenging condition.

Summary

The treatment of pediatric spinal deformity continues to evolve based on knowledge of its natural history. Patients with early-onset spinal deformity are best served by delaying fusion to maximize trunk growth. Cast treatment for progressive early curves is effective, especially for patients with idiopathic deformity. Growth-sparing procedures such as VEPTR are commonly accepted options. Compliance with brace treatment increases control of moderate adolescent idiopathic scoliosis in patients with remaining growth. The Lenke classification system helps standardize surgical treatment for large curves. Posterior fusion with segmental instrumentation is effective for most curves and is also the mainstay of treatment for severe, symptomatic Scheuermann kyphosis. Spondylolysis and spondylolisthesis are initially treated with conservative options, but patients with persistent symptoms are surgical candidates. Fusion in situ or fusion with reduction and instrumentation are options for the management of severe slips.

References

1. Dickson RA, Archer IA: Surgical treatment of late-onset idiopathic thoracic scoliosis: The Leeds procedure. *J Bone Joint Surg Br* 1987; 69(5):709-714.

2. DiMeglio A: Growth in pediatric orthopaedics, in Morrissy RT, Weinstein SL, eds: *Lovell and Winter's Pediatric Orthopaedics.* Philadelphia, PA, Lippincott Williams & Wilkins, 2006, pp 35-65.

3. DiMeglio A, Canavese F, Charles YP: Growth and adolescent idiopathic scoliosis: When and how much? *J Pediatr Orthop* 2011; 31(1, Suppl):S28-S36.

4. Charles YP, Daures JP, de Rosa V, DiMéglio A: Progression risk of idiopathic juvenile scoliosis during pubertal growth. *Spine (Phila Pa 1976)* 2006;31(17):1933-1942.

5. Charles YP, DiMeglio A, Marcoul M, Bourgin JF, Marcoul A, Bozonnat MC: Influence of idiopathic scoliosis on three-dimensional thoracic growth. *Spine (Phila Pa 1976)* 2008; 33(11):1209-1218.

6. Charles YP, DiMeglio A, Marcoul M, Bourgin JF, Marcoul A, Bo-

zonnat MC: Volumetric thoracic growth in children with moderate and severe scoliosis compared to subjects without spinal deformity. *Stud Health Technol Inform* 2008; 140:22-28.

7. Campbell RM Jr, Smith MD, Mayes TC, et al: The characteristics of thoracic insufficiency syndrome associated with fused ribs and congenital scoliosis. *J Bone Joint Surg Am* 2003;85-A(3): 399-408.

8. Pehrsson K, Larsson S, Oden A, Nachemson A: Long-term follow-up of patients with untreated scoliosis: A study of mortality, causes of death, and symptoms. *Spine (Phila Pa 1976)* 1992; 17(9):1091-1096.

9. Canavese F, DiMeglio A, D'Amato C, et al: Dorsal arthrodesis in prepubertal New Zealand white rabbits followed to skeletal maturity: Effect on thoracic dimensions, spine growth and neural elements. *Indian J Orthop* 2010;44(1):14-22.

10. Karol LA, Johnston C, Mladenov K, Schochet P, Walters P, Browne RH: Pulmonary function following early thoracic fusion in nonneuromuscular scoliosis. *J Bone Joint Surg Am* 2008;90(6):1272-1281.

11. Vitale MG, Matsumoto H, Roye DP Jr, et al: Health-related quality of life in children with thoracic insufficiency syndrome. *J Pediatr Orthop* 2008;28(2):239-243.

12. Vitale MG, Gomez JA, Matsumoto H, Roye DP Jr; Chest Wall and Spine Deformity Study Group: Variability of expert opinion in treatment of early-onset scoliosis. *Clin Orthop Relat Res* 2011;469(5):1317-1322.

13. Yang JS, McElroy MJ, Akbarnia BA, et al: Growing rods for spinal deformity: Characterizing consensus and variation in current use. *J Pediatr Orthop* 2010;30(3): 264-270.

14. Dubousset J, Herring JA, Shufflebarger H: The crankshaft phenomenon. *J Pediatr Orthop* 1989; 9(5):541-550.

15. Sankar WN, Acevedo DC, Skaggs DL: Comparison of complications among growing spinal implants. *Spine (Phila Pa 1976)* 2010; 35(23):2091-2096.

16. McCarthy RE, Sucato D, Turner JL, Zhang H, Henson MA, McCarthy K: Shilla growing rods in a caprine animal model: A pilot study. *Clin Orthop Relat Res* 2010; 468(3):705-710.

17. Mehta MH: Growth as a corrective force in the early treatment of progressive infantile scoliosis. *J Bone Joint Surg Br* 2005;87(9): 1237-1247.

18. Sanders JO, D'Astous J, Fitzgerald M, Khoury JG, Kishan S, Sturm PF: Derotational casting for progressive infantile scoliosis. *J Pediatr Orthop* 2009;29(6):581-587.

19. Lloyd-Roberts GC, Pilcher MF: Structural Idiopathic scoliosis in infancy: A study of the natural history of 100 patients. *J Bone Joint Surg Br* 1965;47:520-523.

20. Akel I, Yazici M: Growth modulation in the management of growing spine deformities. *J Child Orthop* 2009;3(1):1-9.

21. Hell AK, Campbell RM, Hefti F: The vertical expandable prosthetic titanium rib implant for the treatment of thoracic insufficiency syndrome associated with congenital and neuromuscular scoliosis in young children. *J Pediatr Orthop B* 2005;14(4):287-293.

22. Samdani AF, St Hilaire T, Emans JB, et al: The usefulness of VEPTR in the older child with complex spine and chest deformity. *Clin Orthop Relat Res* 2010; 468(3):700-704.

23. Harrington PR: The history and development of Harrington instrumentation. *Clin Orthop Relat Res* 1973;93:110-112.

24. Thompson GH, Akbarnia BA, Campbell RM Jr: Growing rod techniques in early-onset scoliosis. *J Pediatr Orthop* 2007;27(3): 354-361.

25. Thompson GH, Akbarnia BA, Kostial P, et al: Comparison of single and dual growing rod techniques followed through definitive surgery: A preliminary study. *Spine (Phila Pa 1976)* 2005; 30(18):2039-2044.

26. Bess S, Akbarnia BA, Thompson GH, et al: Complications of growing-rod treatment for early-onset scoliosis: Analysis of one hundred and forty patients. *J Bone Joint Surg Am* 2010;92(15):2533-2543.

27. Schroerlucke S, Salari P, Pawelek J, Mundis GM, Akbarnia BA; Growing Spine Study Group: Abstract: Preoperative thoracic kyphosis can predict complications in growing rod surgery for early onset scoliosis. American Academy of Pediatrics Website. http://aap.confex.com/aap/2010/ webprogram/Paper9966.html. Accessed June 17, 2011.

28. Sankar WN, Skaggs DL, Yazici M, et al: Lengthening of dual growing rods and the law of diminishing returns. *Spine (Phila Pa 1976)* 2011;36(10):806-809.

29. Myung K, Skaggs DL, Thompson GH, et al: Nutritional improvement following growing rod surgery in children with early onset scoliosis. American Academy of Orthopaedic Surgeons Website. 2010 Annual Meeting podium presentations. http:// www3.aaos.org/education/ anmeet/anmt2010/podium/ podium.cfm?Pevent=185. Accessed August 11, 2011.

30. Miladi L, Dubousset JF: Magnetic powered extensible rod for thorax or spine, in Akbarnia BA, Yazici M, Thompson GH, eds: *The Growing Spine*. New York, NY, Springer, 2011, pp 585-591.

31. Weinstein SL, Dolan LA, Cheng JC, Danielsson A, Morcuende JA: Adolescent idiopathic scoliosis. *Lancet* 2008;371(9623):1527-1537.

32. Ponseti IV, Friedman B: Prognosis in idiopathic scoliosis. *J Bone Joint Surg Am* 1950;32A(2):381-395.

33. Weinstein SL, Ponseti IV: Curve progression in idiopathic scoliosis. *J Bone Joint Surg Am* 1983;65(4):447-455.

34. O'Brien MF, Lenke LG, Bridwell KH, Blanke K, Baldus C: Preoperative spinal canal investigation in adolescent idiopathic scoliosis curves > or = 70 degrees. *Spine (Phila Pa 1976)* 1994;19(14):1606-1610.

35. Lenke LG, Betz RR, Harms J, et al: Adolescent idiopathic scoliosis: A new classification to determine extent of spinal arthrodesis. *J Bone Joint Surg Am* 2001;83-A(8):1169-1181.

36. Lenke LG, Bridwell KH, Erickson MA, et al: Prospective radiographic and clinical outcomes and complications of 756 consecutive operative adolescent idiopathic scoliosis patients. Spine: Affiliated Meeting Abstracts. http://journals.lww.com/spinejournalabstracts/Fulltext/2009/10003/Prospective_Radiographic_and_Clinical_Outcomes_and.3.aspx. Accessed June 17, 2011.

37. Labelle H, Aubin CE, Jackson R, Lenke L, Newton P, Parent S: Seeing the spine in 3D: How will it change what we do? *J Pediatr Orthop* 2011;31(1, Suppl):S37-S45.

38. Sangole AP, Aubin CE, Labelle H, et al: Three-dimensional classification of thoracic scoliotic curves. *Spine (Phila Pa 1976)* 2009;34(1):91-99.

39. Danielsson AJ, Hasserius R, Ohlin A, Nachemson AL: A prospective study of brace treatment versus observation alone in adolescent idiopathic scoliosis: A follow-up mean of 16 years after maturity. *Spine (Phila Pa 1976)* 2007;32(20):2198-2207.

40. Rahman T, Bowen JR, Takemitsu M, Scott C: The association between brace compliance and outcome for patients with idiopathic scoliosis. *J Pediatr Orthop* 2005;25(4):420-422.

41. Nachemson AL, Peterson LE; Brace Study Group of the Scoliosis Research Society: Effectiveness of treatment with a brace in girls who have adolescent idiopathic scoliosis: A prospective, controlled study based on data from the Brace Study of the Scoliosis Research Society. *J Bone Joint Surg Am* 1995;77(6):815-822.

42. Betz RR, Kim J, D'Andrea LP, Mulcahey MJ, Balsara RK, Clements DH: An innovative technique of vertebral body stapling for the treatment of patients with adolescent idiopathic scoliosis: A feasibility, safety, and utility study. *Spine (Phila Pa 1976)* 2003;28(20):S255-S265.

43. Cuddihy L, Danielsson AJ, Cahill PJ, et al: Vertebral body stapling (VBS) vs bracing for patients with high-risk moderate idiopathic scoliosis (IS). http://www.isass.org/pdf/sas11/4-Friday/Innovative-Session/170.pdf. Accessed June 17, 2011.

44. Vedantam R, Lenke LG, Bridwell KH, Haas J, Linville DA: A prospective evaluation of pulmonary function in patients with adolescent idiopathic scoliosis relative to the surgical approach used for spinal arthrodesis. *Spine (Phila Pa 1976)* 2000;25(1):82-90.

45. Yaszay B, Jazayeri R, Lonner B: The effect of surgical approaches on pulmonary function in adolescent idiopathic scoliosis. *J Spinal Disord Tech* 2009;22(4):278-283.

46. Dobbs MB, Lenke LG, Kim YJ, Luhmann SJ, Bridwell KH: Anterior/posterior spinal instrumentation versus posterior instrumentation alone for the treatment of adolescent idiopathic scoliotic curves more than 90 degrees. *Spine (Phila Pa 1976)* 2006;31(20):2386-2391.

47. Luhmann SJ, Lenke LG, Kim YJ, Bridwell KH, Schootman M: Thoracic adolescent idiopathic scoliosis curves between 70 degrees and 100 degrees: Is anterior release necessary? *Spine (Phila Pa 1976)* 2005;30(18):2061-2067.

48. Lenke LG, O'Leary PT, Bridwell KH, Sides BA, Koester LA, Blanke KM: Posterior vertebral column resection for severe pediatric deformity: Minimum two-year follow-up of thirty-five consecutive patients. *Spine (Phila Pa 1976)* 2009;34(20):2213-2221.

49. Murray PM, Weinstein SL, Spratt KF: The natural history and long-term follow-up of Scheuermann kyphosis. *J Bone Joint Surg Am* 1993;75(2):236-248.

50. Sachs B, Bradford D, Winter R, Lonstein J, Moe J, Willson S: Scheuermann kyphosis: Follow-up of Milwaukee-brace treatment. *J Bone Joint Surg Am* 1987;69(1):50-57.

51. Sillence D: Osteogenesis imperfecta: An expanding panorama of variants. *Clin Orthop Relat Res* 1981;159:11-25.

52. Gutowski WT, Renshaw TS: Orthotic results in adolescent kyphosis. *Spine (Phila Pa 1976)* 1988;13(5):485-489.

53. Newton PO, Yaszay B, Upasani VV, et al: Preservation of thoracic kyphosis is critical to maintain lumbar lordosis in the surgical treatment of adolescent idiopathic scoliosis. *Spine (Phila Pa 1976)* 2010;35(14):1365-1370.

54. Fredrickson BE, Baker D, McHolick WJ, Yuan HA, Lubicky JP: The natural history of spondylolysis and spondylolisthesis. *J Bone Joint Surg Am* 1984;66(5):699-707.

55. Harris IE, Weinstein SL: Long-term follow-up of patients with grade-III and IV spondylolisthesis: Treatment with and without posterior fusion. *J Bone Joint Surg Am* 1987;69(7):960-969.

56. Saraste H: Long-term clinical and radiological follow-up of spondylolysis and spondylolisthesis. *J Pediatr Orthop* 1987;7(6): 631-638.

57. Beutler WJ, Fredrickson BE, Murtland A, Sweeney CA, Grant WD, Baker D: The natural history of spondylolysis and spondylolisthesis: 45-year follow-up evaluation. *Spine (Phila Pa 1976)* 2003;28(10):1027-1035.

58. Anderson K, Sarwark JF, Conway JJ, Logue ES, Schafer MF: Quantitative assessment with SPECT imaging of stress injuries of the pars interarticularis and response to bracing. *J Pediatr Orthop* 2000; 20(1):28-33.

59. d'Hemecourt PA, Zurakowski D, Kriemler S, Micheli LJ: Spondylolysis: Returning the athlete to sports participation with brace treatment. *Orthopedics* 2002; 25(6):653-657.

60. McTimoney CA, Micheli LJ: Current evaluation and management of spondylolysis and spondylolisthesis. *Curr Sports Med Rep* 2003; 2(1):41-46.

61. Dubousset J: Treatment of spondylolysis and spondylolisthesis in children and adolescents. *Clin Orthop Relat Res* 1997;337:77-85.

62. McClellan JW, Ryschon K, Stamm S: Healing rate of 124 pars interarticularis fractures treated conservatively. Nebraska Spine Center website. http://www.nebraskaspinecenter.com/Post/sections/34/Files/Healing%20RATE%20FOR%20PARS.pdf. Accessed June 20, 2011.

63. Debnath UK, Freeman BJ, Gregory P, de la Harpe D, Kerslake RW, Webb JK: Clinical outcome and return to sport after the surgical treatment of spondylolysis in young athletes. *J Bone Joint Surg Br* 2003;85(2):244-249.

64. Nozawa S, Shimizu K, Miyamoto K, Tanaka M: Repair of pars interarticularis defect by segmental wire fixation in young athletes with spondylolysis. *Am J Sports Med* 2003;31(3):359-364.

65. Koptan WM, ElMiligui YH, ElSharkawi MM: Direct repair of spondylolysis presenting after correction of adolescent idiopathic scoliosis. *Spine J* 2011;11(2): 133-138.

66. Lenke LG, Bridwell KH, Bullis D, Betz RR, Baldus C, Schoenecker PL: Results of in situ fusion for isthmic spondylolisthesis. *J Spinal Disord* 1992;5(4):433-442.

67. Lamberg T, Remes V, Helenius I, Schlenzka D, Seitsalo S, Poussa M: Uninstrumented in situ fusion for high-grade childhood and adolescent isthmic spondylolisthesis: Long-term outcome. *J Bone Joint Surg Am* 2007;89(3): 512-518.

68. Johnson JR, Kirwan EO: The long-term results of fusion in situ for severe spondylolisthesis. *J Bone Joint Surg Br* 1983;65(1):43-46.

69. Jones AA, McAfee PC, Robinson RA, Zinreich SJ, Wang H: Failed arthrodesis of the spine for severe spondylolisthesis: Salvage by interbody arthrodesis. *J Bone Joint Surg Am* 1988;70(1):25-30.

70. Smith MD, Bohlman HH: Spondylolisthesis treated by a single-stage operation combining decompression with in situ posterolateral and anterior fusion: An analysis of eleven patients who had long-term follow-up. *J Bone Joint Surg Am* 1990;72(3): 415-421.

71. Gaines RW: L5 vertebrectomy for the surgical treatment of spondyloptosis: Thirty cases in 25 years. *Spine (Phila Pa 1976)* 2005; 30(6, Suppl):S66-S70.

72. Mardjetko S, Albert T, Andersson G, et al: Spine/SRS spondylolisthesis summary statement. *Spine (Phila Pa 1976)* 2005; 30(6, Suppl):S3.

73. Schoenecker PL, Cole HO, Herring JA, Capelli AM, Bradford DS: Cauda equina syndrome after in situ arthrodesis for severe spondylolisthesis at the lumbosacral junction. *J Bone Joint Surg Am* 1990;72(3):369-377.

74. Ruf M, Koch H, Melcher RP, Harms J: Anatomic reduction and monosegmental fusion in high-grade developmental spondylolisthesis. *Spine (Phila Pa 1976)* 2006;31(3):269-274.

Video Reference

39.1: Akbarnia BA, Mundis JR GM, Yaszay B: Video. *Dual Growing Rod Surgery for the Surgical Treatment of Infantile Idiopathic Scoliosis*. LaJolla, CA, 2010.

Spine Problems in Young Athletes

Daniel J. Sucato, MD

Lyle J. Micheli, MD

A. Reed Estes, MD

Vernon T. Tolo, MD

Abstract

As the number of young people involved in sports activities increases, acute and chronic back pain has become more common. With a careful medical history and physical examination, along with the judicious use of imaging modalities, the causes of back pain can be correctly diagnosed and treated so that young athletes can quickly return to sports participation.

Although most back pain in these young patients is muscular in origin, findings that should trigger increased concern include night pain, marked hamstring tightness, pain with lumbar spine hyperextension, or any neurologic finding. When recently developed vague back pain is present, a delay in radiographic imaging is warranted. With new back pain after trauma, AP and lateral radiographs of the symptomatic spinal area are indicated. CT, bone scans, and MRI should be reserved for special circumstances.

Spondylolysis is the most common bony cause of back pain in young athletes. Spondylolysis can be treated with activity limitation, a specific exercise program, a thoracolumbar orthosis, and/or surgery. Treatment should be based on the amount of pain as well as the desire of the young athlete to continue in the sports activity that caused the pain. Other significant causes of back pain that require more extensive treatment in these young athletes include spondylolisthesis, lumbar disk disorders, and sacral stress fractures.

It is anticipated that nearly all young athletes can return to sports activity after successful treatment. Even if surgical treatment is needed, return to all sports is expected, with the occasional exception of collision sports.

Instr Course Lect 2012;61:499-511.

As young athletes continue to participate in a variety of sports and succumb to the pressures of more strenuous training regimens, it is common for these young athletes to present for treatment in the orthopaedic clinic with acute and chronic back pain. Many of these disorders can be managed nonsurgically, whereas a smaller number will benefit from surgical treatment.

When evaluating a young athlete with low back pain, consideration must be given to the many differential diagnoses that can produce similar symptoms. Disorders are often chronic by the time the patient presents for professional orthopaedic care. With a careful medical history and physical examination, along with appropriate imaging studies, the causes of back pain can be correctly diagnosed and treated so that these young athletes can quickly return to sports participation.

Dr. Sucato or an immediate family member serves as a board member, owner, officer, or committee member of the American Academy of Orthopaedic Surgeons, the Pediatric Orthopaedic Society of North America, and the Scoliosis Research Society. Dr. Micheli or an immediate family member serves as an unpaid consultant to Carticel (scientific board); has received research or institutional support from Genzyme; and serves as a board member, owner, officer, or committee member of the International Federation of Sports Medicine Executive Committee. Neither of the following authors nor any immediate family member has received anything of value from or owns stock in a commercial company or institution related directly or indirectly to the subject of this chapter: Dr. Estes and Dr. Tolo.

Table 1

Spinal and Nonspinal Causes of Back Pain

Spinal Diagnoses	Nonspinal Diagnoses
Muscle strain/ligament sprain	Intrapelvic, gynecologic conditions (such as ovarian cysts)
Spondylolysis	Renal disease
Spondylolisthesis	Sacroiliac joint dysfunction
Facet syndrome	
Ring apophyseal injury	
Sacral stress fracture	
Central disk herniation	
Sacralization of L5/transverse process impingement	
Facet stress fracture	
Acute traumatic lumbar fracture	
Diskitis/osteomyelitis	
Neoplasm	

Reproduced with permission from Bono CM: Low back pain in athletes. *J Bone Joint Surg Am* 2004;86:382-386.

Epidemiology

Only a few decades ago, back pain in children and adolescents was believed to result from a demonstrable spinal abnormality in approximately 80% to 90% of these patients. Although specific spinal abnormalities are still identified as the source of some cases of back pain, the incidence and prevalence of back pain in young patients has continued to increase, with the rate in adolescents nearly equivalent to that found in adults.

There are multiple and varied risk factors for back pain in children and adolescents.[1] Both too much and too little athletic activity may be factors. Back pain is more prevalent in teenagers than in younger children, and females have back pain more often than males. Back pain is more common in teenagers with a history of headaches or those who have a parent with a history of back pain. Trunk asymmetry and increased sitting height may be associated with back pain, even if no spinal deformity is present.

The incidence of low back pain in pediatric and adolescent patients is between 1% and 30% and is most de-pendent on age (more common in adolescents than in children younger than 12 years), sports participation, time during the rapid growth period, and family history of back pain.[2-4] In adolescent athletes, the incidence of back pain and associated pathologic causes are influenced by the patient's sex, the type of sport played, the training intensity, the frequency of play, and technique. For example, wrestlers have a 59% incidence of low back pain compared with 31% for age-matched subjects, gymnasts 79% versus 38% for age-matched subjects, and adolescent athletes 46% versus 18% for nonathletes.[5,6] A review of collegiate athletes reported 7 of 100 participants had a back injury, with football players and gymnasts having the highest incidence.[7] Injuries occurred during practice in 80% of athletes, during competition in 6%, and during preseason conditioning in 14%.[7]

Back pain is a symptom rather than a diagnosis. It is important to attempt to identify a particular cause for a patient's back pain. There are many differential diagnoses, both spinal and nonspinal, for back pain in athletes (Table 1). Although spinal diagnoses are on the forefront of the orthopaedic surgeon's list, it is important to consider the nonorthopaedic diagnoses, which include intrapelvic conditions (such as ovarian cysts) typically seen by obstetricians or gynecologists. Renal disease or urinary tract infection should be considered in patients who have pain in the flank area.

Medical History

The first step in evaluating the potential sources of back pain is to obtain a careful medical history. Some diagnostic hints can be obtained from a child's response regarding the location of the back pain. If a child points to one particular spot, there is more likely an identifiable underlying cause for the pain than if a vague general area is identified as the pain location. If radiating pain is described, there is usually an identifiable source. If pain is associated with sports participation, the pain may be present during the activity or after the activity is completed. Modification of the activity may help resolve the pain during play. Pain that occurs after completing a sports activity as well as pain with spinal extension during the sport is common in spondylolysis, which should be considered in the differential diagnosis in such instances.

Pain that is present only at night is not sports-related back pain and requires a detailed imaging workup. Pain that is worsening and not intermittent is more indicative of a spinal disorder. Pain that requires narcotic analgesia may indicate a more serious disorder, whereas pain that is treatable with an occasional nonsteroidal anti-inflammatory medication can usually be managed conservatively with periodic follow-up and usually resolves with time. In obtaining the pain history, if the parents talk more about the pain and the effect on the child's sports participation than the patient, the

Physical Examination

physician should consider the possibility that the child is using claimed pain as a method of escape from sporting activities.

The physical examination for young patients with back pain should include general and spine-specific assessments. The sources of back pain in a fit teenager are different from those in an overweight teenager who does not exercise. Once again, if the patient specifies one spot as the location of pain, an identifiable cause is more likely than if the hand is waved over the lower half of the trunk to indicate the location of the pain. The spinal evaluation should include an examination of the trunk and the lower extremities.

Cutaneous abnormalities of the trunk, such as hemangioma, sacral dimples, or café-au-lait spots, may be associated with spinal abnormalities. The back is examined for movement in flexion and extension. Limited forward flexion may be caused by pain or tight hamstring muscles.[8] If the hamstring muscles are tight (particularly in pain with a recent onset), this may be a sign of a spinal cord or neurologic abnormality and should be evaluated with imaging (**Table 2**). Pain with forward flexion is less frequently a specific localizing sign, but pain with hyperextension of the lumbar spine often is associated with spondylolysis. Because pain in the lumbar spine may originate at the sacroiliac joints, this must be assessed with the flexion, abduction, and external rotation (FABER) test, which involves forced abduction and external rotation of the lower limb.

Spinal deformity is evaluated with the Adams forward bend test. If the patient veers to one side during this test instead of bending straight forward, this pathologic finding is usually caused by asymmetric tight hamstrings

and requires advanced imaging evaluations to determine the source of the abnormality. Although scoliosis is generally not a source of pain, the presence of a left thoracic scoliosis and pain is often related to a spinal cord abnormality, and MRI should be done. If increased kyphosis is present, it can be a source of pain in the lower thoracic region. There is an increased incidence of spondylolysis in teenagers (usually boys) with Scheuermann kyphosis.

Imaging Studies

Imaging studies are the key to identifying significant causes of back pain in young patients. When a patient reports the recent onset of back pain, the physician must decide if radiographs are needed. If no traumatic event has occurred and the patient reports vague, generalized low back pain, it is acceptable to delay radiography for 6 weeks, at which time the patient is reevaluated and radiographs are obtained if the back pain persists. In contrast, in cases of recent trauma leading to the onset of back pain, radiographic studies should be strongly considered at the time of the first visit.

AP and lateral lumbar spine radiographs are obtained to assess low back pain. The routine use of oblique lumbar spine radiographs doubles the radiation dose for the young patient and adds little information to aid diagnostic accuracy; all four views are rarely needed in the initial evaluation. Lumbar spine radiographs are excellent for diagnosing spondylolisthesis or disk changes secondary to a vertebral apophyseal rupture. Despite the usefulness of radiographs, they may not provide enough information to confirm a diagnosis of spondylolysis; however, if the AP radiograph shows sclerosis at the pars interarticularis and the lateral radiograph shows a possible radiolucency in the pars interarticularis,

Table 2

Conditions That Lead to Advanced Spinal Imaging Studies

Night pain that occurs more often than day pain

Pain worse with hyperextension

Progressively tight hamstrings

Hyperreflexia or ankle clonus

Pain radiating to lower legs and feet

Cutaneous abnormalities of the truck

Painful scoliosis, especially in the left thoracic area

a presumptive diagnosis of spondylolysis can be made. A CT scan can provide further detail. If scoliosis or excessive kyphosis is present with the pain, long, standing, AP and lateral radiographs of the entire thoracic and lumbar spine should be obtained.

If radiographs are insufficient for the diagnosis of the spinal abnormality, advanced imaging studies including nuclear bone scans, CT, and MRI can be used.[9] Bone scans, usually using technetium-99 as the isotope, are the best imaging modality for localizing an area of abnormal bone activity. They are useful in identifying tumors such as osteoid osteoma that may be impossible to see on radiographs. Bone scans can demonstrate the bone activity at the site of spondylolysis and may be useful in guiding orthopaedic management.[10,11] If a bone scan is obtained to evaluate or diagnose spondylolysis, a single-photon emission computed tomography (SPECT) should be obtained at the same time because it enhances the rate for detecting spondylolysis.[12] In many instances, once the level of increased bone activity has been localized, CT is used to better characterize the bone abnormality. CT is excellent for demonstrating and defining bone lesions, although young patients are exposed to a consid-

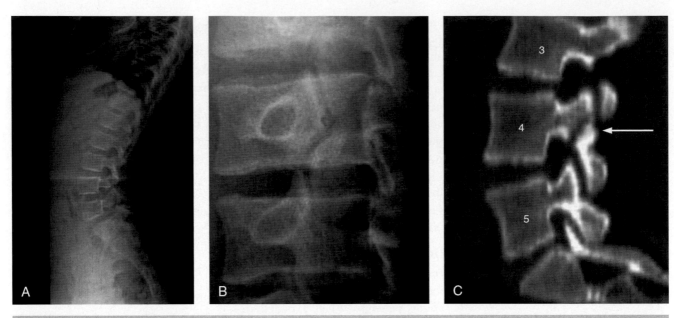

Figure 1 **A,** Lateral radiograph showing a pars interarticularis fracture at L4 and L5. **B,** An oblique radiograph shows the pars defect, as evidenced by the scotty dog sign (the collar of the scotty dog). **C,** CT scan of the defect at L4 (arrow).

erable amount of radiation with this study. CT can clearly identify chronic spondylolysis but is less effective in visualizing an early stress fracture of the pars interarticularis. MRI is the superior imaging study for abnormalities in the spinal cord, the cauda equina, and the intervertebral disks.[13,14] MRI is the primary study to request if there is any neurologic abnormality on physical examination, if painful scoliosis is present, if the hamstrings are excessively tight, or if there is pain radiating into the calf or foot. MRI is not a good diagnostic study for detecting spondylolysis or bone tumors, which are better visualized by CT. Positron emission tomography with CT scanning may be used in complex cases but is generally less available than radiography, bone scanning, CT, and MRI.[15]

Causes of Back Pain

Significant differences exist between the young athlete and the adult with back pain with respect to etiology. A definable cause of the back pain can be determined in approximately 62% of young athletes with pain.[16] Spondylolysis accounts for 47% of back pain in the adolescent athlete, followed by discogenic and muscle-tendon strain. In adult patients, discogenic pain accounts for 48% of the back pain, musculotendon strain for 27%, spinal stenosis or osteoarthritis for 10%, and spondylolysis for 5%.[16]

Muscle Strains

Muscle strain accounts for 20% of the back pain in adolescent athletes and can be defined as a stretch injury at one or more spinal ligaments, with stretching of the interspinous ligament being the most common occurance.[17] Muscle strain can be associated with end-plate changes on lateral radiographs. Lumbar strains and sprains include stretching or disruption of muscle fibers (strain or ligament sprains), usually cause acute pain in the first 24 to 48 hours, and are often associated with spasms that may be localized to a trigger point. Pain is often recurrent with short asymptomatic periods between episodes. Chronic strains

may result in continuous pain. Extensive workups are often obtained, but patients can usually be best treated with a good physical therapy regimen. Muscle strain has been reported to be the most common back injury in college athletes, with acute back injuries more prevalent (59%) than overuse injuries (12%).[17] Treatments generally consist of a short period of rest, the administration of nonsteroidal anti-inflammatory drugs, and ice application. The gradual inclusion of core strengthening and hamstring stretching programs along with conditioning programs and sport-related training has been successful.[18]

Spondylolysis

Spondylolysis is a fracture of the pars interarticularis and has an incidence of 4.4% to 6% in the general population, but it is much more prevalent in athletes[16] (**Figure 1**). Athletes who participate in hyperextension sports, including divers (43%), wrestlers (30%), throwing athletes (27%), weight lifters (23%), gymnasts (17%), and rowers

(17%), have an increased risk for spondylolysis. There is some familial predisposition for spondylolysis. Isthmic spondylolisthesis is associated with spondylolysis and is also commonly seen in patients who perform hyperextension activities (**Figure 2**). The most common level for spondylolisthesis is at L5-S1. For mild grade 1 (< 25% translation) or grade 2 (26% to 50% translation) spondylolisthesis as determined on a lateral radiograph, evaluation, nonsurgical treatment, and observation are the mainstays of treatment.

Lumbar Disk Degeneration and Herniation

Lumbar disk degeneration and herniation are uncommon in adolescents; however, adolescent athletes are more prone to this disorder, with a reported incidence between 30% and 75% compared with 14% to 30% for non-athletes.[13,19] The location of the disk disorder is dependent on the athlete's sport, with disk degeneration in the upper lumbar spine more common in weight lifters, and disk degeneration in the lower lumbar spine more common in soccer players. The incidence appears to be dependent on proper training techniques. A recent study reported that 21% of volleyball players with good technique have disk degeneration compared with 62% with poor technique.[20] The theory that disk degeneration is the pain generator in young athletes is controversial, and treatment is initially aimed at managing symptoms. Disk herniation is best treated nonsurgically, unless worsening neurologic deficits occur or if nonsurgical management is unsuccessful. If the apophyseal disk rupture is anterior, treatment is symptomatic only. If the apophyseal disk rupture is central, a Schmorl node is seen. If the apophyseal rupture is posterior, dural sac compression is common, and MRI is indi-

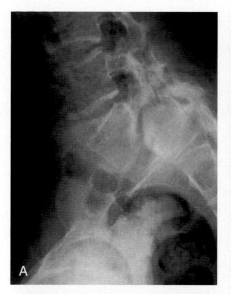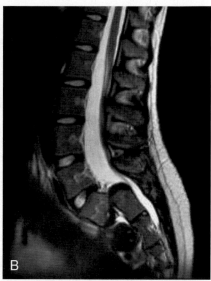

Figure 2   **A,** Lateral radiograph showing an L5-S1 high-grade spondylolisthesis. **B,** MRI scan of the spondylolisthesis.

cated to better characterize the underlying disk pathology, which may require surgical treatment.

Sacral Stress Fractures

Sacral stress fractures are very rare and are nearly exclusively seen in female long-distance runners.[21-23] The clinical presentation is usually an insidious onset of asymmetric low back pain without a history of acute injury. The hopping test, which produces pain with jumping up and down on the affected leg, is often diagnostic for this condition. Radiographs generally fail to show this injury, and early detection is made with MRI, which shows edema in the area of the stress fracture.[22] In patients with prolonged symptoms, a CT scan is diagnostic.

Nonsurgical Treatment
Prevention, Bracing, and Rehabilitation

Spondylolysis is frequently seen in athletes involved in activities that require repetitive hyperextension of the spine, including gymnasts, figure skaters, dancers, and football linemen.[24-27] The repetitive microtrauma caused by

this type of motion places significant stress on the region of the pars interarticularis (the narrow region of the vertebral elements lying between the superior and inferior facets), ultimately culminating in a stress fracture.[28] The suggestion that this injury occurs as a result of fatigue stress at the pars region is supported by the finding that 90% of pars interarticularis lesions heal following nonsurgical posterior spinal stabilization. It appears that controlling the fatiguing forces on this region allows lesions to heal without the need for surgery.[29] With continued activity and repetitive stress to the region, there is little likelihood of healing.

Injury prevention can be addressed by identifying risk factors, such as involvement in sports, that predispose the athlete to injury because of repetitive hyperextension of the lumbar spine. Core strengthening as a part of routine training regimens can help stabilize the lumbar spine by strengthening the surrounding muscular envelope. In athletes willing to consider alternatives, sports modification may allow the athlete to continue to be involved but potentially lessen the risk of

Table 3

Exercise Program for Back Pain Associated With Spondylolysis[a]

Exercise	Day 1	Weeks 4 to 6	
	Level 1	Level 2	Level 3
Abdominal muscles	Trunk rotation, feet down	Trunk rotation, knees to chest	Double knees to chest
	Marching	Bicycles	One half sit-up
	Crunches	One four sit-up	
Lumbar paraspinal muscles	Bridge in neutral pelvic tilt	Bridge with march in neutral with pelvic tilt	Bridge with knee extended in neutral with pelvic tilt
	Seated round overs to neutral	Leaning round overs to neutral	Standing round overs to neutral
Lower extremities	Wall slides or leg press	Wall slides or leg press	
Flexibility[b]	Rectus femoris, iliopsoas, quadriceps, single knee to chest, hamstrings, double knee to chest, and piriformis stretches		

[a]Spondylolysis progression: Before progressing to the next level, the patient should be pain free. The patient should begin with the degree of movement and number of repetitions that are comfortable. The patient should progress to the maximal amount of repetitions prescribed before moving to the next level.

[b]Hold each stretch for 30 seconds, release, and repeat (total, 60 seconds each)

developing a pars interarticularis lesion.

In treating spondylolysis, a successful outcome involves a pain-free return to sports and ideally a bony union at the pars interarticularis site. A stable pain-free fibrous union, however, can be quite functional.[30,31] It was once believed that pars interarticularis lesions did not heal, and management focused on significant activity modification (often the cessation of sports activities) or surgical management involving decompression and posterolateral fusion. After surgical treatment, participation in contact sports was restricted until fusion of the lesions was documented. In treating other spinal disorders, however, it was noted that most incidental pars interarticularis lesions healed following spinal fusion for other disorders; this finding suggested that these lesions could heal without directed surgical management.[29]

Activity modification remains the mainstay of conservative management of pars interarticularis lesions. Restricting activities that cause significant repetitive stress at the pars interarticularis region can lessen the repetitive stresses and provide time for the le-

sions to heal. Athletes treated at Children's Hospital Boston are generally restricted from participating in sports for the initial 4 to 6 weeks following the diagnosis of spondylolysis, after which time they are reassessed and allowed to return to sports with continued bracing if they remain asymptomatic.[32] Return to play without bracing is not considered until the athlete has remained pain free for 4 months from the time of initial treatment.

Muscular imbalances or tightness also can play a role in back pain and should be addressed through a focused physical therapy regimen. In particular, Williams-type flexion-directed spinal exercises in combination with generalized lumbosacral range-of-motion (antilordotic) and strengthening programs can be beneficial. Stretching should focus on the lumbodorsal fascia and the hamstring and abdominal muscles. These therapies are progressed in a pain-free fashion to prevent detrimental effects. The general progression of exercises is shown in **Table 3**.

Bracing for spondylolysis has improved significantly over the years. The underlying goal of brace treatment is

to restrict repetitive hyperextension of the lumbar spine and improve the sagittal alignment of the pars interarticularis by placing an antilordotic force on the lower spine. The braces, constructed of polypropylene or polyethylene, are modular and available in a variety of sizes. Three basic shapes are available that allow for varying degrees (set at 0°, 15°, or 30°) of antilordotic posturing.

Successful nonsurgical management of pars lesions has been reported in multiple studies[30,32-35] (**Table 4**). Although successful healing occurred in some patients, most lesions did not heal and remained symptomatic. Additional modalities, such as electromagnetic field stimulation, have been used in an attempt to improve healing.[36] A prospective, case-controlled study enrolled patients to receive brace treatment alone versus brace treatment with electrical stimulation (PA d'Hemecourt, MD, Boston, MA, unpublished data, 2010). The electrical stimulation treatment was administered for 3 hours daily, and both groups used a 0° modified Boston overlap brace that was to be worn 23 hours per day. Follow-up was performed at 4-month intervals after the initiation of treatment, and crossover was allowed at 4 months in the event of a painful nonunion. Fifty-six adolescent athletes were enrolled in the study. Bony union was documented in 13 of 26 patients in the brace-only group and 20 of 30 patients in the brace plus electrical stimulation group. Of the crossover patients, 6 of 7 progressed to a bony union. The additional effect of electrical stimulation is believed to result from stimulation of angiogenesis and upregulation of bone healing factors, particularly transforming growth factor-β1 and bone morphogenetic proteins 2, 4, 6, and 7.[37]

Management continues to focus on adjuvant therapies in an effort to improve the healing response. Bone stimulation using ultrasound therapy of short duration (20 to 30 minutes per day) and moderate magnitude can act to effect gene expression and increase angiogenesis.[38] There is also speculation regarding the potential benefit of various biologics, such as platelet-rich plasma, in the healing response.[39]

Surgical Treatment

Spondylolysis

Most young patients with spondylolysis do not require surgical treatment; however, in select patients, surgical treatment can provide pain relief and permit return to sports activities. The primary indication for surgical treatment of spondylolysis is unsuccessful relief of back pain with conservative treatment, which generally consists of a trunk and extremity strengthening program under the guidance of a physical therapist, together with a lumbosacral orthosis or thoracolumbosacral orthosis for 3 to 4 months in selected patients. If modification of sports activity is not an acceptable option to the teenage athlete, the pros and cons of surgical treatment should be thoroughly discussed, along with

Table 4

Reports of Success With Nonsurgical Treatment of Spondylolysis

Authors (Year)	Healing
Wiltse et al[33] (1975)	12/17 bone
Steiner and Micheli[30] (1985)	18% bone
Morita et al[35] (1995)	37.9% bone
d'Hemecourt et al[32] (2002)	50% union

the expected natural history (generally favorable through adult life) of spondylolysis without surgical treatment. It is often necessary to reassure the young athlete that continuing sports activities will not necessarily worsen the spondylolysis. With this reassurance, many young athletes will choose to tolerate the mild back pain and decline surgical treatment. If a young athlete is unable to continue to compete in his or her favorite sport because of back pain, surgery may be elected. There is a higher rate of spondylolysis in athletes and a higher rate of surgical treatment in competitive teenage athletes than in the average teenage patient with spondylolysis, at least in part because some athletes will not accept activity limitations.[40,41]

The primary surgical treatment options for spondylolysis are direct repair of the pars interarticularis stress fracture or posterior lumbar fusion. Direct repair can be done at any level but is more often done at the L3 or L4 level than at the L5 level. The advantage of direct repair is that lumbar motion is preserved without fusion. A direct repair is not indicated if spondylolisthesis is present. A preoperative MRI study is needed before direct surgical repair because direct repair is indicated primarily when there is no adjacent disk degeneration or "black disk" on the MRI scan. In general, young adults with spondylolysis have a higher number of black disks on MRI than do young adults without spondylolysis.

Three primary repair methods are generally used if surgical treatment is elected. Each technique includes débridement of the scar tissue in the pars interarticularis defect and repair of this defect with iliac crest autogenous bone graft. The techniques differ in the type of stabilization used to allow bony healing at the pars defect site.

The Buck technique uses intralaminar screw stabilization. A healing success rate of approximately 90% has been reported.[42] The Scott technique, in which wires are placed around the transverse process on each side and through the spinous process to compress the pars defect and bone graft area, is the least rigid of the fixation methods but has been reported to result in healing in 77% of patients.[43] The third fixation method involves the use of pedicle screws and infralaminar hooks attached to a short rod, with compression along the rod to stabilize the pars defect repair.[44] This instrumentation construct provides the most stable fixation and is somewhat bulkier than other implants but does not require removal. In two-level spondylolysis, direct repair may be done for one level and a fusion for the other (**Figure 3**).

One-level posterior or posterolateral fusion is most commonly used at the L5-S1 level. Fusion is indicated if any degree of spondylolisthesis, no matter how small, is present or if there is a degenerated disk at the L5-S1 level. Although posterior fusion can be done

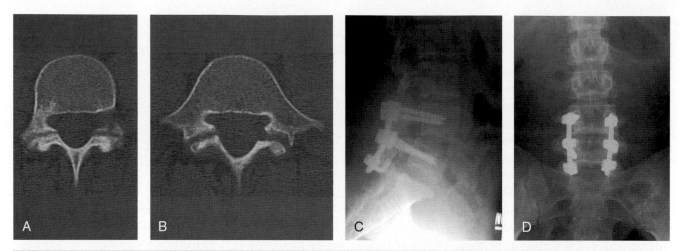

Figure 3 A 14-year-old girl who is a track and field athlete had persistent back pain despite conservative treatment. CT scanning showed a two-level spondylolysis at L4 (**A**) and L5 (**B**). An MRI scan showed a "black disk" at L4-L5. Postoperative lateral (**C**) and AP (**D**) radiographs after surgical treatment with spinal instrumentation and fusion of L4-L5, with direct repair of L5 spondylolysis using a pedicle screw/infralaminar hook construct. Pain was fully relieved, and the patient successfully returned to sports participation.

without spinal instrumentation, pedicle screw instrumentation with connecting rods is the currently preferred method of fixation. If pedicle screw instrumentation is used for this indication, it is important to place the autogenous iliac crest bone graft in the posterolateral position prior to placement of the connecting rod because the bulky nature of the implants makes it difficult to place this bone graft after instrumentation is complete.

Spondylolisthesis

The indications for surgical treatment of spondylolisthesis are more clear-cut than those for spondylolysis.[45] If the slip of the L5 vertebra on S1 is greater than 50% in a skeletally immature patient, surgical treatment is indicated, particularly if a progressive slip has been noted on serial radiographs. If the slip is less than 50%, the primary indication for surgical treatment is the persistence of pain despite conservative treatment. If significant and worsening hamstring tightness is associated with the slip, fusion is usually needed to relieve the hamstring tightness.

Surgical treatment of low lumbar spondylolisthesis always involves pos-

terolateral fusion. Other variable features of this surgery relate to fusing in situ or with partial reduction of the slipped vertebra, the option to include an L5 laminectomy, and the option to include an anterior bone graft through the transforaminal lumbar interbody fusion.[46]

Posterior lumbar fusion without any attempt at correction is generally performed with iliac crest autogenous bone graft placed in a posterolateral or posterior position.[47] Although casts can be used for postoperative stability to allow fusion in younger, slender children, most fusions are stabilized with a pedicle screw construct. Fusion without slip correction carries less risk of iatrogenic neurologic injury than attempted corrective fusion. To avoid unintended correction during pedicle screw instrumentation, the L5 pedicle screw should be left proud as the rod engages the screw heads to prevent pulling the L5 posteriorly. Bone graft should be placed posterolaterally before inserting the rods for final fixation.

Posterior lumbar fusion with correction of the slip deformity has an iat-

rogenic neurologic injury rate of 5% to 10%, with foot drop as the most common complication. Partial slip corrections are safer than attempts at full slip correction, but they still carry a risk of neurologic injury. Spinal cord monitoring, including dermatomal monitoring, is essential. Commonly, in patients with slips greater than 50%, the lamina of L5 should be removed and pedicle screws placed at L4, L5, and the sacrum. In these patients, the fusion must extend proximally into the lumbar lordosis, which means that the upper level is virtually always L4. Prior to correction attempts, it is important to perform foraminotomies to decompress the nerve roots at the level to be reduced in an attempt to limit the risk of neurologic injury. The position of the L5 pedicle screw and how proud it is positioned plays a major role in how much correction is attempted when the rod is engaged. For larger slips, a transforaminal lumbar interbody fusion should be considered to provide some anterior spinal support. Providing anterior column support in transforaminal lumbar interbody fusion is now more common; however, an anterior approach with a fibula strut could be performed in a patient with a severe slip.

Return to Sports

The return of adolescent athletes to sports following the treatment of low back pain is dependent on the spine disorder that caused the pain, the sport played, and whether surgery was required and the specific procedure performed.

After nonsurgical treatment of spondylolysis, most patients return to sports activities in a short period of time. Iwamoto et al[48] reported that 80% of adolescent athletes return to sports at 6 weeks with nonsurgical treatment. Patients who participated in high-risk sports and had an acute onset of symptoms and hamstring tightness had the worst outcomes. Return to sports after surgical treatment of spondylolysis varied. Debnath et al[40] reported on 22 young athletes treated with fusion for spondylolysis with an average duration of symptoms of 9 months and an average radiographic defect size of 3.5 mm. The average Oswestry Disability Index score improved from 39.5 to 10.7, and 82% of athletes returned to their previous sport after a rehabilitation program of 7 months (mean) duration. The Buck direct surgical repair achieved better results with respect to return to sports compared with the Scott wiring technique.

Return to sports following spondylolisthesis surgery is more controversial, and opinions on when athletes can resume activities vary among surgeons. Based on a survey administered to the Scoliosis Research Society membership, whether the spondylolisthesis was low grade (Myerding grades I and II) or high grade (Myerding grades III and IV) was an important consideration for surgeons that affected other criteria when recommending a patient's return

to sports.[49] The time since surgery was a moderately important or important consideration in 94% of the respondents for patients with low-grade slips and 92% of the respondents for patients with high-grade slips. The radiographic appearance of the fusion mass was important to 88% of the respondents for low-grade fusions and 84% for high-grade fusions. The patient's age was rated slightly or moderately important by 72% and 65% of respondents regarding patients with low- and high-grade slips, respectively. The chosen sport was moderately to greatly important for 71% and 68% of the respondents for low- and high-grade spondylolisthesis, respectively; and the surgeon's personal bias on returning the patient to sports was moderately to greatly important for 65% of the respondents treating patients with low-grade and 63% treating high-grade slips.

The patient's level of activities correlated with the timing of return to sports, with return to gym class at 6 months allowed by approximately 40% of the survey respondents, whereas approximately 65% of the respondents allowed patients to return to gym class at 1 year. Low-impact, noncontact sports were allowed at 6 months by 66% of the respondents and at 1 year by 22% of the respondents for athletes with grade I or II spondylolisthesis. Return to other noncontact sports was allowed at 6 months by 66% of the respondents and at 1 year by 22% of the respondents for athletes with grade I or II spondylolisthesis, by 62% for those with grade III spondylolisthesis, and by 23% for athletes with grade IV spondylolisthesis. For contact sports, such as basketball and soccer, 26% of the respondents did not allow return to participation for 6 months for patients with low-grade slips, and 56% of respondents did not allow return for 1

year. In patients with high-grade slips playing those sports, 20% of the respondents allowed return at 6 months, and 51% allowed return at 1 year. Return to collision sports, such as football, was allowed by 11% of the respondents at 6 months and 36% at 1 year for patients with low-grade slips, and by 10% of the respondents at 6 months and 27% at 1 year for their patients with high-grade slips. In some instances, patients were advised not to return to some sports, including gymnastics, football, rugby, wrestling, weight lifting, skydiving, and bungee jumping.[49]

The criteria used by this chapter's authors to return athletes to sports after spondylolisthesis surgery are based on symptoms, strength, and radiographic findings. Patients are allowed to return to sports when they are pain free, when near-normal strength has returned with good flexibility and endurance, and when solid fusion can be identified radiographically on both AP and lateral radiographs (**Figure 4**). In general, more patients are allowed to return to sports at 12 months than 6 months after surgery.

Iwamoto et al[50] reported that 79% of patients return to their original sport by 5 months after nonsurgical treatment for disk herniation. The intensity of the sport did not influence the decision to return to sports; however, the severity of symptoms before treatment inversely correlated with the ability to return to sports. In athletes treated surgically for disk herniation, 89% returned to varsity sports, and Medical Outcomes Study 36-Item Short Form scores improved to the same levels as those of noninjured athletes.[51] In patients treated with epidural injections, 40% to 50% returned to sports.[52]

In general, sports activity is diminished for patients with scoliosis and is dependent on perceived spine func-

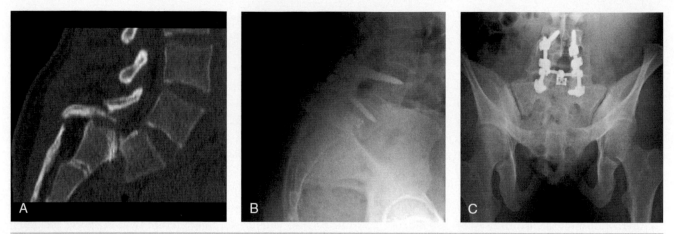

Figure 4 **A,** Preoperative CT scan showing high-grade spondylolisthesis. **B,** Lateral lumbosacral radiograph after all-posterior instrumentation and fusion with a posterior lumbar interbody fusion and translation of L5 on S1. Sagittal alignment was restored. **C,** AP radiograph shows excellent healing, especially between the transverse processes and the ala. The patient was allowed to return to full sports participation 1 year after surgery.

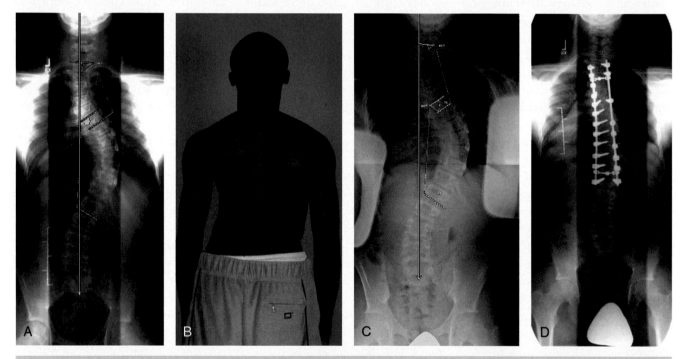

Figure 5 A 17-year-old boy with a 67° right thoracic scoliosis wanted to play contact football during his upcoming senior year. He did not have surgery until the completion of the football season and later had successful posterior fusion and instrumentation when the curve was 74°. **A,** PA standing radiograph showing the 67° curve at the time of diagnosis. **B,** Preoperative clinical photograph of the patient showing the right thoracic curve. **C,** PA standing radiograph showing the 74° curve at the time of surgery. **D,** Postoperative PA radiograph.

tion, back pain, and physical activity.[53] Surgical treatment or the extent of arthrodesis had no effect on participation in sporting activities; however, in surgically treated patients, the higher Cobb angle negatively correlated with

sports participation.[53] Surgeons hold differing opinions on whether patients with scoliosis should return to sporting activities.[49] The most important factors in the decision are the time from surgery, the use of instrumentation,

the chosen sport, the clinical progress of the patient, and the surgeon's habit or bias. A survey of the members of the Scoliosis Research Society showed that gym class activity was allowed at 6 months by 44% of the respondents and at 1 year by 44%. Noncontact sports were allowed at 6 months by 46% of the respondents and 1 year by 34%, whereas contact and collision sports were allowed at 1 year by 61% and 32%, respectively. Some scoliosis patients were told not to return to football, gymnastics, collision sports, and trampoline. The survey respondents also indicated that fusion between L2 and L4 did not influence the recommendation to return to sports, but when fusion was distal to L4, surgeons were unlikely to allow return to sports.

With the increasing use of pedicle screw fixation and the segmental placement of these implants, it is likely that surgeons will allow more widespread participation and earlier return to sporting activity. The greatest influence on the surgeon's decision regarding return to sports is the level of the distal extent of the instrumentation. The decision by one of this chapter's authors (DJS) on when to return patients to sporting activity is largely based on the level of fusion, whether instrumentation of the lumbar spine has occurred, and the chosen sporting activity. In general, patients treated with a thoracic fusion are allowed to return to only light training at 6 weeks, with return to full activities (with the exception of collision sports) at 3 months. For those with lumbar spine fusion, sports training can begin at 3 months, and full sports activity can resume at 6 months. Patients should be advised to avoid participation in collision sports after scoliosis surgery, which may require delaying surgery until the athlete has completed his or her career in the collision sport (**Figure 5**). Despite this recommendation, there is only a single reported case of spine injury during sporting activity in a 14-year-old patient who participated in gymnastics following thoracic scoliosis surgery without neurologic defi-

cit.[54] Other injuries after scoliosis surgery have occurred from high-energy trauma from a motor vehicle crash or a fall from a height;[55-58] no patient had permanent neurologic injury.

Summary

Back pain in adolescents is becoming increasingly common, and the incidence of back pain in young athletes is even greater than in teenagers who do not participate in sports. Most young athletes can be successfully treated conservatively with exercise and trunk strengthening programs, with time allowed for healing. The key to returning the young athlete to his or her sport is establishing an accurate diagnosis of the cause of the back pain through a careful history and physical examination, augmented (as needed) with appropriate imaging studies. Except for muscular disorders, spondylolysis is the most common cause of back pain in young athletes. Although nonsurgical treatment is generally adequate in treating spondylolysis, surgical treatment can be effective if back pain persists despite conservative measures. Whether treatment is nonsurgical or surgical, the goal is to allow young athletes to return to safe participation in their chosen sports activities.

References

1. Jones GT, Watson KD, Silman AJ, Symmons DP, Macfarlane GJ: Predictors of low back pain in British schoolchildren: A population-based prospective cohort study. *Pediatrics* 2003; 111(4 Pt 1):822-828.

2. Duggleby T, Kumar S: Epidemiology of juvenile low back pain: A review. *Disabil Rehabil* 1997; 19(12):505-512.

3. Taimela S, Kujala UM, Salminen JJ, Viljanen T: The prevalence of low back pain among children and adolescents: A nationwide, cohort-based questionnaire survey

in Finland. *Spine (Phila Pa 1976)* 1997;22(10):1132-1136.

4. Kim HJ, Green DW: Adolescent back pain. *Curr Opin Pediatr* 2008;20(1):37-45.

5. Swärd L, Hellstrom M, Jacobsson B, Pëterson L: Back pain and radiologic changes in the thoracolumbar spine of athletes. *Spine (Phila Pa 1976)* 1990;15(2): 124-129.

6. Lundin O, Hellström M, Nilsson I, Swärd L: Back pain and radiological changes in the thoracolumbar spine of athletes: A long-term follow-up. *Scand J Med Sci Sports* 2001;11(2):103-109.

7. Keene JS, Albert MJ, Springer SL, Drummond DS, Clancy WG Jr: Back injuries in college athletes. *J Spinal Disord* 1989;2(3): 190-195.

8. Kayser R, Mahlfeld K, Heyde CE, Grasshoff H, Mellerowicz H: Tight hamstring syndrome and extra- or intraspinal diseases in childhood: A multicenter study. *Eur Spine J* 2006;15(4):403-408.

9. Campbell RS, Grainger AJ, Hide IG, Papastefanou S, Greenough CG: Juvenile spondylolysis: A comparative analysis of CT, SPECT and MRI. *Skeletal Radiol* 2005;34(2):63-73.

10. Connolly LP, d'Hemecourt PA, Connolly SA, Drubach LA, Micheli LJ, Treves ST: Skeletal scintigraphy of young patients with low-back pain and a lumbosacral transitional vertebra. *J Nucl Med* 2003;44(6):909-914.

11. Sanpera I Jr, Beguiristain-Gurpide JL: Bone scan as a screening tool in children and adolescents with back pain. *J Pediatr Orthop* 2006; 26(2):221-225.

12. Anderson K, Sarwark JF, Conway JJ, Logue ES, Schafer MF: Quantitative assessment with SPECT imaging of stress injuries of the pars interarticularis and response to bracing. *J Pediatr Orthop* 2000; 20(1):28-33.

13. Bennett DL, Nassar L, DeLano MC: Lumbar spine MRI in the elite-level female gymnast with low back pain. *Skeletal Radiol* 2006;35(7):503-509.

14. Carrino JA, Lurie JD, Tosteson AN, et al: Lumbar spine: Reliability of MR imaging findings. *Radiology* 2009;250(1):161-170.

15. Ovadia D, Metser U, Lievshitz G, Yaniv M, Wientroub S, Even-Sapir E: Back pain in adolescents: Assessment with integrated 18F-fluoride positron-emission tomography-computed tomography. *J Pediatr Orthop* 2007;27(1):90-93.

16. Micheli LJ, Wood R: Back pain in young athletes: Significant differences from adults in causes and patterns. *Arch Pediatr Adolesc Med* 1995;149(1):15-18.

17. Keene JS, Drummond DS: Mechanical back pain in the athlete. *Compr Ther* 1985;11(1):7-14.

18. Dreisinger TE, Nelson B: Management of back pain in athletes. *Sports Med* 1996;21(4):313-320.

19. Maurer M, Soder RB, Baldisserotto M: Spine abnormalities depicted by magnetic resonance imaging in adolescent rowers. *Am J Sports Med* 2011;39(2):392-397.

20. Bartolozzi C, Caramella D, Zampa V, Dal Pozzo G, Tinacci E, Balducci F: The incidence of disk changes in volleyball players: The magnetic resonance findings. *Radiol Med* 1991;82(6):757-760.

21. McFarland EG, Giangarra C: Sacral stress fractures in athletes. *Clin Orthop Relat Res* 1996;329:240-243.

22. Johnson AW, Weiss CB Jr, Stento K, Wheeler DL: Stress fractures of the sacrum: An atypical cause of low back pain in the female athlete. *Am J Sports Med* 2001;29(4):498-508.

23. Shah MK, Stewart GW: Sacral stress fractures: An unusual cause of low back pain in an athlete. *Spine (Phila Pa 1976)* 2002;27(4):E104-E108.

24. Micheli LJ, McCarthy C: The spine in sports, in Watkins RG, ed: *Figure Skating.* St Louis, MO, Mosby, 1990, pp 557-564.

25. Micheli LJ: Back injuries in gymnastics. *Clin Sports Med* 1985;4(1):85-93.

26. Micheli LJ, Kasser JR: Case report 6: Painful spondylolysis in a young football player, in Hochschuler SH, ed: *The Spine in Sports.* Philadelphia, PA, Hanley and Belfus, 1990, pp 327-330.

27. Micheli LJ, Micheli ER: Back injuries in dancers, in Shell CG, ed: *The 1984 Olympic Scientific Congress Proceedings, Vol 8: The Dancer as Athlete.* Champaign, IL, Human Kinetics, 1986, pp 91-94.

28. Farfan HF, Osteria V, Lamy C: The mechanical etiology of spondylolysis and spondylolisthesis. *Clin Orthop Relat Res* 1976;117:40-55.

29. O'Neill DB, Micheli LJ: Postoperative radiographic evidence for fatigue fracture as the etiology in spondylolysis. *Spine (Phila Pa 1976)* 1989;14(12):1342-1355.

30. Steiner ME, Micheli LJ: Treatment of symptomatic spondylolysis and spondylolisthesis with the modified Boston brace. *Spine (Phila Pa 1976)* 1985;10(10):937-943.

31. Muschik M, Hähnel H, Robinson PN, Perka C, Muschik C: Competitive sports and the progression of spondylolisthesis. *J Pediatr Orthop* 1996;16(3):364-369.

32. d'Hemecourt PA, Zurakowski D, Kriemler S, Micheli LJ: Spondylolysis: Returning the athlete to sports participation with brace treatment. *Orthopedics* 2002;25(6):653-657.

33. Wiltse LL, Widell EH Jr, Jackson DW: Fatigue fracture: The basic lesion is isthmic spondylolisthesis. *J Bone Joint Surg Am* 1975;57(1):17-22.

34. Blanda J, Bethem D, Moats W, Lew M: Defects of pars interarticularis in athletes: A protocol for nonoperative treatment. *J Spinal Disord* 1993;6(5):406-411.

35. Morita T, Ikata T, Katoh S, Miyake R: Lumbar spondylolysis in children and adolescents. *J Bone Joint Surg Br* 1995;77(4):620-625.

36. Fellander-Tsai L, Micheli LJ: Treatment of spondylolysis with external electrical stimulation and bracing in adolescent athletes: A report of two cases. *Clin J Sport Med* 1998;8:232-242.

37. Jervey C, Friedman RJ: Electrical stimulation: Current concepts and indications. *Contemp Orthop* 1990;20(1):61-65.

38. Watanabe Y, Matsushita T, Bhandari M, Zdero R, Schemitsch EH: Ultrasound for fracture healing: Current evidence. *J Orthop Trauma* 2010;24(Suppl 1):S56-S61.

39. Kanthan SR, Kavitha G, Addi S, Choon DS, Kamarul T: Platelet-rich plasma (PRP) enhances bone healing in non-united critical-sized defects: A preliminary study involving rabbit models. *Injury* 2011;42(8):782-789.

40. Debnath UK, Freeman BJ, Gregory P, de la Harpe D, Kerslake RW, Webb JK: Clinical outcome and return to sport after the surgical treatment of spondylolysis in young athletes. *J Bone Joint Surg Br* 2003;85(2):244-249.

41. Rossi F, Dragoni S: Lumbar spondylolysis: Occurrence in competitive athletes: Updated achievements in a series of 390 cases. *J Sports Med Phys Fitness* 1990;30:450-452.

42. Buck JE: Direct repair of the defect in spondylolisthesis: Preliminary report. *J Bone Joint Surg Br* 1970;52(3):432-437.

43. Johnson GV, Thompson AG: The Scott wiring technique for direct repair of lumbar spondylolysis.

J Bone Joint Surg Br 1992;74(3): 426-430.

44. Roca J, Iborra M, Cavanilles-Walker JM, Albertí G: Direct repair of spondylolysis using a new pedicle screw hook fixation: Clinical and CT-assessed study. An analysis of 19 patients. *J Spinal Disord Tech* 2005;18(Suppl): S82-S89.

45. Klein G, Mehlman CT, McCarty M: Nonoperative treatment of spondylolysis and grade I spondylolisthesis in children and young adults: A meta-analysis of observational studies. *J Pediatr Orthop* 2009;29(2):146-156.

46. Lauber S, Schulte TL, Liljenqvist U, Halm H, Hackenberg L: Clinical and radiologic 2-4-year results of transforaminal lumbar interbody fusion in degenerative and isthmic spondylolisthesis grades 1 and 2. *Spine (Phila Pa 1976)* 2006;31(15):1693-1698.

47. Lamberg TS, Remes VM, Helenius IJ, et al: Long-term clinical, functional and radiological outcome 21 years after posterior or posterolateral fusion in childhood and adolescence isthmic spondylolisthesis. *Eur Spine J* 2005; 14(7):639-644.

48. Iwamoto J, Takeda T, Wakano K: Returning athletes with severe low back pain and spondylolysis to original sporting activities with conservative treatment. *Scand J Med Sci Sports* 2004;14(6): 346-351.

49. Rubery PT, Bradford DS: Athletic activity after spine surgery in children and adolescents: Results of a survey. *Spine (Phila Pa 1976)* 2002;27(4):423-427.

50. Iwamoto J, Takeda T, Sato Y, Wakano K: Short-term outcome of conservative treatment in athletes with symptomatic lumbar disc herniation. *Am J Phys Med Rehabil* 2006;85(8):667-674, quiz 675-677.

51. Wang JC, Shapiro MS, Hatch JD, Knight J, Dorey FJ, Delamarter RB: The outcome of lumbar discectomy in elite athletes. *Spine (Phila Pa 1976)* 1999;24(6): 570-573.

52. Jackson DW, Rettig A, Wiltse LL: Epidural cortisone injections in the young athletic adult. *Am J Sports Med* 1980;8(4):239-243.

53. Parsch D, Gärtner V, Brocai DR, Carstens C, Schmitt H: Sports activity of patients with idiopathic

scoliosis at long-term follow-up. *Clin J Sport Med* 2002;12(2): 95-98.

54. Fuchs PD, Bertrand S, Iwinski H, Pellet J: Traumatic C6-C7 dislocation in a 14 year old with posterior spinal fusion for idiopathic scoliosis. *J Trauma* 2001;51(5): 1004-1007.

55. King HA, Bradford DS: Fracture-dislocation of the spine after spine fusion and Harrington instrumentation for idiopathic scoliosis: A case report. *J Bone Joint Surg Am* 1980;62(8):1374-1376.

56. Ebraheim NA, Cecil ML: Seatbelt-type fracture of the lumbar spine following instrumentation and fusion. *Orthopedics* 1995; 18(10):1036-1038.

57. Neyt JG, Weinstein SL: Fracture-dislocation of the lumbar spine after arthrodesis with instrumentation for idiopathic scoliosis. *J Bone Joint Surg Am* 1999;81(1): 111-114.

58. Tuffley DJ, McPhee IB: Fracture of the spine after spinal fusion for idiopathic scoliosis. *Spine (Phila Pa 1976)* 1984;9(5):538-539.

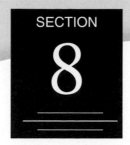

SECTION 8

Sports Medicine

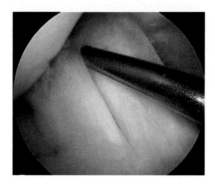

Diagnosis and Management of Patients
With Instability of the Knee

Kelly G. Vince, MD, FRCSC

Abstract

Instability of a total knee arthroplasty is a fundamentally different problem from instability of the knee without an arthroplasty. Revision surgery to correct the inciting forces will usually be necessary, and ligament reconstruction alone is usually unsuccessful. Because it may be the presenting complaint for any of the usual conditions that require revision arthroplasty, instability as reported by a patient should be considered a symptom that requires detailed evaluation rather than immediate surgery. Evaluation should be systematic and comprehensive, meaning that the same algorithm or system should be applied to all knee arthroplasties, and all diagnostic entities should be considered.

There are several common types of instability, each requiring a different surgical strategy. Any dysfunction of the extensor mechanism, including pain inhibition (even from the ipsilateral hip) may result in buckling. Structural recurvatum, often originating from relative quadriceps weakness, may require arthrodesis if extensor function is completely absent. Varus or valgus instability will require stabilization in the form of constrained implants, with or without ligament releases, advancements, or substitution. Realignment will almost always be advantageous. Flexion instability is invariably linked to flexion gaps that are larger or more lax than the extension gap, requiring revision with attention to gap balance, and in many cases, some degree of mechanically constrained devices.

Arthritic knee joints in obese patients and those with severe angular deformity or fixed flexion contractures are at particular risk for instability after total knee arthroplasty. Instability that becomes apparent intraoperatively is a challenging condition, particularly when there is no immediate recourse to using constrained implants.

Instr Course Lect 2012;61:515-524.

The treatment of instability in a total knee arthroplasty (TKA) should differ from approaches to treating an unstable but otherwise normal human knee.

For example, ligament reconstructions without revision arthroplasty tend to be unsuccessful for treating an unstable knee arthroplasty.[1] Krackow[2] clarified the importance of component position and axial alignment in revision knee arthroplasy. Arthroplasty changes the knee in ways (such as excess valgus alignment or a small femoral component) that may destabilize the joint. Unless corrected, the resultant forces overwhelm ligament reconstructions and either break or loosen constrained implants. Similarly, isolated exchange of modular polyethylene inserts usually fails to restore stability.[3]

By definition, a TKA with primary instability has structural failure of supporting soft tissues (plastic deformation) or the inability of these soft tissues to function because of the component size and/or position. Revision TKA for instability can produce the best results for any particular failure mode if an insightful analytical approach is used to plan the reconstruction.[4-10]

Diagnosis

Instability must be carefully evaluated. The patient reporting an unstable arthroplasty is describing a symptom rather than providing a diagnosis.

Dr. Vince or an immediate family member has received royalties from Zimmer; is a member of a speakers' bureau or has made paid presentations on behalf of Zimmer; and serves as a paid consultant to Zimmer.

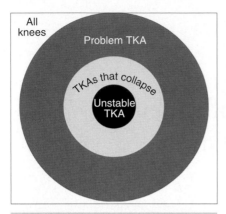

Figure 1 Concentric circle diagram of all "problem TKAs" on the backdrop of all knees. The classification of "TKAs that collapse" is a subset of all "problem TKAs," most of which present with pain. But true primary instability or the classification of "unstable TKAs" (the result of ligaments that have failed or that do not function because of component positioning or size) is a subset of all knees that collapse.

Table 1

Checklist for a Systematic and Comprehensive Approach to Diagnosing a TKA Failure[a]

Sequence	Diagnostic Consideration
1	Infection
2	Extensor mechanism rupture
3	Stiffness
4	Tibial femoral instability
5	Patella and malrotation
6	Loosening
7	Fracture
8	Breakage
9	No diagnosis

[a]Every TKA failure should be subjected to the same algorithmic evaluation or diagnostic system. In this system the presence of infection is considered, then extensor function, etc. Comprehensive implies that even though one diagnosis is identified, all diagnoses must be considered for a complete understanding of the problem.

Before treating instability, the joint should be evaluated in the broad context of all possible TKA complications and then in the more restricted context of TKAs that "give way" (**Figure 1**). A systematic and comprehensive approach is required. According to one diagnostic scheme, eight modes of failure, which are based on the functional elements required by every knee arthroplasty, can reasonably benefit from revision TKA[11-13] (**Table 1**). Systematic evaluation stipulates that the same diagnostic algorithm should be applied to every problem TKA. For example, each diagnostic category should be considered for every knee with instability, preferably in sequence. A knee may collapse because of pain from any of the eight diagnostic categories. Even stiffness may present with instability. Comprehensive means that just because one diagnosis (such as tibial-femoral instability) has been identified, all others must still be considered. The unstable knee might also be infected.

When instability is diagnosed, a thorough mechanical assessment is essential prior to surgery. The obvious distinction is the TKA with grossly loose components or a periprosthetic supracondylar fracture that may be unstable, but is not a case of primary instability (**Figure 2**). The TKA with grossly loose components may be stabilized with well-placed, correctly sized, solidly fixed implants. The TKA with a periprosthetic fracture may be treated with fixation; constrained implants and ligament reconstruction will not be necessary. Distressing varus-valgus instability may result from bone loss, prosthetic breakage, or polyethylene wear; a successful revision must focus on the causes of the instability.

In knees with primary instability, the direction of instability, the deficient structures, and the inciting forces

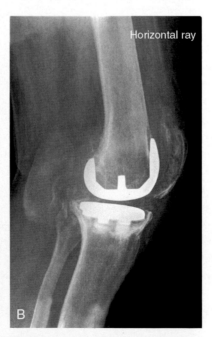

Figure 2 AP (**A**) and lateral (**B**) radiographs of a TKA that the patient described as unstable. This knee can be successfully revised with a nonconstrained implant because the instability primarily results from loosening with subsidence. The ligamentous support structures are intact and can be made to function normally by a revision for loosening.

Table 2
Total Knee Arthroplasty Instability

		Deficiency	Inciting Force
Coronal	Varus	Lateral collateral ligament, iliotibial band	Varus alignment
	Valgus	Medial collateral ligament	Valgus alignment
Sagittal	Buckling (flexion)	Extensor mechanism	Potentially: pain, fixed flexion deformity, recurvatum, maltracking, quadriceps insufficiency
	Recurvatum	Posterior capsule	Extensor insufficiency
Flexion	Posterior subluxation/dislocation	Flexion gap larger than extension gap, extensor mechanism insufficiency (for example, patellectomy)	Potential: hamstring spasticity
	Anterior subluxation/dislocation	Flexion gap larger than extension gap	Excess tibial posterior slope

must be determined. Instability may occur in two directions each for the frontal and sagittal planes: varus, valgus, recurvatum, and buckling (**Table 2**). The load imparted to the joint changes with posture and gait and is the deforming force responsible for joint collapse. The knee, like a four-legged table, requires medial and lateral plus posterior and anterior stabilizers (**Figure 3**). The medial and lateral collateral ligaments stabilize the knee in the frontal plane, and synchronous interaction of the posterior structures with the extensor mechanism provides both motion and stability in the sagittal plane. Stability of a TKA in the plane of joint motion, from full extension to maximum flexion, also depends heavily on the prosthesis size, position, and geometry.

Infection

Infection must be considered in all TKAs prior to revision, with analysis of the erythrocyte sedimentation rate and C-reactive protein level from peripheral blood samples. If these levels are elevated, aspiration of the TKA for white cell count, differential white cell count, and culture with sensitivity will be necessary.[14] Single-leg, weight-bearing, AP and lateral radiographs are helpful. Full-length radiographs, showing the hip, knee, and ankle on

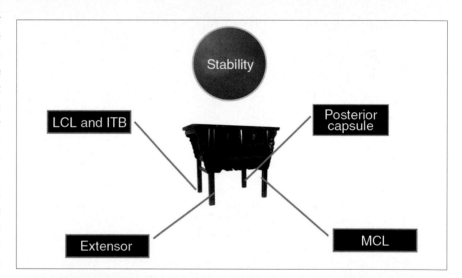

Figure 3   Stability of a TKA is best understood with three-dimensional thinking. Like a four-legged table, the TKA has medial and lateral stabilizers, as well as the extensor mechanism in the front and the posterior soft tissues. Failure to appreciate this relationship can lead to failed treatment plans, such as the misguided insertion of progressively thicker polyethylene as a treatment for an MCL with plastic deformation. As releases are performed on the lateral side to approximate the length of the MCL, thicker polyethylene inserts place the posterior structures under tension until a fixed flexion deformity and persistent valgus deformity result. LCL = lateral collateral ligament, ITB = iliotibial band.

the same image, provide essential information for planning ideal revision alignment and may obviate the need for an AP pelvic radiograph to assess the hip joint. Patellofemoral imaging provides important (albeit static) information about patellar tracking and consequently about the state of tibial and femoral component rotational po-

sitioning (**Figure 4**). CT provides insight regarding component rotation in many complications, including instability.[15,16]

Instability in the Plane of Motion

Patients whose extensor mechanism buckles and those with medial liga-

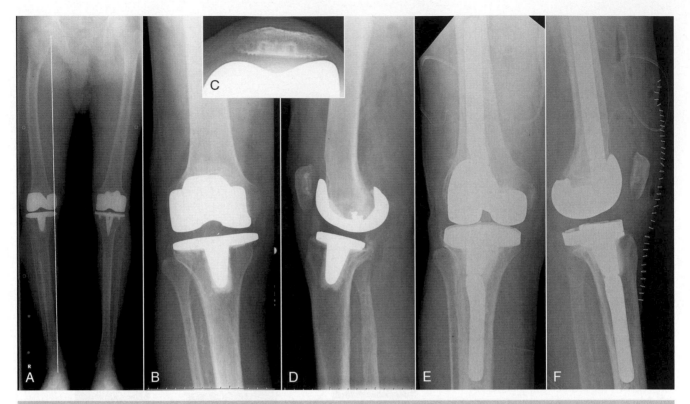

Figure 4   **A,** Full-length AP radiograph showing varus mechanical alignment in a patient with varus instability. **B,** Single-leg, weight-bearing AP radiograph showing varus instability under loading. **C,** Merchant patellofemoral view showing central tracking of the resurfaced patella, indicating correct rotational positioning of the tibial and femoral components. **D,** Lateral, single-leg, weight-bearing radiograph showing full extension under load with neither fixed contracture nor recurvatum, but with a high degree of posterior slope contributing to instability in flexion. **E,** AP radiograph (leg slightly internally rotated) immediately after revision TKA, showing correction of varus alignment with purposeful lateral reaming of the femoral stem extension against the lateral endosteum of the femur with compensatory centralization of the femoral component distally using an offset stem. **F,** Lateral radiograph after revision with reduction of the posterior tibial slope, which indicates the multifactorial assessment necessary in most revision TKAs performed because of instability.

ment failure will report instability; however, it is essential to discriminate between the two disorders. Questioning and attentive listening may help the patient recall if the knee is bending spontaneously or wobbling from side to side. Buckling results from any compromise to the extensor mechanism function, including pain inhibition or muscle shutdown from nociceptive experience. The pain that causes buckling may originate in the knee, the ipsilateral hip, or the spine.

Patients with a fixed flexion TKA deformity may experience quadriceps fatigue and instability. These patients require more energy to walk[17] because stability in midstance depends com-

pletely on quadriceps action. When the muscle inevitably becomes exhausted, the knee collapses. By contrast, the patient with polio, spinal stenosis, or other neurologic compromise of extensor power depends on recurvatum for stability. The knee will buckle if it is not hyperextended and will lock during the stance phase. The cause of recurvatum from extensor paralysis is unknown and is a significant complication of knee arthroplasty surgery. This complication does not respond to ligament reconstruction or prosthetic constraint. As a result, the neurologic contraindications to TKA (genu recurvatum from neurologic origin and gross quadriceps weakness as

enumerated by Insall in 1984) still apply.[18] If these factors are the basis for instability, arthrodesis rather than revision will provide a more reliable outcome for the patient

Although the classic cause of recurvatum deformity is neurologic extensor dysfunction, hyperextension also can occur when the quadriceps has the potential for excellent function. For example, if the patella is a source of chronic pain, patients may adopt a "patellar avoidance" or stiff-legged gait, thrusting the knee backward to maintain extension and minimize patellofemoral joint reaction forces. Eventually, this gait stretches the posterior capsule and creates structural re-

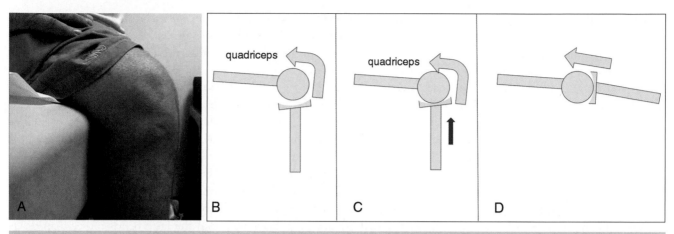

Figure 5   **A,** Photograph of the knee of a patient with a flexion instability seated on the edge of the examination table with the quadriceps muscle relaxed. The tibia has descended and is not in contact with the posterior femoral condyles because the flexion gap is larger than the extension gap and the modular polyethylene was selected to accommodate full extension. Illustrations of the effects of patient-initiated extension: **B,** The quadriceps first pulls the tibia up. **C,** No extension occurs until the tibia is pulled into contact with the femoral condyles (arrow). **D,** After contact, extension is possible. This complication originates in an uncorrected fixed flexion deformity.

curvatum. The quadriceps muscle atrophies. Until the patellofemoral pain is eliminated, the structural deformity corrected with arthroplasty, and the extensor rehabilitated, this deformity will persist or worsen despite TKA.

Recurvatum deformity worsens as the load on the patella increases, such as occurs in obese patients. A telling observation of the deformity in a minority of arthritic knees is hyperextension when a fixed flexion contracture would be expected. These patients should be assessed for patellofemoral pain, and achieving gap balancing may be challenging.

Relative extensor mechanism weakness without anterior knee pain can result from patellectomy; actual muscle strength may be normal or even above average. Without the mechanical advantage of a patella, relative extensor weakness ensues and the patient may adopt back-kneeing and recurvatum as compensatory mechanisms. This situation often accompanies transverse patellar fractures that have been treated unsuccessfully with open reduction and internal fixation, often with multiple attempts that effectively comprise a patellectomy. Extensor mechanism al-

lograft substitution for a missing patella can specifically treat this cause of instability, but concurrent revision will be necessary if recurvatum has occurred[19,20] (M Bedard, MD, K Vince, MD, unpublished data presented at the Canadian Orthopedic Association annual meeting, Whistler, British Columbia, Canada, 2009) (**Figure 5**).

A careful physical examination of patellar tracking, with attention to clues of internal rotation positioning of the tibial and/or femoral components may identify patellar maltracking or even frank dislocation as the source of instability; this can be confirmed with CT.[21] Revision surgery to reorient the patellar track by readjusting the rotational position of the tibial and femoral components will be necessary. Constrained components alone, especially if placed in the same internally rotated position, will not successfully treat patellar maltracking.

In cases in which femoral component subsidence and extensive bone loss result in recurvatum, revision arthroplasty with reconstitution of the defective distal femur will be needed. Linked constrained implants are sometimes considered to treat recurvatum

because they feature a mechanical hyperextension stop as part of the mechanism. Although seemingly reasonable, the hinge is rarely a durable solution to this problem. Removing all recurvatum in a patient with a truly paralyzed extensor will cause the knee to buckle. If some hyperextension is left for stability, the "back knee" gait will increase and break the extension stop or loosen the prosthesis. It is important to consider that the ratio of the lever arms between the tibial shaft and the small internal mechanical stop resembles that of a crowbar.

Varus-Valgus Instability

Instability in the coronal plane typifies the unstable TKA. The resultant gait (usually valgus) includes a medial thrust at the knee with the upper body lurching toward the affected side during the stance phase; this is usually obvious when gait is observed from a distance. Considering ligament reconstruction or hinged arthroplasty to treat the condition may indicate an incomplete assessment of the problem. Although these procedures can provide stability, the forces that lead to the instability must be considered.

For several decades, valgus alignment of approximately 5° of the anatomic axis (defined as the divergence between the intramedullary axes of the femur and tibia) has been the desired alignment for a TKA.[22] This method of alignment has been the standard frame of reference since alignment was first considered important in TKA surgery.[23] It was originally used because standard radiographs are relatively short, and it has remained the frame of reference because of the wide use of intramedullary instrumentation-referenced alignment from the canals.[24] A longer view of the entire lower limb[25] and the spine in cases of scoliosis is useful in understanding a TKA that is unstable in the coronal plane.

There has been a general assumption, facilitated by navigation technology, that ideal TKA alignment of the lower extremity results from achieving collinear lines from the hip to the knee and the knee to the ankle (the neutral mechanical axis). Although achieving a neutral axis may be appealing, it does not correspond to equal loading on the medial and lateral polyethylene surfaces or to equal tension on the medial and lateral collateral ligaments.

The loading situation becomes more complex with the consideration of the dynamism of gait and the location of the body's center of gravity (generally situated just anterior to the sacrum) as it migrates through the gait cycle. If hip pain or abductor weakness necessitates a shift in the center of gravity over the painful joint, this shift has implications for the knee, usually imparting a medial moment and valgus deforming force. Similarly, pathology at the ankle, most commonly a ruptured tibialis posterior tendon and acquired flatfoot deformity, will exacerbate the medial moment at the knee. Although there has been recent debate concerning the importance of the neutral mechanical axis, a strong biomechanical argument can be made that in knee failure caused by coronal instability, overcorrection in the revision arthroplasty may be desirable to mitigate destructive forces.[26]

Soft tissue in a failed TKA will have altered unpredictably as a result of scarring or plastic deformation. Accordingly, the classic techniques that work well in releasing ligaments in a primary arthroplasty are not generally appropriate for revision surgery. Only ligaments that should have been released at the time of the primary TKA, but were not released, will respond. In an unstable knee, the more common scenario is that the soft tissues need to be tighter or shorter. Only ligaments with persistent structural integrity may be advanced through a process of detachment from bone and reattachment at a point more distant from the joint.[2,27] In general a relatively crude isometry prevails—if the joint needs to be tighter in extension it should be reattached more proximally, and if it needs to be tighter in flexion it should be reattached more anteriorly. When global tightening is necessary, the reattachment is done more proximally and more anteriorly. Allograft ligaments (usually the Achilles tendon with a bone block) have been used to supplement deficient collateral ligaments.[28]

TKA with coronal plane instability usually requires revision surgery that reduces and perhaps overcorrects angulation in the direction of the instability with a mechanically constrained implant that substitutes for the failed soft tissues. Ligament allografting may supplement this approach.

Flexion Instability

Some of the earliest experiences with flexion instability involved the posterior tibial dislocation of early cruciate-sacrificing devices implanted in patients with patellectomies. As the hamstring muscles pull on the posterior proximal tibia to flex the knee, the tibia first translates directly posteriorly under the rounded femoral condyles. In the normal human knee joint, the posterior cruciate ligament resists translation and converts this force into flexion. Arthroplasty designs for patients without a posterior cruciate ligament rely on the "uphill principle," that is, as the femoral condyle begins to ride up on the anterior part of the tibia, the collateral ligaments tighten and the knee bends rather than dislocates. The patella helps resist posterior tibial dislocation because it is connected to the anterior tibia and buttressed against the anterior femoral condyles. In one study, the incidence of posterior tibial dislocation with the Total Condylar Prosthesis (Cintor, Raynham, MA) in patients treated with patellectomy was so high that patellectomy was regarded as a contraindication to the use of the prosthesis.[29]

The concept of balanced flexion and extension gaps is fundamental to ensuring that knees flex, extend, and remain stable.[30] The TKA with a flexion gap more spacious (or lax) than the extension gap is at risk for instability. These patients rapidly achieve superior flexion. Within months, laxity becomes troublesome and patients describe knee instability without the knee actually giving way. Recurrent effusions are common, along with soft-tissue tenderness, particularly about the pes anserinus tendon. Positive posterior drawer tests and sag signs are common.[31] A study by Pagnano et al[31] reported that surgery using thicker modular polyethylene inserts was successful in only one of three cases, highlighting the importance of balanced gaps. Even though the authors described success in 19 of 22 knees revised to posterior stabilized implants, a strong argument should be made that a surgical technique that balances flexion and extension gaps is as important as a semiconstrained implant.

Mechanical constraint alone does not guard against flexion instability. Posterior stabilized devices may be characterized by their "jump height" or the flexion gap laxity that can be resisted by the spine and cam mechanism before the tibial spine dislocates and locks behind the femoral cam, without necessarily dislocating the knee joint.[32-34] The knee will be locked painfully in flexion until reduced by hyperflexion and anterior displacement of the proximal tibia.

Posterior stabilized implants may have flexion instability without spine and cam dislocation. The sense of instability without giving way, recurrent effusions and soft-tissue tenderness, and substantial anterior translation at 90° of flexion are reminiscent of instability in the cruciate-retaining device.[35] Flexion instability can be confirmed by carefully observing the patient seated on the edge of the examination table as he or she initiates extension from 90° of flexion (**Figure 5**). Manual distraction of the tibia from the posterior femoral condyle while the patient relaxes with the knee flexed to 90° will confirm laxity more successfully than the posterior drawer test.

The origin of flexion instability is usually simple. Imagine a patient with arthritis and a fixed, flexion deformity. The surgeon who dutifully follows the sequence of bone cuts and applies sizing devices according to the product manual without soft-tissue releases or other adaptations for the contracture will produce a knee with a flexion gap of normal dimensions and a smaller, tight extension gap. If a modular tibial polyethylene insert is selected to permit full extension, flexion instability will result. The physical examination of this TKA can be misleading if the surgeon forgets that in full extension, the posterior structures are tight and give the false impression of stability. As

is the case with the examination of an injured athlete with a suspected medial collateral ligament (MCL) tear, the knee must be assessed in approximately 30° of flexion to relax the posterior structures and reveal instability. This condition is often described incorrectly as midflexion instability when it is simple flexion instability.

Flexion instability is an easily understood condition, resulting from a flexion gap that is larger than the extension gap, with maximal laxity at approximately 90° of flexion. A different condition termed midflexion instability has been described in revision arthroplasty, manifesting as rotational instability to combined external rotation and valgus stress in the position between 45° and 90° of flexion.[36] Another subtle form of flexion instability has been described as condylar liftoff; it usually involves liftoff of the lateral femoral condyle of the flexed knee from the tibial articular surface. This condition has been documented with sophisticated video radiography studies by Dennis et al.[37] Although condylar liftoff may contribute to eccentric wear, only patients with satisfactory knee function were evaluated in this study, and none reported functional instability. It would be inappropriate to recommend revision arthroplasty based on this finding alone.

A surgical technique that evaluates and balances flexion and extension gaps is the key to avoiding flexion instability in primary surgery and preventing it in revision surgery. In a primary arthroplasty, when flexion contractures cannot be corrected with release of the posterior capsule, resection of additional distal femoral bone is appropriate. In revision surgery, a larger femoral component in conjunction with a standard three-step technique will address the problem.[38,39] The first step in the technique requires the establishment of a tibial platform,

which will be common to both the flexion and extension gaps. The flexion gap will be reconstructed during the second step by the selection and positioning of the appropriately sized femoral component. The third step reconstructs the extension gaps as a function of the proximal distal position of the femoral component.[38]

Increased Risk of Instability

Certain clinical factors increase the risk of instability after TKA, including large deformities, valgus deformities, patient obesity, and flexion contractures. Careful preoperative planning helps to avoid complications.[40] Large, angular deformities in an arthritic knee imply significant asymmetry in collateral ligament tension from one side of the knee to the other. It is tempting to believe that the stabilizing structures on the concave side of a deformity have contracted and that classic releases will restore normality. In fact, large deformities are more likely to create disabling pathology from stretching and plastic deformation of soft tissue on the convex side of the joint. In these instances, releases on the inner side cannot lengthen ligaments to the extent that they will balance the outer side of the deformity. Ligament releases (lengthenings) are only effective after a thicker polyethylene insert brings all structures under tension.[41] There are four sides to the knee, and a thicker polyethylene insert eventually tightens the posterior structures, resulting in a flexion contracture. The solution is the preoperative provision of constrained implants when failed ligaments are anticipated in knees with severe angular deformity.

All TKAs in arthritic knees with valgus deformities, with or without patellar tracking problems, appear to be at risk for instability. This is probably because of the osseous pathology, the importance of the MCL for TKA stability, and the stress placed on the MCL by valgus deformity. A smaller, lateral femoral condyle, both distally and posteriorly, is usually part of the valgus deformity. Accordingly, there is a risk that most distal femoral cutting guides will fall into excess valgus during surgery, and rotational guides referencing from the posterior articular surface will fall into internal rotation. Valgus alignment increases potentially destructive tensile loads on the MCL, and internal rotation may cause patellar maltracking. When valgus pathology has damaged the MCL, some degree of constrained component will be essential. Ligament allografting is feasible but more difficult.

The obese patient is probably at greater risk for early instability following TKA than late failure from loosening. The early instability may result from a combination of a difficult exposure where the collateral ligaments may be avulsed and the difficulties in visualizing component positioning.[42] A wide-based gait (and resultant valgus moment on the joint), recurvatum to decrease patellar load (recurvatum), and shifting the center of gravity over the limb in the stance phase to decrease hip abductor load (valgus moment at the knee) result in damaging forces in the knee joint. All of these factors must be considered when revision is planned for TKA instability.

Intraoperative and Late Instability

Intraoperative instability may take the form of patellar maltracking, varus-valgus laxity, and/or inability to balance flexion and extension gaps. Laxity that cannot be corrected with conventional ligament releases can be anticipated in knees with valgus osteoarthritis, especially where the joint space of the medial compartment exceeds 8 mm,[43] which implies failure of the MCL (a type II valgus deformity as de-

scribed by Krackow et al[44]). Access to constrained implants is important, ligament advancements are well described, and imbrication techniques are less reliable for restoring functional tension to the MCL. A more challenging problem is intraoperative rupture of the MCL. Diametrically opposing views have been published regarding the efficacy of intraoperative MCL repair, suggesting variations in the severity of cases treated or the degree of concomitant valgus alignment.[45,46] Well-aligned, mechanically constrained implants provide a reliable treatment option if available. Late instability of a TKA is invariably associated with polyethylene wear and requires revision arthroplasty.

Summary

Revision knee arthroplasty is not one surgical procedure, but several significantly different procedures, depending on the cause of TKA failure. Many complications are associated with instability, but only an insightful evaluation will lead to the correct surgical treatment strategy. Instability in the plane of motion of the joint will be handled differently in patients with referred pain, patellar maltracking, flexion contracture, or extensor rupture. Coronal plane instability requires stabilization and realignment. Flexion instability requires attention to gap balancing. The results of revision arthroplasty for instability are among the best for all revision TKA procedures, provided that the etiology is understood.

References

1. Pritsch M, Fitzgerald RH Jr, Bryan RS: Surgical treatment of ligamentous instability after total knee arthroplasty. *Arch Orthop Trauma Surg* 1984;102(3):154-158.

2. Krackow K: Management of collateral ligament incompetence at revision total knee arthroplasty. *Tech Orthop* 1988;3(2):15-28.

3. Babis GC, Trousdale RT, Morrey BF: The effectiveness of isolated tibial insert exchange in revision total knee arthroplasty. *J Bone Joint Surg Am* 2002;84-A(1):64-68.

4. Parratte S, Pagnano MW: Instability after total knee arthroplasty. *J Bone Joint Surg Am* 2008;90(1):184-194.

5. Niki Y, Mochizuki T, Momohara S, Saito S, Matsumoto H, Tomatsu T: Factors affecting anteroposterior instability following cruciate-retaining total knee arthroplasty in patients with rheumatoid arthritis. *Knee* 2008;15(1):26-30.

6. Naudie DD, Rorabeck CH: Managing instability in total knee arthroplasty with constrained and linked implants. *Instr Course Lect* 2004;53:207-215.

7. Krackow KA: Instability in total knee arthroplasty: Loose as a goose. *J Arthroplasty* 2003;18(3, Suppl 1):45-47.

8. Kelly MA: Ligament instability in total knee arthroplasty. *Instr Course Lect* 2001;50:399-401.

9. Fehring TK, Valadie AL: Knee instability after total knee arthroplasty. *Clin Orthop Relat Res* 1994;299(299):157-162.

10. Vince KG, Abdeen A, Sugimori T: The unstable total knee arthroplasty: Causes and cures. *J Arthroplasty* 2006;21(4, Suppl 1):44-49.

11. Moreland JR. Mechanisms of failure in total knee arthroplasty. *Clin Orthop Relat Res* 1988;226:49-64.

12. Vince K: Modes of failure in total knee arthroplasty, in Lieberman JR, Berry DJ, Azar FM, eds: *Advanced Reconstruction of the Knee*: Rosemont, IL, American Academy of Orthopaedic Surgeons, 2011, pp 341-354.

13. Vince KG: Why knees fail. *J Arthroplasty* 2003;18(3, Suppl 1) 39-44.

14. Parvizi J, Della Valle CJ: AAOS Clinical Practice Guideline: Diagnosis and treatment of periprosthetic joint infections of the hip and knee. *J Am Acad Orthop Surg* 2010;18(12):771-772.

15. Lakstein D, Zarrabian M, Kosashvili Y, Safir O, Gross AE, Backstein D: Revision total knee arthroplasty for component malrotation is highly beneficial: A case control study. *J Arthroplasty* 2010;25(7):1047-1052.

16. Berger RA, Rubash HE: Rotational instability and malrotation after total knee arthroplasty. *Orthop Clin North Am* 2001; 32(4):639-647, ix.

17. Waters RL, Perry J, Conaty P, Lunsford B, O'Meara P: The energy cost of walking with arthritis of the hip and knee. *Clin Orthop Relat Res* 1987;214:278-284.

18. Insall J: Total knee arthroplasty, in Insall J, ed: *Surgery of the Knee.* New York, NY, Churchill Livingstone, 1984, pp 1478-1552.

19. Nazarian DG, Booth RE Jr, Extensor mechanism allografts in total knee arthroplasty. *Clin Orthop Relat Res* 1999;367: 123-129.

20. Vince K, Nakasone C: Extensor mechanism disruption after total knee arthroplasty, in Scott NW, ed: *Surgery of the Knee.* New York, NY, Churchill-Livingstone, 2005.

21. Berger RA, Crossett LS, Jacobs JJ, Rubash HE: Malrotation causing patellofemoral complications after total knee arthroplasty. *Clin Orthop Relat Res* 1998;356:144-153.

22. Moreland JR, Bassett LW, Hanker GJ: Radiographic analysis of the axial alignment of the lower extremity. *J Bone Joint Surg Am* 1987;69(5):745-749.

23. Lotke PA, Ecker ML: Influence of positioning of prosthesis in total knee replacement. *J Bone Joint Surg Am* 1977;59(1):77-79.

24. Hungerford DS, Kenna RV, Krackow KA: The porous-coated anatomic total knee. *Orthop Clin North Am* 1982;13(1):103-122.

25. Hungerford DS: Alignment in total knee replacement. *Instr Course Lect* 1995;44:455-468.

26. Parratte S, Pagnano MW, Trousdale RT, Berry DJ: Effect of postoperative mechanical axis alignment on the fifteen-year survival of modern, cemented total knee replacements. *J Bone Joint Surg Am* 2010;92(12):2143-2149.

27. Krackow KA. Revision total knee replacement ligament balancing for deformity. *Clin Orthop Relat Res* 2002,404:152-157.

28. Peters CL, Dienst M, Erickson J: Reconstruction of the medial femoral condyle and medial collateral ligament in total knee arthroplasty using tendoachilles allograft with a calcaneal bone block. *J Arthroplasty* 2004;19(7):935-940.

29. Vince KG, Insall JN, Kelly MA: The total condylar prosthesis: 10- to 12-year results of a cemented knee replacement. *J Bone Joint Surg Br* 1989;71(5):793-797.

30. Freeman MA, Insall JN, Besser W, Walker PS, Hallel T: Excision of the cruciate ligaments in total knee replacement. *Clin Orthop Relat Res* 1977;126:209-212.

31. Pagnano MW, Hanssen AD, Lewallen DG, Stuart MJ: Flexion instability after primary posterior cruciate retaining total knee arthroplasty. *Clin Orthop Relat Res* 1998;356:39-46.

32. Sharkey PF, Hozack WJ, Booth RE Jr, Balderston RA, Rothman RH: Posterior dislocation of total knee arthroplasty. *Clin Orthop Relat Res* 1992;278:128-133.

33. Galinat BJ, Vernace JV, Booth RE Jr, Rothman RH: Dislocation of

the posterior stabilized total knee arthroplasty: A report of two cases. *J Arthroplasty* 1988;3(4): 363-367.

34. Bindelglass DF, Vince KG: Dislocation following posterior-stabilized TKA. *J Arthroplasty* 1994;9(5):563.

35. Schwab JH, Haidukewych GJ, Hanssen AD, Jacofsky DJ, Pagnano MW: Flexion instability without dislocation after posterior stabilized total knees. *Clin Orthop Relat Res* 2005;440:96-100.

36. McPherson EJ, Cuckler J, Lombardi AV: Midflexion instability in revision total knee arthroplasty. *Surg Technol Int* 2008;17:249-252.

37. Dennis DA, Komistek RD, Walker SA, Cheal EJ, Stiehl JB: Femoral condylar lift-off in vivo in total knee arthroplasty. *J Bone Joint Surg Br* 2001;83(1):33-39.

38. Vince KG, Droll KP, Chivas D: Your next revision total knee arthroplasty: Why start in flexion? *Orthopedics* 2007;30(9):791-792.

39. Vince K, Bedard M: Implanting the revision total knee arthroplasty, in Lotke PA, Lonner J, eds: *Master Techniques in Orthopedic Surgery.* Baltimore, MD, Lippincott Williams and Wilkins, 2008, pp 203-228.

40. Robbins GM, Masri BA, Garbuz DS, Duncan CP: Preoperative planning to prevent instability in total knee arthroplasty. *Orthop Clin North Am* 2001;32(4):611-626, viii.

41. Vince K: Limb length discrepancy after total knee arthroplasty. *Tech Orthop* 1988;3(2):35-43.

42. Winiarsky R, Barth P, Lotke P: Total knee arthroplasty in morbidly obese patients. *J Bone Joint Surg Am* 1998;80(12):1770-1774.

43. Vince KG, Cameron HU, Hungerford DS, Laskin RS, Ranawat CS, Scuderi GR: What would you do? Case challenges in knee sur-

gery. *J Arthroplasty* 2005;20(4, Suppl 2):44-50.

44. Krackow KA, Jones MM, Teeny SM, Hungerford DS: Primary total knee arthroplasty in patients with fixed valgus deformity. *Clin Orthop Relat Res* 1991;273:9-18.

45. Leopold SS, McStay C, Klafeta K, Jacobs JJ, Berger RA, Rosenberg AG: Primary repair of intraoperative disruption of the medical collateral ligament during total knee arthroplasty. *J Bone Joint Surg Am* 2001;83-A(1):86-91.

46. Lee GC, Lotke PA: Management of intraoperative medial collateral ligament injury during TKA. *Clin Orthop Relat Res* 2011; 469(1):64-68.

MRI-Arthroscopy Correlation: The Knee

Matthew D. Milewski, MD

Timothy G. Sanders, MD

Mark D. Miller, MD

Abstract

MRI findings can often be helpful in diagnosing and managing common knee injuries. The association between the normal and pathologic changes in the surgical anatomy of the knee commonly found on MRI and those found at arthroscopy can be demonstrated by examining a series of cases that correlate MRI and arthroscopy findings. Regular interactions are recommended between surgeons and musculoskeletal radiologists to improve MRI interpretation and achieve better surgical outcomes for patients.

Instr Course Lect 2012;61:525-537.

The knee was the first joint to be examined with arthroscopy, and many of the fundamental principles of arthroscopy of all joints were originally developed for the knee. Although knee arthroscopy had its roots in Japan and Europe, it became popular in the United States in the 1960s, and substantial progress has been made over the past five decades.[1] Knee arthroscopy has become the most common orthopaedic procedure performed in the United States.[2] Techniques have evolved allowing a wide range of pathologic conditions of the knee to be

addressed arthroscopically, including meniscal surgery, anterior cruciate ligament (ACL) reconstruction, articular cartilage restoration procedures, and removal of intra-articular pigmented villonodular synovitis.

Although knee arthroscopy predated the development of MRI, the advent of MRI technology in the early 1980s helped orthopaedic surgeons in the treatment of knee disorders in several ways. In the early use of the technology, the improved initial diagnostic accuracy with preoperative MRI proved to be cost effective in reducing

unnecessary surgical interventions and altering treatment plans.[3-7] More recently, it is common practice to acquire an MRI evaluation after clinical examination and radiographs in the workup of potential soft-tissue and articular cartilage abnormality of the knee. When surgical intervention is warranted, the astute orthopaedic surgeon must be able to accurately associate the pathologic condition indicated on the preoperative MRI with the expected findings at the time of surgery, especially arthroscopy. This chapter reviews the association between the normal and pathologic changes in the surgical anatomy of the knee commonly found on MRI and those found at arthroscopy.

It is important to understand the obvious differences between the two modalities because knee arthroscopy provides direct visualization of intra-articular structures, particularly the meniscus, ACL, and articular cartilage surfaces, although it is not as useful in the visualization of extra-articular structures such as the superficial medial collateral ligament or lateral collateral ligament. Although MRI can certainly show both intra-articular and extra-articular anatomy and pathology, it can be less useful than clinical exam-

Neither of the following authors nor any immediate family member has received anything of value from or owns stock in a commercial company or institution related directly or indirectly to the subject of this chapter: Dr. Milewski and Dr. Sanders. Dr. Miller or an immediate family member has received nonincome support (such as equipment or services), commercially derived honoraria, or other non–research-related funding (such as paid travel) from the Miller Orthopaedic Research and Education (MORE) and serves as a board member, owner, officer, or committee member of the American Orthopaedic Society for Sports Medicine.

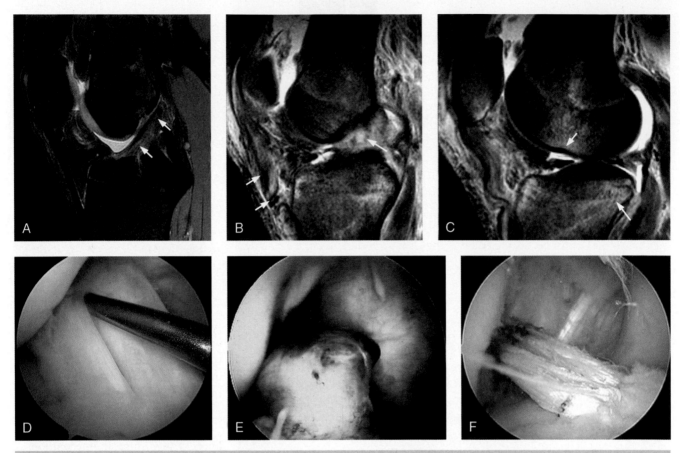

Figure 1   **A,** A normal ACL, which is best depicted in the sagittal imaging plane on MRI. The fibers of the ACL (arrows) appear taut and parallel the roof of the intercondylar notch but should not touch the roof of the notch. **B,** Acute ACL disruption. The sagittal T2-weighted MRI scan shows an edematous mass appearance of the ACL with a complete disruption of the midsubstance (long arrow). Also noted is a high-grade tear of the patellar tendon (short arrows). **C,** A T2-weighted sagittal MRI scan showing the pivot-shift contusion pattern with marrow edema involving the lateral femoral condyle with deepening of the lateral femoral sulcus (short arrow) and a second area of marrow edema involving the posterolateral tibial plateau (long arrow). **D,** Arthroscopic appearance of the normal ACL. **E,** Arthroscopic appearance of ACL stump following a complete ACL disruption. **F,** Arthroscopic appearance following ACL reconstruction.

ination in some patients, such as those with ACL or posterior cruciate ligament (PCL) insufficiency.[3] Preoperative MRI can also direct the surgeon at the time of knee arthroscopy to use additional vigilance and techniques such as additional portals and examination of the posterior aspect of the knee when pathologic changes, such as loose bodies, seen on imaging may not be readily seen at the time of standard diagnostic arthroscopy. The treatment of knee abnormality with both MRI and arthroscopy should be done after both a standardized and a systematic review of preoperative imaging and after a

standard thorough and systematic diagnostic arthroscopic evaluation.

The ACL: Normal and Disrupted

MRI Features

The ACL (**Figure 1**) arises proximally along the medial aspect of the lateral femoral condyle, inserts distally onto the tibia adjacent to the anterior tibial spine, and is composed of two separate bundles (anteromedial and posterolateral). The normal ACL is best evaluated in the sagittal imaging plane with use of a T2-weighted pulse sequence (**Figure 1,** *A*); however, the axial and

coronal imaging planes are also useful in the evaluation of the proximal and distal attachment sites, respectively. With the knee imaged in full extension, the ACL fibers should appear taut with no substantial posterior drooping, and the ACL should parallel the roof of the intercondylar notch but should not touch the roof of the notch.

There are several direct MRI signs that indicate a complete disruption of the ACL.[8] Discontinuity of the ACL fibers seen in any of the three imaging planes is evidence of a complete tear. In the acute setting, the appearance of the disrupted ACL has been described as an edematous mass with increased T2 signal and abnormal morphology (**Figure 1,** *B*). In the subacute setting, the discontinuous ACL fibers demonstrate less of an edematous mass–like appearance and take on a more linear fragmented appearance, whereas in the chronic setting there may be a complete absence or nonvisualization of the ACL fibers. The so-called empty notch sign refers to an MRI finding in which fluid signal rather than normal ACL fibers are seen at the proximal attachment site, usually best depicted on axial T2-weighted images. An avulsion fracture of the anterior tibial spine may be seen with a distal ACL injury.

There are also several indirect MRI signs that may accompany a disruption of the ACL.[9] In the acute setting, a large hemarthrosis, although nonspecific, is often present. The pivot-shift bone contusion pattern (lateral femoral condyle and posterolateral tibial plateau), resulting from a noncontact injury, is often seen following an ACL disruption (**Figure 1,** *C*).[10] Other indirect signs of ACL disruption include the deep sulcus sign (an irregular-appearing lateral femoral sulcus with a depth of > 2 mm), a Segond fracture (a capsular avulsion injury fracture of the lateral tibial plateau), anterior drawer sign (anterior tibial translation), and buckling of the PCL, which is a nonspecific finding.

Arthroscopic Findings

When examined arthroscopically, the normal ACL has a diameter of approximately 11 mm and has broad insertions, which are larger than originally described (**Figure 1,** *D*). Two functional bundles of the ACL have been described and are named for their tibial insertions, which can be observed during arthroscopy.[11] The anteromedial bundle originates more proximally on the femoral insertion and inserts anteromedially on the tibia and is

tighter in flexion.[12] The posterolateral bundle originates more distally on the femoral insertion and inserts posterolaterally on the tibia and is tighter in extension.[12] Although the two bundles appear parallel with the knee in extension, as the knee flexes to 90°, the femoral insertion of the posterolateral bundle moves anteriorly; thus, during knee arthroscopy, the bundles usually appear to cross.[11] The osseous architecture of the lateral wall of the intercondylar notch can also be visualized and used as a guide for the evaluation and treatment of ACL tears. The cruciate ridge (or lateral intercondylar ridge) is a raised area of bone that runs in a proximal-to-distal direction with the ACL fibers inserting posterior to this ridge (when viewed arthroscopically, this ridge is parallel with the floor).[13] The bundle ridge (or bifurcate ridge) lies between the two bundles of the ACL and runs in an anterior-to-posterior direction (more vertical when viewed in the typical arthroscopy position of knee flexion).[13]

Injury to the ACL often results in an obvious "stump" of residual tissue, and direct repair of this tissue is not possible (**Figure 1,** *E*). The empty lateral wall sign indicates a complete ACL tear. Isolated injuries to only one bundle have been described, and treatment options for these partial injuries are controversial. ACL reconstruction can be accomplished with the use of a variety of grafts (hamstring autograft has become the most popular graft in many centers). Recently, an emphasis has been made on placement of the graft in a more anatomic position, with the use of either a single- or double-bundle technique (**Figure 1,** *F*). This involves placement of the graft in the center of the ACL footprint on both the tibia (more anteriorly than previously recommended) and the femur (in a more horizontal and slightly more anterior position).[14]

The PCL: Normal and Disrupted

Although not as common as injury to the ACL, injury to the PCL has been diagnosed more often as clinical examinations, stress radiographs, MRI, and arthroscopy techniques have evolved and improved (**Figure 2**). The PCL is often injured in conjunction with the ACL and, in particular, the lateral collateral ligament and the posterolateral corner. This combination can lead to early osteoarthritis and failure of PCL reconstruction if the associated injuries are not properly managed.[15-17]

MRI Features

The PCL is typically about twice the thickness of the ACL and is best evaluated on MRI with use of the T2-weighted sagittal images. With the knee imaged in full extension, the PCL has an arcuate-shaped bandlike appearance of homogeneous low-signal intensity (**Figure 2,** *A*). The PCL originates along the intercondylar portion of the medial femoral condyle and inserts distally on the slanted portion of the posterior part of the tibia[18] (**Figure 2,** *D*).

The PCL is often injured as a result of a direct trauma to the anterior aspect of the tibia with the knee in flexion, and this injury may result in a bone contusion of the anterior aspect of the proximal part of the tibia[10] (**Figure 2,** *B*). This mechanism of injury places posteriorly directed forces on the proximal part of the tibia, resulting in a PCL injury. The PCL is more often partially torn compared with the ACL, and although injury can occur anywhere along the course of the ligament, most injuries occur within the midsubstance of the PCL (**Figure 2,** *C*). A partial-thickness tear appears as thickening and edema of the ligament, possibly with fluid signal extending partially through the substance of the ligament, but with visualized intact

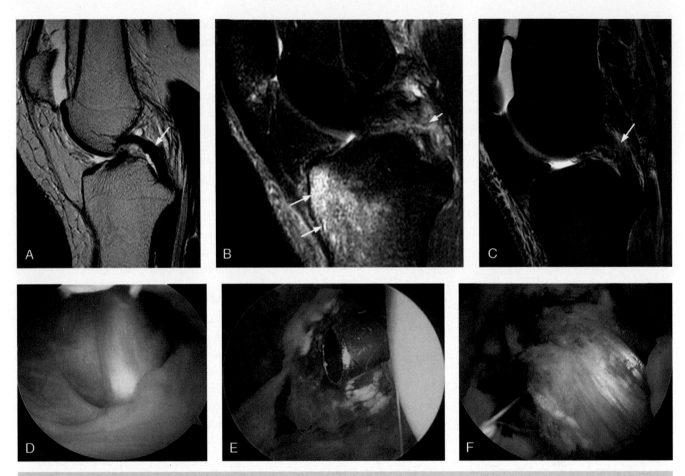

Figure 2 **A,** A sagittal T2-weighted MRI showing the normal appearance of the PCL (arrow) as a low-signal intensity, arcuate-appearing, bandlike structure arising along the intercondylar notch portion of the medial femoral condyle and inserting on the posterior slanted portion of the tibia. **B,** Direct trauma to the anterior aspect of the proximal aspect of the tibia with the knee in flexion can result in an injury to the PCL (short arrow). This injury mechanism often results in a bone contusion (long arrows) isolated to the proximal aspect of the anterior part of the tibia. **C,** A complete tear of the midsubstance of the PCL. A sagittal T2-weighted MRI scan showing a complete disruption of the PCL (arrow) in the midsubstance with a lax-appearing PCL. **D,** A normal PCL as viewed through the posteromedial portal. **E,** A PCL injury viewed through the posteromedial portal. **F,** Arthroscopic view of a reconstructed PCL.

fibers.[19,20] A full-thickness tear demonstrates a complete disruption with discontinuity of the fibers (**Figure 2, C**). A so-called peel-off injury refers to an avulsion injury at the femoral attachment of the PCL. A distal osseous avulsion of the posterior tibial insertion site can also occur and often results in a large avulsion fracture fragment.[21]

Arthroscopic Findings

Fanelli et al[22] described both direct and indirect signs for PCL disruption. Direct signs include a torn graft (**Figure 2, E**). However, more often than not, the findings are subtle and usually involve indirect signs, such as posterior displacement of the tibia in relation to the medial femoral condyle, pseudolaxity of the ACL (the so-called sloppy ACL sign), and late effects of the PCL deficiency, including chondrosis of the medial femoral condyle and patellofemoral joint.

The Posterolateral Corner: Normal and Disrupted

Posterolateral corner (**Figure 3**) injuries are most often associated with combined ligament injuries (especially the PCL) but have been reported in isolated cases. The essential structures in the posterolateral corner include the biceps tendon, iliotibial band, lateral collateral ligament, popliteus musculotendinous unit, popliteofibular ligament, and posterolateral capsule.

MRI Features

The posterolateral corner of the knee is anatomically complex, with several distinct and separate anatomic structures that are responsible for providing stability. These structures include the posterior capsule, arcuate ligament, popliteofibular ligament, popliteomeniscal fascicles, popliteus tendon, fibu-

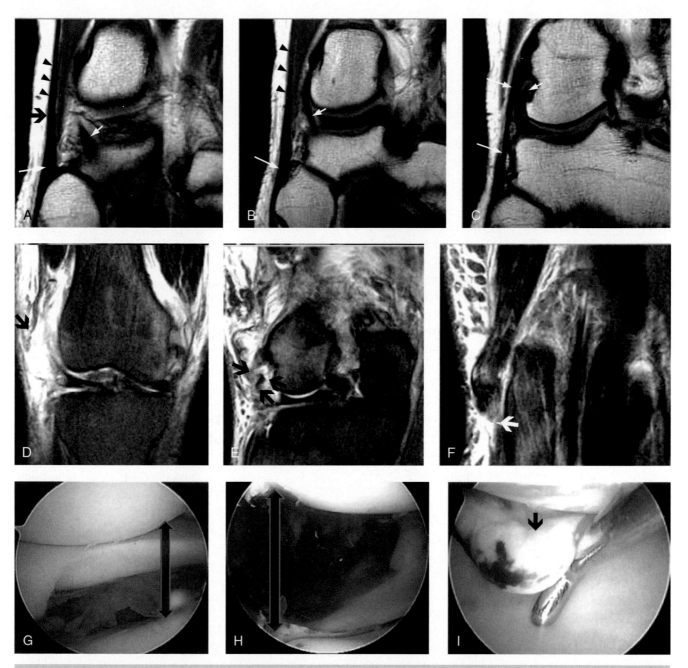

Figure 3 **A** through **C,** Coronal T1-weighted MRI scans through the posterolateral corner of the knee, demonstrating the normal appearance of the distal biceps femoris musculotendinous junction (arrowheads and black arrow), conjoined tendon (long arrows), and popliteus tendon (short arrows). **B** and **C,** Long arrows indicate the fibular collateral ligament. **D** through **F,** Multiple coronal T2-weighted MRI scans through the knee. **D,** The anterior aspect of the knee showing a complete disruption and retraction of the iliotibial band (arrow). **E,** The anterior aspect of the knee showing a complete disruption and retraction of the fibular collateral ligament (single arrow) and the popliteus tendon (two arrows). **F,** The posterior aspect of the knee showing a complete disruption and retracted end of the biceps femoris tendon (arrow). **G** and **H,** Arthroscopic views of the lateral compartment showing a so-called positive drive-through sign (double-headed arrow). **I,** Arthroscopic view of a torn popliteus tendon (arrow) subluxated into the lateral compartment as part of a posterolateral corner injury.

lar collateral ligament, biceps femoris tendon, and the conjoined tendon[23] (**Figure 3,** *A* through *C*). Injury to one or more of these structures can result in posterolateral knee pain, buckling into hyperextension during weight bearing, and instability of the knee on physical examination.

The posterolateral corner structures

are best evaluated with use of T2-weighted sequences, and all three imaging planes (axial, sagittal, and coronal) are required to provide an accurate assessment of each of these individual structures (**Figure 3,** *D* through *F*). Each anatomic structure should be described individually when injury is present. A three-point grading system[24] is used to describe injury to each individual structure: grade I indicates strain; grade II, a partial-thickness tear; and grade III, a complete disruption.

Arthroscopic Findings

Arthroscopic findings of a posterolateral corner injury include excessive opening of the lateral compartment. This has been described by LaPrade[25] as the positive drive-through sign (**Figure 3,** *G* and *H*). Posterolateral corner injuries require open treatment. This is best done with primary repair supplemented by free graft augmentation. The preference of the senior author (MD Miller) is a semitendinosus allograft. Anatomic placement of this graft has shown to be important for good long-term results.[25]

The MCL: Normal and Disrupted

The MCL is the most commonly injured ligament in the knee.[26] Although the MCL provides most of the restraint to valgus stress, additional medial structures are important for stability. The classic description of medial knee structures, by Warren and Marshall,[27] involves three layers. The most superficial layer consists of the fascia investing the sartorius and extending posteriorly to cover the gastrocnemius muscle heads. The next layer consists of the superficial MCL, medial patellofemoral ligament, broad insertions of the semimembranosus tendon, and posteromedial corner ligaments. The deepest layer consists of the true capsule of the knee joint and the deep

MCL with its meniscocapsular connections to the medial meniscus.

MRI Features

The MCL is composed of a superficial and a deep component. The superficial component originates on the adductor tubercle of the medial femoral condyle and inserts distally on the tibia approximately 5 cm distal to the joint line just deep to the insertion of the tendons of the pes anserinus. The ligament measures approximately 1.5 cm in anteroposterior diameter. The deep fibers attach to the medial capsule and medial meniscus. There is a tibial collateral ligament bursa, a potential space between the superficial and deep components of the MCL.[28] The MCL is best evaluated by MRI on coronal T2-weighted images, while the axial imaging plane is complementary. The normal MCL appears as a continuous, low-signal intensity, bandlike structure located along the medial joint line (**Figure 4,** *A*).

MCL injuries occur as a result of valgus stress to the knee. A grade I injury—a sprain of the MCL (**Figure 4,** *B*)—demonstrates soft-tissue edema superficial to the MCL fibers, but the fibers are intact.[29] A grade II injury represents a partial-thickness tear (**Figure 4,** *C*). On MRI, fibers may be thickened and edematous and demonstrate partial disruption, although some fibers remain intact. A grade III injury represents a full-thickness disruption. MRI shows a complete discontinuity of the fibers, with laxity and retraction of the torn ligament ends. A full-thickness tear may occur near the proximal or distal attachment site[30] (**Figure 4,** *D* and *E*). A chronic or old injury demonstrates thickening and fibrosis of the MCL. The term Pellegrini-Stieda refers to calcification or ossification within the substance of the MCL associated with an old injury.

Arthroscopic Findings

Although only the medial capsule and meniscocapsular connection can be directly observed arthroscopically in the normal knee, several observations in the MCL-injured knee can be made at the time of arthroscopy. A corollary to the LaPrade arthroscopic drive-through sign, indicating lateral ligament complex injury, is excessive medial opening with minimal valgus stress as an indicator of MCL injury (**Figure 4,** *F*). Because the meniscus is attached to the deep portion of the MCL, it will often stay with the side where the MCL remains attached. For example, if the MCL is torn from the femoral attachment (the most common pattern of injury), at arthroscopy this would appear as opening more above the medial meniscus because the MCL remains attached distally.

Transient Lateral Dislocation of the Patella

The most common direction of patellar instability is lateral dislocation. This may result in an osteochondral injury to either the medial facet of the patella or the lateral femoral condyle, or both. The medial patellofemoral ligament (**Figure 5**), which is the primary restraint to lateral translation of the patella, may be torn.[31]

MRI Features

The typical MRI findings that indicate a recent transient dislocation of the patella include bone contusions of the anterior peripheral aspect of the lateral femoral condyle and the inferior aspect of the medial patellar facet[32,33] (**Figure 5,** *B*). These MRI findings are often the first clue of the true mechanism of injury, as the patella often reduces spontaneously at the time of injury without the patient realizing that a dislocation occurred. Osteochondral shearing or impaction-type injuries can occur along the midpole to

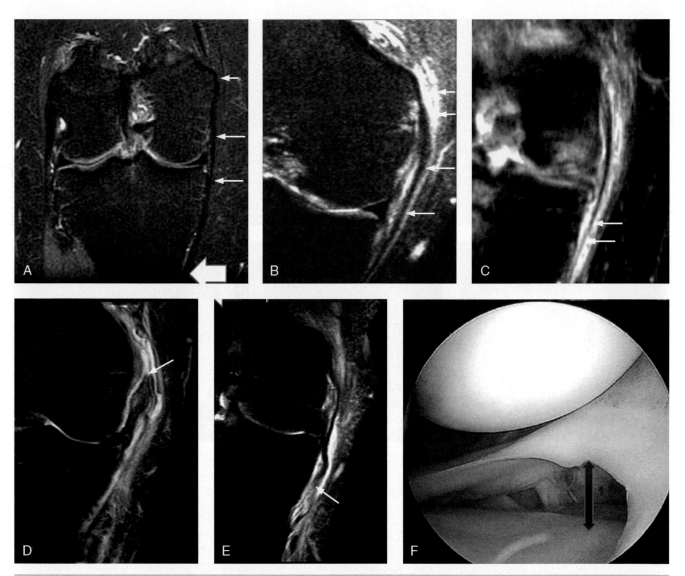

Figure 4 **A,** A coronal T2-weighted MRI scan showing the normal MCL (long arrows), which appears as a low-signal intensity, bandlike structure extending along the medial aspect of the knee. It originates on the adductor tubercle of the medial femoral condyle (short arrow) proximally and extends distally to insert approximately 5 cm below the joint line (large arrow). **B,** Grade I injury: a sprain of the MCL. Coronal T2-weighted MRI scan showing an intact MCL (long arrows) with superficial soft-tissue edema (short arrows). **C,** Grade II injury: a partial-thickness tear of the MCL. Coronal T2-weighted MRI scan showing thinning and attenuation indicating a partial-thickness tear (long arrows) of the distal attachment with overlying soft-tissue edema. **D,** Grade III injury: a complete tear of the MCL. Coronal T2-weighted MRI scan showing a complete disruption and discontinuity (arrow) of the proximal attachment of the MCL. **E,** Grade III injury: A complete tear of the MCL. Coronal T2-weighted MRI scan showing a complete disruption and discontinuity (arrow) of the distal attachment of the MCL. **F,** Arthroscopic view of the medial compartment of the knee with a distal injury to the MCL indicated by the meniscus translated superiorly (arrow).

lower pole of the medial patellar facet or along the peripheral margin of the lateral femoral condyle.[33] A large joint effusion is usually present, and the MRI should be thoroughly evaluated for the presence of an intra-articular loose body (**Figure 5,** *C* and *D*).

The medial soft-tissue restraints include the medial retinaculum, medial patellofemoral ligament, and medial patellotibial ligament. The medial patellofemoral ligament is the most important of the medial patellar stabilizers. Disruption of the medial

patellofemoral ligament most often occurs at the femoral attachment site near the adductor tubercle, but it can also occur in the midsubstance or at the patellar attachment site. Injuries are graded on a three-point grading system.[32] Grade I indicates a sprain,

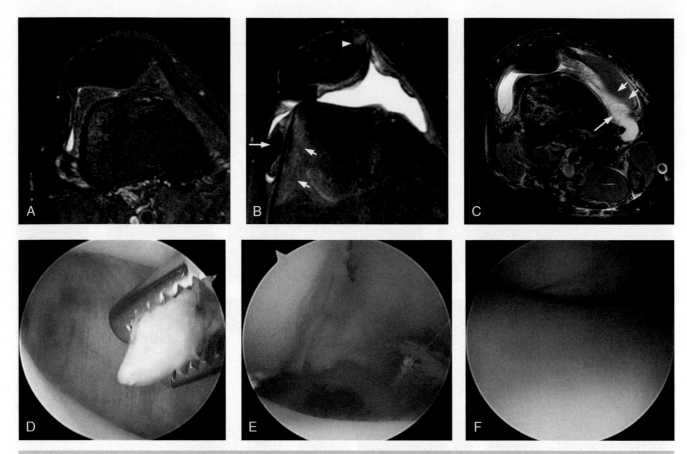

Figure 5   **A,** A normal medial patellofemoral ligament visualized on an axial T2-weighted MRI as the bandlike structure extending from the medial patellar facet, then blending with the deep fibers of the vastus medialis obliquus muscle to insert on the adductor tubercle. **B,** Transient dislocation and osteochondral injury of the patella. Axial T2-weighted MRI scan showing a large loose intra-articular body (long arrow) within the suprapatellar pouch arising from the patella. Bone contusions indicate prior transient dislocation of the patella with contusions of the lateral femoral condyle (short arrows) and medial patellar facet (arrowhead). **C,** Medial patellofemoral ligament disruption following transient patellar dislocation. Axial T2-weighted MRI scan showing a complete disruption of the medial patellofemoral ligament near the medial femoral condyle attachment site with a large adjacent hematoma (long arrow). There is uplifting and displacement of the vastus medialis obliquus muscle (short arrows). **D,** A loose body being removed arthroscopically following a transient dislocation of the patella. Arthroscopic depiction of patellar tracking before (**E**) and after (**F**) medial patellofemoral ligament repair.

seen as adjacent edema but with intact medial patellofemoral ligament fibers; grade II, a partial-thickness tear, seen on MRI as partial disruption of the medial patellofemoral ligament fibers with adjacent soft-tissue edema; and grade III, a full-thickness tear, seen as a complete disruption of the medial patellofemoral ligament with retraction and laxity of the fibers, often associated with an adjacent hematoma and uplifting and displacement of the overlying vastus medialis obliquus muscle[32] (**Figure 5,** *C*).

Arthroscopic Findings

Although the medial patellofemoral ligament is not visible intra-articularly, there are multiple findings during arthroscopy that are consistent with lateral dislocation of the patella. Cartilage damage is most often seen on the medial facet of the patella or on the lateral border of the lateral femoral condyle after patellar dislocation (**Figure 5,** *D*). The superomedial or superolateral portal can be used to evaluate patellar tracking and patellar tilt.[34,35] The lateral facet should engage the trochlea by

20° to 25° of knee flexion and the midpatellar ridge by 35° to 40° of flexion.[35] It is important to check patellar tracking with arthroscopy after either proximal or distal realignment procedures (**Figure 5,** *E* and *F*).

Meniscal Tears

The presence of a meniscal tear is the most common indication for knee arthroscopy, and MRI has evolved into an accurate means of detecting meniscal abnormalities before arthroscopy. Understanding tear patterns and MRI

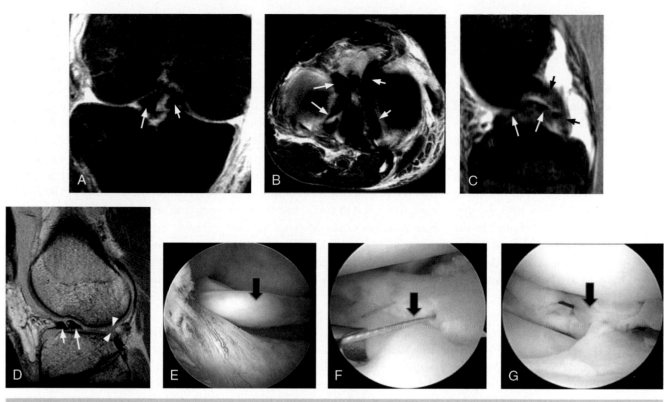

Figure 6   Coronal (**A**) and axial (**B**) T2-weighted MRI scans of the knee showing large bucket-handle fragments of the medial meniscus (short arrows) and lateral meniscus (long arrows), both displaced into the intercondylar notch. **C,** Sagittal T2-weighted MRI scan showing a bucket-handle tear of the medial meniscus with the displaced fragment (long arrows) sitting within the intercondylar notch mimicking a double PCL (short arrows). **D,** A sagittal proton-density MRI scan showing a bucket-handle tear of the lateral meniscus with the meniscal fragment flipped anteriorly (long arrow) behind the native anterior horn (short arrow). Note the small truncated-appearing posterior horn of the lateral meniscus (arrowheads). **E,** Arthroscopic appearance of a displaced bucket-handle tear (arrow). **F,** Arthroscopic appearance of the bucket-handle tear (arrow) after repair. **G,** Arthroscopic appearance of the bucket-handle tear (arrow) after meniscal repair with platelet-rich plasma.

features of menisci can help in surgical planning, especially with regard to possible meniscal repair versus partial meniscectomy.

Bucket-Handle Tear of the Meniscus

MRI Features

The accuracy of MRI in detecting a meniscal tear ranges between 90% and 95%, and the experience level of the MRI reader is one of the most important factors in maximizing diagnostic accuracy. It is critical to assess the meniscus in both the sagittal and coronal imaging planes. Short TE (echo time) sequence imaging (proton density or T1-weighted) is most sensitive for detecting meniscal tears, whereas abnor-

malities seen on T2-weighted images are very specific.[36]

The menisci are composed of fibrocartilage and appear dark on all MRI pulse sequences. On the sagittal images, the peripheral portion of the menisci have been described as demonstrating a bow-tie configuration, although more centrally, the meniscus demonstrates a triangular appearance tapering toward the free edge. The anterior and posterior horns of the lateral meniscus are nearly equivalent in size, whereas the posterior horn of the medial meniscus is nearly twice the size of the anterior horn.[37]

Identifying a displaced meniscal fragment requires a thorough knowledge of the normal MRI appearance of

the menisci in both the sagittal and coronal imaging planes (**Figure 6,** A through D). Direct signs of a meniscal tear include (1) unequivocal surfacing signal, (2) missing meniscal tissue (in the absence of prior surgery), and (3) displaced meniscal fragment. Several MRI signs have been described with regard to the identification of a bucket-handle tear of the menisci. The double PCL sign indicates a bucklehandle tear of the medial meniscus displaced into the intercondylar notch (**Figure 6,** C). The double anterior horn sign indicates a bucket-handle tear of the lateral meniscus that has flipped into the anterior aspect of the lateral compartment of the knee (**Figure 6,** D). The absent bow-tie sign indicates that a meniscal fragment has been displaced and no longer sits in its normal anatomic position.[38-40]

Arthroscopic Findings

The classic arthroscopic appearance of a bucket-handle meniscal tear includes displacement of the torn meniscus into the notch (**Figure 6,** *E*). Bucket-handle tears most commonly occur in the medial meniscus. The meniscus should be reduced back into the medial compartment when found in the notch to allow visualization of the residual peripheral meniscus to decide if a repair is possible. With the meniscus reduced, it is easier to remove if the tear pattern is not amenable to repair and partial meniscectomy is chosen for treatment. If the tear is amenable to repair, the gold standard remains outside-in suture repair that necessitates a separate posteromedial incision for suture removal and protection of the saphenous nerve and vein (**Figure 6,** *F* and *G*). Newer all-inside repair technology and techniques continue to evolve.

Meniscal Tear With Displaced Fragment

MRI Findings

In addition to the bucket-handle tears, several unstable meniscal flap fragments can occur and involve either the medial or lateral meniscus. It is important when evaluating the meniscus on MRI to look for displaced fragments within the various gutters and recesses of the knee to aid in the arthroscopic evaluation of the meniscus. Unstable meniscal flap fragments can be displaced into several locations.[37,41] In the medial compartment, meniscal fragments are most commonly seen along the medial joint line with the fragments displaced into either the superior or inferior recesses. The pattern is more variable in the lateral compartment of the knee, but most fragments are noted in the posterior aspect of the lateral compartment.

Arthroscopic Findings

Both the lateral and medial menisci can be visualized on arthroscopy through standard inferomedial and inferolateral portals. Often it is helpful and sometimes necessary to establish posteromedial and posterolateral portals to ensure that the complete meniscectomy is accomplished and to ensure that there are no residual fragments. Meniscal tears are often classified by their tear pattern, which can be best assessed at the time of arthroscopy. Patterns include bucket-handle longitudinal, radial, oblique, parrot-beak, and complex tear patterns. The location of the tear, particularly a longitudinal tear, should be assessed visually at arthroscopy for its proximity to the periphery because this influences healing rates and can determine whether the tear is repairable. The meniscal roots should also be assessed for tears because these tear patterns have been shown to dramatically change the biomechanics of the meniscus.[42] Often the posteromedial and posterolateral portals are vital to fully visualizing the meniscal root.

Osteochondral Defect

Osteochondritis dissecans refers to a lesion of the articular cartilage and underlying bone typically occurring in adolescents or young adults. Lesions are described as juvenile osteochondritis dissecans if the growth plates are open or as adult osteochondritis dissecans if the growth plates are closed. Juvenile osteochondritis dissecans usually has a better prognosis. In the knee, osteochondritis dissecans most often occurs in the lateral aspect of the medial femoral condyle.

MRI Features

The primary role of imaging is to detect the presence of an osteochondritis dissecans lesion and to determine the stability of the fragment, which guides the need for surgical or nonsurgical treatment. The osteochondritis dissecans should be evaluated in both the sagittal and coronal imaging planes, and the most common sequences used for evaluating the fragment include T2-weighted images with fat saturation or proton density images with fat saturation. The articular cartilage, cortex, and underlying marrow signal all need to be evaluated. The MRI grading system[43] uses a four-point scale, with grade I indicating subchondral bone marrow edema with intact overlying cortex and articular cartilage; grade II, a partially detached osteochondral lesion; grade III, a completely detached fragment in situ (**Figure 7,** *A* through *C*); and grade IV, a completely detached and displaced osteochondral fragment. MRI signs indicating an unstable fragment include (1) linear bands of high T2 signal at the interface of the fragment and the underlying bone measuring more than 5 mm in length, (2) the presence of a subchondral cyst measuring 5 mm or more in diameter underlying the osteochondral fragment, and (3) a focal chondral defect measuring more than 5 mm in diameter. The presence of bright T2 signal undermining the osteochondral fragment is the most common finding indicating an unstable fragment, and sometimes it is difficult to differentiate granulation tissue from fluid undermining the fragment with use of conventional MRI. The presence of contrast completely surrounding the fragment indicates an unstable fragment when magnetic resonance arthrography is used.[43,44]

Arthroscopic Findings

MRI assessment of stability is important for preoperative planning and, combined with arthroscopic findings (**Figure 7,** *D*) and assessment of stabil-

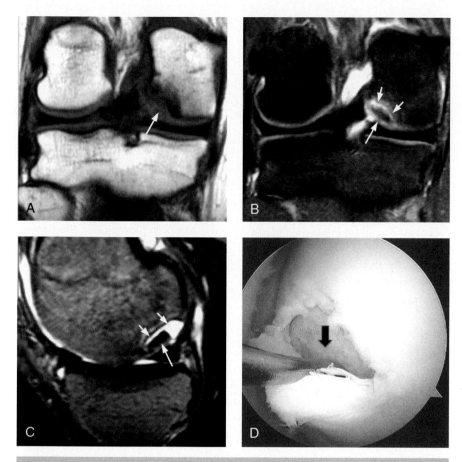

Figure 7 Grade III osteochondral defect of the medial femoral condyle. Coronal T1-weighted MRI scan (**A**), coronal T2-weighted MRI scan with fat saturation (**B**), and sagittal T2-weighted MRI scan without fat saturation (**C**) of the knee, showing an osteochondral defect located in the lateral aspect of the medial femoral condyle. The fragment (long arrows) demonstrates bright T2 signal (short arrows) representing fluid completely undermining the fragment and indicating an unstable fragment. **D,** Arthroscopic appearance of a focal chondral defect within the medial femoral condyle (arrow).

Summary

The use of MRI and arthroscopy of the knee has evolved substantially over the last several decades, and the advancement in surgical treatment of pathologic conditions of the knee has been improved because of both technologies. The astute orthopaedic surgeon must be able to associate the findings on MRI in decision making before and during arthroscopy. An accurate understanding of the surgical anatomy and pathology found on both clinical examination and preoperative imaging will help the surgeon to improve the surgical technique at the time of arthroscopy and ultimately improve patient outcomes.

References

1. Ishibashi Y, Yamamoto Y: The history of arthroscopy, in Miller MD, Cole BJ, eds: *Textbook of Arthroscopy*. Philadelphia, PA, Saunders, 2004, pp 3-7.

2. Garrett WE Jr, Swiontkowski MF, Weinstein JN, et al: American Board of Orthopaedic Surgery Practice of the Orthopaedic Surgeon: Part II. Certification examination case mix. *J Bone Joint Surg Am* 2006;88(3):660-667.

3. Alioto RJ, Browne JE, Barnthouse CD, Scott AR: The influence of MRI on treatment decisions regarding knee injuries. *Am J Knee Surg* 1999;12(2):91-97.

4. Bui-Mansfield LT, Youngberg RA, Warme W, Pitcher JD, Nguyen PL: Potential cost savings of MR imaging obtained before arthroscopy of the knee: Evaluation of 50 consecutive patients. *AJR Am J Roentgenol* 1997;168(4):913-918.

5. Maurer EJ, Kaplan PA, Dussault RG, et al: Acutely injured knee: Effect of MR imaging on diagnostic and therapeutic decisions. *Radiology* 1997;204(3):799-805.

ity, will guide treatment. Understanding the location of the lesion is important for antegrade or retrograde drilling and for being prepared at the time of surgery for potential fixation or salvage options such as osteochondral grafting or autologous chondrocyte implantation. The classic location for osteochondritis dissecans is on the lateral portion of the medial femoral condyle and often bordering the PCL femoral insertion. It is important to know and recognize the location of the lesion at the time of arthroscopy because it can be the only portion of fluid communication underneath an unstable lesion where the remaining cartilage surface appears intact.

In adults with osteochondritis dissecans or other articular cartilage lesions, it is important to know the location of the lesion from the preoperative MRI and whether a loose body might be present. Knee arthroscopy is also crucial in deciding on treatment options for these lesions as their size and depth can be assessed along with whether the other articular cartilage surfaces are involved and whether there is diffuse osteoarthritis.

6. Ruwe PA, Wright J, Randall RL, Lynch JK, Jokl P, McCarthy S: Can MR imaging effectively replace diagnostic arthroscopy? *Radiology* 1992;183(2):335-339.

7. Vincken PW, ter Braak BP, van Erkell AR, et al: Effectiveness of MR imaging in selection of patients for arthroscopy of the knee. *Radiology* 2002;223(3):739-746.

8. Robertson PL, Schweitzer ME, Bartolozzi AR, Ugoni A: Anterior cruciate ligament tears: Evaluation of multiple signs with MR imaging. *Radiology* 1994;193(3): 829-834.

9. Tung GA, Davis LM, Wiggins ME, Fadale PD: Tears of the anterior cruciate ligament: Primary and secondary signs at MR imaging. *Radiology* 1993;188(3): 661-667.

10. Sanders TG, Medynski MA, Feller JF, Lawhorn KW: Bone contusion patterns of the knee at MR imaging: Footprint of the mechanism of injury. *Radiographics* 2000; 20(Spec No):S135-S151.

11. Chhabra A, Starman JS, Ferretti M, Vidal AF, Zantop T, Fu FH: Anatomic, radiographic, biomechanical, and kinematic evaluation of the anterior cruciate ligament and its two functional bundles. *J Bone Joint Surg Am* 2006;88(Suppl 4):2-10.

12. Amis AA, Dawkins GP: Functional anatomy of the anterior cruciate ligament: Fibre bundle actions related to ligament replacements and injuries. *J Bone Joint Surg Br* 1991;73(2): 260-267.

13. Ziegler CG, Pietrini SD, Westerhaus BD, et al: Arthroscopically pertinent landmarks for tunnel positioning in single-bundle and double-bundle anterior cruciate ligament reconstructions. *Am J Sports Med* 2011;39(4):743-752.

14. van Eck CF, Lesniak BP, Schreiber VM, Fu FH: Anatomic single- and double-bundle ante-

rior cruciate ligament reconstruction flowchart. *Arthroscopy* 2010; 26(2):258-268.

15. Strobel MJ, Weiler A, Schulz MS, Russe K, Eichhorn HJ: Arthroscopic evaluation of articular cartilage lesions in posterior-cruciate-ligament-deficient knees. *Arthroscopy* 2003;19(3):262-268.

16. Skyhar MJ, Warren RF, Ortiz GJ, Schwartz E, Otis JC: The effects of sectioning of the posterior cruciate ligament and the posterolateral complex on the articular contact pressures within the knee. *J Bone Joint Surg Am* 1993;75(5): 694-699.

17. Harner CD, Vogrin TM, Höher J, Ma CB, Woo SL: Biomechanical analysis of a posterior cruciate ligament reconstruction: Deficiency of the posterolateral structures as a cause of graft failure. *Am J Sports Med* 2000;28(1):32-39.

18. Gross ML, Grover JS, Bassett LW, Seeger LL, Finerman GA: Magnetic resonance imaging of the posterior cruciate ligament: Clinical use to improve diagnostic accuracy. *Am J Sports Med* 1992; 20(6):732-737.

19. Grover JS, Bassett LW, Gross ML, Seeger LL, Finerman GA: Posterior cruciate ligament: MR imaging. *Radiology* 1990;174(2): 527-530.

20. Rodriguez W Jr, Vinson EN, Helms CA, Toth AP: MRI appearance of posterior cruciate ligament tears. *AJR Am J Roentgenol* 2008;191(4):1031.

21. Sonin AH, Fitzgerald SW, Hoff FL, Friedman H, Bresler ME: MR imaging of the posterior cruciate ligament: Normal, abnormal, and associated injury patterns. *Radiographics* 1995;15(3):551-561.

22. Fanelli GC, Giannotti BF, Edson CJ: The posterior cruciate ligament arthroscopic evaluation and treatment. *Arthroscopy* 1994; 10(6):673-688.

23. Yu JS, Salonen DC, Hodler J, Haghighi P, Trudell D, Resnick D: Posterolateral aspect of the knee: Improved MR imaging with a coronal oblique technique. *Radiology* 1996;198(1):199-204.

24. Vinson EN, Major NM, Helms CA: The posterolateral corner of the knee. *AJR Am J Roentgenol* 2008;190(2):449-458.

25. LaPrade RF: Arthroscopic evaluation of the lateral compartment of knees with grade 3 posterolateral knee complex injuries. *Am J Sports Med* 1997;25(5):596-602.

26. Miyamoto RG, Bosco JA, Sherman OH: Treatment of medial collateral ligament injuries. *J Am Acad Orthop Surg* 2009;17(3): 152-161.

27. Warren LF, Marshall JL: The supporting structures and layers on the medial side of the knee: An anatomical analysis. *J Bone Joint Surg Am* 1979;61(1):56-62.

28. De Maeseneer M, Van Roy F, Lenchik L, Barbaix E, De Ridder F, Osteaux M: Three layers of the medial capsular and supporting structures of the knee: MR imaging-anatomic correlation. *Radiographics* 2000;20(Spec No): S83-S89.

29. Yao L, Dungan D, Seeger LL: MR imaging of tibial collateral ligament injury: Comparison with clinical examination. *Skeletal Radiol* 1994;23(7):521-524.

30. Schweitzer ME, Tran D, Deely DM, Hume EL: Medial collateral ligament injuries: Evaluation of multiple signs, prevalence and location of associated bone bruises, and assessment with MR imaging. *Radiology* 1995;194(3): 825-829.

31. Sallay PI, Poggi J, Speer KP, Garrett WE: Acute dislocation of the patella: A correlative pathoanatomic study. *Am J Sports Med* 1996;24(1):52-60.

32. Sanders TG, Morrison WB, Singleton BA, Miller MD, Cornum

KG: Medial patellofemoral ligament injury following acute transient dislocation of the patella: MR findings with surgical correlation in 14 patients. *J Comput Assist Tomogr* 2001;25(6):957-962.

33. Sanders TG, Paruchuri NB, Zlatkin MB: MRI of osteochondral defects of the lateral femoral condyle: Incidence and pattern of injury after transient lateral dislocation of the patella. *AJR Am J Roentgenol* 2006;187(5):1332-1337.

34. Schreiber SN: Proximal superomedial portal in arthroscopy of the knee. *Arthroscopy* 1991;7(2):246-251.

35. Boden BP, Pearsall AW, Garrett WE Jr, Feagin JA Jr: Patellofemoral instability: Evaluation and management. *J Am Acad Orthop Surg* 1997;5(1):47-57.

36. De Smet AA, Norris MA, Yandow DR, Quintana FA, Graf BK,

Keene JS: MR diagnosis of meniscal tears of the knee: Importance of high signal in the meniscus that extends to the surface. *AJR Am J Roentgenol* 1993;161(1):101-107.

37. Ruff C, Weingardt JP, Russ PD, Kilcoyne RF: MR imaging patterns of displaced meniscus injuries of the knee. *AJR Am J Roentgenol* 1998;170(1):63-67.

38. Rangger C, Klestil T, Kathrein A, Inderster A, Hamid L: Influence of magnetic resonance imaging on indications for arthroscopy of the knee. *Clin Orthop Relat Res* 1996;330:133-142.

39. Wright DH, De Smet AA, Norris M: Bucket-handle tears of the medial and lateral menisci of the knee: Value of MR imaging in detecting displaced fragments. *AJR Am J Roentgenol* 1995;165(3):621-625.

40. Magee TH, Hinson GW: MRI of meniscal bucket-handle tears.

Skeletal Radiol 1998;27(9):495-499.

41. McKnight A, Southgate J, Price A, Ostlere S: Meniscal tears with displaced fragments: Common patterns on magnetic resonance imaging. *Skeletal Radiol* 2010;39(3):279-283.

42. Koenig JH, Ranawat AS, Umans HR, Difelice GS: Meniscal root tears: Diagnosis and treatment. *Arthroscopy* 2009;25(9):1025-1032.

43. De Smet AA, Ilahi OA, Graf BK: Reassessment of the MR criteria for stability of osteochondritis dissecans in the knee and ankle. *Skeletal Radiol* 1996;25(2):159-163.

44. Mosher TJ: MRI of osteochondral injuries of the knee and ankle in the athlete. *Clin Sports Med* 2006;25(4):843-866.

Orthopaedic Medicine

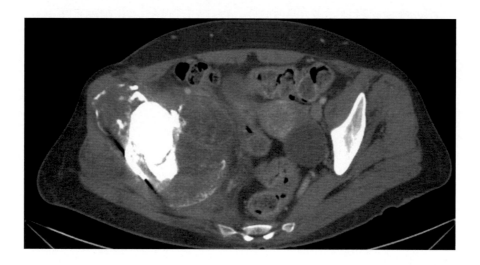

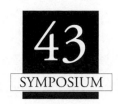

Imaging Interpretation of Oncologic Musculoskeletal Conditions

Carol D. Morris, MD
Theodore W. Parsons III, MD, FACS
Joseph H. Schwab, MD
David M. Panicek, MD

Abstract

There is considerable overlap in the clinical and imaging presentation of general orthopaedic conditions and musculoskeletal neoplasms. At centers that treat orthopaedic oncologic conditions, it is not uncommon to see patients with spine and extremity tumors previously treated for presumed general orthopaedic ailments. It is important for orthopaedic surgeons to understand how to interpret commonly ordered radiographic studies (radiographs, MRIs, and CT scans) as they relate to bone and soft-tissue tumors, to be familiar with the imaging appearance of common musculoskeletal lesions in the extremities and spine, and to understand what imaging findings should trigger a referral to an orthopaedic oncologist.

Instr Course Lect 2012;61:541-551.

Surgeons at centers that treat orthopaedic oncologic conditions often see patients with spine and extremity tumors who were previously treated for presumed general orthopaedic ailments. Almost every subspecialty in orthopaedics is affected because the clinical presentation of bone and soft-tissue tumors often mimics common musculoskeletal symptoms such as limping, a dorsal wrist mass, radiating low back pain, or knee discomfort and swelling. The converse is also true. General orthopaedic conditions, such as fascial herniations and myositis, may be misdiagnosed as a tumor. Given the considerable overlap in symptoms and physical examination findings, understanding the subtleties of commonly ordered imaging studies can be exceedingly valuable.

This chapter discusses the interpretation of commonly ordered imaging studies (radiographs, MRIs, and CT scans) as they relate to bone and soft-tissue tumors, reviews the imaging appearance of common musculoskeletal lesions, and can help surgeons understand imaging findings that require patient referral to an orthopaedic oncologist.

Basics of MRI Interpretation

Musculoskeletal Tumor Appearance

Various extrinsic and intrinsic factors affect the appearance of musculoskeletal tumors on MRIs.[1] The particular magnetic resonance pulse sequence used is the most important extrinsic factor. A pulse sequence is the mechanism by which protons in the patient are interrogated to produce images that emphasize or weight various properties of different tissues or substances. Pulse sequences are loosely analogous to the various stains used by pathologists; each has a different purpose. The two major classes of pulse sequences are spin-echo and gradient echo.

T1-weighted spin-echo images are often described as anatomy images because they depict normal structures

Dr. Morris or an immediate family member serves as a board member, owner, officer, or committee member of the American Academy of Orthopaedic Surgeons. Dr. Parsons or an immediate family member has received research or institutional support from GE Healthcare and serves as a board member, owner, officer, or committee member of the Society of Military Orthopaedic Surgeons, the Musculoskeletal Tumor Society, the Michigan Orthopaedic Society, and the American Orthopaedic Association. Neither of the following authors nor any immediate family member has received anything of value from or owns stock in a commercial company or institution related directly or indirectly to the subject of this chapter: Dr. Schwab and Dr. Panicek.

Table 1

Ranges of Parameters Used to Weight MRI Pulse Sequences

Sequence	Repetition Time (TR) (ms)	Echo Time (TE) (ms)	Inversion Time (TI) (ms)
T1-weighted	400-700	9-15	–
T2-weighted	2,000-6,000	60-120	–
Proton density-weighted	1,800-5,000	10-30	–
STIR	2,000-6,000	20-50	140-160

STIR = Short tau inversion recovery.

with fine detail. T1-weighted images are critical in showing bone tumors against a background of fatty marrow, in distinguishing normal marrow from tumors, and in showing the presence of fat or hemorrhage within a mass. T2-weighted sequences, also referred to as fluid-sensitive sequences, produce "pathology images." In T2-weighted images of bone lesions, fat suppression is essential for distinguishing tumor from surrounding marrow edema and fatty marrow, all of which can show high signal intensity.

Proton density spin-echo images, although widely used in imaging traumatic injuries and internal derangement, are of limited use in musculoskeletal tumor imaging because the signal intensities of tumor, edema, and surrounding marrow are often similar, thereby decreasing the conspicuity of the lesion on such images.

Short tau inversion recovery (STIR) images exhibit uniform fat suppression across the entire image, but this special type of spin-echo image is not recommended for characterizing or staging musculoskeletal tumors. The similarly bright appearance of many tumors on STIR sequences limits their characterization. The actual extent of tumor spread is often overestimated because of the signal produced from even minimal amounts of peritumoral edema. STIR sequences are useful in the presence of surgical hardware because they are less affected by metal artifacts.

Pregadolinium and postgadolinium fat-saturated T1-weighted spin-echo images are often helpful in tumor assessment.[2] Enhancement within a lesion indicates that the lesion is not a cyst but does not distinguish benign from malignant etiologies. Enhancement also may increase the conspicuity of a small tumor recurrence within a background of posttreatment changes.

Gradient-echo images can be obtained more quickly than most spin-echo images but provide different tissue contrast. In tumor imaging, gradient-echo images obtained with long echo times (TE) (> 12 ms) are used to assess for regions of very low signal that appear larger than on other sequences. This finding, called blooming, indicates the presence of metal (such as iron in hemosiderin) and allows considerable narrowing of the differential diagnosis.

An MRI study often includes a printed series descriptor that names the weighting of the pulse sequence used. If not included, the weighting of a spin-echo pulse sequence can be deduced from the combination of repetition time (TR), TE, and for STIR, inversion time (TI) printed on the image. Some typical ranges for these parameters at 1.5 Tesla are shown in **Table 1**.

The selection of various pulse sequences, imaging planes, slice thickness, gadolinium contrast material, and other scan parameters for a particular patient constitutes the scan protocol, which is tailored by the radiologist to optimally answer the questions posed by the referring physician. The chemical and tissue compositions of the tumor are the key intrinsic factors that affect the appearance of tumors on MRI studies. MRI is excellent for identifying various chemicals, such as methemoglobin, hemosiderin, and water. Similarly, MRI can determine the presence of fat (both macroscopic and microscopic) and can suggest the presence of collagen or myxoid matrix within a lesion.

Characterizing Musculoskeletal Tumors

Soft-Tissue Masses

The characterization of a soft-tissue mass as benign or malignant often will be incorrect if the determination relies solely on imaging features such as margin sharpness, local invasion, large size, and internal homogeneity of the lesion. However, if a mass demonstrates certain characteristic imaging features, a specific diagnosis (such as cyst, ganglion, lipoma, fat necrosis, giant cell tumor of the tendon sheath, hemangioma, desmoid/fibromatosis, nerve sheath tumor, subacute hematoma, or elastofibroma) frequently can be made. If such features are not present, the possibility of malignancy should not be dismissed. A specific diagnosis can often be suggested based on the chemical composition (for example, water, hemosiderin, and methemoglobin) of the lesion and/or its tissue composition (for example, fat, collagen, and myxoid matrix) as demonstrated on MRI. Lesion morphology and location can help in lesion characterization.

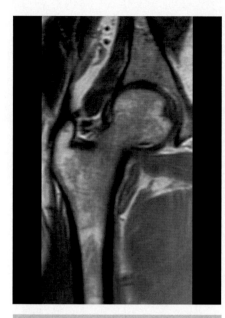

Figure 1 Coronal T1-weighted image of a hip shows the feathery pattern of red marrow, with foci of interspersed fat. Red marrow typically has higher T1-weighted signal than that of nearby muscle, as is seen in this image.

With MRI, sarcomas that are predominantly cystic, myxoid, or hemorrhagic are particularly prone to being misinterpreted as benign cysts or hematomas. Solid elements must be carefully sought and viewed as suspicious for cancer; gadolinium-enhanced imaging is essential in this assessment.

Bone Lesions

Radiographs remain critical in the characterization of bone lesions and should not be neglected in the initial evaluation; however, MRI can provide useful information. Bone tumors (primary or metastatic) replace the normal marrow and typically show signal similar to that of muscle on T1-weighted images.[3,4] Most bone tumors have sharply defined boundaries with surrounding normal marrow on MRI studies; this sharpness should not be misinterpreted as representing a narrow zone of transition; this criterion is only applicable to trabecular altera-

tions at radiography. Similarly, it is important not to mistake red marrow for tumor. Red marrow often has a feathery appearance on T1-weighted images because of foci of interspersed fat and generally shows signal intensity higher than that of muscle on T1-weighted images (**Figure 1**).

MRI generally does not depict calcifications unless they are large and/or very dense, limiting the use of MRI in identifying calcified tumor matrix. On fat-suppressed T2-weighted images, enchondroma and low-grade chondrosarcoma often can be identified because of the presence of multiple small lobules with very high signal intensity caused by the high water content of hyaline cartilage lobules.

Blood-fluid (fluid-fluid) levels have been reported in a wide range of soft-tissue and bone tumors, both benign and malignant. A bone lesion composed solely of blood-fluid levels is consistent with an aneurysmal bone cyst.[5] If thick septa or soft-tissue nodules are present as well, other diagnoses must be considered, such as telangiectatic osteogenic sarcoma, or a secondary aneurysmal bone cyst engrafted on another bone tumor. Gadolinium-enhanced images are useful in assessing soft-tissue elements within an otherwise cystic bone lesion.

Lytic bone metastases generally show moderately increased signal throughout on fat-suppressed T2-weighted images, whereas blastic lesions often show such signal only in a peripheral rim (halo).[6,7] When present, this halo can be helpful in diagnosing a blastic metastasis, which otherwise generally shows low signal on all pulse sequences and might be mistaken for a bone island.

The differential diagnosis for bone lesions surrounded by extensive marrow edema includes osteoid osteoma/osteoblastoma, chondroblastoma, Langerhans cell histiocytosis, and os-

teomyelitis. As a general (but not absolute) guideline, the greater the extent of surrounding marrow edema, the more likely it is that the bone lesion is benign.[8,9]

Extremity Bone Tumors

The discovery of a bone lesion while providing patient care can be an anxiety-provoking event for a surgeon. A basic understanding of how to best interpret the imaging studies associated with these lesions is essential to providing appropriate patient care and arriving at an accurate and timely diagnosis.

Approaches to Identification and Types

Plain radiographs remain the gold standard for evaluating bone lesions, and good quality, orthogonal views should be obtained. The ability to interpret the radiographs generally stems from one of two approaches: the so-called Aunt Minnie approach,[10] where there is general recognition of a certain appearance that leads to the diagnosis (I know my Aunt Minnie when I see her); and the biologic approach as refined by Lodwick et al.[11] The latter approach provides some understanding of the biologic behavior of the lesion and the biologic response of the bone. This method of interpretation is not so dependent on experience but rather allows for the development of a differential diagnosis based on understanding the pathophysiology and significance of the observed radiographic changes. This biologic approach categorizes lesions based on the activity of the lesion in bone and the bone's response to the presence of the lesion (so-called zone of transition), if any. Type I lesions are geographic, and are divided into three subtypes: IA, with sclerotic margin (as in a nonossifying fibroma); IB, with a well-defined margin; and IC, with a poorly defined margin (an active lesion in bone, such as a giant cell tumor or

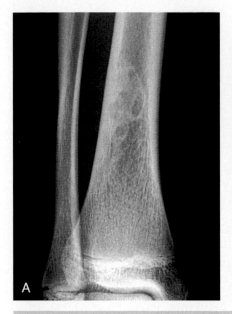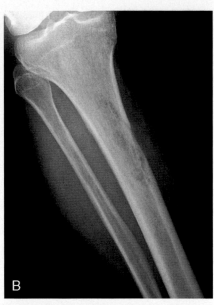

Figure 2 **A,** Radiograph of a distal tibial type IA lesion (sclerotic margins, geographic, and eccentric in the bone). This benign-appearing lesion represents a healing nonossifying fibroma. **B,** Radiograph of a tibial diaphyseal type II lesion with indistinct margins and cortical destruction. This aggressive-appearing lesion represents metastatic carcinoma.

chondroblastoma may appear as a type IB or IC lesion). Type II lesions appear moth eaten and suggest a more aggressive process (such as lymphoma or myeloma). Type III lesions are permeative, destructive lesions that reflect a very aggressive process (such as osteosarcoma or Ewing sarcoma). In general, the higher the classification type, the more aggressive the lesion is in bone (**Figure 2**).

A combination of the two approaches is ideal and generally allows a reasonably accurate diagnosis based on plain radiographs of bone. The more experienced the observer, the greater is his or her comfort level in understanding and recognizing bone lesions.

Aggressiveness of the Lesion

Using a similar approach in identifying the aggressiveness of a bone lesion, the size of the lesion, the zone of transition (margin sclerotic, distinct, or poorly defined), the presence or absence of cortical disruption, and the presence or absence of a soft-tissue mass should

be considered in determining if a lesion is malignant or benign. A malignant lesion is more likely to be large and poorly margined, demonstrate cortical destruction, and manifest soft-tissue extension, whereas a benign lesion is likely to have the opposite appearance (smaller, marginated, intact cortex with no soft-tissue extension).[12] Although this rule generally holds true, there are exceptions. Osteomyelitis, for example, may have a very aggressive appearance and yet is not a malignant lesion (although it may be as difficult to treat as some malignancies), whereas some metastatic lesions to bone may be small and rather indolent in appearance but are by definition malignant.

Other Helpful Diagnostic Factors

The location of the lesion provides additional helpful information because certain lesions have a propensity to appear in specific locations. For example, epiphyseal lesions tend to be subchon-

dral cysts, giant cell tumors, chondroblastomas, or clear cell chondrosarcomas. Most simple bone cysts present in the proximal humerus or the proximal femur, and osteofibrous dysplasia or adamantinoma are generally anterior tibial diaphyseal lesions. Similarly, the transverse location in bone (central, eccentric, cortical, or juxtacortical) aids in the diagnosis. For example, nonossifying fibromas classically present as an eccentric lesion, whereas simple cysts are generally centrally located.

Patient age is another parameter that can provide diagnostic information because certain lesions tend to manifest in specific age groups.[13] Using the appearance of round cell lesions in bone as an example, histocytic lesions (such as eosinophilic granuloma) tend to present in the first decade of life, Ewing sarcoma in the second decade, lymphoma in the fourth or fifth decade, and myeloma or metastatic small cell carcinoma thereafter.

Cortical destruction and new bone formation also provide useful information about the lesion. Periosteal bone patterns, such as the onion skin, sunburst/hair on end, or Codman triangle, indicate an aggressive, usually malignant (or possibly infectious) process (**Figure 3**). Endosteal scalloping is also indicative of an active lesion, although this appearance in bone may form slowly over time.

Matrix production, or the presence of mineral density in a lesion (given most lesions are lytic), provides useful information. Chondroid lesions such as enchondromas, chondroblastomas, or chondromyxoid fibromas may demonstrate a stippled or arcs and rings calcification within the lesion. Intramedullary infarcts generally have a more wispy "smoke up the chimney" appearance. Fibrous dysplasia tends to have a ground glass appearance. Osteosarcoma tends to manifest cloudlike or fluffy mineralization (ossification), whereas chondrosarcoma presents with punctate or stippled mineralization (calcifications).[14]

Bone Scintigraphy

Bone scintigraphy is another useful tool in establishing the differential diagnosis of bone lesions. These scans are extremely sensitive in detecting the presence (or absence) of bone formation in response to a lesion, as well as the vascularity of a lesion. Although nonspecific, this modality is particularly helpful in identifying multiple or metastatic lesions of bone, occult lesions of bone, and, as an adjunct to other imaging modalities, in determining active versus indolent lesions of bone (and as such may help in identifying lesions that have undergone transformation from indolent behavior to aggressive behavior). The surgeon should keep in mind that any rapidly progressive lesion in bone (such as multiple myeloma, renal cell carcinoma, thyroid carcinoma, and aggressive infection with necrosis) may not cause a response in bone that is sufficient to demonstrate significant uptake. Such lesions may give a false-negative result and may be better visualized with other imaging modalities.[15]

Computed Tomography

CT is another useful tool that provides helpful diagnostic information, with superior resolution compared with plain radiographs. It is particularly helpful in identifying and evaluating mineral densities in bone and soft-tissue lesions. Consequently, CT can help identify subtle calcifications within lesions (such as chondroid lesions of bone, or synovial cell sarcomas in soft tissue) or identify the "fluffy" bone formation in osteosarcoma (**Figure 4**). It is an excellent modality for identifying areas of subtle lytic or sclerotic changes in bone, particularly in

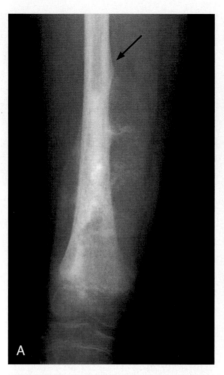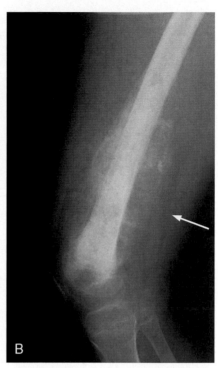

Figure 3   AP (**A**) and lateral (**B**) radiographic views of the femur showing an aggressive bone-forming tumor. The arrow in (A) points to a Codman triangle. The arrow in (B) points to ossified Sharpey fibers. These findings are pathognomonic for high-grade osteosarcoma.

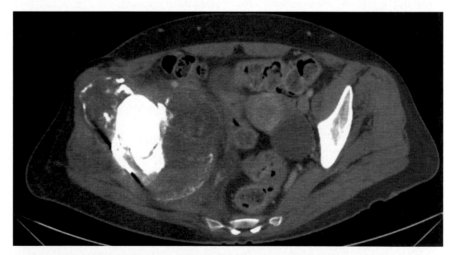

Figure 4   Pelvic CT scan showing a recurrent lesion with punctate calcifications and an extensive soft-tissue mass. Note that the CT scan clearly shows the mineral density in this pelvic chondrosarcoma.

the flat bones.[16] CT can be used to assess areas of cortical thinning or breakthrough that are otherwise difficult to detect. It is superior at identifying the nidus of an osteoid osteoma and can

clearly demonstrate the thin walls of cystic or aneurysmal lesions. CT is useful at visualizing the complex bony anatomy of the axial skeleton and in guiding needle biopsies or radiofre-

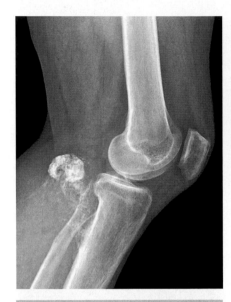

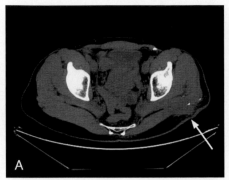

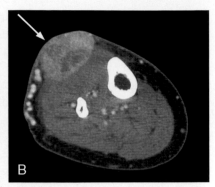

Figure 6 **A,** CT scan of the pelvis without intravenous contrast shows a gluteal mass (arrow). The details of the mass are difficult to see in the absence of contrast. **B,** CT scan of the lower leg with intravenous contrast showing a mass (arrow).

Figure 5 Lateral radiograph of the knee showing the disorganized periarticular calcifications in a synovial sarcoma.

quency thermal ablation of bone lesions. Its relative lack of motion susceptibility makes CT ideal for abdominal imaging. CT scans of the chest, abdomen, and pelvis have become standard imaging studies in the evaluation of patients with metastatic disease to bone, whereas chest CT is a mandatory study for staging known primary malignant bone lesions.[17]

Discussion

The careful evaluation of a bone lesion, including analysis of the plain radiographic features, coupled with additional studies such as MRI, bone scintigraphy, and CT if necessary, will generally lead the surgeon to a limited and accurate differential diagnosis and will expedite appropriate patient care. If a primary malignancy of bone is suspected or there is considerable doubt regarding the diagnosis, patients should be referred to an orthopaedic oncologist for additional evaluation and subsequent treatment.

Extremity Soft-Tissue Tumors

When forming a differential diagnosis for soft-tissue masses, a good first goal is to determine if the lesion is benign or malignant.[18] Several clues are available from imaging studies. The physical examination and clinical suspicion also remain an important part of the evaluation process. As a general rule, any mass that is greater than 5 cm and deep to the fascia must be considered a malignancy until proven otherwise. This is true regardless of whether the mass appears homogeneous or heterogenous on MRI sequences.

Radiography

Plain radiographs can be helpful in the differential diagnosis. Virtually all soft-tissue masses have the potential to develop calcifications or ossification by various mechanisms. Patterns of mineralization as seen on radiographs can be characteristic of certain lesions. For example, phleboliths are seen almost exclusively in soft-tissue hemangiomas. Intra-articular calcifications throughout the joint suggest synovial chondromatosis. Haphazard calcification patterns raise the suspicion of malignancy (for example, up to 20% of synovial sarcomas have areas of mineralization) (**Figure 5**).

Computed Tomography

CT scans are indicated in the workup of soft-tissue masses if there is a contraindication to MRI (such as a pacemaker). When CT is chosen as the primary modality for imaging a soft-tissue mass, the administration of intravenous contrast will make the mass more obvious and aid the radiologist in providing more anatomic and diagnostic details (**Figure 6**). CT is superior to MRI for evaluating areas of mineralization, such as delineating the zonal pattern typically seen in myositis ossificans. CT is also useful for examining the extent of bone involvement adjacent to soft-tissue masses.

Magnetic Resonance Imaging

MRI is the most useful tool for evaluating soft-tissue masses. MRI is an evolving technology, with more sophisticated sequences commonly being used for the delineation of fine anatomic detail. T1-weighted, fat-suppressed T2-weighted, and post-gadolinium sequences are the most informative studies for evaluating soft-tissue tumors. For most tumors, the T1-weighted signal will be isointense to the surrounding skeletal muscle, the fat-suppressed T2-weighted sequence will typically be bright relative to skeletal muscle, and the postcontrast image will show varying degrees of heterogeneity.

Most orthopaedic surgeons will suspect that an obviously large, deeply seated, and heterogeneous mass is likely to be sarcoma (**Figure 7**). Because it is more difficult to diagnose masses that are small and those that have a rather homogeneous appearance on various MRI sequences, the addition of gadolinium can be very helpful. For example, **Figure 8,** *A* and *B* show a small (< 5 cm) periarticular mass with homogeneous signal on both the T1-weighted and fat-suppressed T2-weighted sequences. It would be easy to assume this innocuous-appearing mass represents a cyst. Following the administration of contrast (**Figure 8,** *C*), it can be seen that the mass has central heterogeneous enhancement as opposed to rim enhancement, which is consistent with a solid mass. When the solid nature of the mass is confirmed, the patient should be referred for biopsy. Tissue sampling in this case revealed an extraskeletal myxoid chondrosarcoma. Myxoid is a material composed of glycosaminoglycans, which histologically appear amorphous and semitranspar-

ent (like mucus). The common myxoid-containing tumors are myxoma, myxoid liposarcoma, and myxofibrosarcoma. On MRI, myxoid material has a cystlike appearance that causes diagnostic uncertainty. Gadolinium contrast can help distinguish cysts from myxoid-containing lesions.

Although most superficial masses (those located in the subcutaneous tissue) are likely to be lipomas, up to one third of sarcomas occur in the superficial compartment. These lesions can be easily palpated during a thorough physical examination. Masses that are

hard, fixed to the underlying tissue, or greater that 5 cm should raise the suspicion of malignancy. On MRI, lipomas should have the same signal characteristics as the surrounding subcutaneous fat on all sequences. If the mass in question deviates from this rule even slightly, lipoma should not be presumed, and the patient should be referred for biopsy.

Ultrasound

Ultrasound can be used to distinguish solid and cystic masses. Ultrasound offers many advantages, including cost ef-

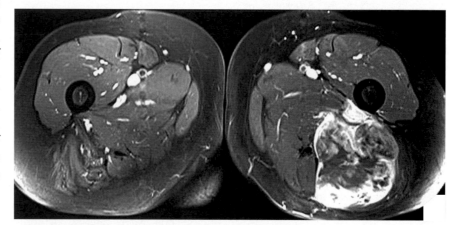

Figure 7   MRI scan of a large heterogeneous mass in the posterior thigh consistent with soft-tissue sarcoma.

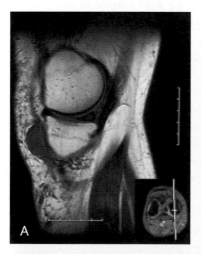 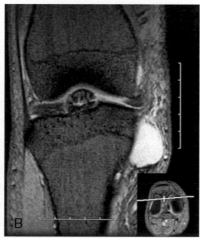 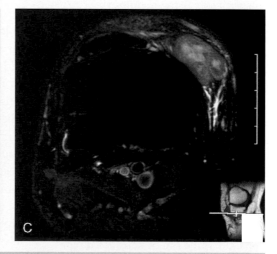

Figure 8   **A,** T1-weighted sagittal MRI scan showing a small periarticular mass in the knee with signal isointense to muscle. **B,** Fat-suppressed, T2-weighted MRI coronal scan showing bright homogeneous signal in the mass. **C,** Post-contrast image demonstrating heterogeneous enhancement of the mass, which confirms its solid nature. A diagnosis of extraskeletal chondrosarcoma was made.

Table 2

Tumors With Their Corresponding Unique Pathopneumonic Imaging Appearance

Tumor Type	Unique Imaging Characteristic
Pigmented villonodular synovitis	Intra-articular; dark signal on T1- and T2-weighted sequences
Intramuscular hemangioma	Does not have the shape of a round mass; serpiginous appearance; contains fat
Elastofibroma	Occurs almost exclusively between the scapula and chest wall
Lipoma	Same signal as subcutaneous fat on all sequences; must uniformly lose signal on fat-suppressed sequences
Neurofibroma	Often associated with a "tail" on sagittal or coronal images

ficiency, portability, and easy side-to-side assessment. It is usually easily available and provides immediate dynamic feedback. Ultrasound is not used as frequently as other imaging modalities because it is operator dependent, resulting in significant variability in imaging.

Discussion

As a general rule, histologic subtypes are not readily identified on imaging. However, there are a few tumor types that have a pathopneumonic appearance on imaging (**Table 2**). It is important to remember that not all neoplastic soft-tissue masses in the extremity are sarcomas. Lymph nodes can reach considerable size in lymphoma and from metastatic disease. Certain carcinomas, such as lung cancer, can present with soft-tissue nodules.

Spine Tumors

Imaging Considerations

The basic concepts of tumor evaluation are the same for the spine as they are in the extremity. The difference is that low back pain is so common that spine imaging is obtained more frequently than extremity imaging. In addition, the predilection for certain tumors to occur in the spine and the anatomic differences found in the spine make it unique. For these reasons, the spine can be considered separately from the remaining skeleton when studying bone tumors.

It is estimated that low back pain costs nearly $100 billion per year in the United States and is one of the most common reasons for a visit to a primary care physician. Imaging studies are often obtained early in the course of managing patients with low back pain despite data suggesting that early imaging does not improve outcomes.[19,20] Obtaining advanced imaging studies can result in the incidental discovery of lesions. Such a finding may prompt further imaging or a referral to a specialist, which further increases costs. Clearly, there are instances in which an aggressive lesion is discovered early in its course with favorable implications. However, it is unclear how many referrals or additional tests are ordered to evaluate benign lesions discovered incidentally. In general, images of the spine should be ordered to help confirm a suspected pathology that is amenable to treatment. Nonspecific low back pain should not prompt imaging studies, particularly when present for less than 6 weeks.

The bones of the spine are unique in that they are separated from the intervertebral disks. As disks show signs of wear, there can be associated commensurate changes in the adjacent vertebral bodies. Abnormal T1- and T2-weighted signal changes along the vertebral end plate are common and are often associated with disk degeneration. Signal changes along the end plate can be associated with increased vascularity, which leads to increased signal on T2-weighted images. Alternatively, as the degeneration proceeds, fat can infiltrate the area and lead to increased T1-weighted signal.[21] It is necessary to look for these changes next to a degenerative disk. If these signal abnormalities are noted in a pristine disk, there may be another underlying cause. The signal changes themselves are nonspecific; it is their association with the degenerative disk that is the key to making a correct diagnosis. The Schmorl node or body, which represents a violation of the vertebral end plate by the intervertebral disk, is another nononcologic finding that might be misinterpreted as an aggressive lesion.

History and Physical Examination

History and physical examination findings are key determinants when advanced imaging studies are being considered and are also helpful in developing a differential diagnosis. The age of the patient can focus the differential diagnoses before imaging studies are obtained. If a patient age 40 to 65 years presents with an unknown lesion in the spine, metastatic disease must be ruled out. More than 1,000,000 new cancer cases are diagnosed in the United States each year,[22] and metastases will develop in more than 50% of patients. Within the skeleton, the spine is the most common site for bone metastasis.

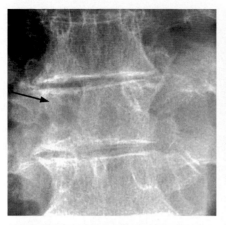

Figure 9 Plain radiograph of the spine showing the winking owl sign, which is the loss of a pedicle (arrow) commonly seen in patients with metastatic disease.

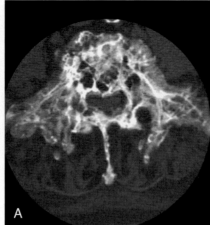
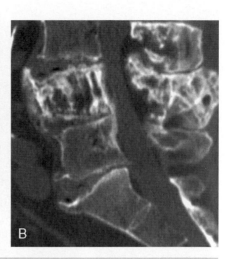

Figure 10 Axial CT view of the cervical spine (**A**) and sagittal CT view of the lumbar spine (**B**) in a patient with Paget disease.

Imaging Findings for Specific Lesions

Plain radiographic images can be helpful in evaluating a patient for a destructive lesion. The so-called winking owl sign is a classic finding indicative of pedicle destruction (**Figure 9**). On an AP radiograph of the spine, the spinous process makes up the nose of the owl. The paired pedicles make up the eyes. When one pedicle is destroyed, then the owl appears to be winking. Metastatic lesions can involve any aspect of the vertebrae.

Hemangiomas are quite common in the spine and are actually hamartomas, not tumors. Hemangiomas can be seen on radiographs but are often seen incidentally on MRI or CT scans. Classic CT findings demonstrate coarsened trabeculae arranged in a vertical direction, and axial imaging demonstrates a polka-dot appearance. The MRI findings reveal increased signal in both T1- and T2-weighted sequences. This is consistent with the fact that blood vessels and fat are both present in most hemangiomas.[23] Hemangiomas typically involved the vertebral body but can involve the posterior elements as well. In fact, one lesion can

involve the entire vertebrae. An abnormality involving the entire vertebrae is suggestive for hemangioma, metastatic disease, or Paget disease.

Certain metabolic bone diseases can mimic neoplastic processes. One example is Paget disease, which typically affects older, white men. Plain radiographs are often diagnostic, and CT can be used to confirm haphazard coarsened trabeculae and bony deformation (**Figure 10**). The lesions are often hot on bone scans, and the alkaline phosphatase level may be elevated. It is important to be aware that Paget disease can dedifferentiate into a Paget sarcoma.

In patients younger than 30 years, the differential diagnosis is less likely metastatic disease and more likely benign entities. Infection and active benign bone tumors such as osteoid osteoma, osteoblastoma, and giant cell tumors are more common. Bacterial infections typically involve the disk space and adjacent vertebral end plates. Local end plate changes and a loss of intervertebral disk height in the setting of normal end plates and well-preserved disk heights can be helpful in making the diagnosis of bacterial infection. Patients typically have pain at

rest in contrast to those with mechanical back pain.

Osteoid osteomas and osteoblastomas typically involve the posterior elements and may be associated with a painful scoliosis (**Figure 11**). Plain radiographs can be useful in identifying these tumors, but advanced imaging is often necessary. Bone scans can be quite useful in detecting these lesions but are nonspecific. MRI will demonstrate low signal intensity on both T1- and T2-weighted images, which is secondary to the bony component of the tumors. These lesions will also demonstrate increased T2-weighted signal in the surrounding tissues, which is indicative of reactive edema. Giant cell tumors often involve the vertebral body rather than the posterior elements. The lesions are lytic and can be quite destructive with associated soft-tissue components.

Summary

Understanding the basic imaging characteristics of bone and soft-tissue tumors can provide the orthopaedic surgeon who does not specialize in oncology with a framework for decision making. Familiarity with radiographic and MRI findings that should

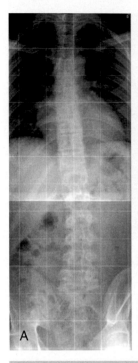
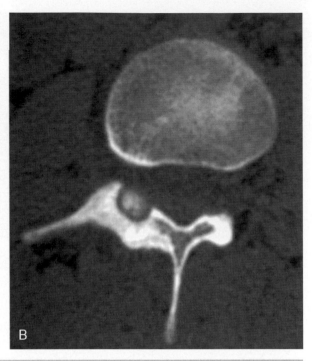

Figure 11 **A,** Scout radiograph shows postural scoliosis, which is often associated with osteoid osteoma. **B,** CT scan shows classic appearance of the nidus of an osteoid osteoma in the posterior spinal elements.

prompt referral to a cancer center is an invaluable diagnostic tool. Continuous review of these imaging characteristics is necessary because musculoskeletal tumors are fairly uncommon.

References

1. Hwang S, Panicek DM: Magnetic resonance imaging, in Davies AM, Sundaram M, James SLJ, eds: *Imaging of Bone Tumors and Tumor-Like Lesions: Techniques and Applications.* Berlin, Germany, Springer-Verlag, 2009, pp 31-52.

2. May DA, Good RB, Smith DK, Parsons TW: MR imaging of musculoskeletal tumors and tumor mimickers with intravenous gadolinium: Experience with 242 patients. *Skeletal Radiol* 1997; 26(1):2-15.

3. Hwang S, Panicek DM: Magnetic resonance imaging of bone marrow in oncology: Part 1. *Skeletal Radiol* 2007;36(10):913-920.

4. Hwang S, Panicek DM: Magnetic resonance imaging of bone marrow in oncology: Part 2. *Skeletal Radiol* 2007;36(11):1017-1027.

5. O'Donnell P, Saifuddin A: The prevalence and diagnostic significance of fluid-fluid levels in focal lesions of bone. *Skeletal Radiol* 2004;33(6): 330-336.

6. Schweitzer ME, Levine C, Mitchell DG, Gannon FH, Gomella LG: Bull's-eyes and halos: Useful MR discriminators of osseous metastases. *Radiology* 1993;188 (1):249-252.

7. Vanel D, Bittoun J, Tardivon A: MRI of bone metastases. *Eur Radiol* 1998;8(8):1345-1351.

8. James SL, Hughes RJ, Ali KE, Saifuddin A: MRI of bone marrow edema associated with focal bone lesions. *Clin Radiol* 2006; 61(12):1003-1009.

9. James SL, Panicek DM, Davies AM: Bone marrow edema associated with benign and malignant

bone tumours. *Eur J Radiol* 2008; 67(1):11-21.

10. Kricun ME: Radiographic evaluation of solitary bone lesions. *Orthop Clin North Am* 1983;14(1): 39-64.

11. Lodwick GS, Wilson AJ, Farrell C, Virtama P, Dittrich F: Determining growth rates of focal lesions of bone from radiographs. *Radiology* 1980;134(3):577-583.

12. Parsons TW III, Frink SJ, Campbell SE: Musculoskeletal neoplasia: Helping the orthopaedic surgeon establish the diagnosis. *Semin Musculoskelet Radiol* 2007; 11(1):3-15.

13. Pettersson H, Springfield DS, Enneking WF: Radiologic diagnosis. *Radiologic Management of Musculoskeletal Tumors.* London, England, Springer-Verlag, 1987, pp 59-86.

14. Sanders TG, Parsons TW III: Radiographic imaging of musculoskeletal neoplasia. *Cancer Control* 2001;8(3):221-231.

15. Weber KL, Peabody T, Frassica FJ, Mott MP, Parsons TW III: Tumors for the general orthopedist: How to save your patients and practice. *Instr Course Lect* 2010;59:579-591.

16. Imhof H, Mang T: Advances in musculoskeletal radiology: Multidetector computed tomography. *Orthop Clin North Am* 2006; 37(3):287-298, v.

17. Parsons TW III, Filzen TW: Evaluation and staging of musculoskeletal neoplasia. *Hand Clin* 2004;20(2):137-145, v.

18. Moulton JS, Blebea JS, Dunco DM, Braley SE, Bisset GS III, Emery KH: MR imaging of soft-tissue masses: Diagnostic efficacy and value of distinguishing between benign and malignant lesions. *AJR Am J Roentgenol* 1995; 164(5):1191-1199.

19. Jarvik JG, Hollingworth W, Martin B, et al: Rapid magnetic reso-

nance imaging vs radiographs for patients with low back pain: A randomized controlled trial. *JAMA* 2003;289(21):2810-2818.

20. Kendrick D, Fielding K, Bentley E, Miller P, Kerslake R, Pringle M: The role of radiography in primary care patients with low back pain of at least 6 weeks duration: A randomised (unblinded) controlled trial. *Health Technol Assess* 2001;5(30):1-69.

21. Modic MT, Steinberg PM, Ross JS, Masaryk TJ, Carter JR: Degenerative disk disease: Assessment of changes in vertebral body marrow with MR imaging. *Radiology* 1988;166(1, Pt 1):193-199.

22. American Cancer Society: *Cancer Facts and Figures 2008*. Atlanta, GA, American Cancer Society, 2008.

23. Wenger DE, Wold LE: Benign vascular lesions of bone: Radiologic and pathologic features. *Skeletal Radiol* 2000;29(2):63-74.

Evaluation of the Patient Presenting
With a Malignant Spinal Tumor

Peter S. Rose, MD

Joseph H. Schwab, MD

Jacob M. Buchowski, MD

Joshua C. Patt, MD, MPH

Abstract

Malignant spinal tumors are frequently encountered in clinical practice. Most of these lesions are caused by metastatic or hematopoietic disease processes. It is useful for the practicing surgeon to have a framework for evaluating and treating these conditions. Equally important is the ability to recognize the rare patient who presents with a primary spinal malignancy, which requires a significantly different treatment protocol.

Instr Course Lect 2012;61:553-565.

Cancer is the second leading cause of death in the United States and the leading cause of death in many industrialized nations.[1,2] There are more than a half million cancer deaths per year in the United States, and up to 70% of patients who die of cancer have spinal metastases present on autopsy.[3,4] It is estimated that more than 20,000 patients per year present with symptomatic epidural spinal cord compression in the United States.[5,6] In contrast, primary spine tumors are extremely rare. Spinal metastases outnumber primary spine tumors by at least 100:1. However, unlike spinal metastases, patients presenting with a primary spinal tumor may potentially be cured with proper treatment.

This chapter discusses the acute presentation and management of patients with primary spinal tumors, the surgical management of patients with metastatic disease, and innovative and minimally invasive treatment options currently available. The proper identification of patients presenting with primary spinal tumors is reviewed because it is critically important to differentiate these patients from those presenting with metastatic spinal disease.

Initial Evaluation

Presentation

Patients presenting with spinal tumors may be symptomatic or asymptomatic. In asymptomatic patients, spinal lesions are generally detected during scans performed for other reasons (such as a CT scan of the abdomen and the pelvis to evaluate pain with a presumptive gastrointestinal etiology) or on staging studies of patients with known oncologic diagnoses but no prior spinal lesions.

Patients with a known oncologic diagnosis and asymptomatic spinal lesions detected on staging studies require careful evaluation. Skeletal metastases are the metastatic lesions initially detected in approximately one third of patients. The identification of these lesions may have profound oncologic implications (upstaging a patient

Dr. Rose or an immediate family member serves as a committee member of the Minnesota Orthopaedic Society and the American Academy of Orthopaedic Surgeons. Dr. Schwab or an immediate family member has received nonincome support (such as equipment or services), commercially derived honoraria, or other non–research-related funding (such as paid travel) from Globus Medical. Dr. Buchowski or an immediate family member is a member of a speakers' bureau or has made paid presentations on behalf of Stryker; serves as a paid consultant to Stryker; and serves as a board member, owner, officer, or committee member of the American Academy of Orthopaedic Surgeons, the Cervical Spine Research Society, the North American Spine Society, the Scoliosis Research Society, and the Spine Arthroplasty Society. Neither Dr. Patt nor any immediate family member has received anything of value from or owns stock in a commercial company or institution related directly or indirectly to the subject of this chapter.

from localized and potentially curable disease to metastatic disease). These patients are generally treated with radiation therapy, chemotherapy, bisphosphonates, and occasionally with careful observation. In highly select patients, solitary lesions may be resected. Patients with incidentally detected spinal tumors and no known history of an oncologic diagnosis require careful staging and evaluation to identify the etiology and rule out a primary spinal neoplasm.

Most patients with spinal tumors usually have pain, which is present in approximately 90% of patients and is often poorly characterized.[7] This neck or back pain may be initially difficult to distinguish from pain caused by typical mechanical causes; however, with time, the pain becomes progressive and unrelenting. The new onset of nonmechanical back pain, especially true night pain, is highly concerning for a malignant etiology. Neurologic signs and symptoms are often present but rarely precede pain symptoms. Although it is rare for patients with a new diagnosis of a spinal tumor to present with frank quadriplegia or paraplegia, many patients have subtle objective neurologic deficits on presentation.[8]

Patients presenting with apparent spinal metastases may be divided into three categories: those with known metastatic disease, those with a history of malignancy without prior metastatic disease, and those with no prior oncologic diagnosis.[9] Patients presenting with characteristic imaging findings of spinal metastases who have established metastatic disease are generally treated without biopsy confirmation. Patients who present with apparent spinal tumors and a history of nonmetastatic cancer require further evaluation before treatment is initiated. New staging studies are obtained in these patients (typically a CT scan of the chest, the abdomen, and the pelvis and a technetium bone scan) to determine the extent of the disease. Biopsy confirmation of metastatic status is usually performed unless miliary, unequivocal metastases are present. These staging studies will often reveal other lesions that may be technically safer and easier to biopsy than a vertebral lesion.

Patients with no prior diagnosis of cancer may present with one or more spinal tumors. Spinal metastases are the first manifestation of malignancy in approximately 20% of patients presenting with vertebral metastases.[10] Biopsy alone will fail to identify a primary tumor in as many as two thirds of these patients. The protocol, described by Rougraff et al,[11] consisting of a patient history and physical examination; routine laboratory studies (complete blood cell count, serum chemistries, inflammatory markers, and myeloma study); a bone scan; and CT of the chest, the abdomen, and the pelvis, will identify the primary site of disease in most patients (approximately 85%) presenting with skeletal lesions from an unknown primary lesion. Many of these patients will not require a biopsy; in those requiring a biopsy, a relatively safely accessed nonspinal lesion for biopsy usually can be identified.

When biopsy is necessary, modern, image-guided, large bore, core needle biopsies are the first-line evaluation of choice.[12] Highly accurate biopsies can be safely performed in the outpatient setting with local analgesia and/or light sedation. Samples are sent for culture and histology to evaluate for possible infectious etiologies. Open biopsy is rarely necessary.

Physical Examination

Patients presenting with a spinal tumor should undergo a complete physical examination to determine their neurologic status and assess evidence of disease spread. The examination should evaluate the entire neurologic axis because patients with spinal tumors may have noncontiguous, clinically significant lesions (present in nearly 15% of patients with metastatic disease) and may have undiagnosed intracranial lesions detected by physical examination findings (for example, cranial nerve deficits).[13]

The physical examination provides key information about the potential for spinal instability from a tumor. At this time, oncologic spinal instability is primarily a clinical rather than a radiologic diagnosis. Although imaging findings provide information to assess stability, these findings are combined with clinical results, information on the nature of the patient's malignancy, and the potential for treatment to determine the need for spinal stabilization. The presence of a clinical deformity, usually kyphosis, suggests present or developing instability. Pain or neurologic signs or symptoms that are exacerbated with position or axial or rotational loading are highly suggestive of local mechanical instability.

Imaging Evaluation

Standing plain radiographs are used to initially assess patients presenting with spinal tumors. Although lacking sensitivity to detect spinal tumors, radiographs are easy to obtain and provide an immediate assessment of alignment, pathologic fractures, and surgical fixation points. Serial radiographs are used to assess disease progression or the response to treatment.

Because as many as 15% of patients presenting with symptomatic spinal metastases will have clinically significant, noncontiguous lesions, it is important to evaluate the full spinal axis (**Figure 1**). MRI provides the most sensitive and specific modality for this evaluation, with sensitivities and specificity for tumor detection of 98.5%

and 98.9%, respectively.[14] CT has decreased sensitivity compared with MRI but provides the highest level of bony detail. CT can be a valuable preoperative study; when combined with myelography, it provides information on neurologic compression in patients unable to undergo MRI. Technetium bone scans are commonly obtained in the staging evaluation of patients with suspected metastatic disease. These studies provide an efficient evaluation of the entire skeleton but may be falsely negative in hematopoietic or aggressive lytic malignancies. Benign conditions (such as osteoporotic fractures) can cloud the interpretation of bone scans in patients with metastatic disease.

The role of positron emission tomography (PET) is currently evolving. PET is commonly used in staging many hematopoietic malignancies as well as carcinomas. However, the sensitivity and specificity of PET is highly dependent on histology and has a low spatial resolution. Relatively lower grade malignancies are not reliably evaluated with PET, and many false positive findings may occur.

Establishing a Diagnosis

Patients who present with a spinal tumor must be evaluated to determine the extent of disease, neurologic status, and the presence of spinal instability. It cannot be overemphasized that even in patients presenting with recent-onset neurologic deficits, diagnostic evaluation is critical before initiating treatment. Treatment strategies are substantially different for patients presenting with metastatic, hematopoietic, malignant primary lesions and benign primary spinal lesions. If treatment strategies are not based on the diagnosis of the underlying condition, the patient may undergo unnecessary procedures, and the opportunity for a cure will be dramatically diminished in patients presenting with primary malignancies.

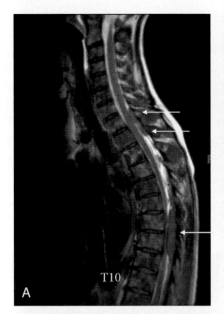
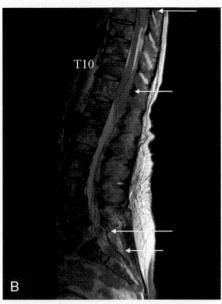

Figure 1   **A** and **B,** Sagittal T2-weighted MRI scans showing seven sites (arrows) of metastatic epidural spinal cord/cauda equina compression.

In practice, basic staging studies (careful history and physical examination; blood tests; and CT of the chest, the abdomen, and the pelvis) can be quickly obtained and will provide a strong indication of whether the spinal tumor has a hematopoietic or a metastatic origin. Hematopoietic tumors rarely require surgical treatment unless pathologic fracture with gross instability is present. Metastatic tumors without clinically important neurologic deficit or spinal instability are often initially treated with chemotherapy and radiation. Primary spinal malignancies require treatment that is dependent on the histology and is highly specialized. In patients treated with surgery, en bloc resection is often necessary to provide the best outcomes. The dramatic variability in the treatment of these conditions highlights the importance of establishing a diagnosis before treatment is initiated.

Corticosteroids are often used in patients who present with spinal tumors. Although widely used in clinical practice, there is relatively modest published evidence to support their

benefit. The existing evidence suggests limited short-term improvement in ambulatory status with adverse side effects in 11% of patients.[15] Doses are generally modest (for example, dexamethasone 6 mg every 6 hours), and any neurologic benefit likely plateaus after 10 to 14 days of treatment. There is little, if any, role for prolonged steroid therapy or for the ultra high-dose steroids used in spinal cord injury protocols for patients with spinal tumors. If the histologic diagnosis has not been established, steroids should not be administered before biopsy. The tumor-lytic effect of steroids can lead to false-negative biopsies in hematopoietic malignancies, and steroid therapy is clearly counterproductive if an occult infection, rather than a tumor, is present.

Treatment of Patients With Metastatic Spinal Tumors

Most patients presenting with spinal tumors will have metastases. The main treatment goal in this population is to maintain or improve the patient's quality of life during a treatable but

Table 1

Radiosensitivity of Common Histologies

Relative Radiosensitivity	Tumor Histology
Sensitive	Hematopoietic Germ cell
Moderately sensitive	Breast
Moderately resistant	Colorectal Lung
Highly resistant	Thyroid Renal cell Sarcoma Melanoma Chordoma

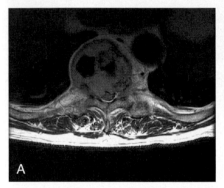 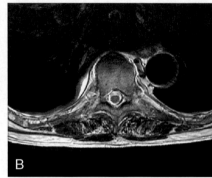

Figure 2   **A,** Fast spin-echo axial MRI showing metastatic epidural spinal cord compression in a patient with multiple myeloma. **B,** MRI showing resolution of tumor mass after treatment with 3,000 cGy radiation in 10 fractions.

ultimately incurable disease process. Treatment should attempt to decrease pain, preserve or improve neurologic function, and maintain mobility. Radiation therapy, chemotherapy, and surgery are used to achieve these goals.

Radiation Therapy

Radiation therapy is indicated in the management of most patients with symptomatic metastatic spinal lesions. Although different histologies have different radiosensitivities (**Table 1**), radiation therapy is still useful in patients to achieve local disease stasis and avoid the need for surgery or as an adjuvant to surgical procedures to minimize the risk of symptomatic local recurrence. A prospective trial by Maranzano and Latini[13] established the efficacy of radiotherapy. Pain relief and maintenance or improvement of neurologic status occurred in approximately 75% of the patients treated with radiotherapy. Most patients are treated with brief courses of conventionally targeted radiotherapy (such as 2,000 cGy in 5 fractions or 3,000 cGy in 10 fractions). Malignancies that are very radiosensitive (hematopoietic tumors, germ cell tumors) rarely require surgical decompression because radiation alone will cause rapid local tumor regression (**Figure 2**). Radiotherapy, however, increases the risk of wound healing complications if surgery is subsequently necessary.[16]

Chemotherapy

Histologic-specific chemotherapy is a key aspect in the treatment of patients with metastatic disease. Surgery and radiotherapy play a strong role in the local control of symptomatic spinal tumors; however, chemotherapy is necessary to treat the overall disease process and is a critical component in prolonging the patient's life. In patients with very chemosensitive malignancies, aggressive chemotherapy may supplant the use of radiotherapy, with or without surgical treatment, to aid in the local control of tumors. Chemotherapy is particularly helpful when patients have tumor- or treatment-related bone marrow suppression, and radiotherapy would expose a large area of hematopoietic marrow to the chronic suppressive effects of radiation.

Careful consideration is needed to weigh the relative timing of chemotherapy and surgery. Patients with ongoing immunosuppressive or other systemic effects of chemotherapy are poor surgical candidates. A minimum 3-week waiting period is generally necessary before chemotherapy is reinitiated after surgical procedures. Particularly powerful agents may necessitate greater restrictions. For example, bevacizumab is a potent angiogenic inhibitor. To decrease the risk of serious wound complications, clinical experience supports a 4- to 6-week delay between the last dose of bevacizumab and surgery, and a similar 4- to 6-week delay after surgery before beginning or continuing this medication.

Surgery

Surgery is used in the treatment of patients with spinal metastases to effect neurologic decompression, stabilization, and/or realignment of the spine (if pathologic deformity is present). Patients are generally considered candidates for spinal surgery if they have a life expectancy of at least 10 to 12 weeks, are able to tolerate surgery, and the surgeon can obtain surgical fixation points. Although there are no absolute indications for surgery, the strongest indications are based on neurologic deficit (progressive greater than fixed), instability, pain, local control (solitary greater than oligo metastases), and, occasionally, the need for diagnostic tissue. Although predicting life expectancy for any individual patient is difficult, Tokuhashi et al[17] created a scoring strategy that integrates histology, extent of disease, and neurologic status to guide physicians in predicting a prognosis and recommending surgical therapy. This framework is useful in evaluating patients; however, one of the most challenging scenarios is the patient who presents with metastatic disease at the time of diagnosis. Estimating survival in a treatment-naïve patient can be very challenging in this evolving age of targeted therapy. Such a situation emphasizes the importance of making surgical decisions on a patient-specific basis after discussions with multidisciplinary treatment teams. Such considerations are the gold standard for selecting patients for surgical treatment rather than reliance on a static scoring system.

The primary consideration for surgical treatment is the presence of a neurologic deficit secondary to a compressive tumor. In patients with a neurologic deficit from a compressive tumor and spinal instability, surgery is the first-line treatment. Radiotherapy and chemotherapy are not expected to restore spinal stability in these patients, even if the local tumor burden and activity are effectively decreased. Patients with a neurologic deficit secondary to compression and no spinal instability should be carefully evaluated for surgical treatment. Patchell et al[8] recently reported on a prospective randomized trial comparing radiation versus surgery followed by radiation for patients presenting with metastatic epidural spinal cord compression originating from a variety of solid organ tumors. In this study (which was halted early by a data safety monitoring board), patients treated

with upfront surgery had improved neurologic status and even improved survival, albeit modest, compared with those treated with radiotherapy alone. Although this study excluded patients with cauda equina or root lesions and those with particularly radiosensitive histologies, it provided level 1 support for early surgical intervention in patients with neurologic signs or symptoms from metastatic disease. A follow-up multinational observational study by Ibrahim et al[18] confirmed these results and the beneficial effect of surgery on quality of life in these patients.

Modern surgical intervention for patients with symptomatic metastatic disease involves direct decompression of the tumor from the nerve structures. Although most metastatic lesions are located anteriorly in the vertebral body, an anterior approach is not necessarily implied. A simple laminectomy, however, is insufficient treatment for these patients.[19,20] If a posterior approach is used, a transpedicular or costotransversectomy-type approach is necessary to provide thorough tumor decompression (**Figure 3**). This decompression is accompanied by spinal instrumentation to maximize stability across segments weakened by disease and the surgical approach.[21]

Except in patients with favorable histology and prognosis (such as a woman with solitary or oligometastatic breast cancer after a long disease-free interval), a formal fusion is not attempted and is not recommended. The process of decortication in preparation for fusion has several drawbacks in this patient population. It removes natural anatomic barriers to tumor extension into adjacent bones that may not currently have tumor involvement. The process of decortication also weakens the bones in preparation for bony fusion. Bony fusion is unlikely to occur

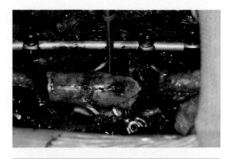

Figure 3   Intraoperative view of a revision circumferential decompression of L1 renal cell metastasis through a posterior transpedicular approach.

in the setting of radiotherapy and chemotherapy. The additional blood loss and surgical time necessary to perform a fusion increases the morbidity for patients and extends the procedure beyond its oncologic goals.

The decision to proceed with an anterior or a posterior approach to the offending tumor mass is highly individualized based on the nature of the compression, the preference of the surgeon, and patient-specific factors. For example, an anterior approach often requires the assistance of an access surgeon who may not be immediately or readily available. In patients with extensive osseous disease, a long posterior approach may allow fixation over a longer segment of diseased bone and achieve stability that cannot be matched by using short segment anterior fixation. In contrast, in patients whose skin has been significantly affected by radiation therapy, the skin is at increased risk of wound-related complications from a posterior approach; an anterior approach may be a better choice. A posterior approach may be preferred when lung metastases or other intrathoracic or intraabdominal disease processes are present.

The surgical approach also can be influenced by the location of disease in the spinal column. Cervical disease is often treated with an anterior approach to address the site of neurologic compression; mechanical factors sometimes necessitate a secondary posterior approach for mechanical support. In general, a single-level and occasionally a two-level corpectomy can stand alone in the presence of normal adjacent and posterior bone on MRI for radiosensitive tumors. A multilevel corpectomy should usually be supplemented by posterior instrumentation. Posterior surgery must always be considered for disease at the cervicothoracic junction or if there is adjacent-level disease.[22]

The thoracic spine represents the most common site of metastatic disease to the spine. Historically, upper thoracic lesions (T1-T5) were difficult to treat, with sternotomy and thoracotomy options presenting significant limitations and excessive morbidity. Posterolateral approaches (costotransversectomy) have evolved to be the most dependable approaches for most experienced spine tumor surgeons and can provide exposure for an extensive anterior column resection with the ability to easily provide mechanical anterior support from this single approach. Lower thoracic lesions (T5-T12) are also effectively treated via these approaches but also can be treated with classic anterior-type approaches.[23]

Lumbar spinal metastases can be treated via direct anterior, retroperitoneal, or transpedicular-style approaches. Disease in the L5 vertebral body is often approached posteriorly to allow fixation to the sacrum and the pelvis.

Some authors have proposed en bloc resection of metastatic disease in carefully selected patients.[24,25] Although a treatment option, these procedures are technically demanding and achieved with high patient morbidity. En bloc excision avoids the need for radiotherapy to decrease the risk of local

recurrence. Although attractive as a hope for cure or to extend life in patients with solitary metastases, the available evidence-based literature does not show a clear survival benefit for these patients. Current data are primarily anecdotal and come from case series. This chapter's authors recommend that such aggressive procedures be performed only by experienced surgeons in carefully selected patients with solitary metastases, favorable histologies, and a long disease-free interval. Advanced radiotherapy techniques are improving local tumor control in patients with adverse histologies, such as renal cell carcinoma, with less aggressive management than en bloc resections.

Surgical management of metastatic disease also should be considered in patients with spinal instability, even those lacking compressive neurologic deficits. In these patients, pathologic fractures or impending fractures may be treated surgically to minimize the risk of the progression of local tumor or deformity, which poses a high threat to neurologic elements.

In all patients treated with less aggressive procedures than an en bloc resection for metastatic disease in the spine, postoperative radiotherapy should be strongly considered to minimize the risk of symptomatic tumor recurrence. In patients with highly chemosensitive malignancies, aggressive medical treatment and careful observation may supplant the need for radiation therapy. The decision to pursue surgical treatment should be made with an understanding of the individual patient's total disease burden, overall performance status, and knowledge of the natural history of the particular tumor.

Complications
Complications are common in patients who receive surgical treatment for spi-

nal metastases.[16] The general medical status of patients is often compromised by the disease and the treatment of the disease. Patients may be malnourished and immunosuppressed. Higher complication rates are seen in patients who had prior radiotherapy. Patients with greater preoperative neurologic deficits of long duration have a higher risk of complications and a lower likelihood of regaining neurologic function from surgical intervention. This highlights the need to consider early surgical intervention in patients presenting with neurologic compromise and exercise careful clinical judgment in selecting candidates for surgery.

Preoperative embolization is used generously in these patients to minimize intraoperative bleeding, which can be substantial[26] (**Figure 4**). In patients with compromised soft tissues from the extraosseous spread of tumor or from prior radiotherapy, local rotational flaps (trapezius or latissimus flaps) should be strongly considered to decrease the risk of wound complications.

Innovative Approaches in Treating Spinal Metastases
Vertebroplasty and Kyphoplasty
Vertebroplasty and kyphoplasty are minimally invasive treatment options in which the vertebral body is accessed percutaneously, generally through the pedicle, and polymethyl methacrylate is injected to strengthen and reconstruct fractured or diseased vertebrae. These procedures are most commonly used in the treatment of osteoporotic fractures; however, they have a role in the treatment of patients with spinal metastatic disease. In the practices of this chapter's authors, the two procedures are quite similar, and a differentiation between the techniques for vertebroplasty and kyphoplasty is not made.

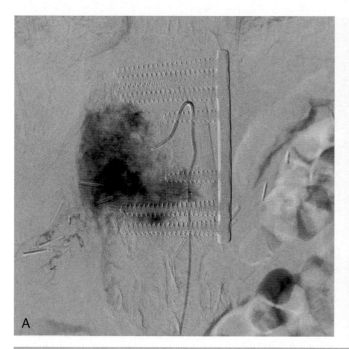
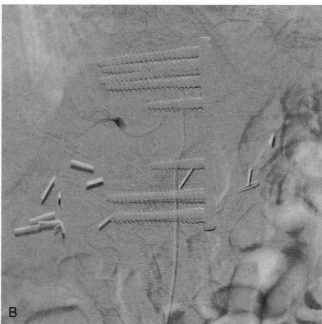

Figure 4 Embolization of a recurrent metastatic renal cell carcinoma after anterior corpectomy. **A,** Angiogram of a hypervascular tumor mass. **B,** The tumor mass after embolization.

These techniques can be helpful in patients with painful compression fractures from lytic metastases. There also may be a role for prophylactic vertebroplasty and/or kyphoplasty in patients at high risk for fracture who are treated with stereotactic radiotherapy of lesions. Care must be taken to minimize the risk of cement extravasation when using these techniques in patients with epidural tumor extension or significant destruction of the posterior vertebral body. This chapter's authors generally prefer that tumors have been initially treated with chemotherapy and/or radiotherapy before initiating vertebroplasty and/or kyphoplasty treatment. Great care should be taken in the treatment of hypervascular metastases (such as renal cell carcinoma) because of the risk of significant epidural hemorrhage and compressive hematoma.

Pain relief is the primary indication for vertebroplasty and/or kyphoplasty procedures in the oncologic population. Several authors have reported on studies of vertebroplasty and/or ky-

phoplasty procedures performed in the oncologic population for multiple myeloma or metastatic spine disease.[27-29] In each of these studies, consistent durable pain relief occurred in most patients. Asymptomatic cement extravasation was seen frequently, but symptoms from cement extravasation were rare. Significant improvements have been reported in Medical Outcomes Study 36-Item Short Form scores following these procedures in the oncologic population, highlighting the objective benefits that vertebroplasty and kyphoplasty can achieve in these patients.

Vertebroplasty and kyphoplasty may also be indicated for patients with early pathologic fractures and imaging evidence suggesting a high risk of progressive fracture with resulting kyphosis and/or neurologic problems (for example, thoracolumbar location and lytic destruction of the anterior vertebral body). Although common in clinical practice, few objective data have been reported in the literature on the use of vertebroplasty and kyphoplasty

for these indications. Although these procedures are generally safely executed, they carry risks of direct neurologic injury, symptomatic cement extravasation, and epidural hematoma. In the oncologic patient population particularly, vertebroplasty and kyphoplasty should be performed by experienced practitioners with access to accurate imaging modalities. When these procedures are performed by skilled physicians in well-selected patients, demonstrable benefits can be realized with low risks and little interruption of adjuvant treatment schedules.

Stereotactic Radiotherapy

Advances in radiation delivery techniques have led to the use of single or hypofractionated delivery of stereotactic radiation to treat patients with relatively radioresistant tumors.[30] These techniques permit the delivery of tightly contoured radiation doses that allows a high-dose intensity over the tumor volume while sparing injury to the adjacent spinal cord and critical organ structures. A targeting precision of

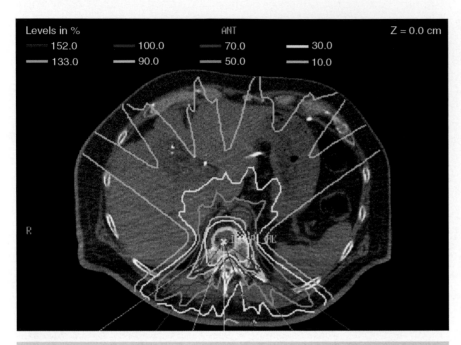

Figure 5   Dose gradations achieved with intensity-modulated radiotherapy.

approximately 2 mm can be achieved (**Figure 5**). This group of techniques is variously called stereotactic body radiotherapy, intensity-modulated radiotherapy, and image-guided (intensity-modulated) radiotherapy.

Because of the tight dose contouring possible with stereotactic radiation therapy, patients previously treated with radiation therapy who have further tumor recurrence are usually candidates for repeat radiation therapy using stereotactic methods.[31] A durable treatment response can be achieved in patients with tumors with traditionally radioresistant histologies, such as sarcoma and renal cell carcinoma, using this method. Because stereotactic radiation treatment is a resource-intensive regimen with limited availability and high costs, its use is restricted to major centers and patients with unique presentations. Conventional external beam radiotherapy remains the standard treatment in patients with spinal metastases. Most patients treated in this manner, even those with tumors with adverse histologies, obtain durable local control.[32]

Patients treated with stereotactic radiation therapy are at risk for the development of pathologic fractures after treatment.[33] Risk factors for collapse appear to be lesions located in the thoracolumbar or lumbar spine, lytic lesions, and those involving increasing amounts of the vertebral body. Fracture development after stereotactic radiation therapy appears to result in increased pain and a worse Karnofsky performance status. Prophylactic vertebroplasty and/or kyphoplasty may be indicated in these select patients.

Minimally Invasive Surgical Procedures

Advances in surgical imaging technologies and instrumentation allow less invasive treatment options for patients presenting with metastatic disease in the spine.[34] For example, patients requiring spinal stabilization, with or without a surgical decompression, may be treated with percutaneous spinal instrumentation coupled with a limited open procedure for spinal decompression (**Figure 6**). These technologies and techniques are still evolving.

Proper patient selection is being refined to understand which patients are good candidates for minimally invasive procedures as opposed to traditional open surgical procedures for the treatment of spinal metastases. The minimally invasive techniques are a surgical treatment option that usually exposes the patient to less physiologic insult and blood loss than traditional open surgical treatments.

Treatment Strategies

Treatment is individualized for patients presenting with metastatic disease to the spine. Patients presenting asymptomatically or with pain and no evidence of fracture or neurologic compromise are usually best treated with systemic chemotherapy and local radiotherapy. A brace may be used to improve comfort during treatment; however, long-term bracing is not recommended in these patients. There are few reasons for brace use for more than approximately 6 weeks because healing of these lesions is not expected. If bracing is needed to obtain adequate spinal stability after that time, surgical treatment should be considered. Patients treated in this manner require careful surveillance for local progression of disease or new spinal metastases.

Patients who present with compressive neurologic deficits are generally candidates for surgical intervention; however, those with exquisitely radiosensitive tumors, such as hematopoietic malignancies or germ cell tumors, can usually be treated with corticosteroids and radiotherapy with excellent results. Vertebroplasty and kyphoplasty may be used to augment these treatments.

Patients presenting with compressive neurologic deficits and/or spinal instability from solid organ metastases will often benefit from surgical intervention. A treatment algorithm to help guide this process is presented in **Fig-**

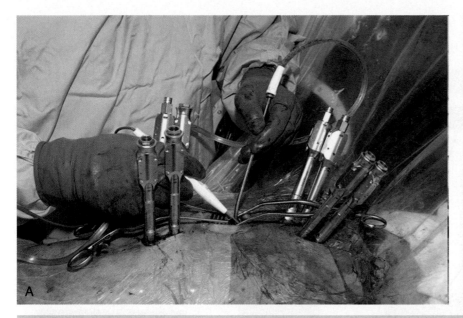
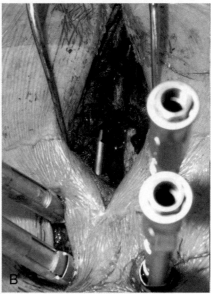

Figure 6 Intraoperative photographs of minimally invasive stabilization and decompression using percutaneous instrumentation and a limited open technique. **A,** A percutaneous approach is used to obtain access to the pedicles above and below the lesion, and a limited midline approach is used for decompression. **B,** Dural decompression and passage of the percutaneous stabilizing rod is shown.

ure 7. The primary considerations in the algorithm include the presence of a compressive neurologic deficit and spinal instability. These two factors, coupled with knowledge of the radiosensitivity of the tumor, help guide the primary indications for surgical treatment in patients with metastatic spinal disease.

Recognition of Primary Spinal Tumors

Primary spinal tumors are very rare. In the United States each year, there are an estimated 560,000 deaths from cancer, of which 390,000 patients are estimated to have spinal metastases.[3,4] In contrast, fewer than 1,000 US patients per year present with a primary spinal tumor; however, proper diagnosis of these patients is critical because primary spinal tumors are potentially curable. The initial treatment will generally determine if a patient can undergo effective curative treatment of a primary spinal malignancy.

The clinical difficulty in assessing these patients is that back and neck pain is nearly universal, and most patients presenting with a primary spinal malignancy do not appear ill. Although the presentation is nonspecific, sporadic pain usually progresses to constant pain, potentially to pathologic fracture, and to true night pain. Neurologic symptoms and deformity are late findings in these patients. Primary spinal tumors are recognized when persistent and unexplained symptoms lead to an imaging study that identifies a solitary spinal lesion. Subsequent staging studies fail to identify any further lesions, and a biopsy confirms a primary tumor histology (such as sarcoma or chordoma).

As with patients presenting with metastatic disease, staging studies consist of a careful history and physical examination; a CT of the chest, abdomen, and pelvis; laboratory studies; and a technetium bone scan. Once a solitary lesion is identified by staging studies, CT-guided core needle biopsy provides a safe, reliable, and excisable biopsy. Unlike in metastatic carci-noma, the biopsy tract of a primary spine tumor is excised at the time of resection; therefore, the nature of the biopsy should be planned in consultation with the resecting surgeon. There is a very limited role for an open biopsy in this setting. Biopsies should be done via a direct near-midline approach to minimize the contamination of tissue (including the epidural plexus) and provide for ready excision (**Figure 8**).

Primary malignant spinal tumors include chordoma, osteosarcoma, chondrosarcoma, and Ewing sarcoma. Paraspinal soft-tissue sarcomas also may invade the spine. The treatment of these malignancies occurs in highly specialized centers with specific chemotherapy and radiotherapy protocols. Surgical management is multidisciplinary and is often much different from the surgical treatment of patients with metastatic disease. Close coordination of the care teams is necessary to maximize the potential for cure. In contrast to patients with metastatic tumors

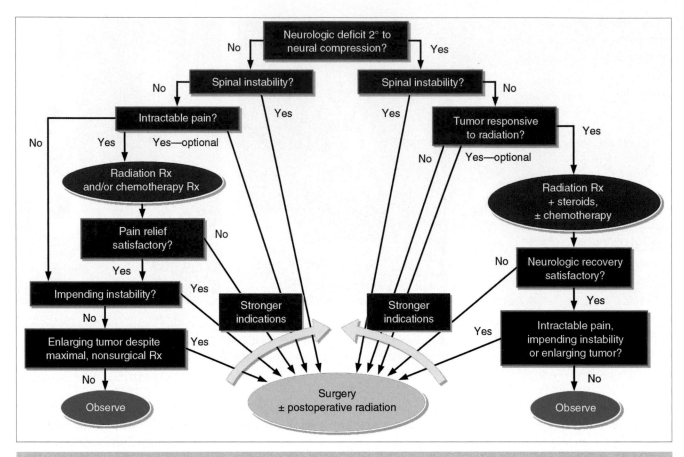

Figure 7 Treatment algorithm for patients presenting with metastatic disease of the spine. Rx = treatment. (Reproduced with permission from Walker MP, Yaszemski MJ, Kim CW, Talac R, Currier BL: Metastatic disease of the spine: Evaluation and treatment. *Clin Orthop Relat Res* 2003;415:S165-S175.)

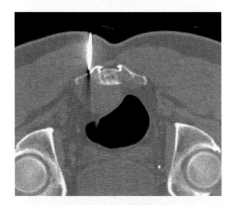

Figure 8 CT scan of a well-planned biopsy of a sacral chordoma. The biopsy approach is direct and near midline without epidural contamination.

in which strong efforts are made to preserve functional outcomes, even at the expense of leaving some residual tumor

behind, patients with primary spine tumors are treated with the goal of curing the patient. To achieve a cure, unpleasant options are sometimes necessary, including procedures that cause loss of bowel, bladder, or sexual function; the resection of adjacent organs; and even concurrent amputation in the case of sacropelvic malignancies. The extensive nature of these surgical procedures requires close coordination between surgical disciplines and the anesthesia and intensive care teams (**Figure 9**). Involvement of the rehabilitation team is important to provide patients with realistic expectations and to maximize their functional outcomes after aggressive tumor resections.

Adjuvant therapy options are dependent on the tumor histology. If the le-

sion is chemosensitive (such as osteosarcoma), chemotherapy is administered preoperatively and postoperatively per standard treatment protocols. When indicated, the choice of preoperative versus postoperative radiotherapy is highly individualized to the nature of the tumor. A primary factor is the extent of vascular dissection necessary. Comparative studies on the relative efficacy of preoperative versus postoperative radiotherapy in the treatment of primary spinal sarcomas are lacking. Clinical experience indicates that patients who require an extensive vascular dissection, particularly around a previously operated field, have a higher risk of complications when preoperative radiotherapy is administered. The use of stereotactic radiotherapy to minimize these risks is still evolving.

In addition to standard staging studies, detailed tumor imaging should be obtained before surgery to maximize the ability to obtain an en bloc resection. Patient outcomes for these tumors are generally governed by two factors: tumor margin and histology. Histology is beyond the control of the surgeon; however, the surgical margin is within the surgeon's control. Data on the surgical treatment of chordoma from the Mayo Clinic shows excellent disease-free survival in patients when a wide margin is achieved.[35] In contrast, disease-free survival is rare in patients if a wide margin is not achieved. Boriani et al[36] reported greatly improved survival for patients with spinal chondrosarcoma after en bloc resection. Thirteen of 14 patients were continuously disease free after an en bloc excision, whereas 8 of 10 patients died of disease after an intralesional procedure. These results highlight the critical aspect of margin status and appropriate initial surgical treatment in this patient population.

Complications are common in patients with spinal sarcomas treated with en bloc resections. Major complications occur in 35% of the patients. Patients undergoing combined approaches and multilevel resections have higher complication rates as would be expected with more extensive surgeries. Patients with prior surgeries have significantly higher rates of complications, emphasizing the need for these patients to be treated in specialized centers.[37]

As treatments advance, new options are becoming available for patients with primary spine tumors. In addition to chemotherapy and conventional and stereotactic radiotherapy, there is an evolving role for particle beam therapy (generally proton beam therapy) in the treatment of patients with spinal sarcomas and chordomas.[38] Proton therapy allows close tar-

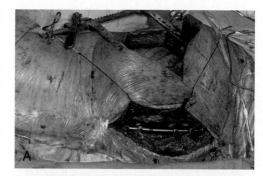

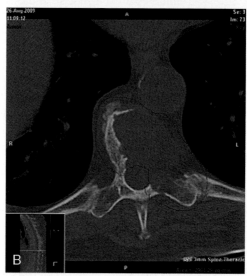

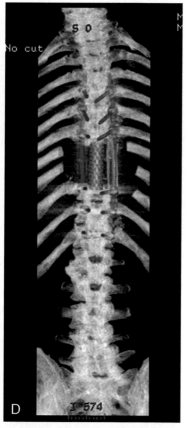

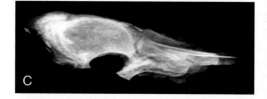

Figure 9 **A,** Intraoperative photograph of an en bloc resection of thoracic sarcoma using a combined surgical approach. **B,** Axial CT scan showing tumor location. **C,** The resected specimen is shown. **D,** Reconstruction after a two-level en bloc vertebrectomy.

geting and high-energy deposition within tumors that traditionally are poorly responsive to radiotherapy. This role is evolving both as an adjuvant to surgery in tumors in which a wide oncologic margin is difficult to achieve and potentially as a primary treatment in patients with malignancies not suited to surgical treatment.

Summary

Spine tumors are frequently seen in clinical practice. Most of these lesions are from metastatic or hematopoietic disease processes. A standardized approach to these patients can confirm the diagnosis (when necessary) and guide treatment decisions. Most patients are treated with chemotherapy and radiotherapy. Surgical intervention is considered for patients with compressive neurologic deficit and/or spinal instability. Novel surgical, percutaneous, and radiotherapy techniques continue to improve the treatment options for these patients.

Primary spinal tumors are rare. A recognition of these processes is critical to preserve the opportunity for curative treatment. The treatment of primary spine tumors is highly specialized and involves the close coordination of many treatment teams to achieve optimal outcomes.

References

1. American Cancer Society: Cancer statistics 2010. http://www.cancer.org/Research/CancerFactsFigures/CancerFactsFigures/cancer-facts-and-figures-2010. Accessed August 29, 2011.

2. World Health Organization: Mortality profiles. http://www.who.int/whosis/mort/profiles/en/. Accessed August 29, 2011.

3. Bach F, Larsen BH, Rohde K, et al: Metastatic spinal cord compression: Occurrence, symptoms, clinical presentations and prognosis in 398 patients with spinal cord compression. *Acta Neurochir (Wien)* 1990;107(1-2):37-43.

4. Perrin RG: Metastatic tumors of the axial spine. *Curr Opin Oncol* 1992;4(3):525-532.

5. Byrne TN, Benzel EC, Waxman SG: Epidural tumors, in Byrne TN, Benzel EC, Waxman SG, eds: *Diseases of the Spine and Spinal Cord.* Oxford, England, Oxford University Press, 2000, pp 166-205.

6. Posner JB: Spinal metastases, in Posner JB, ed: *Neurologic Complications of Cancer.* Philadelphia, PA, FA Davis, 1995, pp 111-114.

7. Gilbert RW, Kim JH, Posner JB: Epidural spinal cord compression from metastatic tumor: Diagnosis and treatment. *Ann Neurol* 1978;3(1):40-51.

8. Patchell RA, Tibbs PA, Regine WF, et al: Direct decompressive surgical resection in the treatment of spinal cord compression caused by metastatic cancer: A randomised trial. *Lancet* 2005;366(9486):643-648.

9. Rose PS, Buchowski JM: Metastatic disease in the thoracic and lumbar spine: Evaluation and management. *J Am Acad Orthop Surg* 2011;19(1):37-48.

10. Schiff D, O'Neill BP, Suman VJ: Spinal epidural metastasis as the initial manifestation of malignancy: Clinical features and diagnostic approach. *Neurology* 1997;49(2):452-456.

11. Rougraff BT, Kneisl JS, Simon MA: Skeletal metastases of unknown origin: A prospective study of a diagnostic strategy. *J Bone Joint Surg Am* 1993;75(9):1276-1281.

12. Lis E, Bilsky MH, Pisinski L, et al: Percutaneous CT-guided biopsy of osseous lesion of the spine in patients with known or suspected malignancy. *AJNR Am J Neuroradiol* 2004;25(9):1583-1588.

13. Maranzano E, Latini P: Effectiveness of radiation therapy without surgery in metastatic spinal cord compression: Final results from a prospective trial. *Int J Radiat Oncol Biol Phys* 1995;32(4):959-967.

14. Buhmann Kirchhoff S, Becker C, Duerr HR, Reiser M, Baur-Melnyk A: Detection of osseous metastases of the spine: Comparison of high resolution multi-detector-CT with MRI. *Eur J Radiol* 2009;69(3):567-573.

15. Sørensen S, Helweg-Larsen S, Mouridsen H, Hansen HH: Effect of high-dose dexamethasone in carcinomatous metastatic spinal cord compression treated with radiotherapy: A randomised trial. *Eur J Cancer* 1994;30A(1):22-27.

16. Wise JJ, Fischgrund JS, Herkowitz HN, Montgomery D, Kurz LT: Complication, survival rates, and risk factors of surgery for metastatic disease of the spine. *Spine (Phila Pa 1976)* 1999;24(18):1943-1951.

17. Tokuhashi Y, Matsuzaki H, Oda H, Oshima M, Ryu J: A revised scoring system for preoperative evaluation of metastatic spine tumor prognosis. *Spine (Phila Pa 1976)* 2005;30(19):2186-2191.

18. Ibrahim A, Crockard A, Antonietti P, et al: Does spinal surgery improve the quality of life for those with extradural (spinal) osseous metastases? An international multicenter prospective observational study of 223 patients: Invited submission from the Joint Section Meeting on Disorders of the Spine and Peripheral Nerves, March 2007. *J Neurosurg Spine* 2008;8(3):271-278.

19. Sørensen S, Børgesen SE, Rohde K, et al: Metastatic epidural spinal cord compression: Results of treatment and survival. *Cancer* 1990;65(7):1502-1508.

20. Young RF, Post EM, King GA: Treatment of spinal epidural metastases: Randomized prospective comparison of laminectomy and radiotherapy. *J Neurosurg* 1980;53(6):741-748.

21. Wang JC, Boland P, Mitra N, et al: Single-stage posterolateral transpedicular approach for resection of epidural metastatic spine tumors involving the vertebral body with circumferential reconstruction: Results in 140 patients. Invited submission from the Joint Section Meeting on Disorders of the Spine and Peripheral Nerves, March 2004. *J Neurosurg Spine* 2004;1(3):287-298.

22. Fehlings MG, David KS, Vialle L, Vialle E, Setzer M, Vrionis FD: Decision making in the surgical treatment of cervical spine metastases. *Spine (Phila Pa 1976)* 2009;34(22, Suppl)S108-S117.

23. Polly DW Jr, Chou D, Sembrano JN, Ledonio CG, Tomita K: An analysis of decision making and treatment in thoracolumbar me-

tastases. *Spine (Phila Pa 1976)* 2009;34(22, Suppl):S118-S127.

24. Tomita K, Kawahara N, Kobayashi T, Yoshida A, Murakami H, Akamaru T: Surgical strategy for spinal metastases. *Spine (Phila Pa 1976)* 2001;26(3):298-306.

25. Yao KC, Boriani S, Gokaslan ZL, Sundaresan N: En bloc spondylectomy for spinal metastases: A review of techniques. *Neurosurg Focus* 2003;15(5):E6.

26. Prabhu VC, Bilsky MH, Jambhekar K, et al: Results of preoperative embolization for metastatic spinal neoplasms. *J Neurosurg* 2003;98(2, Suppl):156-164.

27. Cheung G, Chow E, Holden L, et al: Percutaneous vertebroplasty in patients with intractable pain from osteoporotic or metastatic fractures: A prospective study using quality-of-life assessment. *Can Assoc Radiol J* 2006;57(1):13-21.

28. Dudeney S, Lieberman IH, Reinhardt MK, Hussein M: Kyphoplasty in the treatment of osteolytic vertebral compression fractures as a result of multiple myeloma. *J Clin Oncol* 2002; 20(9):2382-2387.

29. Fourney DR, Schomer DF, Nader R, et al: Percutaneous vertebroplasty and kyphoplasty for painful vertebral body fractures in cancer patients. *J Neurosurg* 2003; 98(1, Suppl):21-30.

30. Yamada Y, Bilsky MH, Lovelock DM, et al: High-dose, single-fraction image-guided intensity-modulated radiotherapy for metastatic spinal lesions. *Int J Radiat Oncol Biol Phys* 2008;71(2): 484-490.

31. Wright JL, Lovelock DM, Bilsky MH, Toner S, Zatcky J, Yamada Y: Clinical outcomes after reirradiation of paraspinal tumors. *Am J Clin Oncol* 2006;29(5):495-502.

32. Moulding HD, Elder JB, Lis E, et al: Local disease control after decompressive surgery and adjuvant high-dose single-fraction radiosurgery for spine metastases. *J Neurosurg Spine* 2010;13(1): 87-93.

33. Rose PS, Laufer I, Boland PJ, et al: Risk of fracture after single fraction image-guided intensity-modulated radiation therapy to spinal metastases. *J Clin Oncol* 2009;27(30):5075-5079.

34. Rose PS, Clarke MS, Dekutoski MB: Minimally invasive treatment of spinal metastases: Techniques. *Int J Surg Oncol* 2011. http://www.hindawi.com/ journals/ijso/2011/494381/. Accessed October 14, 2011.

35. Fuchs B, Dickey ID, Yaszemski MJ, Inwards CY, Sim FH: Operative management of sacral chordoma. *J Bone Joint Surg Am* 2005; 87(10):2211-2216.

36. Boriani S, De Iure F, Bandiera S, et al: Chondrosarcoma of the mobile spine: Report on 22 cases. *Spine (Phila Pa 1976)* 2000;25(7): 804-812.

37. Boriani S, Bandiera S, Donthineni R, et al: Morbidity of en bloc resections in the spine. *Eur Spine J* 2010;19(2):231-241.

38. DeLaney TF, Liebsch NJ, Pedlow FX, et al: Phase II study of high-dose photon/proton radiotherapy in the management of spine sarcomas. *Int J Radiat Oncol Biol Phys* 2009;74(3):732-739.

The Practice of Orthopaedics

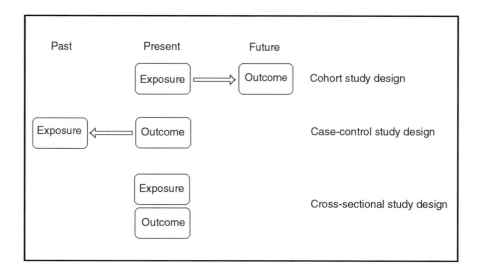

The Practice of Orthopaedics

Communication for All Your Patients

Valerae O. Lewis, MD

Toni McLaurin, MD

Hillard T. Spencer, MD

Norman Y. Otsuka, MD

Ramon L. Jimenez, MD

Abstract

Because communication is something that is often taken for granted, many people do not consciously think about communication habits and behaviors. When patients are questioned concerning important attributes of a doctor, they say they want someone who respects and listens to them. In a time of increasing malpractice litigation, physicians need to examine their communication skills. In an increasingly more diverse world, social and cultural beliefs, attitudes, and behaviors have a considerable effect on the health of communities. Patient safety, satisfaction, and successful outcomes rely on understanding the patient's medical and cultural needs. The concept of becoming a "cultural anthropologist" is improbable, but becoming aware of the demographics of the community in which the physician serves will improve communication and lead to improved patient and physician satisfaction, better patient compliance, and improved health outcomes.

Instr Course Lect 2012;61:569-580.

One aim of the Institute of Medicine as outlined in its 2001 report *Crossing the Quality Chasm*, is the development of a 21st century healthcare system that is safe, effective, timely, efficient, equitable, and patient centered. In 2003, the Institute of Medicine published a report that cataloged healthcare disparities in the United States.[1] This report showed that African-Americans, Hispanics, and Native Americans have 50% to 100% higher rates of illness and mortality from chronic illnesses (such as diabetes and hypertension) than whites, even when insurance status, income, age, education, comorbidities, and the severity of conditions are comparable. This disparity has moral, social, political and economic implications.[2]

The causes of healthcare disparities are multifactorial and include the beliefs and attitudes of the patient and the provider, as well as environmental influences. The role of the environment in shaping healthcare disparities is beyond the scope or intent of this chapter; however, the beliefs and attitudes of both the patient and the provider are two factors that healthcare providers can directly address. Cross-cultural communication is a critical skill for physicians and other healthcare workers to learn to reduce disparities in the access to and the outcomes of medical care.[3] Communication is a key component in patient-centered care. The American Academy of Orthopaedic Surgeons (AAOS) described patient-focused communication as open, honest dialogue that builds trust and promotes healing. Good communication has a favorable impact on patient behavior, outcome, and satisfaction, and, as a consequence, good

Dr. Lewis or an immediate family member has received research or institutional support from Stryker and serves as a board member, owner, officer, or committee member of the Western Orthopaedic Association. Dr. Otsuka or an immediate family member serves as a board member, owner, officer, or committee member of the American Academy of Orthopaedic Surgeons, the American Academy of Pediatrics, Bone and Joint Decade USA, and the Pediatric Orthopaedic Society of North America. Dr. Jimenez or an immediate family member serves as a paid consultant to Zimmer and serves as a board member, owner, officer, or committee member of the J. Robert Gladden Society and the Orthopaedic Research and Education Foundation. Neither of the following authors nor any immediate family member has received anything of value from or owns stock in a commercial company or institution related directly or indirectly to the subject of this chapter: Dr. McLaurin and Dr. Spencer.

communication often reduces the incidence of malpractice lawsuits.

Culturally competent care is synonymous with patient-centered care and is rooted in communication. It is necessary to consider how a patient's concerns might influence communication and clinical assessments. The quality of health care can be compromised when the patient does not understand what the doctor is saying, when the doctor is insensitive to cultural differences, or if there is a language barrier. Providers must enhance their communication skills to negotiate effectively and collaborate with patients.

People of diverse cultures and beliefs perceive health and illness differently and may have different responses to symptoms, diseases, and treatments. It is important that physicians are aware of their patients' attitudes toward health care, modes of communication, and social relationships. Physicians may not change the beliefs of their patients, but with proper knowledge they can collaborate on a mutually acceptable treatment plan.

All people to some extent are consciously or unconsciously biased (attitude) toward members of a group different from themselves.[4] However, the impact of this bias may be more important with physicians because their attitudes can substantially influence their patient and treatment decisions. Many physicians do not realize the discrepancies that exist in health care and outcomes for different ethnic groups. Dogra and Karnik[5] reported that first-year medical students generally disagreed that skin color influenced treatment decisions, and a Kaiser Family Foundation survey of physicians reported that most physicians say the healthcare system "rarely" or "never" treats people unfairly based on monetary resources, fluency in English, education status, racial or ethnic background, sexual orientation, or gender.[6]

There may be some resistance of healthcare providers to acknowledge and discuss issues of culture and diversity in health care. A physician should be aware that his or her own culture, belief systems, and values may affect interactions with patients.[7]

Physicians can improve interactions with a diverse patient population through education in culturally competent care. Cultural competence training has a number of different aspects and has been shown to improve provider knowledge, attitudes, and skills. The education objectives of the Accreditation Council on Graduate Medical Education and the Liaison Committee on Medical Education have incorporated the concept of culturally competent care.[7-9] Gardenswartz and Rowe[10] recommended that physicians consider six "realities of cultural programming" to improve cultural competence. (1) Culture is not obvious. (2) All people believe that their own culture is best. (3) The actions of others are misinterpreted if physicians do not understand their interpretations of observations. (4) We may not know when we are offending others. (5) Awareness of differences and possible barriers improves chances for successful interactions. (6) It is necessary to understand our own "software."

To reduce disparities in access to and outcomes of medical care, cross-cultural communication is a critical skill for physicians and other healthcare workers.

African-American Patients

No discourse on the treatment of the African-American patient can begin without a discussion of the persistence of racial and ethnic disparities in health care. African-American patients wait longer for a diagnosis, receive less aggressive treatment, and have historically been undertreated for pain.[11]

Physicians face greater obstacles in providing treatment for their African-American patients, including increased difficulty in obtaining referrals to subspecialists, obtaining proper imaging, and admitting patients to the hospital for nonemergent reasons.[12] Since the late 1980s, a growing body of literature has shown that African-American patients receive racially disparate care across all fields of medicine, including orthopaedic surgery.[13] Compared with white Americans, African-Americans receive poorer quality health care, have higher morbidity and mortality rates, experience higher rates of major diseases, and are seen less often by specialists.[14,15] They are less likely to receive appropriate preventive care, adequate analgesia in the emergency department (although this may be improving), intensive hospital care, expensive technologic procedures, cardiovascular procedures such as coronary artery bypass graft surgery or angioplasty, lung resections for cancer, kidney and bone marrow transplants, and limb-sparing peripheral vascular procedures.[12,16-24] African-American patients are more likely to receive lower quality hospital and prenatal care, less aggressive treatment of prostate cancer, fewer antidepressants and/or less treatment for depression, fewer admissions for chest pain, and fewer antiretroviral medications for HIV.[1,19,24-27] From an orthopaedic perspective, these patients are less likely to receive adequate physical and occupational therapy after hip fractures or undergo orthopaedic procedures such as joint arthroplasty.[22,28,29] Many studies have evaluated Medicare or Veterans Affairs populations, thus removing insurance and access to health care as variables; race was shown to be an independent variable in the reported disparities.[24,30-33]

The persistence of healthcare disparities has a substantial impact. Despite the overall improvement in health in the United States, the health status of some populations has remained the same or worsened.[34,35] This disparity in health care has moral, social, political, and economic implications.[2] These disparities have multifactorial causes, including the beliefs and attitudes of both the patients and the providers, as well as environmental aspects. The African-American patient may have a certain degree of internalized racism, which causes the patient to develop behaviors and attitudes about his or her health care that are based on mistrust, resignation, helplessness, and hopelessness. These attitudes may have a basis in real or perceived mistreatment,[1,23,36] which can negatively affect interactions with the healthcare system. A patient may have limited health literacy,[37] (the capacity to obtain, process, and understand basic health information and services needed to make appropriate health decisions), despite effectively managing other aspects of life. Although limited health literacy affects nearly 50% of all American adults, it is most common in racial and ethnic minorities.[38] Limited health literacy and cultural differences can compound the likelihood of poor interactions with healthcare providers. African-American patients often have cultural beliefs that may be inconsistent with mainstream American medicine, including the belief that illness is the result of natural causes, exposure to elements, or the will of God for improper behavior.[39] They may also be more likely to recognize barriers to treatment.[40] On a more quantifiable level, numerous studies show African-American patients are less likely to perceive the benefits of certain widely accepted orthopaedic treatments, such as total joint arthroplasty, making them less likely to elect such treatments.[32,40-44]

The role of the environment in shaping healthcare disparities is be-

yond the scope or intent of this chapter, but it is a manifestation of institutionalized racism (defined as the differential access to the goods, services, and opportunities of society according to race and independent of all other factors).[45] Environmental factors contributing to healthcare disparities that are more prevalent in some African-American communities include poverty, limited resources, and limited access to resources.

The role of the provider in permitting healthcare disparities may be difficult for many physicians to accept. All people have some degree of intentional or unintentional prejudice against members of a group different from themselves.[4] If a physician has a negative initial perception of an African-American patient, this perception will affect the patient's satisfaction, compliance, and outcome.[4,14,22,46-48] Race concordance (a physician and patient of the same race) plays a significant role in the physician-patient relationship. African-American patients with African-American physicians are more likely to rate their physicians as excellent and report receiving preventive and all needed medical care than African-American patients with non–African-American physicians. These patients also believe that the physician visit is more participatory and are more likely to describe their physicians as treating them respectfully, listening to their concerns, explaining problems, and being accessible.[49-53] From an orthopaedic perspective, a 2008 report of the American Academy of Orthopaedic Surgeons (AAOS) showed that 1.6% of AAOS fellows are African-American, whereas 12.9% of the US population is identified as African-American.[54] This means there is little chance for race concordance between African-American patients and their orthopaedic physicians and further underscores the need for cul-

turally competent and patient-centered care.

African-Americans are a diverse group of people with different experiences, backgrounds, appearances, religious beliefs, speech patterns, and languages. All geographic and socioeconomic strata are represented. The physician must be aware of both ideologic and practical issues when interacting with an African-American patient and should be aware of the extent and causes of current disparities and of patient and physician conscious and unconscious bias. From a practical standpoint, the physician should develop skills for cross-cultural communication and learn to explore the patient's views of pain, sickness, and treatment. One of the most important things for any provider to understand is that the mistrust of medical care is a major obstacle in establishing an effective provider-patient relationship with African-American patients. This mistrust may originate from the experiences of the patient, friends, or relatives, but it can also arise from a history of societal abuses of trust.

The history of what has been termed medical apartheid in US medicine[55] has created a distrust of medical care that permeates the African-American community. One of the best known and most egregious examples of this distrust is the Tuskegee experiment, in which the US Public Health Service conducted a prospective study from 1931 to 1972 on the effect of untreated syphilis on life expectancy. In an attempt to study the long-term effects and natural history of the disease, African-American men who were known to be infected with syphilis were observed but never treated, even after treatment became widely available.[56] This study was continued for more than 40 years until it was terminated in 1972 after a Senate investigation.[57] Another example of medical care leading to mistrust was a procedure that civil rights activist Fannie Lou Hamer dubbed the "Mississippi appendectomy." In the 1960s and 1970s, federally funded state welfare programs underwrote the coercive sterilization of thousands of poor African-American women in the South. Consent for the procedure was obtained under threat of termination of welfare benefits and/or denial of medical care.[55] Because a basic knowledge of these types of abuses is ingrained in members of the African-American community, physicians treating African-American patients must work against history to establish trust.[58]

This information sets the framework for developing guidelines for the physician treating African-American patients to provide more culturally competent care. It is important to recognize that these guidelines are not meant to stereotype or stigmatize patients but to help treating physicians provide the best possible care based on historic and cultural cues.

Greeting and Communication

History plays a role in an African-American patient's perceptions of his or her care, beginning with how the patient is greeted. African-Americans, especially older patients, should always be greeted by using an appropriate courtesy title and their last name as a show of respect because many older patients lived through the era in which African-Americans were not referred to by name or were addressed only by first name. Some African-Americans were given first names such as Mister, Major, and Doctor to ensure that they would always be referred to by a title.

After greeting the patient, the physician must be aware of both nonverbal and verbal communication. Maintaining eye contact, especially when first meeting and shaking hands, encourages trust and reduces fear and suspicion. Culturally, an African-American patient may be comfortable with a different degree of social distance and space than the provider; therefore, it is important for the physician to allow the patient to define the appropriate social space (too far may be perceived as distaste for the patient and too close may be perceived as overbearing).[59] As with any patient, the physician should try to avoid focusing on time or multitasking because this behavior can be perceived as impersonal, inconsiderate, and unconcerned. Recommendations and instructions may be ignored if the physician is perceived as uninterested.[60]

Appropriate verbal communication requires the physician to allow the patient to tell the story in his or her own way, which may require extra time. The physician should be sensitive to any perceived discrimination on the part of the patient and should avoid any terms (such as "you people") or gestures (such as patting the patient on the head or arm) with possible negative connotations. It is important to provide thorough explanations without the appearance of arrogance.[61] The physician should demonstrate a personal commitment by recognizing a preference for face-to-face rather than electronic or phone interaction, especially with older patients, and by calling personally to answer questions and relay results.

Open-ended questions should be used to ensure a common meaning with the patient, as some terms common in the African-American community may be unfamiliar to the practitioner. Examples include "sugar" for diabetes, "miseries" for pain, "low blood" for anemia, and "high blood" for hypertension.[39] Because the use of such colloquialisms may lead the physician to make assumptions about a patient's level of literacy,[59] it is important to ask the patient to summarize information in his or her own words. If there is a lack of understanding, patients often rely on their own explanations before those of medical professionals. The physician should not be afraid to ask questions such as "What are the main problems your illness has caused you?" "What do you fear most about your illness?" "What kind of treatment would you like to have?"

African-American patients have been shown to be more satisfied with the interaction with their physician if a significant amount of touch is involved; however, before touching the patient, the physician should explain what will be done and why.[39] Patients may prefer that an opposite-sex family member leave the room during the examination, but it is best to ask the patient directly to determine his or her preference.

Family and Community

Although single-parent households, usually headed by a woman, are more common among African-Americans than in any other groups in the United States,[62] it is important to recognize that there are often strong familial ties to a male family member, such as an uncle or a significant other. Grandparents often have combined or sole care of grandchildren, but it is important not to assume a matriarchal family structure, with the mother or grandmother as the ultimate decision-maker, and instead to ask directly about family structure and dynamics. Extended families are common, with multiple generations often living under one roof, providing important support and resources. There is often a strong sense of community among African-Americans, and the physician needs to recognize the importance of family, church, and community when a patient is faced with illness. Friends, neighbors, church members, grandparents, and grandchildren may be active caregivers. It is best to allow the patient to tell the physician whom he or she wishes to be involved in hearing medical information and assisting in medical decision making.

Religion and Spirituality

Religion and spirituality are an integral part of many African-American communities, although they encompass many different belief systems and religious affiliations.[59] Patients may inquire about a provider's religious beliefs and spirituality as a way to make themselves feel more comfortable. The patient's reverend and fellow church members may play significant roles in decision making. The patient's faith is an important factor to consider because faith in God is a strong positive predictor of how a patient will deal with the diagnosis of a disease.[63] The physician should acknowledge the patient's faith and work with it when discussing care. From a surgical standpoint, it is important to recognize that approximately 22% of practicing Jehovah Witnesses are African-Americans who reject blood and blood products as part of treatment.[64]

An important caveat when interacting with African-American patients is that guidelines may differ dramatically for African immigrants compared with those of African descent who have multiple generations of family born and raised in the United States. Although both groups may have deeply rooted traditions, recent immigrants and those who practice some African-American religions may view illness as a supernatural event or the work of the devil and may consult a healer, a member of the clergy, or another spiritual figure along with a medical provider. These beliefs may cause patients to avoid invasive tests or surgery for fear of allowing evil or the devil direct access into the blood and body.[39]

The importance of respecting a patient's religion cannot be overstated because the patient's perception that the physician respects and is involved with the patient's faith leads to increased adherence to treatment plans and can result in earlier consent of elderly patients to undergo surgery.

Nontraditional Medicine

Home remedies, including teas and other concoctions, are common in the African-American community. Poultices may be used around painful or inflamed joints and muscles.[15] These remedies may result in a treatment delay because the patient may seek medical care only after exhausting traditional home remedies.[39] It is necessary to discuss whether these home remedies should be continued or discontinued. Working with the patient by making medically neutral suggestions that fit with the patient's belief system rather than simply discounting nontraditional treatments may help build rapport more quickly.

Treatment Decisions

It is always important to include the patient in the decision-making process, but with the history of paternalistic treatment pervasive throughout many aspects of African-American life, this may be even more important in this population. It is important to understand the anxiety that making treatment decisions may provoke in patients. The physician should allow time to explain the necessity of tests and procedures and acknowledge and understand potential obstacles to the treatment plan, such as available transportation, costs, and personal, family, or community perceptions.[41]

Clinical Research

African-American patients may have significant mistrust or fear about entering clinical studies because of the notable legacy of historic injustices in medical research. To encourage participation in clinical studies, the research should be discussed in detail with patients and their families, with information about the safeguards that are in place to prevent the abuse of research participants.[58] It may require multiple discussions and patience on the part of the physician to convince the patient to participate.

Discussion

Interacting and communicating effectively and in a culturally competent way with African-American patients is in many ways no different from interacting with members of any other patient population. The physician must treat the patient with the dignity and respect that he or she deserves. However, the African-American community as a whole has a long-standing and deep-seated mistrust of the medical community, and it is important that physicians know and understand this background to provide appropriate care. In establishing rapport, the physician should demonstrate a personal commitment by personally calling to give the results of the tests and asking about difficulties with the treatment plans if the physician senses reticence. The physician should allow the patient time to develop trust and respect for the physician's opinions.

Hispanic/Latino Patients

The Hispanic/Latino population in the United States is approximately 48 million and is the largest ethnic minority in this country. It is estimated that by 2040, approximately 25% of the US population will be Hispanic/Latino.[65] Even though 14% of the current population of the United States is Hispanic/Latino, only 2.4% or approximately 400 of 20,000 orthopaedic surgeons are of Hispanic/Latino ethnicity. This constitutes a marked disparity gap. A 2008 study that included 429,000 patients from the National Trauma Bank spanning the years 2001 through 2005 found that Hispanic and African-American patients were less likely to be insured and more likely to sustain penetrating trauma than Caucasian patients.[66] It was also reported that insured Hispanic and African-American patients had increased mortality rates compared with insured Caucasian patients. This effect was more pronounced for uninsured patients across these groups.

The quality of health care can be compromised when the doctor does not speak the patient's language or the patient does not understand what the physician is saying. This is particularly true if the physician is insensitive to cultural differences. A study by Cooper et al[51] concluded that patient-physician race/ethnicity-concordant visits rated higher with patients. Hispanic patients treated by Hispanic physicians rated their medical visits as more satisfying and their physicians as more participatory. Race-concordant visits also last approximately 2.5 minutes longer compared with visits in which the race of the physician and patient differed.

Greeting and Communication

In the United States, approximately 64% of Hispanic and Latino patients are from Mexico, with others from countries throughout Latin America. Hispanics originate from the Iberian Peninsula, and Latinos are from Latin and South America, although the designations are often used interchangeably in the United States.[67,68] It is a cultural courtesy to describe families by their country of origin (such as Cuban, Salvadoran, or Mexican).

Hispanic/Latinos often come from countries that practice paternalistic medicine in which the doctor is esteemed and holds a prestigious posi-

tion. The patient should be greeted with respect, but the physician should not be too familiar at the initial visit. The Spanish language has different words for the formal and informal use of the word you (formally it is usted and informally it is tu). If addressing the patient in Spanish, it is important to use the correct form of the word.

The Hispanic man often is the provider and decision maker in the family. He may manifest a machismo attitude that may affect his decision to consent to surgery; however, fear or risk of disability and/or death may also affect that decision. It is often helpful to arrange a conference with the family to ask for their help in gaining the patient's consent for surgery.

Family

Typically, the Hispanic family is a strong unit, and the support of family members can often overcome cultural taboos. Explaining treatment options and the rationale for recommended treatments will help create advocates of family members and will assist the patient in overcoming his or her health-care biases and fears. If the patriarch of the family is deceased, the eldest son often becomes the decision maker for the family. This is especially important to remember when informed consent is needed for surgery for a widow.

Religion, Spirituality, and Nontraditional Medicine

Religion and spirituality are an integral part of many Hispanic communities. Many Latinos (particularly recent immigrants and older patients) share the belief that the future is preordained and not under human control (fatalismo). Often, Latinos have faith in alternative medicine and may frequent botanicas, which are freestanding stores that sell herbal medications for practically any ailment, diagnosis, or illness. Botanicas are similar to phar-

macies and can be found in most cities or areas with large Latino populations. It is important to ascertain what herbal medications the patient is taking, especially in the perioperative period. A sobador is an individual who treats patients with massage therapy. This type of treatment is often used for sprains and strains of the ankle, knee, shoulder, and elbow. It is believed that massage can be used to "work out" the bunched up nerves, tendons, and muscles.

Asian-American Patients

As the largest continent on earth, encompassing more than 40 nations and approximately 4 billion inhabitants, Asia remains one of the most ethnically and politically diverse regions on the planet. Individuals who identify themselves of Asian ethnicity are a rapidly growing sector of the US population. Understanding the enormous diversity of this population is the first and most important aspect of providing culturally competent care. According to 2007 US Census estimates, this group includes 15.2 million individuals or approximately 5% of the US population, and, of these, 8.9 million people were born outside the United States.[69] Nearly 50% of Asian-Americans make their home within the three most populous US states—5 million in California, 1.4 million in New York, and nearly 1 million in Texas. Hawaii's Asian population almost matches that of Texas. By proportion of state population, Asian-Americans make up a majority of the Hawaiian population (55%), with a significant presence in California (14%), New Jersey (8%), and Washington (8%).

Growth of the Asian-American population from 2006 to 2007 was 2.9%, higher than that of any other ethnic group in the US Census.[69] Numerous national origins and even more numerous ethnic lineages are found within this group. However, certain cultural groups made up a large portion of the 2007 Asian-American population, with 3.54 million Chinese, 3.05 million Filipinos, 2.77 million Asian-Indians, 1.64 million Vietnamese, 1.56 million Koreans, and 1.22 million Japanese. Together, these six groups make up more than 90% of the US Asian population. The fastest growth in the Asian-American population is occurring in the southern and western states, with Nevada, North Carolina, Georgia, Arizona, Nebraska, Tennessee, Florida, Kentucky, Delaware, and Colorado showing the greatest growth.[69] The Asian-American population in those states more than doubled in the decade from 1990 to 2000.[70]

Characterization of such a diverse group is challenging. With countless cultural, religious, and political backgrounds and even certain rare languages beyond the reach of major universities, generalizations often prove inaccurate, and stark contrasts occur in socioeconomic and educational status. However, census statistics shed light on features, such as education level, often overlooked in this population. The Census Bureau estimated that 50% of Asians 25 years or older had a bachelor's degree or higher level of education, compared with 28% of all Americans in the same age range.[69] However, there are wide variations within this group, with 68% of Asian-Indians and 27% of Vietnamese-Americans having higher degrees. Other Asian-American groups, particularly those with high rates of limited English proficiency, may have lower education levels.

Economic Indicators and Access to Care

According to 2007 US Census Bureau estimates, the mean per capita income for the entire population was $26,688, whereas it was $31,138 for non-Hispanic white Americans and $29,466 for Asian-Americans.[71] Living situations also differ between Asian-Americans and the population as a whole, with an average of 2.68 inhabitants per household in the US population, 2.55 among white Americans, and 3.16 among Asian-Americans. This finding probably is related to the higher median household income among Asian-Americans. Cultural tendencies to pool resources and care for elderly family members in the home may add to household size. A markedly higher proportion (6.78%) of Asian households has more than one occupant per room than non-Hispanic white households (1.08%). In addition to the presence of relatives in the home, this finding may also indicate another facet of the socioeconomic status that may have public health implications.

The lack of health insurance coverage in the Asian-American community is 16.8% based on 2007 Census estimates, an increase over the prior year and also higher than the 10.4% for non-Hispanic white Americans but lower than for some other ethnic groups.[69] One final statistic of interest is the proportion of physicians and nurses in certain subgroups of the Asian-American population. Although there is an average of 249 physicians per 100,000 individuals in the US population, Hmong, Laotian, Cambodian, and Malaysian physicians are in short supply with 24, 28, 40, and 84 physicians per 100,000 individuals, respectively.[70] In the nursing workforce, a similar scarcity of Hmong, Bangladeshi, Cambodian, and Laotian nurses suggests that patients with limited English proficiency in these groups may meet language barriers when seeking health care.

Greeting and Communication

Although the physician must keep in mind the extreme diversity in the Asian-American population, certain characteristics appear frequently and should be understood to avoid potential barriers to care. Several of these characteristics were described in a study comparing values espoused by Asians and Caucasians.[72] Asians showed a tendency to be group oriented, considerate of others, modest, hierarchical, and formal, whereas Caucasians tended to be individualistic, assertive, self-confident, egalitarian, and informal. If a white American doctor is caring for an Asian-American patient, there is potential for misunderstanding based on each person's perception of the other. The physician may interpret quietness as lack of assertion, modesty as inability to stand out, formality as being ill at ease, lack of questioning as being noninquisitive, and respect for the doctor as lack of independent thinking.[73] The patient may similarly interpret the doctor's mannerisms as being rude or the emphasis on patient autonomy as showing a lack of consideration for the feelings and decisions of the family group.

The physician should consciously address the patient, especially an elderly patient, with respect and make eye contact to establish trust. Certain Asian cultures place paramount importance on "saving face" and patients may hesitate to disagree with a doctor's recommendations even when they do not intend to follow the treatment plan. A patient who is simply nodding or smiling may not agree with what is presented by the physician, but out of respect may not wish to voice a different point of view. The culturally competent physician will recognize this pitfall and seek to elicit the patient's viewpoint of his or her illness before making recommendations rather than asserting a rigid treatment plan that fails to take into consideration individual cultural elements.

Understanding that many Asian patients, particularly those born outside the United States, may believe in alternative or traditional treatments is important when forming a therapeutic relationship and planning future treatment. The physician should specifically inquire about the patient's other treatments. Alternative medical beliefs can range from the use of herbal supplements to a more holistic belief system relying on balance in nature and leading to misgivings toward invasive modern medical treatments or surgery. An elderly patient may also hesitate to seek medical care out of concern for placing a financial burden on family members.

The physician should be aware of certain gestures that may be interpreted as impolite. Directing the sole of the shoe toward another person is considered rude. A patient might feel lack of respect if the doctor crosses his legs during the interview. It is impossible to describe all points of etiquette for all Asian cultures because there is much variation, but a well-trained physician will be attentive to cues from the patient and will adjust to each situation.

Special Health Considerations

Research has shown considerable variability between ethnic groups when considering risk profiles for metabolic syndrome and cardiovascular disease. It has been shown that Asian-Indians have more than twice the risk of premature coronary artery disease than Caucasians, in addition to higher rates of diabetes and metabolic syndrome,[74] a fact that may affect perioperative risk and influence a surgeon's decision to refer a patient for preoperative medical optimization. Although it is known that the prevalence of metabolic syndrome is increasing worldwide, a North American study demonstrated an odds ratio of 2.0 for metabolic syndrome among Asian patients compared with patients of other ethnicities enrolled in a registry for total knee replacement.[75] Metabolic syndrome is characterized by several factors, including obesity, which has been linked to an increased risk of deep venous thrombosis after total knee arthroplasty and a higher risk of implant failure.[76-78] The surgeon must interpret such data in light of the local population because wide geographic variations are likely.

Increasing awareness of human genetic variation has resulted in a deeper understanding of pathophysiology. Certain Asian populations are known to have a genetic predisposition to orthopaedic conditions. Polymorphisms in both the *COL6A1* gene and the *BMP-2* gene have been shown to increase susceptibility to ossification of the posterior longitudinal ligament in Chinese and Japanese patients.[79,80] Genetic variation also leads to differing responses to pharmacologic treatment. Polymorphisms in the hepatic isoenzyme CYP2D6, responsible for metabolism of 25% to 30% of all clinically administered medications, lead to reductions of enzyme activity in some Asian populations. Variations in the enzyme CYP2C19 place many Asian patients at higher risk for diazepam toxicity;[81] Differences in hepatic glucuronidation leads to variable pharmacologic and toxicologic responses to common medications such as acetaminophen in the Asian population.[82] Findings of genetic variation will undoubtedly expand with further investigation and reinforce the principle that the physician must treat each patient with careful attention to the individual's needs.

Anatomic variation also exists, with important implications for orthopaedic surgeons. A study of Chinese patients found the course of the radial nerve differs from that described as the Caucasian standard, with the nerve traversing the humerus somewhat more distally.[83] Lim and Wong[84] examined cervical spine anatomy in patients of Chinese descent and found such wide variation in sagittal dimensions that they concluded that the Torg ratio, commonly used to predict cervical stenosis, was unreliable in this population. This finding would have important considerations for an orthopaedic surgeon evaluating an Asian patient for cervical stenosis. Researchers in Hong Kong described increased knee joint obliquity in Chinese women compared with Caucasian parameters and suggested increasing the external rotation of the femoral component during total knee arthroplasty to obtain a balanced flexion gap.[85]

Physicians should also be aware of health conditions common to certain ethnic groups, including Asian-Americans. For example, a high rate of hepatitis B has been reported in patients from Southeast Asia, where the disease is endemic; perinatal transmission leads to an increased rate of the disease, even in second-generation Asian-Americans.[73] Because chronic hepatitis may lead to cirrhosis and thus affect hepatic metabolism of multiple drugs, including medications commonly prescribed by orthopaedic surgeons (such as acetaminophen products and warfarin), awareness and screening for hepatitis B can lower a patient's risk for long-term sequelae.

Nontraditional Medicine

Many Asian cultures have a rich heritage of traditional medical philosophies and herbal therapies. An in-depth analysis of the veritable cornucopia of medicinal supplements used in Asian cultures may overwhelm the average American physician, although research is beginning to describe certain desirable and sometimes undesirable effects of these treatments and their interactions with modern pharmaceuticals. The Asian-American patient may be hesitant to discuss or even admit to using these traditional treatments, perhaps because of the perception that many American physicians would discourage or not understand their application. The physician should allow the patient the freedom to discuss traditional Asian treatments, while sharing information on their interaction with proposed pharmaceutical therapies. Many herbal products affect hematologic parameters and coagulation, thus complicating pharmacologic therapies used in orthopaedic surgery. Such herbs include guilinggao, feverfew, qingkailing, and danshen; other medications that may affect coagulation include ginseng, gingko, and ginger. If the patient is taking any form of traditional medicine, the physician should research its effects to provide an informed discussion of the risks and benefits of combining the traditional treatment with modern treatment strategies.

Discussion

Training physicians to work with culturally diverse populations has often been seen as a commendable goal but not as pressing as other issues in medicine. As the world becomes increasingly diverse, social and cultural beliefs, attitudes, and behaviors figure prominently in the health of communities. Patient safety, satisfaction, and successful treatment increasingly depend on understanding patients' medical and cultural needs. An awareness of the patient demographics of the community in which a physician practices offers an opportunity to improve communication and achieve better patient and physician satisfaction, better patient compliance, improved health outcomes, better informed medical deci-

sions, and reduce the likelihood of malpractice lawsuits.[86]

Although it is desirable to change the hearts and minds of caregivers for the purposes of cultural competency alone, the changing face of medicine is mandating this change. Because medicine is becoming more consumer oriented, patients will go elsewhere if a physician is unresponsive to their needs. Poor communication has been linked to poor patient compliance, poor patient satisfaction, and poor outcomes. With the advent of pay for performance, patient satisfaction will affect the income of physicians. In addition, in an attempt to improve health care, seven states (New Jersey, California, Washington, New Mexico, New York, Florida, and Connecticut) have enacted or have pending legislation regarding culturally competent care education.

Summary

Providing culturally competent care to patients involves an understanding of ethnic and cultural diversity, including the history of the ethnic group, socioeconomic status, access to care, cultural etiquette, differing communication styles, beliefs in nontraditional medicine, and biologic and anatomic issues specific to certain ethnic groups. Differences in experiences, appearance, religious beliefs, language, and social organization affect the patient-physician relationship. To provide culturally competent care, physicians should strive to establish trust and a respectful relationship with their patients. Good communications is essential for culturally competent care.

References

1. Smedley BD, Stith AY, Nelson AR, eds: *Unequal Treatment: Confronting Racial and Ethnic Disparities in Health Care*. Washington, DC, National Academies Press, 2003.

2. Satcher D, Pamies RJ, Woelfl NN, eds: *Multicultural Medicine and Health Disparities*. New York, NY, McGraw-Hill, 2006.

3. Tongue JR, Epps HR, Forese LL: Communication skills. *Instr Course Lect* 2005;54:3-9.

4. Burgess DJ, Fu SS, van Ryn M: Why do providers contribute to disparities and what can be done about it? *J Gen Intern Med* 2004;19(11):1154-1159.

5. Dogra N, Karnik N: First-year medical students' attitudes toward diversity and its teaching: An investigation at one U.S. Medical School. *Acad Med* 2003;78(11):1191-1200.

6. The Kaiser Family Foundation: National survey of physicians: Part I. Doctors on disparities in medical care. http://www.kff.org/minorityhealth/20020321a-index.cfm. Accessed October 31, 2011.

7. Hall JA, Horgan TG, Stein TS, Roter DL: Liking in the physician-patient relationship. *Patient Educ Couns* 2002;48(1):69-77.

8. Kutob RM, Senf JH, Harris JM Jr: Teaching culturally effective diabetes care: Results of a randomized controlled trial. *Fam Med* 2009;41(3):167-174.

9. Beach MC, Cooper LA, Robinson KA, et al: Strategies for improving minority healthcare quality. *Evid Rep Technol Assess (Summ)* 2004;90:1-8.

10. Gardenswartz L, Rowe A: *Managing Diversity in Health Care Manual: Proven Tools and Activities for Leaders and Trainers*. San Francisco, CA, Jossey-Bass, 1999.

11. Richardson LD, Babcock IC, Tamayo-Sarver JH: Racial and ethnic disparities in the clinical practice of emergency medicine.

Acad Emerg Med 2003;10(11): 1184-1188.

12. Bach PB, Pham HH, Schrag D, Tate RC, Hargraves JL: Primary care physicians who treat blacks and whites. *N Engl J Med* 2004; 351(6):575-584.

13. Furstenberg A-L, Mezey MD: Differences in outcome between black and white elderly hip fracture patients. *J Chronic Dis* 1987; 40(10):931-938.

14. Becker G, Newsom E: Socioeconomic status and dissatisfaction with health care among chronically ill African Americans. *Am J Public Health* 2003;93(5):742-748.

15. Figaro MK, Russo PW, Allegrante JP: Preferences for arthritis care among urban AfricanAmericans: "I don't want to be cut." *Health Psychol* 2004;23(3):324-329.

16. Todd KH, Deaton C, D'Adamo AP, Goe L: Ethnicity and analgesic practice. *Ann Emerg Med* 2000;35(1):11-16.

17. Quazi S, Eberhart M, Jacoby J, Heller M: Are racial disparities in ED analgesia improving? Evidence from a national database. *Am J Emerg Med* 2008;26(4):462-464.

18. Bijur P, Bérard A, Esses D, Calderon Y, Gallagher EJ: Race, ethnicity, and management of pain from long-bone fractures: A prospective study of two academic urban emergency departments. *Acad Emerg Med* 2008;15(7):589-597.

19. Groeneveld PW, Laufer SB, Garber AM: Technology diffusion, hospital variation, and racial disparities among elderly Medicare beneficiaries: 1989-2000. *Med Care* 2005;43(4):320-329.

20. Hannan EL, van Ryn M, Burke J, et al: Access to coronary artery bypass surgery by race/ethnicity and gender among patients who arc appropriate for surgery. *Med Care* 1999;37(1):68-77.

21. Sedlis SP, Fisher VJ, Tice D, Esposito R, Madmon L, Steinberg

EH: Racial differences in performance of invasive cardiac procedures in a Department of Veterans Affairs Medical Center. *J Clin Epidemiol* 1997;50(8):899-901.

22. Gordon HS, Street RL Jr, Sharf BF, Souchek J: Racial differences in doctors' information-giving and patients' participation. *Cancer* 2006;107(6):1313-1320.

23. Klassen AC, Hall AG, Saksvig B, Curbow B, Klassen DK: Relationship between patients' perceptions of disadvantage and discrimination and listing for kidney transplantation. *Am J Public Health* 2002;92(5):811-817.

24. Gornick ME, Eggers PW, Reilly TW, et al: Effects of race and income on mortality and use of services among Medicare beneficiaries. *N Engl J Med* 1996;335(11): 791-799.

25. SooHoo NF, Farng E, Zingmond DS: Disparities in the utilization of high-volume hospitals for total hip replacement. *J Natl Med Assoc* 2011;103(1):31-35.

26. SooHoo NF, Zingmond DS, Ko CY: Disparities in the utilization of high-volume hospitals for total knee replacement. *J Natl Med Assoc* 2008;100(5):559-564.

27. Strothers HS III, Rust G, Minor P, Fresh E, Druss B, Satcher D: Disparities in antidepressant treatment in Medicaid elderly diagnosed with depression. *J Am Geriatr Soc* 2005;53(3):456-461.

28. Steel N, Clark A, Lang IA, Wallace RB, Melzer D: Racial disparities in receipt of hip and knee joint replacements are not explained by need: The Health and Retirement Study 1998-2004. *J Gerontol A Biol Sci Med Sci* 2008;63(6):629-634.

29. Hoenig H, Rubenstein L, Kahn K: Rehabilitation after hip fracture: Equal opportunity for all? *Arch Phys Med Rehabil* 1996; 77(1):58-63.

30. Aruguete MS, Roberts CA: Participants' ratings of male physicians who vary in race and communication style. *Psychol Rep* 2002;91 (3 Pt 1):793-806.

31. Groeneveld PW, Kruse GB, Chen Z, Asch DA: Variation in cardiac procedure use and racial disparity among Veterans Affairs Hospitals. *Am Heart J* 2007;153(2):320-327.

32. Ibrahim SA, Siminoff LA, Burant CJ, Kwoh CK: Variation in perceptions of treatment and self-care practices in elderly with osteoarthritis: A comparison between African American and white patients. *Arthritis Rheum* 2001; 45(4):340-345.

33. Ibrahim SA, Siminoff LA, Burant CJ, Kwoh CK: Differences in expectations of outcome mediate African American/white patient differences in "willingness" to consider joint replacement. *Arthritis Rheum* 2002;46(9):2429-2435.

34. Williams DR, Rucker TD: Understanding and addressing racial disparities in health care. *Health Care Financ Rev* 2000;21(4): 75-90.

35. Dykes DC, White AA III: Getting to equal: Strategies to understand and eliminate general and orthopaedic healthcare disparities. *Clin Orthop Relat Res* 2009;467(10): 2598-2605.

36. Johnson RL, Saha S, Arbelaez JJ, Beach MC, Cooper LA: Racial and ethnic differences in patient perceptions of bias and cultural competence in health care. *J Gen Intern Med* 2004;19(2):101-110.

37. Health literacy: Report of the Council on Scientific Affairs. Ad Hoc Committee on Health Literacy for the Council on Scientific Affairs, American Medical Association. *JAMA* 1999;281(6):552-557.

38. Schillinger D, Bindman A, Wang F, Stewart A, Piette J: Functional health literacy and the quality of

physician-patient communication among diabetes patients. *Patient Educ Couns* 2004;52(3):315-323.

39. Carter JH: Psychosocial/cultural issues in medicine and psychiatry: Treating African Americans. *J Natl Med Assoc* 1995;87(12): 857-860.

40. Ang DC, Monahan PO, Cronan TA: Understanding ethnic disparities in the use of total joint arthroplasty: Application of the health belief model. *Arthritis Rheum* 2008;59(1):102-108.

41. Groeneveld PW, Kwoh CK, Mor MK, et al: Racial differences in expectations of joint replacement surgery outcomes. *Arthritis Rheum* 2008;59(5):730-737.

42. Figaro MK, Williams-Russo P, Allegrante JP: Expectation and outlook: The impact of patient preference on arthritis care among African Americans. *J Ambul Care Manage* 2005;28(1):41-48.

43. Kroll TL, Richardson M, Sharf BF, Suarez-Almazor ME: "Keep on truckin'" or "It's got you in this little vacuum": Race-based perceptions in decision-making for total knee arthroplasty. *J Rheumatol* 2007;34(5):1069-1075.

44. Blake VA, Allegrante JP, Robbins L, et al: Racial differences in social network experience and perceptions of benefit of arthritis treatments among New York City Medicare beneficiaries with self-reported hip and knee pain. *Arthritis Rheum* 2002;47(4): 366-371.

45. Betancourt JR, Green AR, Carrillo JE, Ananeh-Firempong O II: Defining cultural competence: A practical framework for addressing racial/ethnic disparities in health and health care. *Public Health Rep* 2003;118(4):293-302.

46. van Ryn M, Burke J: The effect of patient race and socio-economic status on physicians' perceptions of patients. *Soc Sci Med* 2000; 50(6):813-828.

47. Street RL Jr, Gordon H, Haidet P: Physicians' communication and perceptions of patients: Is it how they look, how they talk, or is it just the doctor? *Soc Sci Med* 2007; 65(3):586-598.

48. van Ryn M, Burgess D, Malat J, Griffin J: Physicians' perceptions of patients' social and behavioral characteristics and race disparities in treatment recommendations for men with coronary artery disease. *Am J Public Health* 2006;96(2): 351-357.

49. Cooper-Patrick L, Gallo JJ, Gonzales JJ, et al: Race, gender, and partnership in the patient-physician relationship. *JAMA* 1999;282(6):583-589.

50. Saha S, Komaromy M, Koepsell TD, Bindman AB: Patient-physician racial concordance and the perceived quality and use of health care. *Arch Intern Med* 1999;159(9):997-1004.

51. Cooper LA, Roter DL, Johnson RL, Ford DE, Steinwachs DM, Powe NR: Patient-centered communication, ratings of care, and concordance of patient and physician race. *Ann Intern Med* 2003; 139(11):907-915.

52. Ferguson WJ, Candib LM: Culture, language, and the doctor-patient relationship. *Fam Med* 2002;34(5):353-361.

53. Laveist TA, Nuru-Jeter A: Is doctor-patient race concordance associated with greater satisfaction with care? *J Health Soc Behav* 2002;43(3):296-306.

54. *Orthopaedic Practice and Medical Incomes in the U.S. 2008.* Rosemont, IL, American Academy of Orthopaedic Surgeons, 2009. http://testnew.aaos.org/research/opus/2008_CensusMembers.cfm. Accessed November 3, 2011.

55. Washington HA: *Medical apartheid: The Dark History of Medical Experimentation on Black Americans From Colonial Times to the Present.* New York, NY, Doubleday, 2006.

56. Shafer JK, Usilton LJ, Gleeson GA: Untreated syphilis in the male Negro: A prospective study of the effect on life expectancy. *Public Health Rep* 1954;69(7): 684-690.

57. Brawley OW: The study of untreated syphilis in the negro male. *Int J Radiat Oncol Biol Phys* 1998; 40(1):5-8.

58. Hussain-Gambles M, Atkin K, Leese B: Why ethnic minority groups are under-represented in clinical trials: A review of the literature. *Health Soc Care Community* 2004;12(5):382-388.

59. Nápoles-Springer AM, Santoyo J, Houston K, Pérez-Stable EJ, Stewart AL: Patients' perceptions of cultural factors affecting the quality of their medical encounters. *Health Expect* 2005;8(1):4-17.

60. Bogart LM, Bird ST, Walt LC, Delahanty DL, Figler JL: Association of stereotypes about physicians to health care satisfaction, help-seeking behavior, and adherence to treatment. *Soc Sci Med* 2004;58(6):1049-1058.

61. Levinson W, Hudak PL, Feldman JJ, et al: "It's not what you say ...": Racial disparities in communication between orthopedic surgeons and patients. *Med Care* 2008; 46(4):410-416.

62. The Annie E. Casey Foundation: Kids Count Data Center website. Children in single-parent families by race (Percent) - 2009. http://datacenter.kidscount.org/data/acrossstates/Rankings.aspx?ind=107. Accessed November 3, 2011.

63. Jones AC, Kwoh CK, Groeneveld PW, Mor M, Geng M, Ibrahim SA: Investigating racial differences in coping with chronic osteoarthritis pain. *J Cross Cult Gerontol* 2008;23(4):339-347.

64. US Religious Landscape Survey. Portraits: demographics, Jehovah Witnesses. Pew Forum on Religion and Public Life website. http://religions.pewforum.org/portraits#. Accessed November 3, 2011.

65. US Census Bureau: Hispanic population of the United States: A presentation that highlights past, present and future trends of the Hispanic population. http://www.census.gov/population/www/socdemo/hispanic/hispanic_pop_presentation.html. Accessed September 26, 2011.

66. Haider AH, Chang DC, Efron DT, Haut ER, Crandall M, Cornwell EE III : Race and insurance status as risk factors for trauma mortality. *Arch Surg* 2008; 143(10):945-949.

67. US Census Bureau: American fact finder help: Hispanic or Latino origin. http://factfinder2.census.gov/help/en/glossary/s/spanish_hispanic_latino.htm. Accessed September 26, 2011.

68. Statistical Portrait of Hispanics in the United States: 2007. Pew Hispanic Center website. http://pewhispanic.org/files/factsheets/hispanics2007/Table-3.pdf. Accessed May 30, 2009.

69. US Census Bureau News: Facts for features, March 3, 2009. http://www.census.gov/newsroom/releases/archives/facts_for_features_special_editions/cb09-ff06.html. Accessed October 26, 2011.

70. Asian & Pacific Islander American Health Forum: Diverse communities, diverse experiences: The status of Asian Americans & Pacific Islanders in the US. http://www.aapcho.org/altruesite/files/aapcho/Research/Diverse%20Communities%20Diverse%20Experiences.pdf. Accessed: July 14, 2011.

71. US Census Bureau: 2007 American community survey. http://factfinder.census.gov/servlet/DatasetMainPageServlet?_program=ACS&_submenuId=datasets_2&_lang=en. Accessed July 14, 2011.

72. Lin-Fu JS: Ethnocultural barriers to health care: A major problem for Asian and Pacific Islander Americans. *Asian Am Pac Isl J Health* 1994;2(4):290-298.

73. Riew KD, Tsao AK: Asian-American patients, in Jimenez RL, Lewis VO, eds: *The AAOS Culturally Competent Care Guidebook.* Rosemont, IL, American Academy of Orthopaedic Surgeons, 2009, pp 29-36.

74. Enas EA, Mohan V, Deepa M, Farooq S, Pazhoor S, Chennikkara H: The metabolic syndrome and dyslipidemia among Asian Indians: A population with high rates of diabetes and premature coronary artery disease. *J Cardiometab Syndr* 2007;2(4):267-275.

75. Gandhi R, Razak F, Tso P, Davey JR, Mahomed NN: Asian ethnicity and the prevalence of metabolic syndrome in the osteoarthritic total knee arthroplasty population. *J Arthroplasty* 2010; 25(3):416-419.

76. PubMed Health: Metabolic syndrome. http://www.ncbi.nlm.nih.gov/pubmedhealth/PMH0004546/. Accessed September 30, 2011.

77. Kim YH, Kim VE: Factors leading to low incidence of deep vein thrombosis after cementless and cemented total knee arthroplasty. *Clin Orthop Relat Res* 1991;273: 119-124.

78. Gillespie GN, Porteous AJ: Obesity and knee arthroplasty. *Knee* 2007;14(2):81-86.

79. Kong Q, Ma X, Li F, et al: COL6A1 polymorphisms associated with ossification of the ligamentum flavum and ossification of the posterior longitudinal ligament. *Spine (Phila Pa 1976)* 2007;32(25):2834-2838.

80. Wang H, Liu D, Yang Z, et al: Association of bone morphogenetic protein-2 gene polymorphisms with susceptibility to ossification of the posterior longitudinal ligament of the spine and its severity in Chinese patients. *Eur Spine J* 2008;17(7): 956-964.

81. Ma MK, Woo MH, McLeod HL: Genetic basis of drug metabolism. *Am J Health Syst Pharm* 2002; 59(21):2061-2069.

82. Patel M, Tang BK, Kalow W: Variability of acetaminophen metabolism in Caucasians and Orientals. *Pharmacogenetics* 1992; 2(1):38-45.

83. Chou PH, Shyu JF, Ma HL, Wang ST, Chen TH: Courses of the radial nerve differ between Chinese and Caucasians: Clinical applications. *Clin Orthop Relat Res* 2008;466(1):135-138.

84. Lim JK, Wong HK: Variation of the cervical spinal Torg ratio with gender and ethnicity. *Spine J* 2004;4(4):396-401.

85. Tang WM, Zhu YH, Chiu KY: Axial alignment of the lower extremity in Chinese adults. *J Bone Joint Surg Am* 2000;82-A(11): 1603-1608.

86. Frymoyer JW, Frymoyer NP: Physician-patient communication: A lost art? *J Am Acad Orthop Surg* 2002;10(2):95-105.

Practical Research Methods for Orthopaedic Surgeons

Adam S. Dowrick, PhD
Paul Tornetta III, MD
William T. Obremskey, MD
Douglas R. Dirschl, MD
Mohit Bhandari, MD, FRCSC

Abstract

Inherent to understanding an orthopaedic study is a fundamental knowledge of the study's design principles and statistics. Statistics, in part, allow a researcher to sample a portion of the population and use probability to decide whether the findings from the sample are likely to apply to the whole population. Although statistical jargon can be confusing, several simple principles guide the approach to research design. It is helpful for orthopaedic surgeons to review different study designs and their levels of evidence, to understand statistical jargon and the selection of the statistical test that is appropriate for given types of data, and to be familiar with the process of sample size calculations. Knowledge gained from statistical principles and research design is used to interpret study results. Such knowledge is invaluable for judging the value of new clinical evidence and for designing future studies.

Instr Course Lect 2012;61:581-586.

To interpret the quality of the information presented in an orthopaedic study, it is necessary to have a basic knowledge of study design principles and statistics. Similarly, to conduct a study, surgeons need to understand the basic research concepts to consider during the design phase to ensure the results add as much evidence as possible. This chapter presents the basics of study design and statistical concepts relevant to orthopaedic surgical research.

Study Designs

In designing a study protocol, researchers should use the strongest study design that can add the most information to the evidence base in a practical and ethical manner. The study question, the rarity of the condition to be investigated, and the resources available influence the most appropriate design for a given study.[1-3] In general, clinical studies fall into two categories: experimental and observational.[4,5]

In experimental studies, a patient's exposure to an intervention is manipulated by the researcher, and the patient is observed for a period of time to detect the effects of the intervention on predetermined outcome measures. The manipulation involves the random allocation of patients to groups; hence, studies of this type are termed randomized trials. The effect of randomization is to control as many factors as possible so the groups are similar except for the variable of interest.[6] In this way, a causative link can be determined.

Observational studies allow for associations between variables to be investigated, but the evidence is not strong enough to establish a causal link.[5] Because the study is not controlled, there are variables that may influence the results and, therefore, there

Neither of the following authors nor any immediate family member has received anything of value from or owns stock in a commercial company or institution related directly or indirectly to the subject of this chapter: Dr. Dowrick and Dr. Obremskey. Dr. Tornetta or an immediate family member has received royalties from Smith & Nephew; serves as a paid consultant to Smith & Nephew; and serves as a board member, owner, officer, or committee member of the American Orthopaedic Association. Dr. Dirschl or an immediate family member has received royalties from Biomet and serves as a board member, owner, officer, or committee member of the American Orthopaedic Association. Dr. Bhandari or an immediate family member serves as a paid consultant to Amgen, Eli Lilly, Stryker, and Smith & Nephew.

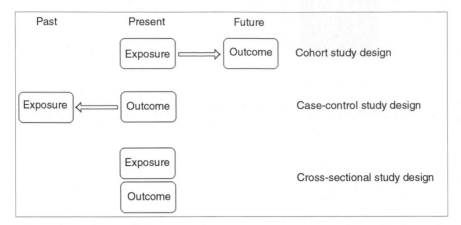

Figure 1 Timing of exposure and outcome for observational study designs.

is inadequate confidence to say that *x* caused *y*. In observational studies, a patient's exposure and outcome status are observed with no influence from the researcher. The timing of the exposure and the outcome defines each observational study design.

In cohort studies, patients are allocated to groups according to their exposure to a treatment or a condition of interest and are followed for a period of time to determine if a specified outcome develops (**Figure 1**). At the end of the study period, the outcome in the exposed group is compared with that in the unexposed group. Cohort studies are not feasible when the condition of interest is rare because the follow-up period required to get a large enough sample size to show an effect is prohibitive. The major difficulty in the cohort study design is that it is not possible to be certain the cohorts were well matched and/or to know what factors influenced the study results (these factors are known as confounders and are defined later in this chapter).

In a case-control study, a group of patients with a defined condition is compared with a group of patients without the condition, and their previous exposure to a risk factor is compared (**Figure 1**). This is a relatively quick and inexpensive study design that is particularly useful for rare con-

ditions or when the time between exposure and outcome is long. Although this study design is also subject to confounding, matching cases and controls on several variables at the time of analysis can help decrease the effect that confounding variables can have on the result. For example, a case patient can be matched with a control patient by sex and age within 5 years (as well as other study-specific variables) to ensure that the two groups are as similar as possible.

Cross-sectional studies analyze patients at a single point in time (**Figure 1**) and are useful in determining what proportion of patients have a condition at that time point (known as prevalence) and what other factors may be associated with the condition. This study design relies on accurate recall by the patient with regard to whether he or she had been exposed to a certain risk factor or had a condition of interest.

Case series and case reports are useful to describe novel conditions or treatments in a small number of patients (generally from a single institution or surgeon). They are useful for conveying information promptly to other surgeons, and the information presented in such reports may be used to generate hypotheses for use with a more robust study design.

Whatever the chosen design, surgeons should be aware of the overall validity of the study in relation to the known hierarchy of evidence.

Levels of Evidence

Keeping up to date with the latest research findings, while also attending to a busy clinical practice, is a time-consuming task that may be difficult for orthopaedic surgeons. In assessing the literature to determine best evidence-based practice, several factors can be taken into account. One of the simplest and most commonly used criteria is the level of evidence. A hierarchy exists that places each study along a continuum based on the likelihood of bias within a given study design. The levels of evidence are different, depending on the primary focus of the study (such as therapy, prognosis, harm, or economic analysis).[5,7] Many different hierarchies are available.[5,8,9]

The gold standard by which clinical research is judged is the randomized controlled trial, which is designated the highest level of evidence. Similarly, meta-analyses or systematic reviews that collate the results of high-quality randomized controlled trials are also designated as level I evidence. Level II evidence includes lesser quality trials (for example, those with less than 80% patient follow-up or improper randomization), systematic reviews or meta-analyses of these second-tier studies, and prospective cohort studies. Level III evidence includes case-control, retrospective cohort, and systematic reviews of these third-tier studies. The lower levels of evidence (levels IV and V) include case series or opinions, respectively.

Level I and II studies should be thoroughly assessed to ensure that the methodology meets all of the criteria for the level assigned.[7,10,11] For example, the authors may have performed a cohort study, but is there a suspicion of bias in the design of the study or are there confounding variables that the authors have not noted and/or accounted for? This additional step of reviewing study methodology is the key to evidence-based practice. A randomized trial with a poor methodology and a relatively small sample size will not necessarily provide more evidence than a well-conducted cohort study. All research has value, and it is up to the clinician to determine the value of each piece of information in a study.[12]

Statistics Simplified

It is generally not logistically possible for a researcher to obtain data from the entire population that he or she wants to study. The role of statistics is to allow a researcher to sample a portion of the population and use probability to decide whether the findings from the sample are likely to apply to the entire population.[13] In this process of research, several jargon terms with specific meanings are used.

Bias is a systematic error in the design or conduct of a study that produces an outcome that is different from the underlying truth.[14] There are several types of bias that need to be considered, depending on the study design. Attrition bias refers to systematic differences between the groups with regard to the number of participants who are lost to follow-up, withdraw consent, or die. Expertise bias exists when a surgeon has a higher competence or familiarity with one study procedure over another, meaning that there is a chance of a better outcome in one group. Recall bias refers to a phenomenon whereby a patient who has an adverse outcome is more likely to recall an exposure than a patient who has a better outcome, independent of the true exposure. Selection bias occurs when the allocation of groups leads to a difference in the baseline characteristics of one study group compared with another.

A confounding variable (or confounder) acts to distort the association between two variables of interest because of its strong relationship with both variables. For example, an association between infection rates and open fractures may be confounded by the severity of the initial soft-tissue injury of the open fracture wound because it would be expected that larger wounds, which require longer and possibly more operations, would be more susceptible to infection. Frequent confounders include sex, age, socioeconomic status, and comorbidities.

The null hypothesis is the default hypothesis that assumes that there are no differences between the groups. The alternative hypothesis suggests that there is a difference between the study groups. The chance of the null hypothesis being true is evaluated by a statistical test.

A type I error, or α error, occurs when the null hypothesis is rejected when in fact it is true, leading to a false-positive result. That is, the researcher concludes that there is a difference between the groups when there is not. The probability of committing such an error, the α level, is generally set at the 0.05 level and assumes that, 5% of the time, the statistical test will find a difference between the groups purely because of chance alone.

A type II error, or β error, occurs when the researcher incorrectly accepts the null hypothesis. The probability of committing such an error, the β level, is generally set at the 0.20 level (20%). This means that the researcher is willing to accept a 20% chance of concluding that there are no differences between the groups when there actually is a difference.

The effect size is the difference between the groups that needs to be detected to establish a true difference and is based on the results of pilot data or values in the literature. It is used in the calculation of the sample size.

Study power refers to the probability of concluding that there are no differences between the groups when there actually is a difference. Study power is equal to 1 minus the value of the β error. By convention, β is set at 0.20, and the power of the study is set at 80% or more, which means that there is a 20% or less chance that the study will demonstrate no significant difference when there is one. Studies are said to be underpowered when the power of the study is less than 80%.

The statistical P value is a measure of the strength of the evidence that is provided by the data that the null hypothesis is true. When the P value is less than α, the researcher can be confident that the evidence is strong enough for the null hypothesis to be rejected and can conclude that the result was significant.

Normality refers to whether the data approximate the shape of a bell curve when plotted as a bar graph. Most statistical tests assume that the data fit the bell curve. When this assumption is broken and the data are skewed, specific types of analyses (known as nonparametric statistics) can be undertaken; otherwise, the conclusions drawn may not be valid. In the frequently reported small samples analyzed in orthopaedic studies, it is rare to obtain normal data.

Categoric data (also known as qualitative data) assign each patient to a single category or type. The simplest example of categoric data is a binary variable consisting of two possible groups (for example, male/female or fracture united/not united). Categoric variables that have three or more groups that have no natural order (for example, blunt/penetrating/burn) are called nominal data, whereas the variables that have a natural progression through the categories that is not to scale (for example, Gustilo open fracture classification) are known as ordi-

Table 1

Which Test Should Be Used?

Desired Analysis	Type of Data	Statistical Test to Use
Comparison of two groups	Comparing means of normally distributed continuous variables	Student t-test
	Comparing medians of not normally distributed continuous variables	Mann-Whitney U test
	Comparing proportions of categoric variables	Chi-square test or Fisher exact test
Comparison of more than two groups	Comparing means of normally distributed continuous variables	Analysis of Variance test (ANOVA)
	Comparing medians of not normally distributed continuous variables	Kruskal-Wallis test
	Comparing proportions of categoric variables	Chi-square test or Fisher exact test
Determination of associations between variables	Normally distributed continuous variables	Pearson correlation (r)
	Ordinal variables	Spearman rank-order correlation (rho) or Kendall rank correlation
Creation of a model to predict y given x	Outcome and single predictor variables are continuous	Simple linear regression
Creation of a model to predict y given two or more variables	Outcome is continuous, and multiple predictor variables are categoric or continuous	Multiple linear regression
	Outcome is binary, and multiple predictor variables are categoric or continuous	Binary logistic regression

nal data. Categoric data are often presented in papers as percentages in tables or bar charts.

In the case of quantitative data, differences between numbers have meaning across a scale (for example, age, height, and weight). When the variable can only have values that are integers, the data are known as discrete. Data that can be recorded to n decimal places are called continuous data. Quantitative data can be condensed to ordinal categoric data; for example, the age of patients participating in a hip fracture study could be broken into categories of 50 years to younger than 60 years, 60 to 70 years, and older than 70 years. In designing a study and planning the data collection methods, it is preferable, when possible, to obtain the data as a continuous variable because this can be changed to discrete or categoric data; however, the reverse is not possible.[15]

Choosing the Statistical Test

Before the statistical tests are performed, it is a good idea to conduct an exploratory data analysis. This simply involves obtaining such values as the mean, median, and range to ensure that all values entered into the database are appropriate values. This helps to detect data entry errors or gross outliers that need to be checked for accuracy. In addition, the bell curve should be plotted to examine the assumption of normality.

In deciding which statistical test to use, the researcher must first define what type of variables he or she wants to analyze. **Table 1** summarizes the tests that are appropriate for specified data types. In basic terms, for comparisons of groups, the test to use is dictated by the type of data and whether the data are normally distributed. For determining associations or creating models, the type of data determines which test to use. Although this information allows for data analysis with the use of the appropriate test, it is very important that the assumptions for each test are examined to ensure that the results and conclusions are valid. For this reason, although current com-

puter programs allow any researcher to obtain a P value for his or her data and present the results to his or her peers, it is always best to consult a statistician to ensure that the correct test is being used and that all assumptions are being met. However, this does not detract from the importance of the clinical researcher having a basic understanding of statistical principles.

As an example, if a researcher wanted to compare hospital lengths of stay (continuous data) for patients having a Gustilo type IIIB open tibial shaft fracture treated with either the principles of early total care or the principles of damage control orthopaedics, a Student t-test would be appropriate when the length-of-stay data are normally distributed. If the data were skewed (as is common for length of stay), the assumption of normality underlying the Student t-test would not be met, and the nonparametric Mann-Whitney U test would be more appropriate. Note that when the Student t-test is used, the results should be summarized with the use of mean and

SD values, and when the Mann-Whitney U test is used, data should be summarized with the use of median and range values. Another alternative is to create a so-called dummy variable by breaking the continuous variable into categoric groups. In this example, one could arbitrarily split the continuous length-of-stay data into weeks (for example, less than 1 week, 7 days to 13 days, 14 days to 20 days, and more than 20 days) and analyze the data with the chi-square test. This should always be defined in the protocol before collecting the data, as so-called data dredging by performing multiple analyses searching for a significant result will find a false-positive significant result by chance in 1 of every 20 comparisons (when α equals 0.05).

The Fundamental Question: How Many Patients Are Needed?

Ideally, a researcher would enroll as many patients as his or her resources, time constraints, and ethics committee would permit. The reality is that a researcher may have only enough funding to hire a research assistant to collect data for 1 year. As such, a sample size calculation early in the process of designing a study is important for several reasons. First, it provides information about the feasibility of the study. If a researcher wanted to conduct a study to investigate the role of pelvic binders, angiographic embolization, pelvic packing, and early internal fixation on reducing mortality after pelvic fracture and the sample size calculation finds that 60 patients are needed to find a significant difference, the study is not feasible if the researcher generally treats 12 patients with pelvic fractures in 1 year. Second, a sample size calculation can provide information on whether the study has enough power to detect a clinically relevant difference. Third, sample size is impor-

tant from an ethical standpoint. An undersized study submits patients to the added burden and to the potentially harmful experimental treatment of a study with no great advance in the evidence base. Fourth, a sample size calculation helps as the researcher finalizes the study protocol and considers writing grant applications because it provides a guide to the resources needed.

Sample size calculation is more of an art than a science, as educated guesses are used to indicate how many patients are required to detect a researcher-defined clinically relevant difference. The particular method used to perform a sample size calculation differs, depending on the type of study being performed. Importantly, although many calculation tools are available in textbooks and on the Internet, they tend to use advanced statistical jargon that can be confusing, and some may require knowledge of how to read statistical tables of distributions that are appropriate in the appendices of statistical textbooks. As such, it is advisable for a researcher, especially one who is new to research methodology, to seek the expertise of a statistician. However, with the following key elements, there are some sample size calculators that may be used with confidence. (1) Type I error (α) is generally set at the 0.05 level. (2) Type II error (β) is generally set at the 0.20 level. (3) Power is generally set at 80%. (4) Effect size melds a thorough literature review, pilot study results, and clinical experience to determine a figure that defines how much of a difference can be expected to be observed between the study groups. For example, a researcher may find a previous study done in another country that observed differences between the groups of 15%; however, in the researcher's experience at his or her institution, the difference is more likely to be 25%. As

such, the researcher may select an effect size of 20% to use in the calculation, remembering that the lower the effect size, the higher the sample size needed to detect a clinical difference. (5) Variability is found by using a review of the literature or the results of a pilot study to help the researcher determine the expected SD within each group.

It is important to remember that the number produced by the sample size calculator is for the minimum number of participants required, given the values for effect size and/or variability that were entered. Extra participants are often added to account for those who drop out or withdraw.

Interpreting the Results: Statistical Versus Clinical Significance

Although the urge to scan a paper looking for significant P values ($P < 0.05$) as the basis for determining the importance of the results is tempting, it is often quite misleading. This approach is equivalent to thinking of the P value as a dichotomous variable rather than a continuous one[16] and fails to recognize the foundation of inferential statistics, whereby a significant finding will be found purely by chance in 1 of 20 analyses. Significant findings may not reflect clinically important outcomes.

The methods section could be considered the most important section of a paper because if the methodology is not sound, then the results of the research will not be valid.[17] One of the simplest things to look at is the number of patients enrolled. Small sample sizes result in underpowered studies that have little chance of finding a clinically relevant effect size. Therefore, studies with small samples that find a larger effect size than would be expected should be suspected of having biased methodology, which should be examined thoroughly.

Summary

The research methodology summarized in this chapter should be considered by orthopaedic surgeons as they read journal articles or listen to conference presentations. The basics of study design and statistics are provided to direct the clinical researcher to pay particular attention to the methodology of orthopaedic investigations. Such knowledge is invaluable for surgeons who want to be able to judge the value of new clinical evidence described in studies and for those who want to develop their own investigations.

References

1. Ward RC, Hruby RJ, Jerome JA, Jones JM, Kappler RE, eds: *Foundations for Osteopathic Medicine*, ed 2. Philadelphia, PA, Lippincott Williams & Wilkins, 2002.

2. Souba WW, Wilmore DW, eds: *Surgical Research*. San Diego, CA, Academic Press, 2001.

3. Gallin JI, Ognibene FP, eds: *Principles and Practice of Clinical Research*, ed 2. Burlington, VT, Elsevier, 2007.

4. Grimes DA, Schulz KF: An overview of clinical research: The lay of the land. *Lancet* 2002;359 (9300):57-61.

5. Bhandari M, Joensson A, eds: *Clinical Research for Surgeons*. New York, NY, Thieme, 2009.

6. Schulz KF, Grimes DA: Generation of allocation sequences in randomised trials: Chance, not choice. *Lancet* 2002;359(9305): 515-519.

7. Guyatt GH, Haynes RB, Jaeschke RZ, et al; Evidence-Based Medicine Working Group: Users' Guides to the Medical Literature: XXV. Evidence-based medicine: Principles for applying the Users' Guides to patient care. *JAMA* 2000;284(10):1290-1296.

8. Atkins D, Eccles M, Flottorp S, et al; GRADE Working Group: Systems for grading the quality of evidence and the strength of recommendations: I. Critical appraisal of existing approaches. *BMC Health Serv Res* 2004; 4(1): 38.

9. Schünemann HJ, Bone L: Evidence-based orthopaedics: A primer. *Clin Orthop Relat Res* 2003;413:117-132.

10. Bhandari M, Guyatt GH, Swiontkowski MF: User's guide to the orthopaedic literature: How to use an article about prognosis. *J Bone Joint Surg Am* 2001;83-A(10): 1555-1564.

11. Bhandari M, Guyatt GH, Swiontkowski MF: User's guide to the orthopaedic literature: How to use an article about a surgical therapy. *J Bone Joint Surg Am* 2001; 83-A(6):916-926.

12. Poolman RW, Petrisor BA, Marti RK, Kerkhoffs GM, Zlowodzki M, Bhandari M: Misconceptions about practicing evidence-based orthopedic surgery. *Acta Orthop* 2007;78(1):2-11.

13. Dowdy S, Weardon S, Chilko D: *Statistics for Research*, ed 3. Hoboken, NJ, John Wiley & Sons, 2004.

14. Bhandari M, Tornetta P III, Guyatt GH: Glossary of evidence-based orthopaedic terminology. *Clin Orthop Relat Res* 2003;413: 158-163.

15. Riffenburgh RH: *Statistics in Medicine*, ed 2. San Diego, CA, Elsevier Academic Press, 2006.

16. Rosnow RL, Rosenthal R: Statistical procedures and the justification of knowledge in psychological science. *Am Psychol* 1989;44: 1276-1284.

17. Urschel JD: How to analyze an article. *World J Surg* 2005;29(5): 557-560.

Maintenance of Certification and Keys to Passing the Recertification Examination

Gregory Katz, BS
Joseph A. Bosco III, MD

Abstract

The American Board of Orthopaedic Surgery requires that each board-certified orthopaedic surgeon recertify every 10 years. This formal procedure of demonstrating competence as a surgeon, which used to be known as recertification, has been replaced by a more comprehensive process termed maintenance of certification (MOC). Even an experienced orthopaedic surgeon may find achieving MOC a daunting prospect. Simply preparing for and taking the recertification examination is an enormous challenge, but it is important to remember that the examination is merely one aspect of maintaining certification. Prior to sitting for the examination, each physician is required to complete the other MOC requirements, including amassing continuing medical education credits, compiling a case list, and soliciting peer recommendations. Familiarity with the MOC process, understanding the details of the examination, and proper preparation techniques will help orthopaedic surgeons gain insights into how to approach MOC.

Instr Course Lect 2012;61:587-593.

The American Board of Orthopaedic Surgery (ABOS) requires that each board-certified orthopaedic surgeon successfully complete a recertification process every 10 years to maintain his or her certification. Achieving ABOS maintenance of certification (MOC) can be a daunting prospect, even for an experienced orthopaedic surgeon. Preparing for and taking the recertification examination is an enormous challenge; however, it is important to remember that the examination is only one aspect of the MOC process. Prior to sitting for the examination, each orthopaedic surgeon is required to complete the other MOC requirements. The goal of this chapter is to serve as a primer for each aspect of the MOC process, with a focus on preparing for and taking the recertification examination. This chapter reviews the MOC requirements, offers insights into how each orthopaedic surgeon should approach recertification, addresses specific concerns regarding the details of the examination, and reviews proper preparation techniques.

Background

The former procedure of demonstrating competence as a surgeon, which

used to be known as recertification, has been replaced by the slightly more demanding process of MOC. The American Board of Medical Specialties (ABMS), of which the ABOS is a member, requires that each specialty board systematically assess the competency of its members as a required part of the MOC process. The ABMS dictates that every physician should be proficient in certain general competencies, including medical knowledge, patient care, interpersonal and communication skills, professionalism, practice-based learning and improvement, and systems-based practice. Changes have been made to the ABOS recertification process to properly comply with ABMS requirements.[1]

Required Competencies

MOC requires more than just sitting for an examination. Whereas the former process of recertification consisted of demonstrating professional standing, acquiring 120 category 1 continuing medical education (CME) credits, and passing a secure examination that quantitatively assessed the orthopaedic surgeon's cognitive knowledge, MOC is slightly more complex. The MOC requirements of the ABOS address the competencies required by the ABMS using four components as specified on the ABOS website:[1] (1) evidence of professional standing, which requires that the diplomate maintain a full and

Neither Mr. Katz nor any immediate family member has received anything of value from or owns stock in a commercial company or institution related directly or indirectly to the subject of this chapter. Dr. Bosco or an immediate family member serves as a board member, owner, officer, or committee member of the American Orthopaedic Society for Sports Medicine and the New York State Society of Orthopaedic Surgeons.

unrestricted license to practice medicine in the United States or Canada; (2) evidence of lifelong learning and self-assessment, which is addressed through requirements for ongoing 3-year cycles of 120 credits of category 1 orthopaedic or relevant CME credits, including a minimum of 20 CME credits from self-assessment examinations; (3) evidence of cognitive expertise, which is demonstrated through a secure examination, as is currently in place for recertification; and (4) evidence of performance in practice, which includes a stringent peer review process and a few performance indicators, namely, compliance with patient safety and best-care initiatives such as the sign your site program, preoperative antibiotics, informed consent, and postoperative anticoagulation.

Each component addresses specific protocols necessary to achieve adequate clinical competence, proof of commitment to learning and self-improvement, and the demonstration of cognitive knowledge. Providing evidence of professional standing requires the orthopaedic surgeon to hold a full and unrestricted license to practice in all locations in which he or she holds a license. Evidence of lifelong learning and self-assessment is proven via documentation of 120 category 1 CME credits. These CME credits are earned via programs certified by the Accreditation Council for Continuing Medical Education (ACCME), which accredits medical organizations and societies to provide continuing education for physicians after their residency training has been completed.

CME Credits

Earning category 1 CME credits requires that the orthopaedic surgeon take an active role in the learning process. The ACCME has specific requirements for acceptable content that can be

certified for credit. The ACCME defines CME as "educational activities which serve to maintain, develop, or increase the knowledge, skills, and professional performance and relationships that a physician uses to provide services for patients, the public, or the profession. The content of CME is that body of knowledge and skills generally recognized and accepted by the profession as within the basic medical sciences, the discipline of clinical medicine, and the provision of health care to the public."[2]

Although the range of learning activities permitted for CME is rather broad, all organizations providing continuing education are required to validate the content of their CME activities. All recommendations involving clinical medicine must be based on evidence accepted by the medical community, and appropriate justification is needed regarding the indications and contraindications for all treatments and procedures. Similarly, the research cited as evidence or justification for the practices advocated from CME activities must conform to the generally accepted standards of scientific method with regard to experimental design, data collection, and analysis. The CME content providers are responsible for validating the content of their activities according to the standards set forth by the ACCME.[3]

Obtaining appropriate verification of CME credits is the responsibility of the surgeon applying for recertification. Written proof of the number of hours/credits earned can be requested from the CME provider, but it is the surgeon's responsibility to provide documentation directly to the ABOS when applying for MOC. This process can be undertaken at the ABOS website, where CME credits can be logged; each entry must be accompanied by a copy of the certificate received from the CME provider or sponsor.[4] There

is a $50.00 fee for submitting CME credits on the ABOS website. Most orthopaedic surgeons take between one and five CME courses during the recertification period.

A minimum of 20 CME credits from self-assessment examinations must be part of the 120 credits taken during the 3-year cycle preceding MOC. The self-assessment examinations must be a minimum of 10 credits each. There is no upper limit to the number of credits that can be achieved via these examinations. The credits are obtained only after both the completion and scoring of appropriate self-assessment examinations. Although the examinations have no passing or failing grade, they are anonymously scored and returned to the surgeon. Currently, four organizations (the American Academy of Orthopaedic Surgeons [AAOS], the American Society for Surgery of the Hand, the American Orthopaedic Society for Sports Medicine, and the *Journal of Bone and Joint Surgery*) offer ABOS-approved self-assessment examinations that count toward CME credits. Self-assessment examinations are required because the goal of the MOC process is ongoing professional improvement. The purpose of the self-assessment program is to direct self-study. It is assumed that these examinations will lead diplomates to areas of study that will guide their continued professional improvement. As with all other CME credits, it is the responsibility of the surgeon to report the completion of self-assessment credits to the ABOS.

The Recertification Examination

Once CME credits have been properly obtained and reported, the next major obligation is to provide evidence of cognitive expertise, a process better known as the recertification examination. Because of the physician's daily responsibilities of an orthopaedic practice, preparing for a standardized examination may be overwhelming and foreign. Learning about the test and preparing for it in advance will lessen anxiety. Attaining knowledge about the examination will maximize the likelihood of passing while minimizing the disruption to the surgeon's life and practice during the preparation process.

As part of the 10-year MOC cycle, the examination can be taken no sooner than 3 years before the certificate expires but after the required 120 CME credits (including at least 20 self-assessment examination credits) have been achieved and reported. Specific deadlines for registration and testing are listed on the ABOS website. The stated goal of the recertification examination is to demonstrate that the diplomate "commands a satisfactory fund of knowledge to practice orthopaedic surgery."[5] The examination takes place in a secure location without the aid of any outside sources.

When enrolling for the examination, the surgeon has two test options: an oral examination or a written examination. Each has a different focus and requires a unique manner of preparation.

Oral Examination

The oral examination is practice based and clinical in nature.[6] It is designed for orthopaedic surgeons who practice in a subspecialty without relevant tests: tumor, foot and ankle, and pediatrics. The applicant must submit a list of all surgical cases during a 6-month period in the 2-year period immediately preceding the test application. The list is submitted to the ABOS, and that organization will choose 12 cases from which the applicant can select 10 to present at the examination. The surgeon must bring all pertinent information regarding the chosen cases. The

oral examination takes approximately 2 hours, is divided into three 35-minute periods, and has two examiners during each session (a total of six examiners). During the testing period, the examiners will ask questions based on the cases presented and the candidate's case list. Each orthopaedic surgeon is evaluated in several domains—data gathering, diagnosis and interpretive skills, treatment planning, technical skills, outcomes, and applied knowledge.[6] Each examiner grades the orthopaedic surgeon on a scale of 0 to 3. The orthopaedic surgeon must achieve an average grade of 2 or greater to pass the examination. Generally, 85% to 95% of orthopaedic surgeons pass the oral examination.[7] The oral examination can be selected as a pathway for MOC only if the diplomate is currently engaged in a practice that includes the surgical care of patients. The oral examination fulfills both the evidence of cognitive expertise and the evidence of performance in practice sections of the MOC process.

Written Examination

The written examination has two categories: (1) general and practice profiled or (2) subspecialty based. The general test consists of 200 questions covering clinical material that "all orthopaedists should know, regardless of their area of expertise."[8] Because 40% of the subspecialty-based test is focused on core orthopaedic knowledge, each orthopaedic surgeon, regardless of his or her specialty, should devote time to all disciplines when preparing for the examination.

The core questions regarding orthopaedic knowledge are taken from a variety of disciplines within the field: general orthopaedics, upper extremity, lower extremity, spine, tumor, and tumor-like conditions. **Table 1** shows the percentage of examination question focusing on each discipline.[9] The

ranges will vary from examination to examination, but the general breakdown remains the same. It is recommended that preparation time be allocated to appropriately reflect the relative importance that the examiners give to each discipline.

The practice-profiled written examination is focused on one of three subspecialty areas: adult reconstruction, sports medicine, or spine surgery. Surgeons who hold a certificate of added qualifications in hand surgery may opt to take a combined hand examination. For each of the three subspecialty tests, there are 80 core questions on general orthopaedics, which make up 40% of the total examination content. The core questions are selected to test the knowledge that a competent orthopaedic surgeon should possess; these questions are the same across all subspecialty examinations. There are 200 questions in total, meaning that 60% of the examination (120 questions) will be based on a subspecialty and will test more focused subspecialty knowledge with increased depth. The combined hand examination contains the same 80 core orthopaedic questions as the other practice-profiled examinations, but the hand section of the test is composed of 160 certificate-of-added-qualification questions on the hand.

To achieve a sense of how to prepare for the examination, it may be helpful to have information regarding the amount of time peers allocate to preparation and the types of resources used. More than 50% of those who prepare for the recertification examination devote at least 60 hours to studying, and approximately two thirds of orthopaedic surgeons use *Orthopaedic Knowledge Update* (OKU), published by the AAOS, as their preferred method of study. The goal of *Orthopaedic Knowledge Update* is to review and condense "the most relevant findings from every

Table 1

Percentage of Written Examination Questions From Each Discipline

Discipline	Examination Questions (%)
General	15-30
Legal or ethical	1-3
Basic science	2-4
Multiple trauma (nonorthopaedic)	10-15
Postoperative complications	1-3
Rheumatology	0-1
Miscellaneous	2-4
Upper extremity	15-30
Fractures of the shoulder girdle	0-2
Shoulder instabilities, arthritis, osteonecrosis	5-7
Elbow: fractures and arthritis	3-5
Radius and ulna: fractures and infection	4-6
Wrist: injury and nerve compression	1-3
Hand: fractures and tendon injuries	5
Lower extremity	35-54
Pelvis and acetabular fractures	3-5
Hip: dislocations/fractures, arthritis, pediatric	8-10
Femur fractures	4
Knee: dislocations/fractures, osteonecrosis, cartilage disorders, patellofemoral problems	10-15
Tibia/fibula injuries	3-5
Ankle	3-5
Foot: arthritis, nerve compression, inflammatory conditions, congenital and developmental disorders	4-6
Spine: fractures, arthritis, stenosis, disk disease	2
Tumor and tumor-like conditions	3-5

major orthopaedic and subspecialty journal" and function as an important resource for both MOC as well as first-time certification.[10] The AAOS also produces self-assessment examinations, some of which are based on material presented in *Orthopaedic Knowledge Update*, which serve the dual purpose of obtaining crucial CME credits and providing an important measuring tool for assessing progress in preparing for the recertification examination. Self-assessment examinations from other approved organizations also can be valuable in obtaining CME credits and preparing for the examination. The AAOS also has addi-tional self-scored examinations; these examinations can be a valuable resource for examination preparation, even if they do not count toward the required CME credits. Adequate preparation is imperative for success, and the self-assessment tests can help to both point out and fill in gaps in clinical knowledge.

Testing Center Procedures

It is helpful to know what to expect on the day of the test. The examination is administered at Prometric testing centers, which are located nationwide. More than 95% of all test takers live within 50 miles of a testing site.

Scheduling a test can be done on the Prometric website, which also provides a listing of all testing centers and links to cancel or reschedule an examination.[11] The term written examination is somewhat of a misnomer because the recertification examination is taken on a computer. There is no test booklet, and paper for taking notes is provided (and must be left) at the testing center. The Prometric testing sites are standardized. The goal is to create an identical testing environment for everyone sitting for the examination regardless of their location in the country. Prometric testing centers have regulations that must be followed by all test takers. For those who have never taken a standardized examination at such a center, the highly structured nature of the experience may be stress provoking.

The orthopaedic surgeon should plan on arriving at the testing center at least 30 minutes before the examination is scheduled to begin. A government-issued photo identification is needed. The test rooms are equipped with standardized computers with the appropriate examination. Although no talking is permitted in the testing rooms, noise-reducing headphones are available to provide an even quieter testing experience.

Each testing center is carefully monitored.[12] The test takers are observed during the examination via video as well as by physical on-site walk-through monitoring by proctors. Communication with outside sources is prohibited during the examination, even during breaks. Test takers are not permitted to speak with other examination candidates in the testing room. Written notes, published materials, or any other testing aids are expressly prohibited. No unauthorized items may be brought into the testing room, including outerwear, hats, food, drinks, briefcases, notebooks, watches, cell phones, recording devices, or photographic equipment. Test takers are given a locker to store any prohibited materials during the examination period. A proctor will ask each test taker to empty and turn out his or her pockets prior to entering the testing room. The test taker will also be required to sign in and out of the testing room on each entrance or exit from the room.[12]

Scoring and Results

The written examination has an average pass rate of 95% to 98%, a rate that is relatively similar from year to year. The range of raw scores on the examination generally ranges from approximately 50% to more than 90% correct. The mean score is usually between 75% and 78%, with an average passing score of 63%.[13]

The process of determining the passing score for the examination is actually quite rigorous. It is not simply a matter of tabulating a raw score. Each question is meticulously reviewed by a team of 10 to 15 physician volunteers to ensure that the question is of high quality and that the correct answer is, in fact, correct. During this review process, an average of 5% to 10% of questions is determined to be poor. These questions are discarded and replaced during subsequent examinations. After each question has been reviewed, the reviewing physicians confer to determine a common passing score.

The goal of any examination question is to separate those who know the information being tested from those who do not. This objective then becomes the prism through which all questions must be reviewed during the assessment process. A question is discarded if it is determined that the question did not adequately fulfill its objective—to separate those with the requisite knowledge from those without it. A bad examination question is not necessarily a question that most test takers answer incorrectly. Indeed, it may simply be a piece of information or an application of knowledge that only a small percentage of the testing population knew or was able to accurately deduce. To distinguish bad questions from those that are merely difficult, the board looks at the population of test takers who correctly answered the questions that had the lowest aggregate percentage of correct answers among all test takers. If those who scored highest on the examination performed better on those questions than those who scored lowest, it is assumed that the question, although challenging, was capable of differentiating high scorers from low scorers. Such a question will be retained. If there is no distinction between high scorers and low scorers for a particular question, it is more likely that the question did not adequately differentiate knowledge; therefore, the question will be discarded. The purpose of the review process is to discard poor questions and determine a passing score.

Testing Strategies

For those who are accustomed to working without time constraints and those who have not taken a standardized test in years, time management is an issue of vital importance. The examination lasts 4 hours with no breaks. There is also a 30-minute tutorial on the testing interface. The tutorial is completed prior to beginning the examination. With the exception of the hand examination, each examination is composed of 200 questions broken down by topic in the manner previously discussed. The 200 questions are divided into two 100-question sections. The surgeon is allotted 2 hours for each question block, which averages to 72 seconds per question. The test taker cannot go back to the previous block of questions once it has been completed. Because no points are deducted for incorrect answers, it is advantageous to answer every question.

The examination has many different types of questions. The question types are best broken down by Bloom question taxonomy, a classification of knowledge acquisition first developed in 1956 by Benjamin Bloom, the famous educational psychologist. Bloom dictated that there are six levels of testing within the cognitive domain (knowledge, comprehension, application, analysis, synthesis, and evaluation), and all test questions fall into one of those six levels. These levels are sometimes more broadly broken down into three levels of question taxonomy. Taxonomy level 1 is knowledge, level 2 is comprehension, and level 3 is application.[14] Knowledge questions test memory of previously learned facts. Comprehension questions test understanding of facts and ideas. Application questions require the use of acquired knowledge to solve a novel problem.[15] Understanding the skill each question is testing can be incredibly helpful both with regard to time management and choosing the correct answer.

For the purpose of time management, it is often unnecessary to classify questions based on Bloom taxonomy. Instead, every question on the examination can be broken down into one of three categories. Category 1 is a question for which the test taker is immediately certain of the answer. For those questions, it is unnecessary for the test taker to look at the answer choices to know his or her selection. Category 2 questions are those that can be narrowed down to two or three possibilities. The last category is composed of questions that the test taker has no idea how to answer. No amount of time will help with those questions.

The goal of a time management strategy is to spend the most time on category 2 questions. Category 1 questions should be answered immediately. There will be no need to revisit those questions during the remainder of the testing period. Category 3 questions should also be answered promptly. Most of these are taxonomy level 1 questions, meaning that answering such questions is dependent on accurately recalling a specific piece of information. These questions often must be answered by random guessing, so it is advantageous to make timely choices and save the bulk of time for questions that can be thought through. Although it can be tempting to spend time obsessing over a difficult-to-recall fact in hopes of having the answer miraculously appear, this practice is an inefficient use of time. It must be remembered that the examination can be passed by correctly answering approximately 63% of the questions, and poor-performing questions are discarded. This knowledge can be used to the test taker's advantage by allocating the most time to score maximization.

Category 2 questions should be approached systematically. Depending on the taxonomic level of the question, the approach will be different. In general, it is best to narrow down answer choices, immediately discarding the answers that are obviously incorrect, and then making an educated guess from the remaining choices. The following is an example of a taxonomy 1, category 2 question and an explanation of the best manner in which to approach the question: The effect of anabolic steroids on lipid and triglyceride profiles is to (1) decrease high-density lipoprotein, (2) increase high-density lipoprotein, (3) increase low-density lipoprotein, (4) decrease low-density lipoprotein, (5) decrease triglycerides.

In reading the question, the test taker may not immediately recall the correct answer but may have enough information to eliminate some of the distracting choices. Keeping in mind that steroids are harmful for long-term health, answers 2, 4, and 5 can be almost immediately discarded as beneficial outcomes. The test taker is now left to choose between answers 1 and 3, increasing the odds of selecting a correct response from 20% to 50%. Taxonomy level 1 questions will often provide clues to increase the odds of selecting the correct answer.

Taxonomy level 3 questions should be approached using the question stem as an important source of information from which to eliminate incorrect choices. The following question offers an example: A healthy 18-year-old man is brought to the trauma unit with an isolated grade 3 open femur fracture. His Glasgow Coma Scale score is 15, and he is moving all of his extremities. His abdominal examination is benign, and his extremities are well perfused. His blood pressure is 80/40, and his pulse is 135. His electrocardiogram is remarkable only for tachycardia. The most likely etiology for his hypotension is (1) cardiogenic shock, (2) neurogenic shock, (3) abdominal bleeding, (4) blood loss from open fracture, or (5) subdural hematoma.

To approach this question, relevant information should be used from the question stem to eliminate obviously wrong answers. The patient's age and the absence of significant pathology on the electrocardiogram indicate cardiogenic shock is an unlikely source of hypotension. Movement in all extremities and the presence of tachycardia indicates that neurogenic shock is also an unlikely answer. A benign abdominal examination eliminates abdominal bleeding as the correct answer. The patient's Glasgow Coma Scale score of 15 makes a subdural hematoma unlikely. The process of elimination and information in the question stem about the presence of an open femur fracture leaves blood loss as the correct answer choice. Even in a straightforward example, the process of using the question stem to guide the correct answer choice should be apparent.

Performance in Practice

After evidence of cognitive expertise has been demonstrated by passing the recertification examination, the final step in the MOC process is the evaluation of performance in practice. The goal of this aspect of the process is to provide the orthopaedic surgeon with a means of assessing the extent to which his or her practices correspond to currently accepted best practices based on available evidence. This evaluation primarily focuses on quality improvement. The list of surgical cases provides the individual orthopaedic surgeon with an opportunity to evaluate his or her own practices and set up a baseline for improvement during the next MOC cycle. As additional best-practice metrics are developed, there will be further opportunity for each orthopaedic surgeon to demonstrate that he or she is practicing competent and safe orthopaedic surgery according to the highest possible standards. Currently, the MOC process is not yet in its final state, with full implementation scheduled for 2016.

Summary

The MOC process is time consuming and complex. Obtaining the requisite CME credits, completing self-assessment examinations, and preparing for and passing the recertification examination are all difficult requirements of MOC. As is the case with mastering most challenges, the first step toward success is proper preparation. The MOC process can be better mastered with requisite knowledge of each step. First, the surgeon must complete the 120 required CME credits, keeping in mind that at least 20 must be earned from provider-scored self-assessment examinations. The surgeon then chooses the preferred type of examination, assesses his or her current readiness, and uses texts such as *Orthopaedic Knowledge Update* and other educational resources to fill in knowledge gaps. Last, testing strategies should be used to maximize the test taker's time so that as many questions as possible can be correctly answered. The orthopaedic surgeon should prepare for the recertification examination with a singular, focused goal.

References

1. Maintenance of Certification (MOC) timeline; Diplomates section. American Board of Orthopaedic Surgeons Website. https://www.abos.org/ModDefault.aspx?module=Diplomates&section=MOCTimeline. Accessed October 30, 2010.

2. CME content. Accreditation Council for Continuing Medical Education Website. http://www.accme.org/index.cfm/fa/Policy.policy/Policy_id/16f1c694-d03b-4241-bd1a-44b2d072dc5e.cfm. Accessed October 30, 2010.

3. Validation of clinical content for CME: The ACCME expectations of providers and of the accreditation process. Accreditation Council for Continuing Medical Education Website. http://www.accme.org/dir_docs/doc_upload/55b39478-d56a-440f-97a3-9272bd906785_uploaddocument.pdf. Accessed October 23, 2010.

4. Instructions for the MOC continuing medical education summary sheet. Diplomates section. American Board of Orthopaedic Surgery Website. https://www.abos.org/ModDefault.aspx?module=Diplomates&section=MOCCMEInstruct. Accessed October 23, 2010.

5. The ABOS responds to questions with answers about MOC. Diplomates section. American Board of Orthopaedic Surgery Website. https://www.abos.org/ModDefault.aspx?module=Diplomates&section=MOCAbout#17. Accessed February 4, 2011.

6. Practice-based oral examination. Diplomates section. American Board of Orthopaedic Surgery Website. https://www.abos.org/ModDefault.aspx?module=Diplomates&section=RecertExamOpOral. Accessed November 3, 2010.

7. Exam statistics. Diplomates section. American Board of Orthopaedic Surgery Website. https://www.abos.org/ModDefault.aspx?module=Diplomates&section=RecertExamStat. Accessed November 1, 2010.

8. Computer administered clinical examination. Diplomates section. American Board of Orthopaedic Surgery Website. https://www.abos.org/ModDefault.aspx?module=Diplomates&section=RecertExamOpCom. Accessed October 27, 2010.

9. Content of "core orthopaedic knowledge" for all ABOS computer recertification examination pathways. American Board of Orthopaedic Surgery Website. https://www.abos.org/documents/Core_Recert_Questions_Content.pdf. Accessed November 5, 2010.

10. Orthopaedic Knowledge Update 10. American Academy of Orthopaedic Surgeons Website. http://www3.aaos.org/product/productpage.cfm?code=05224. Accessed February 4, 2011.

11. Prometric Website. https://www.prometric.com. Accessed February 3, 2011.

12. Prometric testing center regulations. Prometric Website. https://www.prometric.com/TestTakers/FAQs/Regulations.htm. Accessed November 7, 2010.

13. Diplomate newsletter, January 2009. American Board of Orthopaedic Surgery Website. Newsletter archives. https://www.abos.org/documents/Diplomate-2009-Final.pdf. Accessed April 4, 2011.

14. Bloom's taxonomy of educational objectives. Harvard University Website. http://www.laspau.harvard.edu/idia/Taller_Lideres_Seneca/Lecturas_Previas_Silabo/BloomsTaxonomy.pdf. Accessed November 7, 2010.

15. Learning goals and objectives. University of North Carolina-Charlotte Website. http://teaching.uncc.edu/files/file/GoalsAndObjectives/Bloom.pdf. Accessed November 7, 2010.

Real-World Solutions for Orthopaedic On-Call Problems

Samuel G. Agnew, MD, FACS
Robert H. Blotter, MD
Paul K. Kosmatka, MD
Guy J. Rudin, MD

Abstract

An increasing percentage of emergency departments are reporting an inadequate number of on-call specialists. This situation is causing a growing crisis in emergency department on-call coverage for patients requiring orthopaedic care. Many orthopaedic surgeons are electing to opt out of emergency department on-call service. For many reasons, including a dwindling supply of eager participants, more medical groups are finding it difficult to fulfill their on-call obligations. This problem demands a variety of strategies to address the multiple causative factors that occur in practice settings. Initially, it may be necessary to incentivize on-call service so more surgeons are willing to participate. Incentives may include improving the group governance and bylaws to avoid confusion on the rules for providing on-call coverage. The on-call experience may require financial improvements, outsourcing with locum tenens, or a complete restructuring of the on-call arrangement with the formation of a hospitalist program.

Instr Course Lect 2012;61:595-605.

Seventy-five percent of emergency department medical directors report an inadequate number of on-call specialists. This problem has been reported throughout the United States. Forty-two percent of emergency department administrators indicated that the lack of specialty care was putting their patients at significant risk, and the trend is worsening. The on-call coverage problem was first reported nationally (for orthopaedics specifically) in 2002 and has remained a growing problem for the past decade. (SG Agnew, MD, unpublished data presented at the Orthopaedic Trauma Association annual meeting, Toronto, Canada, 2002.) The shortage of orthopaedic surgeons who are willing to provide on-call service is often at the top of the list in terms of problematic areas of on-call staffing.[1-7]

This growing crisis in emergency department on-call coverage has elicited responses from several orthopaedic associations. The American Academy of Orthopaedic Surgeons stated that "orthopaedists are uniquely qualified to provide emergency care for patients with musculoskeletal conditions, including musculoskeletal trauma," and that... "orthopaedic surgeons have a responsibility to work with their communities, with each other and their hospitals to make sure that...emergency patients with musculoskeletal problems receive timely and appropriate care."[8] A position statement by the Orthopaedic Trauma Association states that "orthopaedic surgeons have been trained in basic musculoskeletal care and should maintain the skills needed to provide basic musculoskeletal trauma care services." It also states that "all orthopedic surgeons should make themselves available to their hospital's on-call list during the active years of their practice at their institution." Specialty societies are called on to "work towards mechanisms to assure the sufficient participation of their membership

Dr. Agnew or an immediate family member serves as a paid consultant to Zimmer Delphi HealthCare Partners and serves as an unpaid consultant to Accelero Health Care Partners, Orthopaedic Service Line management, and Select International Executive Search Firm. Dr. Blotter or an immediate family member has stock or stock options held in Pioneer Surgical Alpha Med-Surge. Neither Dr. Kosmatka nor any immediate family member has received anything of value from or owns stock in a commercial company or institution related directly or indirectly to the subject of this chapter. Dr. Rudin or an immediate family member has stock or stock options held in Zimmer and Pfizer.

on-call lists at their institutions, including evidence of such participation as a qualification for membership and certification."[9]

Despite these strong supporting statements, many orthopaedic surgeons are electing to opt out of emergency department on-call service. There are several reasons for the increasing reluctance to participate in on-call coverage. Going off call can often increase productivity and compensation because it results in a more stable elective practice. Regular participation in on-call service requires many physicians to work outside of their normal comfort level in areas outside their regular practices. More physicians are reporting that on-call service disrupts their regular schedule and family life. The number of uninsured patients treated in emergency departments is higher than in regular practices. Eighty-one percent of the patients treated in emergency departments were reported to have Medicaid or self-pay insurance.[10]

Adding to this growing problem is the claim that the graduating population of orthopaedic surgeons is less eager than in the past to assume the heavy workload associated with on-call service, which is often shifted to younger partners in many practices. Many Generation X surgeons are more lifestyle oriented and have experienced a less strenuous residency work environment than older surgeons.[11,12]

Regardless of the reasons, more medical groups are finding it difficult to fulfill their on-call obligations with a dwindling supply of less eager participants. This problem demands a variety of strategies to address the multiple causative factors that occur in the array of practice settings. Initially, it may be necessary to incentivize on-call service so more surgeons are willing to participate. Incentives may include improving the group governance and bylaws

to avoid confusion regarding on-call duty or improving the financial arrangement to make on-call service more attractive. In some situations, it may be necessary to outsource on-call obligations or negotiate a complete restructuring of the on-call arrangement with a hospital.

Group Governance

For many medical groups, the first exposure to an on-call crisis is the day that one of the partners announces his or her intention to cease participation in on-call service. It is often discovered that no prior framework has been established for this inevitable event. Group governance is the establishment and monitoring of policies by a group or its governing body to help balance power in the group while enhancing its primary duties and ensuring prosperity. Properly implemented governance can prevent an impending crisis. The first task in designing an appropriate group governance policy is to answer the following five basic questions concerning on-call service: (1) What is on-call service? (2) Who provides on-call service? (3) What is on-call service worth? (4) Who can go off call and under what circumstances? (5) What is the plan for emergency contingencies? Although these questions are common to all medical practices, every group will have a different answer. In fact, each member within the group may have a different answer. Achieving agreement between all members will require open discussion, compromise, and a commitment to avoid future problems.

What Is On-Call Service?

A clear definition of the responsibilities of on-call service and the duration of the on-call period must be defined and agreed on by all participants. There should be agreement on the timeframe for on-call service, with spe-

cific start and stop times and a description of duties. This agreement should include rules regarding cross coverage of patients in the hospital, on the telephone, and for follow-up visits. Does everyone cover his or her own patients during the normal business day but not nights and weekends, or does a physician always cover his or her own patients? The scope of the needed orthopaedic services should be considered in determining if there is a need for separate hand, pediatric, or trauma on-call participants. Similarly, it should be determined if there is need for a back-up on-call surgeon and if the decisions need to be formalized in a written on-call coverage schedule. For example, it should be decided who will provide subsequent care for a patient with a hip fracture who was admitted through the emergency department the previous night. Will that patient receive continuing care from the surgeon on call at the time of admission or the person on call the next day? If the rules are not clearly established, it may result in "cherry picking" or choosing to care for more desirable surgical patients. The practice geography and logistics may make it necessary to designate one person as the office on-call physician who handles urgent walk-in patients, with a separate physician covering newly admitted hospital patients. If so, who is responsible for the office walk-in patient who needs urgent surgery? It is important to establish specific guidelines to prevent arguments over minor details.

Who Provides On-Call Coverage?

Depending on the on-call volume and intensity, each group will have a critical level of participation before on-call service becomes unbearable. Another variable in this determination is the background of the involved physicians. What is the skill level required to participate in on-call service? If there is a real or perceived inadequacy in skills, will an avenue of continuing medical education be made available to the physician who needs more training? It is important to distinguish between competence and interest level because every board certified/board eligible orthopaedic surgeon is qualified to perform on-call service. It is also important to determine the available options if the pool of on-call participants drops below the previously defined critical threshold. Will this situation require the reactivation of physicians who have been allowed to drop on-call service?

What Is On-Call Service Worth?

Unless everyone in a group is equally participating in on-call service, some monetary value should be assigned to the performance of on-call coverage. The value of on-call service can be difficult to calculate. A good start is calculating the cost of hiring a locum tenens to provide this service. Opportunity costs have to be calculated into the overall cost. Budgeting gaps in a clinic and operating schedule mean a loss of revenue from a surgeon's elective practice, even if some revenue is obtained by performing on-call service. The amount received from the hospital for providing on-call coverage is rarely sufficient to cover the lost practice revenue. Once a value has been determined for on-call service, it must be periodically reevaluated. The final value determined for on-call service will probably never be completely acceptable to everyone; however, if on-call service has no value, participants will be difficult to find.

Who Can Go Off Call?

Nothing can cause more generational conflict in a group than a determination concerning which surgeon can go off call and when he or she can go off

---

Table 1

Sample On-Call Agreement Document

1. On-call coverage consists of providing continuous orthopaedic coverage at ___ hospital.
2. On-call service shall be no more frequent than a critical threshold of one in ___. We agree to provide coverage for the following: emergency department, including unassigned patients, hospital consultations, patient phone calls, hospital rounding. The call day begins at ___ A.M., and ends at ___ A.M.
3. All members of the call pool will maintain sufficient skills to provide on-call coverage. On-call service shall be reimbursed at the following rates: $___ per daytime shift; $___ per nighttime shift; $___ per weekend shift.
4. Call panel members are eligible to go off call after age ___ or after ___ years of service. Members off call shall contribute $___ to the call pool on an annual basis and provide weekend rounding support ___ times per month/year.
5. Once going off call, retirement must occur within ___ years.
6. Emergency on-call coverage shall be provided by all on-call panel members based on a fixed rotation and maintained by the group president/department chief.
7. The group will consider hiring locum tenens coverage for an on-call panel below the critical threshold lasting longer than ___ months.
8. The group will/will not allow individuals to hire locum tenens to satisfy on-call coverage obligations.

---

call. The idea of attained organizational privilege is not recognized by many physicians in the millennial generation or Generation X. However, many older orthopaedic surgeons view ceasing on-call service as an earned privilege and have seen prior partners exercise this benefit. Regardless of a group's current age distribution, the gradual cessation or sunsetting of on-call obligations is a situation best outlined long before a partner exercises the privilege. A sunset on-call plan should consider age of onset, years of service, and the required pool of participants needed to maintain on-call coverage. It is a good idea to have a flexible clause that requires reactivation to the on-call panel if a critically low level of on-call manpower is reached. The length of time a partner can continue a reduced or no-call status should also be determined. Recruiting new partners to a practice is not an easy task if a group has a pool of partners exempt from on-call obligations and no willingess to change that arrangement.

Emergency Contingencies

A good on-call plan should recognize the need to prepare for possible shocks

to the on-call structure or pool. These unexpected variables include illness, injury, or death of a partner. Less dire but also common unplanned events may include a family crisis or sudden resignation. These changes can all be a shock to an already stressed on-call panel, but without any foresight and planning, a crisis can be accelerated. In the short term, enlistment of those in the off-call roster may be considered.

The failure to anticipate and answer questions regarding on-call service is the root of many disagreements. Because it is difficult to set rules in the middle of a crisis, it is advisable to discuss and agree on rules in advance. An example of a group on-call agreement is shown in **Table 1**.

Negotiating On-Call Reimbursement

Medicine has avoided differentiating between work performed during traditional working hours and emergency services rendered during off hours and weekends. For example, many professionals, such as plumbers, charge a different rate for weekend or night work compared with service provided during regular working hours. As traditional sources of income decrease, an increasing number of orthopaedic surgeons are turning to on-call pay as a source of income. In California, the percentage of orthopaedic surgeons reporting compensation for on-call coverage rose from 26% in 2000 to more than 70% in 2010.[13] This growing trend is not limited to California. Most orthopaedic surgeons can expect on-call compensation ranging from $750 to $1,000 per day, but the pay can be much higher.[13] The desire of orthopaedic surgeons to be compensated for their on-call activities is supported by their national organizations; however, this desire is not always met with enthusiasm by hospitals and patients who previously received these services without an extra charge.[6,8,9] Negotiation is generally required to arrive at an arrangement acceptable to the parties involved. Prior consideration of several factors can facilitate this process from the standpoint of the orthopaedic surgeon.

Identify a Need for Service
Ideally, a hospital organization will request an improvement or an enhancement of on-call coverage in their facility, providing an opportunity to request compensation in return. In situations in which no overture has been made for a change in service, orthopaedic surgeons can suggest that services could be improved by, for example, expanding the scope of the service, improving response times, or facilitating transfers when service cannot be provided.

Identify Potential Participants
Participants should be qualified to provide the proposed service. All qualified orthopaedic surgeons on staff, even competitors, should be offered the opportunity to participate in the improved on-call program; this approach will avoid the implication of an unfair business relationship with the hospital.

Participation should be voluntary because volunteers will contribute more enthusiastically than conscripts. A "critical mass" is required, usually at least three providers. Few orthopaedic surgeons will choose to participate more than 120 days per year. It is important to consider an acceptable fee for the requested services because the number of volunteers may depend on the level of compensation.

Identify the Scope of Service
The type of on-call coverage must be discussed with the appropriate hospital administrators. It is important to determine if on-call coverage is limited to emergency department, inpatient, or clinic consultations or will cover all areas. Will on-call coverage be limited to traumatic conditions or include all conditions? Will any conditions be excluded? Who will decide if a condition requires on-call service? What is the role of the orthopaedic surgeon when care cannot be provided at the facility? All these questions should be identified early in the negotiation process. A well-defined scope of service will minimize future misunderstandings and arbitrary decisions.

Identify Compensation
Compensation is more complex than determining a mere dollar amount. Most orthopaedic surgeons would not strive to earn $100 for an additional 10 hours of work unless nonmonetary rewards were part of the package. Factors other than money can increase compensation. A useful mathematical representation of compensation can increase factors in the numerator to increase compensation. For example, the numerator may include factors such as goodwill, which provides benefits from patients, the hospital organization, and other health care providers; satisfaction, which provides fulfillment for the surgeon who is helping patients and

doing a good job; and remuneration, the fair compensation for services. Decreasing factors in the denominator can also increase compensation. For example, the denominator can be decreased by lowering the frustration caused by inefficiency, marginal assistance, and untimely hours; lowering opportunity costs, which result in missed family events, recreational activities, and other employment; and decreasing the time spent in performing on-call service, which can be achieved with priority operating room access or the assistance of advanced practice nurses and physician assistants.

It is important to identify the process by which compensation is paid. Will the on-call surgeon be an employee receiving a wage or salary without the need to bill patients or insurance companies, or will he or she function as an independent contractor who receives a stipend and must bill for services rendered?

After outlining the terms of the proposed on-call program to the expected on-call panel participants, the potential participants can be polled by the chief negotiator to determine the threshold for participation and estimate the available participant pool as the component factors of compensation are negotiated.

Consider the Term of the Contract
The hospital organization may have difficulty providing all the resources promised to support the on-call program, particularly nonmonetary resources such as priority access to the operating room or ancillary help. An initial 6- or 12-month trial can prevent surgeons from being locked into an unfair arrangement. Cost-of-living increases should be considered when long-term contracts are negotiated.

Choose a Spokesperson

A member or representative agent with some discretionary power can negotiate more efficiently than a committee. The spokesperson can inform members or meet with the group regarding pivotal decisions without the frequent need to coordinate busy schedules for large meetings. The spokesperson should be experienced, charismatic, a thoughtful appraiser, innovative, and committed. Having one spokesperson will also avoid the commonly used tool of "divide and conquer." A public unified front is important in any negotiation; disagreements should remain private.

Negotiate

A good negotiating technique is to ask for more than you want but settle for a fair deal. It is wise to avoid the temptation to drive a hard bargain. The incremental gain achieved is not worth the loss of potential future gains that can result from the ill will generated by one transaction. When possible, the on-call spokesperson should negotiate with the administration's decision maker. This technique is more efficient and helps ensure that the group's position is not misrepresented. It is important to be prepared to walk away from an unfair deal; however, walk slowly enough so that a new deal can be tendered.

Renegotiate

It is important to monitor the deal or contract over the period of the arrangement and consider renegotiation at the end of the initial term. If conditions are unfavorable in the short term, the parties should be proactive and willing to approach each other with problems and solutions.

Effective negotiations are fundamental to achieving fair compensation for orthopaedic services. Unfortunately, the art of negotiating is not covered in most medical training and may seem counter to the compassion that

medicine encourages. If no one in the pool of on-call participants is willing and qualified to be an effective negotiator, the help of a professional negotiator should be considered.

Locum Tenens

The term locum tenens comes from Latin and means "one holding the place." Historically, locum tenentes were used primarily in Britain and referred to as substitute physicians. Initially, the use of a locum tenens was popular in primary care specialties but has now become increasingly used by other specialists.[14,15] Often, a physician serving as a locum tenens was believed to be a poor substitute for the physician he or she temporarily replaced, and the service had a poor reputation; however, this perception is changing.

Not all practices have a continuous supply of eager applicants to meet their practice and on-call demands. Some practices may experience an unplanned transition because of the illness, death, retirement, or sudden departure of partners. Unfortunately, these unplanned events may not coincide with a decrease in the on-call demands or responsibilities of the practice members. Locum tenentes can be a part of a valuable contingency plan or a temporary solution to an on-call dilemma. They can provide on-call coverage during a member's absence for continuing medical education, vacations, and holidays. However, the services of a locum tenens may come with a price, both monetarily and in other less obvious forms.

The first and obvious cost to any practice is the monetary cost. Most coverage by locum tenentes is provided through agencies. A substantial fee ranging from $1,650 to more than $2,500 a day can be expected for basic service. Additional fees also can be expected because the practice will be re-

sponsible for the locum tenens' travel, lodging, and local transportation costs. The 2009 agency fees for five companies are shown in **Table 2**.

The members of a medical practice may not be able to cover all the expenses of a locum tenens and should discuss hiring the temporary physician in conjunction with their affiliated hospital. Many hospitals are eager to avoid lapses in on-call coverage and may be open to the opportunity of partnering with a practice in employing a locum tenens.

It is best to obtain quotes from several providers. There are an increasing number of agencies providing locum tenens coverage. The National Association of Locum Tenens had 25 placement agencies in 2004 but currently has 57 member agencies.[16] Some agencies may be more familiar with orthopaedic specialties than others.[17] The agency should request a practice profile to better match the needs of the medical practice and provide the best coverage. The agency normally assists with licensing, preparation, travel, lodging, and credentialing of the locum tenens. To achieve a successful arrangement, the locum tenens' areas of responsibility should be communicated to the agency before the physician is assigned. Responsibilities of the physician in terms of clinic responsibilities and on-call coverage should be specified. It is also important to identify any support that will be available, including physician assistants, nurse practitioners, and the availability of hospital resources. In many rural areas, it is helpful to outline beforehand the capability of the practicing hospital and any agreements for transfers to higher-level facilities. As in any contract situation, the rules should be outlined in advance for all involved parties.

Other nonmonetary costs also should be considered before a locum tenens is employed. How will the locum tenens

Table 2

Locum Tenens Sample Rates

Company	Daily On-Call Only Rate ($)	Hourly On-Call Only Rate ($)	Gratis Hours	Clinic Rate ($)	On-Call After 8 Hours Clinic ($)
A	1,800	230	2	1,700	230
B	2,100 to 2,300	275	4	2,100 to 2,300	275
C	1,900 to 2,300	300 to 400	2	1,900 to 2,300	300 to 400
D	1,650	350	0	1,650	350
E	1,875				275

affect the reputation of the group? The locum tenens physician will be the face of the group during his or her tenure. Because the group usually will provide the follow-up care for the locum tenens' patients, complications and problems will most often be the responsibility of the permanent group members. Negative social or collegial interactions will be transferred to the follow-up care. The mean age of a locum tenens physician is 56 years, and most will have practiced more than 20 years.[18] The pool of locum tenens physicians is largely represented by semiretired physicians (30.1%) and those going through a career transition (29.9%). Locum tenentes are vetted, evaluated, and credentialed by their agencies and also require credentialing by the local hospital.[18] Because this process requires time, planning is required. It is important to realize that the actions of a locum tenens physician are a direct reflection and possible liability to the hiring group.

Hiring a locum tenens is an option for providing on-call coverage and is becoming more popular. Although many groups may be wary of hiring a locum tenens, this option can provide a temporary solution to a sudden on-call problem, although the monetary cost and cost to the group's reputation must be considered.

Hospitalist

It can be argued that enforcing group governance of on-call coverage, negoti-

ating on-call pay, and employing a locum tenens does not solve the on-call crisis but only delays the final solution. Orthopaedic hospitalists may be that final solution. The objective of a well-run hospitalist program is to create a long-term process that will address the burden of providing on-call service specifically and consistently, in much the same manner as seeking any best-practice alliance. With accurate delineation of the areas of burden (both acute and aftercare burdens), the solution or solutions can be derived.

Cost analyses (opportunity cost + recovered losses + new revenue) for both the individual service of trauma care and the global enterprise of orthopaedic surgery should be calculated.[19,20] Investment analysis of the upfront cost and tangible and intangible returns on investment must be included in the groundwork if the transfer of resources from an institution to a practitioner is proposed. With defined areas of intent, estimated costs (investment), a timeline, and a valid return on the investment, the strategy of creating a sustainable solution to the burden of on-call coverage can be undertaken. More sophistication in the process is required than in past years when on-call pay comparisons (for example, the Medical Group Management Association table, the Press Ganey table, and the Sullivan Cotter survey) comprised most of the information used for negotiating a coverage solution to the on-call burden. It is

necessary to move away from processes that attempt to force reluctant orthopaedic surgeons into on-call service, which is perceived as negative, and to begin developing career pathways that solve the problem with dedicated and interested practitioners.[21-23] To maintain sustainability, a long-term hospitalist program must generate mutual deliverable solutions in growth and value for all parties. The strategy crafted between an institution and the providers should demonstrate support for the needs of the community, the involved physicians, and the facility. Any such comprehensive strategy should be designed so that, over a designated period, the provision of on-call coverage would be voluntary and based on overarching performance criteria to ensure growth, value, and global institutional loyalty. A developmental template for a programmatic strategy should be constructed using the following component personnel and processes.

Midlevel Program Providers

Midlevel program providers inevitably will be the core component to any nonuniversity program during the implementation and maturation phases of the program.[24-26] Midlevel providers perform a series of valuable functions for the institution and the physicians. Their roles as first-responders to an emergency or trauma alert and as throughput facilitators (those who accelerate the delivery of care) have proven more valuable than the genera-

Table 2

Locum Tenens Sample Rates (continued)

Malpractice Fee ($)	Administration Daily Fee ($)	Holiday Rate	Agreement Type	Permanent Placement Fee ($)
0	19	½ daily–no work; 1½–work	Contingency	40,000
0	25	½ daily–no work; 1½–work	Contingency	35,000
0	0	$2,500 to $2,900	Contingency	
28.80	18	½ daily–no work; 1½–work	Contingency	40,000
	25	1½ daily	Contingency	30,000

tion of individual or collective professional billing revenues. The additional responsibility of the midlevel provider as a discharge liaison further enhances both the process and the experience of the injured patient and family members. Specific pretraining in the nuances of orthopaedic trauma and fracture care is imperative from an operational standpoint. An environment of mutual trust and professional recognition must be exhibited on an institutional level because midlevel providers serve as patient or process advocates in addition to their roles as physician assistants, regardless of their certification (physician assistant, certified; nurse practitioner; or registered nurse-first assistant). The availability of personnel is a challenge because a sustainable non-physician–provider program will require 3 to 4.5 full-time equivalency non-physician–providers to supply adequate coverage and allow for time off and illness. Currently, orthopaedic trauma is not part of the core education of any of the 130 physician assistant or nurse practitioner educational programs. Once a non-physician–provider program is developed, the retention of personnel must be a part of the institution's plan.

Hospitalist Program

Most nonuniversity trauma programs are based in regional medical centers and care for the specific needs of the community (such as the geriatric population and isolated injuries in patients with multiple comorbidities).[27-31] The collaboration of internal medicine colleagues for concomitant care is paramount for the timely delivery of care to a inpatient surgical population that is anticipated to grow at a rate of 7% annually for any given institution. The immediate incorporation of these internal medicine physicians into a team dedicated to the orthopaedic population will greatly enhance the growth and value of a developing regional orthopaedic program.

Orthopaedic Surgicalist

The designation of orthopaedic surgicalist describes a definable orthopaedic practitioner who is dedicated for a specific time period to the timely delivery of care to an injured patient and does not have confounding clinical or administrative duties.[23,28,30,32-34] This surgeon, whether he or she is part of an existing group, employed by the hospital, or managed by a third party, will have an exclusive and a specific scope of duties pertaining to the timely disposition of and definitive care of injured patients. Ideally, orthopaedic surgicalists should have some formal training or a fellowship in trauma and/or fracture care through an accredited program or significant expertise demonstrated in these types of surgery. In a regional medical center model, these designated orthopaedic surgicalists provide both definitive care for presenting patients and oversee the appropriate "back-triage" of patients to the developing pool of orthopaedic superspecialists who have specific anatomic interests (such as spine, hand, arthroscopy, or pediatrics). This model further enhances value to the institution. The program should be based on prearranged criteria, with the goal of limiting the outmigration of injured patients for definitive care or imaging.[19,20,35] Similarly, the creation of relationships with facilities that provide higher-level care (level I as verified by the American College of Surgeons or accredited by a state's government) will be necessary because a certain percentage of patients will require transfer to other facilities. These roles, responsibilities, and accountabilities are outlined in the Orthopaedic Trauma Association Health Policy position paper[9] and should be officially incorporated into the governance of a program using this on-call solution. With personnel identified and specific roles, responsibilities, and accountabilities outlined, the infrastructure or institutional deliverables can be ascribed accordingly.

Proficiency Benchmarks and Metrics

It is imperative that the result of this collaborative strategy be measurable on many levels because both individual and collective service performance must improve annually. A variety of benchmarks have been developed by accrediting bodies. For example, The Joint Commission developed benchmarks pertaining to acceptable start-time compliance, acceptable turnover time, and other minimum standards for hospital delivery of care; however, metrics specific to institutional performance pertaining to emergent and urgent delivery of musculoskeletal care are still needed.[21,26,31,36] The research evaluating failed trauma programs identified time ÷ work relative value units (RVUs) as a predictable metric for predicting success or failure (SG Agnew, MD, et al, unpublished material presented at the American Academy of Orthopaedic Surgeons annual meeting, San Francisco, CA, 2008; SG Agnew, MD, unpublished material, report to the AAOS Health Care Service Committee, 2009). If a collective institutional quotient (time ÷ wRVUs) does not reflect annual reductions for all trauma and emergency room–related activities, the prognosis for growth or a sustainable orthopaedic hospitalist program is poor. Individually, the lifestyle impact of 3,500 wRVUs (the average aggregate from 0.25 full-time equivalency orthopaedic emergency-room providers) at a typical regional medical center can be calculated if institutional performance is the average of 20 minutes ÷ wRVUs for injury care over the duration of one provider's acute care commitment. Other metrics associated with the total value and hence the sustainability of the enterprise must be delineated inclusive of data consistent with and compliant with US Code Title 42, public health and welfare chapter 7, subchapter XI, part A, § 1320a-7a (Civil Monetary Penalty Act; ancillary revenue + new physician acquisitions + combined value + contribution margin) to highlight the success of this alliance.[19,20]

Growth

Anatomic and geographic growth at the principal institution can be realisti-

cally attained only if the steady flow of fracture and trauma patients does not severely limit the available time and resources for potentially higher margin product lines and drive practitioners to other institutions, specialty care hospitals, or surgical centers.[31] Geographic growth requires predictable access—access of patients to the facility and access of the physicians to the patients at the point of definitive care (operating room). This access strategy may necessitate a more sophisticated plan beyond simple block scheduling. A dedicated orthopaedic trauma operating room at medical centers with a consistent volume of patients has proven valuable.

Discussion

Creating an effective on-call system requires a thorough dissection of the timeline and the priorities (four quadrant analysis) to gain maximum engagement and reduce frustration.[37] Coverage models, despite their popularity, do not address the causes of the on-call burden and may actually mask the problem for too long a period to allow an easy transition to a more comprehensive solution. Outside trained negotiators are a worthwhile investment on behalf of physicians, provided that the institution is willing to allow access to internal data. Negotiating for fair and equitable on-call pay during the maturation phase of a comprehensive programmatic change will have a greater chance of success when tied to significant operational enhancements as were previously outlined.

Realistically, any on-call pay component should be limited in time (with its value based on the defined burden components) and renegotiable if institutional performance or positive programmatic changes have not occurred in a prescribed period of time.[19,27,28,33] Various triggers should be in place to invest additional re-

sources, revenue, and personnel if the volume increases substantially or performance decreases. In 2011, third-party management firms that contract specifically for on-call relief scenarios for physicians and institutions are providing new opportunities.[27,34,38] These firms develop and often employ many surgeons who have an expressed interest in the delivery of fracture and emergent injury care. In many systems, the availability of the necessary practitioners and the presence of dedicated surgeons and infrastructure allow a symbiotic relationship between a medical staff that continues to provide on-call coverage and the institution. In other circumstances, the need for the complete separation of the core medical staff (superspecialists) from the burdens of on-call service may prove to be the most advantageous and sustainable system. Substantial opportunity exists to reduce or eliminate the community practitioner's on-call burden if the value of the orthopaedic enterprise is realized in a valid and reportable fashion (total economic value).[20] As with any business venture, once the intrinsic value of on-call coverage to the institution is ascribed, then the resources necessary to reduce such a burden to the service line can be systematically obtained. Value, performance, and leadership are the pillars of a successful hospital-physician alliance in this type of solution to the on-call problem.

It is important to reflect on the process by which the care of acutely injured patients with musculoskeletal injuries and deformities developed into a burden for the individual practitioner.[9,27,34,38-41] The problem is real. Fewer than one in four respondent providers have a personal or a professional interest in trauma care, and less than 50% of the providers polled considered emergency department coverage a personal or a professional responsibility.[38] This declining pool of willing on-call participants is combined with an increasing number of trauma patients. The Agency for Healthcare Research and Quality and the National Highway Traffic Safety Administration reported injuries per population at 67/1,000 in 2007.[42-44]

The on-call coverage problem appears to stem from the system-wide inability of surgeons to meet the societal demands for musculoskeletal care; this is caused in part by the ever-changing technologic demands that have increased annually without commensurate changes in lifestyle advantages. With the incidence of patients with musculoskeletal injuries presenting for urgent care increasing at an annual rate of 15%, US-based orthopaedic residency and fellowship programs are producing an increasing number of tertiary orthopaedic specialists (super-specialists) who concentrate on specific anatomic areas and specific anatomic problems with specific primary surgical skill sets.[28,32,33,38,42,45] Many newly trained orthopaedic surgeons have the option to practice in specialized care centers that have no relationship with the community institution or its emergency department.[40] Generational differences in the attitude of the workforce must be factored into the on-call problem.[46] These differences have developed, in part, as a direct manifestation of the 2003 restrictions on work hours for residents mandated by the Accreditation Council for Graduate Medical Education Residency Review Committee.

Summary

Providing adequate on-call coverage for orthopaedic injuries has remained a growing problem for the past decade. The delivery of fracture and musculoskeletal injury care is primarily provided by community practitioners; data accrued over the past 20 years consistently has shown that 80% of fracture surgery is performed outside university-affiliated institutions.[42] The number of patients and their treatment expectations are increasing, whereas the performance of community practice centers is not keeping pace. Not all regions or communities are experiencing the same level of problems and are not at the same location on the crisis curve. A host of solutions exist in tackling the problem of providing on-call coverage; however, not all solutions may apply equally to each locale or community. After recognizing the problem, the challenge is to identify the individual solutions that work best for each on-call situation.

References

1. Rudkin SE, Oman J, Langdorf MI, et al: The state of ED on-call coverage in California. *Am J Emerg Med* 2004;22(7):575-581.

2. O'Malley AS, Draper DA, Felland LE: Hospital emergency on-call coverage: Is there a doctor in the house? *Issue Brief Cent Stud Health Syst Change* 2007;115:1-4.

3. Vanlandingham B, Powe NR, Marone B, Diener-West M, Rubin HR: Abstract: The shortage of on-call specialist physician coverage in U.S. hospitals. Academy Health meeting, Boston, MA, 2005. NLM Gateway Website. http://gateway.nlm.nih.gov/MeetingAbstracts/ma?f=103622504.html. Accessed March 17, 2011.

4. Menchine MD, Baraff LJ: On-call specialists and higher level of care transfers in California emergency departments. *Acad Emerg Med* 2008;15(4):329-336.

5. Rudkin SE, Langdorf MI, Oman JA, Kahn CA, White H, Anderson CL: The worsening of ED on-call coverage in California: 6-year trend. *Am J Emerg Med* 2009;27(7):785-791.

6. McConnell KJ, Newgard CD, Lee R: Changes in the cost and management of emergency department on-call coverage: Evidence from a longitudinal statewide survey. *Ann Emerg Med* 2008;52(6):635-642.

7. McConnell KJ, Johnson LA, Arab N, Richards CF, Newgard CD, Edlund T: The on-call crisis: A statewide assessment of the costs of providing on-call specialist coverage. *Ann Emerg Med* 2007;49(6):727-733, e1-e18.

8. AAOS position statement: On-call coverage and emergency care services in orthopaedics. October 2006, volume 54, bulletin No. 5. AAOS Bulletin Archive. http://www2.aaos.org/aaos/archives/bulletin/oct06/cover3.asp. Accessed October 12, 2011. (Position statement retired December 2007.)

9. Orthopaedic Trauma Association: *OTA On-Call Position Statement.* Rosemont, IL, Orthopaedic Trauma Association, December 2005. http://www.ota.org/downloads/PositionStatement12-05.pdf. Accessed March 17, 2011.

10. Bosse MJ, Henley MB, Bray T, Vrahas MS: An AOA critical issue: Access to emergent musculoskeletal care. Resuscitating orthopaedic emergency-department coverage. *J Bone Joint Surg Am* 2006;88(6):1385-1394.

11. Young R M: Young doctors and wish lists: No weekend calls, no beepers. *New York Times.* January 27, 2004.

12. Russell Jr GV: Are you an "old coot" or a young whippersnapper"? *AAOS Now.* July 2009. http://www.aaos.org/news/aaosnow/jul09/managing5.asp. Accessed March 17, 2011.

13. Leahy M: Easing the burden of on-call coverage. *AAOS Now.* June 2010. http://www.aaos.org/news/aaosnow/jun10/

managing2.asp. Accessed March 17, 2011.

14. Schneider FV: Locum tenens. *Bull Am Coll Surg* 2008;93(12):45-46.

15. Smith JD: Locum tenens solve staffing problems. *Physician Exec* 1989;15(4):26-28.

16. National Association of Locum Tenens Organizations (NALTO). http://www.nalto.org. Accessed March 18, 2011.

17. Lowes R: Locum tenens: When you need one, how to get one. *Med Econ* 2007;84(9):38, 40, 42 passim.

18. Simon AB, Alonzo AA: The demography, career pattern, and motivation of locum tenens physicians in the United States. *J Healthc Manag* 2004;49(6):363-375, discussion 375-376.

19. White JA: Putting a dollar figure on a doctor's worth to a hospital. *The Wall Street Journal.* March 17, 2010. http://blogs.wsj.com/health/2010/03/17/putting-a dollar-figure-on-a-doctors-worth-to-a-hospital/. Accessed September 2, 2010.

20. Ziran BH, Barrette-Grischow MK, Marucci K: Economic value of orthopaedic trauma: The (second to) bottom line. *J Orthop Trauma* 2008;22(4):227-233.

21. Gillies RR, Zuckerman HS, Burns LR, et al: Physician-system relationships: Stumbling blocks and promising practices. *Med Care* 2001;39(7, Suppl 1):I92-I106.

22. Hauser M: The ups and downs of managing employed physicians: Medical management. A profession in transition. *Physician Executive.* May 1995. http://findarticles.com/p/articles/mi_m0843/is_n5_v21/ai_16881953/. Accessed March 17, 2011.

23. Warren BJ: Employed specialists: Is it the right service line strategy? Accelero Health Partners White Paper, November 2009. http://www.accelerohealth.com/assets/file/Employed_Specialists11_09(1).pdf. Accessed March 17, 2011.

24. Morgan PA, Strand J, Østbye T, Albanese MA: Missing in action: Care by physician assistants and nurse practitioners in national health surveys. Pub Med Central: Health Services Research. http://www.ncbi.nlm.nih.gov/pmc/articles/PMC2254567/. Accessed March 17, 2011.

25. Rogers C: Easing the strain of a busy practice. *AAOS Now.* July 2007. http://www.aaos.org/news/bulletin/jul07/managing3.asp. Accessed September 1, 2010.

26. Shock LP: Five ways a PA can make your business more profitable. CompHealth, August 6, 2010. http://www.comphealth.com/client-resources/white-papers/five-ways-to-make-pas-profitable. Accessed March 17, 2011.

27. American Hospital Association. 2010 health and hospital trends. http://www.aha.org/aha/research-and-trends/health-and-hospital-trends/2010.html. Accessed March 17, 2011.

28. Berenson RA, Ginsburg PB, May JH: Hospital-physicians relations: Cooperation, competition, or separation? *Health Aff (Millwood)* 2007;(26):w31-w33. http://content.healthaffairs.org/content/26/1/w31.full. Accessed March 17, 2011.

29. Budetti PP, Shortell SM, Waters TM, et al: Physician and health system integration. *Health Aff (Millwood)* 2002;21(1):203-210.

30. Casalino LP, November EA, Berenson RA, Pham HH: Hospital-physician relations: Two tracks and the decline of the voluntary medical staff model. *Health Aff (Millwood)* 2008;27(5):1305-1314.

31. Fabrizio NA, Bohlmann RC: *Integrated Delivery Systems: Ensuring Successful Physician-Hospital Partnerships.* Englewood, CO, Medical Group Management Association, 2010, pp 57-87.

32. Orthopaedic Practice in the US 2008. American Academy of Orthopaedic Surgeons. http://www3.aaos.org/research/opus/2008CensusMembers.cfm. Accessed March 17, 2011.

33. Committee on the Future of Emergency Care in the United States Health System: *Hospital-Based Emergency Care: At the Breaking Point.* Washington, DC, The National Academies Press, 2007.

34. Yamaguchi J: On-call crisis in trauma care: Government responses. Legislative Reference Bureau, January 2006. http://hawaii.gov/lrb/rpts06/traumacare.pdf. Accessed March 17, 2011.

35. Merritt Hawkins: 2010 *Inpatient/Outpatient Revenue Survey.* Irving, TX, Merritt hawkins. http://www.merritthawkins.com/pdf/2010revenuesurvey.pdf. Accessed September 2, 2010.

36. Vallier H, Agnew SA: Career and practice management issues in orthopaedic trauma, in Schmidt AH, Teague DC, eds: *Orthopaedic Knowledge Update Trauma 4.* Rosemont, IL, American Academy of Orthopaedic Surgeons, 2010, pp 19-30.

37. Covey SR: *The 7 Habits of Highly Effective People.* New York, NY, Simon and Schuster, 1994.

38. American Orthopaedic Association. Orthopaedic Institute of Medicine Council report. *Crisis in the delivery of orthopaedic emergency department care: A call to action.* http://www.aoassn.org/media/18119/oiomreport_edcallcoverage_completereport.pdf. Accessed April 13, 2011.

39. Taylor M: On-call coverage: Should hospitals pay orthopedic physicians. July 16, 2009. Becker's Orthopedic and Spine Review. http://www.beckers orthopedicandspine. com/news-analysis/item/87-on-call-coverage-should. Accessed September 1, 2010.

40. American College of Emergency Physicians: On-call specialist coverage in US emergency departments. http://www.acep.org/WorkArea/downloadasset. aspx?id=8974. Accessed September 1, 2010

41. Lott J: On call in crisis. Hospital Association of Southern California. http://www.hasc.org/download.cfm?ID=13604. Accessed September 2, 2010.

42. US Department of Health and Human Services: Agency for Healthcare Research and Quality. http://hcupnet.ahrq.gov/. Accessed March 17, 2011.

43. National Highway Traffic Safety Administration. National Automotive Sampling System. http://www.nhtsa.gov/NASS. Accessed September 1, 2010.

44. National Highway Traffic Safety Administration. Fatality Analysis Reporting System. http://www.nhtsa.gov/FARS. Accessed September 1, 2010.

45. *Occupational Outlook Handbook,* 2010-11 Edition. Physicians and Surgeons. US Department of Labor, Bureau of Labor Statistics. http://www.bls.gov/oco/ocos074.htm. Accessed September 3, 2010.

46. Borges NJ, Manuel RS, Elam CL, Jones BJ: Comparing millennial and generation X medical students at one medical school. *Acad Med* 2006;81(6):571-576.

Index

Page numbers with *f* indicate figures
Page numbers with *t* indicate tables

A

S

T